FOURTH EDITION

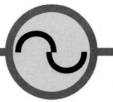

TEXTBOOK OF
GLAUCOMA

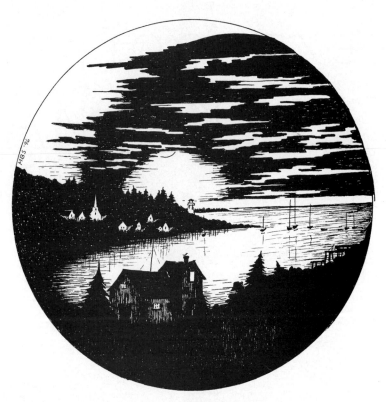

Approaching Darkness IV

Twilight in the Long Island Sound is superimposed on the visual field loss of glaucoma.
Dawn will come again to this New England coast, but not to the person blinded by glaucoma.

FOURTH EDITION

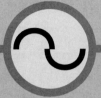

TEXTBOOK OF
GLAUCOMA

M. Bruce Shields, M.D.

Sears Professor and Chairman
Department of Ophthalmology and Visual Science
Yale University School of Medicine
and
Chief of Ophthalmology
Yale-New Haven Hospital

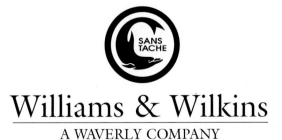

Williams & Wilkins
A WAVERLY COMPANY

BALTIMORE • PHILADELPHIA • LONDON • PARIS • BANGKOK
BUENOS AIRES • HONG KONG • MUNICH • SYDNEY • TOKYO • WROCLAW

Editor: *Darlene Barela Cooke*
Managing Editor: *Frances M. Klass*
Marketing Manager: *Diane Harnish*
Production Coordinator: *Peter J. Carley*
Project Editor: *Thomas Lehr*
Designer: *Susan Blaker*
Illustration Planner: *Peter J. Carley*
Cover Designer: *Susan Blaker*
Typesetter: *Graphic World, Inc.*
Printer: *RR Donnelley & Sons Company*
Digitized Illustrations: *Graphic World*
Binder: *RR Donnelley & Sons Company*

351 West Camden Street
Baltimore, Maryland 21201-2436 USA

Rose Tree Corporate Center
1400 North Providence Road
Building II, Suite 5025
Media, Pennsylvania 19063-2043 USA

Accurate indications, adverse reactions and dosage schedules for drugs are provided in this book, but it is possible that they may change. The reader is urged to review the package information data of the manufacturers of the medications mentioned.

Printed in the United States of America

First Edition, 1982
Second Edition, 1987
Third Edition, 1992

Library of Congress Cataloging-in-Publication Data
Shields, M. Bruce.
    Textbook of glaucoma/M. Bruce Shields, —4th ed.
        p.   cm.
    Includes bibliographical references and index.
    ISBN 0–683–07693–0
    1. Glaucoma.   I. Title.
    (DNLM: 1. Glaucoma. WW 290 S555t 1997)
RE871.S447   1997
617.7′41—dc21
DNLM/DLC   97-983
for Library of Congress   CIP

The publishers have made every effort to trace the copyright holders for borrowed material. If they have inadvertently overlooked any, they will be pleased to make the necessary arrangements at the first opportunity.

To purchase additional copies of this book, call our customer service department at **(800) 638-0672** or fax orders to **(800) 447-8438.** For other book services, including chapter reprints and large quantity sales, ask for the Special Sales department.

Canadian customers should call **(800) 665-1148,** or fax **(800) 665-0103.** For all other calls originating outside of the United States, please call **(410) 528-4223** or fax us at **(410) 528-8550.**

Visit Williams & Wilkins on the Internet: **http://www.wwilkins.com** or contact our customer service department at ***custserv@wwilkins.com.*** Williams & Wilkins customer service representatives are available from 8:30 am to 6:00 pm, EST, Monday through Friday, for telephone access.

97 98 99 00
2 3 4 5 6 7 8 9 10

To

all my

DUKE FRIENDS

Who made the last

25 years so special

PREFACE TO FOURTH EDITION

One impact that the changing healthcare scene does not appear to have had (not yet, at least) is a reduction in the quantity and quality of glaucoma-related articles in peer-reviewed journals. In updating this edition, approximately 2300 original papers were reviewed, which undoubtedly represents only a fraction of the world literature since the last edition was completed about five years ago. Approximately two-thirds of those papers, or 1440 new references, have been incorporated into this edition.

A glance at the distribution of topics in the recent literature provides an indication of where glaucoma research has been focused during the past five years, as well as the principal areas of new information to be found in this edition. Among diagnostic parameters, the optic nerve head and visual function remain the key areas of interest, with 428 papers or 19% of the total glaucoma literature reviewed. Studies of automated image analysis provided 30 of the 208 papers on the optic nerve head, and visual function tests, aside from visual field testing, accounted for 52 of the 220 articles in that category.

The clinical forms of glaucoma were the subjects of 626 (27%) papers, with chronic open-angle glaucoma, at 149 articles, remaining the most commonly studied, but still the most perplexing of the glaucomas. The medical management of glaucoma continues to be an area of keen interest, with 339 (15%) reported studies. Adrenergic antagonists remain the most commonly studied class of drugs at 112 papers, although the 35 and 32 articles on carbonic anhydrase inhibitors and prostaglandins, respectively, reflect the interest in the new topical agents within these drug classes. Not surprisingly, laser and incisional surgery remain the most common subjects of study, with 690 (30%) papers. Filtering surgery accounted for 347 of these, of which 141 dealt with anti-fibrosis agents.

Aside from the updating of the literature and two new chapters on Prostaglandins and Drainage Implant Surgery, the main change in this edition is to be found in a companion volume entitled *Color Atlas of Glaucoma.* This is an attempt to enhance the text in this edition with a series of color photographs ranging from the anatomy of aqueous humor dynamics through the techniques of glaucoma surgical procedures. The text and photographs follow the same order in the two volumes, and cross referencing is provided to facilitate locating corresponding text and color pictures.

With two volumes, I am now twice as indebted to the many kind and talented people who helped me during the preparation of each. First, I again wish to thank Ms. Diane Evans who typed the manuscript for the fourth edition. I never ceased to be amazed at how skillfully she deciphered my chicken scratching, arrows and rearrangements (much of which I couldn't even figure out) from the hard copy of the third edition. I am also again deeply in the debt of my long-time secretary and friend, Ms. Robin Goodwin, who did so many things, from typing the text for the atlas, through proofing the references in the textbook, to serving as a model in both books. I also thank Ms. Cheryl Oplinger, who was extremely helpful in proofing the new references.

My principal gratitude for the atlas, in addition to Ms. Goodwin's typing, goes to our award-winning photographers, Ms. Ruth Schirmer, and her accomplished staff of Ms. Teresa Jackson, Mr. Jeffrey Napoli, and Ms. Kim Salmon. The majority of the photographs in the atlas are the product of their handiwork over the years, and some are from Ms. Schirmer's special collection. Finally, I thank my many friends, who were kind enough to share their excellent photographs to fill in the gaps in my collection, and whose names are listed in the atlas.

I once again have the pleasure of thanking my publisher, Williams and Wilkins, who took a chance on me nearly twenty years ago and have stuck with me through four editions. A special thanks to Ms. Darlene B. Cooke and Ms. Frances M. Klass, who worked most closely with me during the preparation of these two volumes.

As always, however, my greatest thanks goes to you the reader, without whose kind reception of the texts and helpful comments along the way, this work would never have gotten beyond the first edition. My greatest hope remains that this work will prove to be of some benefit as we strive together in our common goal of preventing the blindness of glaucoma.

M. Bruce Shields, M.D.
New Haven, Connecticut

PREFACE TO THE FIRST EDITION

The primary intent of this book is to provide an introduction to the subject of glaucoma, as well as a framework on which to expand the study of that discipline. The content of the text has been organized in modified outline form to facilitate its use as a study guide. Presentation of the material begins with the most fundamental aspects of glaucoma and builds on successive levels of knowledge. In keeping with the simplicity of the format, illustrations have been limited to schematic line drawings and are used only where they are felt to clarify material in the text.

A moderately extensive bibliography has also been included in the study guide, and it is hoped that this may serve at least two purposes. First, it provides the student with a reading list from which he can select material for more detailed study of specific subjects on glaucoma. In addition, it may be of value to the practitioner as a reference source to help him stay abreast of the current concepts regarding the diagnosis and management of the glaucomas. Along with the classic literature on glaucoma, an effort has been made to provide an up-to-date bibliography, insofar as this is possible for a field of medicine in which knowledge is expanding so rapidly.

A valid criticism of this study guide will be the confusion created by attempting to present more than one viewpoint on so many issues. However, the complex nature of glaucoma is such that many questions remain unanswered, and the best one can do is to become familiar with the leading theories. With a few exceptions, an effort has been made to avoid imposing the author's bias into this text, but rather to present as objectively as possible, the various schools of thought in areas where controversy exists.

It is in no way intended that this study guide should compete with the many excellent textbooks that are currently available on the various aspects of glaucoma. Rather, it is hoped that this book may supplement the others by filling what is felt to be a need for a study guide and limited reference source on glaucoma. During the course of initial study or in refreshing oneself on this subject, both student and practitioner are urged to take full advantage of the wealth of outstanding textbooks on glaucoma, most of which are referenced throughout this study guide.

I am deeply indebted to a large number of talented and thoughtful people who helped me in many ways during the preparation of this text. To each of these individuals I wish to express my most sincere gratitude.

The collection and organization of reference materials used in this study guide was started during my time with W. Morton Grant at the Massachusetts Eye and Ear Infirmary. I am grateful to Dr. Grant for allowing access to his files and for the excellent teaching he and his staff provided.

The first several drafts of this book were prepared as outlines to accompany a series of lectures given to the residents at the Duke University Eye Center. The concept of developing this material into a study guide for publication was prompted by the kind words and encouragement of the Duke residents and senior staff. I am very indebted to all of these individuals, and especially to Robert Machemer, who urged me to embark on the project and was a strong source of support throughout its preparation.

The following experts kindly agreed to critically review preliminary drafts of certain chapters in this study guide: A. Robert Bellows, Richard F. Brubaker, David G. Campbell,

David L. Epstein, Keith Green, B. Thomas Hutchinson, Michael Kahn, Gordon K. Klintworth, Marvin L. Kwitko, William E. Layden, Alan I. Mandell, Samuel D. McPherson, Jr., Arthur H. Neufeld, Charles D. Phelps, Irvin P. Pollack, Harry A. Quigley, Robert Ritch, Richard J. Simmons, George L. Spaeth, E. Michael Van Buskirk, David S. Walton, Martin Wand, Myron Yanoff, and Thom J. Zimmerman. Their helpful comments and suggestions were invaluable in preparing the final draft of each chapter.

I was extremely fortunate to receive the highly professional and conscientious assistance of the following individuals: Robert L. Blake, medical illustration; Margaret L. Hayes, manuscript typing; David L. Smith, library research; and Lori S. Fields and Pamela S. Weinert, secretarial assistance. I also wish to thank the publishers, Williams & Wilkins, and especially Barbara C. Tansill for her invaluable help.

M. Bruce Shields, M.D.
Durham, North Carolina

CONTENTS

SECTION III

MANAGEMENT OF GLAUCOMA

CROSS REFERENCES
to M.B. Shields: *Color Atlas of Glaucoma*

SECTION III: MANAGEMENT OF GLAUCOMA

Chapter 1

AN OVERVIEW OF GLAUCOMA

HISTORICAL BACKGROUND

Although our modern understanding of glaucoma dates back only to the mid-19th century, this group of disorders was apparently recognized by the Greeks as early as 400 BC. In Hippocratic writings, it appears as "glaucosis," in reference to the bluish-green hue of the affected eye (1). This term, however, was applied to a larger group of blinding conditions that included cataracts. Although an association with elevated intraocular pressure is found in 10th century Arabian writings, it was not until the 19th century that glaucoma was clearly recognized as a distinct group of ocular disorders.

SIGNIFICANCE OF GLAUCOMA

Glaucoma is a leading cause of irreversible blindness throughout the world. World Health Organization statistics, published in 1995, indicate that glaucoma accounts for blindness in 5.1 million persons, or 13.5% of global blindness (behind cataracts and trachoma at 15.8 million and 5.9 million persons, or 41.8% and 15.5% of global blindness, respectively) (2). In the United States, it is the second leading cause of blindness and the most frequent cause among African-Americans. The U.S. Department of Commerce's Bureau of the Census 1990 population data (provided by the National Society to Prevent Blindness in 1993) estimated the total number of glaucoma cases among those 40 years of age or older to be approximately 1.5 million (1.7%) among Caucasians and others (including Hispanics, Asians and Native Americans) and 0.5 million (5.6%) among African-Americans. Glaucoma is also the second most common reason for ambulatory visits to ophthalmologists in the U.S. by Medicare beneficiaries and the leading cause among African-Americans. An analysis of a random 5% subsample of 1991 Medicare beneficiaries (National Claims History File—Part B) revealed approximately 223 office visits for glaucoma per 1000 Medicare beneficiaries among African-Americans and 154 for Caucasians (compared to 136 and 194 office visits for cataracts, respectively) (3). Although glaucoma more commonly afflicts the elderly, it occurs in all segments of our society with significant health and economic consequences (4), making it a major public health problem.

A DEFINITION OF GLAUCOMA

A Group of Diseases

The most fundamental fact concerning glaucoma is that it is not a single disease process. Rather, it is a large group of disorders that are characterized by widely diverse clinical and histopathologic manifestations. This point is not commonly appreciated by the general public, or even by a portion of the medical community, which frequently leads to confusion. For example, a patient may have difficulty understanding why she has no symptoms with her glaucoma, when a friend experienced sudden pain and redness with a disease of the same name. Another individual may avoid the use of cold medications because the package insert cautions against it in patients with glaucoma, and he was not informed that this only relates to certain types of glaucoma.

Terminology

The term *glaucoma* should only be used in reference to the entire group of disorders, just as the term *cancer* is used to refer to another discipline of medicine that encompasses many diverse clinical entities with certain common denominators. When referring to the diagnosis of a patient, one of the more precise terms, such as chronic open-angle glaucoma, should be used, which relates to the specific type of glaucoma that that individual is believed to have.

Common Denominator

The common denominator of all the glaucomas is a characteristic *optic neuropathy*, which derives from various risk factors including increased *intraocular pressure* (IOP) (5). Although elevated IOP is clearly the most frequent causative risk factor for glaucomatous optic atrophy, it is not the only factor, and attempts to define glaucoma on the basis of ocular tension are no longer advised. Nevertheless, IOP and aqueous humor dynamics, which regulate the pressure, are critical to our understanding of glaucoma, not only because they are the most common and best understood of the causative risk factors for glaucoma, but also because they are presently the only factors that can be controlled to prevent progressive optic neuropathy. Additionally, current classifications of glaucoma are based either on the multitude of initiating events that ultimately lead to elevated IOP, or on the alterations in aqueous humor dynamics that are directly responsible for the pressure rise. As continued research expands our knowledge of the various factors leading to glaucomatous optic neuropathy, both our classifications of glaucoma and approaches to management will undoubtedly change. For now, however, the most important point to recognize is that glaucomatous optic neuropathy is associated with a progressive loss of the *visual field*, which can lead to total, irreversible blindness if the condition is not diagnosed and treated properly. In Section One, therefore, we consider these three crucial parameters as they relate to our current understanding of glaucoma: intraocular pressure, the optic nerve, and the visual field.

PREVENTION OF BLINDNESS FROM GLAUCOMA

Once the blindness of glaucoma has occurred, there is no known treatment that will restore the lost vision. However, in nearly all cases, blindness from glaucoma is preventable. This prevention requires early detection and proper treatment. Detection depends on the ability to recognize the early clinical manifestations of the various glaucomas. In Section Two, we consider the many forms of glaucoma and the clinical and histopathologic features by which they are characterized. Appropriate treatment requires an understanding of the pathogenic mechanisms involved, as well as a detailed knowledge of the drugs and operations that are used to control the IOP. In Section Three, we consider these medical and surgical modalities that are used in the treatment of glaucoma.

REFERENCES

1. Fronimopoulos, J, Lascaratos, J: The terms glaucoma and cataract in the ancient Greek and Byzantine writers. Doc Ophthal 77:369, 1991.
2. Thylefors, B, Négrel, A-D, Pararajasegaram, R, Dadzie, KY: Global data on blindness. Bull World Health Org 73:115, 1995.
3. Javitt, JC: Ambulatory visits for eye care by Medicare beneficiaries. Arch Ophthal 112:1025, 1994.
4. Leske, MC: The epidemiology of open-angle glaucoma. A review. Am J Epidemiol 118:166, 1983.
5. Van Buskirk, EM, Cioffi, GA: Glaucomatous optic neuropathy. Am J Ophthal 113:447, 1992.

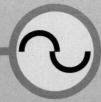

THE BASIC ASPECTS OF
GLAUCOMA

AQUEOUS HUMOR DYNAMICS
I. Anatomy and Physiology

The study of glaucoma deals primarily with the consequences of elevated intraocular pressure (IOP). A logical place to begin this study, therefore, is with the physiologic factors that control the IOP, which are the dynamics of aqueous humor flow.

HOW AQUEOUS HUMOR DYNAMICS INFLUENCE INTRAOCULAR PRESSURE

To reduce a highly complex, and only partially understood, situation to its simplest form, IOP is a function of the rate at which aqueous humor enters the eye (inflow) and the rate at which it leaves the eye (outflow). When inflow equals outflow, a steady state exists, and the pressure remains constant.

Inflow is related to the rate of aqueous humor production, while outflow depends on the resistance to the flow of aqueous from the eye and the pressure in the episcleral veins. The control of IOP, therefore, is a function of (a) production of aqueous humor; (b) resistance to aqueous humor outflow; and (c) episcleral venous pressure.

The remainder of this chapter deals with these three parameters and their complex interrelationship with the IOP.

AN OVERVIEW OF THE ANATOMY

Aqueous humor is involved with virtually all portions of the eye, although the two main structures related to aqueous humor dynamics are the *ciliary body*, the site of aqueous production, and the *limbus*, the principal site of aqueous outflow. The stepwise construction of a schematic model, as shown in Fig. 2.1 (**A–D**), illustrates the close relationship between these two structures and the surrounding anatomy:

1. The limbus is the transition zone between the cornea and the sclera. On the inner surface of the limbus is an indentation, the scleral sulcus, which has a sharp posterior margin, the scleral spur, and a sloping anterior wall that extends to the peripheral cornea.

2. A sieve-like structure, the *trabecular meshwork*, bridges the scleral sulcus and converts it into a tube, called *Schlemm's canal*. Where the meshwork inserts into the peripheral cornea a ridge is created, known as *Schwalbe's line*. Schlemm's canal is connected by intrascleral channels to the episcleral veins. The trabecular meshwork, Schlemm's canal, and the intrascleral channels comprise the main route of aqueous humor outflow.

3. The *ciliary body* attaches to the scleral spur and creates a potential space, the supraciliary space, between itself and the sclera. On cross-section, the ciliary body has the shape of a right triangle, and the *ciliary processes* (the

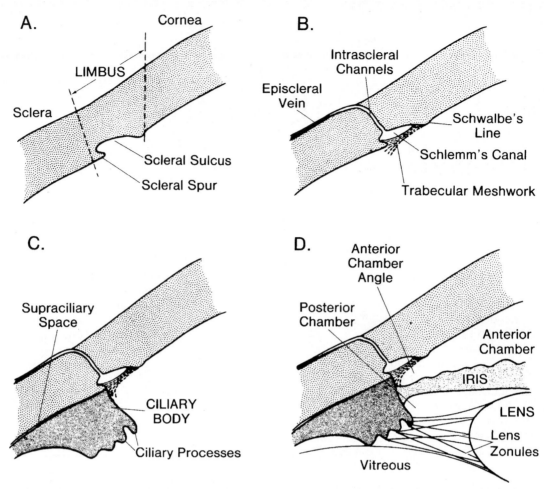

Figure 2.1. Stepwise constuction of a schematic model, depicting the relationship of structures involved in aqueous humor dynamics: A. Limbus. B. Main route of aqueous outflow. C. Ciliary body (site of aqueous production). D. Iris and lens.

actual site of aqueous production) occupy the innermost and anteriormost portion of this structure in the region called the *pars plicata* (or corona ciliaris). The ciliary processes consist of approximately 70 radial ridges (major ciliary processes) between which are interdigitated an equal number of smaller ridges (minor or intermediate ciliary processes) (1) (Fig. 2.2). The posterior portion of the ciliary body, called the *pars plana* (or orbicularis ciliaris), has a flatter inner surface and joins the choroid at the ora serrata.

The anterior-posterior length of the ciliary body in the adult eye ranges from 4.6–5.2 mm nasally to 5.6–6.3 mm temporally, according to various reports, with the pars plana accounting for approximately 75% of this total length. At birth, these measurements are 2.6–3.5 mm nasally and 2.8–4.3 mm temporally, and reach three-fourths of the adult dimensions by 24 months, with a constant ratio between pars plicata and pars plana (2).

4. The *iris* inserts into the anterior side of the ciliary body, leaving a variable width of the latter structure visible between the root of the iris and scleral spur, referred to as

the *ciliary body band*. The *lens* is suspended from the ciliary body by zonules and separates the vitreous, posteriorly, from the aqueous, anteriorly. The iris separates the aqueous compartment into a posterior and an anterior chamber, and the angle formed by the iris and the cornea is called the *anterior chamber angle*. Further details regarding the gonioscopic appearance of the anterior chamber angle are considered in Chapter 3.

PRODUCTION OF AQUEOUS HUMOR[a]

Histology of the Ciliary Body

The ciliary body is one of three portions of the uveal tract, or vascular layer of the eye, the other two structures in

[a]Refer to Shields, MB: Color Atlas of Glaucoma. Baltimore, Williams & Wilkins, 1998, Plate I2.

this system being the iris and choroid. The ciliary body measures 6 mm from the scleral spur to the ora serrata and is composed of (a) muscle, (b) vessels, and (c) epithelia (Fig. 2.3).

Ciliary Muscle

The ciliary muscle consists of two main portions: the longitudinal and the circular fibers. It is the longitudinal fibers which attach the ciliary body to the limbus at the scleral spur. This portion of muscle then runs posteriorly to insert into the suprachoroidal lamina (fibers connecting choroid and sclera) as far back as the equator or beyond. The circular fibers occupy the anterior and inner portion of the ciliary body and run parallel to the limbus. A third portion of the ciliary muscle has been described as radial fibers, which connect the longitudinal and circular fibers.

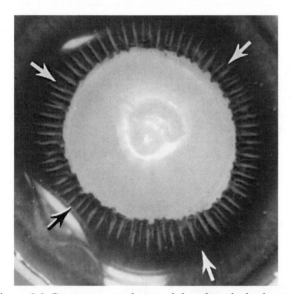

Figure 2.2. Gross anatomical view of the ciliary body showing the radial ridges of the ciliary processes *(arrows)*.

Ciliary Vessels

Traditional teaching holds that the vasculature of the ciliary body is supplied by the *anterior ciliary arteries* and the *long posterior ciliary arteries,* which anastomose near the root of the iris to form the major *arterial circle,* from whence branches supply the iris, ciliary body, and anterior choroid. More recent studies with vascular casting techniques and sequential microdissection in primates have shown this to be a complex vascular arrangement with collateral circulation on at least three levels (3): (a) The anterior ciliary arteries on the surface of the sclera send out lateral branches which supply the episcleral plexus and anastomose with branches from adjacent anterior ciliary arteries to form an *episcleral circle.* (b) The anterior ciliary arteries then perforate the limbal sclera. In the ciliary muscle, branches of these arteries anastomose with each other as well as with branches from the long posterior ciliary arteries to form the *intramuscular circle.* A similar anastomosing circle has been described in the human eye (4). Divisions of the anterior ciliary arteries also provide capillaries to the ciliary muscle and iris, and send recurrent ciliary arteries to the anterior choriocapillaris. (c) The *"major arterial circle,"* which lies near the iris root anterior to the intramuscular circle, is actually the least consistent of the three collateral systems. Although the primate studies reveal a contribution from perforating anterior ciliary arteries, microvascular casting studies of human eyes (4, 5), as well as several nonprimate animals (6, 7), indicate that this circle is formed primarily, if not exclusively, by paralimbal branches of the long posterior ciliary arteries, which begin dividing in the anterior choroid. In any case, the major arterial circle is the immediate vascular supply of the iris and ciliary processes.

There is evidence from human studies that blood in the anterior ciliary arteries, contrary to traditional teaching, flows from the inside of the eye to the outside. This is based on studies with rapid sequence fluorescein angiography (8) and the observations that an increase in IOP is associated

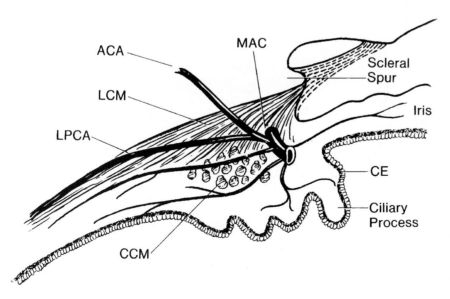

Figure 2.3. Three major components of the ciliary body. *(1)* The ciliary muscle, composed of longitudinal *(LCM)* and circular *(CCM)* fibers. *(2)* The vascular system, formed by branches of the anteior ciliary arteries *(ACA)* and long posterior ciliary arteries *(LPCA),* which form the major arterial circle *(MAC)*. *(3)* The ciliary epithelium *(CE),* composed of an outer pigmented and an inner nonpigmented layer.

with a decrease in anterior ciliary arterial pressure (9, 10) and an increase in the diameter of these vessels (10).

The ciliary processes in primates are supplied by two types of branches from the major arterial circle: the anterior and posterior ciliary process arterioles (11). *Anterior ciliary process arterioles* supply the anterior and marginal (innermost) aspects of the major ciliary processes. These arterioles have luminal constrictions before producing irregularly dilated capillaries within the processes, suggesting precapillary arteriolar sphincters. This may represent the anatomic site of adrenergic neural influence on aqueous humor production by regulation of blood flow through the ciliary processes in response to physiologic and pharmacologic mediators (6, 7). *The posterior ciliary process arterioles* supply the central, basal, and posterior aspects of the major ciliary processes, as well as all portions of the minor processes. These arterioles are of larger caliber than the anterior arterioles and lack the constrictions seen in the latter vessels. Both populations of arterioles have interprocess anastomoses. Venous drainage is into choroidal veins, either from the posterior aspects of the major and minor processes or by direct communication from the interprocess connections (Figs. 2.4 and 2.5).

Vascular casting studies of capillary networks in the ciliary processes of human eyes suggest three different vascular territories with discrete arterioles and venules (4). The first is located in the anterior end of the major ciliary processes and is drained posteriorly by venules without significant connections to other venules in the ciliary processes. The second is in the center of the major processes, while the third capillary network occupies the minor processes and posterior third of the major processes. Both of the latter territories are drained by marginal venules, which are situated at the inner edge of the major processes. It is felt that these three vascular territories may reflect a functional differentiation in the process of aqueous humor production (4).

Ciliary Epithelia

Two layers of epithelium line the inner surface of the ciliary processes and the pars plana: (a) pigmented epithelium comprises the outer layer, adjacent to the stroma, and is composed of low cuboidal cells, while (b) nonpigmented epithelium makes up the inner layer, adjacent to the aqueous in the posterior chamber, and consists of columnar cells (see further details under "Ultrastructure of the Ciliary Processes").

Ultrastructure of the Ciliary Processes

Each ciliary process is composed of (a) capillaries, (b) stroma, and (c) epithelia (Fig. 2.6).

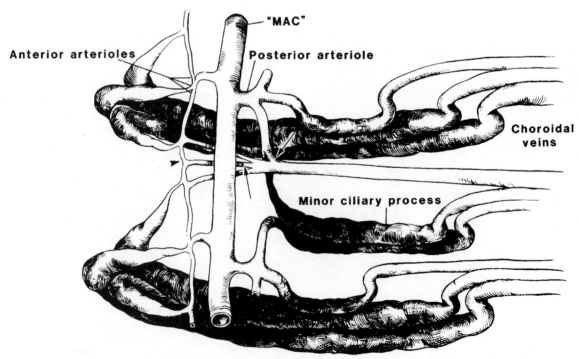

Figure 2.4. Vascular interconnections of two contiguous major ciliary processes. Lateral anterior arteriolar branches join to form interprocess capillary networks *(arrowhead)* which provide communication between major processes. Laterally directed posterior arterioles form posterior interprocess networks through which the minor ciliary processes receive blood. In addition, both anterior and posterior interprocess networks drain directly into the choroidal veins *(arrows)*. MAC, major arterial circle. (Reprinted by permission from Morrison, JC, Van Buskirk, EM: Ciliary process microvasculature of the primate eye. Am J Ophthalmol 97:372, 1984.)

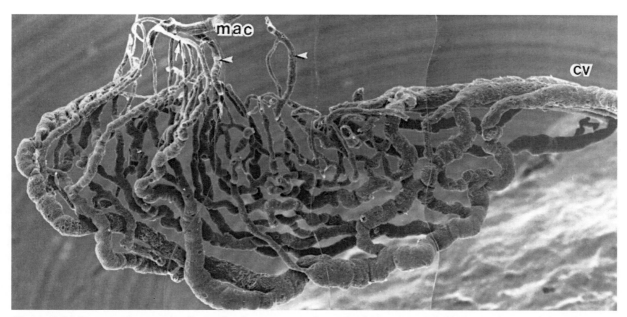

Figure 2.5. Microvascular casting of a single ciliary process. Constricted anterior arterioles *(arrows)* enter the anterior portion of the process to provide large irregular vein-like capillaries that occupy the margins of the process. Posteriorly, larger caliber arterioles *(arrowheads)* originate and enter the middle of the process to divide into smaller capillaries that in general are confined to the base of the process. All capillaries travel posteriorly to drain into the choroidal veins *(CV)*. MAC, major arterial circle. (× 150) (Reprinted by permission from Morrison, JC, Van Buskirk, EM: Ciliary process microvasculature of the primate eye. Am J Ophthalmol 97:372, 1984.)

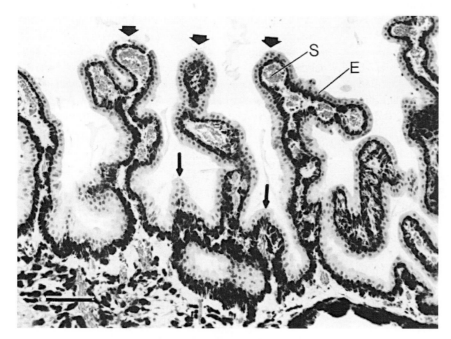

Figure 2.6. Light microscopic view of ciliary processes, sectioned perpendicular to radial ridges, showing major ciliary processes *(large arrows)* and minor ciliary processes *(small arrows)*. Note vascular stroma *(s)* surrounded by outer pigmented and inner nonpigmented epithelium *(E)*. (Hematoxylin & eosin stain; bar = 100 μm)

Ciliary Process Capillaries

The capillary networks occupy the center of each process. The endothelium is very thin with fenestrae, or false "pores," which represent areas of absent cytoplasm with fusion of the plasma membranes, and which may be the site of increased permeability. A basement membrane surrounds the endothelium, and mural cells, or pericytes, are located within the basement membrane (12).

Ciliary Process Stroma

A very thin stroma surrounds the capillary networks and separates them from the epithelial layers. The stroma is composed of ground substance, consisting of mucopolysaccharides, proteins and solute of plasma (except those of large molecular size), a very few collagen connective tissue fibrils, especially collagen type III (13), and wandering cells of connective tissue and blood origin (12). Tubular microfibrils with and without elastin have been demonstrated in bovine ciliary body, especially in the stroma of the pars plana, in relationship to lens zonules (14).

Ciliary Process Epithelia

Two layers of epithelium surround the stroma, with the apical surfaces of the two cell layers in apposition to each other (Fig. 2.7).

PIGMENTED EPITHELIUM. Pigmented epithelium is characterized by numerous melanin granules in the cytoplasm and an atypical basement membrane on the stromal side. The cytoskeletal element, cytokeratin 18, has been observed in the crests of the pars plicata and the posterior pars plana (15).

NONPIGMENTED EPITHELIUM. The basement membrane is composed of fibrils in a glycoprotein with labeling for laminin and collagens I, III, and IV (16). This membrane, which faces the aqueous, is also called the *internal limiting membrane* and fuses with the lens zonules. Numerous mitochondria are seen in the cytoplasm, along with poorly developed, rough and smooth endoplasmic reticulum, and a scant amount of ribosomes. The nonpigmented epithelium stains less intensely than the pigmented layer for cytokeratin 18, but more so for vimentin, with the predominant distribution again in the crests of the pars plicata and the posterior pars plana (15). It also stains with antibodies against S-100 proteins (13). The nucleus has a nucleolus that appears to contain ribosomes. The cell membrane is 200 Å thick and is characterized by infoldings or interdigitations, especially surface infoldings on the free surface and lateral interdigitations, which are actually different cuts of the same structure.

A variety of *intercellular junctions* have been described which connect adjacent cells within each epithelial layer, as well as the apical surfaces of the two layers (17–19). Electrophysiologic studies of rabbit ciliary epithelium suggest that all of the cells in the epithelium function as a syncytium (20). Tight junctions create a permeability barrier between the nonpigmented epithelial cells, which forms part of the *blood-aqueous barrier*. These tight junctions are said to be the "leaky" type, in contrast to the "nonleaky" type in the blood-retinal barrier, and may be the main diffusional pathways for water and ion flow (21, 22). Microvilli separate the two layers of epithelial cells. In addition, "ciliary channels" have been described as spaces between the two epithelial layers (23). They are felt to be related to the formation of aqueous humor since they develop between the fourth and sixth months of gestation, corresponding to the start of aqueous production.

Theories of Aqueous Humor Production

Aqueous humor appears to be derived from plasma within the capillary network of the ciliary processes. To reach the posterior chamber, therefore, the various constituents of aqueous humor must traverse the three tissue layers of the ciliary processes, i.e., the capillary wall, stroma, and epithelia. The principal barrier to transport across these tissues is the cell membrane and related junctional complexes, and substances appear to pass through this structure by one of three mechanisms (24): (a) *diffusion* (lipid-soluble substances are transported through the lipid portions of the membrane proportional to a concentration gradient across the membrane); (b) *ultrafiltration* (water and water-soluble substances, limited by size and charge, flow through theo-

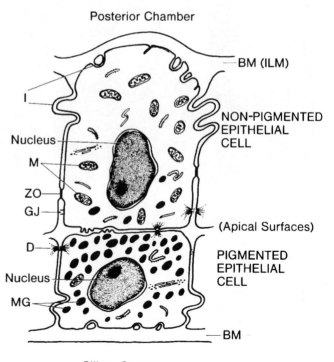

Figure 2.7. The two layers of the ciliary epithelium. Apical surfaces are in apposition to each other. Basement membrane (BM) lines the double-layer and constitutes the internal limiting membrane (ILM) on the inner surface. The nonpigmented epithelium is characterized by mitochondria (M), zonula occludens (ZO), and lateral and surface interdigitations (I). The pigmented epithelium contains numerous melanin granules (MG). Additional intercellular junctions include desmosomes (D) and gap junctions (GJ).

retical "micropores" in the protein of the cell membrane in response to an osmotic gradient or hydrostatic pressure); or (c) *secretion* (water-soluble substances of larger size or greater charge are actively transported across the cell membrane). The latter mechanism is believed to be mediated by globular proteins in the membrane and requires the expenditure of energy. All three transport mechanisms are probably involved in aqueous production, possibly in accordance with the following simplified three-part scheme:

Accumulation of Plasma Reservoir

Tracer studies suggest that most plasma substances pass easily from the capillaries of the ciliary processes, across the stroma, and between the pigmented epithelial cells before accumulating behind the tight junctions of the nonpigmented epithelium (25, 26). Studies with normal rats suggest that pericapillary permeability of the ciliary processes is influenced by the presence of fixed anionic groups which favor the penetration and accumulation of cationic tracers (27). This movement takes place primarily by ultrafiltration, and drugs that alter ciliary perfusion may exert their influence on IOP at this level (5–7, 11, 28).

Transport Across Blood-Aqueous Barrier

The tight junctions between the nonpigmented epithelial cells create part of the blood-aqueous barrier, and certain substances appear to be actively transported across this barrier into the posterior chamber, thereby establishing an osmotic gradient. Studies with isolated rabbit ciliary processes suggest that aqueous humor could be secreted by the generation of a modest osmotic gradient across the nonpigmented cell basal membrane (29). There is a specific secretory pump for sodium ions (30, 31), and approximately 70% of this electrolyte is actively transported into the posterior chamber (32), while the remainder enters by passive ultrafiltration (24) or diffusion (32). The active transport of Na^+ is Na^+K^+-activated ATPase-dependent (33), but does not appear to be related to the concentration of Na^+ in the plasma (34).

A much smaller percentage of the *chloride* ion is actively transported, and this appears to be dependent on the presence of sodium, as well as the pH (35, 36). *Potassium* ions are transported by secretion and diffusion (37). One proposed model for the exit of Na^+ and Cl^- into the aqueous humor is that Na^+K^+-ATPase pumps Na^+ in exchange for K^+ in the aqueous. K^+ recycles through K^+ channels, and Cl^- passively diffuses through Cl^- channels into the aqueous (38). Electrolyte movement across the ciliary epithelium is measured primarily by electrochemical gradients, but studies with rabbit ciliary epithelium have demonstrated electrically silent Na^+ and Cl^- fluxes, suggesting an additional pathway for electrolyte movement (39).

Ascorbic acid is secreted against a large concentration gradient (32), with a probable small contribution from passive diffusion (40). *Amino acids* are secreted by at least three carriers (41). The rapid interconversion between *bicarbonate* and CO_2, which is catalyzed by carbonic anhydrase, makes it difficult to determine the relative proportions of these two substances. However, bicarbonate formation has been shown to influence fluid transport through its effect on Na^+ (42), possibly by regulating the pH for optimum active transport of Na^+ (24).

Osmotic Flow

The osmotic gradient across the ciliary epithelium, which results from the active transport of the above substances, leads to the movement of other plasma constituents by ultrafiltration and diffusion. There is evidence that sodium is the ion primarily responsible for the movement of water into the posterior chamber (28, 30, 43).

The precise location of aqueous humor production appears to be predominantly in the anterior portion of the pars plicata along the tips or crests of the ciliary processes, since this region has been shown to have (a) increased basal and lateral interdigitations, mitochondria, and rough endoplasmic reticulum in the nonpigmented ciliary epithelium, (b) more numerous fenestrations in the capillary endothelium, (c) a thinner layer of ciliary stroma, and (d) an increase in cell organelles and gap junctions between pigmented and nonpigmented epithelia (44, 45). Furthermore, when sodium fluorescein is administered systemically and the ciliary body is observed with a special gonioprism, fluorescein-stained aqueous is seen primarily at the tips of the ciliary processes (46).

The site of active transport is considered to be the nonpigmented epithelial cells, especially in the cell membrane of the lateral interdigitations, since this area has (a) abundant Na^+K^+-activated ATPase and carbonic anhydrase (47), (b) higher specific activity for glycolytic enzymes (48), and (c) preferential incorporation of labeled sulfate into macromolecules (primarily glycolipids and glycoproteins) (49, 50). The ciliary epithelium also contains α- and β-adrenergic receptors, and drugs that act on these receptors or on enzymes, such as carbonic anhydrase, may influence aqueous production, and subsequently IOP, by altering the active transport mechanisms (51).

In addition to actively transporting aqueous humor, ultrastructural studies of primates suggest that the ciliary epithelium produces a secretory material that diffuses into the ciliary body stroma and possibly enters the blood stream (52).

Rate of Aqueous Humor Production

The rate at which aqueous humor is formed (inflow) is measured in microliters per minute (μL/min). The actual value in the human eye varies somewhat according to the measurement techniques, which are discussed in the next chapter. Using a technique of scanning ocular fluorophotometry in more than 300 normal subjects, 3 to 83 years of age, the mean rate of aqueous flow between 8 AM and 4 PM was 2.75 ± 0.63

μL/min (53, 54). The normal range (i.e., 95% of the sample) was 1.8–4.3 μL/min. The flow in the morning, from 8 AM to noon, was higher, at 2.86 ± 0.73, than from noon to 4 PM, which was 2.63 ± 0.57 μL/min. The rates during sleep are approximately one-half of those during the morning (55, 56).

Many factors have been evaluated with regard to an influence on the rate of aqueous production. An elevation of IOP was once thought to be associated with a decline in aqueous production, which was referred to as pseudofacility (57–62). More recent studies, however, indicate that aqueous formation is relatively pressure-insensitive and a possible explanation for conflicting findings is that earlier work involved a relatively short period of observation, whereas a long-standing rise in IOP has less effect on the rate of aqueous flow (63–66).

Fluorophotometric studies support the traditional concept that aqueous production decreases with age (67), although the degree of this change is less than previously thought, amounting to 2.4–3.2% per decade of age after age 10 (53, 68). The formation of aqueous humor is actually much more stable than the IOP or anterior chamber volume with respect to aging changes (68).

The hormonal basis for the diurnal fluctuation in the rate of aqueous flow in humans is unknown (53). It appears to be driven by changes in the concentration of endogenous epinephrine available to the ciliary epithelia, primarily due to the influence on β-adrenergic receptors (69, 70), although chronic topical epinephrine had no measurable effect on the rate of aqueous flow or the circadian rhythm of aqueous flow (71). Nocturnal suppression of aqueous flow is not blocked by bright light, suggesting that it is not driven by systemic melatonin release (72). It is also not dependent on a comparable fall in plasma corticosteroid activity (73), nor is the circadian rhythm influenced by adrenalectomy in humans (74).

Aqueous flow has been shown to be reduced in patients with diabetes mellitus, independent of the type (75), although neither flow, IOP, nor tonographic facility of outflow were found to significantly correlate with the severity of the retinopathy or hemoglobin A_1C in either type 1 or type 2 diabetics (76).

Inflammation (iridocyclitis) causes a decrease in inflow (77), possibly related to a disruption in ciliary epithelium (78). Aqueous production is reduced during the acute phase of hypotony following cyclodialysis but not with chronic cyclodialysis if unassociated with iridocyclitis (77). Choroidal detachment in a hypotonus eye is often associated with, but does not appear to cause, reduced inflow (77). Retinal detachment is commonly associated with a reduction in the IOP, although it is not clear how much of this is due to a decrease in aqueous production (79), or an increase in aqueous outflow by an unconventional, posterior route (77).

Drinking 1000 ml of water is associated with a significant increase in aqueous flow after 90 minutes (80). Caffeine was found to have no clinically significant effect on aqueous flow in the normal human eye (81). Pharmacologic agents that reduce inflow are discussed in Section Three.

FUNCTION AND COMPOSITION OF AQUEOUS HUMOR

Function

In addition to its role in maintaining a proper IOP, aqueous humor has important metabolic requirements in providing substrates and removing metabolites from the avascular cornea and lens. For example, the cornea takes glucose and oxygen from the aqueous and releases lactic acid and a small amount of CO_2 into the aqueous (32). The lens also uses glucose and generates lactate and pyruvate (32). Additionally, it is reported that potassium and amino acids in the aqueous may be taken up by the lens, while sodium moves from the lens to the aqueous (41). The metabolism of the vitreous and retina also appears to be associated with the aqueous humor in that substances such as amino acids and glucose pass into the vitreous from the aqueous (32, 41).

Composition

From the earlier discussion, it may be seen that the composition of aqueous humor depends not only on the nature of its production, but also on the constant metabolic interchanges that occur throughout its intraocular course. However, close similarities in aqueous composition between the phakic and aphakic eye of the same individual suggest that lens metabolism has practically no influence on the composition of aqueous (82). Diffusional exchange across the iris may be a more significant factor in the changing composition of the aqueous between the posterior and anterior chambers, although there appears to be considerable species variation. Studies in rabbit eyes indicate that the total concentration of dissolved substances, pH, and osmotic pressure are the same in the posterior and anterior chambers, while the actual composition of the aqueous in the two chambers is different (83). This difference appears to be related to active transport in the posterior chamber and passive transfer in the anterior chamber, where the iris vessels are permeable to anions and nonelectrolytes (83). Tracer studies in primates suggest that a unidirectional vesicular transport in iris vessels is responsible for the selective movement of anionic substances from the tissues of the eye to the bloodstream (84). In the rhesus monkey, however, the complexity of the interendothelial junctions in the blood vessels of the iris strongly suggests that these vessels participate only minimally in aqueous humor dynamics (85, 86).

The following statements, summarized in Table 2.1, describe only the general character of aqueous humor, expressed relative to plasma. Aqueous of both the anterior and posterior chamber is slightly *hypertonic* compared to plasma. It is *acidic*, with a pH in the anterior chamber of 7.2 (87). The two most striking characteristics of aqueous humor are (a) a marked *excess of ascorbate* (15 times greater

Table 2.1.
GENERAL CHARACTER OF HUMAN AQUEOUS HUMOR (EXPRESSED RELATIVE TO PLASMA)

1. Slightly hypertonic
2. Acidic
3. Marked excess of ascorbate
4. Marked deficit of protein
5. Slight excess of:
    a. Chloride
    b. Lactic acid*
6. Slight deficit of:
    a. Sodium (rabbit study)
    b. Bicarbonate*
    c. Carbon dioxide
    d. Glucose
7. Other reported constituents/features:
    a. Amino acids (variable concentrations)
    b. Sodium hyaluronate
    c. Norepinephrine
    d. Coagulation properties
    e. Tissue plasminogen activator
    f. Latent collagenase activity

*Varies with measurement technique

than that of arterial plasma), and (b) a marked *deficit of protein* (0.02% in aqueous as compared to 7% in plasma). In a study of 22 species of mammals, a wide range of ascorbic acid levels was found, although it was generally higher in diurnal than nocturnal animals, suggesting that it may play a protective role against light-induced damage (88).

Studies in normal rabbit and monkey eyes suggest that a significant amount of plasma protein, normally present in the aqueous, originates in the ciliary body capillaries and diffuses anteriorly through the iris and into the anterior chamber (89, 90). In another study with rabbit eyes, it was concluded that most aqueous proteins are intrinsic glycoproteins of the vitreous, which are secretory products of the inner epithelial layer of the ciliary body (91). Protein content of the aqueous humor has both quantitative and qualitative differences in comparison to that of serum, which may explain the observed characteristic of aqueous to obstruct flow through artificial membranes with pore sizes similar to those found in the aqueous outflow pathway (92, 93). The albumin:globulin ratio is the same as plasma, although there is less γ-globulin. Human aqueous has been found to contain IgG, but no IgD, IgA, or IgM (94). Protein and antibodies in the aqueous equilibrate with those in plasma to form a *plasmoid aqueous* when the eye is inflamed. In addition, following aspiration of aqueous, the newly formed fluid has a high protein content, which is suggested by monkey studies to result from new gaps in the inner wall endothelial lining of Schlemm's canal and enlarged extracellular spaces in the ciliary epithelium of the anterior pars plicata (95, 96). Aque-

ous protein concentration is influenced by aqueous flow in the noninflamed eye, but additional factors affecting protein entry into the aqueous of rabbit eyes prevents a direct reciprocal relationship between aqueous flare and flow (97).

The relative concentrations of free amino acids in human aqueous varies, with aqueous/plasma concentrations ranging from 0.08 to 3.14, supporting the concept of active transport of amino acids (98). The concentrations of most other ions and nonelectrolytes are very close to those in the plasma, and conflicting statements in the literature primarily represent differences with regard to species and measurement techniques. In general, human aqueous has a slight excess of chloride and a deficiency of bicarbonate (87, 99). However, several factors lead to rapid changes in aqueous bicarbonate levels, and the concentrations measured may not accurately reflect the relative concentration of bicarbonate transported by the ciliary epithelia. Lactic acid is reported to be in relative excess in human aqueous (99), although this determination varies widely with the technique of measurement. Sodium in rabbits and glucose in human eyes show a relative deficiency in the aqueous (99). The total CO_2 content in aqueous has considerable species variation, with a deficiency in man (100).

Sodium hyaluronate in human aqueous humor, obtained before cataract extraction, is reported to have a mean value of 1.14 ± 0.46 mg/g, with no substantial difference in patients with diabetes or glaucoma (101). Norepinephrine was found consistently in human aqueous and was higher in patients undergoing cataract surgery than those with glaucoma (102). Human aqueous also appears to have coagulation properties as demonstrated by its ability to shorten ear lobe puncture bleeding time, prothrombin time, and partial thromboplastin time (103). However, tissue plasminogen activator activity is also present in normal human aqueous, and the ratio to total protein is about 30 times greater than that in plasma, suggesting an important role in intraocular fibrinolysis (104). In addition, a relatively high concentration of urokinase-type plasminogen activator indicates a shift in the proteolytic balance of aqueous in the anterior chamber toward fibrinolysis (106).

Several additional factors have been identified in the aqueous which may influence the trabecular meshwork activity and subsequently the IOP. For example, a latent collagenase activity may participate in the extracellular matrix metabolism of the meshwork (107). A number of growth factors, which are polypeptides involved in the homeostatic balance of cells in a tissue, have been observed in human aqueous, and receptors for many of these factors have been identified on trabecular cells in tissue culture (108). Among these growth-promoting factors in the aqueous is transferrin, which has been demonstrated in the tau fraction (109) and which may be related to a breakdown of the blood-aqueous barrier with implications in the pathogenesis of various intraocular disorders (110). Transforming growth factor β is also present in high concentrations in normal aqueous and may contribute to immunosuppressive properties of aqueous (111). Other factors in aqueous that may influence trabecular meshwork formation are endothelin-1, a

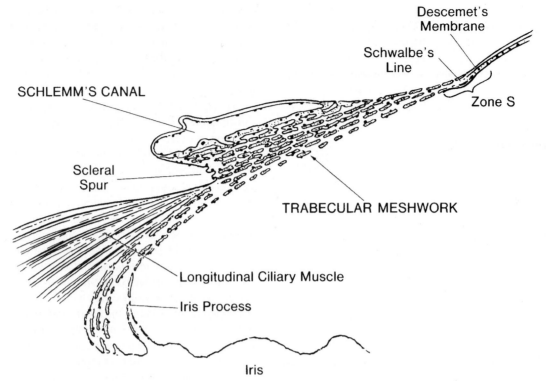

Figure 2.8. The trabecular meshwork extends from iris, ciliary body, and scleral spur to the sloping anterior wall of the scleral sulcus, converting the sulcus into Schlemm's canal.

potent vasoconstrictive peptide that may mediate contraction in meshwork cells or ciliary muscle (112), and indoleamine 2,3-dioxygenase, an important enzyme in the protection against free oxygen radical damage (113).

AQUEOUS HUMOR OUTFLOW[b]

As noted earlier in this chapter, most of the aqueous humor leaves the eye at the anterior chamber angle through the system consisting of trabecular meshwork, Schlemm's canal, intrascleral channels, and episcleral and conjunctival veins. It has been estimated that this pathway, referred to as the *conventional* or *canalicular system,* accounts for 83% (114) to 96% (115) of aqueous outflow in human eyes under normal circumstances. The other 5–15% of the aqueous leaves the eye by a number of systems that are only partially understood, but include *uveoscleral* (115–117) and *uveo-vortex* (118) systems. Collectively, these alternate aqueous outflow pathways may be referred to as the *unconventional* (119) or *extracanalicular system,* or secondary pathways (120). (The terms canalicular, referring to involvement of Schlemm's canal, and extracanalicular were proposed by Richard F. Brubaker, M.D., personal communication, 1981.)

[b]Refer to Shields, MB: Color Atlas of Glaucoma. Baltimore, Williams & Wilkins, 1998, Plate I3.

Histology of the Conventional Aqueous Outflow System

The reader may wish to refer back to "An Overview of the Anatomy," at the outset of this chapter, before proceeding with the following details of the outflow system.

Scleral Spur

The posterior wall of the scleral sulcus is formed by a group of fibers, the scleral roll, which run parallel to the limbus and project inward to form the *scleral spur* (Fig. 2.1) (121). The scleral spur-roll is composed of 75–80% collagen and 5% elastic tissue (122). It has been suggested that this circular structure prevents the ciliary muscle from causing Schlemm's canal to collapse (121). Myofibroblast-like scleral spur cells (123), in close association with varicose axons characteristic of mechanoreceptor nerve endings, (124) suggest a mechanism for measuring stress or strain in the scleral spur, as might occur with ciliary muscle contraction or changes in IOP.

Schwalbe's Line

Just anterior to the apical portion of the trabecular meshwork is a smooth area, which varies in width from 50–150 μm and has been called *Zone S* (125). The anterior border of this zone consists of the transition from trabecular to corneal endothelium and the thinning and termination of Descemet's membrane. The posterior border is demarcated by a discontinuous elevation, called *Schwalbe's line,* that appears to be formed by the oblique insertion of uveal trabeculae into limbal stroma. Clusters of secretory cells, called *Schwalbe line's cells,* have been observed just beneath this ridge in monkey eyes, and are believed to produce a phospholipid material that facilitates aqueous flow through the canalicular system (126).

Trabecular Meshwork

As previously discussed, the scleral sulcus is converted into a circular channel, called Schlemm's canal, by the trabecular meshwork. This tissue consists of a connective tissue core surrounded by endothelium and may be divided into three portions: (a) uveal meshwork, (b) corneoscleral meshwork, and (c) juxtacanalicular tissue (Figs. 2.8–2.10).

UVEAL MESHWORK. The portion adjacent to the aqueous in the anterior chamber is arranged in bands or rope-like trabeculae that extend from the iris root and ciliary body to the peripheral cornea. The arrangement of the trabecular bands creates irregular openings that vary in size from 25–75 μm across (127).

CORNEOSCLERAL MESHWORK. This portion extends from the scleral spur to the anterior wall of the scleral sulcus and consists of sheets of trabeculae that are perforated by elliptical openings. These holes become progressively smaller as the trabecular sheets approach Schlemm's canal, with a diameter range of 5–50 μm (127). The ciliary muscle extends anterior to the scleral spur well into the corneoscleral meshwork, suggesting potential contractile properties in this portion of the meshwork (128).

JUXTACANALICULAR TISSUE. The outermost portion of the meshwork (adjacent to Schlemm's canal) consists of a layer

of connective tissue lined on either side by endothelium (129). The outer endothelial layer comprises the inner wall of Schlemm's canal, while the inner layer is continuous with the remainder of the trabecular endothelium.

Schlemm's Canal

This 360° endothelial-lined channel averages 190–370 mm in diameter (130, 131). It may be a single channel, but occasionally branches into a plexus-like system.

Intrascleral Channels

Schlemm's canal is connected to episcleral and conjunctival veins by a complex system of vessels. Intrascleral aqueous vessels, the *aqueous veins of Ascher* (132), have been defined as originating at the outer wall of Schlemm's canal and terminating in episcleral and conjunctival veins in a lamination of aqueous and blood, referred to as the *laminated vein of Goldmann* (133). However, others refer to the proximal portion of these vessels as *outflow channels* (131, 134), or *collector channels* (130), since the structural pattern of the outer wall of Schlemm's canal extends into the first third of these channels (134). Two systems of intrascleral vessels have been identified: (a) a direct system of large caliber vessels which run a short intrascleral course and drain directly into the episcleral venous system, and (b) an indirect system of more numerous, finer channels, which form an intrascleral plexus before eventually draining into the episcleral venous system (130, 131, 134–136). The intrascleral aqueous channels do not connect with vessels of the uveal system, except for occasional fine communications with the ciliary muscle (137). There are no arterial communications (135–137), although arteriovenous anastomotic vessels may occur in the anterior episcleral system (135–140).

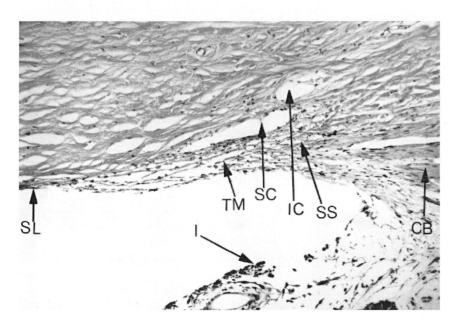

Figure 2.9. Light microscopic view of conventional aqueous outflow system: iris (*I*), ciliary body (*CB*), scleral spur (*SS*), trabecular meshwork (*TM*), Schlemm's canal (*SC*), intrascleral channels (*IC*), Schwalbe's line (*SL*). (Hematoxylin & eosin stain, ×128)

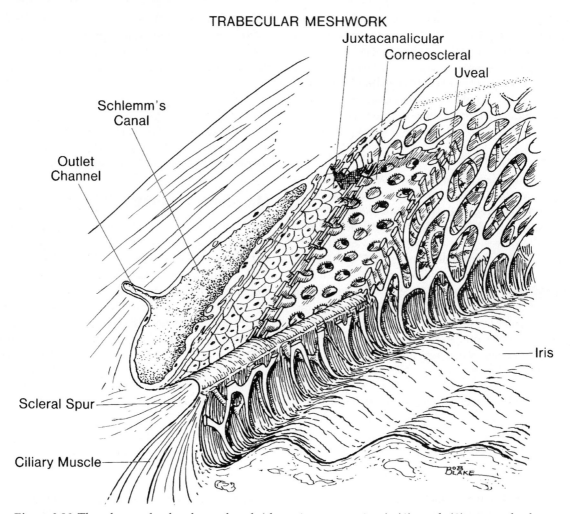

Figure 2.10. Three layers of trabecular meshwork (shown in cutaway views): (1) uveal; (2) corneoscleral; and (3) juxtacanalicular.

Episcleral and Conjunctival Veins

The aqueous vessels join the episcleral venous system by several routes (132). Most aqueous vessels are directed posteriorly with the majority of these draining into episcleral veins, while a few cross the subconjunctival tissue and drain into conjunctival veins. Some aqueous vessels proceed anteriorly to the limbus, with most of these running a short course parallel to the limbus before turning posteriorly to conjunctival veins. Other vessels make a sharp loop to join conjunctival veins or rarely extend a short distance into the cornea before turning posteriorly (Figs. 2.11 and 2.12). Casting studies in rabbit and dog eyes revealed a wide venous plexus in the limbic region of the episcleral vasculature anastomosing with a small arteriolar segment, the latter of which contains smooth muscle cells that may have a role in regulating aqueous humor drainage by the episcleral venous plexus and subsequently influencing the IOP (139, 140). In the rhesus monkey, the conjunctival vessels have a diameter consistent with that of capillaries, while most of the vessels in the episcleral plexus are the size of venules (141). Both types of vessels have simple walls composed of endothelium and a discontinuous layer of pericytes, through which horse-radish peroxidase (and presumably aqueous) freely diffuse into subconjunctival and episcleral loose connective tissue (141). The episcleral veins drain into the cavernous sinus via the anterior ciliary and superior ophthalmic veins, while the conjunctival veins drain into superior ophthalmic or facial veins via the palpebral and angular veins (133).

Ultrastructure of Trabecular Meshwork and Schlemm's Canal

Uveal and Corneoscleral Meshwork

Although the gross structure of these two trabecular subunits differs, as previously discussed, their ultrastructure is similar. Each trabecular band or sheet is composed of four concentric layers (142).

INNER CONNECTIVE TISSUE CORE. An inner connective tissue core is composed of typical collagen fibers, with the usual 640

Å periodicity (142). Indirect immunofluorescent studies of human trabecular meshwork indicate that the central core contains collagen types I and III and elastin (143, 144).

"ELASTIC" FIBERS. "Elastic" fibers are actually composed of otherwise typical collagen, arranged in a spiraling pattern with an apparent periodicity of 1000 Å (145). These spiral fibrils may wind loosely or tightly, and may provide flexibility to the trabeculae (146).

GLASS MEMBRANE. Glass membrane is a name given to the layer between the spiraling collagen and the basement membrane of the endothelium (142). It is a broad zone composed of delicate filaments embedded in a ground substance (144).

ENDOTHELIAL LAYER. An endothelial layer provides a continuous covering over the trabeculae. The cells are larger, more irregular, and have less prominent borders than corneal endothelial cells (125). They are joined by gap junctions and desmosomes, which provide stability, but allow aqueous humor to freely traverse the patent endothelial clefts (146, 147). Two types of microfilaments have been found in the cytoplasm of human trabecular endothelium (148, 149). Six-nanometer filaments are located primarily in the cell periphery, around the nucleus, and in cytoplasmic processes. These appear to be actin filaments (149) which are involved in cell contraction and motility, phagocytosis and pinocytosis, and cell adhesion. Tissue culture studies suggest that actin filaments are important in regulating the shape and cytoskeletal organization of human (150), monkey (151), and bovine (152) trabecular cells. Intermediate filaments of 10 nm are more numerous in the cells and are composed of vimentin and desmin, according to immunocytochemical studies of cultured human trabecular cells, suggesting that these cells possess muscle cell-like functions (153).

Animal studies of trabecular meshwork tissue indicate that the cells synthesize a heterogenous mixture of glycosaminoglycans and glycoproteins (154, 155), which are distributed throughout the trabecular meshwork (154–161). Human trabecular meshwork contains hyaluronic acid, chondroitin sulfate, dermatan sulfate, keratan sulfate (160), and heparan sulfate (143, 162–166). Other components of the extracellular matrix of human trabecular meshwork includes fibronectin and laminin (glycoprotein basement membrane components) and collagen types III, IV, and V in the basement membrane (143, 167–169). Human trabecular meshwork has also been shown to contain cells that express class II glycoproteins of the major histocompatibility complex, suggesting an important role in the initiation and regulation of ocular immunity (170, 171). Neuron-specific eno-

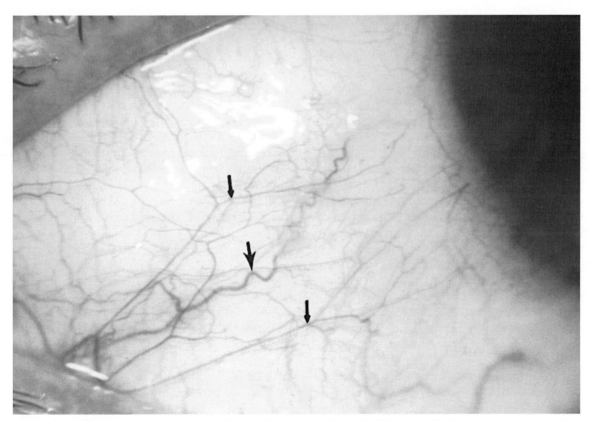

Figure 2.11. Slit-lamp view of normal episcleral and conjunctival vessels. Note typically large, serpiginous anterior ciliary artery (*large arrow*) and thinner, straighter episcleral and conjunctival veins (*small arrows*). (Courtesy of Douglas E. Gaasterland, M.D.)

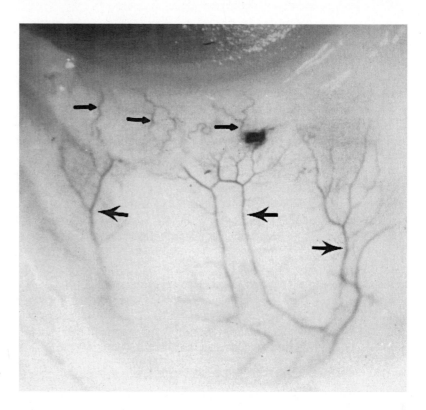

Figure 2.12. India ink perfusion of anterior chamber in human autopsy eye demonstrates filling of episcleral (*large arrows*) and conjunctival (*small arrows*) veins from aqeuous veins.

lase has been found in the trabecular meshwork of monkey eyes, which may be evidence of neuroregulatory cells (172).

As discussed earlier in this chapter under "Function and Composition of Aqueous Humor," the aqueous contains a wide variety of polypeptides, referred to as cytokines, which are involved in cell-to-cell communication. Trabecular cells have been found to have receptors to several of these growth-promoting substances, including transforming growth factor β1 (173) and transferrin (174), suggesting an influence of these aqueous components on the homeostasis of trabecular cells.

The trabecular endothelial cells have been shown to phagocytize and degrade foreign material (175–179), or to engulf debris, detach from the trabecular core, and leave in Schlemm's canal (180). Phagocytically challenged bovine trabecular meshwork cells in tissue culture revealed a transient increase in sensitivity to trypsin and reduced amounts of fibronectin and laminin, suggesting short-term loss of cell-matrix cohesiveness (181). The amount of pigment in the trabecular meshwork, however, does not appear to correlate with the cellularity or morphology of the tissue (182).

Juxtacanalicular Tissue

The portion of the trabecular meshwork adjacent to Schlemm's canal (and which actually makes up the inner wall of the canal) differs histologically from the other parts of the meshwork and has been given various names, e.g., *juxtacanalicular connective tissue, pore tissue,* and *endothelial meshwork,* depending on how one defines the anatomi-

cal limits of the tissue. In the broadest sense, this structure has three layers, discussed here beginning with the innermost portion (Figs. 2.13 and 2.14).

TRABECULAR ENDOTHELIAL LAYER. A trabecular endothelial layer is continuous with the endothelium of the corneoscleral meshwork and might be considered as a part of this layer.

CENTRAL CONNECTIVE TISSUE LAYER. A central connective tissue layer of variable thickness is unfenestrated and has several layers of parallel, spindle-shaped cells loosely arranged in a connective tissue ground substance (129, 145, 183). This tissue contains collagen type III, but no collagen type I or elastin (143). Connective tissue cells in human and rabbit trabecular meshwork have been shown to contain coated pits and coated vesicles in the plasma membrane which are involved in receptor-mediated endocytosis (184, 185).

INNER WALL ENDOTHELIUM OF SCHLEMM'S CANAL. The inner wall endothelium of Schlemm's canal is also the outermost portion of the trabecular meshwork, i.e., the last tissue that aqueous must traverse before entering the canal. This endothelial layer has significant morphological characteristics, which distinguish it from the rest of the endothelium in both the trabecular meshwork and in Schlemm's canal. The surface is bumpy due to protruding nuclei (183), cyst-like vacuoles (186), and finger-like projections (187) bulging into the canal. The finger-like projections have been described as endothelial tubules with patent lumens, although there is lack of agreement as to whether they communicate between the anterior chamber and Schlemm's canal (187) or have no significant openings (188). Actin filaments, as previously described in the uveal and corneoscleral trabecular endothelium, are also present in the inner wall endothelium of Schlemm's canal (149).

The intercellular spaces are 150–200 Å wide and the adjacent cells are connected by a variety of intercellular junctions (145, 183). It is not clear as to how tightly these junctions maintain the intercellular connections, although it has been shown that they will open to permit the passage of red blood cells (183). Zonulae occludentes have been demonstrated in primate studies, which are traversed by meandering channels of extracellular space or slit pores, although it is estimated that this accounts for only a small fraction of the aqueous humor that leaves the eye by the conventional route (147). In the human eye, the overall structure of the interendothelial junctions is more complex and less permeable than in the monkey eye (189). The endothelial cells are anchored by cytoplasmic processes to underlying subendothelial cells and trabecular meshwork (190).

Openings in the endothelial cells have been described by many investigators. Considerable controversy has arisen as to the morphology and function of these structures. In general, the openings consist of minute *pores* and large or *giant vacuoles*. The reported sizes of the pores vary considerably, although most are in the range of 0.5 to 2.0 μm (127, 130, 191–197). Tracer studies have shown that these pores communicate between the intertrabecular spaces and Schlemm's canal (195, 196). In one study, the giant vacuoles of the endothelial cells were felt to be postmortem artifacts (198), while other studies were believed to confirm their existence and suggest that they are involved in aqueous outflow (199–202). It may be that the pores and vacuoles represent different parts of the same transcellular channels (195). The possible significance of these structures in resistance to aqueous outflow is discussed later in this chapter.

Sonderman's "canals," although originally described as endothelial-lined channels communicating between Schlemm's canal and intertrabecular spaces (203), have subsequently been interpreted as tortuous communications wandering irregularly and obliquely through the meshwork

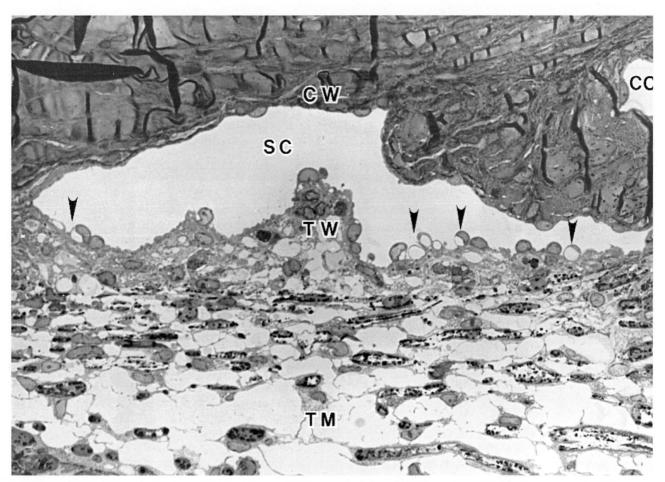

Figure 2.13. Light microscopic view of Schlemm's canal (SC) and adjacent trabecular meshwork (TM) of normotensive Rhesus monkey eye. Trabecular wall of Schlemm's cannal (TW) with prominent vacuolated cells (*arrows*); corneoscleral wall of Schlemms' canal (CW); collector channel (CC). (Toluidine blue stain; ×1030) (Reprinted with permission from Tripathi, RC: Ultrastructure of the trabecular wall of Schlemm's canal in relation to aqueous outflow. Exp Eye Res 7:335, 1968.)

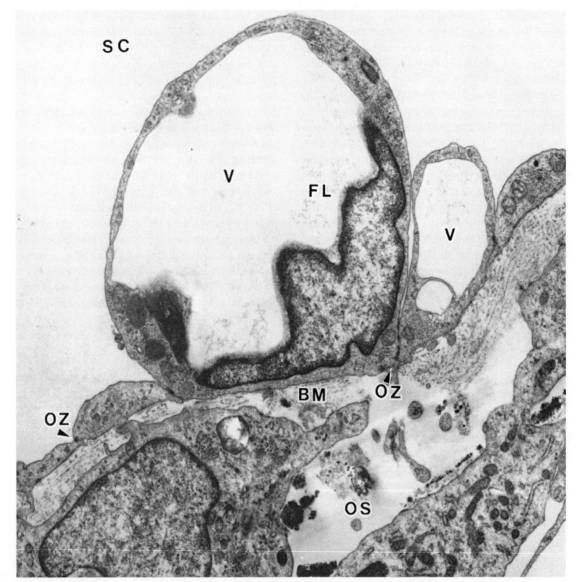

Figure 2.14. Electron microscopic view of trabecular wall of Schlemm's canal (SC) of normotensive human eye, showing vacuolated endothelial cells (V) containing flocculent material (FL). Occluding zonules (OZ), basement membrane (BM), open spaces in endothelial meshwork (OS). (×15,000) (Reprinted with permission from Tripathi, RC: Ultrastructure of the trabecular wall of Schlemm's canal. (A study of normotensive and chronic simple glaucomatous eyes). Trans Ophthalmol Soc UK 89:449, 1970.)

(204), or as deep grooves on cross-section (202), slit-like spaces between cells (205), or artifacts (127). It is unlikely that the structures, if they exist, have a significant role in aqueous outflow.

Outer Wall of Schlemm's Canal

The endothelium of the outer wall is a single cell layer that is continuous with the inner wall endothelium (145). The surface is smoother than that of the inner wall and has larger, less numerous cells (206) and no pores (191, 192), but numerous, large *outlet channels*, as previously described. Smooth muscle myosin-containing cells have been localized in the human aqueous outflow pathway adjacent to the col-

lector channels, slightly distal to the outer wall of Schlemm's canal (207). Torus or lip-like thickenings have been observed around the openings of the outlet channels (131, 134), and septa have been noted to extend from these openings to the inner wall of Schlemm's canal, which presumably help to keep the canal open (130, 131, 134). The endothelium is separated from the collagenous bundles of the limbus by a basement membrane (145) and layers of fibrocytes and fibroblasts (134).

Age-Related Changes

The normal human trabecular meshwork undergoes several changes with age. The general configuration changes from a long, wedge shape to a shorter, more rhomboidal form (208). The scleral spur becomes more prominent, the uveal meshwork becomes more compact, and localized closures in Schlemm's canal become more common (208). The trabecular beams progressively thicken, and the endothelial cellularity declines (208, 209) at the rate of approximately 0.58% of cells per year (210), occasionally leading to trabecular denuding (208). A decrease in the number of giant vacuoles and of the cell count in Schlemm's canal are both explained by an age-related reduction in the size of Schlemm's canal (211). A narrowing of the intertrabecular spaces and an increase in extracellular material, especially of electron-dense plaques near the juxtacanalicular tissue, is also seen with increasing age (208, 209). Immunogold labeling of human trabecular tissue of enucleated eyes from subjects 52–75 years of age revealed collagen types I, III, V, and VI, but no type II, and no long-spacing collagen or elastin-like material (212). Alpha-smooth muscle actin decreased with age in both normal and glaucomatous eyes (213).

Additional observations regarding the trabecular meshwork and Schlemm's canal that may relate to aqueous outflow resistance are considered later in this chapter, while those associated with possible drug responses are discussed in the pharmacology chapters in Section Three.

Unconventional Aqueous Outflow Pathways

As discussed earlier in this chapter, aqueous humor diffuses throughout virtually every portion of the eye. It is likely, therefore, that many ocular tissues, such as retina and cornea, participate in unconventional outflow by absorbing small quantities of aqueous. However, the only structure in which this has been studied in detail is the uveal tract. Two pathways have been identified whereby aqueous leaves the eye following absorption by the anterior uvea.

Uveoscleral Outflow

Tracer studies in human (114) and animal (115–119) eyes suggest that aqueous may pass through the root of the iris and interstitial spaces of the ciliary muscle to reach the suprachoroidal space. From there it passes to episcleral tissue via scleral pores surrounding ciliary arteries and nerves, vessels of optic nerve membranes, or through the actual collagen substance of the sclera. Studies with cynomolgus monkeys revealed a lower hydrostatic pressure in the suprachoroidal space as compared to that in the anterior chamber, and it was suggested that this pressure differential is the driving force for uveoscleral outflow (214). The extracellular matrix of normal human ciliary muscle contains collagen types I, III, and IV, fibronectin, and laminin in association with muscle fibers and blood vessels, and it has been suggested that the biosynthesis and turnover of these glycopro-

teins may play an important role in the function of the non-conventional outflow pathways and in mediating the action of certain pharmacological agents (215).

Uveovortex Outflow

It has also been demonstrated by tracer studies in primates that iris vessels allow unidirectional flow into the lumen of the vessel by vesicular transport, which is not energy dependent (216). The tracer can penetrate vessels of the iris, ciliary muscle, and anterior choroid to eventually reach the vortex veins (117).

A computed tomographic study of perfused radiopaque contrast media in Rhesus monkeys suggested that the unconventional aqueous drainage pathways are cleared immediately by circulating blood in the uvea and possibly the extraocular muscles, since posterior movement of contrast media through the globe wall was not seen in the living animal, but appeared immediately after death when the IOP was maintained artificially (217).

Normal Resistance to Aqueous Outflow

Assuming an average normal IOP of 15 mm Hg and an episcleral venous pressure of approximately 10 mm Hg, a resistance to aqueous outflow of 5 mm Hg must be accounted for to explain the equilibrium between inflow and outflow in the normal steady state. Grant (218, 219) demonstrated that a 360° incision in the trabecular meshwork of nonglaucomatous, enucleated human eyes eliminated 75% of the resistance to aqueous outflow. The exact site and nature of this resistance within the conventional outflow system is uncertain. The following observations, however, provide some insight into this important question.

Resistance in the Trabecular Meshwork

Studies with tracer elements show relatively free flow through the trabecular spaces and juxtacanalicular connective tissue until reaching the inner surface of the inner wall endothelium of Schlemm's canal (183, 195, 196, 200). It would appear, therefore, that this endothelial layer accounts for the majority of any resistance to outflow that the meshwork may provide, although results of studies are not conclusive and other portions of the system may also contribute to the regulation of aqueous outflow.

PORES AND GIANT VACUOLES. Pores and giant vacuoles in the inner wall endothelium of Schlemm's canal, as previously discussed, appear to be parts of a transcellular system for aqueous outflow, since tracer elements injected into the anterior chamber are seen in the vacuoles and pores (183, 195, 196, 200, 220). The observation that the concentration of tracer material in the giant vacuoles is not always the same as in the juxtacanalicular connective tissue (183) suggests a dynamic system in which the vacuoles intermittently open and close to transport aqueous from the juxtacanalicular tissue to Schlemm's canal (Fig. 2.15) (200). Whether this transport is active or passive is controversial.

Indirect evidence for a theory of active transport includes the demonstration of enzymes (221) and electron microscopic structures (222) compatible with an active transport system in or near the endothelial layer. However, the bulk of evidence supports the theory of passive (pressure-dependent) transport, since the number and size of the vacuoles have been shown to increase with progressive elevation of the IOP (223–226). Furthermore, this phenomenon is reversible in the enucleated eye (223), and hypothermia has no effect on the development of the vacuoles in the enucleated eye (227). It

may be, therefore, that potential transcellular spaces exist in the inner wall endothelium of Schlemm's canal, which open as a system of vacuoles and pores, primarily in response to pressure, to transport aqueous from the juxtacanalicular connective tissue to Schlemm's canal.

An alternative theory to that of intracellular transport is paracellular routes through the inner wall endothelium. Perfusion of monkey eyes with cationized ferritin revealed separation of adjacent cell membranes between tight junctions forming openings and tunnel-like channels, which stained with the tracer indicating intercellular passage (228). These paracellular pathways were larger at higher perfusion pressure, and apparent giant vacuoles were often dilatations of the paracellular spaces.

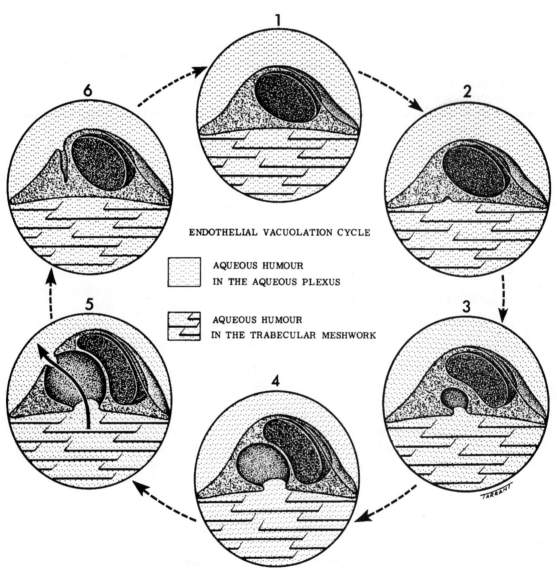

Figure 2.15. Theory of transcellular aqueous transport in which series of pores and giant vacuoles open (probably in response to transendothelial hydrostatic pressure) on connective tissue side of juxtacanalicular meshwork (2–4). Fusion of basal and apical cell plasmalemma creates a temporary transcellular channel (5) that allows bulk flow of aqueous into Schlemm's canal. (Reprinted with permission from Tripathi, RC: Mechanism of the aqueous outflow across the trabecular wall of Schlemm's canal. Exp Eye Res 11:116, 1971.)

If intracellular transport through the inner wall endothelium of Schlemm's canal exists, it has been calculated, based on the estimated size and total number of pores, that resistance to outflow through this system accounts for only a small fraction of the total resistance to aqueous outflow (229, 232). Several possibilities have been considered to explain the inability of the observed morphology of the inner wall endothelium of Schlemm's canal to account for the 5 mm Hg pressure drop across this tissue. It may be that the major resistance is located elsewhere in the trabecular meshwork, although there is no strong evidence for this theory (231). Shrinkage of tissue during preparation for electron microscopy might cause artificial enlargement of the natural lumina (231), which is taken into account in most theoretical models. Tissue preparation might also alter or remove extracellular materials (231, 232). Proteins or glycoproteins in the aqueous humor might cause a greater resistance to flow than isotonic saline (233). It is also possible that only a portion of the juxtacanalicular tissue actually filters (231). It has been suggested that aqueous humor flows preferentially through those regions of the juxtacanalicular connective tissue nearest the inner wall pores creating a "funneling effect," which increases apparent flow resistance in the connective tissue by approximately 30-fold (234). It has also been shown that microspheres that are smaller than the morphologically determined flow dimensions of a perfused eye are captured by "sticky wall" interactions, so that filtration studies provide limited information concerning the dimensions of the flow-limiting passages in the aqueous outflow system (235).

GLYCOSAMINOGLYCANS. Glycosaminoglycans (acid mucopolysaccharides), which are present in large concentration within the trabecular beams, on the surface of the trabecular endothelial cells, and in the juxtacanalicular tissue (162–164), may contribute significantly to aqueous outflow resistance in the trabecular meshwork (231, 232). These polysaccharide chains in covalent association with protein form highly polymerized complexes, which exert osmotic forces that may help to maintain hydration of the trabecular meshwork. In addition, a strong negative charge influences electromagnetic properties of tissues, which may determine the directional transport of ions in the aqueous humor. It has been proposed that trabecular cells can modulate flow by changing the ionic microenvironment of the extracellular matrices near their surfaces within the flow channels (236).

The precise mechanism by which glycosaminoglycans contribute to the resistance and regulation of aqueous humor flow through the trabecular meshwork is not clear. It has been suggested that enzymes which catabolize glycosaminoglycans are released by lysosomes in the meshwork, to depolymerize the glycosaminoglycans, thereby reducing this cause of resistance to outflow (237, 238). Hyaluronidase has been shown to decrease aqueous outflow resistance in nonprimate species (219, 239, 240), and similar results were reported with chondroitinase ABC in cynomolgus monkeys (241), suggesting a glycosaminoglycans barrier to aqueous outflow.

However, perfusion studies with enucleated monkey eyes, using a trabeculotomy and hyaluronidase, suggest that outflow resistance due to glycosaminoglycans is only slightly related to the trabecular meshwork (242).

It has been shown that prolonged perfusion of canine and monkey eyes causes a time-dependent increase in outflow facility, apparently due to a "washout" of a hyaluronidase-sensitive component of the barrier to aqueous outflow (243–245). The washout effect, however, is not observed in either the adult or infant human enucleated eye, and it is felt that this difference in washout behavior may signify a potentially important fundamental difference in the biology of the outflow pathways between human and other primate eyes (245).

GLUCOCORTICOID RECEPTORS. Glucocorticoid receptors have been demonstrated in the trabecular meshwork of trabeculectomy specimens from human glaucomatous eyes, nonglaucomatous autopsy eyes (246), and cultured human trabecular cells (247), suggesting that glucocorticoids may influence the outflow facility by a direct effect on the metabolism of these cells. This effect may be on the incorporation of precursors of extracellular matrix components, leading to an increase in collagen synthesis or a decreased synthesis of glycosaminoglycans, glycoproteins, or possibly glycolipids (248). Glucocorticoids also inhibit the synthesis of prostaglandins (249), production of which has been seen in cultured human trabecular cells (249, 250). Prostaglandins have been shown to cause increased IOP in high doses, but reduced ocular tension in moderate to low concentrations (251).

CONTRACTILE MICROFILAMENTS. Contractile microfilaments, as previously described, occur in the inner wall endothelium of Schlemm's canal, as well as the endothelium lining the trabeculae. Perfusing monkey eyes with substances that are known to disrupt the microfilaments, such as cytochalasin B (252–255), cytochalasin D (255), or EDTA (256, 257), significantly reduces the resistance to aqueous outflow, and histologic studies suggest that this is primarily due to an alteration in the trabecular meshwork or inner wall of Schlemm's canal (253, 254, 256, 257).

SULFHYDRYL GROUPS. Sulfhydryl groups in trabecular cells also appear to modulate aqueous outflow by several mechanisms. Perfusion with certain sulfhydryl reagents, including iodoacetic acid (258), iodoacetamide (259), and N-ethylmaleimide (260), increases facility of outflow. This is apparently not due to a metabolic inhibitory action, but to an alteration of cell membrane sulfhydryl groups at multiple sites in the endothelial lining of Schlemm's canal (261). Conversely, mercurial sulfhydryl agents cause a decrease in aqueous outflow, presumably due to cellular swelling of the trabecular meshwork (262).

Ethacrynic acid is a sulfhydryl-reactive drug, which has been shown to increase facility of outflow in the human eye (263). This was originally felt to be related to alterations of trabecular cytoskeletal elements (264). However, three agents known to react with cytoskeletal components had no significant influence on outflow facility (265), and subsequent studies suggested that the action of ethacrynic acid was through separation between inner wall endothelial cells (266).

Another mechanism by which sulfhydryl groups modulate aqueous outflow may involve hydrogen peroxide, a normal constituent of aqueous humor which may reduce outflow through oxidative damage of the trabecular meshwork. Bovine trabecular meshwork cells have significant antioxidant activity with a major contribution provided by the glutathione redox cycle (267). Calf trabecular meshwork has been shown to contain the sulfhydryl compound, glutathione (268), as well as the enzyme glutathione peroxidase (269), which catalyses the reaction between glutathione and hydrogen peroxide, thereby detoxifying the latter and presumably protecting the meshwork from its harmful effects (270). In the pig eye, oxidative damage increases outflow facility at normal pressure but decreases it with elevated IOP, suggesting that elevated pressure may increase susceptibility of the outflow pathway to this form of insult (271).

FIBRINOLYTIC ACTIVITY. Fibrinolytic activity has been demonstrated in the endothelium of Schlemm's canal (272), but no evidence of coagulation factors has been found (273). Tissue plasminogen activator, which is responsible for the conversion of plasminogen to plasmin, thereby mediating the lysis of formed fibrin, has been demonstrated in many ocular tissues, including the trabecular meshwork of human and animal eyes (274–276). This suggests that a hemostatic balance, displaced towards fibrinolysis, protects this portion of the outflow system from occlusion by fibrin and platelets (272–276). In addition to facilitating the resolution of hyphema, tissue plasminogen activator may also influence resistance to aqueous outflow under normal circumstances by altering the glycoprotein content of the extracellular matrix (231, 232).

Studies with cultured bovine trabecular meshwork cells suggest that endothelin-1 may be involved in regulating aqueous humor dynamics by changing the intracellular Ca^{2+} and pH (277). It has also been shown that the human outflow pathway and ciliary muscle are enriched sites of nitric oxide synthesis, which may have a role in modulating outflow resistance (278).

Resistance in Schlemm's Canal

Once aqueous has entered Schlemm's canal, resistance to continued flow into the intrascleral outlet channels may depend on the spatial configuration of the canal. There is controversy as to whether the canal is normally entirely open and whether it allows circumferential flow. Perfusion studies in enucleated human adult eyes suggest that aqueous cannot flow more than 10° within the canal (279), although there is

less resistance to circumferential flow in infant eyes (280). However, studies of segmental blood reflux into Schlemm's canal imply that the canal is normally entirely open and that there is circumferential flow (281).

PRESSURE-DEPENDENT CHANGES. Pressure-dependent changes in aqueous outflow facility appears to be related to a collapse of Schlemm's canal. Elevation of IOP is associated with increased resistance to outflow (223, 282–284), which is most likely due to collapse of the canal. Histological studies of eyes perfused at different pressures suggest that compromise of the canal lumen with elevated IOP is due to distention of the trabecular meshwork (223, 285, 286), an increase in endothelial vacuoles (224–226), and a ballooning of the inner wall endothelial cells into the canal (190). Perfusion studies also suggest that the resistance to aqueous outflow may normally depend in part on an intact, unyielding outer wall of Schlemm's canal against which the intact inner wall is pressed by the IOP (287), probably due to blockage of the intrascleral outlet (collector) channels by the canal's inner wall (288). However, significant differences in the response to elevated perfusion pressure have been found among different mammalian eyes, and it has been suggested that factors other than, or in addition to, collapse of Schlemm's canal may be important regarding the influence of elevated IOP on resistance to outflow (289).

As might be expected from these observations, resistance to outflow is decreased by expanding Schlemm's canal. The trabecular meshwork has been described as a three-dimensional set of diagonally crossing collagen fibers, which respond to backward, inward displacement with a widening of Schlemm's canal (290). The effect of tensing the meshwork has been demonstrated by deepening of the anterior chamber during perfusion studies when an iridectomy is not made (218), by posterior depression of the lens (279, 288, 291–294), or by tension on the choroid (295). With each experimental model, the tension on the trabecular meshwork is associated with increased outflow facility, which appears to be due to widening of Schlemm's canal (292, 294) and an increase in canal inner wall porosity (292).

As previously noted, a 360° incision of the trabecular meshwork (trabeculotomy) eliminates approximately 75% of the normal outflow resistance (218, 219). However, when such an eye is perfused at 7 mm Hg, the trabeculotomy only eliminates half the resistance, with further decrease in resistance of 2% per mm Hg rise in the IOP (296). This suggests that a significant fraction of aqueous outflow resistance is in the distal aspects of the outflow system, and that this resistance decreases with increasing IOP.

Resistance in the Intrascleral Outflow Channels

The remainder of the resistance to aqueous outflow appears to be within the intrascleral outflow channels. One monkey study has suggested that 60–65% of outflow resistance is in the trabecular meshwork, 25% is in the inner $\frac{1}{3}$ to $\frac{1}{2}$ of the sclera, and 15% is in the outer $\frac{1}{2}$ to $\frac{2}{3}$ of the sclera (297).

Resistance to Unconventional Outflow

Unlike the conventional outflow system, unconventional outflow has been reported to improve with an elevation of the IOP, presumably due to ultrafiltration of aqueous into uveal vessels (115). It has also been shown that outflow by this route is reduced by miotics (114). It should be noted that our understanding of the unconventional outflow system is based more on physiology than on anatomy, and further study is needed to correlate function and anatomy in this system.

Episcleral Venous Pressure

As discussed earlier in this chapter, another factor which contributes to the IOP is the episcleral venous pressure. The precise interrelationship between episcleral venous pressure and aqueous humor dynamics is complex and only partially understood. It has been commonly held that the IOP rises mm Hg for mm Hg with an increase in episcleral venous pressure, although it may be that the magnitude of IOP rise is greater than the rise in venous pressure (299). The normal episcleral venous pressure is reported to be within the range of 8–11 mm Hg (300–303), and one study found that this does not vary with age (303). However, these values are influenced considerably by the particular technique of measurement (304), which is discussed in the next chapter.

SUMMARY

Intraocular pressure is the result of a complex interplay of the components of aqueous humor dynamics, especially the rate of aqueous production, the resistance to aqueous outflow, and the episcleral venous pressure. Aqueous humor is produced by the ciliary processes through ultrafiltration of plasma from capillaries, active transport of certain constituents of the plasma across an epithelial barrier, and flow of other plasma components across the epithelium due to an osmotic gradient that is created by the active transport. The aqueous enters the posterior chamber, between the iris and lens, and undergoes metabolic interchanges with virtually all ocular structures, especially the cornea, iris, lens, vitreous, and retina. The bulk of aqueous, however, flows through the pupil into the anterior chamber and leaves the eye via structures in the anterior chamber angle, primarily through the trabecular meshwork and Schlemm's canal (conventional outflow) with a small contribution from anterior uveal absorption. From Schlemm's canal, aqueous passes through intrascleral channels to reunite with the blood system in the episcleral veins.

REFERENCES

1. Hogan, MF, Alvarado, JA, Weddell, JE: Histology of the Human Eye. Philadelphia, WB Saunders, 1971, p. 269.
2. Aiello, AL, Tran, VT, Rao, NA: Postnatal development of the ciliary body and pars plana. A morphometric study in childhood. Arch Ophthalmol 110:802, 1992.
3. Morrison, JC, Van Buskirk, EM: Anterior collateral circulation in the primate eye. Ophthalmology 90:707, 1983.
4. Funk, R, Rohen, JW: Scanning electron microscopic study on the vasculature of the human anterior eye segment, especially with respect to the ciliary processes. Exp Eye Res 51:651, 1990.
5. Woodlief, NF: Initial observations on the ocular microcirculation in man. I. The anterior segment and extraocular muscles. Arch Ophthalmol 98:1268, 1980.
6. Morrison, JC, DeFrank, MP, Van Buskirk, EM: Regional microvascular anatomy of the rabbit ciliary body. Invest Ophthalmol Vis Sci 28:1314, 1987.
7. Morrison, JC, DeFrank, MP, Van Buskirk, EM: Comparative microvascular anatomy of mammalian ciliary processes. Invest Ophthalmol Vis Sci 28:1325, 1987.
8. Talusan, ED, Schwartz, B: Fluorescein angiography. Demonstration of flow patterns of anterior ciliary arteries. Arch Ophthalmol 99:1074, 1981.
9. Sakimoto, G, Schwartz, B: Decrease of anterior ciliary arterial pressure with increased ocular pressure. Invest Ophthalmol Vis Sci 25:992, 1984.
10. Nanba, K, Schwartz, B: Increased diameter of the anterior ciliary artery with increased intraocular pressure. Arch Ophthalmol 104:1652, 1986.
11. Morrison, JC, Van Buskirk, EM: Ciliary process microvasculature of the primate eye. Am J Ophthalmol 97:372, 1984.
12. Smelser, GK: Electron microscopy of a typical epithelial cell and of the normal human ciliary process. Trans Am Acad Ophthalmol Otolarynol 70:738, 1966.
13. Kitada, S, Shapourifar-Tehrani, S, Smyth, RJ, Lee, DA: Characterization of human and rabbit pigmented and nonpigmented ciliary body epithelium. Eye Res 10:409, 1991.
14. Streeten, BW, Licari, PA: The zonules and the elastic microfibrillar system in the ciliary body. Invest Ophthalmol Vis Sci 24:667, 1983.
15. Eichhorn, M, Flügel, C, Lütjen-Drecoll, E: Regional differences in the distribution of cytoskeletal filaments in the human and bovine ciliary epithelium. Graefe's Arch Ophthalmol 230:385, 1992.
16. Marshall, GE, Konstas, AGP, Abraham, S, Lee, WR: Extracellular matrix in aged human ciliary body: an immunoelectron microscope study. Invest Ophthalmol Vis Sci 33:2546, 1992.
17. Raviola, G, Raviola, E: Intercellular junctions in the ciliary epithelium. Invest Ophthalmol Vis Sci 17:958, 1978.
18. Smith, RL, Raviola, G: The structural basis of the blood-aqueous barrier in the chicken eye. Invest Ophthalmol Vis Sci 24:326, 1983.
19. Oh, J, Krupin, T, Tang, L-Q, et al: Dye coupling of rabbit ciliary epithelial cells in vitro. Invest Ophthalmol Vis Sci 35:2509, 1994.
20. Green, K, Bountra, C, Georgiou, P, House, CR: An electrophysiologic study of rabbit ciliary epithelium. Invest Ophthalmol Vis Sci 26:371, 1985.
21. Cunha-Vas, JG: The blood-ocular barriers. Invest Ophthalmol Vis Sci 17:1037, 1978.
22. Pederson, JE: Fluid permeability of monkey ciliary epithelium in vivo. Invest Ophthalmol Vis Sci 23:176, 1982.
23. Wulle, KG: Zelldifferenzierungen im Ciliarepithel wahrend der menschlichen Fetalentwicklung und ihre Beziehungen zur Kammerwasserbildung. Graefe's Arch Clin Exp Ophthalmol 172:170, 1967.
24. Richardson, KT: Cellular response to drugs affecting aqueous dynamics. Arch Ophthalmol 89:65, 1973.
25. Uusitalo, R, Palkama, A, Stjernschantz, J: An electron microscopical study of the blood-aqueous barrier in the ciliary body and iris of the rabbit. Exp Eye Res 17:49, 1973.

26. Smith, RS, Rudt, LA: Ultrastructural studies of the blood-aqueous barrier. 2. The barrier to horseradish peroxidase in primates. Am J Ophthalmol 76:937, 1973.

27. Peress, NS, Tompkins, DC: Pericapillary permeability of the ciliary processes. Role of molecular charge. Invest Ophthalmol Vis Sci 23:168, 1982.

28. Macri, JF, Cevario, SJ: The formation and inhibition of aqueous humor production. Arch Ophthalmol 96:1664, 1978.

29. Farahbakhsh, NA, Fian, GL: Volume regulation of non-pigmented cells from ciliary epithelium. Invest Ophthalmol Vis Sci 28:934, 1987.

30. Becker, B: The effect of hypothermia on aqueous humor dynamics. III. Turnover of ascorbate and sodium. Am J Ophthalmol 51:1032, 1961.

31. Berggren, L: Effect of composition of medium and of metabolic inhibitors on secretion in vitro by the ciliary processes of the rabbit eye. Invest Ophthalmol 4:83, 1965.

32. Sears, ML: The aqueous. In Adler's Physiology of the Eye, 6th edition. Moses, RA, ed. St Louis, CV Mosby Co, 1975, p. 232.

33. Bonting, SL, Becker, B: Studies on sodium-potassium activated adenosinetriphosphatase. XIV. Inhibition of enzyme activity and aqueous humor flow in the rabbit eye after intravitreal injection of ouabain. Invest Ophthalmol 3:523, 1964.

34. Cole, DF: Some effects of decreased plasma sodium concentration on the composition and tension of the aqueous humor. Br J Ophthalmol 43:268, 1959.

35. Holland, MG, Gipson, CC: Chloride ion transport in the isolated ciliary body. Invest Ophthalmol 9:20, 1970.

36. Holland, MG: Chloride ion transport in the isolated ciliary body. II. Ion substitution experiments. Invest Ophthalmol 9:30, 1970.

37. Bito, L, Davson, H: Steady-state concentrations of potassium in the ocular fluids. Exp Eye Res 3:283, 1964.

38. Helbig, H, Korbmacher, C, Wohlfarth, J, et al: Electrical membrane properties of a cell clone derived from human nonpigmented ciliary epithelium. Invest Ophthalmol Vis Sci 30:882, 1989.

39. Chu, T-C, Candia, OA: Electrically silent Na^+ and Cl^- fluxes across the rabbit ciliary epithelium. Invest Ophthalmol Vis Sci 29:594, 1988.

40. Chu, T-C, Candia, OA: Active transport of ascorbate across the isolated rabbit ciliary epithelium. Invest Ophthalmol Vis Sci 29:594, 1988.

41. Reddy, VN: Dynamics of transport systems in the eye. Invest Ophthalmol Vis Sci 18:1000, 1979.

42. Maren, TH: The rates of movement of Na^+, Cl^-, and HCO^-_3 from plasma to posterior chamber: effect of acetazolamide and relation to the treatment of glaucoma. Invest Ophthalmol 15:356, 1976.

43. Cole, DF: Effects of some metabolic inhibitors upon the formation of the aqueous humor in rabbits. Br J Ophthalmol 44:739, 1960.

44. Hara, K, Lutjen-Drecoll, E, Prestele, H, Rohen, JW: Structural differences between regions of the ciliary body in primates. Invest Ophthalmol Vis Sci 16:912, 1977.

45. Ober, M, Rohen, JW: Regional differences in the fine structure of the ciliary epithelium related to accommodation. Invest Ophthalmol Vis Sci 18:655, 1979.

46. Mizuno, K, Asaoka, M: Cycloscopy and fluorescein cycloscopy. Invest Ophthalmol 15:561, 1976.

47. Lutjen-Drecoll, E, Lonnerholm, G, Eichhorn, M: Carbonic anhydrase distribution in the human and monkey eye by light and electron micorscopy. Graefe's Arch Clin Exp Ophthalmol 220:285, 1983.

48. Russman, W: Levels of glycolytic enzyme activity in the ciliary epithelium prepared from bovine eyes. Ophthalmic Res 2:205, 1971.

49. Feeney, L, Mixon, R: Localization of [35]sulfated macromolecules at the site of active transport in the ciliary processes. Invest Ophthalmol 13:882, 1974.

50. Feeney, L, Mixon, RN: Sulfate and galactose metabolism in differentiating ciliary body and iris epithelia: autoradiographic and ultrastructural studies. Invest Ophthalmol 14:364, 1975.

51. Krupin, T, Wax, M, Moolchandani, J: Aqueous production. Trans Ophthalmol Soc UK 105:156, 1986.

52. Raviola, G: Evidence for a secretory process, distinct from that of the aqueous humour, in the ciliary epithelium of Macaca mulatta. Trans Ophthalmol Soc UK 105:140, 1986.

53. McLaren, JW, Brubaker, RF: A scanning ocular fluorophotometer. Invest Ophthalmol Vis Sci 29:1285, 1988.

54. Brubaker, RF: Flow of aqueous humor in humans. Invest Ophthalmol Vis Sci 32:3145, 1991.

55. Reiss, GR, Lee, DA, Topper, JE, Brubaker, RF: Aqueous humor flow during sleep. Invest Ophthalmol Vis Sci 25:776, 1984.

56. McLaren, JW, Trocme, SD, Relf, S, Brubaker, RF: Rate of flow of aqueous humor determined from measurements of aqueous flare. Invest Ophthalmol Vis Sci 31:339, 1990.

57. Brubaker, RF, Kupfer, C: Determination of pseudofacility in the eye of the rhesus monkey. Arch Ophthalmol 75:693, 1966.

58. Kupfer, C, Sanderson, P: Determination of pseudofacility in the eye of man. Arch Ophthalmol 80:194, 1968.

59. Bill, A: Aspects on suppressability of aqueous humour formation. Doc Ophthalmol 26:73, 1969.

60. Brubaker, RF: The measurement of pseudofacility and true facility by constant pressure perfusion in the normal rhesus monkey eye. Invest Ophthalmol 9:42, 1970.

61. Leydhecker, W, Rehak, S, Mathyl, J: Investigations on homeostasis: the effect of experimental changes of pressure on the production of aqueous humour in the living rabbit eye. Klin Monatsbl Augenheilkd 159:427, 1971.

62. Kupfer, C, Ross, K: Studies of aqueous humor dynamics in man. 1. Measurements in young normal subjects. Invest Ophthalmol 10:518, 1971.

63. Bill, A: Effects of longstanding stepwise increments in eye pressure on the rate of aqueous humor formation in a primate (cercopithecus ethiops). Exp Eye Res 12:184, 1971.

64. Carlson, KH, McLaren, JW, Topper, JE, Brubaker, RF: Effect of body positions on intraocular pressure and aqueous flow. Invest Ophthalmol Vis Sci 28:1653, 1985.

65. Moses, RA, Grodzki, WJ, Jr., Carras, PL: Pseudofacility. Arch Ophthalmol 103:1653, 1985.

66. Brown, JD, Brubaker, RF: A study of the relation between intraocular pressure and aqueous humor flow in the pigment dispersion syndrome. Ophthalmology 96:1468, 1989.

67. Becker, B: The decline in aqueous secretion and outflow facility with age. Am J Ophthalmol 46:731, 1958.

68. Brubaker, RF, Nagtaki, S, Townsend, DJ, et al: The effect of age on aqueous humor formation in man. Ophthalmology 88:283, 1981.

69. Topper, JE, Brubaker, RF: Effects of timolol, epinephrine, and acetazolamide on aqueous flow during sleep. Invest Ophthalmol Vis Sci 26:1315, 1985.

70. Gharagozloo, NZ, Larson, RS, Kullerstrand, LJ, Brubaker, RF: Terbutaline stimulates aqueous humor flow in human during sleep. Arch Ophthalmol 106:1218, 1988.

71. Schneider, RL, Brubaker, RF: Effect of chronic epinephrine on aqueous humor flow during the day and during sleep in normal healthy subjects. Invest Ophthalmol Vis Sci 32:2507, 1991.

72. Koskela, T, Brubaker, RF: The nocturnal suppression of aqueous humor flow in humans is not blocked by bright light. Invest Ophthalmol Vis Sci 32:2504, 1991.

73. Sheridan, PT, Brubaker, RF, Larsson, L-I, et al: The effect of oral dexamethasone on the circadian rhythm of aqueous humor flow in humans. Invest Ophthalmol Vis Sci 35:1150, 1994.

74. Maus, TL, Young, WF Jr., Brubaker, RF: Aqueous flow in humans after adrenalectomy. Invest Ophthalmol Vis Sci 35:3325, 1994.

75. Hayashi, M, Yablonski, ME, Boxrud, C, et al: Decreased formation of aqueous humour in insulin-dependent diabetic patients. Br J Ophthalmol 73:621, 1989.

76. Larsson, L-I, Pach, JM, Brubaker, RF: Aqueous humor dynamics in patients with diabetes mellitus. Am J Ophthalmol 120:362, 1995.

77. Pederson, JE: Ocular Hypotony. Trans Ophthalmol Soc UK 105:220, 1986.

78. Howes, EL, Cruse, VK: The structural basis of altered vascular permeability following intraocular inflammation. Arch Ophthalmol 96:1668, 1978.

79. Dobbie, JG: A study of the intraocular fluid dynamics in retinal detachment. Arch Ophthalmol 69:53, 1963.

80. Diestelhorst, M, Krieglstein, GK: The effect of the water-drinking test on aqueous humor dynamics in healthy volunteers. Graefe's Arch Exp Clin Ophthalmol 232:145, 1994.

81. Adams, BA, Brubaker, RF: Caffeine has no clinically significant effect on aqueous humor flow in the normal human eye. Ophthalmology 97:1030, 1990.

82. De Berardinis, E, Tieri, O, Iuglio, N, Polzella, A: The composition of the aqueous humour of man in aphakia. Acta Ophthalmol 44:64, 1966.

83. Kinsey, VE: Comparative chemistry of aqueous humor in posterior and anterior chamber of rabbit eye. Its physiologic significance. Arch Ophthalmol 50:401, 1953.

84. Raviola, G, Butler, JM: Asymmetric distribution of charged domains on the two fronts of the endothelium of iris blood vessels. Invest Ophthalmol Vis Sci 26:597, 1985.

85. Freddo, TF, Raviola, G: The homogeneous structure of blood vessels in the vascular tree of Macaca mulatta iris. Invest Ophthalmol Vis Sci 22:279, 1982.

86. Freddo, TF, Raviola, G: Freeze-fracture analysis of the interendothelial junctions in the blood vessels of the iris in Macaca mulatta. Invest Ophthalmol Vis Sci 23:154, 1982.

87. Becker, B: Chemical composition of human aqueous humor. Effects of acetazoleamide. Arch Ophthalmol 57:793, 1957.

88. Reiss, GR, Werness, PG, Zollman, PE, Brubaker, RF: Ascorbic acid levels in the aqueous humor of nocturnal and diurnal mammals. Arch Ophthalmol 104:753, 1986.

89. Freddo, TF, Bartels, SP, Barsotti, MF, Kamm, RD: The source of proteins in the aqueous humor of the normal rabbit. Invest Ophthalmol Vis Sci 31:125, 1990.

90. Barsotti, MF, Barteles, SP, Freddo, TF, Kamm, RD: The source of protein in the aqueous humor of the normal monkey eye. Invest Ophthalmol Vis Sci 33:581, 1992.

91. Haddad, A, Laicine, EM, de Almeida, JC: Origin and renewal of the intrinsic glycoproteins of the aqueous humor. Graefe's Arch Clin Exp Ophthalmol 229:371, 1991.

92. Pavao, AF, Lee, DA, Ethier, CR, et al: Two-dimensional gel electrophoresis of calf aqueous humor, serum, and filter-bound proteins. Invest Ophthalmol Vis Sci 30:731, 1989.

93. Ethier, CR, Kamm, RD, Johnson, M, et al: Further studies on the flow of aqueous humor through microporous filters. Invest Ophthalmol Vis Sci 30:739, 1989.

94. Sen, DK, Sarin, GS, Saha, K: Immunoglobulins in human aqueous humour. Br J Ophthalmol 61:216, 1977.

95. Okisaka, S: Effects of paracentesis on the blood-aqueous barrier: a light and electron microscopic study on cynomolgus monkey. Invest Ophthalmol 15:824, 1976.

96. Bartels, SP, Pederson, JE, Gaasterland, DE, Armaly, MF: Sites of breakdown of the blood-aqueous barrier after paracentesis of the rhesus monkey eye. Invest Ophthalmol Vis Sci 18:1050, 1979.

97. Murray, DL, Bartels, SP: The relationship between aqueous humor flow and anterior chamber protein concentration in rabbits. Invest Ophthalmol Vis Sci 34:370, 1993.

98. Dickinson, JC, Durham, DG, Hamilton, PB: Ion exchange chromatography of free amino acids in aqueous fluid and lens of the human eye. Invest Ophthalmol 7:551, 1968.

99. De Berardinis, E, Tieri, O, Polzella, A, Iuglio, N: The chemical composition of the human aqueous humour in normal and pathological conditions. Exp Eye Res 4:179, 1965.

100. Davson, H., Luck CP: A comparative study of the total carbon dioxide in the ocular fluids, cerebrospinal fluid, and plasma of some mammalian species. J Physiol 132:454, 1956.

101. Laurent, UBG: Hyaluronate in human aqueous humor. Arch Ophthalmol 101:129, 1983.

102. Trope, GE, Rumley, AG: Catecholamines in human aqueous humor. Invest Ophthalmol Vis Sci 26:399, 1985.

103. Khodadoust, AA, Stark, WJ, Bell, WR: Coagulation properties of intraocular humors and cerebrospinal fluid. Invest Ophthalmol Vis Sci 24:1616, 1983.

104. Tripathi, RC, Park, JK, Tripathi, BJ, Millard, CB: Tissue plasminogen activator in human aqueous humor and its possible therapeutic significance. Am J Ophthalmol 106:719, 1988.

105. Smalley, DM, Fitzgerald, JE, Taylor, DM, et al: Tissue plasminogen activator activity in human aqueous humor. Invest Ophthalmol Vis Sci 35:48, 1994.

106. Bernatchez, S, Tabatabay, C, Belin, D: Urokinase-type plasminogen activator in human aqueous humor. Invest Ophthalmol Vis Sci 33:2687, 1992.

107. Vadillo-Ortega, F, Gonzalez-Avila, G, Chevez, P, et al: A latent collagenase in human aqueous humor. Invest Ophthalmol Vis Sci 30:332, 1989.

108. Tripathi, RC, Borisuth, NSC, Li, J, Tripathi, BJ: Growth factors in the aqueous humor and their clinical significance. J Glauc 3:248, 1994.

109. Tripathi, RC, Millard, CB, Tripathi, BJ, Noronha, A: Tau fraction of transferrin is present in human aqueous humor and is not unique to cerebrospinal fluid. Exp Eye Res 50:541, 1990.

110. Tripathi, RC, Borisuth, NSC, Tripathi, BJ, Gotsis, SS: Quantitative and qualitative analyses of transferrin in aqueous humor from patients with primary and secondary glaucomas. Invest Ophthalmol Vis Sci 33:2866, 1992.

111. Cousins, SW, McCabe, MM, Danielpour, D, Streilen, JW: Identification of transforming growth factor-beta as an immunosuppressive factor in aqueous humor. Invest Ophthalmol Vis Sci 32:2201, 1991.

112. Lepple-Wienhues, A, Becker, M, Stahl, F, et al: Endothelin-like immunoreactivity in the aqueous humour and conditioned medium from cultured ciliary epithelial cells. Eye Res 11:1041, 1992.

113. Malina, HZ, Martin, XD: Indoleamine 2,3–dioxygenase activity in the aqueous humor, iris/ciliary body, and retina of the bovine eye. Graefe's Arch Exp Clin Ophthalmol 231:482, 1993.

114. Jocson, VL, Sears, ML: Experimental aqueous perfusion in enucleated human eyes. Arch Ophthalmol 86:65, 1971.

115. Bill, A, Phillips, CI: Uveoscleral drainage of aqueous humour in human eyes. Exp Eye Res 12:275, 1971.

116. Pederson, JE, Gaasterland, DE, MacLellan, HM: Uveoscleral aqueous outflow in the rhesus monkey: importance of uveal reabsorption. Invest Ophthalmol Vis Sci 16:1008, 1977.

117. Inomata, H, Bill, A: Exit sites of uveoscleral flow of aqueous humor in cynomolgus monkey eyes. Exp Eye Res 25:113, 1977.

118. Sherman, SH, Green, K, Laties, AM: The fate of anterior chamber fluorescein in the monkey eye. I. The anterior chamber outflow pathways. Exp Eye Res 27:159, 1978.

119. Inomata, H, Bill, A, Smelser, GK: Unconventional routes of aqueous humor outflow in cynomolgus monkey (Macaca irus). Am J Ophthalmol 73:893, 1972.

120. McMaster, PRB, Macri, FJ: Secondary aqueous humor outflow pathways in the rabbit, cat, and monkey. Arch Ophthalmol 79:297, 1968.

121. Moses, RA, Grodzki, WF Jr: The scleral spur and scleral roll. Invest Ophthalmol Vis Sci 16:925, 1977.

122. Moses, RA, Grodzki, WJ Jr, Starcher, BC, Galione, MJ: Elastin content of the scleral spur, trabecular mesh, and sclera. Invest Ophthalmol Vis Sci 17:817, 1978.

123. Tamm, ER, Koch, TA, Mayer, B, et al: Innervation of myofibroblast-like scleral spur cells in human and monkey eyes. Invest Ophthalmol Vis Sci 36:1633, 1995.

124. Tamm, ER, Flügel, C, Stefani, FH, Lütjen-Drecoll, E: Nerve endings with structural characteristics of mechanoreceptors in the human scleral spur. Invest Ophthalmol Vis Sci 35:1157, 1994.

125. Spencer, WH, Alvarado, J, Hayes, TL: Scanning electron microscopy of human ocular tissues: Trabecular meshwork. Invest Ophthalmol 7:651, 1968.

126. Raviola, G: Schwalbe line's cells: a new cell type in the trabecular meshwork of Macaca mulatta. Invest Ophthalmol Vis Sci 22:45, 1982.

127. Flocks, M: The anatomy of the trabecular meshwork as seen in tangential section. Arch Ophthalmol 56:708, 1957.

128. de Kater, AW, Shahsafaei, A, Epstein, DL: Localization of smooth muscle and nonmuscle actin isoforms in the human aqueous outflow pathway. Invest Ophthalmol Vis Sci 33:424, 1992.

129. Fine, BS: Observations on the drainage angle in man and rhesus monkey: A concept of the pathogenesis of chronic simple glaucoma. A light and electron microscopic study. Invest Ophthalmol 3:609, 1964.

130. Hoffmann, F, Dumitrescu, L: Schlemm's canal under the scanning electron microscope. Ophthalmic Res 2:37, 1971.

131. Rohen, JW, Rentsch, FJ: Morphology of Schlemm's canal and related vessels in the human eye. Graefe's Arch Exp Clin Ophthalmol 176:309, 1968.

132. Ascher, KW: The Aqueous Veins. Biomicroscopic Study of the Aqueous Humor Elimination. Springfield, IL, Charles C Thomas, 1961.

133. Last, RJ: Wolff's Anatomy of the Eye and Orbit, Fifth edition. Philadelphia, WB Saunders, 1961, p. 49.

134. Rohen, JW, Rentsch, FJ: Electronmicroscopic studies on the structure of the outer wall of Schlemm's canal, its outflow channels and age changes. Graefe's Arch Exp Clin Ophthalmol 177:1, 1969.

135. Jocson, VL, Sears, ML: Channels of aqueous outflow and related blood vessels. I. Macaca mulatta (rhesus). Arch Ophthalmol 80:104, 1968.

136. Jocson, VL, Sears, ML: Channels of aqueous outflow and related blood vessels. II. Cercopithecus ethiops (Ethiopian green or green vervet). Arch Ophthalmol 81:244, 1969.

137. Jocson, VL, Grant, WM: Interconections of blood vessels and aqueous vessels in human eyes. Arch Ophthalmol 73:707, 1965.

138. Gaasterland, DE, Jocson, VL, Sears, ML: Channels of aqueous outflow and related blood vessels. III. Episcleral arteriovenous anastomoses in the rhesus monkey eye (Macaca mulatta). Arch Ophthalmol 84:770, 1970.

139. Funk, RHW, Rohen, JW: In vivo observations of the episcleral vasculature in the albino rabbit. J Glauc 3:44, 1994.

140. Rohen, JW, Funk, RHW: Functional morphology of the episcleral vasculature in rabbits and dogs: presence of arteriovenous anastomoses. J Glauc 3:51, 1994.

141. Raviola, G: Conjunctival and episcleral blood vessels are permeable to blood-borne horseradish peroxidase. Invest Ophthalmol Vis Sci 24:725, 1983.

142. Ashton, N: The exit pathway of the aqueous. Trans Ophthalmol Soc UK 80:397, 1960.

143. Murphy, CG, Yun, AJ, Newsome, DA, Alvarado, JA: Localization of extracellular proteins of the human trabecular meshwork by indirect immunofluorescence. Am J Ophthalmol 104:33, 1987.

144. Gong, H, Trinkaus-Randall, V, Freddo, TF: Ultrastructural immunocytochemical localization of elastin in normal human trabecular meshwork. Curr Eye Res 8:1071, 1989.

145. Fine, BS: Structure of the trabecular meshwork and the canal of Schlemm. Trans Am Acad Ophthalmol Otolaryngol 70:777, 1966.

146. Yi, Y, Li, Y: Histochemical and electron microscopic studies of the trabecular meshwork in normal human eyes. Eye Sci 1:9, 1985.

147. Raviola, G, Raviola, E: Paracellular route of aqueous outflow in the trabecular meshwork and canal of Schlemm. A freeze-fracture study of the endothelial junctions in the sclerocorneal angle of the macaque monkey eye. Invest Ophthalmol Vis Sci 21:52, 1981.

148. Grierson, I, Rahi, AHS: Microfilaments in the cells of the human trabecular meshwork. Br J Ophthalmol 63:3, 1979.

149. Gipson, IK, Anderson, RA: Actin filaments in cells of human trabecular meshwork and Schlemm's canal. Invest Ophthalmol Vis Sci 18:547, 1979.

150. Ryder, MI, Weinreb, RN, Alvarado, J, Polansky, JR: The cytoskeleton of the cultured human trabecular cell. Characterization and drug response. Invest Ophthalmol Vis Sci 29:251, 1988.

151. Weinreb, RN, Ryder, MI, Polansky, JR: The cytoskeleton of the cynomolgus monkey trabecular cell. Invest Ophthalmol Vis Sci 27:1312, 1986.

152. Grierson, I, Miller, L, Yong, JD, et al: Investigations of cytoskeletal elements in cultured bovine meshwork cells. Invest Ophthalmol Vis Sci 27:1318, 1986.

153. Iwamoto, Y, Tamura, M: Immunocytochemical study of intermediate filaments in cultured human trabecular cells. Invest Ophthalmol Vis Sci 29:244, 1988.

154. Knepper, PA, Collins, JA, Weinstein, HG, Breen, M: Aqueous outflow pathway complex carbohydrate synthesis in vitro. Invest Ophthalmol Vis Sci 24:1546, 1983.

155. Ohnishi, Y, Taniguchi, Y: Distributions of ^{35}S-sulfate and ^{3}H-glucosamine in the angular region of the hamster: Light and electron microscopic autoradiography. Invest Ophthalmol Vis Sci 24:697, 1983.

156. Richardson, TM: Distribution of glycosaminoglycans in the aqueous outflow system of the cat. Invest Ophthalmol Vis Sci 22:319, 1982.

157. Rohen, JW, Schachtschabel, DO, Berghoff, K: Histoautoradiographic and biochemical studies on human and monkey trabecular meshwork and ciliary body in short-term explant culture. Graefe's Arch Exp Clin Ophthalmol 221:199, 1984.

158. Schachtschabel, DO, Berghoff, K, Rohen, JW: Synthesis and composition of glycosaminoglycans by explant cultures of human ciliary body and ciliary processes in serum-containing and serum-free defined media. Graefe's Arch Exp Clin Ophthalmol 221:207, 1984.

159. Polansky, JR, Wood, IS, Maglio, MT, Alvarado, JA: Trabecular meshwork cell culture in glaucoma research: Evaluation of biological activity and structural properties of human trabecular cells in vitro. Ophthalmology 91:580, 1984.

160. Acott, TS, Westcott, M, Passo, MS, Van Buskirk, EM: Trabecular meshwork glycosaminoglycans in human and cynomolgus monkey eye. Invest Ophthalmol Vis Sci 26:1320, 1985.

161. Yue, BYJT, Elvart, JL: Biosynthesis of glycosaminoglycans by trabecular meshwork cells in vitro. Curr Eye Res 6:959, 1987.

162. Berggren, L, Vrabec, F: Demonstration of a coating substance in the trabecular meshwork of the eye and its decrease after perfusion experiments with different kinds of hyaluronidase. Am J Ophthalmol 44:200, 1957.

163. Armaly, MF, Wang, Y: Demonstration of acid mucopolysaccharides in the trabecular meshwork of the rhesus monkey. Invest Ophthalmol 14:507, 1975.

164. Grierson, I, Lee, WR: Acid mucopolysaccharides in the outflow apparatus. Exp Eye Res 21:417, 1975.

165. Mizokami, K: Demonstration of masked acidic glycosaminoglycans in the normal human trabecular meshwork. Jpn J Ophthalmol 21:57, 1977.

166. Tawara, A, Varner, HH, Hollyfield, JG: Distribution and characterization of sulfated proteoglycans in the human trabecular tissue. Invest Ophthalmol Vis Sci 30:2215, 1989.

167. Worthen, DM, Cleveland, PH: Fibronectin production by cultured human trabecular meshwork cells. Invest Ophthalmol Vis Sci 23:797, 1985.

168. Floyd, BB, Cleveland, PH, Worthen, DM: Fibronectin in human trabecular drainage channels. Invest Ophthalmol Vis Sci 26:797, 1985.

169. Hernandez, MR, Weinstein, BI, Schwartz, J, et al: Human trabecular meshwork cells in culture: Morphology and extracellular matrix components. Invest Ophthalmol Vis Sci 28:1655, 1987.

170. Lynch, MG, Peeler, JS, Brown, RH, Niederkorn, JY: Expression of HLA class I and II antigens on cells of the human trabecular meshwork. Ophthalmology 94:851, 1987.

171. Latina, M, Flotte, T, Crean, E, et al: Immunohistochemical staining of the human anterior segment. 106:95, 1988.

172. Stone, RA, Kuwayama, Y, Laties, AM, Marangos, PJ: Neuron-specific enolase-containing cells in the rhesus monkey trabecular meshwork. Invest Ophthalmol Vis Sci 25:1332, 1984.

173. Borisuth, NSC, Tripathi, BJ, Tripathi, RC: Identification and partial characterization of TGF-1 receptors on trabecular cells. Invest Ophthalmol Vis Sci 33:596, 1992.

174. Tripathi, RC, Kolli, SP, Borisuth, NSC, Tripathi, BJ: Identification and quantification of transferrin receptors on trabecular cells. Invest Ophthalmol Vis Sci 33:3449, 1992.

175. Grierson, I, Chisholm, IA: Clearance of debris from the iris through the drainage angle of the rabbit's eye. Br J Ophthalmol 62:694, 1978.

176. Grierson, I, Day, J, Unger, WG, Ahmed, A: Phagocytosis of latex microspheres by bovin meshwork cells in culture. Graefe's Arch Exp Clin Ophthalmol 224:536, 1986.

177. Barak, MH, Weinreb, RN, Ryder, MI: Quantitative assessment of cynomolgus monkey trabecular cell phagocytosis and absorption. Curr Eye Res 7:445, 1988.

178. Shirato, S, Murphy, CG, Bloom, E, et al: Kinetics of phagocytosis in trabecular meshwork cells. Flow cytometry and morphometry. Invest Ophthalmol Vis Sci 30:2499, 1989.

179. Johnson, DH, Richardson, TM, Epstein, DL: Trabecular meshwork recovery after phagocytic challenge. Curr Eye Res 8:1121, 1989.

180. Grierson, I, Lee, WR: Erythrocyte phagocytosis in the human trabecular meshwork. Br J Ophthalmol 57:400, 1973.

181. Zhou, L, Fukuchi, T, Kawa, JE, et al: Loss of cell-matrix cohesiveness after phagocytosis by trabecular meshwork cells. Invest Ophthalmol Vis Sci 36:787, 1995.

182. Johnson, DH: Does pigmentation affect the trabecular meshwork? Arch Ophthalmol 107:250, 1989.

183. Feeney, L, Wissig, S: Outflow studies using an electron dense tracer. Trans Am Acad Ophthalmol Otolaryngol 70:791, 1966.

184. Diaz, G, Orzalesi, N, Fossarello, M, et al: Coated pits and coated vesicles in the endothelial cells of trabecular meshwork. Exp Eye Res 35:99, 1982.

185. Diaz, G, Carta, S, Orzalesi, N: Nonrandom distribution of coated pits and vesicles in the connective tissue cells of the trabecular meshwork of rabbit. Graefe's Arch Exp Clin Ophthalmol 224:147, 1986.

186. Anderson, DR: Scanning electron microscopy of primate trabecular meshwork. Am J Ophthalmol 71:90, 1971.

187. Johnstone, MA: Pressure-dependent changes in configuration of the endothelial tubules of Schlemm's canal. Am J Ophthalmol 78:630, 1974.

188. Svedbergh, B: Protrusions of the inner wall of Schlemm's canal. Am J Ophthalmol 82:875, 1976.

189. Bhatt, K, Gong, H, Freddo, TF: Freeze-fracture studies of interendothelial junctions in the angle of the human eye. Invest Ophthalmol Vis Sci 36:1379, 1995.

190. Johnstone, MA: Pressure-dependent changes in nuclei and the process origins of the endothelial cells lining Schlemm's canal. Invest Ophthalmol Vis Sci 18:44, 1979.

191. Segawa, K: Electron microscopic observations on the replicas of Schlemm's canal. Acta Soc Ophthalmol Jpn 73:2013, 1969.

192. Segawa, K: Scanning electron microscopic studies on the iridocorneal angle tissue in normal human eyes. Acta Soc Ophthalmol Jpn 76:659, 1972.

193. Holmberg, A: The fine structure of the inner wall of Schlemm's canal. Arch Ophthalmol 62:956, 1959.

194. Holmberg, A: Schlemm's canal and the trabecular meshwork. An electron microscopic study of the normal structure in man and monkey (cercopithecus ethiops). Doc Ophthalmol 19:339, 1965.

195. Inomata, H, Bill, A, Smelse, GK: Aqueous humor pathways through the trabecular meshwork and into Schlemm's canal in the cynomolgus monkey (Macaca irus). Am J Ophthalmol 73:760, 1972.

196. Segawa, K: Pores of the trabecular wall of Schlemm's canal. Ferritin perfusion in enucleated human eyes. Acta Soc Ophthalmol Jpn 74:1240, 1970.

197. Segawa, K: Pore structures of the endothelial cells of the aqueous outflow pathway: scanning electron microscopy. Jpn J Ophthalmol 17:133, 1973.

198. Shabo, AL, Reese, TS, Gaasterland, D: Postmortem formation of giant endothelial vacuoles in Schlemm's canal of the monkey. Am J Ophthalmol 76:896, 1973.

199. Tripathi, RC: Ultrastructure of the trabecular wall of Schlemm's canal in relation to aqueous outflow. Exp Eye Res 7:335, 1968.

200. Tripathi, RC: Mechanism of the aqueous outflow across the trabecular wall of Schlemm's canal. Exp Eye Res 11:116, 1971.

201. Tripathi, RC: Ultrastructure of the exit pathway of the aqueous in lower mammals (a preliminary report on the "angular aqueous plexus"). Exp Eye Res 12:311, 1971.

202. Speakman, JS: Drainage channels in the trabecular wall of Schlemm's canal. Br J Ophthalmol 44:513, 1960.

203. Sondermann, R: Beitrag zur entwicklung und morphologie des Schlemmschen kanals. Graefe's Arch Exp Clin Ophthalmol 124:521, 1930.

204. Ashton, N, Brini, A, Smith, R: Anatomical studies of the trabecular meshwork of the normal human eye. Br J Ophthalmol 40:257, 1956.

205. Iwamoto, T: Further observation on Sondermann's channels of the human trabecular meshwork. Graefe's Arch Exp Clin Ophthalmol 172:213, 1967.

206. Lutjen-Drecoll, E, Rohen, JW: Uber die endotheliale auskleidung des Schlemmschen kanals im silberimprägnationsbild. Graefe's Arch Clin Ophthalmol 180:249, 1970.

207. de Kater, AW, Spurr-Michaud, SJ, Gipson, IK: Localization of smooth muscle myosin-containing cells in the aqueous outflow pathway. Invest Ophthalmol Vis Sci 31:347, 1990.

208. McMenamin, PG, Lee, WR, Aitken, DAN: Age-related changes in the human outflow apparatus. Ophthalmology 93:194, 1986.

209. Miyazaki, M, Segawa, K, Urakawa, Y: Age-related changes in the trabecular meshwork of the normal human eye. Jpn J Ophthalmol 31:558, 1987.

210. Alvarado, J, Murphy, C, Polansky, J, Juster, R: Age-related changes in trabecular meshwork cellularity. Invest Ophthalmol Vis Sci 21:714, 1987.

211. Ainsworth, JR, Lee, WR: Effects of age and rapid high-pressure fixation on the morphology of Schlemm's canal. Invest Ophthalmol Vis Sci 31:745, 1990.

212. Marshall, GE, Konstas, AGP, Lee, WR: Immunogold ultrastructural localization of collagens in the aged human outflow system. Ophthalmology 98:692, 1991.

213. Flügel, C, Tamm, E, Lütjen-Drecoll, E, Stefani, FH: Age-related loss of smooth muscle actin in normal and glaucomatous human trabecular meshwork of different age groups. J Glauc 1:165, 1992.

214. Emi, K, Pederson, JE, Toris, CB: Hydrostatic pressure of the suprachoroidal space. Invest Ophthalmol Vis Sci 30:233, 1989.

215. Weinreb, RN, Lindsey, JD, Luo, X-X, Wang, T-H: Extracellular matrix of the human ciliary muscle. J Glauc 3:70, 1994.

216. Raviola, G, Butler, JM: Unidirectional transport mechanism of horseradish peroxidase in the vessels of the iris. Invest Ophthalmol Vis Sci 25:827, 1984.

217. Butler, JM, Raviola, G, Beers GJ, Carter AP: Computed tomography of aqueous humor outflow pathways. Exp Eye Res 39:709, 1984.

218. Grant, WM: Further studies on facility of flow through the trabecular meshwork. Arch Ophthalmol 60:523, 1958.

219. Grant, WM: Experimental aqueous perfusion in enucleated human eyes. Arch Ophthalmol 69:783, 1963.

220. Tripathi, RC, Tripathi, BJ: The mechanism of aqueous outflow in lower mammals. Exp Eye Res 14:73, 1972.

221. Tarkkanen, A, Niemi, M: Enzyme histochemistry of the angle of the anterior chamber of the human eye. Acta Ophthalmol 45:93, 1987.

222. Vegge, T: Ultrastructure of normal human trabecular endothelium. Acta Ophthalmol 41:193, 1963.

223. Johnstone, MA, Grant, WM: Pressure-dependent changes in structure of the aqueous outflow system of human and monkey eyes. Am J Ophthalmol 75:365, 1973.

224. Grierson, I, Lee, WR: Changes in the monkey outflow apparatus at graded levels of intraocular pressure: a qualitative analysis by light microscopy and scanning electron microscopy. Exp Eye Res 19:21, 1974.

225. Grierson, I, Lee, WR: Pressure-induced changes in the ultrastructure of the endothelium lining Schlemm's canal. Am J Ophthalmol 80:863, 1975.

226. Kayes, J: Pressure gradient changes on the trabecular meshwork of monkeys. Am J Ophthalmol 79:549, 1975.

227. Van Buskirk, EM, Grant, WM: Influence of temperature and the question of involvement of cellular metabolism in aqueous outflow. Am J Ophthalmol 77:565, 1974.

228. Epstein, DL, Rohen, JW: Morphology of the trabecular meshwork and inner-wall endothelium after cationized ferritin perfusion in the monkey eye. Invest Ophthalmol Vis Sci 32:160, 1991.

229. Bill, A, Svedbergh, B: Scanning electron microscopic studies of the trabecular meshwork and the canal of Schlemm—An attempt to localize the main resistance to outflow of aqueous humor in man. Acta Ophthalmol 50:295, 1972.

230. Moseley, H, Grierson, J, Lee, W: Mathematical modeling of aqueous humor outflow from the eye through the pores in the lining endothelium of Schlemm's canal. Clin Phys Physiol Meas 4:47, 1983.

231. Seiler, T, Wollensak, J: The resistance of the trabecular meshwork to aqeuous humor outflow. Graefe's Arch Exp Clin Ophthalmol 223:88, 1985.

232. Ethier, CR, Kamm, RD, Palaszewski, BA, et al: Calculations of flow resistance in the juxtacanalicular meshwork. Invest Ophthalmol Vis Sci 27:1741, 1986.

233. Johnson, M, Ethier, CR, Kamm, RD, et al: The flow of aqueous humor through micro-porous filters. Invest Ophthalmol Vis Sci 27:92, 1986.

234. Johnson, M, Shapiro, A, Ethier, CR, Kamm, RD: Modulation of outflow resistance by the pores of the inner wall endothelium. Invest Ophthalmol Vis Sci 33:1670, 1992.

235. Johnson, M, Johnson, DH, Kamm, RD, et al: The filtration characteristics of the aqueous outflow system. Exp Eye Res 50:407, 1990.

236. Gard, TL, Van Buskirk, EM, Acott, TS: Ionic modulation of flow resistance in an immobilized proteoglycan model of the trabecular meshwork. J Glauc 2:183, 1993.

237. Francois, J: The importance of the mucopolysaccharides in intraocular pressure regulation. Invest Ophthalmol Vis Sci 14:173, 1975.

238. Hayasaka, S, Sears, ML: Distribution of acid phosphatase, betaglucuronidase, and lysosomal hyaluronidase in the anterior segment of the rabbit eye. Invest Ophthalmol Vis Sci 17:982, 1978.

239. Grierson, I, Lee, WR, Abraham, S: A light microscopic study of the effects of testicular hyaluronidase on the outflow system of a baboon (Papio cynocephalus). Invest Ophthalmol Vis Sci 18:356, 1979.

240. Knepper, PA, Farbman, AI, Telser, AG: Exogenous hyaluronidase and degradation of hyaluronic acid in the rabbit eye. Invest Ophthalmol Vis Sci 25:286, 1984.

241. Sawaguchi, S, Yue, BYJT, Yeh, P, Tso, MOM: Effects of intracameral injection of chondroitinase ABC in vivo. Arch Ophthalmol 110:110, 1992.

242. Peterson, WS, Jocson, VL: Hyaluronidase effects of aqueous outflow resistance. Quantitative and localizing studies in the rhesus monkey eye. Am J Ophthalmol 77:573, 1974.

243. Van Buskirk, EM, Brett, J: The canine eye: in vitro dissolution of the barriers to aqueous outflow. Invest Ophthalmol Vis Sci 17:258, 1978.

244. Van Buskirk, EM, Brett, J: The canine eye: in vitro studies of the intraocular pressure and facility of aqueous outflow. Invest Ophthalmol Vis Sci 17:373, 1978.

245. Erickson-Lamy, K, Schroeder, AM, Bassett-Chu, S, Epstein, DL: Absence of time-dependent facility increase ("washout") in the perfused enucleated human eye. Invest Ophthalmol Vis Sci 31:2384, 1990.

246. Hernandez, MR, Wenk, EJ, Weinstein, BI, et al: Glucocorticoid target cells in human outflow pathway: autopsy and surgical specimens. Invest Ophthalmol Vis Sci 24:1612, 1983.

247. Weinreb, RN, Bloom E, Baxter, JD, et al: Detection of glucocorticoid receptors in cultured human trabecular cells. Invest Ophthalmol Vis Sci 21:403, 1981.

248. Hernandez, MR, Weinstein, BI, Wenk, EJ, et al: The effect of dexamethasone on the in vitro incorporation of precursors of extracellular matrix components in the outflow pathway region of the rabbit eye. Invest Ophthalmol Vis Sci 24:704, 1983.

249. Weinreb, RN, Mitchell, MD, Polansky, JR: Prostaglandin production by human trabecular cells: in vitro inhibition by dexamethasone. Invest Ophthalmol Vis Sci 24:1541, 1983.

250. Weinreb, RN, Polansky, JR, Alvarado, JA, Mitchell, MD: Arachidonic acid metabolism in human trabecular meshwork. Invest Ophthalmol Vis Sci 29:1708, 1988.

251. Bito, LZ, Draga, A, Blanco, J, Camras, CB: Long-term maintenance of reduced intraocular pressure by daily or twice daily topical application of prostaglandins to cat or rhesus monkey eyes. Invest Ophthalmol Vis Sci 24:312, 1983.

252. Kaufman, PL, Bárány, EH: Cytochalasin B reversibly increases outflow facility in the eye of the cynomolgus monkey. Invest Ophthalmol Vis Sci 16:47, 1977.

253. Svedbergh, B, Lutjen-Drecoll, E, Ober, M, Kaufman, PL: Cytochalasin B-induced structural changes in the anterior ocular segment of the cynomologus monkey. Invest Ophthalmol Vis Sci 17:718, 1978.

254. Johnstone, M, Tanner, D, Chau, B, Kopecky, K: Concentration-dependent morphologic effects of cytochalasin B in the aqueous outflow system. Invest Ophthalmol Vis Sci 19:835, 1980.

255. Kaufman, PL, Erickson, KA: Cytochalasin B and D dose-outflow facility response relationships in the cynomolgus monkey. Invest Ophthalmol Vis Sci 23:646, 1982.

256. Kaufman, PL, Svedbergh, B, Lutjen-Drecoll, E: Medical trabeculocanalotomy in monkeys with cytochalasin B or EDTA. Ann Ophthalmol 11:795, 1979.

257. Bill, A, Lutjen-Drecoll, E, Svedbergh, B: Effects of intracameral Na2EDTA and EGTA on aqueous outflow routes in the monkey eye. Invest Ophthalmol Vis Sci 19:492, 1980.

258. Barany, EH: In vitro studies of the resistance to flow through the angle of the anterior chamber. Acta Soc Med Uppsal 59:260, 1954.

259. Epstein, DL, Hashimoto, JM, Anderson, PJ, Grant, WM: Effect of iodoacetamide perfusion on outflow facility and metabolism of the trabecular meshwork. Invest Ophthalmol Vis Sci 20:625, 1981.

260. Epstein, DL, Patterson, MM, Rivers, SC, Anderson, PJ: N-ethylmaleimide increases the facility of aqueous outflow of excised monkey and calf eyes. Invest Ophthalmol Vis Sci 22:752, 1982.

261. Lindenmayer, JM, Kahn, MG, Hertzmark, E, Epstein, DL: Morphology and function of the aqueous outflow system in monkey eyes perfused with sulfhydryl reagents. Invest Ophthalmol Vis Sci 24:710, 1983.

262. Freddo, TF, Patterson, MM, Scott, DR, Epstein, DL: Influence of mercurial sulfhydryl agents on aqueous outflow pathways in enucleated eyes. Invest Ophthalmol Vis Sci 25:278, 1984.

263. Epstein, DL, Freddo, TF, Bassett-Chu, S, et al: Influence of ethacrynic acid on outflow facility in the monkey and calf eye. Invest Ophthalmol Vis Sci 28:2067, 1987.

264. Erickson-Lamy, K, Schroeder, A, Epstein, DL: Ethacrynic acid induces reversible shape and cytoskeletal changes in cultured cells. Invest Ophthalmol Vis Sci 33:2631, 1992.

265. Quinn, RF, Tingey, DP: Effects of cytoskeleton-reactive agents on aqueous outflow facility in a porcine ocular anterior segment preparation. Can J Ophthalmol 30:4, 1995.

266. Liang, L-L, Epstein, DL, de Kater, AW, et al: Ethacrynic acid increases facility of outflow in the human eye in vitro. Arch Ophthalmol 110:106, 1992.

267. Padgaonkar, V, Giblin, FJ, Leverenz, V, et al: Studies of H_2O_2-induced effects on cultured bovine trabecular meshwork cells. J Glauc 3:123, 1994.

268. Kahn, MG, Giblin, FJ, Epstein, DL: Glutathione in calf trabecular meshwork and its relation to aqueous humor outflow facility. Invest Ophthalmol Vis Sci 24:1283, 1983.

269. Scott, DR, Karageuzian, LN, Anderson, PJ, Epstein, DL: Glutathione peroxidase of calf trabecular meshwork. Invest Ophthalmol Vis Sci 25:599, 1984.

270. Nguyen, KPV, Chung, ML, Anderson, PJ, et al: Hydrogen peroxide removal by the calf aqueous outflow pathway. Invest Ophthalmol Vis Sci 29:976, 1988.

271. Yan, DB, Trope, GE, Ethier, CR, et al: Effects of hydrogen peroxide-induced oxidative damage on outflow facility and washout in pig eyes. Invest Ophthalmol Vis Sci 32:2515, 1991.

272. Pandolfi, M, Kwaan, HC: Fibrinolysis in the anterior segment of the eye. Arch Ophthalmol 77:99, 1967.

273. Pandolfi, M: Coagulation Factor VIII localization in the aqueous outflow pathways. Arch Ophthalmol 94:656, 1976.

274. Tripathi, BJ, Geanon, JD, Tripathi, RC: Distribution of tissue plasminogen activator in human and monkey eyes. Ophthalmology 94:1434, 1987.

275. Park, JK, Tripathi, RC, Tripathi, BJ, Barlow, GH: Tissue plasminogen activator in the trabecular endothelium. Invest Ophthalmol Vis Sci 28:1341, 1987.

276. Shuman, MA, Polansky, JR, Merkel, C, Alvarado, JA: Tissue plasminogen activator in cultured human trabecular meshwork cells. Predominance of enzyme over plasminogen activator inhibitor. Invest Ophthalmol Vis Sci 29:401, 1988.

277. Kohmoto, H, Matsumoto, S, Serizawa, T: Effects of endothelin-1 on $[Ca^{2+}]_i$ and pH_i in trabecular meshwork cells. Curr Eye Res 13:197, 1994.

278. Nathanson, JA, McKee, M: Identification of an extensive system of nitric oxide-producing cells in the ciliary muscle and outflow pathway of the human eye. Invest Ophthalmol Vis Sci 36:1765, 1995.

279. Van Buskirk, EM, Grant, WM: Lens depression and aqueous outflow in enucleated primate eyes. Am J Ophthalmol 76:632, 1973.

280. Van Buskirk, EM: Trabeculotomy in the immature, enucleated human eye. Invest Ophthalmol Vis Sci 16:63, 1977.

281. Moses, RA, Hoover, GS, Oostwouder, PH: Blood reflux in Schlemm's canal. I. Normal findings. Arch Ophthalmol 97:1307, 1979.

282. Ellingsen, BA, Grant, WM: The relationship of pressure and aqueous outflow in enucleated human eyes. Invest Ophthalmol 10:430, 1971.

283. Ellingsen, BA, Grant, WM: Influence of intraocular pressure and trabeculotomy on aqueous outflow in enucleated monkey eyes. Invest Ophthalmol 10:705, 1971.

284. Brubaker, RF: The effect of intraocular pressure on conventional outflow resistance in the enucleated human eye. Invest Ophthalmol 14:286, 1975.

285. Grierson, I, Lee, WR: The fine structure of the trabecular meshwork at graded levels of intraocular pressure. (1) Pressure effects within the near-physiological range (8–30 mm Hg). Exp Eye Res 20:505, 1975.

286. Grierson, I, Lee, WR: The fine structure of the trabecular meshwork at graded levels of intraocular pressure. (2) Pressure outside the physiological range (0 and 50 mm Hg). Exp Eye Res 20:523, 1975.

287. Ellingsen, BA, Grant, WM: Trabeculotomy and sinusotomy in enucleated human eyes. Invest Ophthalmol 11:21, 1972.

288. Moses, RA: The conventional outflow resistances. Am J Ophthalmol 92:804, 1981.

289. Hashimoto, JM, Epstein, DL: Influence of intraocular pressure on aqueous outflow facility in enucleated eyes of different mammals. Invest Ophthalmol Vis Sci 19:1483, 1980.

290. Moses, RA, Arnzen, RJ: The trabecular mesh: a mathematical analysis. Invest Ophthalmol Vis Sci 19:1490, 1980.

291. Van Buskirk, EM: Changes in the facility of aqueous outflow induced by lens depression and intraocular pressure in excised human eyes. Am J Ophthalmol 82:736, 1976.

292. Moses, RA, Etheridge, EL, Grodzki, WJ Jr: The effect of lens depression on the components of outflow resistance. Invest Ophthalmol Vis Sci 22:37, 1982.

293. Van Buskirk, EM: Anatomic correlates of changing aqueous outflow facility in excised human eyes. Invest Ophthalmol Vis Sci 22:625, 1982.

294. Rosenquist, RC Jr, Melamed, S, Epstein, DL: Anterior and posterior axial lens displacement and human aqueous outflow facility. Invest Ophthalmol Vis Sci 29:1159, 1988.

295. Moses, RA, Grodzki, WJ Jr: Choroid tension and facility of aqueous outflow. Invest Ophthalmol Vis Sci 16:1062, 1977.

296. Rosenquist, R, Epstein, D, Melamed, S, et al: Outflow resistance of enucleated human eyes at two different perfusion pressures and different extents of trabeculotomy. Curr Eye Res 8:1233, 1989.

297. Peterson, WS, Jocson, VL, Sears, ML: Resistance to aqueous outflow in the rhesus monkey eye. Am J Ophthalmol 72:445, 1971.

298. Kollarits, CR, Gaasterland, D, Di Chiro, G, et al: Management of a patient with orbital varices, visual loss, and ipsilateral glaucoma. Ophthalmic Surg 8:54, 1977.

299. Brubaker, RF: Determination of episcleral venous pressure in the eye. A comparison of three methods. Arch Ophthalmol 77:110, 1967.

300. Podos, SM, Minas, TF, Macri, FJ: A new instrument to measure episcleral venous pressure. Comparison of normal eyes and eyes with primary open-angle glaucoma. Arch Ophthalmol 80:209, 1968.

301. Krakau, CET, Widakowich, J, Wilke, K: Measurements of the episcleral venous pressure by means of an air jet. Acta Ophthalmol 51:185, 1973.

302. Phelps, CD, Armaly, MF: Measurement of episcleral venous pressure. Am J Ophthalmol 85:35, 1978.

303. Zeimer, RC, Gieser, DK, Wilensky, JT, et al: A practical venomanometer. Measurement of episcleral venous pressure and assessment of the normal range. Arch Ophthalmol 101:1447, 1983.

304. Gaasterland, DE, Pederson, JE: Episcleral venous pressure: A comparison of invasive and noninvasive measurements. Invest Ophthalmol Vis Sci 24:1417, 1983.

Chapter 3

AQUEOUS HUMOR DYNAMICS
II. Techniques for Evaluating

EVALUATION OF AQUEOUS PRODUCTION

Cycloscopy

This technique allows direct visualization of ciliary processes under special circumstances, such as the presence of an iridectomy, wide iris retraction, aniridia, and some cases of aphakia (Fig. 3.1). Although special contact prisms with scleral indentors have been developed for cycloscopy (Fig. 3.2) (1, 2), the procedure is still limited by the small percentage of eyes in which circumstances are favorable for good visualization of the ciliary processes. The main value of the technique thus far has been in research studies of the ciliary processes (1, 2), and in conjunction with laser therapy to the ciliary processes (transpupillary cyclophotocoagulation), which is discussed in Section Three.

Measuring the Rate of Aqueous Production

Fluorophotometry

Fluorescein techniques involve instillation of fluorescein into the anterior chamber by iontophoresis with subsequent measurement of either (a) the flow of unstained aqueous from the posterior to anterior chamber using photogrammetric methods (3), or (b) the change in concentration of fluorescein in the anterior chamber by fluorophotometry (4–9). Of these two approaches, fluorophotometry has become the most commonly used and is currently the standard research technique by which the rate of aqueous humor flow is calculated in normal human subjects and glaucoma patients under various circumstances including the response to glaucoma drugs (9).

Other Techniques for Calculating Inflow

Radioactive-labeled isotopes have been used to measure inflow in animals by observing either (a) the accumulation of the isotope in the anterior chamber (10), or (b) the decay rate of the intracamerally injected isotope (11). Perfusion of eyes at a constant pressure can also be used to determine the inflow in animals (12).

EVALUATION OF AQUEOUS OUTFLOW

Gonioscopy[a]

Gonioscopy is a clinical technique that is used to examine structures in the anterior chamber angle. In the management

---

[a]Refer to Shields, MB: Color Atlas of Glaucoma. Baltimore, Williams & Wilkins, 1998, Plates I4–6.

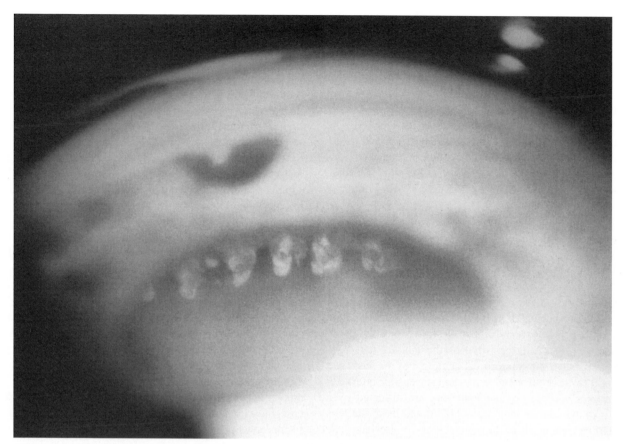

Figure 3.1. Transpupillary view of ciliary processes as seen by cycloscopy in eye with neovascular glaucoma in which fibrovascular membrane has caused dilatation and anterior displacement of iris.

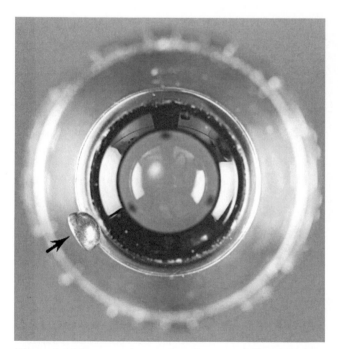

Figure 3.2. Mizuno cycloscopy lens (*arrow* indicates scleral indentor).

of glaucoma, gonioscopic assessment is necessary to establish the type of glaucoma. This is essential in planning the appropriate therapy since the treatment for one type of glaucoma may be ineffective or contraindicated in another form. The present discussion is limited to technique and normal anatomic findings, while the gonioscopic alterations associated with the various forms of glaucoma are considered in Section Two.

Historical Background (13)

In 1907, Trantas visualized the angle in an eye with keratoglobus by indenting the limbus. He later coined the term gonioscopy. Salsmann introduced the goniolens in 1914, and Koeppe improved it 5 years later by designing a steeper lens. Troncoso also contributed to gonioscopy by developing the gonioscope for magnification and illumination of the angle. In 1938, Goldmann introduced the gonioprism, and Barkan established the use of gonioscopy in the management of glaucoma.

Principle of Gonioscopy (Fig. 3.3) (14)

The problem is the *critical angle.* When light passes from a medium with a greater index of refraction to one with a lesser index, the angle of refraction *(r)* will be larger than the angle of incidence *(i).* When r equals 90°, *i* is said to have attained the critical angle. When *i* exceeds the critical angle, the light is reflected back into the first medium. The critical angle for the cornea-air interface is approximately 46°. Light rays coming from the anterior chamber angle exceed this critical angle and are therefore reflected back into the anterior chamber, preventing visualization of the angle.

The solution to this problem is to eliminate the cornea (optically). Since the index of refraction of a contact lens approaches that of the cornea, there is minimal refraction at the interface of these two media, which eliminates the optical effect of the front corneal surface. Therefore, light rays from the anterior chamber angle enter the contact lens and are then made to pass through the new contact lens-air interface by one of two basic designs. In *direct gonioscopy,* the anterior curve of the contact lens (goniolens) is such that the critical angle is not reached, and the light rays are refracted at the contact lens-air interface. In *indirect gonioscopy,* the light rays are reflected by a mirror in the contact lens (gonioprism) and leave the lens at nearly a right angle to the contact lens-air interface. The more commonly used goniolenses and gonioprisms are listed in Table 3.1.

Direct Gonioscopy

INSTRUMENTS. The *Koeppe* lens is the prototype diagnostic goniolens and is available in different diameters and radii of posterior curvature (Fig. 3.4). A gonioscope, or hand biomicroscope, provides 15–20× magnification. It may be hand-held or suspended from the ceiling with a counterbalance, or on an elastic belt (15). The light source is usually a separate hand-held unit, such as the Barkan focal illuminator, although it may be attached to the gonioscope.

TECHNIQUE. Direct gonioscopy is performed with the patient in a supine position, preferably on a movable diagnostic table. After applying a topical anesthetic, the goniolens is positioned on the cornea, using a bridge of balanced salt solution, a viscous preparation such as methylcellulose, or the patient's own tears. The examiner usually holds the gonioscope in one hand and a light source in the other (Fig. 3.5). Occasionally, an assistant may be needed to move the goniolens to the desired position. Alternatively, a gonioscope with mounted light source may be used, which allows the examiner to control the goniolens with the other hand. In either case, the examiner scans the anterior chamber angle by shifting his or her position until all 360° have been studied.

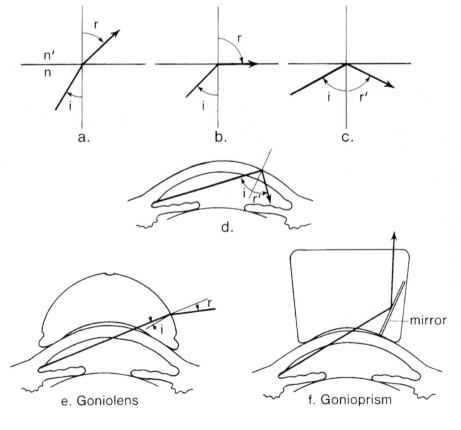

Figure 3.3. Principle of gonioscopy: **A.** Light ray is refracted when angle of incidence (*i*) at interface of two media with different indices of refraction (*n* and *n'*) is less than the critical angle. **B.** Angle of refraction (*r*) is 90° when *i* equals the critical angle. **C.** Light is reflected when *i* exceeds the critical angle. **D.** Light from anterior chamber angle exceeds the critical angle at the cornea-air interface and is reflected back into the eye. **E** and **F.** Contact lenses have an index of retraction (*n*) similar to that of the cornea, allowing light to enter the lens and then be refracted (goniolens) or reflected (gonioprism) beyond contact lens-air interface.

Table 3.1.

CONTACT LENSES FOR GONIOSCOPY

	Lens	Description/Use
I. Goniolenses (Direct Gonioscopy)	1. Koeppe	1. Prototype diagnostic goniolens
	2. Richardson-Schaffer	2. Small Koeppe lens for infants
	3. Layden	3. For premature infant gonioscopy
	4. Barkan	4. Prototype surgical goniolens
	5. Thorpe	5. Surgical and diagnostic lens for operating room
	6. Swan-Jacob	6. Surgical goniolens for children
II. Gonioprisms (Indirect Gonioscopy)	1. Goldmann single-mirror	1. Mirror inclined at 62° for gonioscopy
	2. Goldmann three-mirror	2. One mirror for gonioscopy; two for retina; coated front surface available for laser use
	3. Zeiss four-mirror	3. All four mirrors inclined at 64° for gonioscopy; requires holder (Unger); fluid bridge not required
	4. Posner four-mirror	4. Modified Zeiss four-mirror gonioprism with attached handle
	5. Sussman four-mirror	5. Hand-held Zeiss-type gonioprism
	6. Thorpe four-mirror	6. Four gonioscopy mirrors, inclined at 62°; requires fluid bridge
	7. Ritch Trabeculoplasty Lens	7. Four gonioscopy mirrors; two inclined at 59° and two at 62° with convex lens over two

Indirect Gonioscopy

INSTRUMENTS. The gonioprism and a slitlamp are the only instruments needed for indirect gonioscopy. The *Goldmann* single-mirror lens is the prototype gonioprism (Fig. 3.6). The mirror in this lens has a height of 12 mm and a tilt of 62° from the plano front surface. The central well has a diameter of 12 mm and a posterior radius of curvature of 7.38 mm. A Goldmann three-mirror lens has two mirrors for examination of the fundus and one for the anterior chamber angle, which is tilted at 59°. The posterior radius of curvature of both standard Goldmann diagnostic gonioprisms is such that a viscous material must be used to fill the space between cornea and lens. However, a modified Goldmann-type lens has been developed with an 8.4-mm radius of curvature, which eliminates the need for a viscous bridge (16). Goldmann-type lenses have also been modified with antireflection coating for use with laser trabeculoplasty.

In the *Zeiss four-mirror* lens, all four mirrors are tilted at 64° for evaluation of the angle, thereby eliminating the need to rotate the lens. The original four-mirror lens is mounted on a holding fork (Unger holder), while newer models have a permanently attached holding rod (Posner lens) or are held directly (Sussman lens) (Fig. 3.7) (17). An adjustable slitlamp mount has also been developed for the Zeiss four-mirror gonioprism (18). The posterior curvature

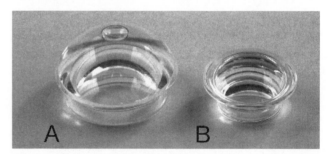

Figure 3.4. Koeppe goniolenses. **A.** Adult lens. **B.** Infant lens.

of each of these four-mirror lenses is similar to that of the cornea, which allows the patient's own tears to be used as the fluid bridge.

The Ritch trabeculoplasty lens has four gonioscopy mirrors, two of which are tilted at 59° and two at 62°, with a convex lens over one mirror of each set (19). Another four-mirror lens, referred to as the "trabeculens," has a 30-diopter convex contact lens in a hollow funnel, with four mirrors at 62° angles (20). It can be used as a diagnostic gonioprism, as well as for laser trabeculoplasty and iridotomy. The use of gonioprisms in laser therapy is discussed further in Section Three.

With both Goldmann- and Zeiss-type instruments, the anterior chamber angle is viewed "indirectly" through a mirror 180° from the quadrant being viewed. A new gonio-prism has been developed, however, with double mirrors that allow direct viewing (21).

TECHNIQUE. The cornea is anesthetized and, with the patient positioned at the slitlamp, the gonioprism is placed against the cornea with or without a fluid bridge, depending on the posterior radius of curvature of the instrument (Figs. 3.8 and 3.9). The lens is then rotated to allow visualization of all 360° of the angle, or the quadrants are studied with the four mirrors. Visualization into a narrow angle can be enhanced by manipulating the gonioprism, e.g., asking the patient to look in the direction of the mirror being used, although such maneuvers must be used with caution, since they can distort the appearance of the angle depth (22).

Comparison of Direct and Indirect Gonioscopy

There is no unanimity of opinion as to which basic method of gonioscopy is best. Advantages have been suggested for both approaches. With *direct gonioscopy,* the height of the ob-server may be changed to look deeper into a narrow angle,

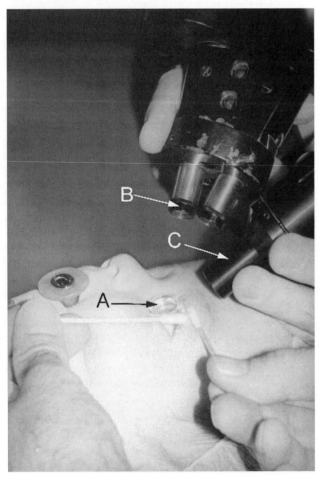

Figure 3.5. Technique of direct gonioscopy during examina-tion of infant under anesthesia. **A.** Koeppe goniolens. **B.** Gonioscope. **C.** Focal illuminator.

while the gonioprism is limited in this regard by the height of the mirror. In addition, the goniolens may cause less distor-tion of the anterior chamber. Both features make it desirable when assessing the true depth of the anterior chamber angle (23, 24). A major advantage of direct gonioscopy, especially with the infant Koeppe lenses, is its use in sedated or anes-thetized patients, as in the examination of children. These lenses are also useful in examining the fundus through a small pupil with a direct ophthalmoscope.

In *indirect gonioscopy,* the slitlamp may provide better optics and lighting, which could be an advantage when look-ing for subtle details in the angle (25). Furthermore, the method requires less additional instrumentation and space (assuming the slitlamp is already a part of the routine office examination) and is probably faster than direct gonioscopy. The latter is particularly true of the Zeiss four-mirror lenses and modified Goldmann-type lenses in which a viscous bridge is not required. Gonioprisms with a posterior radius of curvature closer to that of the anterior corneal surface may also reduce corneal distortion (22, 26). In addition, gonioprisms with taller mirrors facilitate visualization of narrow angles (22). The Zeiss four-mirror lens, because of the smaller diameter of corneal contact, also has the advan-tage of use in "compressive gonioscopy," which is explained in Section Two under "Angle Closure Glaucoma" (27).

Cleaning of Diagnostic Contact Lenses

Any instrument that contacts the eye creates the potential haz-ard of transmitting bacterial and viral infection. This problem is considered in more detail in the next chapter with regard to tonometry, although the basic principles of instrument clean-ing also apply to diagnostic contact lenses. In addition, a con-tainer has been developed which allows the diagnostic lens to stay in contact with a disinfectant solution (28).

Gonioscopic Appearance of the Normal Anterior Chamber Angle

Starting at the root of the iris and progressing anteriorly toward the cornea, the following structures can be identi-

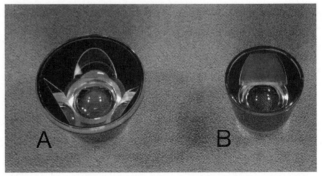

Figure 3.6. Goldmann gonioprisms. **A.** Three-mirror lens (domed mirror used for gonioscopy). **B.** Single-mirror lens.

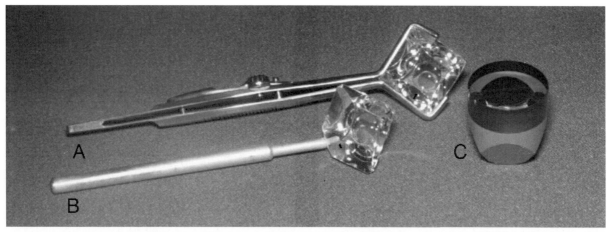

Figure 3.7. Four-mirror gonioprisms (all four mirrors for gonioscopy). **A.** Zeiss four-mirror lens with Unger holder. **B.** Posner lens. **C.** Sussman lens.

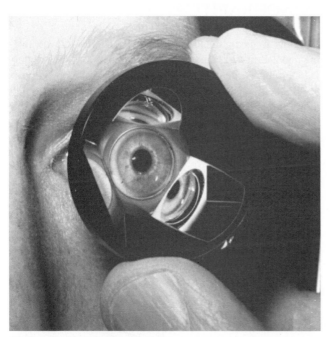

Figure 3.8. Technique of indirect gonioscopy with a Goldmann three-mirror lens.

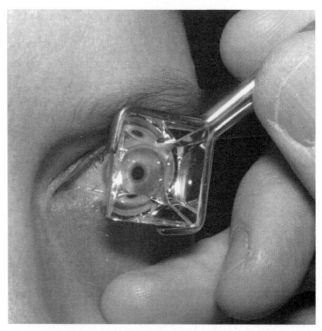

Figure 3.9. Technique of indirect gonioscopy with a Zeiss four-mirror lens.

fied by gonioscopy in a normal open adult angle (Figs. 3.10 and 3.11).

CILIARY BODY BAND. This structure is the portion of ciliary body which is visible in the anterior chamber as a result of the iris insertion into the ciliary body. The width of the band depends on the level of iris insertion, and tends to be wider in myopia and narrower in hyperopia. The color of the band is usually gray or dark brown.

SCLERAL SPUR. This is the posterior lip of the scleral sulcus, which is attached to the ciliary body posteriorly and the corneoscleral meshwork anteriorly. It is usually seen as a prominent white line between the ciliary body band and functional trabecular meshwork, unless it is obscured by

dense uveal meshwork or excessive pigment dispersion. Variable numbers of fine, pigmented strands may frequently be seen crossing the scleral spur from the iris root to the functional meshwork. These are referred to as *iris processes,* and represent thickenings of the posterior uveal meshwork.

FUNCTIONAL TRABECULAR MESHWORK. This is seen as a pigmented band just anterior to the scleral spur. Although the trabecular meshwork actually extends from the iris root to Schwalbe's line, it may be considered in two portions: (a) the anterior part, between Schwalbe's line and the anterior edge of Schlemm's canal, which is involved to a lesser degree in aqueous outflow, and (b) the posterior (or functional) part which is the remainder of the meshwork and is the primary site of aqueous outflow (especially that portion immediately adjacent to Schlemm's canal) (29).

The appearance of the functional meshwork varies considerably depending upon the amount and distribution of pigment deposition. It has no pigment at birth, but develops color with age from faint tan to dark brown, depending on the degree of pigment dispersion in the anterior chamber. The distribution of pigment may be homogeneous for 360° in some eyes and irregular in others. In the functional portion of the meshwork, especially when lightly pigmented, blood reflux in Schlemm's canal may sometimes be seen as a red band.

SCHWALBE'S LINE. This is the junction between the anterior chamber angle structures and the cornea. It is a fine ridge just anterior to the meshwork and is often identified by a small buildup of pigment, especially inferiorly.

NORMAL BLOOD VESSELS. Blood vessels are normally not seen in the angle, although loops from the major arterial circle may appear in front of the ciliary body band and less commonly over the scleral spur and trabecular meshwork. These vessels typically take a circumferential route in the angle.

In addition, an anterior ciliary artery may occasionally be seen as a more radially-oriented vessel in the ciliary body band of lightly pigmented eyes. Circumferential and radial vessels may also occasionally be seen in the peripheral iris of lightly colored eyes. In a study of 100 patients with no known cause for abnormal anterior chamber angle vascularization, 16 had normal angle vessels in both eyes and 10 more had them in one eye (30). Radial vessels were more common in the peripheral iris, while the circumferential type were more common on the ciliary body band.

Recording Gonioscopic Findings

A variety of classifications have been suggested for describing the width and appearance of the anterior chamber angle. These are discussed in Section Two under "Angle Closure Glaucoma." However, descriptive words and drawings are probably the most useful technique for recording gonioscopic findings. The recorded data should include: (a) configuration of the angle, (b) depth of the angle on the basis of the most posterior structure that can be seen, (c) degree of pigmentation, and (d) presence of abnormal structures. For example, a normal angle might be recorded as "wide open, with visualization to a wide ciliary body band for 360° and moderate trabecular meshwork pigmentation." Drawings can also be placed on a chart with concentric circles to document more specific details.

TONOGRAPHY

Tonography is a clinical, noninvasive technique for estimating the facility of aqueous outflow. It has been extremely valuable in advancing our understanding of the mechanisms of glaucoma and the actions of antiglaucoma drugs, although its clinical usefulness in the detection and management of glaucoma remains a matter of controversy. Nevertheless, it is worth considering tonography in some detail, since an understanding of the involved physiology provides insight into the complex interplay of factors related to aqueous humor dynamics.

Historical Background

The 19th century French physician and physiologist, Poiseuille (pronounced "pwah zoo' e"), pursued his interest

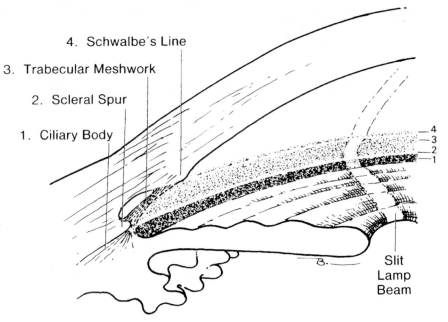

Figure 3.10. Normal adult anterior chamber angle showing gonioscopic appearance *(right)* and cross-section of corresponding structures *(left)*: *1.* Ciliary body band; *2.* Scleral spur; *3.* Trabecular meshwork (degree of pigmentation varies); *4.* Schwalbe's line.

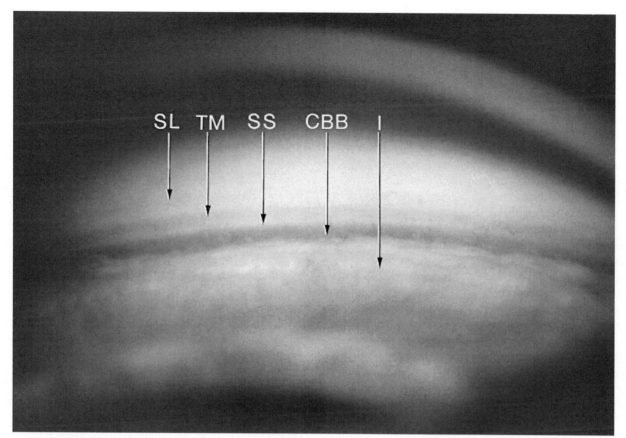

Figure 3.11. Gonioscopic view of normal anterior chamber angle, showing iris (I), ciliary body band (CBB), scleral spur (SS), trabecular meshwork (TM), and Schwalbe's line (SL).

in the circulation of blood by studying the flow of liquids in tubes of very small diameter (31). This work led to the formulation of an equation, *Poiseuille's law,* that relates the velocity of flow *(F)* of fluid in a rigid tube to (a) the radius of the tube *(r),* (b) the pressure drop per length of tube (P1 − P2/1), and (c) the coefficient of viscosity *(n)* of the fluid (32):

$$F = \frac{\pi r^4}{8n} \cdot \frac{P1 - P2}{1}$$

In 1949, Goldmann sought to apply Poiseuille's law to aqueous outflow, suggesting that the rate of aqueous flow through the trabecular meshwork *(F)* is directly proportional to the intraocular pressure *(Po)* minus the episcleral venous pressure *(Pv)* and inversely proportional to the resistance to outflow *(R)* (33):

$$F = \frac{Po - Pv}{R}$$

The equation implied that aqueous flow in living ocular tissue could be expressed in the same linear terms as that of fluid in rigid tubes, a belief that would subsequently be proven inaccurate. Nevertheless, it was modifications of Poiseuille's law that led to the mathematical foundation for tonography.

At approximately the same time that Poiseuille was conducting his studies, Pagenstecher, in 1878, observed that massage of the eye lowered the intraocular pressure (IOP). In 1905, Schiøtz reported that repeated tonometry also lowered the pressure, although less so in eyes with glaucoma. Polak-van Gelder, applying these observations, in 1911, described a technique of repeated tonometer applications for 1–2 minutes to differentiate normal and glaucomatous eyes. Schoenberg modified this technique the following year by using a continuous application of the tonometer while reading the pressure fall on the scale of the instrument (34).

In 1950, Grant (35) introduced the modern concept of tonography by combining a modification of Poiseuille's law with electronic techniques of continuous IOP measurement.

Mathematical Basis

RELATIONSHIP OF INTRAOCULAR PRESSURE TO OUTFLOW. As Goldmann (33) suggested, the rate of aqueous outflow *(F),* which is expressed in μL/min, is proportional to the IOP *(Po),* minus the episcleral venous pressure *(Pv)*:

$$F \; \gamma \; (Po - Pv)$$

Grant (35, 36) proposed that the factors which convert this proportionality to equality be expressed collectively as the *coefficient of outflow facility (C),* which is given in μL/min/mm Hg:

$$F = C \, (Po - Pv)$$

The C-value is an expression of the degree to which a change in the IOP will cause a change in the rate of aqueous outflow, which is an indirect expression of the patency of the aqueous outflow system.

ESTIMATION OF THE C-VALUE (35). Tonography is a means of estimating the C-value by raising the IOP with the weight of an indentation tonometer and observing the subsequent decay curve in the IOP. (This discussion presupposes an understanding of indentation tonometry, and the reader may wish to see the next chapter for an explanation of that technique.) The weight of the tonometer plunger on the cornea raises the IOP from the baseline *(Po)* to a new, higher level *(Pt).* The elevated pressure causes an increased rate of aqueous outflow, leading to a change in the aqueous volume *(V),* which is inferred from Friedenwald's tables relating volume change to Schiøtz scale readings (37). Direct measurements of intraocular fluid volume change in enucleated eyes have supported Friedenwald's calculations (38). Assuming for the moment that the elevated pressure does not alter other ocular parameters, the rate of volume decrease *(ΔV/T)* equals the rate of outflow.

The standard tonographic technique is to measure the IOP for 4 minutes, i.e., T = 4. The change in IOP during this time is computed as an arithmetical average of pressure increments for successive half-minute intervals (Ave. Pt − Po). The C-value is then derived from Grant's equation:

$$C = \frac{V}{T \, (\text{Ave. Pt} - Po)}$$

Perfusion studies of enucleated human eyes have supported Grant's equation, although newer tables used in the formula have given C-values far higher than those generally accepted (39).

Ocular Parameters That Influence Tonography

The tonographic calculation assumes that only the rate of aqueous outflow changes in response to a change in IOP. However, there are many other ocular parameters that respond to a pressure change, all of which can influence the tonographic result.

AQUEOUS PRODUCTION. Aqueous production may decrease during the early phase of a rise in IOP, primarily due to an alteration in ultrafiltration (40). Any subsequent IOP drop in response to reduced production of aqueous creates an impression of increased outflow and is called *pseudofacility.* This accounts for up to 20% of the total C-value (40). Tonography measures the total C-value, without distinguishing between true facility and pseudofacility. More recent fluo-

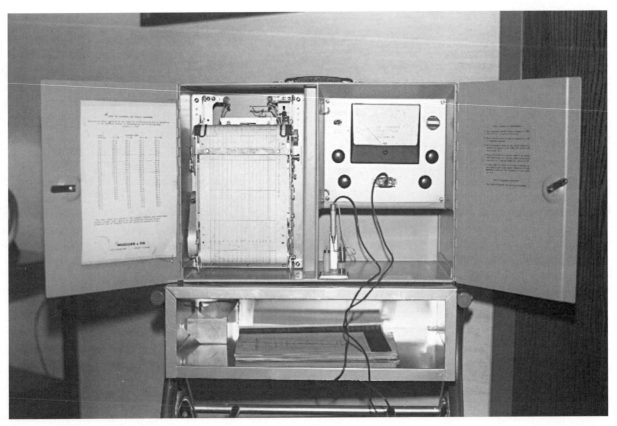

Figure 3.12. Tonography unit.

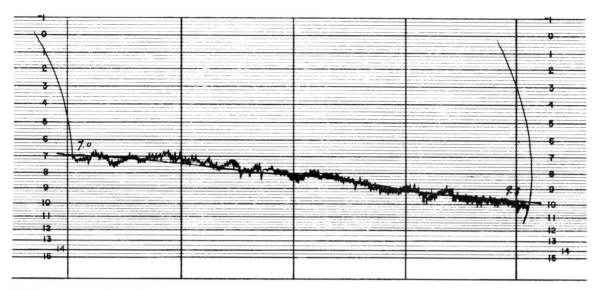

Figure 3.13. Tonographic tracing.

rophotometric studies suggest that aqueous production is relatively insensitive to long-term changes in IOP (41).

RESISTANCE TO AQUEOUS OUTFLOW. Resistance to aqueous outflow increases with an increase in the IOP, the physiologic basis of which was discussed in Chapter 2. The tonographic result is that the C-value of an eye decreases with increasing IOP (42). This phenomenon relates to the conventional route of aqueous outflow. The influence of unconventional outflow on the tonographic results is not fully understood.

EPISCLERAL VENOUS PRESSURE. Episcleral venous pressure rises an average of 1.25 mm Hg with the pressure elevation during tonography (43), which is usually corrected for in the formula by adding 1.25 to Po. Episcleral venous pressure measurements throughout tonography indicate that the rise is greatest during the first half of tonography, with a return to a nearly pretonographic level by the end of the procedure and a mean change in episcleral venous pressure during this time of 0.44 mm Hg (44).

OCULAR RIGIDITY. Ocular rigidity is an expression of the "stretchability" of the eye in response to an increase in IOP and probably represents several characteristics of the eye. An average ocular rigidity of 0.0125 is used in calculating the tonographic C-value, although there is significant interpatient variation in this parameter, which leads to a potential source of error in tonography. For this reason it is useful to check the pressure by applanation tonometry before performing the tonography and to compare this with the Po obtained with the indentation tonometer, as a means of identifying any major discrepancy in ocular rigidity.

EXPULSION OF UVEAL BLOOD. The expulsion of uveal blood in response to elevated IOP probably influences tonography, although the actual effect is uncertain (45).

Technique of Tonography (34)

The standard tonography unit consists of an electronic indentation tonometer, which continuously records IOP on a paper strip (Fig. 3.12). With the recorder running, the tonometer is calibrated at scale readings of 0 and 7. The recording needle is then set at 0 for the subsequent readings. The patient is in a supine position, fixing on a target overhead. After instilling a topical anesthetic on the cornea, the IOP is measured with two brief applications of the electronic tonometer.

The 4-minute pressure tracing is then made by gently applying the tonometer to the cornea and maintaining this position until a smooth tracing has been obtained for a full 4 minutes. A good tracing will have fine oscillations and a gentle downward slope. If the slope is steeper or irregular during the first few seconds, which is not uncommon, the study should be continued until a smooth 4-minute tracing has been obtained. The slope of the tracing is then estimated by placing a free-hand line through the middle of the oscillations (Fig. 3.13). The scale readings are noted at the beginning and end of the 4-minute tracing. Po and the change in scale readings over four minutes *(R)* are then used to obtain the C-value from special tonographic tables.

A basic assumption of tonography is that C-value calculations from each minute of the clinical tonogram do not differ significantly, although this has been shown to be invalid, with a trend toward highest values in the first minute and progressive reduction in the ensuing minutes (46). A computer program has been developed to evaluate tonograms and assess the findings (47), and a computerized tonography instrument has been devised, which has been shown to give outflow facilities that do not differ statistically significantly from those obtained with a standard tonography unit (48).

Applanation tonometers cause less change in IOP, resulting in less effect on outflow resistance and on the other parameters influenced by pressure change. The use of applanation tonometers in tonography has been evaluated by using instruments that maintain a constant IOP level (49, 50), or a constant diameter of tonometer contact with the cornea (51). These techniques are still investigational. Tonography with a pneumatic tonometer (pneumotonography, described in Chapter 4) was compared to that with a Schiøtz tonometer in normal and glaucomatous subjects and was found to give virtually identical average C-values, but had significantly higher intrasubject and interobserver variability (52).

Sources of Error in Tonographic Technique

VARIATIONS IN CORNEAL CURVATURE. Variations in corneal curvature from the assumed average of 7.8 mm may significantly influence the pressure measurements (34).

MOSES EFFECT. The hole in the tonometer footplate must be slightly larger in electronic tonometers to prevent sticking. At low scale readings, the cornea may mold into the space between the plunger and hole, pushing the plunger up and leading to falsely high pressure readings (53).

VARIATIONS IN LINE VOLTAGE. Variations in line voltage may produce an apparent drift in the IOP measurements, which can be minimized with line voltage stabilizers and by avoiding magnetic fields (34).

CONSENSUAL PRESSURE DROP. The IOP has been shown to drop approximately 1 mm Hg in the fellow eye while tonography is being performed on the first eye. A neural etiology was once postulated for this phenomenon, but it was subsequently found to be secondary to the evaporation that results from keeping the eye open for fixation during the 4-minute test (54). The problem can be eliminated by draping a plastic sheet over the fellow eye while the first eye is being tested (54).

EYE MOVEMENT. Eye movement under the tonometer can also influence the tonographic tracing.

PATIENT RELAXATION EFFECT. During the first 15–20 seconds after the tonometer is placed on the cornea, the IOP will fall as the patient relaxes. Time should be allowed for this before starting the 4-minute tracing.

OPERATOR ERROR. Operator error, including improper cleaning, calibration, or positioning of the instrument, as well as improper calculation of the tracing, can also lead to inaccurate results.

Interpreting Tonographic Results

Despite the many potentials for error in tonography and the possibility that currently accepted values may be grossly inaccurate, it is, nevertheless, necessary to be familiar with the values that might be anticipated with current techniques.

From a study of 1379 eyes, Becker (55) reported the following values.

C-Value: The mean in 909 normal eyes was 0.28 μL/min/mm Hg, and the prevalence of low C-values was:

C-Value	Normals (n = 909)	Glaucoma Patients (n = 250)	Family History of Glaucoma (n = 220)
< 0.18	2.5%	65%	20%
< 0.13	0.15%	43%	11%

Po/C Ratio: The mean of the normal population was 56, and the prevalence of high Po/C ratios was:

C-Value	Normals	Glaucoma Patients	Family History of Glaucoma
> 100	2.5%	73%	21%
> 138	0.15%	50%	14%

In a study of 7577 eyes, the C-value was found to decrease with age, with an average of 0.2932 for ages 41–45 years, compared to 0.2518 in the 81–85-year-old group. There was no sex difference at any age level (56).

When the C-value and Po do not seem to correlate, the following possibilities should be considered (34). A low C with a normal Po may be due to: (a) a sticky tonometer, (b) low ocular rigidity, or (c) hyposecretion. A normal C with elevated Po may be due to: (a) an artificially elevated Po, (b) high ocular rigidity, (c) high pseudofacility, (d) elevated episcleral venous pressure, (e) angle-closure glaucoma (the force of the tonometer may open the angle), or (f) the Moses effect.

The wave components of a tonographic tracing include: (a) fine oscillations, which reflect the cardiac pulse; (b) large waves, which reflect the respiratory movement; and (c) still larger, irregular waves (Traube-Hering waves), which reflect periodic oscillations in the systemic blood pressure. Cardiac irregularities, e.g., extrasystoli, bigeminy, etc., can also cause irregularities in the tonographic tracing (57).

Clinical Value of Tonography

As previously noted, there is controversy regarding the value of tonography in the detection and management of glaucoma. The following are the main situations in which tonography is felt by some physicians to have clinical value.

As an adjunct in diagnosing open-angle glaucoma, tonography is suggested to have predictive value regarding the development of nerve damage in patients with elevated IOP (58, 59), although this has not been confirmed in all studies (60). The Po/C ratio is generally felt to be the more sensitive parameter in this situation (58, 59), and a prior water-drinking test (discussed in Chapter 9) has been suggested

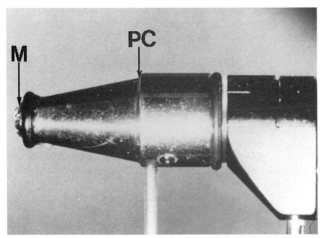

Figure 3.14. Head of instrument for measuring episcleral venous pressure showing flexible membrane (M), which presses against episcleral vessel, and pressure chamber (PC), which transfers pressure to membrane. (Courtesy of Douglas E. Gaasterland, M.D.)

to further enhance the predictive value of tonography (58). However, it has been stressed that abnormal tonometric and tonographic results do not make the diagnosis of glaucoma, but alert the ophthalmologist to follow the patient more closely (61).

A wide diurnal fluctuation in IOP was felt to correlate with a low C-value, but a study of 388 eyes showed that a single tonometric reading correlated with the diurnal curve better than did the tonographic results (62).

In angle-closure glaucoma, a 25–30% fall in the C-value may be used as adjunctive confirmation of a positive provocative test. In addition, once an acute attack is broken, a C-value of 0.10 or less suggests that a peripheral iridotomy alone may be insufficient (34).

Ocular inflammation, as with surgery, trauma, disease, etc., may mask a compromised outflow system by temporarily reducing aqueous production, and tonography during this time can disclose the abnormal outflow (34).

Myasthenia gravis may also be evaluated with tonography by observing a rise in IOP of 2–5 mm Hg in response to intravenous tensilon (63).

Since both aqueous and blood are expelled from the eye in variable amounts during tonography, it may be that a future value of tonography lies in its ability to assess the posterior half of the eye, the portion directly related to visual loss, by measuring the blood-ejection coefficient (45, 64).

MEASUREMENT OF EPISCLERAL VENOUS PRESSURE

A variety of techniques have been developed for measuring the pressure in the episcleral veins. All of these work on the principle of correlating partial collapse of the vein with the force required to achieve the alteration in blood flow. A *pres-*

sure chamber technique utilizes a thin membrane stretched over the tip of a hollow applanating head, which is filled with air (65–67) or saline (68) (Fig. 3.14). The pressure in the chamber is raised until the bulging membrane produces the desired visible change in the adjacent vessel. Most of these instruments are mounted on a slitlamp, although a portable pressure transducer has been developed to measure espiscleral venous pressure with a subject in various body positions (69). A *torsion balance* instrument utilizes a clear plastic applanating head, attached to a torsion rod (65, 70). The applanating head is placed over a vein, and the pressure of the applanating head against the vessel is raised until the desired endpoint in blood flow change is achieved. An *air jet* technique uses a stream of air to collapse the vessel (71). When the first two methods were compared to direct cannulation of the episcleral vein, the pressure chamber method was found to be superior to the torsion technique (65).

As noted in Chapter 2, the normal episcleral venous pressure is generally considered to be between 8 and 11 mm Hg. Two features that significantly influence the measured pressure are the selected endpoint and the choice of vessel. When a pressure chamber technique was compared to direct cannulation, a slight indentation, rather than an intermittent or sustained collapse of the vein lumen, gave the most accurate reading (68). It has been suggested that the best point of measurement is just distal to the junction of aqueous and episcleral veins, although this junction is often difficult to ascertain and it may be more practical to take all measurements 3 mm from the limbus (67).

SUMMARY

Instruments and techniques have been developed for evaluating aqueous humor inflow by directly visualizing the ciliary processes (cycloscopy) and by measuring the actual rate of aqueous production (fluorophotometry). Other instruments can be used to study aqueous humor outflow by direct visualization of the anterior chamber angle (gonioscopy), estimation of the resistance to aqueous outflow (tonography), and the measurement of episcleral venous pressure. Of these techniques, only gonioscopy is commonly used in daily clinical practice, with the others currently having primary value as research tools.

REFERENCES

1. Mizuno, K, Asaoka, M: Cycloscopy and fluorescein cycloscopy. Invest Ophthalmol 15:561, 1976.
2. Mizuno, K, Asaoka, M, Muroi, S: Cycloscopy and fluorescein cycloscopy of the ciliary process. Am J Ophthalmol 84:487, 1977.
3. Holm, O: A photogrammetric method for estimation of the pupillary aqueous flow in the living human eye. I. Acta Ophthalmol 46:254, 1968.
4. Brubaker, RF, Nagtaki, S, Townsend, DJ, et al: The effect of age on aqueous humor formation in man. Ophthalmology 88:283, 1981.
5. Jones, RF, Maurice, DM: New methods of measuring the rate of aqueous flow in man with fluorescein. Exp Eye Res 5:208, 1966.

6. Bloom, JN, Levene, RZ, Thomas, G, Kimura, R: Fluorophotometry and the rate of aqueous flow in man. Arch Ophthalmol 94:435, 1976.

7. Coakes, RL, Brubaker, RF: Method of measuring aqueous humor flow and corneal endothelial permeability using a fluorophotometry nomogram. Invest Ophthalmol Vis Sci 18:288, 1979.

8. Brubaker, RF, Coakes, RL: Use of xenon flash tube as the excitation source in new slit-lamp fluorophotometer. Am J Ophthalmol 86: 474, 1978.

9. Brubaker, RF, McLaren, JW: Uses of fluorophotometry in glaucoma research. Ophthalmology 92:884, 1985.

10. Becker, B: The measurement of rate of aqueous flow with iodide. Invest Ophthalmol 1:52, 1962.

11. Macri, JF, Cevario, SJ: The formation and inhibition of aqueous humor production. Arch Ophthalmol 96:1664, 1978.

12. Wickham, MG, Worthen, DM, Downing, D: A randomized technique of constant pressure infusion. Invest Ophthalmol 15:1010, 1976.

13. Becker, S: Clinical Gonopscopy—A Text and Stereoscopic Atlas. St. Louis, CV Mosby, 1972.

14. Rubin, ML: Optics for Clinicians, 2nd ed. Gainsesville, FL, Triad Scientific Publishing, 1974, p. 56.

15. O'Rourke, J, Lal, M, Kalwat, W: Weightless Koeppe gonioscopy. Arch Ophthalmol 99:1646, 1981.

16. Kapetansky, FM: A bubble-free goniolens. Ophthalmic Surg 19: 414, 1988.

17. Sussman, W: A new instrument for gonioscopy. Ophthalmology 86:130, 1979.

18. Kaufman, PL, Neider, MW, Pankonin, WH: Slitlamp mount for Zeiss gonioscopy lens. Arch Ophthalmol 99:1455, 1981.

19. Ritch, R: A new lens for argon laser trabeculoplasty. Ophthalmic Surg 16:331, 1985.

20. Mizuno, K: A new multipurpose goniolens. Arch Ophthalmol 106:1309, 1988.

21. Kapetansky, FM, Johnstone, MA: A direct-view goniolens. Am J Ophthalmol 93:242, 1982.

22. Becker, SC: Unrecognized errors induced by present-day gonioprisms and a proposal for their elimination. Arch Ophthalmol 82:160, 1969.

23. Hetherington, J Jr: Koeppe lens gonioscopy. In Controversy in Ophthalmology. Brockhurst, FJ, Boruchoff, SA, Huctchinson, BT, Lessell, S, eds. Philadelphia, WB Saunders, 1977, p. 142.

24. Campbell, DG: A comparison of diagnostic techniques in angle-closure glaucoma. Am J Ophthalmol 88:197, 1979.

25. Schwartz, B: Slit lamp gonioscopy. In Controversy in Ophthalmology. Brockhurst, FJ, Boruchoff, SA, Huctchinson, BT, Lessell, S, eds. Philadelphia, WB Saunders, 1977, p. 146.

26. Smith, RJH: An improved diagnostic contact lens. Br J Ophthalmol 63:482, 1979.

27. Forbes, M: Gonioscopy with corneal indentation. Arch Ophthalmol 76:488, 1966.

28. Vijfvinkel, G, de Jong, PTVM: Disinfectant container for diagnostic lenses. Am J Ophthalmol 99:600, 1985.

29. Inomata, H, Tawara, A: Anterior and posterior parts of human trabecular meshwork. Jpn J Ophthalmol 28:339, 1984.

30. Shihab, ZM, Lee, P-F: The significance of normal angle vessels. Ophthalmic Surg 16:382, 1985.

31. Bingham, EC: Biography of Dr. Jean Leonard Marie Poiseuille. Rheological Memoirs 1:vii, 1940.

32. Frank, NH: Introduction to Mechanics and Heat, 2nd ed. New York, McGraw-Hill, 1939, p. 246.

33. Goldmann, H: Augendruck and gluakom. Die Kammerwasservenen und das Poiseuille'sche Gesetz. Ophthalmologica 118:496, 1949.

34. Drews, RC: Manual of tonography. St Louis, CV Mosby, 1971.

35. Grant, WM: Tonographic method for measuring the facility and rate of aqueous flow in human eyes. Arch Ophthalmol 44:204, 1950.

36. Grant, WM: Clinical measurements of aqueous outflow. Arch Ophthalmol 46:113, 1951.

37. Friedenwald, JS: Some problems in the calibration of tonometers. Am J Ophthalmol 31:935, 1948.

38. Hetland-Eriksen, J, Odberg, T: Experimental tonography on enucleated human eyes. II. The loss of intraocular fluid caused by tonography. Invest Ophthalmol 14:944, 1975.

39. Hetland-Eriksen, J, Odberg, T: Experimental tonography on enucleated human eyes. I. The validity of Grant's tonography formula. Invest Ophthalmol 14:199, 1975.

40. Kupfer, C: Clinical significance of pseudofacility. Am J Ophthalmol 75:193, 1973.

41. Carlson, KH, McLaren, JW, Topper, JE, Brubaker, RF: Effect of body position on intraocular pressure and aqueous flow. Invest Ophthalmol Vis Sci 28:1346, 1987.

42. Moses, RA: Constant pressure applanation tonography. III. The relationship of tonometric pressure to rate of loss of ocular volume. Arch Ophthalmol 77:181, 1967.

43. Linnér, E: Episcleral venous pressure during tonograpy. Acta XVII Cong Ophthalmol 3:1532, 1955.

44. Leith, AB: Episcleral venous pressure in tonography. Br J Ophthalmol 47:271, 1963.

45. Fisher, RF: Value of tonometry and tonography in the diagnosis of glaucoma. Br J Ophthalmol 56:200, 1972.

46. Armaly, MF: On the consistency of tonography. II. One minute analysis of clinical tonogram. Klin Monatsbl Augenheilkd 184: 299, 1984.

47. Strobel, J: A new method of evaluating tonograms. Klin Monatsbl Augenheilkd 183:301, 1983.

48. Teitelbaum, CS, Podos, SM, Lustgarten, JS: Comparison of standard and computerized tonography instruments on human eyes. Am J Ophthalmol 99:403, 1985.

49. Moses, RA: Constant pressure applanation tonography with the Mackay-Marg tonometer. I. A preliminary report. Arch Ophthalmol 76:20, 1966.

50. Moses, RA: Constant pressure applanation tonography with the Mackay-Marg tonometer. II. Limits of the instrument. Arch Ophthalmol 77:45, 1967.

51. Moses, RA, Grodzki, WJ Jr, Arnzen, RJ: Constant-area applanation tonography. Invest Ophthalmol Vis Sci 20:722, 1981.

52. Feghali, JG, Azar, DT, Kaufman, PL: Comparative aqueous outflow facility measurements by pneumatonography and Schiøtz tonography. Invest Ophthalmol Vis Sci 27:1776, 1986.

53. Moses, R: Tonometry-effect of tonometer footplate hole on scale reading. Further studies. Arch Ophthalmol 61:373, 1959.

54. Grant, WM, English, FP: An explanation for so-called consensual pressure drop during tonography. Arch Ophthalmol 69:314, 1963.

55. Becker, B: Tonography in the diagnosis of simple (open angle) glaucoma. Trans Am Acad Ophthalmol Otolaryngol 65:156, 1961.

56. Johnson, LV: Tonographic survey. Am J Ophthalmol 61:680, 1966.

57. Haik, GM, Perez, LF, Reitman, HS, Massey, JY: Tonographic tracings in patients with cardiac rhythm disturbances. Am J Ophthalmol 70:929, 1970.

58. Becker, B, Christensen, RE: Water-drinking and tonography in the diagnosis of glaucoma. Arch Ophthalmol 56:321, 1956.

59. Portney, GL, Krohn, M: Tonography and projection perimetry. Relationship according to receiver operating characteristic curves. Arch Ophthalmol 95:1353, 1977.

60. Pohjanpelto, PEJ: Tonography and glaucomatous optic nerve damage. Acta Ophthalmol 52:817, 1974.

61. Podos, SM, Becker, B: Tonography-current thoughts. Am J Ophthalmol 75:733, 1973.

62. Phelps, CD, Woolson, RF, Kolker, AE, Becker, B: Diurnal variation in intraocular pressure. Am J Ophthalmol 77:367, 1974.

63. Wray, SH, Pavan-Langston, D: A reevaluation of edrophonium chloride (Tensilon) tonography in the diagnosis of myasthenia gravis: With observations on some other defects of neuromuscular transmission. Neurology 21:586, 1971.

64. Spaeth, GL: Tonography and tonometry. In Clinical Ophthalmology. Vol. 3, Chap. 47. Duane, TD, ed. Hagerstown, MD, Harper & Row, 1976.

65. Brubaker, RF: Determination of episcleral venous pressure in the eye. A comparison of three methods. Arch Ophthalmol 77:110, 1967.
66. Phelps, CD, Armaly, MF: Measurement of episcleral venous pressure. Am J Ophthalmol 85:35, 1978.
67. Zeimer, RC, Gieser, DK, Wilensky, JT, et al: A practical venomanometer. Measurement of episcleral venous pressure and assessment of the normal range. Arch Ophthalmol 101:1447, 1983.
68. Gaasterland, DE, Pederson, JE: Episcleral venous pressure: A comparison of invasive and noninvasive measurements. Invest Ophthalmol Vis Sci 24:1417, 1983.
69. Friberg, TR: Portable transducer for measurement of episcleral venous pressure. Am J Ophthalmol 102:396, 1986.
70. Podos, SM, Minas, TF, Macri, FJ: A new instrument to measure episcleral venous pressure. Comparison of normal eyes and eyes with primary open-angle glaucoma. Arch Ophthalmol 80:209, 1968.
71. Krakau, CET, Widakowich, J, Wilke, K: Measurements of the episcleral venous pressure by means of an air jet. Acta Ophthalmol 51:185, 1973.

Chapter 4

INTRAOCULAR PRESSURE AND TONOMETRY

INTRAOCULAR PRESSURE

What is Normal?

Within the context of a discussion on glaucoma, "normal" intraocular pressure (IOP) might be defined as that pressure which does not lead to glaucomatous damage of the optic nerve head. Unfortunately, such a definition cannot be expressed in precise numerical terms, since all eyes do not respond the same to given pressure levels. The best we can do is to describe the distribution of IOP in general populations and in groups of individuals with glaucomatous damage to establish levels of risk for glaucoma within different pressure ranges. In this chapter, we consider the distribution of IOP in the general population and the factors, other than glaucoma, that may influence IOP. In Section Two, the significance of various pressure levels within populations of patients with specific types of glaucoma are considered.

Distribution in General Populations

The most frequently cited population study is that by Leydhecker and associates (1) in which 10,000 persons with no known eye disease were tested with Schiøtz tonometers. These investigators obtained a distribution of pressures that resembled a Gaussian curve, but was skewed toward the higher pressures. They interpreted these findings to represent two subpopulations: a large, "normal" group and a smaller group that was felt to represent previously unrecognized glaucoma (this included individuals with and without established glaucomatous optic nerve damage). In the "normal" group, the mean IOP was 15.5 ± 2.57 mm Hg. Two standard deviations (2SD) above the mean was approximately 20.5 mm Hg, which the authors interpreted as the upper limit of "normal," since approximately 95% of the area under a Gaussian curve lies between the mean ± 2SD. However, the latter principle does not apply when a frequency distribution is skewed, and the concept of "normal" IOP limits must be viewed as only a rough approximation (2).

Subsequent IOP screening studies, using either indentation or applanation tonometry (these techniques are explained later in this chapter), have generally agreed with Leydhecker's findings regarding pressure distribution in general populations, with small differences probably related to population selection and testing techniques (Table 4.1) (3–11). However, the division of IOP groups into normal and abnormal is not as simple as Leydhecker and associates (1) originally suspected since

Table 4.1.

REPORTED IOP DISTRIBUTIONS IN GENERAL POPULATIONS

A. Tested with Schiøtz Tonometers

Investigators	Number of Individuals	Ages (years)	IOP (mm Hg) Mean	SD
Leydhecker, et al. (1958) (1)	10,000	10–69	15.8	2.57
Johnson (1966) (3)	7577	>41	15.4	2.65
Seal & Skwierczyriska (1967) (4)	15,695	>30	15.3–15.9 (women) 15.0–15.2 (men)	

B. Tested with Applanation Tonometers

Investigators	Number of Individuals	Ages (years)	IOP (mm Hg) Mean	SD
Armaly (1965) (5)	2316	20–79	15.91	3.14*
Perkins (1965) (6)	2000	>40	15.2 14.9	2.5 (OD) 2.5 (OS)
Loewen, et al. (1976) (7)	4661	9–89	17.18	3.78
Ruprecht, et al. (1978) (8)	8899	5–94	16.25	3.45
Shiose & Kawase (1986) (9)	75,545 (men) 18,158 (women)	<70	14.60 15.04	2.52 2.33
David, et al. (1987) (10)	2504	40–70+	14.93	4.04
Klein, et al. (1992) (11)	4856	43–86	15.4	3.35

*Computed from data reported according to sex and age groups.

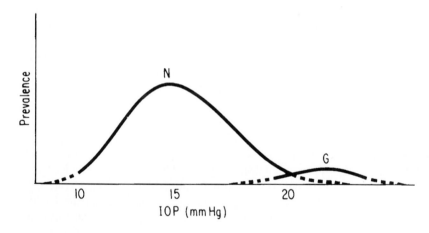

Figure 4.1. Theoretical distribution of intraocular pressures in nonglaucoma (N) and glaucoma (G) populations, showing overlap between the two groups (*dotted lines* represent uncertainty of extreme values in both populations).

there are many factors which influence the IOP. Furthermore, as previously noted, all eyes do not respond the same to given pressure levels. This leads to an overlapping of IOP distributions within nonglaucoma and glaucoma populations, which can only be illustrated theoretically (Fig. 4.1) since the precise boundaries of both groups are not known.

Factors Exerting Long-term Influence on Intraocular Pressure

The following factors are felt to exert, to variable degrees, a sustained influence on IOP throughout the lifetime of the individual.

Genetics

The IOP within the general population appears to be under hereditary influence, possibly through a polygenic, multifactorial mode (12–14). In addition, the IOP tends to be higher in individuals with an enlarged cup-disc ratio (10) and those who have relatives with open-angle glaucoma (5, 15).

Age

There is, in general, an increase in IOP with age. Most studies indicate that young children have significantly lower pressures than the rest of the normal population, although tonometric measurements may be influenced by the level of cooperation of the child if they are awake, or the anesthetic or other agents when they are asleep or sedated. The mean IOP, using only topical anesthesia for the tonometry, has been reported to be 11.4 ± 2.4 mm Hg in newborns (16) and 8.4 ± 0.6 mm Hg in infants under 4 months of age (17). In a study of 460 children between birth and 16 years using a noncontact tonometer, the mean IOP rose from 9.59 ± 2.3 mm Hg at birth to 13.73 ± 2.05 mm Hg at 3–4 years, with more stable measurements thereafter (18). Results of studies in premature infants have been conflicting, with mean IOPs of 18 mm Hg in one study (19) and 10.13–10.17 mm Hg in another (20). The tonometer may also influence the results, with mean IOPs in 50 supine children under 5 years of age of 5.89 mm Hg with a hand-held applanation tonometer and 14.76 mm Hg with a pneumotonometer (21). The use of general anesthesia or a hypnotic agent in children may artificially lower the IOP (17). This is discussed later in this chapter under "General Anesthesia."

In the adult population, the IOP distribution is Gaussian between 20 and 40 years of age (5). Thereafter, the curve begins to shift toward the higher pressures with advancing age (5, 7, 8). Some investigators feel this is due to a positive independent correlation between IOP and age (5, 10, 22, 23). Others, however, have found a weak (24, 25) or negative (9, 26) correlation, and suggest that other factors such as pulse rate (24), obesity (9), or blood pressure (9, 25, 26) may be responsible for the apparent rise in IOP with increasing age. If there is a true positive correlation between IOP and age, it may be related to reduced facility of aqueous outflow since aqueous production actually appears to decrease slightly with increasing age (27–29).

Sex

IOP is equal between the sexes in ages 20–40 years. In older age groups, the apparent increase in the mean IOP with age is greater in females and coincides with the onset of menopause, while the increase in the standard deviation of the IOP distribution is equal between the sexes (5).

Refractive Error

A positive correlation between IOP and both axial length of the globe (30) and increasing degrees of myopia (10, 15, 31, 32) has been reported. Increasing IOP was also related to myopia in a study of 321 children with a mean age of 9.8 years (33). However, another study of patients with anisometropic myopia found no difference in IOP between the two eyes (34). Myopes also have a higher incidence of chronic open-angle glaucoma, and it is hard to know whether the higher pressures in this group are a reflection of the early glaucoma cases or a truly higher IOP distribution throughout the myopic population.

Race

Race may occasionally influence IOP distribution. For example, full-blood Indians in a New Mexican tribe were found to have a significantly lower mean IOP than a control population (35). Blacks have been reported to have slightly higher pressures than whites (22, 23), and persons born in Africa or Asia were found to have higher mean IOPs than those born in Europe or America (10).

Factors Exerting Short-term Influence on Intraocular Pressure

The following are factors that have been associated with a rise or fall in IOP, lasting from seconds to months.

Diurnal Variation

Like many biological parameters, the IOP is subject to cyclic fluctuations throughout the day. The reported mean amplitude of the daily fluctuation ranges from approximately 3 mm Hg (36) to 6 mm Hg (37). An amplitude greater than 10 mm Hg is generally considered to be pathologic (38), and glaucomatous eyes have been reported to exceed 30 mm Hg of diurnal variation (38). The pattern of the daily cycle has classically been described as having the peak IOP in the morning hours (36). This may, in fact, be the most common pattern, with one study of 690 diurnal curves showing the highest IOP in the early morning in 40% of cases and before noon in 65% (39). However, other studies have revealed frequent peak pressures in the afternoon, as well as short-term fluctuations throughout the day (37, 38, 40–42). Patients with open-angle glaucoma or ocular hypertension, as compared to normal controls, appear to have more variability in their diurnal curves, with one study showing a high percentage with no diurnal rhythm, with frequent differences between the two eyes, and with differences in diurnal curve patterns from one day to the next (42).

The obvious primary clinical value of measuring diurnal IOP variation is to avoid the risk of missing a pressure elevation with single readings. In addition, patients with IOP peaks of 6 mm Hg or more above the daytime average are more likely to have progressive visual field loss, than those with a lower amplitude of diurnal fluctuation (43). A practical concern, however, is the logistics of obtaining the diurnal measurements. In one study using a self-tonometer (described later in this chapter) to obtain 24-hour diurnal curves, half of the IOP peaks occurred at times outside of normal office hours (44). Using the same self-tonometry, the authors found that many patients have a significant drop in IOP between the time they awake and 30 minutes later (45), suggesting that either the act of waking is associated with a transient pressure rise or significant IOP peaks may disappear before the patient is seen in the clinic. In any case, nighttime measurements are not only hard to obtain, but also difficult to interpret, and many physicians use a modified diurnal curve, by measuring the IOP in the office approximately every 2 hours from early morning to late afternoon or early evening. This at least has the benefit of establishing the best time of day for future pressure checks, i.e., when the IOP is highest.

The mechanism of diurnal IOP variation is uncertain. Results of tonographic studies have been conflicting, with one showing an inverse relationship between IOP and outflow facility (46), and another showing no relationship (38). A relationship between adrenocortical steroids and diurnal IOP variation has been suggested, since the diurnal variation of plasma cortisol has been observed to parallel that of the IOP, peaking 3–4 hours before the latter (46, 47). Furthermore, interruption of the normal daily corticosteroid cycle has been shown to alter the diurnal IOP curve (46, 48), and oral administration of metyrapone, an inhibitor of adrenal cortical biosynthesis, is associated with a decrease in IOP (49). However, the reduction of aqueous humor flow during sleep has been shown to occur in the absence of a comparable fall in plasma corticosteroid activity (50). The circadian rhythm of aqueous flow also does not appear to be influenced by plasma melatonin levels (51). Rabbits have a circadian rhythm in a light-dark environment, with a low IOP in the light and a high IOP in the dark (52, 53). The pressure elevation appears to be related to both increased aqueous outflow resistance and increased aqueous flow (54), which in turn appears to be related to increased adrenergic activity during the dark phase (55–57).

Postural Variation

Most studies show that the IOP increases when changing from the sitting to the supine position, with reported average pressure differences of 0.3–6.0 mm Hg (58–60). Some investigators, however, have been unable to confirm these findings in normal eyes (61, 62), and one study showed poor reproducibility of postural changes in IOP among subjects without glaucoma (63). The postural influence on IOP is greater in eyes with glaucoma (58, 60, 64), and persists even after a successful trabeculectomy (64). One study suggested that the postural variation is greatest in patients with low tension glaucoma (65), while another found that 15% of ocular hypertensives had an IOP rise of 5–9 mm Hg when going from the sitting to supine position, which was sustained throughout 4 hours of observation (66). In a study of ocular hypertensives, normal controls, and patients with low tension glaucoma, all had an average IOP rise of 4 mm Hg in changing from the sitting to supine position, which remained stable after 30 minutes in the low tension and normal groups, but rose an additional 1.6 mm Hg in the ocular hypertensives, associated with an equally significant decrease in blood pressure (67). Postural variation is also higher in patients with central retinal vein occlusion (62), and patients with systemic hypertension have a significantly higher IOP rise after 15 minutes in the supine position, than normotensive controls (68). These observations may explain why retinal vascular occlusive events are most often discovered in the morning.

Whole-body, head-down tilt leads to a further increase in IOP, which correlates with the degree of inversion (69). In one study, after 5 minutes of total inversion, the mean pressure rose from 16.8 ± 2.8 to 32.9 ± 7.9 mm Hg in normal eyes, and from 21.3 ± 2.3 to 37.6 ± 5 mm Hg in glaucomatous eyes (70). The mechanism of this phenomenon appears to be elevated episcleral venous pressure (71).

Exertional Influences

Exertion may lead to either a lowering or an elevation of the IOP, depending on the nature of the activity. Both prolonged exercise, such as running or bicycling (72–76), as well as brief exercise, such as six deep knee bends (77), have been reported to lower the IOP. Reports vary regarding the magnitude of this pressure response, but in general it appears to be greater in glaucoma patients than in normal individuals. The effect was also found to be minimal in elderly (66–85 years) nonglaucomatous subjects (78). Reports also differ regarding the effect of exercise over longer periods of time, e.g., 3–4 months, on IOP with some showing a significant reduction in both normotensive individuals (76) and glaucoma suspects (79), while another study of 80 healthy volunteers found no effect on either IOP or aqueous flow (80).

Theories of mechanism for exercise-induced IOP reduction include increased serum osmolarity (73, 81), metabolic acidosis (74), hypocapnia (82), blood lactate levels (83), and sympathetic activity (77, 82). Salt-loading in patients on a bicycle ergometer was associated with only a 1 mm Hg decrease in IOP (84). These differences may be influenced by the type of exercise, although it appears that many factors are probably involved in the influence of exercise on IOP.

Straining, as associated with Valsalva's maneuver (85, 86) or electroshock therapy (87) has been reported to elevate the IOP. Mechanisms for this phenomenon likely include elevated episcleral venous pressure, especially with Valsalva's maneuver, and increased orbicularis tone.

Lid and Eye Movement

Blinking has been shown to raise the IOP 10 mm Hg, while hard lid squeezing may raise it as high as 90 mm Hg (88). It has also been shown that repeated lid squeezing will lead to a slight reduction in IOP, although less so in glaucomatous eyes (89). Voluntary lid fissure widening causes an increase in IOP of about 2 mm Hg, which may relate to an increased orbital volume from retraction of the upper lid into the orbit (90). Reports differ as to whether decreased orbicularis tone, as with Bell's palsy or local facial nerve block, reduces IOP (91, 92). Patients with third neuron Horner's syndrome were found to have a slight reduction in IOP without alterations in aqueous humor dynamics (93). Contraction of extraocular muscles also influences the IOP. There is an increase in IOP on upgaze in normal individuals, which is augmented by Graves infiltrative ophthalmopathy (94). Intraocular pressure has been shown to increase slightly in horizontal gaze position (95), especially when full duction is restricted in patients with noncomitant strabismus (96), and it has been suggested that a rise of more than 5 mm Hg may distinguish restrictive from paretic strabismus (97). During strabismus surgery, especially for eyes with thyroid ophthalmopathy, the IOP has been recorded to rise as high as 84 mm Hg (98).

Intraocular Conditions

In addition to the many ocular conditions that can lead to elevated IOP with associated glaucoma (discussed in Section Two), there are some intraocular conditions that may lead to a reduction in IOP. *Anterior uveitis,* as noted in Chapter 2, often leads to a slight reduction in IOP, due to a decrease in aqueous humor formation. *Rhegmatogenous retinal detachment* may also be associated with a reduced IOP, apparently due to reduced aqueous flow (99), as well as a shunting of aqueous from the posterior chamber, through the vitreous and retinal hole, into the subretinal space, and across the retinal pigment epithelium (100).

Systemic Conditions

Most studies have revealed a positive correlation between *systemic hypertension,* especially the systolic level, and IOP (9, 15, 22–24, 26, 101–104). During cardiopulmonary bypass surgery there is reduced ocular perfusion and a slight increase in IOP, possibly due to hemodilution (105). The risk of IOP elevation may be minimized by using colloid solution rather than crystalloid solution during the bypass surgery (106), and by administering mannitol 30 minutes prior to the surgery, rather than at the start of the procedure (107). A slight IOP elevation may persist for the first 2 days after cardiopulmonary bypass surgery (108). This does not correlate with weight gain or hemodilution, and may be associated with postoperative medications.

Systemic hyperthermia has been shown to cause an increased IOP in rabbits (109) and man (110). Other systemic factors reported to have a positive correlation with IOP include obesity (9, 26), pulse rate (24), and hemoglobin concentration (24, 111).

In addition to the possible *hormonal influence* on diurnal fluctuation in IOP, as previously discussed, preliminary evidence suggests that the IOP may increase in response to ACTH, glucocorticoids, and growth hormone, and decrease in response to progesterone, estrogen, chorionic gonadotropin, and relaxin (112, 113). The IOP does not appear to be influenced by the menstrual cycle in humans (114, 115), although it has been shown to be significantly reduced during pregnancy (116, 117), which may be due to blocking of the ocular hypertensive effect of endogenous corticosteroids by excess progesterone (117). Topical antidiuretic hormone (vasopressin) lowers IOP in human eyes, while intravenous administration in rabbits increases the pressure (118). Intravenous pituitary hormone releasing factors variably influence the IOP in rabbits, with corticotropin releasing factor and luteinizing hormone releasing factor causing a decrease and thyrotropin releasing hormone causing a rise in pressure (119).

The IOP has also been reported to be lower with hyperthyroidism and higher in patients with hypothyroidism (120), and treatment of the hypothyroidism has been reported to improve IOP and facility of outflow (121). Patients with acromegaly were found to have slight IOP elevation, although this was apparently due to the influence of increased central corneal thickness on the tonometric measurement (122). In myotonic dystrophy the IOP is markedly low, which may be partially due to reduced aqueous production (123), but also to increased outflow, possibly by the uveoscleral route from atrophy of the ciliary muscles (124). Diabetic patients have been reported to have higher pressures than the general population (102, 125), while a fall in IOP has been noted during acute hypoglycemia in patients with insulin-dependent diabetes (126).

Environmental Conditions

Exposure to cold air reduces IOP, apparently due to a decrease in episcleral venous pressure (127). Reduced gravity causes a sudden, marked increase in IOP, apparently due to cephalad shifts in intravascular and extravascular body fluids (128, 129).

General Anesthesia

General anesthesia is usually associated with a reduction in the IOP (130), although there are exceptions, such as with trichloroethylene (131) and ketamine (132), which are reported to elevate the ocular pressure. In two situations, the physician must be particularly concerned about alterations in IOP during general anesthesia.

In *infants* and *children* who are examined under anesthesia for suspicion of congenital glaucoma, the main concern is to avoid the artificial reduction of IOP, as discussed earlier in this chapter, which could mask a pathologic pressure elevation. In one study, the mean IOP for children measured under halothane anesthesia was 7.8 ± 0.4 mm Hg at age 1 year, with a gradual increase of about 1 mm Hg per year of age to 11.7 ± 0.6 mm Hg at age 5 years (17). However other studies showed no significant difference from pressures recorded in newborns and infants using only topical anesthesia (133, 134). Hypnotics that are used to produce unconsciousness, such as 4-hydroxybutyrate, are also reported to reduce the IOP (135), and barbiturates and tranquilizers may, in some cases, cause a transient pressure reduction (136). High-dose oral chloral hydrate sedation (100 mg/kg for the first 10 kg and then 50 mg/kg) did not significantly alter the IOP in children under 6 years of age, as compared to measurements in the same children without sedation (137).

When operating on an *open eye,* as following penetrating injury or during intraocular surgery, the primary concern is to avoid sudden elevations of IOP that might lead to extrusion of ocular contents. Depolarizing muscle relaxants, such as succinylcholine (138) and suxamethonium (139), cause a transient rise in IOP possibly due to a combination of extraocular muscle contraction and intraocular vasodilation. Pretreatment with nondepolarizing muscle relaxants, such as D-tubocurarine and gallamine (138, 139), or with a subparalytic dose of succinylcholine prior to the full paralyzing dose (140) has not been proven to prevent IOP elevation during endotracheal intubation. However, pretreatment with diazepam (141), fazadinium (142), or atracurium (143) has been reported to eliminate the risk of IOP elevation. It has also been suggested that intramuscular succinylcholine will cause less IOP rise than intravenous (144). Tracheal intubation may also cause an IOP rise, and neither intravenous lignocaine (147) nor atracurium (143) have been found to prevent this.

Elevated pCO_2 causes a rise in IOP (148, 149), while reduced pCO_2 (150) or increased concentration of O_2 (151) is associated with an IOP reduction. Rabbit studies suggest that the latter phenomenon may be due to a decrease in episcleral venous pressure (152).

Foods and Drugs

The following drugs and other substances have been studied for their effect on the IOP. This list is exclusive of antiglaucoma drugs, which are discussed in Section Three.

Alcohol has been shown to lower the IOP, although more so in patients with glaucoma (153). In another study, populations of individuals who abstained from liquor had a higher prevalence of ocular hypertensives than those who drank liquor on a daily basis (15). The pressure reduction is not associated with a change in facility of aqueous outflow (153), and it has been suggested that the mechanism may be a combination of suppressed circulating antidiuretic hormone, leading to a reduction of net water movement into the eye, and direct inhibition of aqueous secretion (154).

Caffeine may cause a slight, transient rise in IOP, although in the levels associated with customary coffee drinking, this does not appear to cause a significant, sustained pressure elevation (136, 155). The effect does not appear to be related to aqueous flow (156). Herbal tea caused significantly less pressure rise than regular coffee in glaucoma patients (155).

A fat free diet has been shown to reduce IOP, which may be related to a concomitant reduction in plasma prostaglandin levels (157).

Tobacco smoking may cause a transient rise in the IOP (158), although another study revealed no association of cigarette-smoking history with open-angle glaucoma or ocular hypertension (159).

Heroin and *marijuana* lower the IOP (the latter is discussed further in Section Three), while *LSD* causes an IOP elevation (160). *Corticosteroids* may also cause IOP elevation and are discussed in detail in Section Two.

Systemic *vasodilators,* including glyceryl trinitrate (nitroglycerine) (161, 162), pentaerythritol tetranitrate (161), isosorbide dinitrate (162), becyclan (162), nicotinic acid (163), and cyclandelate (163), are all reported to have no influence on IOP in normal or glaucomatous eyes with open angles. However, one study revealed that nitroglycerin, when administered by perfusion techniques, and isosorbide dinitrate lower the IOP in normal individuals as well as in patients with open-angle or angle-closure glaucoma (164). A systemic digitalis preparation, β-methyldigoxin, has also been shown to cause a decrease in IOP (165).

Systemic *anticholinergics,* such as atropine (166, 167), propantheline (168), and pizotifen (169) have been found to have no influence on IOP in normal or glaucomatous eyes with open anterior chamber angles, especially with short-term therapy. However, topical cyclopentolate will elevate the IOP in some patients with open-angle glaucoma (166, 170), and it has been suggested that these patients may also manifest a slight pressure rise in response to long-term administration of systemic anticholinergics (167). Scopolamine dermal patches were found to have no significant IOP effect in open-angle glaucoma patients (171). Drugs that may precipitate angle-closure attacks of glaucoma are discussed in Section Two.

Anticonvulsants, e.g, diphenylhydantoin (136), amphetamines, e.g, dextroamphetamines (136), and antihistamines, e.g, cimetidine, a histamine-2 receptor antagonist (172), have not been found to influence the IOP in eyes with open angles.

Prostaglandins, when administered topically, may either increase or decrease IOP, depending on the dosage used, which is discussed further in Section Three. In women undergoing prostaglandin-induced abortion, no significant effect on IOP was observed (173).

TONOMETERS AND TONOMETRY[a]

Classification of Tonometers

All clinical tonometers measure the IOP by relating a deformation of the globe to the force responsible for the deformation. The two basic types of tonometers differ according to the shape of the deformation: indentation and applanation (flattening).

Indentation Tonometers

The shape of the deformation with this type of tonometer is a truncated cone (Fig. 4.2**A**). The precise shape, however, is variable and unpredictable. In addition, these instruments displace a relatively large intraocular volume. As a result of these characteristics, conversion tables based on empirical data from in vitro and in vivo studies must be used to estimate the IOP. The prototype of this group is the Schiøtz tonometer, which was introduced in 1905.

[a]Refer to Shields, MB: Color Atlas of Glaucoma. Baltimore, Williams & Wilkins, 1998, Plates I7–9.

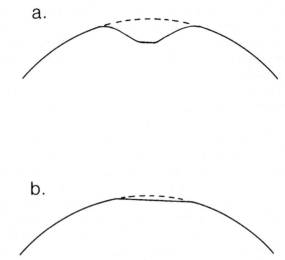

Figure 4.2. Corneal deformation created by (**A**) indentation tonometers (a truncated cone) and (**B**) applanation tonometers (simple flattening).

Applanation Tonometers

The shape of the deformation with these tonometers is a simple flattening (Fig. 4.2**B**), and, because the shape is constant, its relationship to the IOP can, in most cases, be derived from mathematical calculations. The applanation tonometers are further differentiated on the basis of the variable that is measured.

VARIABLE FORCE. This type of tonometer measures the force that is required to applanate (flatten) a standard area of the corneal surface. The prototype is the *Goldmann* applanation tonometer, which was introduced in 1954.

VARIABLE AREA. Other applanation tonometers measure the area of the cornea that is flattened by a known force (weight). The prototype in this group is the *Maklakov* tonometer, which was introduced in 1885. The division between indentation and applanation tonometers, however, does not correlate entirely with the magnitude of intraocular volume displacement. In the case of Maklakov-type tonometers, the volume displacement is sufficiently large to require the use of conversion tables.

Noncontact Tonometer

A third type of tonometer uses a puff of air to deform the cornea and measures either the time or force of the air puff that is required to create a standard amount of corneal deformation. The prototype was introduced by *Grolman* in 1972.

We will first consider the descriptions and techniques of these various tonometers, and then compare their relative values and limitations.

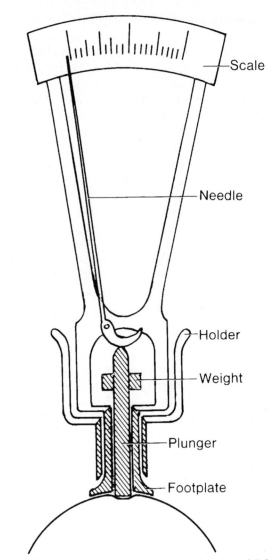

Figure 4.3. Cut-away view showing basic features of Schiøtz-type indentation tonometer.

Schiøtz Indentation Tonometry

Description of Tonometer

The body of the tonometer has a footplate, which rests on the cornea. A plunger moves freely (except for the effect of friction) within a shaft in the footplate, and the degree to which it indents the cornea is indicated by the movement of a needle on a scale. A 5.5-gram weight is permanently fixed to the plunger, which can be increased to 7.5, 10, or 15 grams by adding additional weights (Fig. 4.3).

Basic Concept of Indentation Tonometry

When the plunger indents the cornea, the baseline or resting pressure (P_o) is artificially raised to a new value (P_t). Since the tonometer actually measures P_t, it is necessary to estimate

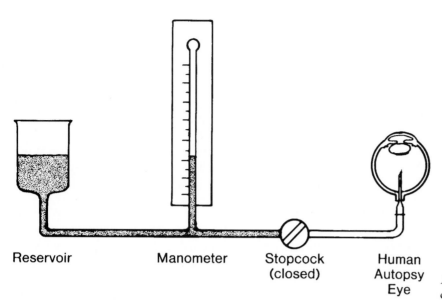

Reservoir Manometer Stopcock (closed) Human Autopsy Eye

Figure 4.4. Apparatus used in manometric calibration of Schiøtz tonometer.

P_o for each scale reading and weight. Schiøtz estimated P_o by experiments in which a manometer was attached to enucleated eyes by a cannula inserted through the optic nerve. A stopcock was placed between the cannula and manometer, and a reservoir was used to adjust the pressure in the eye (Fig. 4.4). He then made two sets of readings. In one set (open manometer), the stopcock was left open when the tonometer was placed on the cornea, which allowed correlation of P_t with the scale reading and weight. In the second set (closed manometer), the desired pressure was introduced in the eye and the stopcock was closed before placing the tonometer on the cornea, thereby allowing correlation of P_o with the scale reading and weight. It was the data from these sets of readings that were used to calibrate the tonometer.

The change in pressure from P_o to P_t is an expression of the resistance an eye offers to the displacement of a volume of fluid (V_c). In the early days of indentation tonometry, the IOP values that were considered to be normal were considerably higher than today's accepted range, and it was not until Friedenwald's work, beginning in the late 1930s, that indentation tonometry acquired a mathematical basis. Friedenwald (174) developed an empirical formula for the linear relationship between the logarithm of the pressure and the volume change in a given eye. The formula has a single numerical constant, the *coefficient of ocular rigidity (K)*, which is roughly an expression of the distensibility of the eye. He developed a nomogram for estimating K based on two tonometric readings with different weights, and subsequent studies using applanation tonometry with different sized applanating areas have supported the accuracy of his formulations (175). Based on this formula and additional experiments, Friedenwald (176) calculated an average K of 0.0245 and used this to develop a set of conversion tables, referred to as the 1948 tables. He later revised the average K to a value of 0.0215 (177), on which he based a new set of tables that became known as the 1955 tables (178). Subse-

quent studies, however, indicate that the 1948 tables agree more closely with measurements by Goldmann applanation tonometry (179, 180).

Technique of Schiøtz Indentation Tonometry

With the patient in a supine position and fixing on a target just overhead, the examiner separates the eyelids and gently rests the tonometer footplate on the anesthetized cornea in a position that allows free vertical movement of the plunger (Fig. 4.5). When the tonometer is properly positioned, the examiner will observe a fine movement of the indicator needle on the scale in response to the ocular pulsations. The scale reading should be taken as the average between the extremes of these excursions. It is customary to start with the fixed 5.5-gram weight. However, if the scale reading is 4 or less, additional weight should be added to the plunger. A conversion table is then used to derive the IOP in millimeters of mercury (mm Hg) from the scale reading and plunger weight. The scale reading, weight, IOP, and conversion table from which the pressure value was derived should all be recorded. For example, a scale reading of 7, using a 5.5-gram weight, which corresponds to an IOP of 12 mm Hg according to the 1955 conversion tables, would be written as *7/5.5 = 12 mm Hg ('55).*

Sources of Error with Indentation Tonometry

The accuracy of indentation tonometry depends on the assumption that all eyes respond the same to the external force of indentation, which is not the case. The following are some of the more common variables that introduce potential for error.

OCULAR RIGIDITY. Since conversion tables are based on an "average" coefficient of ocular rigidity (K), eyes that deviate significantly from this K value will give false IOP measurements. A high K will cause a falsely high IOP, while a low K will lead to a falsely low reading. Factors that have been associated with abnormally *high ocular rigidity* include high hyperopia (181), extreme myopia (174), long-standing glaucoma (174), age-related macular degeneration (182), and vasoconstrictor therapy (174). Conditions associated with a *reduction in K* include high myopia (181), elevated IOP (183) (which may explain the lower K values during water provocative testing), osteogenesis imperfecta (184), miotic therapy, especially with cholinesterase inhibitors (181), vasodilator therapy (174), and retinal detachment surgery utilizing cryopexy (185), scleral buckling (186, 187), vitrectomy (187), or intravitreal injection of a compressible gas (186–188). Keratoconus was once thought to be associated with an abnormally low K, but this may be an artifact due to the thin cornea, since it is not seen after keratoplasty for this condition (189). Reports on the relationship of age to ocular rigidity are conflicting (174, 181, 190).

The technique for determining K is based on the concept of differential tonometry, using two indentation tonometric readings with different weights and Friedenwald's nomo-

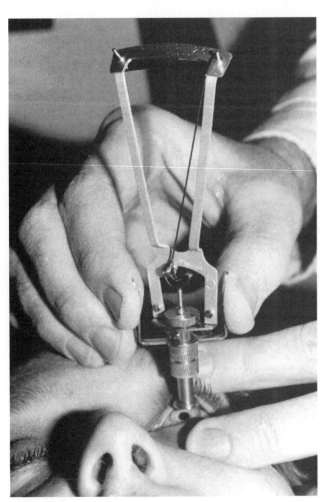

Figure 4.5. Technique of indentation tonometry with Schiøtz tonometer.

gram as previously discussed (174). It may be more accurate, however, to obtain one reading with a Schiøtz tonometer using a 10-gram weight and the second with an applanation tonometer and to plot these readings on Friedenwald's nomogram (191). Chandler and Grant (192) suggested that the estimation of ocular rigidity by any method is premature and of little value until more accurate calibrations are achieved. Attempts to more accurately represent the pressure-volume relationship of the corneoscleral coat over a wide range have included a single-parameter ocular rigidity function in which the proportionality constant K is insensitive to changes in IOP (193).

BLOOD VOLUME ALTERATION. The variable expulsion of intraocular blood during indentation tonometry may also influence the IOP measurement (194).

CORNEAL INFLUENCES. Either a steeper or thicker cornea will cause a greater displacement of fluid during indentation tonometry, which leads to a falsely high IOP reading (176).

MOSES EFFECT. The Moses effect on indentation tonometry was discussed under "Tonography" in Chapter 3.

Electronic Indentation Tonometers

Grant combined the concept of Schiøtz tonometry with continuous electronic monitoring of the pressure for use in tonography (discussed in Chapter 3), and similar instruments were subsequently designed, although none are commonly used at this time.

Goldmann Applanation Tonometry

Basic Concept

Goldmann based his concept of tonometry on a modification of the *Maklakov-Fick Law* (also referred to as the *Imbert-Fick Law*) (195, 196). This law states that an external force *(W)* against a sphere equals the pressure in the sphere *(P_t)* times the area flattened (applanated) by the external force *(A)* (Fig. 4.6A):

$$W = P_t \times A$$

The validity of the law requires that the sphere is (a) perfectly spherical, (b) dry, (c) perfectly flexible, and (d) infinitely thin. The cornea fails to satisfy any of these requirements, since it is aspherical and wet, and neither perfectly flexible, nor infinitely thin. The moisture creates a surface tension *(S)*, while the lack of flexibility requires a force to bend the cornea *(B)*, which is independent of the internal pressure. In addition, since the cornea has a central thickness of approximately 0.55 mm, the outer area of flattening *(A)* is not the same as the inner area (A_1). It was, therefore, necessary to modify the Imbert-Fick Law in the following

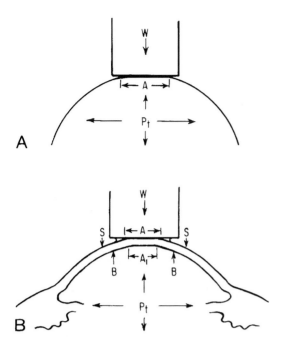

Figure 4.6. **A.** The Imbert-Fick Law ($W = P_t \times A$). **B.** Modification of Imbert-Fick Law for the cornea ($W + S = P_t \times A_1 + B$).

manner to account for these characteristics of the cornea (Fig. 4.6B):

$$W + S = P_t A_1 + B$$

When $A_1 = 7.35$ mm², S balances B and $W = P_t$. This internal area of applanation is obtained when the diameter of the external area of corneal applanation is 3.06 mm, which is used in the standard instrument. An external diameter of 3.53 mm has been reported to be equally acceptable (197). The volume displacement produced by applanating an area with a diameter of 3.06 mm is approximately 0.50 mm³, so that P_t is very close to P_o, and ocular rigidity does not significantly influence the measurement.

Description of Tonometer (198)

The instrument is mounted on a standard slitlamp in such a way that the examiner's view is directed through the center of a plastic biprism, which is used to applanate the cornea. Two beam-splitting prisms within the applanating unit optically convert the circular area of corneal contact into semicircles. The prisms are adjusted so that the inner margins of the semicircles overlap when 3.06 mm of cornea is applanated. In a variation of this design, the prisms are located near the slitlamp objective and the image is doubled and then displaced (199). The biprism is attached by a rod to a housing, which contains a coil spring and series of levers that are used to adjust the force of the biprism against the cornea (Fig. 4.7).

Technique

The cornea is anesthetized with a topical preparation, and the tear film is stained with sodium fluorescein. With the cornea and biprism illuminated by a cobalt blue light from the slitlamp, the biprism is brought into gentle contact with the apex of the cornea (Fig. 4.8). The fluorescence of the stained tears facilitates visualization of the tear meniscus at the margin of contact between cornea and biprism. The fluorescent semicircles are viewed through the biprism, and the force against the cornea is adjusted until the inner edges overlap (Fig. 4.9). As with the indentation tonometer, the influence of the ocular pulsations is seen when the instrument is properly positioned, and the excursions must be averaged to give the desired endpoint. The IOP is then read directly from a scale on the tonometer housing.

The staining of the tear film may be accomplished by instilling a drop of topical anesthetic and touching a fluorescein-impregnated paper strip to the tears in the lower cul-de-sac. However, a 0.25% solution of sodium fluorescein has been shown to produce the optimum fluorescent semicircles (200), and commercial solutions are available in combination with topical anesthetics (201). Studies have shown that the preservative in these commercial preparations imparts a satisfactory degree of resistance to bacterial contamination, especially when a pipette-type dispenser is used (201–205). However, the cap of a squeeze bottle may be a reservoir for bacterial contamination (203), and all commercial preparations do not appear to impart the same degree of resistance to bacterial contamination. When contaminated with *Pseudomonas* or *Staphylococcus*, a fluorescein preparation with the anesthetic, benoxinate, and the preservative, chlorobutanol (Fluress), regained sterility in the solution in 1 minute and on the dropper tip in 5 minutes, while preparations with proparacaine and thimerosal took at least 1 hour (204). The former preparation also performed as well as proparacaine with benzalkonium chloride and a fluorescein paper strip in the same experiment (205). Some physicians have felt that Goldmann applanation tonometry could be performed without fluorescein, but this has been shown to give a significant underestimation of the IOP and is not recommended (206).

Sources of Error with Goldmann Tonometry

SEMICIRCLES. The width of the meniscus may influence the reading slightly, with wider menisci causing falsely higher pressure estimates (196). Improper vertical alignment (one semicircle larger than the other) will also lead to a falsely high IOP estimate (Fig. 4.9) (198).

CORNEAL VARIABLES. The thickness of the cornea has been shown to influence the pressure estimate, with thin corneas producing falsely low readings (207). A thick cornea causes a falsely high measurement if the thickness is due to increased collagen fibrils (207, 208), whereas low readings occur if the thickness is due to edema (207). Corneal curvature has also been shown to influence IOP measurements, with an increase of approximately 1 mm Hg for each 3 diopters of increase in corneal power (209). Marked corneal astigmatism will produce an elliptical area of corneal contact. When the biprism is in the usual orientation, with the mires displaced horizontally, the IOP will be underestimated for with-the-rule and overestimated for against-the-rule astigmatism, with approximately 1 mm Hg of error for every 4 diopters of astigmatism (210). To minimize this error, the biprism may be rotated until the dividing line between the prisms is 45% to the major axis of the ellipse (198), or an average may be taken of horizontal and vertical readings (209). An irregular cornea will also distort the semicircles and interfere with the accuracy of the IOP estimates (198).

PROLONGED CONTACT. Prolonged contact of the biprism with the cornea leads to corneal injury, as manifested by staining, which makes multiple readings unsatisfactory (198). In addition, prolonged contact causes a decrease in IOP over a period of minutes, which is less pronounced in eyes with carotid occlusive disease, suggesting that it may be related to intraocular blood (211).

CALIBRATION. It is also essential that the Goldmann tonometer be calibrated periodically. Instructions for quick, simple calibration come with the instrument, and this should be performed at least monthly. If the tonometer does not meet calibration specifications, it should be returned to the manufacturer or distributor for correction.

Disinfection of Goldmann (and Other) Tonometers

With all tonometers, especially those that contact the eye, there is the risk of transmitting infection, such as the adenovirus of epidemic keratoconjunctivitis (EKC) and herpes simplex virus type 1. In addition, there is the potential for transmitting more serious diseases, such as hepatitis and acquired immunodeficiency syndrome (AIDS). Hepatitis B virus (HBV) surface antigen DNA polymerase and hepatitis B virus DNA have been found in the tears of a high percentage of hepatitis B carriers (212, 213), and the antigen was detected on the tonometer tip in one-fourth of the patients in one series (212). Human T-cell lymphotropic virus type III (HTLV-III), the causative agent of AIDS, has been isolated from the tears in 5 of 16 patients with AIDS or AIDS-related

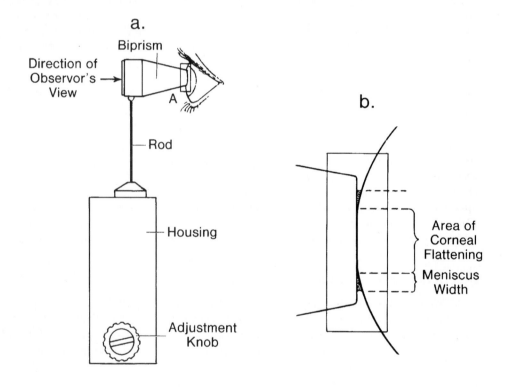

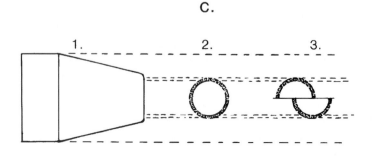

Figure 4.7. Goldmann-type applanation tonometry. **A.** Basic features of tonometer, shown in contact with patient's cornea. **B.** Enlargement shows tear film meniscus created by contact of biprism and cornea. **C.** View through biprism (*1*) reveals circular meniscus (*2*), which is converted into semicircles (*3*) by prisms.

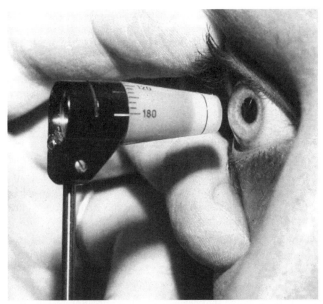

Figure 4.8. Technique of applanation tonometry with Goldmann tonometer.

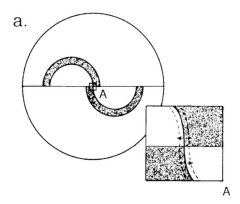

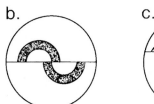

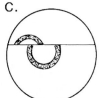

Figure 4.9. Semicircles of Goldmann-type applanation tonometry. **A.** Proper width and position. Enlargement (A) depicts excursions of semicircles caused by ocular pulsations. **B.** Semicircles are too wide. **C.** Improper vertical and horizontal alignment.

complex (214, 215). Although there is no evidence to suggest transmission of HTLV-III by contact with tears, precautions are needed to minimize this possibility, as well as the spread of other microbial pathogens that might be present in tears.

A variety of techniques has been described for disinfecting tonometer tips. Adenovirus type 8 was removed or inactivated by soaking the applanation tip for 5–15 minutes in diluted sodium hypochlorite (1:10 household bleach), 3% hydrogen peroxide, or 70% isopropyl alcohol, or by wiping with alcohol, hydrogen peroxide, iodophor (providone-iodine), 1:1000 merthiolate, or dry tissues (216, 217). Herpes simplex virus type 1 was eliminated by swabbing the applanation tonometer head with 70% isopropyl alcohol (218). Ten minutes of continuous rinsing in running tap water was reported to remove all detectable HBV surface antigen from contaminated tonometers (212), although another study showed that soap and water wash was the only disinfection method that removed all HBV DNA (219). Wiping with 3% hydrogen peroxide or 70% isopropyl alcohol swabs completely disinfected tonometer tips contaminated with the human immunodeficiency virus type 1 of AIDS (220). Other techniques for preventing spread of infection include disposable film covers for applanation tips (221, 222) and sterilization by exposure to ultraviolet light (223). A disinfectant receptacle has also been described for applanation tonometer heads utilizing a plastic Petri dish with 11-mm holes in the cover (224).

In August 1988, a Clinical Alert was issued jointly by the American Academy of Ophthalmology, the National Society to Prevent Blindness, and the Contact Lens Association of Ophthalmologists, with updated recommendations for ophthalmic practice in relation to AIDS and other infectious diseases (225). Wiping with an alcohol sponge was felt to be an adequate disinfection procedure for Goldmann-type

applanation tips, as well as Schiøtz tonometers, digital pneumotonometers, and noncontact tonometers. Alternative measures for disinfecting applanation tips, as previously recommended by the Centers for Disease Control (226), involve soaking in 1:10 household bleach, 3% hydrogen peroxide, or 70% isopropyl alcohol for 5 minutes. With any technique, it is important to carefully remove the disinfectant from the contact surface before the next use since both alcohol (227) and hydrogen peroxide (228) have been shown to cause transient corneal defects.

OTHER APPLANATION TONOMETERS WITH VARIABLE FORCE

Hand-held Goldmann-type Tonometers

PERKINS APPLANATION TONOMETER (229). This instrument utilizes the same biprism as the Goldmann applanation tonometer. The light source is powered by a battery and the force is varied manually. A counterbalance makes it possible to use the instrument in either the vertical or horizontal position (Fig. 4.10).

DRAEGER APPLANATION TONOMETER. This instrument is similar to the Perkins tonometer, but utilizes a different biprism and has an electric motor which varies the force (230, 231).

Mackay-Marg Tonometer

Although the original instrument is no longer available, newer models have been developed that utilize the same basic principle. We first consider the original unit and then the newer Mackay-Marg-type tonometers.

BASIC CONCEPT (232). The force measured is that which is required to keep the flat plate of a plunger flush with a surrounding sleeve against the pressure of corneal deformation. The effect of corneal rigidity, i.e, the force required to bend the cornea, is transferred to the sleeve, so the plate reads only the IOP.

DESCRIPTION OF INSTRUMENT (233). The plate has a diameter of 1.5 mm and is surrounded by a rubber sleeve. The force required to keep the plate flush with the sleeve is electronically monitored and recorded on a paper strip.

TECHNIQUE (233). As the instrument tip momentarily touches the cornea, the tracing (representing the force required to keep the plate flush with the sleeve) rises until the applanated area reaches a diameter of 1.5 mm. At this point (the crest), the pressure against the plate represents the IOP plus the force required to bend the cornea. The tracing then falls as the effect of corneal rigidity is transferred to the surrounding sleeve. When a corneal diameter of 3 mm is flattened (the initial trough), the plate is considered to be reading only the IOP. The tracing then rises due to artificial elevation of the IOP (Fig. 4.11). Since the tonometer records IOP instantaneously, several readings

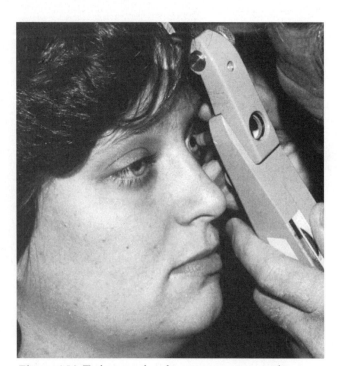

Figure 4.10. Technique of applanation tonometry with Perkins tonometer.

should be averaged to compensate for fluctuations due to ocular pulsation.

Mackay-Marg-Type Tonometers

The newer models differ from the Mackay-Marg tonometer in having an internal logic program that automatically selects the acceptable measurements and rejects the inappropriate ones. Three or more good IOP readings are averaged and displayed on a digital readout. Among those that have been clinically evaluated are the *CAT 100* applanation tonometer (234), the *Challenger* digital electronic applanation tonometer (outcome of the redesigned EMT-20) (235), and the *Biotronics* tonometer (236). None of these has yet been shown to be sufficiently accurate for clinical use.

TONO-PEN. This hand-held Mackay-Marg-type tonometer has a strain gauge that creates an electrical signal as the foot plate flattens the cornea (Fig. 4.12) (237). A built-in single chip microprocessor senses the proper force curves and averages 4–10 readings to give a final digital readout. It also provides the percentage of variability between the lowest and highest acceptable readings from 5–20%. A similar instrument, the ProTon tonometer utilizes the same basic Mackay-Marg principle, but differs from the Tono-Pen in that the probe and display unit are separated (238). The Tono-Pen has had the most extensive clinical evaluation of any Mackay-Marg-type tonometer although the reported results have been conflicting (these are discussed later in the chapter under "Comparison of Tonometers").

Pneumatic Tonometers (Pneumotonometer) (239, 240)

BASIC CONCEPT. The concept of this tonometer is similar to that of the Mackay-Marg in that a central sensing device measures the IOP, while the force required to bend the cornea is transferred to a surrounding structure. The sensor in this case, however, is air pressure, rather than an electronically controlled plunger.

DESCRIPTION OF INSTRUMENT. At one end of a pencil-like holder is a sensing nozzle, which has a 0.25-inch outer diameter and a 2.0-mm central chamber. The nozzle is covered with a silastic diaphragm, and pressurized air in the central chamber exhausts at the face of the nozzle between the orifice of the central chamber and the diaphragm. The air pressure is dependent on the resistance to the exhaust, and a pneumatic-to-electronic transducer converts the air pressure to a recording on a paper strip.

TECHNIQUE. As the sensing nozzle touches the cornea, the tracing rises as an increasing area of corneal surface comes in contract with the diaphragm (Fig. 4.13). When the area of

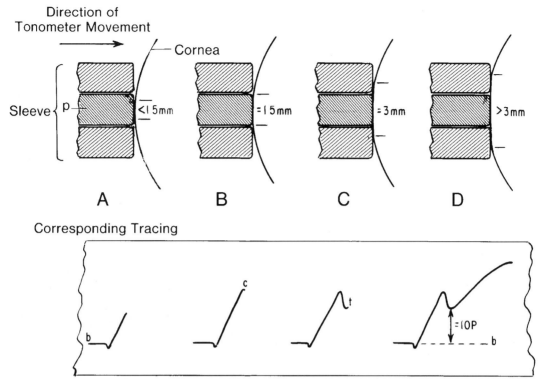

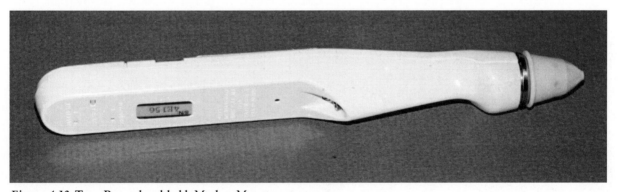

Figure 4.11. Mackay-Marg tonometry (modified from Marg, E, Mackay, RS, Oechsli, R: Trough height, pressure and flattening in tonometry. Vision Res 1:379, 1962). **A.** As plate *(p)* contacts cornea, tracing begins to rise. **B.** Crest *(c)* is reached when diameter of contact equals that of plate surface (1.5 mm). **C.** With further corneal flattening, force of bending cornea is transferred to sleeve, and tracing falls to trough *(t)* when diameter of contact equals 3 mm. **D.** Still further corneal flattening leads to artificial elevation of intraocular pressure *(IOP)*. Distance from baseline *(b)* of tracing to trough is read as the IOP.

Figure 4.12. Tono-Pen; a hand-held, Mackay-Marg-type tonometer.

contact equals that of the central chamber, an initial inflection is recorded, which represents the IOP and the force required to bend the cornea. With further enlargement of the corneal contact, the bending force is transferred to the face of the nozzle and the tracing falls to a trough, which is interpreted as the actual IOP. Still further contact leads to artificial pressure elevation and a second inflection (Fig. 4.14). The instrument can also be used for continuous IOP monitoring. As with applanation tonometers, sterile, single-use, latex covers can be placed over the pneumotonometer tip to avoid conta-

mination between patients, and one study showed that they did not significantly influence the pressure reading (241).

Maklakov Applanation Tonometry

Basic Concept

Maklakov introduced the concept in which IOP is estimated by measuring the area of cornea that is flattened by a known weight (242). It is still popular in Russia.

Instrument and Technique (242, 243)

A dumbbell-shaped metal cylinder has flat endplates of polished glass on either end with diameters of 10 mm. A set of four such instruments are available, weighing 5, 7.5, 10, and 15 grams, and a cross-action wire handle is supplied to support the instrument on the cornea. A layer of dye (a suspension of argyrol, glycerin, and water) is applied to either endplate and, with the patient in a supine position and the cornea anesthetized, the instrument is allowed to rest vertically on the cornea for 1 second. This produces a circular white imprint on the endplate, which corresponds to the area of cornea that was flattened. The diameter of the white area is measured with a transparent plastic measuring scale to 0.1 mm, and the IOP is read from a conversion table in the column corresponding to the weight used.

Conversion Tables

Although the volume displacement with Maklakov-type applanation tonometry is less than with indentation

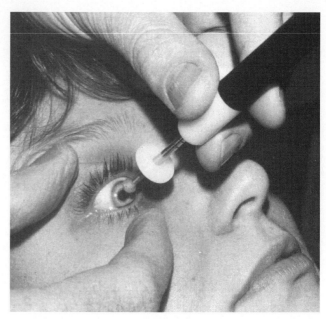

Figure 4.13. Technique of tonometry with the Pneumotonometer.

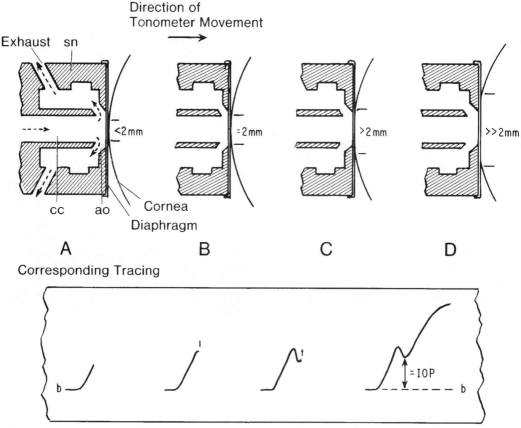

Figure 4.14. Pneumatic tonometry (modified from Durham, DG, Bigliano, RP, Masino, JA: Pneumatic applanation tonometer. Trans Am Acad Ophthalmol Otol 69:1029, 1965). **A.** As sensing nozzle (*sn*) touches cornea, resistance to air flow (*dotted lines*) begins to increase at annular opening (*ao*), with corresponding rise in tracing. **B.** When diameter of corneal contact equals 2 mm, an initial inflection (*i*) is recorded. **C.** With further corneal flattening, force of bending cornea is transferred to face of sensor, and air pressure in central chamber (*cc*) measures IOP, represented by distance from baseline (*b*) to trough (*t*) of tracing. **D.** Further corneal compression by tonometer leads to artificial IOP rise.

Table 4.2.

APPLANATION TONOMETERS WITH VARIABLE AREA

Tonometer	Description/Use
1. Maklakov-Kalfa (242)	1. Prototype
2. Applanometer (246)	2. Ceramic endplates
3. Tonomat (247)	3. Disposable endplates
4. Halberg tonometer (248)	4. Transparent endplate for direct reading: multiple weights
5. Barraquer tonometer (249)	5. Plastic tonometer for use in operating room
6. Ocular Tension Indicator (250)	6. Utilizes Goldmann biprism and standard weight, for screening (measures above or below 21 mm Hg)
7. GlaucoTest (251)	7. Screening tonometer with multiple endplates for selecting different "cutoff" pressures

tonometry, it is large enough that ocular rigidity must be considered in computing the IOP. Kalfa recognized this problem at approximately the same time that Friedenwald was applying the concept of ocular rigidity to Schiøtz tonometry (244). He, too, used different weights to estimate the average ocular rigidity of the eyeball, which he called an "elastometric rise." New conversion tables have been developed which provide nomograms for the differential tonometry (245).

Other Maklakov-type tonometers are listed in Table 4.2 (242, 246–251).

Noncontact Tonometer

The noncontact tonometer (NCT) was introduced by Grolman (252) and has the unique advantage over other tonometers of not touching the eye, other than with a puff of air. This instrument should not be confused with the pneumatic tonometers previously discussed.

Basic Concept

A puff of room air creates a constant force, which momentarily deforms the cornea. It is difficult to determine the exact nature of the corneal deformation, although it is postulated that the central cornea is flattened at the moment the pressure measurement is made. The time from an internal reference point to the moment of presumed flattening is measured and converted to IOP based on prior comparisons with readings from Goldmann applanation tonometers.

Description of Instrument (252–254)

The original NCT is mounted on a table and consists of three subsystems: (a) an alignment system allows the operator to optically align the patient's cornea in three dimensions (axial, vertical, and lateral); (b) an optoelectronic applanation monitoring system consists of a transmitter, which directs a collimated beam of light at the corneal vertex, and a receiver and detector, which accepts only parallel, coaxial rays reflected from the cornea; and (c) a pneumatic system generates a puff of room air, which is directed against the cornea. A newer, hand-held NCT, the *Pulsair* tonometer, is also commercially available (255, 256).

Technique (252–254)

The patient observes an internal target while the operator aligns the cornea by superimposing a reflection of the target from the patients cornea on a stationary ring (Fig. 4.15). During this time, light from the transmitter is reflected from the undisturbed cornea, which allows only a small number of rays to enter the receiver. When the cornea is properly aligned, the operator depresses a trigger which causes a puff of air to be directed against the cornea. At the moment that the central cornea is flattened, the greatest number of reflected light rays are received, which is recorded as the peak intensity of light detected. The time from an internal reference point to the moment of maximum light detection is converted to IOP and displayed on a digital readout. In a subsequent version of the table-mounted NCT, the *X-Pert NCT*, the air puff is automatically triggered when alignment criteria are satisfied and the force of air to achieve peak light detection is the measured variable (Fig. 4.16).

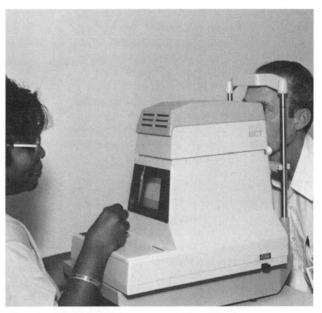

Figure 4.15. The X-Pert noncontact tonometer.

The time interval for an average NCT measurement is 1–3 milliseconds (1/500 of the cardiac cycle) and is random with respect to the phase of the cardiac cycle so that the ocular pulse becomes a significant variable, i.e., it cannot be averaged as with some tonometers. Furthermore, glaucomatous eyes have a significantly greater range of momentary fluctuations in IOP (257). The probability that an instantaneous pressure measurement will lie within a given range of mean IOP increases as the number of tonometric measurements, averaged together, increases (258). For this reason, it is recommended that a minimum of three readings within 3 mm Hg be taken and averaged as the IOP.

Miscellaneous Tonometers

Continuous IOP Monitoring Devices

In the diagnosis and management of glaucoma, there is need for a tonometer that can continuously monitor the IOP for hours, days, or indefinitely without artificially altering the pressure. Preliminary laboratory studies have investigated the feasibility of remote IOP monitoring with telemetric devices. Strain gauges can be used to drive the monitor. The strain gauge can be placed in a contact lens to measure changes in the meridional angle of the corneoscleral junc-

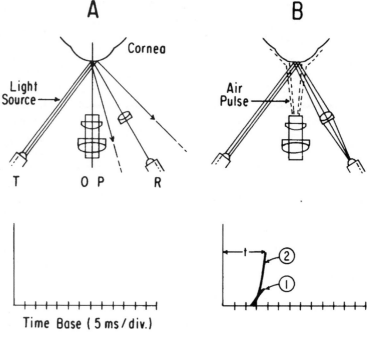

Figure 4.16. Noncontact tonometry (modified from Grolman, B: A new tonometer system. Am J Optom & Arch Am Acad Optom 49:646, 1972). **A.** Light source from transmitter (T) is reflected from undisturbed cornea toward receiver (R), while cornea is aligned by optical system (O). **B.** Air puff (1) from pneumatic system (P) deforms cornea, which increases the number of light rays (2) received and detected by R. Time (t) from internal reference point to moment of maximum light detection (which presumably corresponds to applanation of the cornea) is converted to IOP (based on calibrations with Goldmann applanation tonometer) and displayed on digital readout. **C.** Continued air pulse produces momentary concavity of cornea, causing sharp reduction in light rays received by R. **D.** As cornea returns to undisturbed state, a second moment of applanation causes another light peak (3). (Reprinted from Shields, MB: The non-contact tonometer. Its value and limitations. Surv Ophthalmol 24:211, 1980, by permission.)

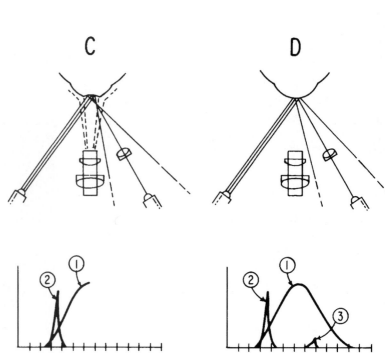

tion (259), or it can be embedded in an encircling scleral band to measure the distention of the globe (260). Another approach is to use a scleral applanating device attached to a passive radio telemetric pressure transducer (261, 262). An instrument with applanating suction cups has also been devised, which allows bilateral recoding of IOP for up to 1 hour in supine subjects (263).

HOME TONOMETRY. Another approach to obtaining multiple IOP measurements at various times of day and night (aside from admission to the hospital for tonometry by a physician, nurse, or technician), is to have the measurements made at home. This has been done by teaching a family member to perform Schiøtz tonometry on their relative, although the accuracy of the results are highly variable. A new device, the *self-tonometer,* which utilizes the applanation principle and can be used by the patient without assistance, has shown promise in preliminary studies (42–45, 264, 265).

Attempts have also been made to estimate the IOP by measuring the duration of contact of a spring driven hammer with the eye (impact tonometer) (266), or the frequency of a vibrating probe in contact with the cornea (Vibra-Tonometer) (267).

Comparison of Tonometers

Comparison with Goldmann Tonometer in Eyes with Regular Corneas

The most precise method for evaluating the accuracy of a tonometer is to compare it with manometric measurements of the cannulated anterior chamber. While this technique is frequently used with animal and autopsy eyes, it has obvious limitations in large scale human studies. The alternative is to compare the tonometer in question against the instrument which previous studies have shown to be the most accurate. In eyes with regular corneas, the Goldmann applanation tonometer is generally accepted as the standard against which other tonometers must be compared. Even with this instrument, however, inherent variability must be taken into account. When two readings were taken on the same eye with Goldmann tonometers within a short time frame, using either one instrument and one examiner (268), or two instruments and two examiners (269), at least 30% of the paired readings differed by 2 and 3 mm Hg or more, respectively. In another study, intraobserver variation was 1.5 ± 1.96 mm Hg and interobserver variation was 1.79 ± 2.41 mm Hg, which could be reduced 9% and 11%, respectively, by using the median value of three consecutive measurements (270).

SCHIØTZ TONOMETER. Studies consistently indicate that the Schiøtz tonometer reads lower than the Goldmann (271–273), even when the postural influence on IOP is eliminated by performing both measurements in the supine posi-

tion (176, 274, 275). In one study, age was found to be the most important source of variation, with the greatest discrepancies occurring in the 50s and 60s (276). The magnitude of disagreement between the two tonometers and the influence of ocular rigidity are such that the Schiøtz tonometer is felt to indicate only that the IOP is within a certain range (176) and is of limited value even for screening purposes (272, 273, 277). The Schiøtz tonometer is particularly unsuitable for situations in which ocular rigidity is known to be significantly altered, such as following retinal detachment surgery (185–187), or in eyes containing compressible gas (186–188, 278). In eye-bank eyes with manometrically determined IOP, the Schiøtz tonometer artificially raised the pressure a mean of 16.5 mm Hg, compared to 0.7 mm Hg and 12.1 mm Hg with Perkins and Tono-Pen tonometers, respectively (279).

PERKINS APPLANATION TONOMETER. This instrument has compared favorably against the Goldmann tonometer (280, 281). In one study, the difference between readings with the two instruments, expressed as the root mean square difference, was 1.4 mm Hg (280). It is subject to the same influence of corneal thickness as the Goldmann tonometer, with thin corneas producing underestimations and thick corneas causing overestimation of the IOP (282). The Perkins tonometer is especially useful in infants and children and is accurate in the horizontal, as well as the vertical, position. It is, therefore, an excellent tonometer to use in the operating room for examinations under anesthesia, as well as on the ward or wherever a Goldmann applanation tonometer is not available.

DRAEGER APPLANATION TONOMETER. Comparative studies with Goldmann tonometry have given inconsistent results, with one showing satisfactory agreement (281), while another found the Draeger instrument to be no better than a properly-used Schiøtz tonometer (283). Because of its more complex design, the Draeger tonometer is more difficult to use than the Perkins, and patient acceptance tends to be worse.

MACKAY-MARG TONOMETER. A highly significant correlation was found between IOP readings with the Mackay-Marg and Goldmann tonometers using topical anesthesia for both instruments, with the Mackay-Marg reading systematically higher and the Goldmann systematically lower than their mean results (284). When the Mackay-Marg was used without anesthesia, the mean IOP was approximately 2 mm Hg higher than that obtained by the same instrument with anesthesia (284). One study showed significant discrepancies between Mackay-Marg and Goldmann measurements when the former was used by a technician (285).

MACKAY-MARG-TYPE TONOMETERS. As previously noted, most of the newer instruments that utilize the Mackay-Marg principle (e.g., CAT 100, Challenger, EMT-20, and the

Biotronics tonometers) have not been found to be sufficiently accurate for clinical use (234–236). The *Tono-Pen* has compared favorably against manometric readings in human autopsy eyes (286, 287), although it may cause, as previously noted, a significant increase in the IOP during the measurement (279). In clinical comparisons with Goldmann applanation readings, some studies found a good correlation, especially within the normal IOP range (287–289), although most studies agree that it underestimates Goldmann IOP in the higher range and overestimates in the lower range (237, 288, 289). One study found an average absolute deviation of 2.70 mm Hg between paired Goldmann and Tono-Pen readings, with a difference of more than 5 mm Hg in 7% of the readings (290). In another study, the discrepancy was not sufficiently systematic to allow the application of a correction factor for measurement of diurnal curves (291). Readings obtained from the midperipheral and clear limbal cornea did not differ significantly from those taken in the central cornea, although readings taken from the sclera were 8.8–17 mm Hg higher than those taken from the central cornea (292). In one comparison against Goldmann applanation tonometry, the ProTon had a higher level of accuracy than the Tono-Pen XL (238).

PNEUMATIC TONOMETERS. Comparative studies with one pneumatic tonometer, the pneumatonograph, showed close correlations with Goldmann tonometers (293, 294), even when the pneumatic tonometer was operated by a technician (273). However, the pneumatonograph tends to read statistically higher (293, 294).

HALBERG APPLANATION TONOMETER. This instrument compared more favorably with the Goldmann tonometer than did the Schiøtz (273, 295), although it compared less favorably than the pneumatonograph in one study (273). Its use was felt to be easier to learn than Perkins hand-held tonometry (296), although medical students in another study preferred, and were more accurate with, a Schiøtz tonometer (297).

GLAUCOTEST. Evaluations of this tonometer suggest that it is a good screening instrument (251), even when used by a technician (273).

NONCONTACT TONOMETER. In most studies, comparisons against Goldmann applanation tonometers indicate that the NCT is reliable within the normal IOP range, although the reliability is reduced in the higher pressure ranges and is limited by an abnormal cornea or poor fixation (252–254, 298). One study found a close correlation between the mean IOP obtained by the two instruments, but considerable individual patient variation (299). Corneal thickness has a greater influence on noncontact tonometry than on Goldmann tonometry (300).

The hand-held Pulsair NCT has compared favorably with Goldmann readings in normal and glaucomatous eyes (255), and was effective in identifying ocular hypertension in postoperative eyes (256). One study, however, revealed an average absolute deviation of 2.49 mm Hg between paired Goldmann and Pulsair readings, with 8% differing by more than 5 mm Hg (290). Another study showed a strong linear correlation between readings with the two instruments, although the Pulsair tended to read lower at pressures above the normal range (301).

A significant advantage of the NCT is the elimination of potential hazards associated with all contact tonometers, including (a) abrasion of the cornea, (b) reactions to topical anesthetics, and (c) spread of infection. In addition, the instrument can be used reliably by paramedical personnel and has particular value in mass screening and possibly in studies of topical antiglaucoma drugs. Caution should be advised with abnormal corneas, however, since subepithelial bubbles have been seen after NCT measurements (302). In addition, there is the remote chance that infection could be spread by contamination of the front surface of the instrument with tear film at the time of air impact (303), and it should be cleaned after use with an alcohol swab.

Tonometry on Irregular Corneas

The accuracy of Goldmann- and Maklakov-type applanation tonometers and the noncontact tonometers is limited in eyes with irregular corneas. In cases of scarred or edematous corneas, the Mackay-Marg tonometer is generally considered to be the most accurate (304–306). However, the pneumatic tonometer has also been shown to be useful in eyes with diseased corneas (306, 307). One study, using cannulated eye-bank eyes with abnormal corneas, showed that the pneumatonograph gave more consistent and objective measurements than the Mackay-Marg (308). The Tono-Pen compared favorably with Makay-Marg tonometry on irregular corneas in one study (309). In eyes following penetrating keratoplasty, the TonoPen significantly overestimated Goldmann readings (310), and in another study, a minified Goldmann tonometer (applanating head reduced from 7 to 4 mm) was felt to be equal or superior to the pneumotonometer and TonoPen (311).

Tonometry Over Soft Contact Lenses

It has been claimed that the Mackay-Marg (312), the pneumatonograph (307, 313), and the Tono-Pen (314, 315) can measure the IOP through bandage contact lenses with reasonable accuracy, although soft contact lenses of different powers created a bias with the Tono-Pen (315). In cadaver eyes with four different brands of therapeutic contact lenses, the pneumotonometer correlated well with manometrically-determined IOP, while the Tono-Pen consistently underestimated the pressure (316). Applanation measurements are said to be affected by the power of the contact lenses with high water content, and correction tables have been developed to compensate for this (317). An evaluation of

NCT readings on eyes with and without soft contact lenses indicated that the power of the lens influenced the difference in IOP between the paired readings, with hyperopic lenses giving the greatest difference (318). Waiting 5 minutes after removing a bandage contact lens may improve the accuracy of the IOP reading (319).

Tonometry with Gas-filled Eyes

As previously noted, intraocular gas significantly influences scleral rigidity, rendering indentation tonometry particularly unsatisfactory in such cases. One pneumatic tonometer underestimated Goldmann IOP measurements in eyes with intravitreal gas (278), while the Tono-Pen was reported to compare favorably with Goldmann readings in eyes following pars plana vitrectomy and gas-fluid exchange (320). In another study of 50 eyes with irregular corneas following vitrectomy and air/gas-fluid exchange, readings with the Tono-Pen and pneumotonometer were highly correlated, although there was a mean difference of 1.4 mmHg, with the Tono-Pen usually reading lower (321). A manometric study with human autopsy eyes indicated that both instruments significantly underestimated the IOP at pressures above 30 mmHg (321).

Other Ocular Conditions

In premature infants with Stage V retinopathy of prematurity, applanation tonometry was preferable to indentation tonometry (323). In eye-bank eyes with flat anterior chambers, neither the Goldmann applanation tonometer, pneumotonometer, nor Tono-Pen provided IOP readings that correlated well with the manometrically-determined pressure (324).

SUMMARY

The distribution of IOP within the general population is almost Gaussian except for a slight skew toward higher pressures. The mean value is approximately 15 mm Hg, and 2 standard deviations to either side of the mean gives a "normal" range of roughly 10–20 mm Hg. Many factors, in addition to glaucoma, influence the IOP and can be divided into two categories: (a) those which exert a long-term influence, and (b) those which cause short-term fluctuations in the pressure. The former group includes genetics, age, sex, refractive error, and race, while the latter includes time of day, body position, exertion, lid and eye movement, various ocular and systemic conditions, general anesthesia, and some food and drugs.

Tonometers measure the IOP by relating a deformation of the globe to the force responsible for the deformation. Some tonometers indent the cornea, such as the Schiøtz tonometer, while others flatten or applanate the cornea. Within the latter group, some instruments measure the force

required to flatten a standard area, of which the Goldmann tonometer is an example, while others measure the area that is applanated by a standard force. Other instruments, such as the Mackay-Marg and pneumatic tonometers, employ a modified applanation principle with electronic recording of the pressure. Yet another, the noncontact tonometer, deforms the eye with a puff of air and automatically records the IOP.

REFERENCES

1. Leydhecker, W, Akiyama, K, Neumann, HG: Der intraokulare Druck gesunder menschlicher Augen. Klin Monatsbl Augenheilkd 133:662, 1958.
2. Colton, T, Ederer, F: The distribution of intraocular pressures in the general population. Surv Ophthalmol 25:123, 1980.
3. Johnson, LV: Tonographic survey. Am J Ophthalmol 61:680, 1966.
4. Segal, P, Skwierczynska, J: Mass screening of adults for glaucoma. Ophthalmologica 153:336, 1967.
5. Armaly, MF: On the distribution of applanation pressure. I. Statistical features and the effect of age, sex, and family history of glaucoma. Arch Ophthalmol 73:11, 1965.
6. Perkins, ES: Glaucoma screening from a public health clinic. Br J Ophthalmol 1:417, 1965.
7. Loewen, U, Handrup, B, Redeker, A: Results of a glaucoma mass screening program. Klin Monatsbl Augenheilkd 169:754, 1976.
8. Ruprecht, KW, Wulle, KG, Christl, HL: Applanation tonometry within medical diagnostic "check-up" programs. Klin Monatsbl Augenheilkd 172:332, 1978.
9. Shiose, Y, Kawase, Y: A new approach to stratified normal intraocular pressure in a general population. Am J Ophthalmol 101:714, 1986.
10. David, R, Zangwill, L, Stone, D, Yassur, Y: Epidemiology of intraocular pressure in a population screened for glaucoma. Br J Ophthalmol 71:766, 1987.
11. Klein, BEK, Klein, R, Linton, KLP: Intraocular pressure in an American community. The Beaver Dam eye study. Invest Ophthalmol Vis Sci 33:2224, 1992.
12. Armaly, MF: The genetic determination of ocular pressure in the normal eye. Arch Ophthalmol 78:187, 1967.
13. Armaly, MF, Monstavicius, BF, Sayegh, RE: Ocular pressure and aqueous outflow facility in siblings. Arch Ophthalmol 80:354, 1968.
14. Levene, RZ, Workman, PL, Broder, SW, Hirschhorn, K: Heritability of ocular pressure in normal and suspect ranges. Arch Ophthalmol 84:730, 1970.
15. Seddon, JM, Schwartz, B, Flowerdew, G: Case-control study of ocular hypertension. Arch Ophthalmolmol 101:891, 1983.
16. Radtke, ND, Cohan, BE: Intraocular pressure measurement in the newborn. Am J Ophthalmol 78:501, 1974.
17. Goethals, M, Missotten, L: Intraocular pressure in children up to five years of age. J Pediatr Ophthalmol Strabismus 20:49, 1983.
18. Pensiero, S, Da Pozzo, S, Perissutti, P, et al: Normal intraocular pressure in children. J Ped Ophthalmol Strabismus 29:79, 1992.
19. Musarella, MA, Morin, JD: Anterior segment and intraocular pressure measurements of the unanesthetized premature infant. Metab Pediatr Syst Ophthalmol 8:53, 1985.
20. Spierer, A, Huna, R, Hirsh, A, Chetrit, A: Normal intraocular pressure in premature infants. Am J Ophthalmol 117:801, 1994.
21. Jaafar, MS, Kazi, GA: Normal intraocular pressure in children: a comparative study of the Perkins applanation tonometer and the pneumotonometer. J Pediatr Ophthalmol Strabismus 30:284, 1993.
22. Klein, BE, Klein, R: Intraocular pressure and cardiovascular risk variables. Arch Ophthalmol 99:837, 1981.
23. Hiller, R, Sperduto, RD, Krueger, DE: Race, iris pigmentation, and intraocular pressure. Am J Epidemiol 115:674, 1982.

24. Carel, RS, Korczyn, AD, Rock, M, Goya, I: Association between ocular pressure and certain health parameters. Ophthalmology 91:311, 1984.

25. Schulzer, M, Drance, SM: Intraocular pressure, systemic blood pressure, and age: a correlation study. Br J Ophthalmol 71:245, 1987.

26. Shiose, Y: The aging effect on intraocular pressure in an apparently normal population. Arch Ophthalmol 102:883, 1984.

27. Becker, B: The decline in aqueous secretion and outflow facility with age. Am J Ophthalmol 46:731, 1958.

28. Gartner, J: Aging changes of the ciliary epithelium border layers and their significance for intraocular pressure. Am J Ophthalmol 72:1079, 1971.

29. Brubaker, RF, Nagataki, S, Townsend, DJ, Burns, RR, Higgins, RG, Wentworth, W: The effect of age on aqueous humor formation in man. Ophthalmology 88:283, 1981.

30. Tomlinson, A, Phillips, CI: Applanation tension and axial length of the eyeball. Br J Ophthalmol 54:548, 1970.

31. Deodati, F, Fontan, P, Mouledous, J-M: La tension oculaire du grand myope. Arch D'Ophthalmologie 34:77, 1974.

32. David, R, Zangwill, LM, Tessler, Z, Yassur, Y: The correlation between intraocular pressure and refractive status. Arch Ophthalmol 103:1812, 1985.

33. Quinn, GE, Berlin, JA, Young, TL, et al: Association of intraocular pressure and myopia in children. Ophthalmology 102:180, 1995.

34. Bonomi, L, Mecca, E, Massa F: Intraocular pressure in myopic anisometropia. Int Ophthalmol 5:145, 1982.

35. Kass, MA, Zimmerman, TJ, Alton, E, Lemon, L, Becker, B: Intraocular pressure and glaucoma in the Zuni Indians. Arch Ophthalmol 96:2212, 1978.

36. Katavisto, M: The diurnal variations of ocular tension in glaucoma. Acta Ophthalmologica Suppl 78, 1964.

37. Kitazawa, Y, Horie, T: Diurnal variation of intraocular pressure in primary open-angle glaucoma. Am J Ophthalmol 79:557, 1975.

38. Newell, FW, Krill, AE: Diurnal tonography in normal and glaucomatous eyes. Trans Am Ophthalmol Soc 62:349, 1964.

39. David, R, Zangwill, L, Briscoe, D, et al: Diurnal intraocular pressure variations: an analysis of 690 diurnal curves. Br J Ophthalmol 76:280, 1992.

40. Henkind, P, Leitman, M, Weitzman, E: The diurnal curve in man: new observations. Invest Ophthalmol 12:705, 1973.

41. Smith, J: Diurnal intraocular pressure: correlation to automated perimetry. Ophthalmology 92:858, 1985.

42. Wilensky, JT, Gieser, DK, Dietsche, ML, et al: Individual variability in the diurnal intraocular pressure curve. Ophthalmology 100:940, 1993.

43. Zeimer, RC, Wilensky, JT, Gieser, DK, Viana, MAG: Association between intraocular pressure peaks and progression of visual field loss. Ophthalmology 98:64, 1991.

44. Wilensky, JT, Gieser, DK, Mori, MT, et al: Self-tonometry to manage patients with glaucoma and apparently controlled intraocular pressure. Arch Ophthalmol 105:1072, 1987.

45. Zeimer, RC, Wilensky, JT, Gieser, DK: Presence and rapid decline of early morning intraocular pressure peaks in glaucoma patients. Ophthalmology 97:547, 1990.

46. Boyd, TAS, McLeod, LE: Circadian rhythms of plasma corticoid levels, intraocular pressure and aqueous outflow facility in normal and glaucomatous eyes. Ann NY Acad Sci 117:597, 1964.

47. Weitzman, ED, Henkind, P, Leitman, M, Hellman, L: Correlative 24-hour relationships between intraocular pressure and plasma cortisol in normal subjects and patients with glaucoma. Br J Ophthalmol 59:566, 1975.

48. Kimura, R, Maekawa, N: Effect of orally administered hydrocortisone on the ocular tension in primary open-angle glaucoma subjects. Preliminary report. Acta Ophthalmologica 54:430, 1976.

49. Levi, L, Schwartz, B: Decrease of ocular pressure with oral metyrapone: a double-masked crossover trial. Arch Ophthalmol 105:777, 1987.

50. Sheridan, PT, Brubaker, RF, Larsson, L-I, et al: The effect of oral dexamethasone on the circadian rhythm of aqueous humor flow in humans. Invest Ophthalmol Vis Sci 35:1150, 1994.

51. Viggiano, SR, Koskela, TK, Klee, GG, et al: The effect of melatonin on aqueous humor flow in humans during the day. Ophthalmology 101:326, 1994.

52. Rowland, JM, Sawyer, WK, Tittel, J, Ford, CJ: Studies on the circadian rhythm of IOP in rabbits: correlation with aqueous inflow and cAMP content. Curr Eye Res 5:201, 1986.

53. Smith, SD, Gregory, DS: A circadian rhythm of aqueous flow underlies the circadian rhythm of IOP in NZW Rabbits. Invest Ophthalmol Vis Sci 30:775, 1989.

54. Liu, JHK, Dacus, AC, Bartels, SP: Adrenergic mechanism in circadian elevation of intraocular pressure in rabbits. Invest Ophthalmol Vis Sci 32:2178, 1991.

55. Liu, JHK, Dacus, AC: Endogenous hormonal changes and circadian elevation of intraocular pressure. Invest Ophthalmol Vis Sci 32:496, 1991.

56. Yoshitomi, T, Gregory, DS: Ocular adrenergic nerves contribute to control of the circadian rhythm of aqueous flow in rabbits. Invest Ophthalmol Vis Sci 32:523, 1991.

57. Yoshitomi, T, Horio, B, Gregory, DS: Changes in adqueous norepinephrine and cyclic adenosine monophosphate during the circadian cycle in rabbits. Invest Ophthalmol Vis Sci 32:1609, 1991.

58. Anderson, DR, Grant, WM: The influence of position on intraocular pressure. Invest Ophthalmol 12:204, 1973.

59. Krieglstein, GK, Brethfeld, V, Collani, EV: Comparative intraocular pressure measurements with position independent hand-applanation tonometers. Graefes Arch Clin Exp Ophthalmol 199:101, 1976.

60. Jain, MR, Marmion, VJ: Rapid pneumatic and Mackay-Marg applanation tonometry to evaluate the postural effect on intraocular pressure. Br J Ophthalmol 60:687, 1976.

61. Kindler-Loosli, C, Schmidt, T: Intraocular pressure after changing the patient's position. Graefes Arch Clin Exp Ophthalmol 194:17, 1975.

62. Williams, BI, Peart, WS: Effect of posture on the intraocular pressure of patients with retinal vein obstruction. Br J Ophthalmol 62:688, 1978.

63. Wilson, MR, Baker, RS, Mohammadi, P, et al: Reproducibility of postural changes in intraocular pressure with the Tono-Pen and Pulsair tonometers. Am J Ophthalmol 116:479, 1993.

64. Parsley, J, Powell, RG, Keightley, SJ, Elkington, AR: Postural response of intraocular pressure in chronic open-angle glaucoma following trabeculectomy. Br J Ophthalmol 71:494, 1987.

65. Tsukahara, S, Sasaki, T: Postural change of IOP in normal persons and in patients with primary wide open-angle glaucoma and low-tension glaucoma. Br J Ophthalmol 68:389, 1984.

66. Leonard, TJK, Kerr-Muir, MG, Kirkby, GR, Hitchings, RA: Ocular hypertension and posture. Br J Ophthalmol 67:362, 1983.

67. Yamabayashi, S, Aguilar, RN, Hosoda, M, Tsukahara, S: Postural change of intraocular and blood pressures in ocular hypertension and low tension glaucoma. Br J Ophthalmol 75:652, 1991.

68. Williams, BI, Peart, WS, Letley, E: Abnormal intraocular pressure control in systemic hypertension and diabetes mellitus. Br J Ophthalmol 64:845, 1980.

69. Linder, BJ, Trick, GL, Wolf, ML: Altering body position affects intraocular pressure and visual function. Invest Ophthalmol Vis Sci 29:1492, 1988.

70. Cook, J, Friberg, TR: Effect of inverted body position on intraocular pressure. Am J Ophthalmol 98:784, 1984.

71. Friberg, TR, Sanborn, G, Weinreb, RN: Intraocular and episcleral venous pressure increase during inverted posture. Am J Ophthalmol 103:523, 1987.

72. Lempert, P, Cooper, KH, Culver, JF, Tredici, TJ: The effect of exercise on intraocular pressure. Am J Ophthalmol 63:1673, 1967.

73. Stewart, RH, LeBlanc, R, Becker, B: Effects of exercise on aqueous dynamics. Am J Ophthalmol 69:245, 1970.

74. Kypke, W, Hermannspann, U: Glaucoma physical activity and sport. Klin Monatsbl Augenheilkd 164:321, 1974.

75. Shapiro, A, Shoenfeld, Y, Shapiro, Y: The effect of standardised submaximal work load on intraocular pressure. Br J Ophthalmol 62:679, 1978.

76. Passo, MS, Goldberg, L, Elliot, DL, Van Buskirk, EM: Exercise conditioning and intraocular pressure. Am J Ophthalmol 103:754, 1987.

77. Orgül, S, Flammer, J: Moderate exertion lasting only seconds reduces intraocular pressure. Graefes Arch Clin Exp Ophthalmol 232:262, 1994.

78. Era, P, Parssinen, O, Kallinen, M, Suominen, H: Effect of bicycle ergometer test on intraocular pressure in elderly athletes and controls. Acta Ophthalmol 71:301, 1993.

79. Passo, MS, Goldberg, L, Elliot, DL, Van Buskirk, EM: Exercise training reduces intraocular pressure among subjects suspected of having glaucoma. Arch Ophthalmol 109:1096, 1991.

80. Dolan, JW, Kacere, RD, Squires, RW, Brubaker, RF: Effects of exercise conditioning on aqueous humor flow. J Glau 2:21, 1993.

81. Ashkenazi, I, Melamed, S, Blumenthal, M: The effect of continuous strenous exercise on intraocular pressure. Invest Ophthalmol Vis Sci 33:2874, 1992.

82. Harris, A, Malinovsky, VE, Cantor, LB, et al: Isocapnia blocks exercise-induced reductions in ocular tension. Invest Ophthalmol Vis Sci 33:2229, 1992.

83. Harris, A, Malinovsky, V, Martin, B: Correlates of acute exercise-induced ocular hypotension. Invest Ophthalmol Vis Sci 35:3852, 1994.

84. Shapiro, A, Shapiro, Y, Udassin, R, et al. The effect of salt loading diet on the intraocular pressure. Acta Ophthalmol 60:35, 1982.

85. Oggel, K, Sommer, G, Neuhann, Th, Hinz, J: Variations of intraocular pressure during Valsalva's maneuver in relation to body position and length of the bulbus in myopia. Graefes Arch Clin Exp Ophthalmol 218:51, 1982.

86. Rafuse, PE, Mills, DW, Hooper, PL, et al: Effects of Valsalva's manoeuvre on intraocular pressure. Can J Ophthalmol 29:73, 1994.

87. Epstein, HM, Fagman, W, Bruce, DL, Abram, A: Intraocular pressure changes during anesthesia for electroshock therapy. Anesth Anal 54:479, 1975.

88. Coleman, DJ, Trokel, S: Direct-recorded intraocular pressure variations in a human subject. Arch Ophthalmol 82:637, 1969.

89. Green, K, Luxenberg, MN: Consequences of eyelid squeezing on intraocular pressure. Am J Ophthalmol 88:1072, 1979.

90. Moses, RA, Carniglia, PE, Grodzki, WJ Jr, Moses, J: Proptosis and increase of intraocular pressure in voluntary lid fissure widening. Invest Ophthalmol Vis Sci 25:989, 1984.

91. Losada, F, Wolintz, AH: Bell's palsy: a new ophthalmologic sign. Ann Ophthalmol 5:1093, 1973.

92. Starrels, ME, Krupin, T, Burde, RM: Bell's palsy and intraocular pressure. Ann Ophthalmol 7:1067, 1975.

93. Wentworth, WO, Brubaker, RF: Aqueous humor dynamics in a series of patients with third neuron Horner's Syndrome. Am J Ophthalmol 92:407, 1981.

94. Spierer, A, Eisenstein, Z: The role of increased intraocular pressure on upgaze in the assessment of Graves ophthalmopathy. Ophthalmology 98:1491, 1991.

95. Moses, RA, Lurie, P, Wette, R: Horizontal gaze position effect on intraocular pressure. Invest Ophthalmol Vis Sci 22:551, 1982.

96. Saunders, RA, Helveston, EM, Ellis, FD: Differential intraocular pressure in strabismus diagnosis. Ophthalmology 87:59, 1981.

97. Muñoz, M, Capó, H: Differential intraocular pressure in restrictive strabismus. Am J Ophthalmol 112:352, 1991.

98. Raizman, MB, Beck, RW: Sustained increases in intraocular pressure during strabismus surgery. Am J Ophthalmol 101:308, 1986.

99. Pederson, JE: Experimental retinal detachment: IV. Aqueous humor dynamics in rhegmatogenous detachments. Arch Ophthalmol 100:1814, 1982.

100. Pederson, JE, Cantrill, HL: Experimental retinal detachment: V. Fluid movement through the retinal hole. Arch Ophthalmol 102:136, 1984.

101. Bulpitt, CJ, Hodes, C, Everitt, MG: Intraocular pressure and systemic blood pressure in the elderly. Br J Ophthalmol 59:717, 1975.

102. Leske, MC, Podgor, MJ: Intraocular pressure, cardiovascular risk variables, and visual field defects. Am J Epidemiol 118:280, 1983.

103. Williams, BI, Ledingham, JG: Significance of intraocular pressure measurement in systemic hypertension. Br J Ophthalmol 68:383, 1984.

104. McLeod, SD, West, SK, Quigley, HA, Fozard, JL: A longitudinal study of the relationship between intraocular and blood pressures. Invest Ophthalmol Vis Sci 31:2361, 1990.

105. Larkin, DFP, Connolly, P, Magner, JB, et al: Intraocular pressure during cardiopulmonary bypass. Br J Ophthalmol 71:177, 1987.

106. Abbott, MA, McLaren, AD, Algie, T: Intra-ocular pressure during cardiopulmonary bypass. A comparison of crystalloid and colloid priming solutions. Anaesthesia 49:353, 1994.

107. Larkin, DFP, Murphy, R, Magner, JB, Eustace, P: Management of intraocular pressure during cardiopulmonary bypass. Acta Ophthalmol 65:591, 1988.

108. Deutch, D, Lewis, RA: Intraocular pressure after cardiopulmonary bypass surgery. Am J Ophthalmol 107:18, 1989.

109. Krupin, T, Bass, J, Oestrich, C, et al: The effect of hyperthermia on aqueous humor dynamics in rabbits. Am J Ophthalmol 83:561, 1977.

110. Shapiro, A, Shoenfeld, Y, Konikoff, F, et al: The relationship between body temperature and intraocular pressure. Ann Ophthalmol 13:159, 1981.

111. Broekema, N, van Bijsterveld, OP, de Bos Kuil, RJC: Intraocular pressure during hemodialysis. Ophthalmologica 197:60, 1988.

112. Kass, MA, Sears, ML: Hormonal regulation of intraocular pressure. Surv Ophthalmol 22:153, 1977.

113. Elman, J, Caprioli, J, Sears, M, et al: Chorionic gonadotropin decreases intraocular pressure and aqueous humor flow in rabbit eyes. Invest Ophthalmol Vis Sci 28:197, 1987.

114. Feldman, F, Bain, J, Matuk, AR: Daily assessment of ocular and hormonal variables throughout the menstrual cycle. Arch Ophthalmol 96:1835, 1978.

115. Green, K, Cullen, PM, Phillips, CI: Aqueous humour turnover and intraocular pressure during menstruation. Br J Ophthalmol 68:736, 1984.

116. Green, K, Phillips, CI, Cheeks, L, Slagle, T: Aqueous humor flow rate and intraocular pressure during and after pregnancy. Ophthalmic Res 20:353, 1988.

117. Ziai, N, Ory, SJ, Khan, AR, Brubaker, RF: β-Human chorionic gonadotropin, progesterone, and aqueous dynamics during pregnancy. Arch Ophthalmol 112:801, 1994.

118. Wallace, I, Moolchandani, J, Krupin, T, et al: Effects of systemic desmopressin on aqueous humor dynamics in rabbits. Invest Ophthalmol Vis Sci 29:406, 1988.

119. Liu, JHK, Dacus, AC, Bartels, SP: Thyrotropin-releasing hormone increases intraocular pressure. Mechanism of action. Invest Ophthalmol Vis Sci 30:2200, 1989.

120. Aziz, MA: The relationship of IOP to hormonal disturbance. Bull Ophthalmol Soc Egypt 60:303, 1967.

121. Smith, KD, Tevaarwerk, GJM, Allen, LH: An ocular dynamic study supporting the hypothesis that hypothyroidism is a treatable cause of secondary open-angle glaucoma. Can J Ophthalmol 27:341, 1992.

122. Bramsen, T, Klauber, A, Bierre, P: Central corneal thickness and intraocular tension in patients with acromegaly. Acta Ophthalmol 58:971, 1980.

123. Walker, SD, Brubaker, RF, Nagataki, S: Hypotony and aqueous humor dynamics in myotonic dystrophy. Invest Ophthalmol Vis Sci 22:744, 1982.

124. Khan, AR, Brubaker, RF: Aqueous humor flow and flare in patients with myotonic dystrophy. Invest Ophthalmol Vis Sci 34:3131, 1993.

125. Klein, BEK, Klein, R, Moss, SE: Intraocular pressure in diabetic persons. Ophthalmology 91:1356, 1984.

126. Frier, BM, Hepburn, DA, Fisher, BM, Barrie, T: Fall in intraocular pressure during acute hypoglycaemia in patients with insulin dependent diabetes. Br Med J 294:610, 1987.

127. Ortiz, GJ, Cook, DJ, Yablonski, ME, et al: Effect of cold air on aqueous humor dynamics in humans. Invest Ophthalmol Vis Sci 29:138, 1988.

128. Wirt, H, Draeger, J: Tonometry in microgravity. Klin Mbl Augenheilk 188:505, 1986.

129. Mader, TH, Gibson, CR, Caputo, M, et al: Intraocular pressure and retinal vascular changes during transient exposure to microgravity. Am J Ophthalmol 115:347, 1993.

130. Duncalf, D: Anesthesia and intraocular pressure. Trans Am Acad Ophthalmol Otol 79:562, 1975.

131. Schreuder, M, Linssen, GH: Intra-ocular pressure and anaesthesia. Direct measurements by needling the anterior chamber in the monkey. Anaesthesia 27:165, 1972.

132. Maddox, TS Jr, Kielar, RA: Comparison of the influence of ketamine and halothane anesthesia on intraocular tensions of nonglaucomatous children. J Ped Ophthalmol 11:90, 1974.

133. Ausinsch, B, Graves, SA, Munson, ES, Levy, NS: Intraocular pressures in children during isoflurane and halothane anesthesia. Anesthesiology 42:167, 1975.

134. Dominguez, A, Banos, MS, Alvarez, MG, et al: Intraocular pressure measurement in infants under general anesthesia. Am J Ophthalmol 78:110, 1974.

135. Wyllie, AM, Beveridge, ME, Smith, I: Intraocular pressure during 4-hydroxy-butyrate narcosis. Br J Ophthalmol 56:436, 1972.

136. Peczon, JD, Grant, WM: Sedatives, stimulants, and intraocular pressure in glaucoma. Arch Ophthalmol 72:178, 1964.

137. Jaafar, MS, Kazi, GA: Effect of oral chloral hydrate sedation on the intraocular pressure measurement. J Ped Ophthalmol Strabismus 30:372, 1993.

138. Meyers, EF, Krupin, T, Johnson, M, Zink, H: Failure of nondepolarizing neuromuscular blockers to inhibit succinylcholine-induced increased intraocular pressure, a controlled study. Anesthesiology 48:149, 1978.

139. Bowen, DJ, McGrand, JC, Hamilton, AG: Intraocular pressures after suxamethonium and endotracheal intubation. Anaesthesia 33:518, 1978.

140. Meyers, EF, Singer, P, Otto, A: A controlled study of the effect of succinylcholine self-taming on intraocular pressure. Anesthesiology 53:72, 1980.

141. Cunningham, AJ, Albert, O, Cameron, J, Watson, AG: The effect of intravenous diazepam on rise of intraocular pressure following succinylcholine. Am J Ophthalmol 93:536, 1982.

142. Couch, JA, Eltringham, RJ, Magauran, DM: The effect of thiopentone and fazadinium on intraocular pressure. Anaesthesia 34:586, 1979.

143. Murphy, DF, Eustace, P, Unwin, A, Magner, JB: Atracurium and intraocular pressure. Br J Ophthalmol 69:673, 1985.

144. Goldstein, JH, Gupta, MK, Shah, MD: Comparison of intramuscular and intravenous succinylcholine on intraocular pressure. Ann Ophthalmol 13:173, 1981.

145. Moreno, RJ, Kloess, P, Carlson, DW: Effect of succinylcholine on the intraocular contents of open globes. Ophthalmology 98:636, 1991.

146. Wang, ML, Seiff, SR, Drasner, K: A comparison of visual outcome in open-globe repair: succinylcholine with D-tubocurarine vs. nondepolarizing agents. Ophthalmic Surg 23:746, 1992.

147. Murphy, DF, Eustace, P, Unwin, A, Magner, JB: Intravenous lignocaine pretreatment to prevent intraocular pressure rise following suxamethonium and tracheal intubation. Br J Ophthalmol 70:596, 1986.

148. Kielar, RA, Teraslinna, P, Kearney, JT, Barker, D: Effect of changes in PCO_2 on intraocular tension. Invest Ophthalmol Vis Sci 16:534, 1977.

149. Petounis, AD, Chondreli, S, Vadaluka-Sekioti, A: Effect of hypercapnea and hyperventilation on human intraocular pressure during general anaesthesia following acetazolamide administration. Br J Ophthalmol 64:422, 1980.

150. Harris, A, Malinovsky, V, Martin, BJ: Ocular hypotension during short- and long-term hypocapnia. J Glau 3:226, 1994.

151. Gallin-Cohen, PF, Podos, SM, Yablonski, ME: Oxygen lowers intraocular pressure. Invest Ophthalmol Vis Sci 19:43, 1980.

152. Yablonski, ME, Gallin, P, Shapiro, D: Effect of oxygen on aqueous humor dynamics in rabbits. Invest Ophthalmol Vis Sci 26:1781, 1985.

153. Peczon, JD, Grant, WM: Glaucoma, alcohol, and intraocular pressure. Arch Ophthalmol 73:495, 1965.

154. Houle, RE, Grant, WM: Alcohol, vasopressin, and intraocular pressure. Invest Ophthalmol 6:145, 1967.

155. Higginbotham, EJ, Kilimanjaro, HA, Wilensky, JT, et al: The effect of caffeine on intraocular pressure in glaucoma patients. Ophthalmology 96:624, 1989.

156. Adams, BA, Brubaker, RF: Caffeine has no clinically significant effect on aqueous humor flow in the normal human eye. Ophthalmology 97:1030, 1990.

157. Naveh-Floman, N, Belkin, M: Prostaglandin metabolism and intraocular pressure. Br J Ophthalmol 71:254, 1987.

158. Shephard, RJ, Ponsford, E, Basu, PK, LaBarre, R: Effects of cigarette smoking on intraocular pressure and vision. Br J Ophthalmol 62:682, 1978.

159. Stewart, WC, Crinkley, CMC, Murrell, HP: Cigarette-smoking in normal subjects, ocular hypertensive, and chronic open-angle glaucoma patients. Am J Ophthalmol 117:267, 1994.

160. Green, K: Ocular effects of diacetyl morphine and lysergic acid diethylamide in rabbit. Invest Ophthalmol 14:325, 1975.

161. Whitworth, CG, Grant, WM: Use of nitrate and nitrite vasodilators by glaucomatous patients. Arch Ophthalmol 71:492, 1964.

162. Leydhecker, W, Waller, W, Krieglstein, G: The effect of vasodilators on the intraocular pressure. Klin Monatsbl Augenheilkd 164:293, 1974.

163. Peczon, JD, Grant, WM, Lambert, BW: Systemic vasodilators, intraocular pressure, and chamber depth in glaucoma. Am J Ophthalmol 72:74, 1971.

164. Wizemann, AJS, Wizemann, V: Organic nitrate in glaucoma. Am J Ophthalmol 90:106, 1980.

165. Hardt, BW, Johnen, R, Fahle, M: The influence of systemic digitalis application on intraocular pressure. Graefes Arch Clin Exp Ophthalmol 219:76, 1982.

166. Lazenby, GW, Reed, JW, Grant, WM: Short-term tests of anticholinergic medication in open-angle glaucoma. Arch Ophthalmol 80:443, 1968.

167. Lazenby, GW, Reed, JW, Grant, WM: Anticholinergic medication in open-angle glaucoma. Long-term tests. Arch Ophthalmol 84:719, 1970.

168. Hiatt, RL, Fuller, IB, Smith, L, et al: Systemically administered anticholinergic drugs and intraocular pressure. Arch Ophthalmol 84:735, 1970.

169. Stelzer, R, Wohlzogen, FX: Anticholinergic drugs in open-angle glaucoma. Klin Monatsbl Augenheilkd 177:151, 1980.

170. Valle, O: Effect of cyclopentolate on the aqueous dynamics in incipient or suspected open-angle glaucoma. Acta Ophthalmolmologica: XXI Meeting of Nordic Ophthalmologists June 13–16, 1973, p. 52.

171. Maus, TL, Larsson, L-I, Brubaker, RF: Ocular effects of scopolamine dermal patch in open-angle glaucoma. J Glau 3:190, 1994.

172. Feldman, F, Cohen, MM: Effect of histamine-2 receptor blockade by cimetidine on intraocular pressure in humans. Am J Ophthalmol 93:351, 1982.

173. Ober, M, Scharrer, A: Changes in intraocular pressure during prostaglandin-induced abortion. Klin Monatsbl Augenheilkd 180:230, 1982.

174. Friedenwald, JS: Contribution to the theory and practice of tonometry. Am J Ophthalmol 20:985, 1937.

175. Moses, RA, Tarkkanen, A: Tonometry: the pressure-volume relationship in the intact human eye at low pressures. Am J Ophthalmol

47:557, 1959.

176. Friedenwald, JS: Some problems in the calibration of tonometers. Am J Ophthalmol 31:935, 1948.

177. Friedenwald, JS: Tonometer calibration: An attempt to remove discrepancies found in the 1954 calibration scale for Schiøtz tonometers. Trans Am Acad Ophthalmol Otol 61:108, 1957.

178. Kronfeld, PC: Tonometer calibration empirical validation. The committee on standardization of tonometers. Trans Am Acad Ophthalmol Otol 61:123, 1957.

179. Anderson, DR, Grant, WM: Re-evaluation of the Schiøtz tonometer calibration. Invest Ophthalmol 9:430, 1970.

180. Bayard, WL: Comparison of Goldmann applanation and Schiøtz tonometry using 1948 and 1955 conversion scales. Am J Ophthalmol 69:1007, 1970.

181. Drance, SM: The coefficient of scleral rigidity in normal and glaucomatous eyes. Arch Ophthalmol 63:668, 1960.

182. Friedman, E, Ivry, M, Ebert, E, et al: Increased scleral rigidity and age-related macular degeneration. Ophthalmology 96:104, 1989.

183. Draeger, J: Die Abhangigkeit des Rigiditatskoeffizienten von der Hohe des intraokularen Druckes. Ophthalmologica 140:55, 1960.

184. Kaiser-Kupfer, MI, McCain, L, Shapiro, JR, et al: Low ocular rigidity in patients with ostoegenesis imperfecta. Invest Ophthalmol Vis Sci 20:807, 1981.

185. Harbin, TS Jr, Laikam, SE, Lipsitt, K, et al: Applanation-Schiøtz disparity after retinal detachment surgery utilizing cryopexy. Ophthalmology 86:1609, 1979.

186. Johnson, MW, Han, DP, Hoffman, KE: The effect of scleral buckling on ocular rigidity. Ophthalmology 97:190, 1990.

187. Simone, JN, Whitacre, MM: The effect of intraocular gas and fluid volumes on intraocular pressure. Ophthalmology 97:238, 1990.

188. Aronowitz, JD, Brubaker, RF: Effect of intraocular gas on intraocular pressure. Arch Ophthalmol 94:1191, 1976.

189. Foster, CS, Yamamoto, GK: Ocular rigidity in keratoconus. Am J Ophthalmol 86:802, 1978.

190. Draeger, J: Untersuchungen uber den rigiditatskoeffizienten. Doc Ophthalmol 13:431, 1959.

191. Goldmann, H, Schimdt, TH: Der rigiditatskoeffizient (Friedenwald). Ophthalmologica 133:330, 1957.

192. Chandler, PA, Grant, WP: Glaucoma, 2nd ed. Philadelphia, Lea and Febiger, 1979, p. 16.

193. van der Werff, TJ: A new single-parameter ocular rigidity function. Am J Ophthalmol 92:391, 1981.

194. Hetland-Eriksen, J: On tonometry. 2. Pressure recordings by Schiøtz tonometry on enucleated human eyes. Acta Ophthalmol 44:12, 1966.

195. Goldmann, MH: Un nouveau tonometre a aplanation. Bull Soc Fr Ophthalmol 67:474, 1954.

196. Goldmann, H, Schmidt, TH: Uber applanationstonometrie. Ophthalmologica 134:221, 1957.

197. Stepanik, J: Tonometry results using a corneal applanation 3.53 mm in diameter. Klin Monatsbl Augenheilkd 184:40, 1984.

198. Moses, RA: The Goldmann applanation tonometer. Am J Ophthalmol 46:865, 1958.

199. Koester, CJ, Campbell, CJ, Donn, A: Ophthalmic optical instruments: Two recent developments. Jpn J Ophthalmol 24:1, 1980.

200. Grant, WM: Fluorescein for applanation tonometry. More convenient and uniform application. Am J Ophthalmol 55:1252, 1963.

201. Quickert, MH: A fluorescein-anesthetic solution for applanation tonometry. Arch Ophthalmol 77:734, 1967.

202. Stewart, HL: Prolonged antibacterial activity of a fluorescein-anesthetic solution. Arch Ophthalmol 88:385, 1972.

203. Coad, CT, Osato, MS, Wilhelmus, KR: Bacterial contamination of eyedrop dispensers. Am J Ophthalmol 98:548, 1984.

204. Duffner, LR, Pflugfelder, SC, Mandelbaum, S, Childress, LL: Potential bacterial contamination in fluorescein-anesthetic solutions. Am J

Ophthalmol 110:199, 1990.

205. Palmberg, R, Gutierrez, YS, Miller, D, et al: Potential bacterial contamination of eyedrops used for tonometry. Am J Ophthalmol 117:578, 1994.

206. Roper, DL: Applanation tonometry with and without fluorescein. Am J Ophthalmol 90:668, 1980.

207. Ehlers, N, Bramsen, T, Sperling, S: Applanation tonometry and central corneal thickness. Acta Ophthalmol 53:34, 1975.

208. Johnson, M, Kass, MA, Moses, RA, Grodzki, WJ: Increased corneal thickness simulating elevated intraocular pressure. Arch Ophthalmol 96:664, 1978.

209. Mark, HH: Corneal curvature in applanation tonometry. Am J Ophthalmol 76:223, 1973.

210. Holladay, JT, Allison, ME, Prager, TC: Goldmann applanation tonometry in patients with regular corneal astigmatism. Am J Ophthalmol 96:90, 1983.

211. Bynke, H, Wilke, K: Repeated applanation tonometry in carotid occlusive disease. Acta Ophthalmol 52:125, 1974.

212. Moniz, E, Feldman, F, Newkirk, M, et al: Removal of hepatitis B surface antigen from a contaminated applanation tonometer. Am J Ophthalmol 91:522, 1981.

213. Gastaud, P, Baudouin, CH, Ouzan, D: Detection of HBs antigen, DNA polymerase activity, and hepatitis B virus DNA in tears: relevance to hepatitis B transmission by tears. Br J Ophthalmol 73:333, 1989.

214. Fujikawa, LS, Salahuddin SZ, Palestine AG, et al: Isolation of the human T-lymphotropic virus type III from the tears of a patient with the acquired immunodeficiency syndrome. Lancet 2:529, 1985.

215. Fujikawa, LS, Salahuddin, SZ, Ablashi, D, et al: HTLV-III in the tears of AIDS patients. Ophthalmology 93:1479, 1986.

216. Craven, ER, Butler, SL, McCulley, JP, Luby, JP: Applanation tonometer tip sterilization for adenovirus type 8. Ophthalmology 94:1538, 1987.

217. Threlkeld, AB, Froggatt, JW, Schein, OD, Forman, MS: Efficacy of a disinfectant wipe method for the removal of adenovirus 8 from tonometer tips. Ophthalmology 100:1841, 1993.

218. Ventura, LM, Dix, RD: Viability of herpes simplex virus type 1 on the applanation tonometer. Am J Ophthalmol 103:48, 1987.

219. Su, CS, Bowden, S, Fong, LP, Taylor, HR: Current tonometer disinfection may be inadequate for hepatitis B virus. Arch Ophthalmol 112:1406, 1994.

220. Pepose, JS, Linnette, G, Lee, SF, MacRae, S: Disinfection of Goldmann tonometers against human innumodeficiency virus type 1. Arch Ophthalmol 107:983, 1989.

221. Nardi, M, Bartolomei, MP, Falco, L, Carelli, F: Disposable film cover for the tip of Goldmann's tonometer. Graefe`s Arch Ophthalmol 223:109, 1985.

222. Assia, E, Bartov, E, Blumenthal, M: Disposable parafilm cover for the applanation tonometer. Am J Ophthalmol 102:397, 1986.

223. Wizemann, A: Modified version of UV sterilizer to disinfect Goldmann tonometer heads, gonioscopes and fundus contact lenses. Klin Monatsbl Augenheilkd 181:40, 1982.

224. Van buskirk, EM: Disinfectant receptacle for applanation tonometers. Am J Ophthalmol 104:307, 1987.

225. American Academy of Ophthalmology: Clinical Alert 2/4. Updated recommendations for ophthalmic practice in relation to the human immunodeficiency virus, August 1988.

226. Centers for Disease Control. Recommendations for preventing possible transmission of human T-lymphotropic virus type III/lymphadenopathy-associated virus in tears. MMWR Morb Mortal Wkly Rep 34:533, 1985.

227. Soukiasian, SH, Asdourian, GK, Weiss, JS, Kachadoorian, HA: A complication from alcohol-swabbed tonometer tips. Am J Ophthalmol 105:424, 1988.

228. Pogrebniak, AE, Sugar, A: Corneal toxicity from hydrogen peroxide-soaked tonometer tips. Arch Ophthalmol 106:1505, 1988.

229. Perkins, ES: Hand-held applanation tonometer. Br J Ophthalmol 49:591, 1965.

230. Draeger, J: Simple hand applanation tonometer for use on the seated as well as on the supine patient. Am J Ophthalmol 62:1208, 1966.

231. Draeger, J: Principle and clinical application of a portable applanation tonometer. Invest Ophthalmol 6:132, 1967.

232. Mackay, RS, Marg, E: Fast, automatic, electronic tonometers based on an exact theory. Acta Ophthalmol 37:495, 1959.

233. Marg, E, Mackay, RS, Oechsli, R: Trough height, pressure and flattening in tonometry. Vision Res 1:379, 1962.

234. Blondeau, P: Clinical evaluation of the Dicon CAT 100 applanation tonometer. Am J Ophthalmol 99:708, 1985.

235. Lim, JI, Ruderman, JM: Comparison of the Challenger digital applanation tonometer and the Goldmann applanation tonometer. Am J Ophthalmol 102:154, 1986.

236. Miller, K, Sanborn, GE, Jennings, LW: Clinical evaluation of the Cavitron biotronics tonometer. Arch Ophthalmol 106:1210, 1988.

237. Kao, SF, Lichter, PR, Bergstrom, TJ, et al: Clinical comparison of the Oculab Tono-Pen to the Goldmann applanation tonometer. Ophthalmology 94:1541, 1987.

238. Midelfart, A, Wigers, A: Clinical comparison of the ProTon and Tono-Pen tonometers with the Goldmann applanation tonometer. Br J Ophthalmol 78:895, 1994.

239. Durham, DG, Bigliano, RP, Masino, JA: Pneumatic applanation tonometer. Trans Am Acad Ophthalmol Otol 69:1029, 1965.

240. Langham, ME, McCarthy, E: A rapid pneumatic applanation tonometer. Comparative findings and evaluation. Arch Ophthalmol 79:389, 1968.

241. Hodkin, MJ, Pavilack, MA, Musch, DC: Pneumotonometry using sterile single-use tonometer covers. Ophthalmology 99:688, 1992.

242. Posner, A: An evaluation of the Maklakov applanation tonometer. EENT Monthly 41:377, 1962.

243. Posner, A: Practical problems in the use of the Maklakov tonometer. EENT Monthly 42:82, 1963.

244. Friedenwald, JS: Contribution to the theory and practice of tonometry. II. An analysis of the work of Professor S. Kalfa with the applanation tonometer. Am J Ophthalmol 22:375, 1939.

245. Schmidt, TFA: Calibration of the Maklakoff tonometer. Am J Ophthalmol 77:740, 1974.

246. Posner, A: A new portable applanation tonometer. EENT Monthly 43:88, 1964.

247. Posner, A, Inglima, R: The Tonomat applanation tonometer. EENT Monthly 46:996, 1967.

248. Halberg, GP: Hand applanation tonometer. Trans Am Acad Ophthalmol Otol 72:112, 1968.

249. Barraquer, JI: New applanation tonometer for operating room. Ophthalmologica 153:225, 1967.

250. Jensen, JB: An ocular tension indicator of the applanation type. Acta Ophthalmol 45:546, 1967.

251. Kaiden, JS, Zimmerman, TJ, Worthen, DM: An evaluation of the GlaucoTest screening tonometer. Arch Ophthalmol 92:195, 1974.

252. Grolman, B: A new tonometer system. Am J Optom & Arch Am Acad Optom 49:646, 1972.

253. Forbes, M, Pico, G, Grolman, B: A noncontact applanation tonometer description and clinical evaluation. Arch Ophthalmol 91:134, 1974.

254. Shields, MB: The non-contact tonometer. Its value and limitations. Surv Ophthalmol 24:211, 1980.

255. Fisher, JH, Watson, PG, Spaeth, G: A new hand-held air impulse tonometer. Eye 2:238, 1988.

256. Vernon, SA: Non-contact tonometry in the postoperative eye. Br J Ophthalmol 73:247, 1989.

257. Piltz, JR, Starita, R, Miron, M, Henkind, P: Momentary fluctuations of intraocular pressure in normal and glaucomatous eyes. Am J Ophthalmol 99:333, 1985.

258. Moses, RA, Arnzen, RJ: Instantaneous tonometry. Arch Ophthalmol 101:249, 1983.

259. Greene, ME, Gilman, BG: Intraocular pressure measurement with instrumented contact lenses. Invest Ophthalmol 13:299, 1974.

260. Wolbarsht, ML, Wortman, J, Schwartz, B, Cook, D: A scleral buckle pressure gauge for continuous monitoring of intraocular pressure. Int Ophthalmol 3:11, 1980.

261. Cooper, RL, Beale, DG, Constable, IJ: Passive radiotelemetry of intraocular pressure in vivo: calibration and validation of continual scleral guard-ring applanation transensors in the dog and rabbit. Invest Ophthalmol Vis Sci 18:930, 1979.

262. Cooper, RL, Beale, DG, Constable, IJ, Grose, GC: Continual monitoring of intraocular pressure: effect of central venous pressure, respiration, and eye movements on continual recordings of intraocular pressure in the rabbit, dog, and man. Br J Ophthalmol 63:799, 1979.

263. Nissen, OI: Bilateral recording of human intraocular pressure with an improved applanating suction cup tonograph. Acta Ophthalmol 58:377, 1980.

264. Zeimer, RC, Wilensky, JT, Gieser, DK, et al: Evaluation of a self tonometer for home use. Arch Ophthalmol 101:1791, 1983.

265. Zeimer, RC, Wilensky, JT, Gieser, DK, et al: Application of a self-tonometer to home tonometry. Arch Ophthalmol 104:49, 1986.

266. Dekking, HM, Coster, HD: Dynamic tonometry. Ophthalmologica 154:59, 1967.

267. Roth, W, Blake, DG: Vibration tonometry—principles of the vibra-tonometer. J Am Optom Assoc 34:971, 1963.

268. Moses, RA, Liu, CH: Repeated applanation tonometry. Am J Ophthalmol 66:89, 1968.

269. Phelps, CD, Phelps, GK: Measurement of intraocular pressure: a study of its reproducibility. Graefes Arch Clin Exp Ophthalmol 198:39, 1976.

270. Dielemans, I, Vingerling, JR, Hofman, A, et al: Reliability of intraocular pressure measurement with the Goldmann applanation tonometer in epidemiological studies. Graefes Arch Clin Exp Ophthalmol 232:141, 1994.

271. Smith, JL, et al. The incidence of Schiøtz-applanation disparity. Cooperative study. Arch Ophthalmol 77:305, 1967.

272. Bengtsson, B: Comparison of Schiøtz and Goldmann tonometry in a population. Acta Ophthalmol 50:445, 1972.

273. Krielgstein, GK: Screening tonometry by technicians. Graefes Arch Clin Exp Ophthalmol 194:221, 1975.

274. Armaly, MF, Salamoun, SG: Schiøtz and applanation tonometry. Arch Ophthalmol 70:603, 1963.

275. Schwartz, JT, Dell'Osso, GG: Comparison of Goldmann and Schiøtz tonometry in a community. Arch Ophthalmol 75:788, 1966.

276. Bengtsson, B: Some factors affecting the relationship between Schiøtz and Goldmann readings in a population. Acta Ophthalmol 51:798, 1973.

277. Stepanik, J: Why is the Schiøtz tonometer not suitable for measuring intraocular pressure? Klin Monatsbl Augenheilkd 176:61, 1980.

278. Del Priore, LV, Michels, RG, Nunez, MA, et al: Intraocular pressure measurement after pars plana vitrectomy. Ophthalmology 96:1353, 1989.

279. Whitacre, MM, Emig, M, Hassanein, K: The effect of Perkins, Tono-Pen, and Schiötz tonometry on intraocular pressure. Am J Ophthalmol 111:59, 1991.

280. Dunn, JS, Brubaker, RF: Perkins applanation tonometer clinical and laboratory evaluation. Arch Ophthalmol 89:149, 1973.

281. Krieglstein, GK, Waller, WK: Goldmann applanation versus hand-applanation and Schiøtz indentation tonometry. Graefes Arch Clin Exp Ophthalmol 194:11, 1975.

282. Whitacre, MM, Stein, RA, Hassanein, K: The effect of corneal thickness on applanation tonometry. Am J Ophthalmol 115:592, 1993.

283. Finlay, RD: Experience with the Draeger applanation tonometer. Trans Ophthalmol Soc UK 90:887, 1970.

284. Moses, RA, Marg, E, Oechsli, R: Evaluation of the basic validity and clinical usefulness of the Mackay-Marg tonometer. Invest Ophthalmol 1:78, 1962.

285. Petersen, WC, Schlegel, WA: Mackay-Marg tonometry by technicians. Am J Ophthalmol 76:933, 1973.

286. Hessemer, V, Rösler, R, Jacobi, KW: Comparison of intraocular pressure measurements with the Oculab Tono-Pen vs manometry in humans shortly after death. Am J Ophthalmol 105:678, 1988.

287. Boothe, WA, Lee, DA, Panek, WC, Pettit, TH: The Tono-Pen. A manometric and clinical study. Arch Ophthalmol 106:1214, 1988.

288. Frenkel, REP, Hong, YJ, Shin, DH: Comparison of the Tono-Pen to the Goldmann applanation tonometer. Arch Ophthalmol 106:750, 1988.

289. Hessemer, V, Rossler, R, Jacobi, KW: Tono-Pen, a new hand-held tonometer: comparison with the Goldmann applanation tonometer. Klin Monatsb Augenheilkd 193:420, 1988.

290. Armstrong, TA: Evaluation of the Tono-Pen and the Pulsair tonometers. Am J Ophthalmol 109:716, 1990.

291. Farrar, SM, Miller, KN, Shields, MB, Stoup, CM: An evaluation of the Tono-Pen for the measurement of diurnal intraocular pressure. Am J Ophthalmol 107:411, 1989.

292. Khan, JA, Davis, M, Graham, CE, et al: Comparison of Oculab Tono-Pen readings obtained from various corneal and scleral locations. Arch Ophthalmol 109:1444, 1991.

293. Quigley, HA, Langham, ME: Comparative intraocular pressure measurements with the pneumatonograph and Goldmann tonometer. Am J Ophthalmol 80:266, 1975.

294. Jain, MR, Marmion, VJ: A clinical evaluation of the applanation pneumatonograph. Br J Ophthalmol 60:107, 1976.

295. Francois, J, Vancea, P, Vanderkerckhove, R: Halberg tonometer. An evaluation. Arch Ophthalmol 86:376, 1971.

296. Zimmerman, TJ, Worthen, DM: A comparison of two hand-applanation tonometers. Arch Ophthalmol 88:421, 1972.

297. Kaiden, JS, Zimmerman, TJ, Worthen, DM: Hand-held tonometers. An evaluation by medical students. Arch Ophthalmol 89:110, 1973.

298. Jessen, K, Hoffmann, F: Current standardization of air-pulse tonometers and methods of testing them, taking the non-contact tonometer II as an example. Klin Monatsbl Augenheilkd 183:296, 1983.

299. Derka, H: The American Optical non-contact tonometer and its results compared with the Goldmann applanation tonometer. Klin Monatsbl Augenheilkd 177:634, 1980.

300. Gräf, M: The effect of corneal thickness on non contact tonometry. Klin Mbl Augenheilk 199:183, 1991.

301. Sponsel, WE, Kaufman, PL, Strinden, TI, et al: Evaluation of the Keeler Pulsair non-contact tonometer. Acta Ophthalmol 67:567, 1989.

302. Insler, MS: Acute corneal bullae produced during noncontact tonometry. Am J Ophthalmol 101:375, 1986.

303. Britt, JM, Clifton, BC, Barnebey, HS, Mills, RP: Microaerosol formation in noncontact "air-puff" tonometry. Arch Ophthalmol 109:225, 1991.

304. Kaufman, HE, Wind, CA, Waltman, SR: Validity of Mackay-Marg electronic applanation tonometer in patients with scarred irregular corneas. Am J Ophthalmol 69:1003, 1970.

305. McMillan, F, Forster, RK: Comparison of MacKay-Marg, Goldmann, and Perkins tonometers in abnormal corneas. Arch Ophthalmol 93:420, 1975.

306. West, CE, Capella, JA, Kaufman, HE: Measurement of intraocular pressure with a pneumatic applanation tonometer. Am J Ophthalmol 74:505, 1972.

307. Krieglstein, GK, Waller, WK, Reimers, H, Langham, ME: Intraocular pressure measurements on soft contact lenses. Graefes Arch Clin Exp Ophthalmol 199:223, 1976.

308. Richter, RC, Stark, WJ, Cowan, C, Pollack, IP: Tonometry on eyes with abnormal corneas. Glaucoma 2:508, 1980.

309. Rootman, DS, Insler, MS, Thompson, HW, et al: Accuracy and precision of the Tono-Pen in measuring intraocular pressure after keratoplasty and epikeratophakia and in scarred corneas. Arch Ophthalmol 106:1697, 1988.

310. Geyer, O, Mayron, Y, Loewenstein, A, et al: Tono-Pen tonometry in normal and in post-keratoplasty eyes. Br J Ophthalmol 76:538, 1992.

311. Ménage, MJ, Kaufman, PL, Croft, MA, Landay, SP: Intraocular pressure measurement after penetrating keratoplasty: minified Goldmann applanation tonometer, pneumatonometer, and Tono-Pen versus manometry. Br J Ophthalmol 78:671, 1994.

312. Meyer, RF, Stanifer, RM, Bobb, KC: MacKay-Marg Tonometry over therapeutic soft contact lenses. Am J Ophthalmol 86:19, 1978.

313. Rubenstein, JB, Deutsch, TA: Pneumatonometry through bandage contact lenses. Arch Ophthalmol 103:1660, 1985.

314. Khan, JA, LaGreca, BA: Tono-Pen estimation of intraocular pressure through bandage contact lenses. Am J Ophthalmol 108:422, 1989.

315. Panek, WC, Boothe, WA, Lee, DA, et al: Intraocular pressure measurement with the Tono-Pen through soft contact lenses. Am J Ophthalmol 109:62, 1990.

316. Mark, LK, Asbell, PA, Torres, MA, Failla, SJ: Accuracy of intraocular pressure measurements with two different tonometers through bandage contact lenses. Cornea 11:277, 1992.

317. Draeger, J: Applanation tonometry on contact lenses with high water content: Problems, results, correction factors. Klin Monatsbl Augenheilkd 176:38, 1980.

318. Insler, MS, Robbins, RG: Intraocular pressure by noncontact tonometry with and without soft contact lenses. Arch Ophthalmol 105:1358, 1987.

319. Khan, JA, Graham, CE: Effect of contact lens removal or displacement on intraocular pressure. Arch Ophthalmol 109:825, 1991.

320. Hines, MW, Jost, BF, Fogelman, KL: Oculab Tono-Pen, Goldmann applanation tonometery, and pneumatic tonometry for intraocular pressure assessment in gas-filled eyes. Am J Ophthalmol 106:174, 1988.

321. Lim, JI, Blair, NP, Higginbotham, EJ, et al: Assessment of intraocular pressure in vitrectomized gas-containing eyes. A clinical and manometric comparison of the Tono-Pen to the pneumotonometer. Arch Ophthalmol 108:684, 1990.

322. Hartnett, ME, Hirose, T, Richardson, TM, et al: Intraocular pressure determination in infants with severe retinopathy of prematurity. Graefes Arch Clin Exp Ophthalmol 230:406, 1992.

323. Wright, MM, Grajewski, AL: Measurement of intraocular pressure with a flat anterior chamber. Ophthalmology 98:1854, 1991

Chapter 5

OPTIC NERVE HEAD AND PERIPAPILLARY RETINA

The primary consequence of elevated intraocular pressure (IOP) in an eye with glaucoma is progressive atrophy of the optic nerve head. Since it is this pathologic alteration which leads to the irreversible loss of vision, an understanding of glaucomatous optic atrophy is essential in the diagnosis and management of glaucoma.

ANATOMY AND HISTOLOGY[a]

Terminology

Within the context of a discussion on glaucoma, the optic nerve head is defined as the distal portion of the optic nerve

[a]Refer to Shields, MB: Color Atlas of Glaucoma. Baltimore, Williams & Wilkins, 1998, Plate I10.

that is directly susceptible to elevated IOP. In this sense, the optic nerve head extends from the retinal surface to the myelinated portion of the optic nerve that begins just behind the sclera. The term "optic nerve head" is generally preferred over "optic disc" since the latter suggests a flat structure without depth. However, the terms "disc" and "papilla" are frequently used when referring to the portion of the optic nerve head that is clinically visible by ophthalmoscopy.

General Description

The optic nerve head is composed of the nerve fibers which originate in the ganglion cell layer of the retina and converge upon the nerve head from all points in the fundus. At the surface of the nerve head, these axons bend acutely to leave the globe through a fenestrated scleral canal, called the *lamina cribrosa*. Within the nerve head,

Optic Nerve Head

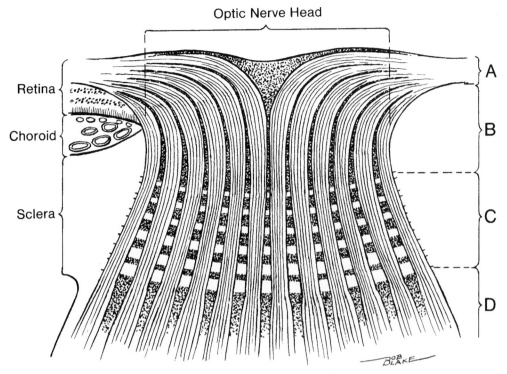

Retina

Choroid

Sclera

A

B

C

D

Figure 5.1. Divisions of the optic nerve head: **A.** Surface nerve fiber layer; **B.** Prelaminar region; **C.** Lamina cribrosa region; **D.** Retrolaminar region.

the axons are grouped into approximately 1000 fascicles, or bundles, and are supported by astrogliocytes. There is considerable variation in the size of the optic nerve head. In one study, the diameter varied from 1.18 to 1.75 mm (1). Other studies have revealed ranges of 0.85–2.43 mm in the shortest diameter and 1.21–2.86 mm in the longest (2), or a mean of 1.88 mm vertically and 1.77 horizontally (3). The disc area may range from 0.68 mm² to 4.42 mm² (2). The diameter of the nerve expands to approximately 3 mm just behind the sclera, where the neurons acquire a myelin sheath. The optic nerve head is also the site of entry and exit of the retinal vessels. This vascular system supplies some branches to the optic nerve head, although the predominant blood supply for the nerve head comes from the ciliary circulation.

Divisions of the Optic Nerve Head

The nerve head may be arbitrarily divided into four portions from anterior to posterior (Fig. 5.1) (4).

Surface Nerve Fiber Layer

The innermost portion of the optic nerve head is composed predominantly of neurons. In the Rhesus monkey, this layer is 94% neurons and 5% astrocytes (5). The axonal bundles

acquire progressively more interaxonal glial tissue within the intraocular portion of the nerve head as this structure is followed posteriorly (5).

Prelaminar Region

The prelaminar region is also called the anterior portion of the lamina cribrosa (6). The predominant structures at this level are neurons and astrocytes, with a significant increase in the quantity of astroglial tissue.

Lamina Cribrosa Region

This portion contains fenestrated sheets of scleral connective tissue and occasional elastic fibers. Astrocytes separate the sheets and line the fenestrae (6), and the fascicles of neurons leave the eye through these openings.

Retrolaminar Region

This area is characterized by a decrease in astrocytes and the acquisition of myelin, that is supplied by oligodendrocytes. The axonal bundles are surrounded by connective tissue septa.

The posterior extent of the retrolaminar region is not clearly defined. An India ink study of monkey eyes showed nonfilling for 3–4 mm behind the lamina cribrosa, when the

IOP was elevated (7). However, a similar study with unlabeled microspheres showed an increased flow in the retrolaminar region close to the lamina even when the pressure was elevated high enough to stop retinal flow (8).

Vasculature

Arterial Supply

The four divisions of the optic nerve head correlate roughly with a four-part vascular supply (Fig. 5.2).

The surface nerve fiber layer is mainly supplied by arteriolar branches of the central retinal artery (9), which anastomose with vessels of the prelaminar region (10) and are continuous with the peripapillary retinal and long radial peripapillary capillaries (4). One or more of the ciliary-derived vessels from the prelaminar region may occasionally enlarge to form cilioretinal arteries (4).

The prelaminar and laminar regions are supplied primarily by short posterior ciliary arteries which form a peri-

neural, circular arterial anastomosis at the scleral level, called the circle of Zinn-Haller (4, 9–11). Branches from this circle penetrate the optic nerve to supply the prelaminar and laminar regions and the peripapillary choroid. The circle is not present in all eyes, in which case direct branches from the short posterior ciliary arteries supply the anterior optic nerve. The peripapillary choroid may also make a minimal contribution to anterior optic nerve (4, 9–11).

The retrolaminar region is supplied by both the ciliary and retinal circulations, with the former coming from recurrent pial vessels. Medial and lateral paraoptic short posterior ciliary arteries anastomose to form an elliptical arterial circle around the optic nerve, which has also been referred to as the circle of Zinn-Haller (12). This perioptic nerve arteriolar anastomoses, which supplies the retrolaminar optic nerve, was found to be complete in 75% of 18 human eyes in one study (12). The central retinal artery provides centripetal branches from the pial system and frequently, but not always, gives off centrifugal vessels (13). A "central optic nerve artery" was once described as a branch of the ophthalmic artery, supplying the axial portion of the optic nerve

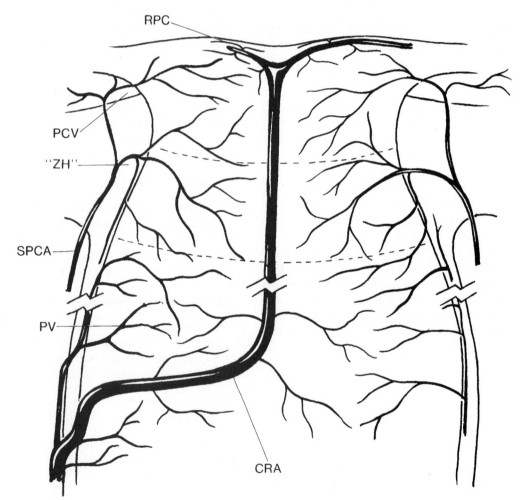

Figure 5.2. Vascular supply of the optic nerve head: central retinal artery (CRA); radial peripapillary capillaries (RPC); pial vessels (PV); short posterior ciliary arteries (SPCA); peripapillary choroidal vessels (PCV); "circle" of Zinn-Haller (ZH).

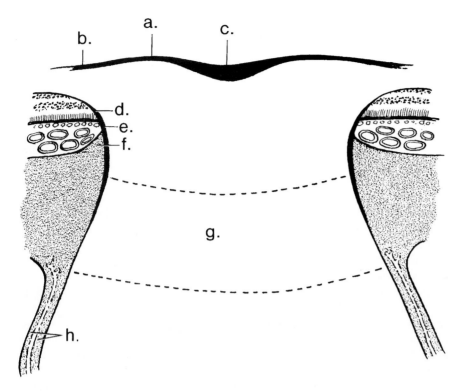

Figure 5.3. Supportive structures of the optic nerve head: internal limiting membrane of Elschnig *(a)*; continuous with the internal limiting membrane of the retina *(b)*; central meniscus of Kuhnt *(c)*; intermediary tissue of Kuhnt *(d)*; border tissue of Jacoby *(e)*; border tissue of Elschnig *(f)*; lamina cribrosa *(g)*; meningeal sheaths *(h)*.

(14). This structure has not been confirmed in subsequent studies, but may represent a rare variant of the normal anatomy (13).

A continuity between small vessels from the retrolaminar region to the retinal surface has been observed (10), and the optic nerve head microvasculature is said to represent an integral part of the retina-optic nerve vascular system (11).

Capillaries

Although derived from both the retinal and ciliary circulations, the capillaries of the optic nerve head resemble more closely the features of retinal capillaries than of the choriocapillaris. These characteristics include (a) tight junctions, (b) abundant pericytes, and (c) nonfenestrated endothelium (11). They do not leak fluorescein and may represent a nerve-blood barrier, supporting the concept of the retina-nerve vasculature as a continuous system with the central nervous system (10, 11). The capillaries become fewer behind the lamina, especially along the margins of the larger vessels (15).

Venous Drainage

The venous return in the optic nerve head is almost entirely by the central retinal vein (9), although some blood may enter the choroidal system, thereby establishing another communication between the retina and choroid (4). Occasionally, these communications are enlarged as retinociliary veins, which drain from the retina to the choroidal circulation, or cilio-optic veins, which drain from the choroid to the central retinal vein (16).

Astroglial Support

Astrocytes provide a continuous layer between the neurons and blood vessels in the optic nerve head (17). In the Rhesus monkey, astrocytes occupy 5% of the nerve fiber layer, but increase to 23% of the laminar region, and then decrease to 11% in the retrolaminar area (5). The astrocytes are joined by "gap junctions," which resemble tight junctions, but have minute gaps between the outer membrane leaflets (18).

The astroglial tissue also provides a covering for portions of the optic nerve head (Fig. 5.3). The *internal limiting membrane of Elschnig* separates the nerve head from the vitreous and is continuous with the internal limiting membrane of the retina (17, 19–21). The central portion of the internal limiting membrane is referred to as the *central meniscus of Kuhnt* (20). Although the central meniscus of Kuhnt is traditionally described as a central thickening of the internal limiting membrane, ultrastructural studies of the monkey optic nerve head revealed a thinning of 20 nm centrally, which thickened to 70 nm peripherally (21). The *intermediary tissue of Kuhnt* separates the nerve from the retina, while the *border tissue of Jacoby* separates the nerve from the choroid (6, 20).

Collagen Support

Lamina Cribrosa

This structure consists of fenestrated sheets of connective tissue and occasional elastic fibers lined by astrocytes (6).

There are regional differences in the fenestration or pores through which the axons pass. The superior and inferior portions, as compared to the nasal and temporal regions, have larger single pore areas, summed pore areas, thinner connective tissue, and glial cell support (Fig. 5.4) (22–25). The ratio of single and summed pore areas between the laminar regions decreases with increasing lamina cribrosa size, but does not correlate with age or sex (25). The possible significance of these regional differences to the mechanism of glaucomatous optic atrophy is discussed later in this chapter. The size of the laminar openings for the retinal vessels does not correlate with the lamina cribrosa size (25).

The lamina cribrosa of the human optic nerve head contains a specialized *extracellular matrix* composed of collagen types I through VI, laminin, and fibronectin (26–28). Studies of young human donor eyes show that the cribriform plates are composed of a core of elastin fibers with a sparse, patchy distribution of collagen type III, coated with collagen type IV and laminin (29). Cell cultures of human lamina cribrosa revealed two cell types, which appear to synthesize this extracellular matrix (30). The expression of mRNA for collagen types I and IV in both fetal and adult human optic nerve heads suggests that these extracellular matrix proteins are synthesized in this tissue throughout life (31). Proteoglycans, which are macromolecular components of connective tissue, believed to have a role in the organization of other extracellular matrix components and in the hydration and rigidity of tissue, have been identified within the cores of the laminar plates in association with collagen fibers (32, 33). Abnormalities of this extracellular matrix in the lamina cribrosa may influence optic nerve function and its susceptibility to glaucomatous damage by elevated IOP.

A rim of connective tissue, the *border tissue of Elschnig,* occasionally extends between the choroid and optic nerve tissues, especially temporally (Fig. 5.3) (20). Posterior to the globe, the optic nerve is surrounded by meningeal sheaths (pia, arachnoid, and dura), which consist of connective tissue lined by meningothelial cells, or mesothelium (34). Vascularized connective tissue extends from the undersurface of the pia mater to form longitudinal septa, which partially separate the axonal bundles in the intraorbital portion of the optic nerve (20).

Axons

Retinal Nerve Fiber Layer

As the axons traverse the nerve fiber layer from the ganglion cell bodies to the optic nerve head, they are distributed in a characteristic pattern (Fig. 5.5). Fibers from the temporal periphery originate on either side of a horizontal dividing line, the median raphe, and arch above or below the fovea as the *arcuate nerve fibers,* while those from the central retina, the *papillomacular fibers,* and the nasal fibers take a more direct path to the nerve head. The significance of this anatomy to the visual field defects of glaucoma is discussed in Chapter 6. The axons in monkeys and rabbits are grouped into fiber bundles by tissue tunnels composed of elongated processes of Muller cells (35–37). These bundles, especially on the temporal side, become larger as they approach the nerve head, primarily due to lateral fusion of bundles (38), and are normally visible by ophthalmoscopy as retinal striations (37). The axons within the bundles vary in size, with larger fibers coming from the more peripheral retina (38).

Axons in Optic Nerve Head

The arcuate nerve fibers occupy the superior and inferior temporal portions of the optic nerve head, with axons from the peripheral retina taking a more peripheral position in the nerve head (Fig. 5.6) (39). The arcuate fibers are the most susceptible to early glaucomatous damage. The papillomacular fibers spread over approximately one-third of the distal optic nerve, primarily inferior temporally where the axonal density is higher (40, 41). They intermingle with extramacular fibers, which may explain the retention of central vision during early glaucomatous optic atrophy.

Reports of the mean axonal population in the normal human optic nerve head range from 693,316 to 1,158,000 when using computerized image analysis of sections throughout the nerve (41–44). All studies agree that there is a large variability of axonal numbers among normal eyes of

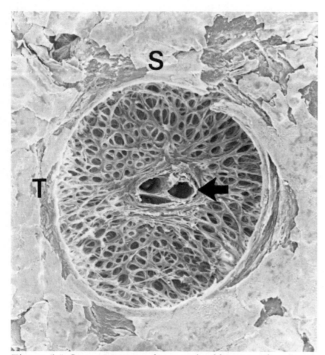

Figure 5.4. Gross anatomic photograph of lamina cribrosa showing central openings for central retinal vessels *(arrow)* and surrounding fenestrae of lamina for passage of axon bundles. Note larger size of fenestrae in superior and inferior quadrants. Superior *(S)*, temporal *(T)*. (Courtesy of Harry A. Quigley, M.D.)

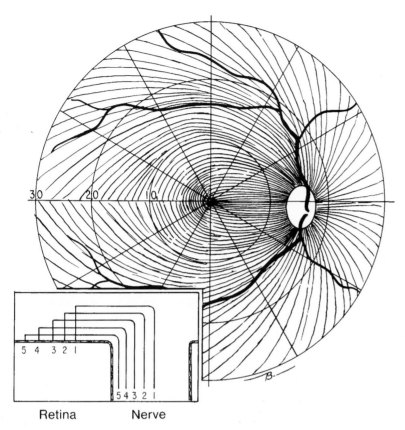

Figure 5.5. Distribution of retinal nerve fibers. Note arching above and below the fovea of fibers temporal to the optic nerve head. Inset depicts cross-sectional arrangement of axons, with fibers originating from peripheral retina running closer to choroid and periphery of optic nerve, while fibers originating nearer to the nerve head are situated closer to the vitreous and occupy a more central portion of the nerve.

approximately $\pm$ 200,000 fibers. The optic nerve fiber count has been shown to increase significantly with the optic nerve area in human (44) and monkey (45) eyes, although another study of human eyes failed to show such a correlation (43). A positive correlation has also been demonstrated between the retinal photoreceptor count and optic nerve area (46). The reported mean axonal fiber diameter ranges from 0.65 to 1.10 μm (41, 42, 47). Axons of all sizes are mixed throughout the nerve area, although higher mean diameters appear to be more common in the nasal segment (41).

Influence of Age

The optic nerve cross-sectional area reaches 50% of the adult size by 20 weeks gestation, 75% at birth, and 95% before 1 year of age (48). At birth, the optic nerve is nearly unmyelinated (49), and myelination, which proceeds from the brain to the eye during gestation, is largely completed in the retrolaminar region of the optic nerve by the first year of life (50). The connective tissue of the lamina cribrosa is also incompletely developed at birth, which may account for the greater susceptibility of the infant nerve head to glaucomatous cupping, as well as its potential for reversible cupping (51). With increasing age, the cores of the cribriform plates enlarge, and there is an increase in the apparent density of collagen types I, III, and IV and elastin (52, 53). Not only does elastin increase with age, but elastic fibers become

thicker, tubular, and surrounded by densely packed collagen fibers (53). Proteoglycans filaments in the human lamina cribrosa also decrease in length and diameter with age (54). Also with increasing age, there appears to be a progressive loss of axons and a corresponding increase in the cross-sectional area occupied by the leptomeninges and fibrous septa (41–44). The loss of axons has been estimated to be between 4000 and 12,000 per year, with most studies nearer the lower figure (41, 43, 44). One study suggested a selective loss of large nerve fibers with age (42), although this has not been confirmed by others (41, 47).

PATHOGENESIS OF GLAUCOMATOUS OPTIC ATROPHY[b]

Theories

The pathogenesis of glaucomatous optic atrophy has remained a matter of controversy since the mid-19th century when two concepts were introduced in the same year. In 1858, Muller (55) proposed that the elevated IOP led to direct compression and death of the neurons (the mechanical theory), while von Jaeger (56) suggested that a vascular

[b]Refer to Shields, MB: Color Atlas of Glaucoma. Baltimore, Williams & Wilkins, 1998, Plates II1–23.

abnormality was the underlying cause of the optic atrophy (the vascular theory). In 1892, Schnabel (57) proposed another concept in the pathogenesis of glaucomatous optic atrophy, suggesting that atrophy of neural elements created empty spaces, which pulled the nerve head posteriorly (Schnabel's cavernous atrophy).

Initially, the mechanical theory received the greatest support (58–60). This concept held sway through the first quarter of the 20th century until LaGrange and Beauvieux (61) popularized the vascular theory in 1925. In general, this belief held that glaucomatous optic atrophy was secondary to ischemia, whether the primary result of the elevated IOP or an unrelated vascular lesion (62–64). In 1968, however, the role of axoplasmic flow in glaucomatous optic atrophy was introduced (65), which revived support for the mechanical theory, but did not exclude the possible influence of ischemia.

Evidence

Continued investigation into the pathogenesis of glaucomatous optic atrophy has led to the following bodies of information.

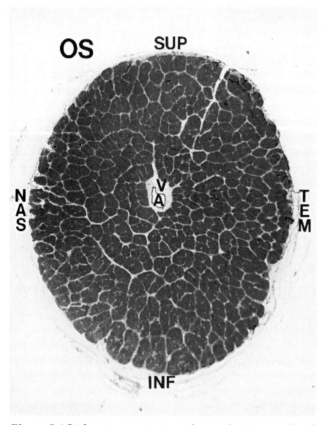

Figure 5.6. Light microscopic view of normal optic nerve head on cross-section with darkly-staining axon bundles and intervening glial supportive tissue surrounding openings for central retinal vessels. Superior *(SUP)*; temporal *(TEM)*. (Courtesy of Harry A. Quigley, M.D.)

Anatomic and Histopathologic Studies

Histopathologic observations of human eyes with glaucoma provide the most direct method of studying the alterations associated with glaucomatous optic atrophy, although they do not fully explain the mechanisms that caused the damage. One of the limiting factors has been that many of the specimens studied have come from eyes with advanced glaucomatous change, which led to possible misconceptions regarding the early pathogenic features. More recent studies, which have attempted to correlate clinical observations with histopathologic changes in optic nerve heads from eyes with varying stages of glaucoma, appear to clarify many of these points.

GLIAL ALTERATIONS. It was once suggested that loss of astroglial supportive tissue precedes neuronal loss (66), which was thought to explain the early and reversible cupping in infants (67). However, subsequent studies have shown that glial cells are not selectively lost in early glaucoma and are actually the only remaining cells after loss of axons in advanced cases (68, 69).

VASCULAR ALTERATIONS. It was also once proposed that loss of small vessels in the optic nerve head accompanies atrophy of axons (70), and one histologic study suggested a selective loss of retinal radial peripapillary capillaries in eyes with chronic glaucoma (71). However, subsequent investigations revealed neither a correlation between atrophy of this vascular system and visual field loss (72), nor a major selective loss of optic nerve head capillaries in human eyes with glaucoma (68, 69, 73). In animal models of optic atrophy, created by either sustained IOP elevation (73), sectioning of the optic nerve (74–76) or photocoagulation of the retinal nerve fiber layer (77), the resulting disc pallor was not associated with a decrease in the ratio of capillaries to neural tissue, although the caliber of the vessels diminished (76). Instead, these studies showed a proliferation (75) or reorganization (74, 77) of glial tissue, which obscures ophthalmoscopic visualization of the vessels.

ALTERATIONS OF LAMINA CRIBROSA. Backward bowing of the lamina cribrosa has long been recognized as a characteristic feature of late glaucomatous optic atrophy (78, 79), as well as an early change in the infant eye with glaucoma (51). Further study, however, has suggested that alterations in the lamina may actually be a primary event in the pathogenesis of glaucomatous optic atrophy. In enucleated human eyes, acute IOP elevation caused a backward bowing of the lamina (80, 81), and similar changes have been observed in primate glaucoma models (82, 83). The majority of the posterior displacement occurred in the peripheral lamina cribrosa, corresponding to the region of early axonal loss (81). In a histopathologic evaluation of 25 glaucomatous human eyes, compression of successive lamina cribrosa sheets was the earliest detected abnormality, while backward bowing of the

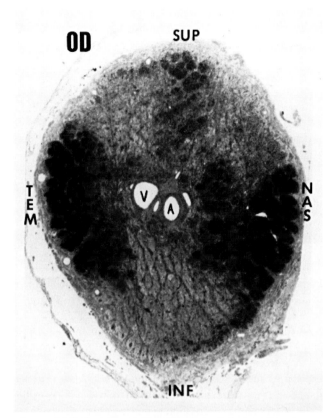

Figure 5.7. Light microscopic cross-sectional view of optic nerve head with glaucomatous atrophy showing loss of axon bundles predominantly in the inferior and superior quadrants (compare with normal nerve head in Fig. 5.6). Superior *(SUP)*; temporal *(TEM)*. (Courtesy of Harry A. Quigley, M.D.)

entire lamina occurred later and involved primarily the upper and lower poles (84).

In the early stages of adult glaucoma, the magnitude of backward bowing is not sufficient to explain the ophthalmoscopically observed cupping, but may be enough to cause compression of the axons, and it has been suggested that the structure of the lamina cribrosa may be an important determinant in the susceptibility of the optic nerve head to damage from elevated IOP (68, 69). A racial comparison of the relative connective tissue support and regional pore size of the lamina cribrosa did not explain the greater susceptibility of blacks to glaucomatous damage (85). The extracellular matrix of the lamina cribrosa may play an important role in the progression of glaucomatous damage (86–88). In glaucomatous monkey eyes, increased collagen type IV and laminin lined the margins of the laminar beams (87, 88), and collagen types I, III, and IV were found in the pores of the beams (87). Elastin, which is the major protein of elastic fibers and responsible for elastic recoil, appeared curled instead of straight and seemed disconnected from other elements of the connective tissue matrix in glaucomatous eyes of humans and monkeys (89), and elastin mRNA expression in human eyes with open-angle glaucoma suggests synthesis

of abnormal elastic fibers (90). These changes may be secondary to long-standing elevation of IOP and may modify the course of glaucomatous optic atrophy.

AXONAL ALTERATIONS. The actual cause of early optic nerve head cupping in glaucoma is loss of axonal tissue (68, 69, 91). Experimental models of primate eyes exposed to chronic IOP elevation suggest that the damage is associated with a posterior and lateral displacement of the lamina cribrosa, which compresses the axons (92). The damage first involves axonal bundles throughout the nerve with somewhat greater involvement of the inferior and superior poles (84). With continued nerve damage, the susceptibility of the polar zones becomes more prominent (Fig. 5.7) (68, 69, 84, 91). Histologic studies of both monkey (93) and human (94) optic nerves indicate that nerve fibers larger than the normal mean diameter atrophy more rapidly in glaucomatous eyes, although no fiber size is spared from damage. This preferential loss of large fibers appears to be due to a higher proportion of the fibers in the inferior and superior poles, as well as an inherent susceptibility to injury by glaucoma (93, 94).

In the retina of glaucomatous monkey eyes, there is also a selective loss of the larger ganglion cells in both the midperiphery (95) and fovea (96), and it has been suggested that psychophysical testing should be aimed at these cells in the early stages of glaucoma (95, 96). The same animal studies suggest that some retinal ganglion cells in glaucoma die by apoptosis, a genetically programmed process of cell death, possibly related to loss of trophic influences due to inhibited transmission of neurotrophic signals from axon terminals to neuronal cell bodies, and characterized histologically by chromatin condensation and intracellular fragmentation (97). Histologic studies have also shown a significant decrease of corpora amylacea, homogeneous oval bodies believed to correlate with axonal degeneration, in retinal ganglion cells and the optic nerve of human eyes with advancing stages of glaucoma (98, 99). One study revealed a significant reduction in photoreceptor count in human eyes with angle closure glaucoma associated with trauma (100), although this was not observed in human eyes with chronic open-angle glaucoma (101) nor in monkey eyes with experimental glaucoma (102).

Studies of Blood Flow

Blood flow in the optic nerve head of cats is relatively high compared to that in more posterior portions of the nerve, and autoregulation appears to compensate for alterations in mean arterial blood pressure (103). With elevation of IOP, blood flow in the optic nerve head, retina, and choroid of cat eyes is only slightly affected before the pressure is within 25 mm Hg of the mean arterial blood pressure, and flow in the lamina cribrosa is reduced only with extreme pressure elevations, again suggesting autoregulation in the optic nerve head (104). Another study, however, suggests that the electrical function of ganglion cell axons in cat eyes depends on the perfusion pressure and not on the absolute height of the IOP

(105). Real-time analysis of optic nerve head oxidative metabolism in cats indicates that the metabolic response is dependent on IOP and/or mean arterial pressure and that lowering the IOP can reverse metabolic dysfunction (106).

Short-term IOP elevation in monkey eyes did not alter optic nerve head blood flow until it exceeded 75 mm Hg, and long-term glaucoma in monkeys had no apparent influence on mean blood flow in the nerve head (107). A study of oxygen tension in the monkey optic nerve head suggested that autoregulation compensates for changes in perfusion pressure (108), and a noninvasive phosphorescence imaging technique in cats revealed well maintained oxygen tension in the optic nerve head and retina despite increasing IOP, until blood flow to the eye was stopped (109). Blood flow measurements in the optic nerve head of human eyes, using laser Doppler, also demonstrated autoregulatory compensation to reduced perfusion pressure secondary to elevated IOP (110). In glaucomatous eyes, however, Doppler studies show reduced flow velocity in the nerve head (111–114). A technique of continuously monitoring disc brightness during and after an abrupt artificial elevation of IOP also showed that the extent to which a glaucomatous eye can adjust to the pressure changes is significantly reduced from that of nonglaucomatous eyes (115). Age may influence the vascular responses to IOP. One study showed that major retinal vessels at the disc border increased in caliber in response to IOP reduction in patients with chronic open-angle glaucoma who were 55 years or younger, but not after that age (116). It may be, therefore, that ischemia of the optic nerve head in glaucoma involves faculty autoregulation, which may worsen with age.

Fluorescein Angiographic Observations

NORMAL FLUORESCEIN PATTERN. The normal fluorescein pattern of the optic nerve head is usually described as having three phases (4): (a) An initial filling, or preretinal arterial, phase is felt to represent filling of the prelaminar and lamina cribrosa regions by the posterior ciliary arteries. Fluorescein in the retrobulbar vessels may also contribute to this phase (117). (b) The peak fluorescence, or retinal arteriovenous phase, is primarily due to filling of the dense capillary plexus on the nerve head surface from retinal arterioles. With increasing age, there is a decrease in the filling time of both the retinal and choroidal circulations (118). (c) A late phase consists of 10–15 minutes of delayed staining of the nerve head, which is probably due to fluorescein in the connective tissue of the lamina cribrosa. Tracer studies in monkeys suggest the leakage may come from the adjacent choroid (119).

EFFECT OF ARTIFICIALLY ELEVATED INTRAOCULAR PRESSURE. The effect of artificially elevated IOP on the fluorescein angiographic pattern has provided an understanding of the relative vulnerability of ocular vessels to elevated pressure in the normal and glaucomatous eye. There is a general delay in the entire ocular circulation in response to an elevation of the IOP. The prelaminar portion of the nerve head appears to be the most vulnerable portion of the ocular vascular system to elevated pressure in monkeys (4, 120).

Studies regarding the vulnerability of the peripapillary choroid to IOP elevation have provided conflicting results. Fluorescein angiography of monkey eyes has suggested a marked susceptibility of this vascular system to elevated pressure (4, 120) and fluorescein studies of human eyes with glaucoma have shown similar delays in peripapillary choroidal filling (120–124). The delay appears to be sensitive to elevated IOP (121). It has been suggested that this vascular disturbance of the peripapillary choroid contributes to glaucomatous optic atrophy (123). However, fluorescein angiographic studies of normal human eyes have shown similar delayed or irregular choroidal filling at normal pressures (125, 126), and the peripapillary choroidal capillaries of normal human eyes were relatively resistant to artificial pressure elevations (127). Furthermore, a fluorescein study of patients with low-tension or chronic open-angle glaucoma provided no evidence that hypoperfusion of the peripapillary choroid contributed to optic nerve hypoperfusion (128).

A selective nonfilling of the retinal radial peripapillary capillaries during India ink perfusion has been demonstrated in cats (129). As previously discussed, however, histopathologic observations are conflicting with regard to alterations of this vascular system in glaucomatous eyes (71, 72). Most studies of monkey (4, 120) and normal human eyes (130, 131) have shown the choroidal circulation in general to be more vulnerable than that of the retina to elevated IOP, although one study found the two systems to fill at the same level of increased pressure (132).

STUDIES OF GLAUCOMATOUS EYES. Fluorescein angiographic studies of glaucomatous and nonglaucomatous eyes have revealed two types of filling defects of the optic nerve head: (a) persisting hypoperfusion and (b) transient hypoperfusion (133, 134).

Persisting hypoperfusion, or absolute filling defects, are more common in eyes with glaucoma, especially low-tension glaucoma, and are said to correlate with visual field loss (133–135). The characteristics of a filling defect include decreased blood flow, a smaller vascular bed, narrower vessels, and increased permeability of the vessels (136). The filling defect may be either focal or diffuse. The former is felt to reflect susceptible vasculature with or without elevated IOP and is the typical defect in low-tension glaucoma (128). Focal defects occur primarily in the inferior and superior poles of the optic nerve head (133–135, 137). In glaucomatous eyes, they are most often seen in the wall of the cup, while in normal eyes they occur more commonly in the floor of the cup (138). The diffuse defect is felt to represent prolonged pressure elevation (128).

Patients with ocular hypertension (elevated IOP, but normal optic nerve heads and visual fields) have more filling defects than the normal population, although fewer than in eyes with glaucoma (135, 139). The only other condition reported to give absolute filling defects is sectorial ischemic optic neuropathy (140). However, the nature of the defect in open-angle glaucoma is felt to be specific, and it has been suggested that fluorescein angiography of the optic nerve head may help to differentiate open-angle glaucoma from other conditions that have similar clinical changes in the optic disc (140). A correlation between vascular changes of the optic nerve head and visual field loss in glaucoma has not been fully established. However, it has been reported that the development of new visual field defects is associated with changes in the optic nerve head circulation, as determined by fluorescein angiography (141). Computerized image analysis has been used to objectively quantify fluorescein angiograms of the optic disc and has shown that increases in fluorescein-filling defect areas correlate with glaucomatous progression (142).

Transient hypoperfusion, or relative (delayed) filling defects, are seen in the normal population and do not correlate with optic nerve head or visual field changes (133–135). However, it has been postulated that they may progress to absolute defects, which is felt to provide a sign of impending field loss (135). One fluorescein angiographic study revealed fluorescein leakage of the optic nerve head associated with advanced glaucomatous optic atrophy in 9 of 150 patients with chronic open-angle glaucoma (143). Staining of the nerve head was seen in 30% of glaucomatous eyes in another fluorescein study (133, 134). Fluorescein angiograms have also been used to study blood flow in glaucomatous eyes, which revealed decreased flow in eyes with elevated IOP and also in two cases of low tension glaucoma (144).

Observations of Axoplasmic Flow

PHYSIOLOGY OF AXOPLASMIC FLOW. Axoplasmic flow, or axonal transport, refers to the movement of material (axoplasm) along the axon of a nerve (the dendrite may also have transport) in a predictable, energy-dependent manner. This movement has been characterized as having fast and slow components, although numerous intermediate rates may also exist (145). The fast phase moves approximately 410 mm/day in various species and may supply material to synaptic vesicles, the axolemma, and agranular endoplasmic reticulum of the axon, while the slow phase moves at 1–3 mm/day and is believed to subserve growth and maintenance of axons (145). The flow of axoplasm may be orthograde (from retina to lateral geniculate body) or retrograde (lateral geniculate body to retina) (146).

EXPERIMENTAL MODELS OF AXOPLASMIC FLOW. Animal models (usually in monkeys) have been developed for studying axoplasmic flow by injecting radioactive amino acids, such as tritiated leucine, into the vitreous. The amino acid is incorporated into the protein synthesis of retinal ganglion cells and then moves down the ganglion cell axon into the optic nerve, allowing histologic study of the orthograde movement of radioactively-labeled protein (147). In addition, retrograde flow can be studied by observing the accumulation of certain unlabeled neuronal components such as mitochondria by electron microscopy (148), or by injecting tracer elements such as horseradish peroxidase into the lateral geniculate body and studying its movement toward the retina (149). These models can be used to study factors that cause abnormal blockade of axoplasmic flow, which may relate to glaucomatous optic atrophy in the human eye.

INFLUENCE OF INTRAOCULAR PRESSURE ON AXOPLASMIC FLOW. Elevated IOP in monkey eyes causes obstruction of axoplasmic flow at the lamina cribrosa (146, 150–155) and the edge of the posterior scleral foramen (155). Axonal transport in monkey eyes with chronic IOP elevation is also preferentially decreased in the magnocellular layers of the dorsal lateral geniculate nucleus, to which the large retinal ganglion cells project (156). The obstruction in general involves both the fast (151, 154) and slow (151) phases, as well as the orthograde and retrograde components (146, 153). In monkey eyes, the obstruction to fast axonal transport preferentially involves the superior, temporal, and inferior portions of the optic nerve head (157). The height and duration of pressure elevation influence the onset, distribution, and degree of axoplasmic obstruction in the optic nerve head (154, 158, 159). The mechanism by which elevated IOP leads to obstruction of axoplasmic flow is uncertain, but there are two popular theories: mechanical and vascular.

The mechanical theory suggests that physical alterations in the optic nerve head, such as a misalignment of the fenestrae in the lamina cribrosa due to its backbowing, may lead to the axoplasmic flow obstruction (65, 79, 154). In support of this hypothesis is the observation that elevated IOP leads to blockage of axonal transport despite an intact nerve head capillary circulation and an elevated arterial pO$_2$ (146, 160). Furthermore, obstruction of axoplasmic flow has also been reported in response to ocular hypotony (151, 153, 161), leading some investigators to suggest that a pressure differential across the optic nerve head, whether due to a relative increase or decrease in IOP, causes mechanical changes with compression of the axonal bundles (151, 153, 161, 162).

In conflict with the mechanical theory is the observation that elevated intracranial pressure in monkeys neither caused obstruction of rapid axoplasmic flow, nor prevented it in response to elevated IOP despite reduction in the pressure gradient across the lamina (163). This suggests that more than a simple mechanical or hydrostatic mechanism may be involved with obstruction of axoplasmic flow in response to elevated IOP (163). Also against the simple mechanical theory are the observations that axon damage is diffuse within bundles, rather than focal as might be expected with a kinking effect (164), and the location of transport interruption does not correlate with the cross-section area of fiber bundles, the shape of the laminar pores, nor the density of interbundle septa (165, 166).

The vascular theory suggests that ischemia at least plays a role in the obstruction of axoplasmic flow in response to elevated IOP. Interruption of the short posterior ciliary arteries in monkeys has been reported to block both slow (167, 168) and fast (169) axoplasmic flow, although it did not cause glaucomatous cupping (167, 168). Central retinal artery occlusion has been associated with obstruction of both rapid orthograde and retrograde axonal transport (170). Furthermore, accumulation of tracer at the lamina cribrosa was inversely proportional to the perfusion pressure in cat eyes (171), and IOP-induced blockage of axonal transport was greater in eyes with angiotensin-induced systemic hypertension (172). It has also been noted in monkey eyes with elevated IOP that leakage from microvasculature of the nerve head was associated with blockade of axonal transport at the lamina cribrosa (173).

Against a vascular mechanism for pressure-induced obstruction of axoplasmic flow is the observation that ligation of the right common carotid artery in monkeys, which reduced the estimated ophthalmic artery pressure by 10–20 mm Hg below the left side, did not significantly affect the extent to which IOP elevation interrupted axonal transport (174). When obstruction to retrograde axoplasmic flow was studied in enucleated rat eyes, a direct relationship with IOP was still found despite removing the influence of the blood circulation and the fact that the lamina cribrosa is only a single laminar sheet (149). It may be, therefore, that factors other than, or in addition to, ischemia and kinking of axons by a multilayered lamina cribrosa are involved in the intraocular pressure-induced obstruction to axoplasmic flow.

Electrophysiologic Studies

When the intraocular tension is artificially elevated in normal human eyes, a significant reduction in the amplitudes of electroretinographic components (175, 176) and visual-evoked potentials (176) occurs only when the pressure approaches or exceeds the ophthalmic blood pressure. However, the perfusion-pressure amplitude curve of the visual evoked potential in normal eyes showed a kink, suggestive of vascular autoregulation, which was not observed in glaucoma patients (177), again pointing to a possible deficiency in autoregulation in glaucoma. As previously noted, the electrical function of retinal ganglion cells in cat eyes was found to depend more on perfusion pressure than the absolute height of the IOP (105).

Comparison with Nonglaucomatous Disorders

Studies of other ocular disorders provide some indirect insight into the possible mechanism of glaucomatous optic atrophy. For example, a histopathologic study of severe peripapillary choroidal atrophy revealed a normal optic nerve head, suggesting that the vascular supply of these two structures may be independent (178). Studies of nonglaucomatous optic atrophy have been used both to support and to refute an ischemic basis for glaucomatous optic atrophy. In

patients with *anterior ischemic optic neuropathy,* cupping similar to that seen in glaucoma is frequently observed when the ischemia is due to giant cell arteritis, but is less common in nonarteritic cases (179–181). These observations have led to the suggestion that glaucoma and anterior ischemic optic neuropathy have the same vasogenic basis of optic nerve damage, but differ according to the rate of change (179). It has also been suggested that acute ischemic optic neuropathy may be one of several mechanisms of optic nerve disease in chronic glaucoma (182). If this is true, the difference in visual field loss suggests that there is also a difference in the nature or distribution of the ischemia (181). In addition, the pattern of optic nerve fiber loss in nonarteritic anterior ischemia optic neuropathy involves primarily the superior half of the nerve and is unlike that found in glaucoma (183).

In contrast to the above studies, a review of 170 eyes with nonglaucomatous optic atrophy of various etiologies revealed a small, but significant increase in cupping (184). However, the cups were morphologically different than those seen in glaucoma, which was suggested as evidence against a vascular etiology in glaucomatous cupping. Furthermore, a study of 18 patients with vasogenic shock and poor peripheral tissue perfusion revealed no evidence of glaucomatous optic nerve head or visual field change (185).

Cavernous atrophy of the optic nerve, as originally described by Schnabel (57), has been considered to be a form of glaucomatous optic atrophy due to severe elevations of IOP. However, this also occurs in patients with normal pressures, in which case it may represent an aging change associated with generalized arteriosclerosis (186).

Conclusions

The present evidence suggests that obstruction to axoplasmic flow may be involved in the pathogenesis of glaucomatous optic atrophy. However, it is still not clear as to whether mechanical or vascular factors are primarily responsible for this obstruction, and whether other alterations are also important in the ultimate loss of axons. It may be that all of these factors are involved to some degree or, as Spaeth (133, 134) has suggested, that there is more than one mechanism of optic atrophy in eyes with glaucoma. For example, the observed differences in glaucomatous visual field defects between patients with low-tension and high-tension glaucomas has led to the suggestion that ischemia may be the predominant factor in those glaucomas at the lower end of the IOP scale, while a more direct mechanical effect of the pressure may prevail in cases with higher IOP (Fig. 5.8) (187).

CLINICAL APPEARANCE OF GLAUCOMATOUS OPTIC ATROPHY

While investigators continue to study the pathophysiology of glaucomatous optic atrophy, the practicing physician has

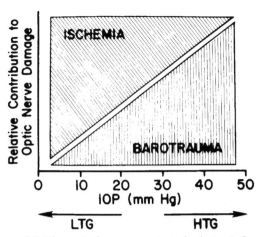

Figure 5.8. Theoretical representation of relative influence exerted by mechanical and vascular forces on the development of glaucomatous optic atrophy at different levels of intraocular pressure. (Reprinted with permission from Caprioli, J, Spaeth, GL: Comparison of visual field defects in the low-tension glaucomas with those in the high-tension glaucomas. Am J Ophthalmol 97:730, 1984.)

a responsibility to become thoroughly familiar with the clinical morphology of this condition, since it provides the most reliable early evidence of damage in glaucoma.

Morphology of the Normal Optic Nerve Head

In order to recognize pathologic alterations of the optic nerve head, one must first be familiar with the wide range of normal variations.

General Features

The ophthalmoscopic appearance of the optic nerve head is generally that of a vertical oval, although there is considerable variation in size and shape. Clinical studies have revealed a greater than six-fold difference in the area of normal nerve heads (188, 189), which is consistent with histologic studies cited earlier (1–3). The central portion of the disc usually contains a depression, the *cup,* and an area of *pallor,* which represents a partial or complete absence of axons, with exposure of the lamina cribrosa. While the size and location of cup and pallor are normally the same, it is important to note that this is not always the case, especially in disease states (190), and these two parameters should not be thought of as being synonymous. The tissue between the cup and disc margins is referred to as the *neural rim.* It represents the location of the bulk of the axons and normally has an orange-red color, due to the associated capillaries. Retinal vessels ride up the nasal wall of the cup, often kinking at the cup margin before crossing the neural rim to the retina (Figs. 5.9 and 5.10).

Physiologic Cup

SIZE. The size of the optic nerve head cup, which is commonly described as the horizontal cup/disc ratio (C/D), varies considerably within the normal population, which appears to be explained by the normal variation in disc diameter (3). Reports of C/D distribution within the general population differ according to examination techniques. When the discs were studied by direct ophthalmoscopy, the distribution was found to be non-Gaussion with most eyes having a C/D of 0.0–0.3 and only 1–2% being 0.7 or greater (191). However, when stereoscopic views were utilized, a Gaussian distribution was found with a mean C/D of 0.4 and approximately 5% with 0.7 (192). In another study, the two techniques of optic nerve head evaluation were compared, and stereoscopic examination with a Hruby lens gave consistently larger C/D estimates with a mean of 0.38 as compared to 0.25 by direct ophthalmoscopy (193). These authors noted, however, that the disparity between estimated C/D for the same eye at different times seldom exceeds 0.2, so that the documentation of such a difference over time should be viewed with suspicion (193). It is also important to note that physiologic cups tend to be symmetrical between the two eyes of the same individual (191, 192, 194, 195), with a C/D difference of greater than 0.2 between fellow eyes occurring in only 1% of the normal population (191).

The size of the physiologic cup is frequently similar to that of the individual's parents and siblings (191, 196, 197), and is felt to be genetically determined on a polygenic, multifactorial basis (191, 198). The heritability has been estimated at $\frac{2}{3}$, with the remaining variance attributed to errors of development (197). It is helpful, therefore, to examine other members of the family when attempting to distinguish between a large physiologic cup and glaucomatous cupping. The physiologic C/D does not appear to correlate with a family history of open-angle glaucoma (191, 199), although some studies have suggested a weak correlation with higher IOPs (192, 199–201), abnormal tonographic outflow facilities (199, 200), or highly positive pressure responses to topical corticosteroids (202). Other studies, looking primarily at disc area, showed significantly larger discs in patients with normal-tension glaucoma, as compared to open-angle glaucoma patients or normal controls (203), and suggested that larger discs are more susceptible to glaucomatous damage at normal pressures (204).

Most studies have shown no significant correlation between age and the size of the physiologic cup (189, 191, 196, 199, 205, 206), while other investigations suggest that both the cup (192, 193, 201, 207) and pallor (208) do enlarge slightly with increasing age. One study revealed an age-related decline in disc rim area, consistent with the histologic evidence of the age-related decline of ganglion cell axons, as discussed earlier (41–44), while the C/D and rim area/disc ratios remain relatively constant throughout adult life (209). It is important to note that any enlargement of the

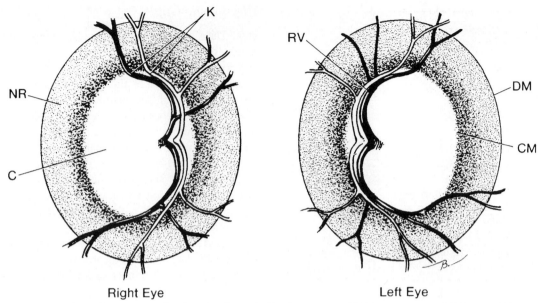

Right Eye   Left Eye

Figure 5.9. Normal optic nerve heads: neural rim (NR); disc margin (DM); cup margin (CM); cup (C); retinal vessels (RV); kinking of vessels at cup margin (K). Note that size of cups is symmetrical between the two eyes and that neural rims are even for 360°.

cup with age is gradual and should not be confused with the more rapid progression of glaucomatous cupping.

Racial differences in optic nerve head parameters have been shown, with black individuals having a larger disc and C/D than whites (206, 210–212). This racial difference has also been demonstrated in children (213). Most studies have found no correlation between cup size and sex (191, 192, 196, 197), although one investigation revealed larger relative areas of pallor in white males than in white females (208), and another showed that men have 2–3% larger discs than women (206). Refractive errors do not appear to correlate with the diameter of the physiologic cup (189, 191, 196, 201, 206), although a study of highly myopic eyes (more than 8.00 diopters) revealed a significant correlation between refraction and disc size (214).

In the differential diagnosis of glaucomatous optic atrophy, it is important to distinguish between a large physiologic cup and glaucomatous enlargement of the cup (Fig. 5.11). One distinguishing feature is symmetry of cup size between right and left eye in the physiologic state, taking into consideration the normal variations as previously discussed. Another helpful feature is the configuration of the cup and neural rim, as well as the appearance of the peripapillary pigmentation and retinal nerve fiber layer (all discussed later in this chapter), which are the same in eyes with either large or normal size physiologic cups (215). The most important feature, however, is the documentation of progressive cup enlargement, which is highly suggestive of glaucoma.

SHAPE. The shape of the physiologic cup is roughly correlated with the shape of the disc, which means that the margins of cup and disc tend to run more or less parallel with each other (216). However, the inferior neural rim is the

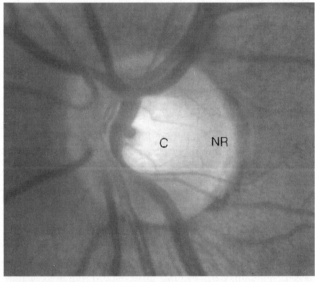

Figure 5.10. Fundus photo of normal optic nerve head. Neural rim (NR); cup (C).

broadest of the four quadrants, followed by the superior, nasal, and temporal rims (189). Consequently, the cup has a horizontally oval shape in the majority of normal eyes, so that a vertical C/D greater than the horizontal C/D should be looked upon with suspicion (189, 193). The three-dimensional contour of the cup varies even more than the two-dimensional configuration in normal eyes. In 1899, Elschnig grouped physiologic cups into the following categories on the basis of configuration, and this classification has subsequently been supported by contour mapping of the optic nerve head surface (Fig. 5.12) (217, 218).

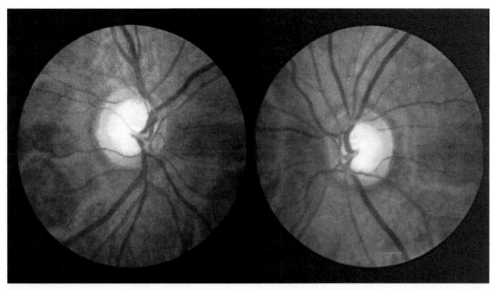

Figure 5.11. Large, physiologic optic nerve head cups, characterized by symmetrical size of cups and intact, even neural rims.

Type I: Small cup with funnel-shaped walls.

Type II: Temporal, cylindrical (steep-walled) cup.

Type III: Central, trough-shaped cup.

Type IV: Temporal or central cup with a well-developed nasal wall, but a temporal wall that gradually slopes to disc margin. This is particularly common along the inferotemporal margin and can be confused with early glaucomatous cupping (219).

Type V: Developmental anomalies (discussed later in this chapter).

The contour of the cup appears to influence the C/D in that cups with steep margins appear to have larger areas than those with temporal flat slopes (189).

Physiologic Neural Rim

By tradition, more is said about the cup than the neural rim of both normal and glaucomatous optic nerve heads. However, it is actually alterations in the neural rim of an eye with glaucoma that leads to changes in the cup as well as to loss of visual field. The C/D is only an indirect measure of the amount of neural tissue in the optic nerve head and may be misleading, since an increasing diameter of the nerve head may be associated with decreasing neural rim width and increasing cup size, despite a stable area of neural tissue (201, 220). It is important, therefore, to pay close attention to the appearance of the neural rim.

As previously noted, the neural rim of the normal optic nerve head is typically broadest in the inferior quadrant, followed by the superior and then the nasal rims, with the temporal rim being the thinnest (189). Several studies have attempted to correlate the area of the neural rim with that of the disc, and there is general agreement that the two are positively correlated, i.e., larger discs have larger neural rim ar-

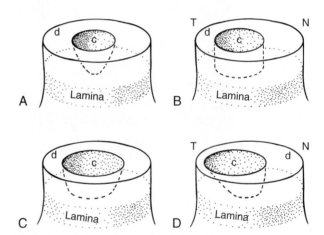

Figure 5.12. Variation in shape of physiologic cups based on classification of Elschnig and subsequent contour mapping (160, 161): A. small funnel-shaped; B. temporal, cylindrical; C. central, trough-shaped; D. steep nasal wall with sloping of temporal wall toward disc margin. Disc (*d*); cup (*c*); temporal (*T*); nasal (*N*).

eas (189, 221–223). However, the contour of the cup influences this correlation, in that the rim area increases by a greater factor with the disc area in discs having cups with flat temporal slopes than those with circular steep cups (223). The increase in neural rim area with increasing disc area appears to be due, at least in part, to a greater number of ganglion cell axons (3).

There are several factors that can interfere with the interpretation of the neural rim width. *A gray crescent in the optic nerve head* has been described, which typically is slate gray and located in the temporal or inferotemporal periphery of the neural rim (224). It is more common in blacks and apparently represents a variation of the normal anatomy. However, mistaking the gray crescent for a peripapillary pigmented crescent could result in the physiologic neural rim being misinterpreted as pathologically thin in that area (Fig. 5.13).

Another source of error in interpreting the neural rim is the *optic nerve head in myopia,* in which the oblique insertion of the nerve may lead to obstruction of the temporal neural rim from ophthalmoscopic view, suggesting pathologic thinning of this tissue (Fig. 5.14). Other features of highly myopic discs that may interfere with interpretation include a larger disc area, a shallower than usual cup, which

may mask the deepening of the cup in glaucoma, and a temporal peripapillary crescent, which may be confused with peripapillary pigmentary changes that are seen more frequently around some glaucomatous discs (214).

As previously noted, the disc rim area declines with age, while the rim area/disc area ratio remains relatively constant (209). In addition, the neural rim declined with increasing IOP in one population-based study (225). It has also been observed that patients with diabetes mellitus may have an increase in the neural rim over time, which the authors felt could be due to nerve swelling (226).

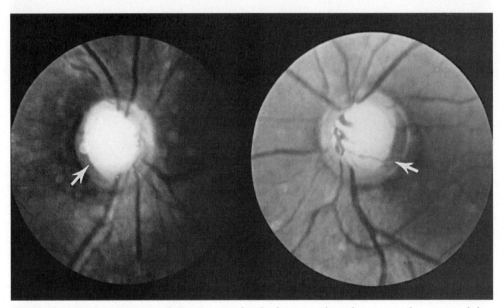

Figure 5.13. Gray crescents in the optic nerve head, obscuring the inferotemporal portions of the neural rims *(arrows).* (Reprinted with permission from Shields, MB: Gray crescent in the optic nerve head. Am J Ophthalmol 89:238, 1980.)

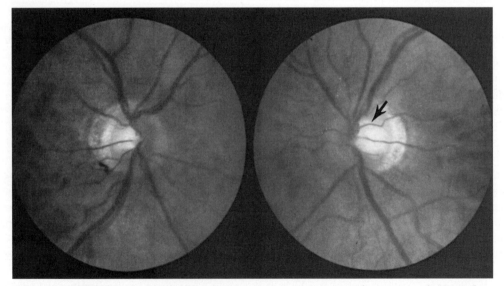

Figure 5.14. Oblique insertion of optic nerve heads in myopic patient obscures visualization of temporal neural rim and creates wide temporal peripapillary crescent, which interferes with distinguishing between physiologic and glaucomatous cupping. In this case, larger cup with baring of circumlinear vessels in left eye *(arrow)* indicates glaucomatous damage.

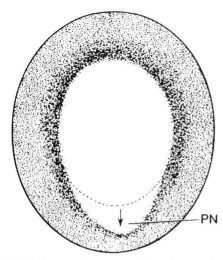

Figure 5.15. Inferior enlargement of cup *(arrow)* from original cup margin *(dotted line)* in glaucomatous optic atrophy, creating a polar notch *(PN)*.

Physiologic Peripapillary Retina

RETINAL NERVE FIBER LAYER. Striations in the retinal nerve fiber layer are normally seen ophthalmoscopically as light reflexes from bundles of nerve fibers (37, 227). They are only visible after the bundles reach a critical thickness, and are consequently seen best in the posterior pole and peripapillary regions, especially at the vertical poles of the disc and extending temporally from them (228). In one large study, the retinal nerve fiber layer was most visible in the inferior temporal arcade, followed by the superior temporal arcade, then the temporal macular area, and finally the nasal area (229). The nerve fiber layer has been noted to decrease with age (229). The visibility of the nerve fiber layer has been shown to correlate with the width of the neural rim and the caliber of the retinal artery (230), and the relative nerve fiber layer height, especially when combined with visual field mean defect, has been shown to discriminate best between normal and glaucomatous eyes (231).

PARAPAPILLARY PIGMENTARY VARIATIONS. The normal optic nerve head may be surrounded by zones that vary in width, circumference and pigmentation. A clinicopathologic study has revealed several clinical configurations with anatomic correlations (232, 233). A *scleral lip,* which appears commonly as a thin, even, white rim that marks the disc margin, usually for the full 360°, represents an anterior extension of sclera between the choroid and optic nerve head. A *chorioscleral crescent,* also called *zone beta,* is a broader but more irregular and incomplete area of depigmentation, which represents a retraction of retinal pigment epithelium from the disc margin, often associated with a thinning or absence of choroid next to the disc, with exposure of the sclera. It is commonly seen with a tilted scleral canal, as in myopia. A parapapillary crescent of increased pigmentation has been called *zone alpha* and may represent

a malposition of the embryonic fold with a double layer or irregularity of retinal pigment epithelium. It may be peripheral to zone beta or may be adjacent to the disc if the latter zone is absent.

Morphology of Glaucomatous Optic Atrophy

The disc changes of glaucoma are typically progressive and asymmetric and present in a variety of characteristic clinical patterns. It may be helpful to think of these in three categories: (a) disc patterns; (b) vascular signs; and (c) parapapillary changes.

Disc Patterns of Glaucomatous Optic Atrophy

As bundles of axons are destroyed in an eye with glaucoma, the neural rim begins to thin in one of several patterns.

FOCAL ATROPHY. Selective loss of neural rim tissue in glaucoma occurs primarily in the inferotemporal region of the optic nerve head and, to a somewhat lesser extent, in the superotemporal sector in the early stages of damage, which leads to enlargement of the cup in a vertical or oblique direction (Fig. 5.15) (234–243). In contrast to the normal optic nerve head, the inferior temporal rim in the glaucomatous eye is usually thinner than the superior temporal area, and the quotient of horizontal to vertical C/D is lowered (241, 242). The mean neural rim area is typically smaller than that of normal discs and is a better parameter than C/D in separating eyes with early glaucoma from normals (241, 244, 245). As previously noted, however, the wide range of neural rim areas in normal eyes even limits the usefulness of this parameter. As the glaucomatous process continues, the temporal neural rim is typically involved after the vertical poles, with the nasal quadrant being the last to go (242).

The focal atrophy of the neural rim often begins as a small, discrete defect, usually in the inferotemporal quadrant, which has been referred to as *polar notching* (236, 237), *focal notching* (238), or *pit-like changes* (239). As the focal defect enlarges and deepens, it may develop a sharp nasal margin, often adjacent to a major retinal vessel, a sign referred to as the *sharpened polar nasal edge* (236). When the local thinning of neural rim tissue reaches the disc margin (i.e., no visible neural rim remains in that area), a *sharpened rim* is said to be produced (236). If a retinal vessel crosses the sharpened rim, it will bend sharply at the edge of the disc, creating what has been termed *bayoneting at the disc edge* (236).

CONCENTRIC ATROPHY. In contrast to focal atrophy, glaucomatous damage may less commonly lead to enlargement of the cup in concentric circles, which are sometimes horizontal, but are more often directed inferotemporally or superotemporally (237). Since the loss of neural rim tissue usually begins temporally and then progresses circumferentially toward these poles, this has been called *temporal unfolding* (236, 237). In one study, this generalized expansion of the cup, with retention of its "round" appearance, was the most common form of early glaucomatous damage (246). Since it is difficult to distinguish this type of glaucomatous cup from a physiologic cup, it is important to compare the cup in the fellow eye for symmetry and to study serial photographs for evidence of progressive change.

A *thinning of the neural rim* may be seen as a crescentic shadow adjacent to the disc margin as the intense beam of a direct ophthalmoscope passes across the neural rim (247). The histologic explanation for this phenomenon is uncertain, but is felt to be associated with early glaucomatous damage (248), and should not be confused with the previously discussed gray crescent in the optic nerve head (224).

DEEPENING OF THE CUP. In some cases, the predominant pattern of early glaucomatous optic atrophy is a deepening of the cup, which has been said to occur only when the lamina is not initially exposed (249). This may produce the picture of *overpass cupping,* in which vessels initially bridge the deepened cup and later collapse into it (236, 237). Exposure of the underlying lamina cribrosa by the deepening cup is often recognized by the gray fenestra of the lamina, which has been referred to as the *laminar dot sign* (236). In most cases, the fenestra of the lamina cribrosa have a dot-like appearance by ophthalmoscopy, although some are more striate, and the latter configuration is said to have a much higher association with glaucomatous damage (250, 251).

PALLOR/CUP DISCREPANCY. In the early stages of glaucomatous optic atrophy, enlargement of the cup may progress ahead of that of the area of pallor. This biphasic pattern differs from other causes of optic atrophy in which the area of pallor is typically larger than the cup (190). A potential pitfall in interpreting optic nerve head cupping is to look only at the area of pallor and miss the larger area of cupping. The latter can usually be recognized by observing kinking of vessels at the cup margin or by examining the disc with stereoscopic techniques. Although the pallor/cup discrepancy is typical and strongly suggestive of glaucomatous cupping, it may also be seen in some normal optic nerve heads (219).

Pallor/cup discrepancy may occur with diffuse or focal enlargement of the cup. *Saucerization* refers to a pattern of early glaucomatous change in which diffuse, shallow cupping extends to the disc margins with retention of a central pale cup (Figs. 5.16 and 5.17) (252) and may be an early sign of glaucoma (252, 253). *Focal saucerization* refers to a more localized shallow, sloping cup, usually in the inferior temporal quadrant (237). The retention of normal neural rim color in the area of focal saucerization has been called the *tinted hollow* (236). As the glaucomatous damage progresses, the color is replaced by a grayish hue, termed the *shadow sign,* or by the *laminar dot sign* (Figs. 5.18 and 5.19) (236).

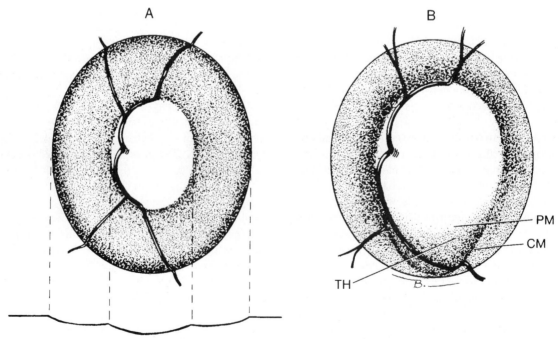

Figure 5.16. Glaucomatous optic atrophy. Pallor/cup discrepancy: A. Saucerization with corresponding cross-sectional view; B. Focal saucerization with tinted hollow *(TH)* between pallor margin *(PM)* and cup margin *(CM)*. Note kinking of vessels in both cases.

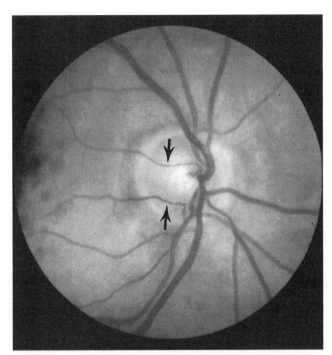

Figure 5.17. Saucerization of optic nerve head, evidenced by gradual sloping of vessels *(arrows)* with kinking at disc margin.

ADVANCED GLAUCOMATOUS CUPPING. If the progressive changes of glaucomatous optic atrophy are not arrested by appropriate measures to reduce the IOP, the typical course is eventual loss of all neural rim tissue. The ultimate result is total cupping, which is seen clinically as a white disc with loss of all neural rim tissue and bending of all vessels at the margin of the disc (Fig. 5.20). This has also been called *bean-pot cupping,* because the cross-section of a histologic specimen reveals extreme posterior displacement of the lamina cribrosa and undermining of the disc margin (Fig. 5.21) (237, 238).

Vascular Signs of Glaucomatous Optic Atrophy

OPTIC DISC HEMORRHAGES. Splinter hemorrhages, usually near the margin of the optic nerve head (Figs. 5.22 and 5.23), are a common feature of glaucomatous damage (254–257). They occur more commonly in patients with normal-tension glaucoma as compared to chronic open-angle glaucoma and glaucoma suspects, with cumulative incidences of 35.3%, 10.3%, and 10.4%, respectively (256). They tend to come and go, so that they may be seen on one visit and gone the next, only to reappear at a later date in the same or new location (258). Although they typically cross the disc margin, the papillary portion often disappears first during resorption, leaving the appearance of an extrapapillary hemorrhage (258). The most common location is the inferior quadrant, although they may be seen superiorly or at any other point around the disc margin. They are seen most often in the early to middle stages of glaucomatous damage

and decline in frequency with advanced damage, rarely appearing in quadrants with absent neural rim (257). While not pathognomonic of glaucoma, disc hemorrhages are a significant finding, since they may be the first sign of glaucomatous damage, often preceding retinal nerve fiber layer defects (259), notches in the neural rim (260), and glaucomatous visual field defects (261–263). They are especially suggestive of glaucoma when associated with high IOP (264). However, as previously noted, disc hemorrhages commonly occur with minimal pressure elevation or in eyes with normal-tension glaucoma (256, 265). They occur more commonly in diabetic patients with glaucoma (266, 267). Although they are not invariably associated with an increased rate of disc damage (267, 268), they should be viewed as a sign that the glaucoma may be out of control (254, 255, 264). It has also been noted that high-tension glaucoma patients with disc hemorrhages have a significantly higher prevalence of neurosensorial dysacousia than those without hemorrhages, which was felt to suggest a common vascular denominator in both conditions (269).

TORTUOSITY OF RETINAL VESSELS. Tortuosity of retinal vessels on the disc may be seen with advanced glaucomatous optic atrophy, and in some cases with only moderate damage. It is believed to represent loops of collateral vessels in response to chronic central retinal vessel occlusion (270). Venovenous anastomoses associated with chronic branch retinal vessel occlusion, as well as the typical picture of acute central retinal vessel occlusion with massive flame hemorrhages, also occur with increased frequency in eyes with chronic glaucoma (270). Asymptomatic venous stasis

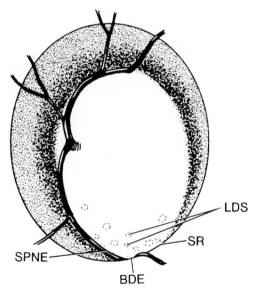

Figure 5.18. Inferior-temporal loss of neural rim in glaucomatous optic atrophy, creating a sharpened rim *(SR)* at the disc margin, a sharpened polar nasal edge *(SPNE)* along the cup margin, bayoneting at the disc edge *(BDE)* where the vessels cross the sharpened rim, and laminar dot sign *(LDS)* due to exposure of fenestrae in lamina cribrosa.

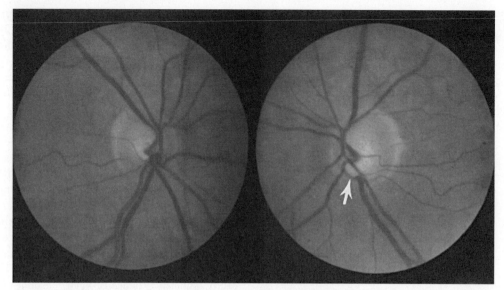

Figure 5.19. Glaucomatous optic atrophy evidenced by a larger left optic nerve head cup with a sharpened rim and bayoneting of the vessels inferiorly *(arrow).*

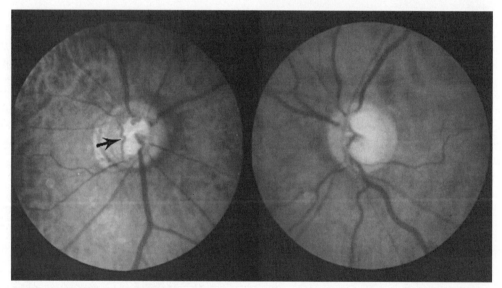

Figure 5.20. Advanced glaucomatous optic atrophy with nearly total cupping of both optic nerve heads and a shunt vessel on the right disc *(arrow).*

changes on the disc, which are seen as enlargement of collateral vessels, have been estimated to occur in 3% of patients with early to moderate glaucoma and may be associated with progression of glaucomatous optic atrophy (271).

CILIORETINAL ARTERIES. One study of 20 patients with bilateral, symmetrical open-angle glaucoma and unilateral cilioretinal arteries revealed a larger C/D and more visual field damage in the eye with the cilioretinal artery (272). However, a similar study did not support this observation (273), while another suggested that glaucomatous eyes with one or more temporal cilioretinal arteries were more likely to retain central visual field than similar eyes with no cilioretinal artery (274).

LOCATION OF RETINAL VESSELS. The location of retinal vessels in relation to the cup may also have some diagnostic value. The significance of *overpass cupping,* in which vessels bridge a cup that is becoming deeper (236, 237), was previously mentioned. Another vessel sign with some diagnostic value has been called *baring of the circumlinear vessel* (275, 276). In many normal optic nerve heads, one or two vessels may curve to outline a portion of the physiologic cup. With glaucomatous enlargement of the cup, these circumlinear vessels may be "bared" from the margin of the cup (Fig. 5.22). This sign may occasionally be seen with nonglaucomatous disorders of the optic nerve (276) and in some individuals with physiologic cups (277), although its presence in a glaucoma suspect group was significantly associated with the development of visual field loss (278). It was once taught that nasal displacement of the retinal vessels on the optic nerve head was a sign of glaucomatous cupping. However, since these vessels enter and leave the eye along the nasal margin of the cup, their location on the disc is a function of cup size, whether physiologic or glaucomatous, and does not provide a useful diagnostic parameter (200). On the other hand, the vertical eccentricity of the central retinal vessel trunk (where the vessels enter and leave through the disc) may be related to the course of glaucomatous optic atrophy. In one study, neural rim loss was more likely to occur in the vertical quadrant that was further from the trunk (279).

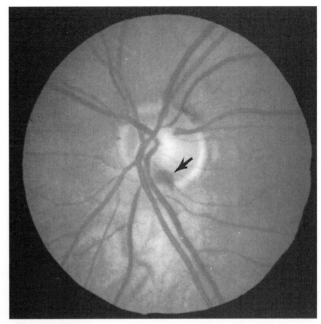

Figure 5.23. Splinter hemorrhage *(arrow)* in glaucomatous optic atrophy.

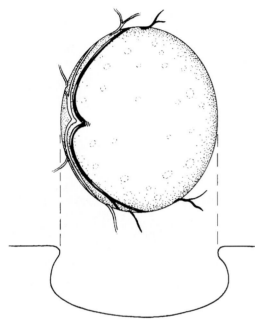

Figure 5.21. Advanced glaucomatous optic atrophy with total (bean-pot) cupping, shown best in cross-sectional view.

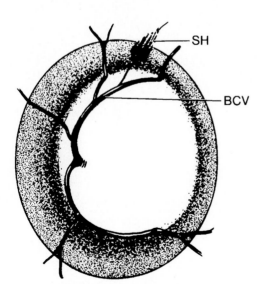

Figure 5.22. Vascular changes in glaucomatous optic atrophy: splinter hemorrhage *(SH)* and baring of circumlinear vessel *(BCV).*

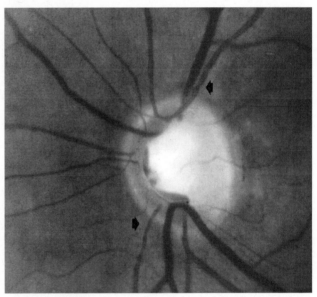

Figure 5.24. Proximal constriction of retinal arteries *(arrows)* in eye with glaucomatous optic atrophy.

Retinal vessels beyond the disc margins may also undergo changes in glaucoma. One study showed *proximal constriction* (narrowing of retinal arteries near the disc) in 42% of both high-tension and normal-tension glaucoma patients, which correlated with the sectors of greatest cupping (Fig. 5.24) (280). *General arterial narrowing* (throughout the retinal course) was seen in 52–78%, corresponding to the overall severity of optic nerve damage (280). However, similar findings were also seen in patients with nonarteritic anterior ischemic optic neuropathy.

Peripapillary Changes Associated with Glaucomatous Optic Atrophy

NERVE FIBER BUNDLE DEFECTS. The loss of axonal bundles, which leads to the neural rim changes of glaucomatous optic atrophy, also produces visible defects in the retinal nerve fiber layer. These appear either as dark stripes or wedge shaped defects of varying width in the peripapillary area, paralleling the normal retinal striations, or as diffuse loss of the striations (Fig. 5.25) (281–284). They often follow disc hemorrhages (259, 284, 285) and correlate highly with visual field changes (281–283), neural rim area (286), and fluorescein filling defects (287). Retinal nerve fiber layer defects are also seen in many neurological disorders, as well as in ocular hypertensive and normal individuals. However, attention to the appearance of the defects in glaucoma has improved the sensitivity and specificity of this finding, and several studies have shown retinal nerve fiber layer defects to be the most

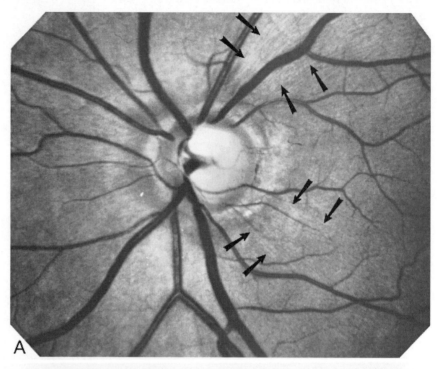

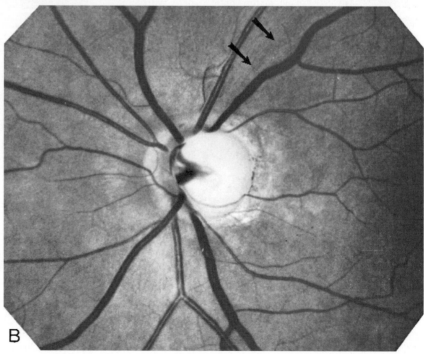

Figure 5.25. Nerve fiber bundle defects of glaucoma. **A.** Normal striations of arcuate nerve fiber bundles, seen best in superior-temporal and inferior-temporal quadrants (*arrows*). **B.** Same eye after extensive glaucomatous damage, showing slit-like defect superiorly (*arrows*) and diffuse loss of nerve fiber bundles inferiorly. (Reprinted with permission from Sommer, A, Miller, NR, Pollack, I, et al: The nerve fiber layer in the diagnosis of glaucoma. Arch Ophthalmol 95:2149, 1977.)

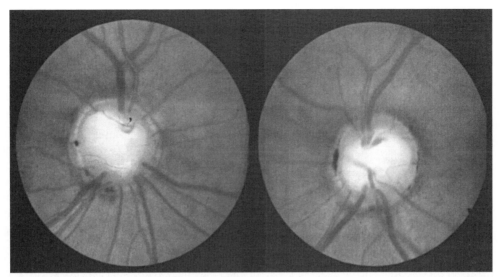

Figure 5.26. Colobomas of the optic nerve heads, as an example of developmental anomalies that may be confused with glaucomatous optic atrophy.

useful parameter in the early detection of glaucomatous damage (288–291). The diffuse loss is more common in glaucoma patients than in ocular hypertensives (292), but also more common among ocular hypertensives than normotensive individuals (293). Localized defects are more directly associated with localized visual field loss than is the case with diffuse nerve loss (294). Either localized or diffuse loss may be the initial sign of glaucomatous damage (295).

PARAPAPILLARY DEPIGMENTATION. Parapapillary depigmentation is frequently associated with glaucomatous optic atrophy, but is also seen with other conditions, such as myopia and aging changes. As previously noted, several variations of peripapillary pigmentary change may be seen in normal eyes. The scleral lip, or *peripapillary halo,* is a narrow, homogenous light band at the edge of the disc. The incidence of prominent halos is higher in glaucoma, although the average degree of halos is statistically the same as in nonglaucomatous eyes (296). *Parapapillary atrophy* (both zone beta and zone alpha, as previously described) occurs more frequently and is larger in eyes with glaucomatous damage, as compared to normal eyes (297–299), and has been observed to progressively enlarge in eyes with glaucoma (300). It increases with decreasing neural rim area and correlates with the quadrants of greatest rim loss (301). There is preliminary evidence that the absence of parapapillary atrophy may reduce the risk of glaucomatous damage among ocular hypertensives (302).

Reversal of Glaucomatous Damage

It is generally taught that glaucomatous damage of the optic nerve head and visual field is an irreversible process. While this may be true in many cases, especially when associated with actual loss of axons, there are situations in which glaucomatous damage may be reversible. This is seen most com-

monly in children with early stages of glaucoma, particularly during the first year of life, when the IOP is successfully lowered surgically (303, 304). However, improvement in the cup, neural rim, and even the nerve fiber layer height have been described in adults following a marked reduction in IOP by surgical or medical means (305–311).

DIFFERENTIAL DIAGNOSIS OF GLAUCOMATOUS OPTIC ATROPHY

Normal Variations

Normal variations in the physiologic cup, the neural rim, and the peripapillary retina, as discussed earlier in this chapter, may be confused with the changes of glaucoma. In addition, developmental anomalies and nonglaucomatous optic atrophies may be sources of diagnostic confusion.

Developmental Anomalies

Colobomas of the optic nerve head can simulate glaucomatous cupping. The defect may involve the entire disc, which is enlarged and excavated (Fig. 5.26) (312, 313). In some cases, the diagnostic problem is compounded by associated field defects, which may resemble those of glaucoma, but are typically not progressive. A variation of optic nerve head colobomas, called the *morning glory syndrome,* is characterized by a large funnel-shaped staphylomatous coloboma of the nerve head and peripapillary region with white central tissue, elevated peripapillary pigment disturbance, and multiple radially-oriented retinal vessels (314–316). Yet another optic nerve head anomaly, which may represent an atypical coloboma, is the *congenital pit* (315, 316). This is a localized, pale depression, usually near the temporal or inferotemporal margin of the disc, although they may be found in any area of the nerve head, and there may be two, or even three, pits in some eyes. These anomalies may have associated visual disturbance due to macular or extramacular serous detachment (317). Cases have also been reported in which congenital pits were noted to enlarge when observed for many years (318). *Tilted disc syndrome* is a congenital anomaly in which the optic disc is tilted on its horizontal axis, with inferior chorioretinal hypoplasia (319). While it is less likely than the colobomas to be confused with glaucoma, it can interfere with the recognition of glaucomatous damage, which is compounded by superotemporal visual field loss (319).

Nonglaucomatous Causes of Acquired Cupping

Studies have shown that ophthalmologists are not always able to distinguish between glaucomatous and nonglaucomatous optic atrophy on the basis of the optic disc appearance alone (320). Parameters that are most useful in making this differentiation include pallor of the neural rim in nonglaucomatous cases and obliteration of the rim in glaucoma (321). Nonglaucomatous conditions that may cause acquired cupping include anterior ischemic optic neuropathy, as previously discussed, especially when the ischemia is due to arteritis (179–181). A similar entity has been described in which infarction of the optic nerve head caused shallow cupping inferotemporally, associated with arcuate field defects (322). This differed from glaucoma in that it was not progressive. Acquired cupping may also occur with compressive lesions of the optic nerve, such as an intracranial aneurysm, which was reported to cause cupping indistinguishable from that of early glaucoma (323).

CLINICAL TECHNIQUES FOR EVALUATING THE OPTIC NERVE HEAD[c]

Progressive cupping of the optic nerve head in a patient with glaucoma is the most reliable indicator that the IOP is not being adequately controlled. It is essential, therefore, to evaluate and record the appearance of the nerve head in a way that will accurately reveal subtle glaucomatous changes over the course of followup evaluations. In current practice, this involves careful evaluation in the office combined with photographic documentation. In addition, there are newer, automated techniques which may provide more precise methods of observation.

[c]Refer to Shields, MB: Color Atlas of Glaucoma. Baltimore, Williams & Wilkins, 1998, Plate I24.

Techniques of Office Evaluation and Recording

In the clinical evaluation of the optic nerve head, the direct ophthalmoscope is occasionally useful, especially when looking through a small pupil or evaluating the nerve fiber layer with a red-free filter. However, this technique does not permit detection of many of the glaucomatous changes in the nerve head and peripapillary area, and the most useful office approach is to carefully study these structures with stereoscopic methods. The most useful stereoscopic technique is with a slitlamp and an auxiliary fundus lens such as the Goldmann contact lens, the hand-held 90-diopter lens (Fig. 5.27), or the Hruby lens slitlamp attachment (Fig. 5.28). Each of these systems provides the advantages of magnification and stereopsis. However, since the lateral and axial magnifications are unequal, there is a certain amount of image distortion, with the Goldmann and 90-diopter lenses producing a decrease in apparent depth and the Hruby lens producing a slight increase (324). Several methods have been described for estimating the size of the disc and neural rim. These include use of: (a) a direct ophthalmoscope, using either the graticule incorporated in the instrument (325) or the smallest round white light spot of the Welch Allyn direct ophthalmoscope, which projects a 1.5-mm diameter spot on the retina in most eyes (326); (b) an indirect ophthalmoscope with a spacing device on the condensing lens that allows measurement of the disc image with calipers (327, 328); and (c) a Haag-Streit slitlamp with a 90-diopter lens (329) or contact lens (330, 331), in which the height of the slit-beam is adjusted to coincide with the

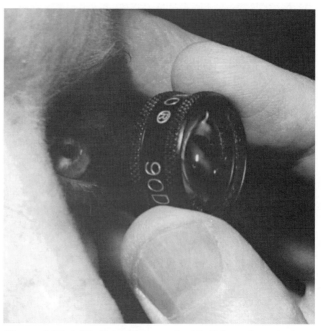

Figure 5.27. A 90-diopter lens used with slitlamp for stereoscopic indirect ophthalmoscopic evaluation of optic nerve head.

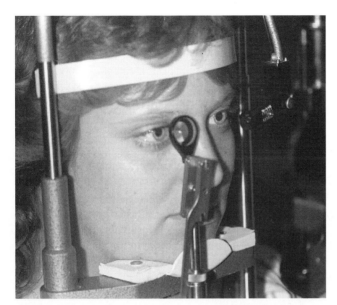

Figure 5.28. Hruby lens attachment to the slitlamp for stereoscopic evaluation of the optic nerve head.

disc edges and then read off the scale. When compared to more quantitative measurements such as planimetry, these techniques provide reasonably accurate estimates, especially when appropriate correction factors are considered.

Subjective estimates of cup dimensions have been shown to vary greatly, even among expert observers (332–335). These can be improved by paying attention to the many complex optic nerve head and peripapillary retinal parameters associated with glaucomatous damage (336), and the need for standardized methods for interobserver evaluation of the optic disc in glaucoma has been emphasized (335). Detailed drawings should be made that include the area of cupping and pallor in all quadrants, the position and kinking of major vessels, splinter hemorrhages, and peripapillary changes (Fig. 5.29). However, no degree of attention to detail is sufficient to detect subtle changes in all cases, and the office evaluation should be considered only an adjunct to the indispensable use of photographic records.

Photographic and Other Techniques

Two-Dimensional Photos

Two-dimensional photos, whether color or black-and-white, have the advantages of simplicity and lower cost as compared to stereophotos. In addition, the relative dimensions of the pallor and cup can be measured directly on the photograph (337, 338). Although one study found monocular and stereoscopic photographs to afford similar levels of accuracy (339), the former technique is frequently limited by the inability to precisely determine the cup margins. The projections of fine, parallel lines onto the disc have been suggested as a way to improve recognition of the cup contours on both two-dimensional and stereophotographs (340, 341). Techniques have also been developed to electronically scan black-and-white disc photos to obtain an objective measure of the amount of optic disc pallor (342, 343). The main value of two-dimensional photos in the future may be to document the *retinal nerve fiber layer*. Special techniques to enhance the subtle details of this parameter include monochromatic (red-free) filters and high resolution film (344–348), cross-polarization photography (349), a wide-angle fundus camera (350), a spectral reflectance (351), and a charge-coupled device with digital filtering (352). The use of nerve fiber layer photography compared favorably with other glaucoma-screening methods in a general medical clinic setting (348).

Stereoscopic Photographs

A method that may be more reliable for recording disc cupping, as well as the other aspects of glaucomatous optic atrophy, is the use of color stereophotographs. Stereophotographs can be obtained by taking two photos in sequence, either by manually repositioning the camera or by using a sliding carriage adapter (Allen separator) (353), or by taking simultaneous photos with two cameras that utilize the indirect ophthalmoscopic principle (Donaldson stereoscopic fundus camera) (354) or a twin-prism separator (355). In an early study, these three techniques were compared for reproducibility, and the Donaldson camera was found to be superior (356). However, a more recent simultaneous stereo-camera, which provides the stereo pair on two halves of the

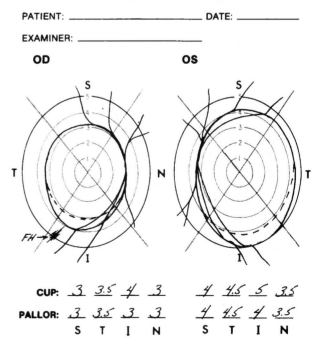

Figure 5.29. Example of optic nerve head drawing made at time of stereoscopic evaluation of the disc as adjunct to disc photos.

same frame (Nidek 3Dx) was found to have significantly better overall mean stereoscopic quality than the Donaldson camera (357). Transparencies from the Nidek camera can also be used to create "lenticular images," which are single prints on a unique, photosensitized plastic base that produces a three-dimensional image without use of a stereoviewer (358).

Serial Comparisons

Stereochronoscopy utilizes the stereoscopic principle to detect subtle changes in photographs of a disc taken at different times (359, 360). If there has been any progression of the cupping, the disparity in the cup margins of the superimposed photographs will produce a stereoscopic effect. A modification of this concept, referred to as *stereochronometry,* uses a stereoplotter to measure the changes created by the two photos (361). Other techniques for detecting differences in serial fundus photographs involve analysis of *flicker* while alternately viewing one photograph and then the other (362), and *electronic subtraction,* in which areas of disparity between the two images will be enhanced (363).

Colorimetric Measurements

Colorimetric measurements have also been studied in an effort to detect reduced or changing color intensity of the optic nerve head (364–366). A photographic technique has also been developed to permit quantitative evaluation of the relative brightness of the illuminated optic nerve head (367).

Fluorescein Angiographic Studies

Fluorescein angiographic studies of the optic nerve head were discussed earlier in this chapter and may one day have practical clinical application in the detection and management of glaucoma.

Ultrasonography

It has been shown that ultrasound can be used to detect glaucomatous cupping of 0.7 cup/disc ratio or greater (368), and high-resolution contact B-scan echography may one day provide a reliable estimate of the optic cup size in eyes with opaque media (369).

COMPUTERIZED IMAGE ANALYSIS OF THE OPTIC NERVE HEAD AND RETINAL NERVE FIBER LAYER[d]

Even the most sophisticated fundus photographs are limited in their clinical value by the qualitative, subjective interpre-

[d]Refer to Shields, MB: Color Atlas of Glaucoma. Baltimore, Williams & Wilkins, 1998, Plates I25–26.

tation of the images. Efforts to refine the assessment of these subtle findings have included quantitative analyses of optic nerve head topography and pallor and retinal nerve fiber layer height or thickness. These techniques were initially performed manually (370–374), which was time consuming and impractical for routine clinical practice. With the advent of computer and newer imaging technologies, however, there is now the possibility of applying these concepts to the clinical management of glaucoma.

The concept of computerized image analysis of the optic nerve head was pioneered by Dr. Bernard Schwartz, who developed prototypes for analysis of both contour and pallor of the disc (Fig. 5.30) (375, 376). Since then several commercial instruments have been described in the literature, which utilize a variety of principles, including stereophotogrammetry, confocal laser scanning, rasterstereography, and optical coherence tomography.

Stereophotogrammetry

Principle

These instruments utilize the basic principle of stereopsis, in which disparity between corresponding points of stereo pair images are used to generate contour lines and three-dimensional contour maps.

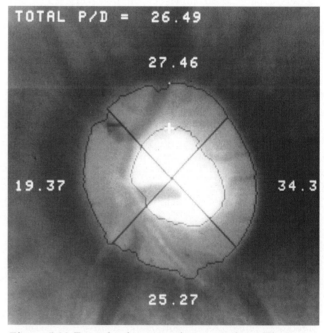

Figure 5.30. Example of automated image analysis. The computer has delineated the optic disc and area of pallor *(black lines),* as well as the disc quadrants. *Numbers* indicate the percentage of pallor found across the total disc area *(Total P/D),* as well as each of the disc quadrants. (Reprinted with permission from Nagin P, Schwartz B, Nanba K: The reproducibility of computerized boundary analysis for measuring optic disc pallor in the normal optic disc. Ophthalmology 92:243, 1985).

Instruments

The *Rodenstock Optic Nerve Head Analyzer* (ONHA) has probably had the most extensive evaluation within this group of instruments (377–392). It measures optic nerve head contour by projecting vertical light stripes on the disc and peripapillary retina and then obtaining simultaneous stereovideo images, which are processed by a microcomputer. Disparity between corresponding points along the light stripes of stereo pairs is used to generate vertical contour lines and three-dimensional contour maps. A pallor map of the disc can also be generated by obtaining video images with both red and green wavelengths and computing the ratio of color reflectance at various points in the image. In addition, a method has been developed to make height measurements of the peripapillary surface relative to a retinal reference plane, which is established in the peripheral portions of the videographic image (389–392).

Two other commercial instruments in this category are the *Topcon Imagenet* (formerly the PAR IS 2000) (393–398) and the *Humphrey Retinal Analyzer* (RA) (399, 400). These instruments differ from the ONHA by using disparity between existing structures in the stereo images, rather than projected light stripes. They can also analyze data from either simultaneous stereovideo images or stereophotographs.

Evaluations

To have practical clinical application, any image analyzer must provide information that is both reproducible and accurate. Reproducibility, or variability, studies typically involve obtaining multiple measurements of the same eye within a short time frame and calculating the variance of intrapatient results. Ideally, there should be no variation in the measurements, and that which is calculated provides an indication of the inherent testing variability that must be factored in when assessing real change over time. Several such studies have shown that contour measurements by the ONHA have acceptable reproducibility, especially for cup/disc ratio and neural rim area (377–381), and comparable results have been reported for the Imagenet (394) and the RA (399, 400). Reproducibility studies of pallor measurements with the ONHA have been somewhat conflicting. Variation was acceptably low when the distribution of pallor values throughout the image was calculated (382, 383), but was inadequate when an area of specific pallor values within the disc was compared between measurements of the same eye (384). Accuracy of topographic measurements with the ONHA was evaluated with a plastic model eye and was felt to be clinically acceptable when appropriate correction factors for magnification error were used (385).

Despite reasonable reproducibility and accuracy, these instruments never achieved widespread clinical use primarily because of technical complexity, the size and cost of the instruments, and the need for relatively wide pupillary dilatation and clear media. At the time of this writing, the Imagenet was the only stereophotogrammetry unit still commercially available. Nevertheless, the experience gained through the study of these instruments has provided the basis for much of our understanding of computerized image analysis of the optic nerve head and of the potential for clinical application of newer instruments and techniques in the management of glaucoma.

Confocal Laser Scanning

Principle

This is a technique for obtaining high resolution images by using a focused laser beam to scan over the area of the fundus to be imaged. Only a small spot on the fundus is illuminated at any instant, and the light reflected determines the brightness of the corresponding *pixel* on a TV monitor. To improve contrast, a pinhole, or *confocal aperture,* is placed in front of the photodetector to eliminate scattered light. The aperture is conjugate to the laser focus, and the image so obtained is said to be *confocal.* The instantaneous volume of tissue from which reflected light is accepted by the confocal aperture is called a *voxel,* and the smaller the aperture, the smaller the voxel and the higher the confocality of the image. By scanning the fundus with the laser, a two-dimensional image can be built up as an array of pixels (*confocal scanning laser ophthalmoscopy*). If a series of such images are obtained at successive planes of depth in the tissue, these can be used to construct a three-dimensional image (*confocal scanning laser tomography*).

Instruments

The prototype within this category of instruments is the *Laser Tomographic Scanner* (LTS) (401–404). Although it is no longer commercially available, two second-generation units that are on the market, the *Heidelberg Retina Tomograph* (HRT) and the *Laser Diagnostic Technologies TOPss,* were both developed directly from the original LTS and are very similar in basic design. The HRT, which has had the most extensively reported evaluation, uses a 670-nm diode laser and performs 32 consecutive scans in 1.6 seconds. The first section image is located above the reflection of the first retinal vessel, and the last is beyond the bottom of the optic nerve head cup (405–408). An integrated computer calculates the height position for each of 256×256 pixels in the whole images within a $10° \times 10°$ area. From these data, the instrument provides a wide range of two-dimensional and three-dimensional information on the disc and peripapillary retina, which is displayed on a monitor and in hard copy.

Other confocal laser scanners that have been described in the literature, include the *Rodenstock 101 Confocal Scanning Laser Ophthalmoscope* (cSLO), which can be used to obtain high resolution two-dimensional fundus images (409), as well as three-dimensional topography of the optic disc (410, 411). Another prototype confocal laser scanning ophthalmoscope was by *Carl Zeiss, Inc.* (412). The principle employed in these two instruments is similar to that described for the HRT.

Another confocal laser scanning is the *Nerve Fiber Analyzer* (NFA), which combines the concept of scanning laser polarimetry to measure the nerve fiber layer thickness (413). Based on the assumption that the nerve fiber layer is birefringent, a polarized diode laser light penetrates the tissue, which changes the state of polarization of the reflected light. This change in the state of polarization is referred to as *retardation* and is linearly related to the thickness of the retinal nerve fiber layer. The computer provides thickness data for concentric circles around the disc margin.

Confocal scanning laser ophthalmoscopy has also been evaluated as a means of enhancing angiographic examination of small vessels of the optic nerve head using fluorescein or indocyanine green (414).

Evaluations

Numerous reproducibility studies have been reported for the LTS (401, 404) and HRT (405–408, 415, 416). In general, these have revealed acceptably low variability, with one study showing the HRT to be superior to the ONHA (415). Highly reproducible topographic data can be obtained with an undilated pupil (407), although one study showed reduced reproducibility in patients using pilocarpine (416), and it has been suggested that reproducibility can be improved in general by using a series of three examinations (405). Studies with the Rodenstock (411) and Zeiss (412) instruments were also felt to demonstrate acceptable reproducibility.

An accuracy study was performed with the LTS, using the same plastic model eye as previously described with the ONHA, and revealed low average relative errors for diameter and depth (402). However, vertical disc diameter measurements with the HRT were significantly smaller than those obtained with planimetric methods (417).

One lesson that has been learned from the study of image analysis of the optic nerve head is that traditional parameters, such as cup/disc ratio and neural rim area, are no longer adequate for interpreting the subtle findings in the disc and peripapillary retina in normal and diseased states. To address this problem, 14 predefined stereometric-shaped parameters were incorporated into the software of the HRT. One of these parameters is referred to as the *third moment,* which relates to the frequency distribution of depth values relative to the curved surfaces inside the disc area and is a function of the overall shape of the optic nerve head. This parameter was found to be the most useful indicator of the degree of glaucomatous nerve damage (418) and early glaucomatous visual field loss (419). Other important parameters were maximum depth in the disc contour and height variation in contour (419).

Rasterstereography
Principle

"Raster" simply refers to a scanning pattern that moves from side-to-side and from top-to-bottom (actually the same scanning pattern used in confocal laser scanning). In rasterstereography, a series of horizontal dark/light line pairs are projected on the disc and peripapillary retina at a fixed angle, and the computer scans a video image of the lines in a raster fashion. Since the lines are deflected proportional to the height or depth of the disc and retinal surfaces, a computer algorithm can translate the deflections into depth numbers and create a topographic map.

Instrument

At the present time, the only image analyzer that utilizes the rasterstereography concept is the *Glaucoma-Scope* (420, 421). It projects a near infrared light (750 nm) in 25 parallel stripes at a 9° angle to the nerve head. The computer analyzes approximately 8750 data points to generate approximately 760 depth measures, which are displayed in microns relative to reference planes, 350 microns nasal and temporal to the disc. In the initial set of measurements, the actual depth measures are provided, while followup studies show only change of more than 50 microns from baseline. Other disc and peripapillary parameters are also provided in the printout.

Evaluations

Two reproducibility studies have been reported, both of which showed acceptably low variability and suggested that any change greater than 50 microns could represent true progressive damage (420, 421).

Optical Coherence Tomography

The principle of optical coherence tomography (OCT) involves a low-coherence infrared (843-nm) diode light source, which is divided into reference and sample paths. Reflected sample light from the subject's eye creates an interference signal with the reference beam, which is detected in a fiberoptic interferometer. Cross-sectional images of the retina and disc are then constructed from a sequence of signals, similar to an ultrasound B mode (422). Preliminary studies have demonstrated that nerve fiber layer thickness can be measured using the OCT (423).

SUMMARY

The optic nerve head is composed of axons from the retinal ganglion cells, blood vessels, and astroglial and collagen support. The normal optic nerve head has considerable variation in size and surface contour. The pathogenesis of glaucomatous optic atrophy appears to involve obstruction of axoplasmic flow, although it is not clear whether this is a direct mechanical effect of elevated IOP or secondary to vascular changes. Glaucomatous optic atrophy is characterized clinically by a progressive, asymmetric loss of neural rim tissue, which is manifested by an enlargement in the area of cupping and pallor. This most often extends in a focal direction, producing early thinning of the inferior and superior portions of the neural rim. Enlargement of the cup often precedes that of the area of pallor, creating a pallor/cup discrepancy. Other important signs of glaucomatous optic atrophy are disc hemorrhages and peripapillary nerve fiber bundle defects. The differential diagnosis of glaucomatous optic atrophy includes normal variations, developmental anomalies, and nonglaucomatous causes of acquired cupping. Techniques for evaluating the optic nerve head include a careful office examination and photographic documentation, although newer techniques such as computerized imaging analysis are being developed that may soon provide more precise methods of observation in the clinical management of glaucoma.

REFERENCES

1. Kronfeld, PC: Normal variations of the optic disc as observed by conventional ophthalmoscopy and their anatomic correlations. Trans Am Acad Ophthalmol Otol 81:214, 1976.

2. Jonas, JB, Gusek, GC, Guggenmoos-Holzmann, I, Naumann, GOH: Size of the optic nerve scleral canal and comparison with intravital determination of optic disc dimensions. Graefes Arch Clin Exp Ophthalmol 226:213, 1988.

3. Quigley, HA, Brown, AE, Morrison, JD, Drance, SM: The size and shape of the optic disc in normal human eyes. Arch Ophthalmol 108:51, 1990.

4. Hayreh, SS: Anatomy and physiology of the optic nerve head. Trans Am Acad Ophthalmol Otol 78:240, 1974.

5. Minckler, DS, McLean, IW, Tso, MOM: Distribution of axonal and glial elements in the rhesus optic nerve head studied by electron microscopy. Am J Ophthalmol 82:179, 1976.

6. Anderson, DR: Ultrastructure of human and monkey lamina cribrosa and optic nerve head. Arch Ophthalmol 82:800, 1969.

7. Hamasaki, DI, Fujino, T: Effect of intraocular pressure on ocular vessels. Arch Ophthalmol 78:369, 1967.

8. Geijer, C, Bill, A: Effects of raised intraocular pressure on retinal, prelaminar, laminar, and retrolaminar optic nerve blood flow in monkeys. Invest Ophthalmol Vis Sci 18:1030, 1979.

9. Onda, E, Cioffi, GA, Bacon, DR, Van Buskirk, EM: Microvasculature of the human optic nerve. Am J Ophthalmol 120:92, 1995.

10. Liebermann, MF, Maumenee, AE, Green, WR: Histologic studies of the vasculature of the anterior optic nerve. Am J Ophthalmol 82:405, 1976.

11. Anderson, DR, Braverman, S: Reevaluation of the optic disc vasculature. Am J Ophthalmol 82:165, 1976.

12. Olver, JM, Spalton, DJ, McCartney, ACE: Quantitative morphology of human retrolaminar optic nerve vasculature. Invest Ophthalmol Vis Sci 35:3858, 1994.

13. Hayreh, SS: The central artery of the retina: Its role in the blood supply of the optic nerve. Br J Ophthalmol 47:651, 1963.

14. Francois, J, Neetens, A: Vascularization of the optic pathway. I. Lamina cribrosa and optic nerve. Br J Ophthalmol 38:472, 1954.

15. Goder, G: The capillaries of the optic nerve. Am J Ophthalmol 77:684, 1974.

16. Zaret, CR, Choromokos, EA, Meisler, DM: Cilio-optic vein associated with phakomatosis. Ophthalmology 87:330, 1980.

17. Anderson, DR, Hoyt, WF, Hogan, MJ: The fine structure of the astroglia in the human optic nerve and optic nerve head. Trans Am Ophthalmol Soc 65:275, 1967.

18. Quigley, HA: Gap junctions between optic nerve head astrocytes. Invest Ophthalmol Vis Sci 16:582, 1977.

19. Anderson, DR: Ultrastructure of the optic nerve head. Arch Ophthalmol 83:63, 1970.

20. Anderson, DR, Hoyt, WF: Ultrastructure of intraorbital portion of human and monkey optic nerve. Arch Ophthalmol 82:506, 1969.

21. Heegaard, S, Jensen, OA, Prause, JU: Structure of the vitread face of the monkey optic disc (Macacca mulatta). Graefes Arch Clin Exp Ophthalmol 226:377, 1988.

22. Quigley, HA, Addicks, EM: Regional differences in the structure of the lamina cribrosa and their relation to glaucomatous optic nerve damage. Arch Ophthalmol 99:137, 1981.

23. Radius, RL, Gonzales, M: Anatomy of the lamina cribrosa in human eyes. Arch Ophthalmol 99:2159, 1981.

24. Radius, RL: Regional specificity in anatomy at the lamina cribrosa. Arch Ophthalmol 99:478, 1981.

25. Jonas, JB, Mardin, CY, Schlötzer-Schrehardt, U, Naumann, GOH: Morphometry of the human lamina cribrosa surface. Invest Ophthalmol Vis Sci 32:401, 1991.

26. Hernandez, MR, Igoe, F, Neufeld, AH: Extracellular matrix of the human optic nerve head. Am J Ophthalmol 102:139, 1986.

27. Rehnberg, M, Ammitzboll, T, Tengroth, B: Collagen distribution in the lamina cribrosa and the trabecular meshwork of the human eye. Br J Ophthalmol 71:886, 1987.

28. Goldbaum, MH, Jeng, S, Logemann, R, Weinreb, RN: The extracellular matrix of the human optic nerve. Arch Ophthalmol 107:1225, 1989.

29. Hernandez, MR, Luo, XX, Igoe, F, Neufeld, AH: Extracellular matrix of the human lamina cribrosa. Am J Ophthalmol 104:567, 1987.

30. Hernandez, MR, Igoe, F, Neufeld, AH: Cell culture of the human lamina cribrosa. Invest Ophthalmol Vis Sci 29:78, 1988.

31. Hernandez, MR, Wang, N, Hanley, NM, Neufeld, AH: Localization of collagen types I and IV mRNAs in human optic nerve head by in situ hybridization. Invest Ophthalmol Vis Sci 32:2169, 1991.

32. Caparas, VL, Cintron, C, Hernandez-Neufeld, MR: Immunohistochemistry of proteoglycans in human lamina cribrosa. Am J Ophthalmol 112:489, 1991.

33. Sawaguchi, S, Yue, BYJT, Fukuchi, T, et al: Sulfated proteoglycans in the human lamina cribrosa. Invest Ophthalmol Vis Sci 33:2388, 1992.

34. Anderson, DR: Ultrastructure of meningeal sheaths. Normal human and monkey optic nerves. Arch Ophthalmol 82:659, 1969.

35. Radius, RL, Anderson, DR: The histology of retinal nerve fiber layer bundles and bundle defects. Arch Ophthalmol 97:948, 1979.

36. Radius, RL, Anderson, DR: The course of axons through the retina and optic nerve head. Arch Ophthalmol 97:1154, 1979.

37. Radius, RL, de Bruin, J: Anatomy of the retinal nerve fiber layer. Invest Ophthalmol Vis Sci 21:745, 1981.

38. Ogden, TE: Nerve fiber layer of the primate retina: morphometric analysis. Invest Ophthalmol Vis Sci 25:19, 1984.

39. Minckler, DS: The organization of nerve fiber bundles in the primate optic nerve head. Arch Ophthalmol 98:1630, 1980.

40. Hoyt, WF, Luis, O: Visual fiber anatomy in the infrageniculate pathway of the primate. Arch Ophthalmol 68:94, 1962.

41. Mikelberg, FS, Drance, SM, Schulzer, M, et al: The normal human optic nerve. Ophthalmology 96:1325, 1989.

42. Repka, MX, Quigley, HA: The effect of age on normal human optic nerve fiber number and diameter. Ophthalmology 96:26, 1989.

43. Mikelberg, FS, Yidegiligne, HM, White, VA, Schulzer, M: Relation between optic nerve axon number and axon diameter to scleral canal area. Ophthalmology 98:60, 1991.

44. Jonas, JB, Schmidt, AM, Müller-Bergh, JA, et al: Human optic nerve fiber count and optic disc size. Invest Ophthalmol Vis Sci 33:2012, 1992.

45. Quigley, HA, Coleman, AL, Dorman-Pease, ME: Larger optic nerve heads have more nerve fibers in normal monkey eyes. Arch Ophthalmol 109:1441, 1991.

46. Panda-Jonas, S, Jonas, JB, Jakobczyk, M, Schneider, U: Retinal photoreceptor count, retinal surface area, and optic disc size in normal human eyes. Ophthalmology 101:519, 1994.

47. Johnson, BM, Miao, M, Sadun, AA: Age-related decline of human optic nerve axon populations. Age 10:5, 1987.

48. Rimmer, S, Keating, C, Chou, T, et al: Growth of the human optic disk and nerve during gestation, childhood, and early adulthood. Am J Ophthalmol 116:748, 1993.

49. Dolman, CL, McCormick, AQ, Drance, SM: Aging of the optic nerve. Arch Ophthalmol 98:2053, 1980.

50. Magoon, EH, Robb, RM: Development of myelin in human optic nerve and tract: A light and electron microscopic study. Arch Ophthalmol 99:655, 1981.

51. Quigley, HA: The pathogenesis of reversible cupping in congenital glaucoma. Am J Ophthalmol 84:358, 1977.

52. Hernandez, MR, Luo, XX, Andrzejewska, W, Neufeld, AH: Age-related changes in the extracellular matrix of the human optic nerve head. Am J Ophthalmol 107:476, 1989.

53. Hernandez, MR: Ultrastructural immunocytochemical analysis of elastin in the human lamina cribrosa. Invest Ophthalmol Vis Sci 33:2891, 1992.

54. Sawaguchi, S, Yue, BYJT, Fukuchi, T, et al: Age-related changes of sulfated proteoglycans in the human lamina cribrosa. Curr Eye Res 12:685, 1993.

55. Müller, H: Anatomische Beitrage zur Ophthalmologie: Ueber Nervean-Veranderungen an der Eintrittsstelle des Schnerven. Arch Ophthalmol 4:1, 1858.

56. von Jaeger, E: Ueber Glaucom und seine Heilung durch Iridectomie. Z Ges der Aerzte zu Wien 14:465, 484, 1858.

57. Schnabel, J: Das glaucomatose Sehnervenleiden. Archiv fur Augenheilkunde XXIV:18, 1892.

58. Laker, C: Ein experimenteller Beitrag zur Lehre von der glaukomatosen Excavation. Klin Monatsble Augenheilkd 24:187, 1886.

59. Schreiber, L: Ueber Degeneration der Netzhaut naut experimentellen und pathologisch-anatomischen Untersuchungen. Graefes Arch Clin Exp Ophthalmol 64:237, 1906.

60. Fuchs, E: Ueber die Lamina cribrosa. Graefes Arch Clin Exp Ophthalmol 91:435, 1916.

61. LaGrange, F, Beauvieux, J: Anatomie de l'excavation glaucomateuse. Arch Ophthalmol (Paris) 42:129, 1925.

62. Duke-Elder, S: Fundamental concepts in glaucoma. Arch Ophthalmol 42:538, 1949.

63. Gafner, F, Goldmann, H: Experimentelle Untersuchungen uber den Zusammenhang von Augendrucksteigerung und Gesichtsfeldschadigung. Ophthalmologica 130:357, 1955.

64. Duke-Elder, S: The problems of simple glaucoma. Trans Ophthalmol Soc UK 82:307, 1962.

65. Lampert, PW, Vogel, MH, Zimmerman, LE: Pathology of the optic nerve in experimental acute glaucoma. Electron microscopic studies. Invest Ophthalmol 7:199, 1968.

66. Shaffer, RN: The role of the astroglial cells in glaucomatous disc cupping. Doc Ophthalmol 26:516, 1969.

67. Shaffer, RN, Hetherington, J Jr: The glaucomatous disc in infants. A suggested hypothesis for disc cupping. Trans Am Acad Ophthalmol Otol 73:929, 1969.

68. Quigley, HA, Green, WR: The histology of human glaucoma cupping and optic nerve damage: Clinicopathologic correlation in 21 eyes. Ophthalmology 86:1803, 1979.

69. Quigley, HA, Addicks, EM, Green, WR, Maumenee, AE: Optic nerve damage in human glaucoma. II. The site of injury and susceptibility to damage. Arch Ophthalmol 99:635, 1981.

70. Schwartz, B: Cupping and pallor of the optic disc. Arch Ophthalmol 89:272, 1973.

71. Kornzweig, AL, Eliasoph, I, Feldstein, M: Selective atrophy of the radial peripapillary capillaries in chronic glaucoma. Arch Ophthalmol 80:696, 1968.

72. Daicker, B: Selective atrophy of the radial peripapillary capillaries and visual field defects in glaucoma. Graefes Arch Clin Exp Ophthalmol 195:27, 1975.

73. Quigley, HA, Hohman, RM, Addicks, EM, Green, WR: Blood vessels of the glaucomatous optic disc in experimental primate and human eyes. Invest Ophthalmol Vis Sci 25:918, 1984.

74. Quigley, HA, Hohman, RM, Addicks, EM: Quantitative study of optic nerve head capillaries in experimental optic disc pallor. Am J Ophthalmol 93:689, 1982.

75. Quigley, HA, Anderson, DR: The histologic basis of optic disk pallor in experimental optic atrophy. Am J Ophthalmol 83:709, 1977.

76. Henkind, P, Bellhorn, R, Rabkin, M, Murphy, ME: Optic nerve transection in cats. II. Effect on vessels of optic nerve head and lamina cribrosa. Invest Ophthalmol Vis Sci 16:442, 1977.

77. Radius, RL, Anderson, DR: The mechanism of disc pallor in experimental optic atrophy. A fluorescein angiographic study. Arch Ophthalmol 97:532, 1979.

78. Hayreh, SS: Pathogenesis of cupping of the optic disc. Br J Ophthalmol 58:863, 1974.

79. Emery, JM, Landis, D, Paton, D, et al: The lamina cribrosa in normal and glaucomatous human eyes. Trans Am Acad Ophthalmol Otol 78:290, 1974.

80. Levy, NS, Crapps, EE: Displacement of optic nerve head in response to short-term intraocular pressure elevation in human eyes. Arch Ophthalmol 102:782, 1984.

81. Yan, DB, Coloma, FM, Metheetrairut, A, et al: Deformation of the lamina cribrosa by elevated intraocular pressure. Br J Ophthalmol 78:643, 1994.

82. Radius, RL, Pederson, JE: Laser-induced primate glaucoma. II. Histopathology. Arch Ophthalmol 102:1693, 1984.

83. Coleman, AL, Quigley, HA, Vitale, S, Dunkelberger, G: Displacement of the optic nerve head by acute changes in intraocular pressure in monkey eyes. Ophthalmology 98:35, 1991.

84. Quigley, HA, Hohman, RM, Addicks, EM, et al: Morphologic changes in the lamina cribrosa correlated with neural loss in open-angle glaucoma. Am J Ophthalmol 95:673, 1983.

85. Dandona, L, Quigley, HA, Brown, AE, Enger, C: Quantitative regional structure of the normal human lamina cribrosa. A racial comparison. Arch Ophthalmol 108:393, 1990.

86. Hernandez, MR, Andrzejewska, WM, Neufeld, AH: Changes in the extracellular matrix of the human optic nerve head in primary open-angle glaucoma. Am J Ophthalmol 109:180, 1990.

87. Morrison, JC, Dorman-Pease, ME, Dunkelberger, GR, Quigley, HA: Optic nerve head extracellular matrix in primary optic atrophy and experimental glaucoma. Arch Ophthalmol 108:1020, 1990.

88. Fukuchi, T, Sawaguchi, S, Hara, H, et al: Extracellular matrix changes of the optic nerve lamina cribrosa in monkey eyes with experimentally chronic glaucoma. Graefes Arch Clin Exp Ophthalmol 230:421, 1992.

89. Quigley, HA, Brown, A, Dorman-Pease, ME: Alterations in elastin of the optic nerve head in human and experimental glaucoma. Br J Ophthalmol 75:552, 1991.

90. Hernandez, MR, Yang, J, Ye, H: Activation of elastin mRNA expression in human optic nerve heads with primary open-angle glaucoma. J Glau 3:214, 1994.

91. Vrabee, F: Glaucomatous cupping of the human optic disk. A neurohistologic study. Graefes Arch Clin Exp Ophthalmol 198:223, 1976.

92. Quigley, HA, Addicks, EM: Chronic experimental glaucoma in primates. II. Effect of extended intraocular pressure elevation on optic nerve head and axonal transport. Invest Ophthalmol Vis Sci 19:137, 1980.

93. Quigley, HA, Sanchez, RM, Dunkelberger, GR, et al: Chronic glaucoma selectively damages large optic nerve fibers. Invest Ophthalmol Vis Sci 23:913, 1987.

94. Quigley, HA, Dundelberger, GR, Green, WR: Chronic human glaucoma causing selectively greater loss of large optic nerve fibers. Ophthalmology 95:357, 1988.

95. Glovinsky, Y, Quigley, HA, Dunkelberger, GR: Retinal ganglion cell loss is size dependent in experimental glaucoma. Invest Ophthalmol Vis Sci 32:484, 1991.

96. Glovinsky, Y, Quigley, HA, Pease, ME: Foveal ganglion cell loss is size dependent in experimental glaucoma. Invest Ophthalmol Vis Sci 34:395, 1993.

97. Quigley, HA, Nickells, RW, Kerrigan, LA, et al: Retinal ganglion cell death in experimental glaucoma and after axotomy occurs by apoptosis. Invest Ophthalmol Vis Sci 36:774, 1995.

98. Kubota, T, Holbach, LM, Naumann, GOH: Corpora amylacea in glaucomatous and non-glaucomatous optic nerve and retina. Graefes Arch Clin Exp Ophthalmol 231:7, 1993.

99. Kubota, T, Naumann, GOH: Reduction in number of corpora amylacea with advancing histological changes of glaucoma. Graefes Arch Clin Exp Ophthalmol 231:249, 1993.

100. Panda, S, Jonas, JB: Decreased photoreceptor count in human eyes with secondary angle-closure glaucoma. Invest Ophthalmol Vis Sci 33:2532, 1992.

101. Kendell, KR, Quigley, HA, Kerrigan, LA, et al: Primary open-angle glaucoma is not associated with photoreceptor loss. Invest Ophthalmol Vis Sci 36:200, 1995.

102. Wygnanski, T, Desatnik, H, Quigley, HA, Glovinsky, Y: Comparison of ganglion cell loss and cone loss in experimental glaucoma. Am J Ophthalmol 120:184, 1995.

103. Weinstein, JM, Duckrow, RB, Beard, D, Brennant, RW: Regional optic nerve blood flow and its autoregulation. Invest Ophthalmol Vis Sci 24:1559, 1983.

104. Sossi, N, Anderson, DR: Effect of elevated intraocular pressure on blood flow. Occurrence in cat optic nerve head studied with Iodoantipyrine I 125. Arch Ophthalmol 101:98, 1983.

105. Grehn, F, Prost, M: Function of retinal nerve fibers depends on perfusion pressure: Neurophysiologic investigations during acute intraocular pressure elevation. Invest Ophthalmol Vis Sci 24:347, 1983.

106. Novack, RL, Stefánsson, E, Hatchell, DL: Intraocular pressure effects on optic nerve-head oxidative metabolism measured in vivo. Graefes Arch Clin Exp Ophthalmol 228:128, 1990.

107. Quigley, HA, Hohman, RM, Sanchez, R, Addicks, EM: Optic nerve head blood flow in chronic experimental glaucoma. Arch Ophthalmol 103:956, 1985.

108. Ernest, JT: Pathogenesis of glaucomatous optic nerve disease. Trans Am Ophthalmol Soc LXXIII:366, 1975.

109. Shonat, RD, Wilson, DF, Riva, CE, Cranstoun, SD: Effect of acute increases in intraocular pressure on intravascular optic nerve head oxygen tension in cats. Invest Ophthalmol Vis Sci 33:3174, 1992.

110. Riva, CE, Grunwald, JE, Sinclair, SH: Laser doppler measurement of relative blood velocity in the human optic nerve head. Invest Ophthalmol Vis Sci 22:241, 1982.

111. Rojanapongpun, P, Drance, SM, Morrison, BJ: Ophthalmic artery flow velocity in glaucomatous and normal subjects. Br J Ophthalmol 77:25, 1993.

112. Costa, VP, Sergott, RC, Smith, M, et al: Color Doppler imaging in glaucoma patients with asymmetric optic cups. J Glau 3:S91, 1994.

113. Hamard, P, Hamard, H, Dufaux, J, Quesnot, S: Optic nerve head blood flow using a laser Doppler velocimeter and haemorheology in primary open-angle glaucoma and normal pressure glaucoma. Br J Ophthalmol 78:449, 1994.

114. Rankin, SJA, Walman, BE, Buckley, AR, Drance, SM: Color Doppler imaging and spectral analysis of the optic nerve vasculature in glaucoma. Am J Ophthalmol 119:685, 1995.

115. Robert, Y, Steiner, D, Hendrickson, P: Papillary circulation dynamics in glaucoma. Graefes Arch Clin Exp Ophthalmol 227:436, 1989.

116. Shin, DH, Tsai, CS, Parrow, KA, et al: Intraocular pressure-dependent retinal vascular change in adult chronic open-angle glaucoma patients. Ophthalmology 98:1087, 1991.

117. Ernest, JT, Archer, D: Fluorescein angiography of the optic disk. Am J Ophthalmol 75:973, 1973.

118. Schwartz, B, Kern, J: Age, increased ocular and blood pressures, and retinal and disc fluorescein angiogram. Arch Ophthalmol 93:1980, 1980.

119. Tso, MOM, Shih, C-Y, McLean, IW: Is there a blood-brain barrier at the optic nerve head? Arch Ophthalmol 93:815, 1975.

120. Hayreh, SS: Optic disc changes in glaucoma. Br J Ophthalmol 56:175, 1972.

121. Rosen, ES, Boyd, TAS: New method of assessing choroidal ischemia in open-angle glaucoma and ocular hypertension. Am J Ophthalmol 70:912, 1970.

122. Raitta, C, Sarmela, T: Fluorescein angiography of the optic disc and the peripapillary area in chronic glaucoma. Acta Ophthalmol 48:303, 1970.

123. Blumenthal, M, Best, M, Galin, MA, Toyofuku, H: Peripapillary choroidal circulation in glaucoma. Arch Ophthalmol 86:31, 1971.

124. Hayreh, SS: The pathogenesis of optic nerve lesions in glaucoma. Trans Am Acad Ophthalmol Otol 81:197, 1976.

125. Oosterhuis, JA, Boen-Tan, TN: Choroidal fluorescence in the normal human eye. Ophthalmologica 162:246, 1971.

126. Evans, PY, Shimizu, K, Limaye, S, et al: Fluorescein cineangiography of the optic nerve head. Trans Am Acad Ophthalmol Otol 77:260, 1973.

127. Best, M, Toyofuke, H: Ocular hemodynamics during induced ocular hypertension in man. Am J Ophthalmol 74:932, 1972.

128. Hitchings, RA, Spaeth, GL: Fluorescein angiography in chronic simple and low-tension glaucoma. Br J Ophthalmol 61:126, 1977.

129. Alterman, M, Henkind, P: Radial peripapillary capillaries of the retina. II. Possible role in Bjerrum scotoma. Br J Ophthalmol 52:26, 1968.

130. Blumenthal, M, Gitter, KA, Best, M, Galin, MA: Fluorescein angiography during induced ocular hypertension in man. Am J Ophthalmol 69:39, 1970.

131. Blumenthal, M, Best, M, Galin, MA, Gitter, KA: Ocular circulation: Analysis of the effect of induced ocular hypertension on retinal and choroidal blood flow in man. Am J Ophthalmol 71:819, 1971.

132. Archer, DB, Ernest, JT, Krill, AE: Retinal, choroidal, and papillary circulations under conditions of induced ocular hypertension. Am J Ophthalmol 73:834, 1972.

133. Spaeth, GL: Fluorescein angiography: Its contributions towards understanding the mechanisms of visual loss in glaucoma. Trans Am Ophthalmol Soc LXXIII:491, 1975.

134. Spaeth, GL: The Pathogenesis of Nerve Damage in Glaucoma: Contributions of Fluorescein Angiography. New York, Grune & Stratton, 1977.

135. Schwartz, B, Rieser, JC, Fishbein, SL: Fluorescein angiographic defects of the optic disc in glaucoma. Arch Ophthalmol 95:1961, 1977.

136. Sonty, S, Schwartz, B: Two-point fluorophotometry in the evaluation of glaucomatous optic disc. Arch Ophthalmol 98:1422, 1980.

137. Fishbein, SL, Schwartz, B: Optic disc in glaucoma. Topography and extent of fluorescein filling defects. Arch Ophthalmol 95:1975, 1977.

138. Adam, G, Schwartz, B: Increased fluorescein filling defects in the wall of the optic disc cup in glaucoma. Arch Ophthalmol 98:1590, 1980.

139. Loebl, M, Schwartz, B: Fluorescein angiographic defects of the optic disc in ocular hypertension. Arch Ophthalmol 95:1980, 1977.

140. Talusan, E, Schwartz, B: Specificity of fluorescein angiographic defects of the optic disc in glaucoma. Arch Ophthalmol 95:2166, 1977.

141. Talusan, ED, Schwartz, B, Wilcox, LM Jr: Fluorescein angiography of the optic disc. A longitudinal follow-up study. Arch Ophthalmol 98:1579, 1980.

142. Tuulonen, A, Nagin, P, Schwartz, B, Wu, D-C: Increase of pallor and fluorescein-filling defects of the optic disc in the followup of ocular hypertensives measured by computerized image analysis. Ophthalmology 94:558, 1987.

143. Tsukahara, S: Hyperpermeable disc capillaries in glaucoma. Adv Ophthalmol 35:65, 1978.

144. Moses, RA: Intraocular blood flow from analysis of angiograms. Invest Ophthalmol Vis Sci 24:354, 1983.

145. Minckler, DS, Tso, MOM: A light microscopic, autoradiographic study of axoplasmic transport in the normal rhesus optic nerve head. Am J Ophthalmol 82:1, 1976.

146. Minckler, DS, Bunt, AH, Johanson, GW: Orthograde and retrograde axoplasmic transport during acute ocular hypertension in the monkey. Invest Ophthalmol Vis Sci 16:426, 1977.

147. Taylor, AC, Weiss, P: Demonstration of axonal flow by the movement of tritium-labeled protein in mature optic nerve fibers. Proc Natl Acad Sci USA 54:1521, 1965.

148. Weiss, P, Pillai, A: Convection and fate of mitochondria in nerve fibers: axonal flow as vehicle. Proc Natl Acad Sci USA 54:48, 1965.

149. Johansson, J-O: Inhibition of retrograde axoplasmic transport in rat optic nerve by increased IOP in vitro. Invest Ophthalmol Vis Sci 24:1552, 1983.

150. Anderson, DR, Hendrickson, A: Effect of intraocular pressure on rapid axoplasmic transport in monkey optic nerve. Invest Ophthalmol 13:771, 1974.

151. Minckler, DS, Tso, MOM, Zimmerman, LE: A light microscopic, autoradiographic study of axoplasmic transport in the optic nerve head during ocular hypotony, increased intraocular pressure, and papilledema. Am J Ophthalmol 82:741, 1976.

152. Quigley, HA, Anderson, DR: The dynamics and location of axonal transport blockade by acute intraocular pressure elevation in primate optic nerve. Invest Ophthalmol 15:606, 1976.

153. Minckler, DS, Bunt, AH, Klock, IB: Radioautographic and cytochemical ultrastructural studies of axoplasmic transport in the monkey optic nerve head. Invest Ophthalmol Vis Sci 17:33, 1978.

154. Quigley, HA, Guy, J, Anderson, DR: Blockage of rapid axonal transport. Effect of intraocular pressure elevation in primate optic nerve. Arch Ophthalmol 97:525, 1979.

155. Sakugawa, M, Chihara, E: Blockage at two points of axonal transport in glaucomatous eyes. Graefes Arch Clin Exp Ophthalmol 223:214, 1985.

156. Dandona, L, Hendrickson, A, Quigley, HA: Selective effects of experimental glaucoma on axonal transport by retinal ganglion cells to the dorsal lateral geniculate nucleus. Invest Ophthalmol Vis Sci 32:1593, 1991.

157. Radius, RL: Distribution of pressure-induced fast axonal transport abnormalities in primate optic nerve. Arch Ophthalmol 99:1253, 1981.

158. Quigley, HA, Anderson, DR: Distribution of axonal transport blockade by acute intraocular pressure elevation in the primate optic nerve head. Invest Ophthalmol Vis Sci 16:640, 1977.

159. Gaasterland, D, Tanishima, T, Kuwabara, T: Axoplasmic flow during chronic experimental glaucoma. I. Light and electron microscopic studies of the monkey optic nerve head during development of glaucomatous cupping. Invest Ophthalmol Vis Sci 17:838, 1978.

160. Quigley, HA, Flower, RW, Addicks, EM, McLeod, DS: The mechanism of optic nerve damage in experimental acute intraocular pressure elevation. Invest Ophthalmol Vis Sci 19:505, 1980.

161. Minckler, DS, Bunt, AH: Axoplasmic transport in ocular hypotony and papilledema in the monkey. Arch Ophthalmol 95:1430, 1977.

162. Tso, MOM: Axoplasmic transport in papilledema and glaucoma. Trans Am Acad Ophthalmol Otol 83:771, 1977.

163. Anderson, DR, Hendrickson, AE: Failure of increased intracranial pressure to affect rapid axonal transport at the optic nerve head. Invest Ophthalmol Vis Sci 16:423, 1977.

164. Radius, RL, Anderson, DR: Rapid axonal transport in primate optic nerve. Distribution of pressure-induced interruption. Arch Ophthalmol 99:650, 1981.

165. Radius, RL, Bade, B: Axonal transport interruption and anatomy at the lamina cribrosa. Arch Ophthalmol 100:1661, 1982.

166. Radius, RL: Pressure-induced fast axonal transport abnormalities and the anatomy at the lamina cribrosa in primate eyes. Invest Ophthalmol Vis Sci 24:343, 1983.

167. Levy, NS, Adams, CK: Slow axonal protein transport and visual function following retinal and optic nerve ischemia. Invest Ophthalmol 14:91, 1975.

168. Levy, NS: The effect of interruption of the short posterior ciliary arteries on slow axoplasmic transport and histology within the optic nerve of the rhesus monkey. Invest Ophthalmol 15:495, 1976.

169. Radius, RL: Optic nerve fast axonal transport abnormalities in primates. Occurrence after short posterior ciliary artery occlusion. Arch Ophthalmol 98:2018, 1980.

170. Radius, RL, Anderson, DR: Morphology of axonal transport abnormalities in primate eyes. Br J Ophthalmol 65:767, 1981.

171. Radius, RL, Bade, B: Pressure-induced optic nerve axonal transport interruption in cat eyes. Arch Ophthalmol 99:2163, 1981.

172. Sossi, N, Anderson, DR: Blockage of axonal transport in optic nerve induced by elevation of intraocular pressure. Effect of arterial hypertension induced by Angiotensin I. Arch Ophthalmol 101:94, 1983.

173. Radius, RL, Anderson, DR: Breakdown of the normal optic nerve head blood-brain barrier following acute elevation of intraocular pressure in experimental animals. Invest Ophthalmol Vis Sci 19:244, 1980.

174. Radius, RL, Schwartz, EL, Anderson, DR: Failure of unilateral carotid artery ligation to affect pressure-induced interruption of rapid axonal transport in primate optic nerves. Invest Ophthalmol Vis Sci 19:153, 1980.

175. Sipperley, J, Anderson, DR, Hamasaki, D: Short-term effect of intraocular pressure elevation on the human electroretinogram. Arch Ophthalmol 90:358, 1973.

176. Bartl, G: The electroretinogram and the visual evoked potential in normal and glaucomatous eyes. Graefes Arch Clin Exp Ophthalmol 207:243, 1978.

177. Pillunat, LE, Stodtmeister, R, Wilmanns, I, Christ, TH: Autoregulation of ocular blood flow during changes in intraocular pressure. Preliminary results. Graefes Arch Clin Exp Ophthalmol 223:219, 1985.

178. Weiter, J, Fine, BS: A histologic study of regional choroidal dystrophy. Am J Ophthalmol 83:741, 1977.

179. Hayreh, SS: Anterior Ischemic Optic Neuropathy. New York, Springer-Verlag, 1975.

180. Quigley, H, Anderson, DR: Cupping of the optic disc in ischemic optic neuropathy. Trans Am Acad Ophthalmol Otol 83:755, 1977.

181. Sebag, J, Thomas, JV, Epstein, DL, Grant, WM: Optic disc cupping in arteritic anterior ischemic optic neuropathy resembles glaucomatous cupping. Ophthalmology 93:357, 1986.

182. Hitchings, RA: The optic disc in glaucoma, III: Diffuse optic disc pallor with raised intraocular pressure. Br J Ophthalmol 62:670, 1978.

183. Quigley, HA, Miller, NR, Green, WR: The pattern of optic nerve fiber loss in anterior ischemic optic neuropathy. Am J Ophthalmol 100:769, 1985

184. Radius, RL, Maumenee, AE: Optic atrophy and glaucomatous cupping. Am J Ophthalmol 85:145, 1978.

185. Jampol, LM, Board, RJ, Maumenee, AE: Systemic hypotension and glaucomatous changes. Am J Ophthalmol 85:154, 1978.

186. Brownstein, S, Font, RL, Zimmerman, LE, Murphy, SB: Nonglaucomatous cavernous degeneration of the optic nerve. Report of two cases. Arch Ophthalmol 98:345, 1980.

187. Caprioli, J, Spaeth, GL: Comparison of visual field defects in the low-tension glaucomas with those in the high-tension glaucomas. Am J Ophthalmol 97:730, 1984.

188. Jonas, JB, Gusek, GC, Guggenmoos-Holzmann, I, Naumann, GOH: Variability of the real dimensions of normal human optic discs. Graefes Arch Clin Exp Ophthalmol 226:332, 1988.

189. Jonas, JB, Gusek, GC, Naumann GOH: Optic disc, cup and neuroretinal rim size, configuration and correlations in normal eyes. Invest Ophthalmol Vis Sci 29:1151, 1988.

190. Schwartz, B: Cupping and pallor of the optic disc. Arch Ophthalmol 89:272, 1973.

191. Armaly, MF: Genetic determination of cup/disc ratio of the optic nerve. Arch Ophthalmol 78:35, 1967.

192. Schwartz, JT, Reuling, FH, Garrison, RJ: Acquired cupping of the optic nerve head in normotensive eyes. Br J Ophthalmol 59:216, 1975.

193. Carpel, EF, Engstrom, PF: The normal cup-disk ratio. Am J Ophthalmol 91:588, 1981.
194. Fishman, RS: Optic disc asymmetry. A sign of ocular hypertension. Arch Ophthalmol 84:590, 1970.
195. Holm, OC, Becker, B, Asseff, CF, Podos, SM: Volume of the optic disk cup. Am J Ophthalmol 73:876, 1972.
196. Hollows, FC, McGuiness, R: The size of the optic cup. Trans Ophthalmol Soc Aust NZ 19:33, 1966.
197. Bengtsson, B: The inheritance and development of cup and disc diameters. Acta Ophthalmol 58:733, 1980.
198. Teikari, JM, Airaksinen, JP: Twin study on cup/disc ratio of the optic nerve head. Br J Ophthalmol 76:218, 1992.
199. Armaly, MF, Sayegh, RE: The cup/disc ratio. The findings of tonometry and tonography in the normal eye. Arch Ophthalmol 82:191, 1969.
200. Armaly, MF: The optic cup in the normal eye. I. Cup width, depth, vessel displacement, ocular tension and outflow facility. Am J Ophthalmol 68:401, 1969.
201. Bengtsson, B: The alteration and asymmetry of cup and disc diameters. Acta Ophthalmol 58:726, 1980.
202. Becker, B: Cup/disk ratio and topical corticosteriod testing. Am J Ophthalmol 70:681, 1970.
203. Jonas, JB: Size of glaucomatous optic discs. Ger J Ophthalmol 1:41, 1992.
204. Burk, ROW, Rohrschneider, K, Noack, H, Völcker, HE: Are large optic nerve heads susceptible to glaucomatous damage at normal intraocular pressure? A three-dimensional study by laser scanning tomography. Graefes Arch Clin Exp Ophthalmol 230:552, 1992.
205. Snydacker, D: The normal optic disc. Ophthalmoscopic and photographic studies. Am J Ophthalmol 58:958, 1964.
206. Varma, R, Tielsch, JM, Quigley, HA, et al: Race-, age-, gender-, and refractive error-related differences in the normal optic disc. Arch Ophthalmol 112:1068, 1994.
207. Schwartz, B: Optic disc changes in ocular hypertension. Surv Ophthalmol 25:148, 1980.
208. Schwartz, B, Reinstein, NM, Lieberman, DM: Pallor of the optic disc. Quantitative photographic evaluation. Arch Ophthalmol 89:278, 1973.
209. Tsai, CS, Ritch, R, Shin, DH, et al: Age-related decline of disc rim area in visually normal subjects. Ophthalmology 99:29, 1992.
210. Beck, RW, Messner, DK, Musch, DC, et al: Is there a racial difference in physiologic cup size? Ophthalmology 92:873, 1985.
211. Chi, T, Ritch, R, Stickler, D, et al: Racial differences in optic nerve head parameters. Arch Ophthalmol 107:836, 1989.
212. Tsai, CS, Zangwill, L, Gonzalez, et al: Ethnic differences in optic nerve head topography. J Glau 4:248, 1995.
213. Mansour, AM: Racial variation of optic disc parameters in children. Ophthalmic Surg 23:469, 1992.
214. Jonas, JB, Gusek, GC, Naumann, GOH: Optic disc morphometry in high myopia. Graefes Arch Clin Exp Ophthalmol 226:587, 1988.
215. Jonas, JB, Zach, F-M, Gusek, GC, Naumann, GOH: Pseudoglaucomatous physiologic large cups. Am J Ophthalmol 107:137, 1989.
216. Tomlinson, A, Phillips, CI: Ovalness of the optic cup and disc in the normal eye. Br J Ophthalmol 58:543, 1974.
217. Portney, GL: Qualitative parameters of the normal optic nerve head. Am J Ophthalmol 76:655, 1973.
218. Portney, GL: Photogrammetric categorical analysis of the optic nerve head. Trans Am Acad Ophthalmol Otol 78:275, 1974.
219. Shields, MB: Problems in recognizing non-glaucomatous optic nerve head cupping. Perspect Ophthalmol 2:129, 1978.
220. Balazsi, AG, Drance, SM, Schulzer, M, Douglas, GR: Neuroretinal rim area in suspected glaucoma and early chronic open-angle glaucoma. Correlation with parameters of visual function. Arch Ophthalmol 102:1011, 1984.
221. Caprioli, J, Miller, JM: Optic disc rim area is related to disc size in normal subjects. Arch Ophthalmol 105:1683, 1987.
222. Britton, RJ, Drance, SM, Schulzer, M, et al: The area of the neuroretinal rim of the optic nerve in normal eyes. Am J Ophthalmol 103:497, 1987.
223. Jonas, JB, Gusek, GC, Guggenmoos-Holzmann, I, Naumann, GOH: Correlations of the neuroretinal rim area with ocular and general parameters in normal eyes. Ophthalmic Res 20:298, 1988.
224. Shields, MB: Gray crescent in the optic nerve head. Am J Ophthalmol 89:238, 1980.
225. Varma, R, Hilton, SC, Tielsch, JM, et al: Neural rim area declines with increased intraocular pressure in urban Americans. Arch Ophthalmol 113:1001, 1995.
226. Klein, BEK, Moss, SE, Klein, R, et al: Neuroretinal rim area in diabetes mellitus. Invest Ophthalmol Vis Sci 31:805, 1990.
227. Radius, RL: Thickness of the retinal nerve fiber layer in primate eyes. Arch Ophthalmol 100:807, 1982.
228. Quigley, HA, Addicks, EM: Quantitative studies of retinal nerve fiber layer defects. Arch Ophthalmol 100:807, 1982.
229. Jonas, JB, Nguyen, NX, Naumann, GOH: The retinal nerve fiber layer in normal eyes. Ophthalmology 96:627, 1989.
230. Jonas, JB, Schiro, D: Visibility of the normal retinal nerve fiber layer correlated with rim width and vessel caliber. Graefes Arch Clin Exp Ophthalmol 231:207, 1993.
231. Caprioli, J: Discrimination between normal and glaucomatous eyes. Invest Ophthalmol Vis Sci 33:153, 1992.
232. Fantes, FE, Anderson, DR: Clinical histologic correlation of human peripapillary anatomy. Ophthalmology 96:20, 1989.
233. Jonas, JB, Königsreuther, KA, Naumann, GOH: Optic disc histomorphometry in normal eyes and eyes with secondary angle-closure glaucoma. II. Parapapillary region. Graefes Arch Clin Exp Ophthalmol 230:134, 1992.
234. Kirsch, RE, Anderson, DR: Clinical recognition of glaucomatous cupping. Am J Ophthalmol 75:442, 1973.
235. Weisman, RL, Asseff, DF, Phelps, CD, et al: Vertical elongation of the optic cup in glaucoma. Trans Am Acad Ophthalmol Otol 77:157, 1973.
236. Read, RM, Spaeth, GL: The practical clinical appraisal of the optic disc in glaucoma: the natural history of cup progression and some specific disc-field correlations. Trans Am Acad Ophthalmol Otol 78:255, 1974.
237. Spaeth, GL, Hitchings, RA, Sivalingam, E: The optic disc in glaucoma: Pathogenetic correlation of five patterns of cupping in chronic open-angle glaucoma. Trans Am Acad Ophthalmol Otol 81:217, 1976.
238. Hitchings, RA, Spaeth, GL: The optic disc in glaucoma. I: classification. Br J Ophthalmol 60:778, 1976.
239. Radius, RL, Maumenee, AE, Green, WR: Pit-like changes of the optic nerve head in open-angle glaucoma. Br J Ophthalmol 62:389, 1978.
240. Betz, PH, Camps, F, Collignon-Brach, J, et al: Biometric study of the disc cup in open-angle glaucoma. Graefes Arch Clin Exp Ophthalmol 218:70, 1982.
241. Jonas, JB, Gusek, GC, Naumann, GOH: Optic disc morphometry in chronic primary open-angle glaucoma: I. Morphometric intrapapillary characteristics. Graefes Arch Clin Exp Ophthalmol 226:522, 1988.
242. Jonas, JB, Fernández, MC, Stürmer, J: Pattern of glaucomatous neuroretinal rim loss. Ophthalmology 100:63, 1993.
243. Shin, DH, Lee, MK, Briggs, KS, et al: Intraocular pressure-related pattern of optic disc cupping in adult glaucoma patients. Graefes Arch Clin Exp Ophthalmol 230:542, 1992.
244. Airaksinen, PJ, Drance, SM, Schulzer, M: Neuroretinal rim area in early glaucoma. Am J Ophthalmol 99:1, 1985.
245. Drance, SM, Balazsi, G: The neuro-retinal rim area in early glaucoma. Klin Monatsbl Augenheilkd 184:271, 1984.
246. Pederson, JE, Anderson, DR: The mode of progressive disc cupping in ocular hypertension and glaucoma. Arch Ophthalmol 98:490, 1980.
247. Cher, I, Robinson, LP: "Thinning" of the neural rim of the optic nerve-head. An altered state, providing a new ophthalmoscopic sign associated with characteristics of glaucoma. Trans Ophthalmol Soc UK 93:213, 1973.

248. Cher, I, Robinson, LP: Thinning of the neural rim: a simple new sign on the optic disc related to glaucoma—statistical considerations. Aust J Ophthalmol 2:27, 1974.

249. Portney, GL: Photogrammetric analysis of the three-dimensional geometry of normal and glaucomatous optic cups. Trans Am Acad Ophthalmol Otol 81:239, 1976.

250. Susanna, R Jr: The lamina cribrosa and visual field defects in open-angle glaucoma. Can J Ophthalmol 18:124, 1983.

251. Miller, KM, Quigley, HA: The clinical appearance of the lamina cribrosa as a function of the extent of glaucomatous optic nerve damage. Ophthalmology 95:135, 1988.

252. Chandler, PA, Grant, WM: Glaucoma, 2nd ed. Philadelphia, Lea and Febiger, 1977.

253. Phillips, CI, Tsukahara, S, Makino, F, et al: Saucerisation (recession) of neuro-retinal rim is characteristic of glaucoma. Jpn J Ophthalmol 37:171, 1993.

254. Drance, SM, Fairclough, M, Butler, DM, Kottler, MS: The importance of disc hemorrhage in the prognosis of chronic open angle glaucoma. Arch Ophthalmol 95:226, 1977.

255. Susanna, R, Drance, SM, Douglas, GR: Disc hemorrhages in patients with elevated intraocular pressure. Occurrence with and without field changes. Arch Ophthalmol 97:284, 1979.

256. Hendrickx, KH, van den Enden, A, Rasker, MT, Hoyng, PFJ: Cumulative incidence of patients with disc hemorrhages in glaucoma and the effect of therapy. Ophthalmology 101:1165, 1994.

257. Jonas, JB, Xu, L: Optic disk hemorrhages in glaucoma. Am J Ophthalmol 118:1, 1994.

258. Sonnsjö, B: Glaucomatous disc haemorrhages photographed at short inervals. Acta Ophthalmol 64:263, 1986.

259. Airaksinen, PJ, Mustonen, E, Alanko, HI: Optic disc hemorrhages precede retinal nerve fiber layer defects in ocular hypertension. Acta Ophthalmol (Copenh) 59:627, 1981.

260. Bengtsson, B, Holmin, C, Krakau, CET: Disc hemorrhage and glaucoma. Acta Ophthalmol 59:1, 1981.

261. Shihab, ZM, Lee, P-F, Hay, P: The significance of disc hemorrhage in open-angle glaucoma. Ophthalmology 89:211, 1982.

262. Bengtsson, B: Characteristics of manifest glaucoma at early stages. Graefes Arch Clin Exp Ophthalmol 227:241, 1989.

263. Bengtsson, B: Optic disc haemorrhages preceding manifest glaucoma. Acta Ophthalmol 68:450, 1990.

264. Diehl, DLC, Quigley, HA, Miller, NR, et al: Prevalence and significance of optic disc hemorrhage in a longitudinal study of glaucoma. Arch Ophthalmol 108:545, 1990.

265. Gloster, J: Incidence of optic disc hemorrhages in chronic simple glaucoma and ocular hypertension. Br J Ophthalmol 65:452, 1981.

266. Poinoosawmy, D, Gloster, J, Nagasubramanian, S, Hitchings, RA: Association between optic disc haemorrhages in glaucoma and abnormal glucose tolerance. Br J Ophthalmol 70:599, 1986.

267. Tuulonen, A, Takamoto, T, Wu, D-C, Schwartz, B: Optic disc cupping and pallor measurements of patients with a disk hemorrhages. Am J Ophthalmol 103:505, 1987.

268. Heijl, A: Frequent disc photography and computerized perimetry in eyes with optic disc haemorrhage. Acta Ophthalmol 64:274, 1986.

269. Susanna, R Jr, Basseto, FL: Hemorrhage of the optic disc and neurosensorial dysacousia. J Glau 1:248, 1992.

270. Hitchings, RA, Spaeth, GL: Chronic retinal vein occlusion in glaucoma. Br J Ophthalmol 60:694, 1976.

271. Tuulonen, A: Asymptomatic miniocclusions of the optic disc veins in glaucoma. Arch Ophthalmol 107:1475, 1989.

272. Shihab, ZM, Beebe, WE, Wentlandt, T: Possible significance of cilioretinal arteries in open-angle glaucoma. Ophthalmology 92:880, 1985.

273. Lindenmuth, KA, Skuta, GL, Musch, DC, Bueche, M: Significance of cilioretinal arteries in primary open angle glaucoma. Arch Ophthalmol 106:1691, 1988.

274. Lee, SS, Schwartz, B: Role of the temporal cilioretinal artery in retaining central visual field in open-angle glaucoma. Ophthalmology 99:696, 1992.

275. Herschler, J, Osher, RH: Baring of the circumlinear vessel. An early sign of optic nerve damage. Arch Ophthalmol 98:865, 1980.

276. Osher, RH, Herschler, J: The significance of baring of the circumlinear vessel. A prospective study. Arch Ophthalmol 99:817, 1981.

277. Sutton, GE, Motolko, MA, Phelps, CD: Baring of a circumlinear vessel in glaucoma. Arch Ophthalmol 101:739, 1983.

278. Kasner, O, Balazsi, AG: Glaucomatous optic nerve atrophy: the circumlinear vessel revisited. Can J Ophthalmol 26:264, 1991.

279. Jonas, JB, Fernández, MC: Shape of the neuroretinal rim and position of the central retinal vessels in glaucoma. Br J Ophthalmol 78:99, 1994.

280. Rader, J, Feuer, WJ, Anderson, DR: Peripapillary vasoconstriction in the glaucomas and the anterior ischemic optic neuropathies. Am J Ophthalmol 117:72, 1994.

281. Sommer, A, Miller, NR, Pollack, I, et al: The nerve fiber layer in the diagnosis of glaucoma. Arch Ophthalmol 95:2149, 1977.

282. Sommer, A, Pollack, I, Maumenee, AE: Optic disc parameters and onset of glaucomatous field loss. II. Static screening criteria. Arch Ophthalmol 97:1449, 1979.

283. Quigley, HA, Miller, NR, George, T: Clinical evaluation of nerve fiber layer atrophy as an indicator of glaucomatous optic nerve damage. Arch Ophthalmol 98:1564, 1980.

284. Jonas, JB, Schiro, D: Localised wedge-shaped defects of the retinal nerve fibre layer in glaucoma. Br J Ophthalmol 78:285, 1994.

285. Airaksinen, PJ, Tuulonen, A: Early glaucoma changes in patients with and without optic disc hemorrhage. Acta Ophthalmol 62:197, 1984.

286. Airaksinen, PJ, Drance, SM: Neuroretinal rim area and retinal nerve fiber layer in glaucoma. Arch Ophthalmol 103:203, 1985.

287. Nanba, K, Schwartz, B: Nerve fiber layer and optic disc fluorescein defects in glaucoma and ocular hypertension. Ophthalmology 95:1227, 1988.

288. Quigley, HA, Katz, J, Derick, RJ, et al: An evaluation of optic disc and nerve fiber layer examinations in monitoring progression of early glaucoma damage. Ophthalmology 99:19, 1992.

289. Jonas, JB, Königsreuther, KA: Optic disk appearance in ocular hypertensive eyes. Am J Ophthalmol 117:732, 1994.

290. Sommer, A, Katz, J, Quigley, HA, et al: Clinically detectable nerve fiber atrophy precedes the onset of glaucomatous field loss. Arch Ophthalmol 109:77, 1991.

291. Jonas, JB, Fernandez, MC, Naumann, GOH: Glaucomatous optic nerve atrophy in small discs with low cup-to-disc ratios. Ophthalmology 97:1211, 1990.

292. Airaksinen, PJ, Drance, SM, Douglas, GR, et al: Diffuse and localized nerve fiber loss in glaucoma. Am J Ophthalmol 98:566, 1984.

293. Sommer, A, Quigley, HA, Robin, AL, et al: Evaluation of nerve fiber layer assessment. Arch Ophthalmol 102:1766, 1984.

294. Airaksinen, PJ, Drance, SM, Douglas, GR, et al: Visual field and retinal nerve fiber layer comparisons in glaucoma. Arch Ophthalmol 103:205, 1985.

295. Tuulonen, A, Airaksinen, PJ: Initial glaucomatous optic disk and retinal nerve fiber layer abnormalities and their progression. Am J Ophthalmol 111:485, 1991.

296. Wilensky, JT, Kolker, AE: Peripapillary changes in glaucoma. Am J Ophthalmol 81:341, 1976.

297. Jonas, JB, Naumann, OH: Parapapillary chorioretinal atrophy in normal and glaucoma eyes. II. Correlations. Invest Ophthalmol Vis Sci 30:919, 1989.

298. Buus, DR, Anderson, DR: Peripapillary crescents and halos in normal-tension glaucoma and ocular hypertension. Ophthalmology 96:16, 1989.

299. Jonas, JB, Fernández, MC, Naumann, GOH: Parapapillary atrophy and retinal vessel diameter in nonglaucomatous optic nerve damage. Invest Ophthalmol Vis Sci 32:2942, 1991.

300. Rockwood, EJ, Anderson, DR: Acquired peripapillary changes and progression in glaucoma. Graefes Arch Clin Exp Ophthalmol 226:510, 1988.

301. Jonas, JB, Fernández, MC, Naumann, GOH: Glaucomatous parapapillary atrophy. Occurrence and correlations. Arch Ophthalmol 110:214, 1992.

302. Kasner, O, Feuer, WJ, Anderson, DR: Possibly reduced prevalence of peripapillary crescents in ocular hypertension. Can J Ophthalmol 24:211, 1989.

303. Kessing, SV, Gregersen E: Distended disk in early stages of congenital glaucoma. Acta Ophthalmol 55:431, 1977.

304. Quigley, HA: Childhood glaucoma. Results with trabeculotomy and study of reversible cupping. Ophthalmology 89:219, 1982.

305. Pederson, JE, Herschler, J: Reversal of glaucomatous cupping in adults. Arch Ophthalmol 100:426, 1982.

306. Schwartz, B, Takamoto, T, Nagin, P: Measurements of reversibility of optic disc cupping and pallor in ocular hypertension and glaucoma. Ophthalmology 92:1396, 1985.

307. Greenidge, KC, Spaeth, GL, Traverso, CE: Change in appearance of the optic disc associated with lowering of intraocular pressure. Ophthalmology 92:897, 1985.

308. Katz, LJ, Spaeth, GL, Cantor, LB, et al: Reversible optic disk cupping and visual field improvement in adults with glaucoma. Am J Ophthalmol 107:485, 1989.

309. Funk, J: Increase of neuroretinal rim area after surgical intraocular pressure reduction. Ophthalmic Surg 21:585, 1990.

310. Parrow, KA, Shin, DH, Tsai, CS, et al: Intraocular pressure-dependent dynamic changes of optic disc cupping in adult glaucoma patients. Ophthalmology 99:36, 1992.

311. Sogano, S, Tomita, G, Kitazawa, Y: Changes in retinal nerve fiber layer thickness after reduction of intraocular pressure in chronic open-angle glaucoma. Ophthalmology 100:1253, 1993.

312. Jensen, PE, Kalina, RE: Congenital anomalies of the optic disk. Am J Ophthalmol 82:27, 1976.

313. Pagon, RA: Ocular coloboma. Surv Ophthalmol 25:223, 1981.

314. Kindler, P: Morning glory syndrome: Unusual congenital optic disk anomaly. Am J Ophthalmol 69:376, 1970.

315. Apple, DJ, Rabb, MF, Walsh, PM: Congenital anomalies of the optic disc. Surv Ophthalmol 27:3, 1982.

316. Brodsky, MC: Congenital optic disk anomalies. Surv Ophthalmol 39:89, 1994.

317. Brown, GC, Shields, JA, Goldberg, RE: Congenital pits of the optic nerve head. II. Clinical studies in humans. Ophthalmology 87:51, 1980.

318. Theodossiadis, G: Evolution of congenital pit of the optic disk with macular detachment in photocoagulated and nonphotocoagulated eyes. Am J Ophthalmol 84:620, 1977.

319. Brazitikos, PD, Safran, AB, Simona, F, Zulauf, M: Threshold perimetry in tilted disc syndrome. Arch Ophthalmol 108:1698, 1990.

320. Trobe, JD, Glaser, JS, Cassady, J, et al: Optic atrophy. Differential diagnosis by fundus observation alone. Arch Ophthalmol 98:1040, 1980.

321. Trobe, JD, Glaser, JS, Cassady, J, et al: Nonglaucomatous excavation of the optic disc. Arch Ophthalmol 98:1046, 1980.

322. Lichter, PR, Henderson, JW: Optic nerve infarction. Am J Ophthalmol 85:302, 1978.

323. Portney, GL, Roth, AM: Optic cupping caused by an intracranial aneurysm. Am J Ophthalmol 84:98, 1977.

324. Repka, MX, Uozato, H, Guyton, DL: Depth distortion during slit-lamp biomicroscopy of the fundus. Ophthalmology 93(S):47, 1986.

325. Romano, JH: Graticule incorporated into an ophthalmoscope for the clinical evaluation of the cup/disc ratio. Br J Ophthalmol 67:214, 1983.

326. Gross, PG, Drance, SM: Comparison of a simple ophthalmoscopic and planimetric measurement of glaucomatous neuroretinal rim areas. J Glau 4:314, 1995.

327. Montgomery, DMI: Measurement of optic disc and neuroretinal rim areas in normal and glaucomatous eyes. A new clinical method. Ophthalmology 98:50, 1991.

328. Montgomery, DMI: Clinical disc biometry in early glaucoma. Ophthalmology 100:52, 1993.

329. Ruben, S: Estimation of optic disc size using indirect biomicroscopy. Br J Ophthalmol 78:363, 1994.

330. Spencer, AF, Vernon, SA: Optic disc measurement with the Zeiss four mirror contact lens. Br J Ophthalmol 78:775, 1994.

331. Jonas, JB, Papastathopoulos, K: Ophthalmoscopic measurement of the optic disc. Ophthalmology 102:1102, 1995.

332. Shaffer, RN, Ridgway, WL, Brown, R, Kramer, SG: The use of diagrams to record changes in glaucomatous disks. Am J Ophthalmol 80:460, 1975.

333. Lichter, PR: Variability of expert observers in evaluating the optic disc. Trans Am Ophthalmol Soc LXXIV:532, 1976.

334. Schwartz, JT: Methodologic differences and measurement of cup-disc ratio. An epidemiologic assessment. Arch Ophthalmol 94:1101, 1976.

335. Varma, R, Steinmann, WC, Scott, IU: Expert agreement in evaluating the optic disc for glaucoma. Ophthalmology 99:215, 1992.

336. Tielsch, JM, Katz, J, Quigley, HA, et al: Intraobserver and interobserver agreement in measurement of optic disc characteristics. Ophthalmology 95:350, 1988.

337. Gloster, J, Parry, DG: Use of photographs for measuring cupping in the optic disc. Br J Ophthalmol 58:850, 1974.

338. Hitchings, RA, Genio, C, Anderton, S, Clark, P: An optic disc grid: Its evaluation in reproducibility studies on the cup/disc ratio. Br J Ophthalmol 67:356, 1983.

339. Sharma, NK, Hitchings, RA: A comparison of monocular and "stereoscopic" photographs of the optic disc in the identification of glaucomatous visual field defects. Br J Ophthalmol 67:677, 1983.

340. Cohan, BE: Multiple-slit illumination of the optic disc. Arch Ophthalmol 96:497, 1978.

341. Kennedy, SJ, Schwartz, B, Takamoto, T, Eu, JKT: Interference fringe scale for absolute ocular fundus measurement. Invest Ophthalmol Vis Sci 24:169, 1983.

342. Schwartz, B, Kern, J: Scanning microdensitometry of optic disc pallor in glaucoma. Arch Ophthalmol 95:2159, 1977.

343. Rosenthal, AR, Falconer, DG, Barrett, P: Digital measurement of pallor-disc ratio. Arch Ophthalmol 98:2027, 1980.

344. Frisen, L: Photography of the retinal nerve fibre layer: An optimised procedure. Br J Ophthalmol 64:641, 1980.

345. Sommer, A, D'Anna, SA, Kues, HA, George, T: High-resolution photography of the retinal nerve fiber layer. Am J Ophthalmol 96:535, 1983.

346. Airaksinen, PJ, Nieminen, H: Retinal nerve fiber layer photography in glaucoma. Ophthalmology 92:877, 1985.

347. Peli, E, Hedges, TR, III, McInnes, T, et al: Nerve fiber layer photography. A comparative study. Acta Ophthalmol 65:71, 1987.

348. Wang, F, Quigley, HA, Tielsch, JM: Screening for glaucoma in a medical clinic with photographs of the nerve fiber layer. Arch Ophthalmol 112:796, 1994.

349. Sommer, A, Kues, HA, D'Anna, SA, et al: Cross-polarization photography of the nerve fiber layer. Arch Ophthalmol 102:864, 1984.

350. Airaksinen, PJ, Nieminen, H, Mustonen, E: Retinal nerve fibre layer photography with a wide angle fundus camera. Acta Ophthalmol 60:362, 1982.

351. Knighton, RW, Jacobson, SG, Kemp, CM: The spectral reflectance of the nerve fiber layer of the macaque retina. Invest Ophthalmol Vis Sci 30:2393, 1989.

352. Richards, DW, Janesick, JR, Elliot, ST, et al: Enhanced detection of normal retinal nerve-fiber striations using a charge-coupled device and digital filtering. Graefes Arch Clin Exp Ophthalmol 231:595, 1993.

353. Allen, L: Stereoscopic fundus photography with the new instant positive print films. Am J Ophthalmol 57:539, 1964.

354. Donaldson, DD: A new camera for stereoscopic fundus photography. Arch Ophthalmol 73:253, 1965.

355. Saheb, NE, Drance, SM, Nelson, A: The use of photogrammetry in evaluating the cup of the optic nervehead for a study in chronic simple glaucoma. Can J Ophthalmol 7:466, 1972.

356. Rosenthal, AR, Kottler, MS, Donaldson, DD, Falconer, DG: Comparative reproducibility of the digital photogrammetric procedure utilizing three methods of stereophotography. Invest Ophthalmol Vis Sci 16:54, 1977.

357. Greenfield, DS, Zacharia, P, Schuman, JS: Comparison of Nidek 3Dx and Donaldson simultaneous stereoscopic disk photography. Am J Ophthalmol 116:741, 1993.

358. Minckler, DS, Nichols, T, Morales, RB: Preliminary clinical experience with the Nidek 3Dx camera and lenticular stereo disc images. J Glau 1:184, 1992.

359. Schirmer, KE, Kratky, V: Stereochronoscopy of the optic disc with stereoscopic cameras. Arch Ophthalmol 98:1647, 1980.

360. Goldmann, H, Lotmar, W, Zulauf, M: Quantitative studies in stereochronoscopy (Sc): application to the disc in glaucoma. II. Statistical evaluation. Graefes Arch Clin Exp Ophthalmol 222:82, 1984.

361. Takamoto, T, Schwartz, B: Stereochronometry: quantitative measurement of optic disc cup changes. Invest Ophthalmol Vis Sci 26:1445, 1985.

362. Heijl, A, Bengtsson, B: Diagnosis of early glaucoma with flicker comparisons of serial disc photographs. Invest Ophthalmol Vis Sci 30:2376, 1989.

363. Alanko, H, Jaanio, E, Airaksinen, PJ, Nieminen, H: Demonstration of glaucomatous optic disc changes by electronic subtraction. Acta Ophthalmol 58:14, 1980.

364. Gloster, J: The colour of the optic disc. Doc Ophthalmol 26:155, 1969.

365. Davies, EWG: Quantitative assessment of colour of the optic disc by a photographic method. Exp Eye Res 9:106, 1970.

366. Berkowitz, JS, Balter, S: Colorimetric measurement of the optic disk. Am J Ophthalmol 69:385, 1970.

367. Hendrickson, P, Robert, Y, Stockli, HP: Principles of photometry of the papilla. Arch Ophthalmol 102:1704, 1984.

368. Cohen, JS, Stone, RD, Hetherington, J Jr, Bullock, J: Glaucomatous cupping of the optic disk by ultrasonography. Am J Ophthalmol 82:24, 1976.

369. Darnley-Fisch, DA, Byrne, SF, Hughes, JR, et al: Contact B-scan echography in the assessment of optic nerve cupping. Am J Ophthalmol 109:55, 1990.

370. Kottler, MS, Rosenthal, AR, Falconer, DG: Analog vs. digital photogrammetry for optic cup analysis. Invest Ophthalmol 15:651, 1976.

371. Krohn, MA, Keltner, JL, Johnson, CA: Comparison of photographic techniques and films used in stereophotogrammetry of the optic disk. Am J Ophthalmol 88:859, 1979.

372. Schirmer, KE: Simplified photogrammetry of the optic disc. Arch Ophthalmol 94:1997, 1976.

373. Rosenthal, AR, Falconer, DG, Pieper, I: Photogrammetry experiments with a model eye. Br J Ophthalmol 64:881, 1980.

374. Johnson, CA, Keltner, JL, Krohn, MA, Portney, GL: Photogrammetry of the optic disc in glaucoma and ocular hypertension with simultaneous stereo photography. Invest Ophthalmol Vis Sci 18:1252, 1979.

375. Schwartz, B: New techniques for the examination of the optic disc and their clinical application. Trans Am Acad Ophthalmol Otol 81:227, 1976.

376. Nagin, P, Schwartz, B: Detection of increased pallor over time. Computerized image analysis in untreated ocular hypertension. Ophthalmology 91:252, 1984.

377. Mikelberg, FS, Douglas, GR, Schulzer, M, et al: Reliability of optic disk topographic measurements recorded with a video-ophthalmograph. Am J Ophthalmol 98:98, 1984.

378. Caprioli, J, Klingbeil, U, Sears, M, Pope, B: Reproducibility of optic disc measurements with computerized analysis of stereoscopic video images. Arch Ophthalmol 104:1035, 1986.

379. Shields, MB, Martone, JF, Shelton, AR, et al: Reproducibility of topographic measurements with the Optic Nerve Head Analyzer. Am J Ophthalmol 104:581, 1987.

380. Tomita, G, Goto, Y, Yamada, T, Kitazawa, Y: Reliability of optic measurement with computerized stereoscopic video image analyzer. Acta Soc Ophthalmol Jpn 90:1317, 1986.

381. Bishop, KI, Werner, EB, Krupin, T, et al: Variability and reproducibility of optic disk topographic measurements with the Rodenstock optic nerve head analyzer. Am J Ophthalmol 106:696, 1988.

382. Miller, JM, Caprioli, J: Videographic quantification of optic disc pallor. Invest Ophthalmol Vis Sci 29:320, 1988.

383. Mikelberg, FS, Douglas, GR, Drance, SM, et al: Reproducibility of computerized pallor measurements obtained with the Rodenstock disk analyzer. Graefes Arch Clin Exp Ophthalmol 226:269, 1988.

384. Miller, KN, Shields, MB, Ollie, AR: Reproducibility of pallor measurements with the Optic Nerve Head Analyzer. Graefes Arch Clin Exp Ophthalmol 227:562, 1989.

385. Shields, MB, Tiedeman, JS, Miller, KN, et al: Accuracy of topographic measurements with the Optic Nerve Head Analyzer. Am J Ophthalmol 107:273, 1989

386. Mikelberg, FS, Airaksinen, PJ, Douglas, GR, et al: The correlation between optic disk topography measured by the video-ophthalmograph (Rodenstock Analyzer) and clinical measurement. Am J Ophthalmol 100:417, 1985.

387. Mikelberg, FS, Douglas, GR, Schulzer, M, et al: The correlation between cup-disk ratio, neuroretinal rim area, and optic disk area measured by the video-ophthalmograph (Rodenstock Analyzer) and clinical measurement. Am J Ophthalmol 101:7, 1986.

388. Caprioli, J, Miller, JM: Videographic measurements of optic nerve topography in glaucoma. Invest Ophthalmol Vis Sci 29:1294, 1988.

389. Caprioli, J, Miller, JM: Measurement of relative nerve fiber layer surface height in glaucoma. Ophthalmology 96:633, 1989.

390. Caprioli, J, Ortiz-Colberg, R, Miller, JM, Tressler, C: Measurements of peripapillary nerve fiber layer contour in glaucoma. Am J Ophthalmol 108:404, 1989.

391. Miller, E, Caprioli, J: Regional and long-term variability of fundus measurements made with computer-image analysis. Am J Ophthalmol 112:171, 1991.

392. Miller, JM, Caprioli, J: An optimal reference plane to detect glaucomatous nerve fiber layer abnormalities with computerized image analysis. Graefes Arch Clin Exp Ophthalmol 230:124, 1992.

393. Varma, R, Spaeth, GL: The PAR IS 2000: a new system for retinal digital image analysis. Ophthalmic Surg 19:183, 1988.

394. Varma, R, Steinmann, WC, Spaeth, GL, Wilson, RP: Variability in digital analysis of optic disc topography. Graefes Arch Clin Exp Ophthalmol 226:435, 1988.

395. Varma, R, Spaeth, GL, Hanau, C, et al: Positional changes in the vasculature of the optic disk in glaucoma. Am J Ophthalmol 104:457, 1987.

396. Varma, R, Spaeth, GL, Steinmann, WC, Katz, LJ: Agreement between clinicians and an image analyzer in estimating cup-to-disc ratios. Arch Ophthalmol 107:526, 1989.

397. Burgoyne, CF, Varma, R, Quigley, HA, et al: Global and regional detection of induced optic disc change by digitized image analysis. Arch Ophthalmol 112:261, 1994.

398. Burgoyne, CF, Quigley, HA, Varma, A: Comparison of clinician judgment with digitized image analysis in the detection of induced optic disk change in monkey eyes. Am J Ophthalmol 120:176, 1995.

399. Dandona, L, Quigley, HA, Jampel, HD: Reliability of optic nerve head topographic measurements with computerized image analysis. Am J Ophthalmol 108:414, 1989.

400. Dandona, L, Quigley, HA, Jampel, HD: Variability of depth measurements of the optic nerve head and peripapillary retina with computerized image analysis. Arch Ophthalmol 107:1786, 1989.

401. Dreher, AW, Tso, PC, Weinreb, RN: Reproducibility of topographic measurements of the normal and glaucomatous optic nerve head with the laser tomographic scanner. Am J Ophthalmol 111:221, 1991.

402. Dreher, AW, Weinreb, RN: Accuracy of topographic measurements in a model eye with the laser tomographic scanner. Invest Ophthalmol Vis Sci 32:2992, 1991.

403. Burk, ROW, Rohrschneider, K, Takamoto, T, et al: Laser scanning tomography and stereophotogrammetry in three-dimensional optic disc analysis. Graefes Arch Clin Exp Ophthalmol 231:193, 1993.

404. Rohrschneider, K, Burk, ROW, Völcker, HE: Reproducibility of topometric data acquisition in normal and glaucomatous optic nerve heads with the laser tomographic scanner. Graefes Arch Clin Exp Ophthalmol 231:457, 1993.

405. Weinreb, RN, Lusky, M, Bartsch, D-U, Morsman, D: Effect of repetitive imaging on topographic measurements of the optic nerve head. Arch Ophthalmol 111:636, 1993.

406. Mikelberg, FS, Wijsman, K, Schulzer, M: Reproducibility of topographic parameters obtained with the Heidelberg retina tomograph. J Glau 2:101, 1993.

407. Lusky, M, Bosem, ME, Weinreb, RN: Reproducibility of optic nerve head topography measurements in eyes with undilated pupils. J Glau 2:104, 1993.

408. Rohrschneider, K, Burk, ROW, Kruse, FE, Völcker, HE: Reproducibility of the optic nerve head topography with a new laser tomographic scanning device. Ophthalmology 101:1044, 1994.

409. Woon, WH, Fitzke, FW, Bird, AC, Marshall, J: Confocal imaging of the fundus using a scanning laser ophthalmoscope. Br J Ophthalmol 76:470, 1992.

410. Fitzke, FW, Masters, BR: Three-dimensional visualization of confocal sections of in vivo human fundus and optic nerve. Curr Eye Res 12:1015, 1993.

411. Chihara, E, Takahashi, F, Chihara, K: Assessment of optic disc topography with scanning laser ophthalmoscope. Graefes Arch Clin Exp Ophthalmol 231:1, 1993.

412. Cioffi, GA, Robin, AL, Eastman, RD, et al: Confocal laser scanning ophthalmoscope. Reproducibility of optic nerve head topographic measurements with the confocal laser scanning ophthalmoscope. Ophthalmology 100:57–62, 1993.

413. Weinreb, RN, Shakiba, S, Zangwill, L: Scanning laser polarimetry to measure the nerve fiber layer of normal and glaucomatous eyes. Am J Ophthalmol 119:627, 1995.

414. Weinreb, RN, Bartsch, D-U, Freeman, WR: Angiography of the glaucomatous optic nerve head. J Glau 3:S55, 1994.

415. Janknecht, P, Funk, J: Optic nerve head analyser and Heidelberg retina tomograph: accuracy and reproducibility of topographic measurements in a model eye and in volunteers. Br J Ophthalmol 78:760, 1994.

416. Tomita, G, Honbe, K, Kitazawa, Y: Reproducibility of measurements by laser scanning tomography in eyes before and after pilocarpine treatment. Graefes Arch Clin Exp Ophthalmol 32:406, 1994.

417. Spencer, AF, Sadiq, SA, Pawson, P, Vernon, SA: Vertical optic disk diameter: discrepancy between planimetric and SLO measurements. Invest Ophthalmol Vis Sci 36:796, 1995.

418. Brigatti, L, Caprioli, J: Correlation of visual field with scanning confocal laser optic disc measurements in glaucoma. Arch Ophthalmol 113:1191, 1995.

419. Mikelberg, FS, Parfitt, CM, Swindale, NV, et al: Ability of the Heidelberg retina tomograph to detect early glaucomatous visual field loss. J Glau 4:242, 1995.

420. Hoskins, HD, Hetherington, J, Glenday, M, et al: Repeatability of the glaucoma-scope measurements of optic nerve head topography. J Glau 3:17, 1994.

421. Pendergast, SD, Shields, MB: Reproducibility of optic nerve head topographic measurements with the glaucoma-scope. J Glau 4:170, 1995.

422. Hee, MR, Izatt, JA, Swanson, EA, et al: Optical coherence tomography of the human retina. Arch Ophthalmol 113:325, 1995.

423. Schuman, JS, Hee, MR, Puliafito, CA, et al: Quantification of nerve fiber layer thickness in normal and glaucomatous eyes using optical coherence tomography. Arch Ophthalmol 113:586, 1995.

Chapter 6

VISUAL FUNCTION IN GLAUCOMA

Advances in the technology of visual field testing are changing our clinical perception of normal and abnormal fields of vision. For example, the familiar two-dimensional presentation of concentric lines around the point of fixation is giving way to three-dimensional displays in symbols and numerical values. It is important to keep in mind, however, that the normal field of vision and the changes created by glaucoma are just the same as when Bjerrum discovered the arcuate scotoma using the back of his consulting room door as a background for his field testing nearly 100 years ago. We begin this chapter, therefore, by considering the normal field of vision and how it is altered by glaucomatous damage and then review the instruments and techniques by which these parameters can be measured.

NORMAL VISUAL FIELD

A helpful way to begin the study of visual fields and the methods by which they are measured is to consider Traquair's classic analogy of "an island of vision surrounded by a sea of blindness" (Fig. 6.1). This three-dimensional concept can be reduced to quantitative values by plotting lines (isopters) at various levels around the island, or by measuring the height (sensitivity) at different points within the island of vision.

Boundaries

The shoreline of the island corresponds to the peripheral limits of the visual field, which normally measure, with maximum target stimulation, approximately 60° above and nasal, 70–75° below, and 100–110° temporal to fixation (1). The typical configuration of the normal visual field, therefore, is a horizontal oval, often with a shallow inferonasal depression (Fig. 6.1). The shape is usually of greater diagnostic significance than the absolute size of the visual

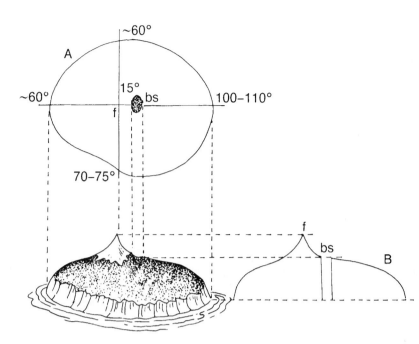

Figure 6.1. The normal visual field is depicted as Traquair's "island of vision surrounded by a sea of blindness," with projections showing the peripheral limits (**A**) and the profile (**B**). Fixation *(f)* corresponds to the foveola of the retina, and the blind spot *(bs)*, to the optic nerve head. The approximate dimensions of the absolute peripheral boundary of the visual field and the location of the blind spot are shown (*A*).

field, since the latter is influenced by many physiologic variables.

Contour

The peaks and valleys on the island correspond to areas of increased or decreased vision within the peripheral limits of the visual field. These contours can by mapped by recording the relative visual sensitivities at specific points in the field of vision, or by using test objects with reduced stimulus value to plot smaller isopters within the absolute boundaries. The area of maximum visual acuity in the normal field is at the point of fixation, corresponding to the foveola of the retina, and appears as a smoothly rising peak surrounded by a high plateau (2). The visual sensitivity then tapers down more gradually until it again falls abruptly at the peripheral limits.

Blind Spot

Within the boundaries of the normal visual field is a deep depression, or blind spot, which corresponds to the region of the optic nerve head. It is located approximately 15% temporal to fixation and has two portions: (a) an absolute scotoma and (b) a relative scotoma (3). The absolute scotoma corresponds to the actual optic nerve head and is seen as a vertical oval. Since there are no photoreceptors in the nerve head, this portion of the blind spot is independent of the test object stimulus value. The relative scotoma surrounds the absolute portion and corresponds to peripapillary retina, which has reduced visual sensitivity, especially inferiorly and superiorly. In a study correlating the blind spot size to the area of the optic disc and parapapillary atrophy, the ab-

solute scotoma included the peripapillary scleral ring and the parapapillary zone Beta (see definitions in Chapter 5), while zone Alpha was attributed to the relative scotoma (4).

The relative portion of the blind spot is dependent on the stimulus value and varies with different testing methods. If the temporal margin of the relative blind spot comes close to the corresponding isopter, the two boundaries may artifactually become confluent, creating *false baring of the blind spot*. In addition, because the reduced sensitivity of the peripapillary retina is greater in the upper and lower poles, test objects with small stimulus value may cause vertical elongation of the blind spot, which can break through the isopter causing *true baring of the blind spot* (Fig. 6.2).

GLAUCOMATOUS INFLUENCES ON VISUAL FUNCTION[a]

Diffuse Visual Field Loss

The increased sensitivity with which newer instruments allow evaluation of vision is changing our understanding of the natural history of progressive visual field loss in glaucoma. While defects related to loss of retinal nerve fiber bundles are the most familiar visual field changes induced by glaucoma, and central vision is typically one of the last regions to be totally lost, studies are now showing mild central and diffuse reduction in the visual field even in the early stages of glaucoma (5–12). The mechanism for this is uncertain, although it appears to represent pressure-induced damage (9, 10) with diffuse nerve-fiber loss, as evidenced by abnormal

[a]Refer to Shields, MB: Color Atlas of Glaucoma. Baltimore, Williams & Wilkins, 1998, Plate I27.

light-sense and flicker perimetry, which have been shown to accompany diffuse retinal nerve-fiber layer loss (11, 12).

Although most studies agree that some patients with early glaucoma can have purely diffuse loss in the absence of other causes (5–12) other investigators have challenged this concept, suggesting that these patients have other causes for the diffuse loss of perimetric sensitivity, such as media opacity, miosis, or retinal dysfunction (13, 14). In any case, the diagnostic value of this finding is currently limited by its nonspecific nature, but it should still be looked for and noted in the course of visual field testing and analysis. The following are some of the perimetric and other measures that can be used to evaluate generalized visual impairment in glaucoma. In the future, they may acquire greater diagnostic significance as our knowledge of glaucomatous visual dysfunction expands.

Concentric Contraction

Generalized reduction in the visual field may become manifest as a decrease in sensitivity for specific retinal locations

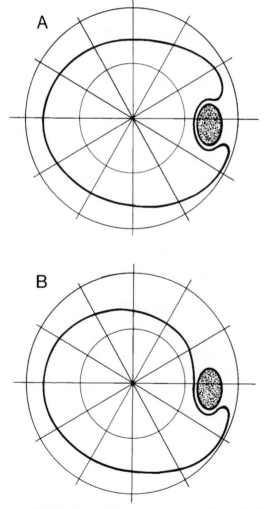

Figure 6.2. False baring (**A**) and true baring (**B**) of the blind spot.

or as a concentric constriction of the visual field, both of which have been noted to precede other detectable glaucomatous field defects in many patients (15, 16). Isopter contraction, as an early field defect of glaucoma, is often more marked in the nasal field, which has been called "crowding of the peripheral nasal isopters" (17).

Enlargement of the Blind Spot

Enlargement of the blind spot, due to depression of peripapillary retinal sensitivity, is also considered to be an early glaucomatous field change. However, it may be seen with other optic nerve or retinal disorders. One example has been called "acute idiopathic blind spot enlargement," and is related to multiple evanescent white dot syndrome and possible other retinal diseases (18). Enlargement of the blind spot can also be produced in normal individuals with threshold targets, so that it is not a pathognomonic sign of glaucoma (19).

Angioscotomata

Angioscotomata are long, branching scotomas above and below the blind spot, which are presumed to result from shadows created by the large retinal vessels. This finding is felt to represent an early glaucomatous field defect (20), although it is technically difficult to demonstrate and not highly diagnostic.

Other Measures of Generalized Visual Impairment in Glaucoma

In addition to the diffuse reduction in retinal sensitivity that can be demonstrated by visual field changes in early glaucoma, there are other psychophysical tests which support the concept that a generalized decrease in visual function may be the earliest visual change in glaucoma.

Color Vision

Reduced sensitivity to colors has been described in various forms of glaucoma, and may precede any detectable loss of peripheral or central vision by standard acuity or visual field testing. Most studies agree that the color vision deficit is associated primarily with blue-sensitive pathways (6, 21–30). This is consistent with the observation that blue signals travel in larger diameter axons, which are more susceptible than small fibers to increased intraocular pressure (IOP) (31). Blue cones contribute little to the sensation of brightness or to visual acuity, which may explain why standard visual acuity tests, perimetry, or contrast sensitivity studies might miss such a color vision loss. The visual dysfunction is significantly more common in high-tension glaucoma as compared to low-tension glaucoma (28) and is strongly related to higher IOP levels (29), suggesting that the damage is pressure induced.

It is not clear as to whether the loss of color vision and the visual field changes associated with nerve fiber bundle loss share the same mechanism. Ocular hypertensives with yellow-blue and blue-green defects were found to have diffuse early changes in visual field sensitivity (24) as well as an increased chance of developing glaucomatous visual field loss as compared to similar patients without these color vision disturbances (21). The same color abnormalities in patients with early glaucoma correlated significantly with diffuse retinal nerve fiber loss (30). However, no significant correlation between color vision scores and visual field performance was found among ocular hypertensives when age correction was applied to the color variable (32), and another study revealed no clear association between early glaucomatous cupping and color vision anomalies (25). Specificity is limited by the fact that the tritan deficit is also the one most frequently seen with age-related changes. When study populations were matched for age and lens density, however, color vision loss in glaucoma was still attributable in part to the disease process (33).

In most reported studies, the color vision testing was performed with the Farnsworth-Munsell 100-hue test, dichotomous (D-15) tests, or variants of these, all of which are laborious and of questionable precision. Several new tests have been devised to overcome these limitations, including computer-driven monitors that present flickering color contrasts (34) or peripheral color contrasts (35), an automatic anomaloscope (36), and a color contrast sensitivity test in which the target and surround have the same luminance, but different chromaticity (37). Even with the most sensitive, precise system, however, not all glaucoma patients are detected, suggesting that some patients with glaucoma have true preservation of color vision (37). Later in this chapter, we consider how color vision deficits are being used to enhance perimetry.

Contrast Sensitivity

Subtle loss of both central and peripheral vision can be demonstrated in some patients with glaucoma, prior to detectable visual field changes with standard techniques, by measuring the amount of contrast required for a patient to discriminate between adjacent visual stimuli. Tests to measure contrast sensitivity may use either spatial or temporal strategies.

SPATIAL CONTRAST SENSITIVITY. Sine wave gratings of parallel light and dark bands (Arden gratings), in which the patient must detect the striped pattern at various levels of contrast and spatial frequencies, have had the most extensive evaluation within this group of psychophysical tests (38). The original Arden gratings were limited by the subjectivity of the required responses (39, 40). A modification, in which the patient must indicate the orientation of the gratings, is reported to minimize the latter limitation (40). The two testing methods most commonly used are microprocessor-controlled video displays and photographically reproduced grating patterns, both of which have been shown to give good approximations of the spatial contrast sensitivity function (41).

Impaired contrast sensitivity by this testing method has been reported among glaucoma patients (38, 42–48). In some studies, the impairment correlates with visual field (43–45), especially with the central visual field (49), and optic nerve head (45) damage. The yield of detecting glaucoma may be increased by measuring peripheral contrast sensitivity, 20–25% eccentrically (50). While spatial contrast sensitivity may be a useful adjunct, caution has been advised in interpreting the results without considering additional clinical data (48). The overlap with other causes of reduced spatial contrast sensitivity, including age, create high false-negative and false-positive rates (45, 46, 51–54). Spatial contrast sensitivity has been shown to decrease in normal subjects after 50 years of age (55), which appears to be independent of the crystalline lens (56).

Visual function in glaucoma patients, as measured by contrast sensitivity, has been shown to improve after β-blocker therapy (57), and it may be that this, or some other visual function test, will one day prove useful in judging the efficacy of glaucoma therapy.

TEMPORAL CONTRAST SENSITIVITY. Temporal contrast sensitivity, in which the patient must detect a visual stimulus flickering at various frequencies, provides another measure of contrast sensitivity. The stimulus may be presented either as a homogeneous flickering field (flicker fusion frequency) (1) or as a counterphase flickering grating of low spatial frequency (spatiotemporal contrast sensitivity) (55, 58). Glaucoma patients may have reduced function with either method, although the latter appears to be a more sensitive test (58, 59). One study found peripheral flicker testing to be more sensitive than threshold perimetry in detecting nasal arcuate loss in glaucoma patients (60). Spatiotemporal contrast sensitivity was also found to be more useful in detecting glaucoma than spatial contrast sensitivity testing of the central retina, although age influence again limited the usefulness of the test to those under 50 (55). Other studies have found age to be a less significant factor in sensitivity loss (61, 62), although one study suggested that cardiovascular disease may be associated with foveal dysfunction (63). There is also a question as to whether temporal contrast sensitivity loss among ocular hypertensives represents early glaucomatous damage or a transient influence of raised IOP. One study suggested that either mechanism may be found within subsets of this population (64).

Several techniques have been evaluated to improve contrast sensitivity testing. One study suggested that the determination of a ratio between spatial contrast sensitivity and flicker sensitivity is a more precise measure of visual pathology than the absolute value of either test (65). Another test of temporal contrast sensitivity, in which the patient must discriminate two rapidly successive pulses of light from a single pulse, is reported to be highly sensitive and specific in separating glaucomatous from normal eyes (66). Another test, the *whole-field scotopic retinal sensitivity test,* uses a flashlight-sized device in which the patient views a white light in the entire visual field and is asked to detect alternating illuminated and dark fields at one second intervals (67). It may be useful as a screening tool (67, 68), although one study found too much overlap between normal and ocular hypertensive individuals (69), and another study showed that cataracts may alter the results (70).

Electrophysiologic Studies

The measures of visual function described above are all dependent on the patients subjective response. Work is also being done in this area on alternative, objective methods.

ELECTRORETINOGRAMS. Electroretinograms (ERG) evoked by reversing checkerboard or grating patterns *(pattern ERG)* are sensitive to retinal ganglion cell and optic nerve dysfunction and have reduced amplitudes in glaucoma patients (71–78). Reduced pattern ERG amplitudes appear in the early stages of glaucoma (79, 80) and in some ocular hypertensives (77–82), especially those at higher risk of developing glaucoma (81, 84). These findings suggest that pattern ERG may be useful in discriminating between ocular hypertensives who will develop visual field loss and those who will not.

Studies differ as to whether pattern ERG correlates with IOP and disc topography, with one study showing no correlation (82), and others showing an association with IOP control (87) and with computerized disc analysis (88). The pattern ERG has been shown to correlate with visual field indices (89), and visual field defects are associated with ERG reduction in the corresponding hemisphere (90). However, no precise correlation was found with color vision deficits (83). Decreased amplitude and an increase in peak latency was found to correlate with increasing age (76), paralleling the estimated normal loss of ganglion cells. Indeed, reduction in pattern ERG was directly related to histologically defined optic nerve damage in a monkey model (91).

The electroretinogram evoked by a flash of light *(flash ERG)* is effected more by outer retinal elements and is not typically abnormal in glaucoma. Acute IOP elevation in cats, however, caused a reduction in both pattern and flash ERG, proportional to the reduction in perfusion pressure and irrespective of the absolute IOP, suggesting a vascular mechanism to which the ganglion cells are less likely to recover (92). Glaucoma patients in one study had reduced ERG amplitudes in response to a flickering stimulus *(flicker ERG)* (78).

VISUAL EVOKED POTENTIALS. Visual evoked potentials (VEP) may also be abnormal in patients with chronic (22, 71, 75, 93–95) or acute glaucoma (96), although this is more variable than the pattern ERG response (74, 91). However, larger diameter axons, which are preferentially damaged in glaucoma, correlate with fast, transiently responding retinal

ganglion cells, and a reduced response to high-frequency flicker VEP (above 13 Hz) correlated with the degree of glaucomatous damage (97–99). It has also been suggested that blue-on-yellow VEP may be a useful test in glaucoma research (100).

Glaucoma patients were also found in one study to have increased baseline values with *electro-oculography* (101).

Miscellaneous Tests

Patients with glaucomatous optic atrophy have decreased light sensitivity when dark adapted, which correlates with the degree of nerve damage (102), and *dark adaptation,* tested with chromatic stimuli, has been reported to be abnormal in populations of ocular hypertensives (103). Light sensitivity can also be evaluated with a *brightness ratio test,* in which the patient discriminates the difference in sensitivity of the two eyes to light (104), and it has been suggested that tests of this type may be useful in glaucoma screening (104, 105). *Dichoptic testing,* in which one-half of a test object is presented to one eye, and the other half to the fellow eye, as an aid to determining the location of a defect in the visual pathway, was found in preliminary studies to give abnormal responses in patients with open-angle glaucoma (106). The eye with glaucomatous damage also has reduced ability to perceive motion, both centrally (107) and peripherally (108, 109), which may be related to the preferential damage to larger retinal ganglion cells, and *motion perception tests* may prove to be a useful tool in the detection of early glaucoma (107–109). The detection of vernier offsets is also affected in glaucoma, but it is not sensitive enough to distinguish glaucoma patients from controls (110).

A *relative afferent pupillary defect* offers yet another measure of visual pathway disturbance in glaucoma (111). It has been shown to be proportional to the amount of visual field loss (112–114), and may precede detectable field loss by static automated perimetry (114). When pupillary status, such as marked miosis, prevents determination of relative afferent pupillary defect, it has shown that brightness comparison testing, as described above, correctly predicts the presence of a relative afferent pupillary defect in 92% of glaucoma patients (115).

Nerve Fiber Bundle Defects

While the measures of generalized reduction in visual function, as considered above, may one day be important in the early detection of glaucoma, they are too inconsistent and nonspecific at the present time to be of highly significant clinical value. Focal defects due to loss or impairment of retinal nerve fiber bundles are more specific for glaucoma and constitute the most definitive early evidence of visual field loss from these disorders. The nature of the nerve fiber bundle defects relates to the retinal topography of these fibers as discussed in Chapter 5.

Scatter

Before considering the specific forms of visual field loss associated with nerve fiber bundle defects, it is important to note that discrete scotomas may be preceded by variable threshold responses to repeated testing in the same area (116–119). This has been referred to as scatter, fluctuation, or localized minor disturbances. The phenomenon has been studied with the *differential light threshold,* which is the basis of threshold static perimetry (discussed later in this chapter) and is defined as the light stimulus that can be recognized above background with a probability of 50% in a given retinal location (120). Studies with this technique show that patients with glaucoma have substantially greater scatter during one examination *(short-term fluctuation),* as well as from one test to another *(long-term fluctuation)* (120–123). While scatter is not a definitive sign of glaucomatous visual field damage, it should be looked upon with suspicion as an early warning sign of impending absolute field loss. Further details regarding the interpretation of these and other visual field observations are discussed later in this chapter.

Arcuate Defects

The arcuate or Bjerrum (pronounced "Bee yer' um") area within the visual field arches above and below fixation from the blind spot to the median raphe, corresponding to the arcuate retinal nerve fibers (Fig. 6.3**A**). The nasal extreme of the arcuate area along the median raphe may come within 1° of fixation and extends nasally for 10–20° (124). Early visual loss in glaucoma commonly occurs within this arcuate area, especially in the superior half, which correlates with the predilection of the inferior and superior temporal poles of the optic nerve head for early glaucomatous damage (124, 125). As field defects develop within the arcuate area, they most often appear first as one or more localized defects, or *paracentral scotomas* (Fig. 6.3**B**). The typical pattern of progression of glaucomatous visual field defects is for a shallow paracentral depression to become denser and larger (126), eventually forming a central absolute defect, surrounded by a relative scotoma (118, 127, 128). The relative scotoma represents fluctuation (as described earlier) and can be seen at the border of the physiologic blind spot and glaucomatous defects, but is significantly larger and more sloping in the latter (129). Occasionally, the early arcuate defect may connect with the blind spot and taper to a point in a slightly curved course, which has been referred to as a *Seidel scotoma* (Fig. 6.3**C**). As the isolated defects enlarge and coalesce, they form an arching scotoma that eventually fills the entire arcuate area from the blind spot to the median raphe, which is called an *arcuate* or *Bjerrum scotoma* (Fig. 6.3**D**). With further progression, a double arcuate (or ring) scotoma will develop (Fig. 6.3**E**). The rate of visual field loss correlates with the size of the scotoma, in that the larger the scotoma the more rapidly it is likely to enlarge (130).

Differential Diagnosis of Arcuate Scotomas

Although the arcuate defect is probably the most reliable early form of glaucomatous field loss, it is not pathognomonic, and the following additional causes must be considered, especially when the field and disc changes do not seem to correlate: chorioretinal lesions, optic nerve head lesions, anterior optic nerve lesions, and posterior lesions of the visual pathway (Table 6.1) (124, 131).

Nasal Steps (Fig. 6.3E)

The loss of retinal nerve fibers rarely proceeds at the same rate in the upper and lower portions of an eye. Consequently, a step-like defect is frequently created where the nerve fibers meet along the median raphe. Since the superior field is involved somewhat more frequently than the inferior portion in the early stages of glaucoma, the nasal step more often results from a greater defect above the horizontal midline, which is referred to as a superior nasal step. However, inferior nasal steps are not uncommon. Nasal steps are also distinguished by their central or peripheral location (132). A *central nasal step* is created at the nasal termination of an unequal double arcuate scotoma. Unequal contraction of the peripheral isopters due to loss of corresponding bundles of peripheral arcuate nerve fibers produces a defect that has been called the *peripheral nasal step of Ronne.* It may begin as an isolated scotoma in the nasal periphery (133). The shape of the peripheral nasal step differs according to its distance from fixation, and is not necessarily found in all isopters (127, 128).

Vertical Step (Fig. 6.3F)

A stepwise defect along the vertical midline, referred to as a vertical step or *hemianopic offset,* is a less common feature of glaucomatous field loss than the nasal step, but has been reported to occur in approximately 20% of cases (134, 135). The mechanism of this field defect is not fully understood, although it may relate to a segregation within the optic nerve head of axons from either side of the vertical midline (134). The defect more often appears on the nasal side of the vertical midline. However, studies of normal subjects have also revealed greater sensitivity temporal to the hemianopic border, and it has been suggested that a small peripheral step at the vertical midline should arouse suspicion of glaucoma only if the defect is located temporally (136, 137). It also has limited diagnostic value because most are associated with other glaucomatous field changes (135), and the main significance of the observation is in distinguishing glaucomatous vertical midline defects from those caused by neurologic lesions.

Temporal Sector Defect

Since the retinal nerve fibers nasal to the optic nerve head converge on the disc by a direct route, a lesion involving these fiber bundles produces a sector defect temporal to the blind

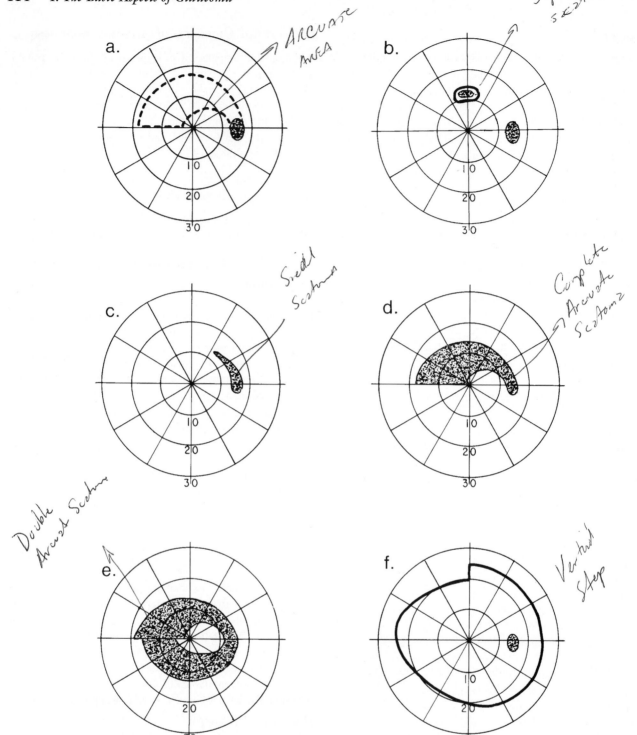

Figure 6.3. Arcuate nerve fiber bundle defects. **A.** The arcuate (or Bjerrum) area is shown within the dotted lines. **B.** Superior paracentral scotoma, with central absolute defect surrounded by a relative scotoma. **C.** Seidel scotoma. **D.** Complete arcuate (Bjerrum) scotoma. **E.** Double arcuate (ring) scotoma with superior central nasal step. **F.** Vertical step (or hemianopic offset).

spot (127, 128). This defect usually appears later in the course of glaucomatous field loss (138). With automated perimetry, glaucomatous defects temporal to the blind spot are not uncommon, but usually add significant information over central field testing only in patients with late visual field loss (139).

VALUE OF PERIPHERAL FIELD TESTING. Defects along the peripheral boundaries of the visual field, as described earlier, i.e., peripheral nasal steps, vertical steps, and temporal sector defects, are most often found in association with scotomas in the arcuate area, although in some patients with

Table 6.1.
DIFFERENTIAL DIAGNOSIS OF ARCUATE SCOTOMAS

A. Chorioretinal lesions
   1. Juxtapapillary choroiditis and retinochoroiditis
   2. Myopia with peripapillary atrophy
   3. Retinal pigment epithelium and photoreceptor degeneration
   4. Retinal artery occlusions
B. Optic nerve head lesions
   1. Drusen
   2. Retinal artery plaques
   3. Chronic papilledema
   4. Papillitis
   5. Colobomas (including optic nerve pit)
C. Anterior optic nerve lesions
   1. Carotid and ophthalmic artery occlusion
   2. Ischemic infarct
   3. Cerebral arteritis
   4. Retrobulbar neuritis
   5. Electric shock
   6. Exophthalmos
D. Posterior lesions of the visual pathway
   1. Pituitary adenoma
   2. Opticochiasmatic arachnoiditis
   3. Meningiomas of the dorsum sella or optic foramen
   4. Progressive external ophthalmoplegia
   5. Pseudotumor cerebri

Modified from Harrington, DO: Differential diagnosis of the arcuate-scotoma. Invest Opthal 8:96, 1969.

early glaucomatous visual field loss, they may be the only detectable abnormality (132, 133, 140, 141). With automated static perimetry (discussed later in this chapter), it has become common practice to measure only the central 24–30° of the visual field due to the increased time requirement with this technique. The question arises, therefore, as to how much information is being missed by ignoring the more peripheral portions of the field. In the presence of paracentral scotomas, peripheral isopters do not appear to add significant information regarding the progression of visual field damage (142). In the initial diagnosis, however, a peripheral field defect, usually a nasal step, may be the only abnormality detected by automated perimetry in 3–11% of patients, depending on the testing method (143–146). To be clinically useful, the time required to obtain this information must not add excessively to the overall testing time and further study is needed to determine whether this can be achieved with newer programs for automated perimetry.

Advanced Glaucomatous Field Defects

The natural history of progressive glaucomatous field loss is eventual development of a complete double arcuate scotoma with extension to the peripheral limits in all areas except temporally. This results in a *central island* and a *temporal island* of vision in advanced glaucoma. With continued damage these islands of vision progressively diminish in size until the tiny central island is totally extinguished, which may occur abruptly. Glaucoma surgery appears to accelerate the loss of the small central island in some patients, possibly due to the sudden change in IOP, although the frequency with which this surgical complication occurs is not large enough to constitute a contraindication to surgery in these patients (147). The temporal island of vision is more resistant and may persist long after central vision is lost. However, it, too, will eventually be destroyed if the IOP is not controlled, leaving the patient with no light perception.

Visual Field Changes in Normal-Tension Glaucoma

The nature of visual field defects may be influenced by the level of the IOP, although the reports are somewhat conflicting. One study of open-angle glaucoma patients with early visual field loss showed that those with diffuse depression had higher pressures than those with localized defects (148). In addition, open-angle glaucoma patients whose IOP has never exceeded approximately 21 mm Hg, commonly referred to as normal-tension (or low-tension) glaucoma, were found in some studies to have scotomas with steeper slopes, greater depth, and closer proximity to fixation than chronic glaucoma patients with higher IOP (149, 150). Others, however, found no significant difference between these two groups when the same degree of optic nerve damage was present (151, 152). Another study of normal-tension and high-tension glaucoma patients whose automated visual fields were matched to within a 0.3-dB mean deviation (explained later in this chapter) revealed no significant difference in focal defects in the overall field or superior hemifield, but did show significantly more localized loss in the inferior hemifield among the normal-tension patients, supporting the hypothesis of a vascular mechanism in that group (153).

Visual Field Changes with Acute Pressure Elevation

The preceding discussions have dealt with field changes that are associated primarily with chronic forms of glaucoma. When the IOP elevation is sudden and marked, as in acute angle-closure glaucoma, a variety of associated field changes has been reported, including general depression, early loss of central vision, arcuate scotomas, and enlargement of the blind spot (154). After the acute attack is brought under control, the fields will return to normal in some patients, while others may have reduced color vision, generalized decreased sensitivity, or constriction of isopters, especially superiorly (155).

When the IOP is artificially elevated, either by compression of the globe (156–158) or administration of topical steroids (159–162), typical glaucomatous field defects (156–161), or constriction of central isopters (162), occur in some eyes. The changes are reversible when the IOP returns to normal (160, 161). This response to artificial pressure elevation is said to occur more commonly in glaucoma patients (156, 157), especially those with normal-tension glaucoma (154), although one study found no significant difference between glaucoma and nonglaucoma patients (158).

Reversibility of Glaucomatous Field Defects

Although visual field loss from glaucoma has traditionally been felt to be irreversible, it has been reported that both central visual acuity and the field of vision may improve if the IOP is reduced in the early stages of the disease (163–166). Visual field global indices with automated perimetry (explained later in this chapter) improved proportional to the amount of IOP reduction in two studies (167, 168). Other investigators, however, were unable to demonstrate reversibility following pressure reduction achieved by argon-laser trabeculoplasty (169, 170). These conflicting findings may indicate that a critical level of pressure reduction and/or intervention at a critical time in the disease process is needed to achieve reversal of field loss.

Correlation Between Optic Nerve Head and Visual Field Defects

In most patients with glaucoma, clinically recognizable disc changes precede detectable field loss (171, 172), and the presence or absence of glaucomatous field defects can usually, but not always, be predicted from the appearance of the optic nerve head (171–177). Quigley and coworkers (178, 179) attempted to correlate axon loss in the optic nerve head with visual field defects. Although limited by small sample sizes, their work did suggest that, not only does nerve fiber loss occur prior to reproducible field defects in some patients with elevated IOP, but that the extent of axonal loss may be much greater than the corresponding visual field change. With standard manual perimetric techniques as many as 35% of the fibers may be gone in an eye with a normal field, while more than half the fibers may be lost by the time reproducible early field defects are found, and 10% or fewer axons may remain by the stage of severe field loss (178). When correlating retinal ganglion cell atrophy with automated perimetry in glaucoma patients, a 20% loss of cells, especially large ganglion cells in the central 30° of the retina, correlated with a 5-dB sensitivity loss (discussed later in this chapter), while a 40% loss corresponded with a

10-dB decrease, and some ganglion cells remained in areas with 0-dB sensitivity (179).

The nature of optic nerve head cupping can also be used to predict the type (in addition to the presence) of field loss. Extensive or focal absence of neural rim tissue, especially at the inferior or superior poles, is the most reliable indicator of visual field disturbance (173, 180–183), and is usually associated with a field defect in the corresponding arcuate area. In some cases, field loss may occur before the pallor reaches the disc margin (180), and unusual cases have been reported with field damage despite round, symmetric cups (173). Quantitative measures of the retinal nerve fiber layer have also been shown to correlate with the visual field loss in glaucoma patients (184).

The ability to predict impending glaucomatous visual field loss by the appearance of the optic nerve head is less accurate than correlating disc damage with established field loss. No single parameter or combination of parameters in glaucomatous optic atrophy has been found to be totally satisfactory for this purpose. The parameters which correlate best with visual field loss are magnification-corrected measurements of neuroretinal rim area (185–188) and defects in the retinal nerve fiber layer (189–193). Diffuse structural changes in the optic nerve head or retinal nerve fiber layer are more often associated with diffuse depression of visual function, while localized changes correlate more with localized visual field changes (192). In some cases, the early field loss associated with retinal nerve fiber layer defects can be detected with automatic perimetry when it has been missed with manual perimetry (194, 195).

The correlation between optic nerve head and visual field defects in glaucoma is close enough to prompt a search for other underlying disease processes, such as neurologic disorders, if a correlation is not found. Nevertheless, the absence of a perfect correlation indicates that both disc and field examinations are essential in managing the glaucoma patient (196). In general, optic nerve head and retinal nerve fiber layer changes have their greatest value in the early stages of glaucoma, while progressive visual field loss becomes the more useful guide to therapy in advanced cases (171, 197).

TECHNIQUES AND INSTRUMENTS FOR MEASURING THE FIELD OF VISION

Basic Principles

Just as a cartographer maps the boundaries and topography of an island, so the perimetrist can measure both the peripheral limits of a visual field and the relative visual acuity of areas within those limits. This may be accomplished by using kinetic and/or static techniques with instruments that are either manually operated or computer-assisted (automatic).

Kinetic Techniques

This method involves moving the test object from a nonseeing to a seeing area and recording the point at which it is first seen in relation to fixation (Fig. 6.4**A**). The procedure documents the boundaries of the visual field, for both the absolute limits as well as areas of relative differences in visual acuity within the field (Fig. 6.5). As previously noted, the boundaries, or contour lines, are called isopters. The size and shape of a particular isopter depends, in part, on the stimulus value of the corresponding test object.

Static Techniques

This approach involves the presentation of stationary test objects utilizing either suprathreshold or threshold presentations. *Suprathreshold static presentation* is an "on-off" technique in which a test object that is just above the anticipated threshold for the corresponding portion of the visual field is momentarily presented and the points at which the patient fails to recognize the target are noted. It is a way of "spot checking" for areas of relative or absolute blindness, usually within the central visual field. *Threshold static (profile) perimetry* measures the relative intensity thresholds for the visual acuity of individual retinal points within the field of vision. The technique involves gradually increasing the target light from subthreshold intensity and recording the level at which the patient first indicates recognition of the target (Fig. 6.4**B**), or decreasing it from a suprathreshold level and recording the lowest stimulus value seen. The points tested can be along one meridian, either radiating from fixation or along a circular line around a fixed point from fixation, and displayed on a flat abscissa or a circular chart (Fig. 6.6) (1).

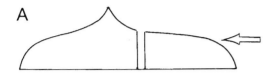

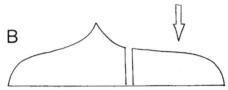

Figure 6.4. Standard techniques for measuring the visual field. In kinetic technique (**A**), test object moves from non-seeing to seeing area. Static technique (**B**) measures sensitivity of retina at a given point.

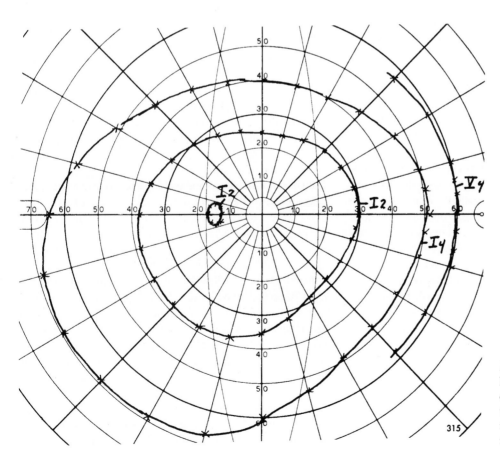

Figure 6.5. Example of manual kinetic perimetry showing two complete isopters (I₂ and I₄) and third partial isopter (V₄) in nasal periphery with blind spot measured by I₂ target.

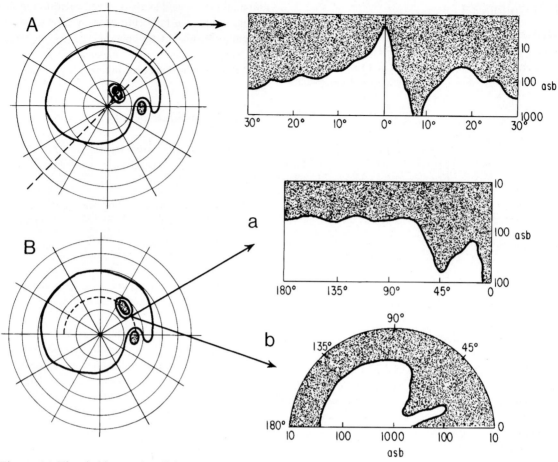

Figure 6.6. Threshold static (profile) perimetry. **A.** Meridian static perimetry. **B.** Circular static perimetry on flat abscissa *(a)* and circular chart *(b).* The *dotted lines* indicate the cuts through the fields that are being displayed in profile.

The more common technique with automated perimetry, however, is to test retinal points distributed throughout a portion of the visual field and record the visual thresholds as symbols or numerical values (Fig. 6.7).

Threshold static perimetry has been shown to be more sensitive than kinetic perimetry in detecting glaucomatous field loss (198). In one study of patients with open-angle glaucoma, a defect was found in one-third of the cases with static circular perimetry that was missed by kinetic perimetry (199). In a long-term study of ocular hypertensive patients, 75% of those who developed glaucomatous damage had an abnormality by automated static perimetry (using a hemifield test, which is explained later) 1 year before field loss was detected by manual perimetry, using a combination of kinetic and static presentations (200).

Test Objects

The standard target for both kinetic and static perimetry is a white disc, the stimulus value of which can be adjusted by varying the target size and/or luminosity relative to that of the background. In normal subjects, the mean retinal sensi-

tivity has been shown to increase with the increasing size of the test object (201). The following modifications in the test object have also been evaluated in an effort to increase the sensitivity of the testing procedure.

COLOR STIMULI. As compared to white targets, color stimuli may influence the visual field results in one of two ways. With targets that reflect light, as used with tangent screen testing, color targets have less luminance and a lower stimulus value than white. More significantly, if the luminance is kept constant and the color saturation is varied, the stimulus value might be more sensitive to specific color vision defects, as in some patients with glaucoma (202). Early studies suggested that such a technique could reveal field defects that are larger than those obtained with conventional luminance perimetry (203, 204). Other studies found color targets to be no more sensitive than white ones in detecting glaucomatous defects (205–207). These conflicting results may be related to the colors selected for the test and continued study has led to the following observations with new test objects.

Short-wavelength automated perimetry (SWAP) takes advantage of glaucoma-induced color vision deficits (dis-

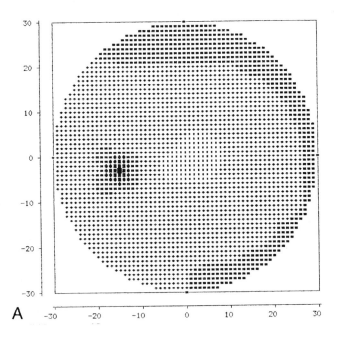

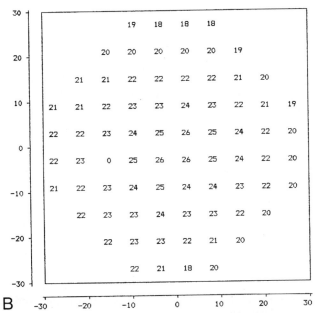

Figure 6.7. Examples of threshold static (computer-assisted) perimetry. Retinal sensitivity is measured at points throughout a portion of the visual field (central 30° in this example). Results can be displayed with symbols (**A**) and/or in numerical values (**B**).

cussed earlier in this chapter) by presenting short-wavelength blue targets on a bright yellow background (208). Preliminary studies indicate that SWAP deficits represent early glaucomatous damage (209, 210), and that the test may indicate significant change in visual function before it is apparent on standard white-on-white visual fields (211). Several longitudinal studies have demonstrated the ability of blue-on-yellow to predict the development of glaucoma in ocular hypertensives (212, 213), as well as which patients with early glaucomatous visual field loss are most

likely to progress (214). However, the test is influenced by age and cataracts, necessitating stringent statistical analysis in interpreting the results (215–217).

CONTRAST SENSITIVITY. Another modification of test objects has been the utilization of contrast sensitivity, such as sine wave gratings of low spatial frequency and laser interference fringes, in an effort to increase sensitivity to peripheral defects (218–220). However, these techniques, such as the use of sinusoidal grating targets, are difficult and time-consuming. An effort to minimize these limitations has led to the development of *high-pass resolution perimetry* (or ring perimetry) in which the target is a ring of light outlined by narrow, dark bands that have a contrast of 25% within the target and give a space-average luminance across the target that is equal to the background value. By also using high-pass spatial filtering, the targets can be detected and resolved at the same ring size, in an effect known as vanishing optotype, allowing rapid definition of the resolution threshold. Normal subjects showed increased resolution threshold toward the periphery, a slight but significant decline in sensitivity with age, and high repeatability (221), as well as reliability indices comparable to standard automated perimetry (222). In glaucoma patients it showed significant reduction in overall resolution threshold (223) and was comparable to standard perimetry in sensitivity and specificity (224, 225).

Another attempt to incorporate the advantages of contrast sensitivity into perimetry has been the use of a temporal contrast or flickering target, which has been called *temporal modulation perimetry* (226) or *flicker perimetry* (227, 228). In normal subjects there is an age-related loss of temporal modulation sensitivity (226). It appears to be less affected by visual acuity (227) or retinal degradation (228) than either light-sense or resolution perimetry, and is more sensitive than light-sense perimetry to increasing IOP (229).

Different target *shapes and patterns,* which the patient must distinguish, are also reported to be of particular values in detecting optic nerve disease (230, 231). In one study with *pattern discrimination perimetry,* long-term and short-term fluctuation were clinically significant, but did not prevent adequate separation between normal and abnormal measurements (232).

Yet another technique, *random dot motion perimetry,* takes advantage of reduced motion sense in glaucoma patients by presenting a shift in position of dots within a defined circular area against a background of fixed dots. A preliminary study showed that open-angle glaucoma patients manifest abnormal motion perception with the test as compared to normal subjects (233).

Presentation of Test Objects

To minimize the patient's anticipation of when or where the next test object will appear, the presentation should be random, rather than following a predictable pattern, and the time between stimuli should be varied slightly. To avoid patient anxiety when testing in a nonseeing area, the examination should return periodically to a previously seen area. For kinetic targets, a stimulus velocity of 4° per second appears to be optimal for all targets in the central and peripheral visual field (234). The test object should always be moved from a nonseeing to a seeing area, i.e., from the periphery toward fixation when outlining an isopter and from the center of the blind spot or a scotoma. Suprathreshold static targets should be presented for a consistent duration of time, usually 0.5–1 second, and test objects should be just above threshold for the area being tested.

Background Illumination

Background illumination for manual perimetric techniques has traditionally been mesopic to stimulate both rods and cones. The adapting field luminances currently used in static and kinetic perimetry range from photopic to mesopic (4–31.5 apostilbs), although the optimum luminance has yet to be established. One study suggested that the lower levels of background illumination may allow minor reductions in light transmission by the ocular media to produce significant changes in the recorded threshold sensitivity (235). In a comparison of scotopic and photopic fields, localized scotomas in glaucoma patients were of equal depth, but diffuse scotopic defects significantly exceeded the photopic, supporting the concept that not all ganglion cell types are equally susceptible to glaucomatous damage (236).

With bowl perimeters, photometric adjustment should be made with the patient in place, since facial coloring effects luminosity. The most important principle regarding illumination is to keep both target and background constant and reproducible from one examination to the next.

Physiologic Factors that Influence Visual Fields

The following factors should be compensated for if possible, or otherwise should be considered when interpreting the fields.

CLARITY OF OCULAR MEDIA. *Cataracts,* especially if associated with miosis, can cause or exaggerate central or peripheral field defects, which could be mistaken for the development or progression of glaucomatous field loss. Even minimal light scattering, as may be caused by an early cataract that has a relatively insignificant effect on visual acuity, may influence threshold measurements (237). As previously noted, this effect may be greater with lower levels of background illumination (235). In a study of 90 eyes with open-angle glaucoma and cataracts, 41% had reversal of a partial or complete scotoma after cataract extraction (238). Nuclear cataracts depress central perimetric sensitivity more than peripheral sensitivity with both large and small targets, while nonnuclear cataracts influence central sensitivity more for small targets and peripheral sensitivity for large

targets (239). Attempts have been made to correlate visual field damage with lens opacity (240) and visual acuity (241) to aid clinicians in determining the significance of field change in patients with glaucoma and cataracts. Reduced clarity of the ocular media from other causes, such as a corneal disturbance, a cloudy posterior lens capsule after cataract surgery, or vitreous opacities, may also effect the visual fields. Applanation tonometry prior to automated static threshold perimetry was found in one study to have no detrimental effect on the visual field results (242).

PUPIL SIZE. *Miosis* alone may depress central and peripheral threshold sensitivities and exaggerate field defects (243), even after correction of induced myopia (244). One study utilized neutral density filters to reduce the retinal illumination the equivalent of halving the pupillary diameter, which reduced the mean threshold with two automated perimeters by 1.1–1.7 dB (245). For this reason, the pupil size should be recorded with each field, and the influence of miosis should be considered when a field change is detected. Mydriasis has less influence on the visual field, although pupillary dilation with tropicamide 1% in healthy subjects on no ocular medication was shown in one study to significantly reduce threshold sensitivity with automated perimetry (246).

REFRACTIVE ERRORS. Refractive errors primarily influence the central field. Myopia does not require correction when using a 300-mm perimeter, unless the refractive error exceeds 3 diopters. Posterior staphylomas can create areas of relative myopia, called *refraction scotomas,* which may be confused with glaucomatous field defects, but can usually be eliminated with an appropriate refractive correction. *Hyperopia* has a greater influence on perimetric results, especially for the central field, and even small refractive errors can significantly alter threshold sensitivity (247–249). Age tables are available to aid in determining the appropriate correction for presbyopia. A contact lens provides the best correction for the aphakic eye, although spectacle correction can be used for the central 25–30° with no correction for the peripheral field. Astigmatism should be corrected unless the cylinder is under 1 diopter, in which case it can be included as the spherical equivalent.

INCREASING AGE. Increasing age is also associated with a reduction in retinal threshold sensitivity. This effect starts as early as 20 years of age, progresses linearly throughout life, and involves the peripheral and superior areas more than the pericentric and inferior portions of the field (246, 250, 251). This age-related visual field sensitivity appears to be primarily due to neural loss rather than preretinal factors (252).

Psychologic Factors that Influence Visual Fields

The patient's understanding of the test and his or her alertness, concentration, fixation, and cooperation all influence the results of visual field testing (253). A learning effect with automated perimetry may influence the results of a patient's first or second field, suggesting that an initial field that does not agree with the clinical findings should be repeated (254–256). Another study found that moderate alcohol ingestion did not influence differential light sensitivity as tested by automated perimetry (257). With manual perimetry, the skill of the perimetrist will, of course, significantly influence the visual field results (258).

Manual Perimetry

Although automated perimeters are being used with increasing frequency in clinical practice, the older, manual perimeters still provide valuable information, especially when the test is performed by a skilled observer. Therefore, we first consider those units before discussing automated perimetry.

Tangent Screens

The tangent screen is a flat square of black felt or flannel with a central white fixation target on which 30° of the visual field can be studied. The test should be performed in mesopic lighting of approximately 7 footcandles with the patient seated either 1 or 2 meters from the screen. Both kinetic and suprathreshold static techniques can be used with the tangent screen. With the kinetic approach, the examiner moves a test object from the periphery toward fixation until the patient indicates recognition of the target. The procedure is repeated at various intervals around fixation until the isopter has been mapped. The stimulus value of the test objects can be changed by varying the size and/or color. The corresponding isopter is designated by the ratio of target diameter to the distance between patient and target, with both expressed in millimeters, e.g., "2/1000 white" for a 2-mm white test object at 1 meter (when the color is not indicated it is understood to be white).

Suprathreshold static perimetry can be performed by turning the disc-shaped test object from the black to the white side or by using a self-illuminating target with an on-off switch. Specific locations at which the patient fails to see the target are then evaluated further with kinetic techniques.

The tangent screen has the advantages of low cost and simplicity of operation. However, reproducibility of the fields, which is essential in managing patients with glaucoma, is limited by variations in background lighting and stimulus value of the targets and by difficulty in monitoring fixation. Furthermore, it does not include the peripheral field, where early glaucomatous defects may appear.

Arc and Bowl Perimeters

With these instruments, both the central and peripheral fields of vision can be examined. The screen of the perimeter may be either a curved ribbon of metal (arc perimeter) or bowl-shaped. The latter is preferable for glaucoma examinations, and the prototype is the *Goldmann perimeter* (Fig. 6.8) (259). Other similar instruments have been compared with the Goldmann unit with variable results (260). The bowl of the Goldmann perimeter has a radius of 300 mm and extends 95% to each side of fixation. The target is projected onto the bowl, and the stimulus value of the test object can be varied by changing (a) the size, (b) the intensity, or (c) the light transmission. The latter variable merely provides finer intensity adjustment for the stimulus. Arbitrary designations for each value variable are usually printed on the visual field chart, with O–V for size, 1–4 for intensity, and a-e for transmission. An isopter, therefore, might be designated as "I2e," which indicates a test object size of 0.25 mm², an intensity of 10 millilamberts, and 100% transmission of the light source. The patient's fixation can be monitored by the examiner through a telescope in the center of the bowl.

The Goldmann perimeter can be used for both kinetic and static visual field testing. Other perimeters have been designed exclusively for the measurement of static threshold (profile) fields. The prototype instrument in the latter group is the *Tübingen perimeter,* which consists of a bowl-type screen and stationary test objects with variable light intensity (261).

Specific Techniques for Manual Perimetry

Within the context of glaucoma detection and management, visual field testing has two basic aspects: (a) screening techniques to detect the presence of glaucomatous field loss, and (b) in-depth techniques to more accurately determine the extent of the damage and to follow the fields for evidence of progressive change.

SCREENING TECHNIQUES. Armaly (262) developed a method of visual field screening for glaucoma which was modified by Drance and associates (263–265), and is commonly referred to as *selective perimetry* or the Armaly-Drance technique. The basic concept is to test those areas in the visual field that have the highest probability of showing glaucomatous defects. The technique utilizes a Goldmann-type perimeter with suprathreshold static perimetry to test for central field defects and both suprathreshold static and kinetic perimetry to examine the peripheral field, with emphasis on the nasal and temporal periphery (Fig. 6.9). An evaluation of the technique in 106 normal individuals and 49 with glaucomatous defects revealed a high sensitivity and specificity, which made it suitable for clinical and survey screening (263, 265). An additional modification is to use the V4e isopter nasally to rule out crowding of the peripheral nasal isopters (17). Another technique for use with Goldmann-type perimeters utilizes three suprathreshold targets within three concentric zones from fixation in accordance with the normal physio-

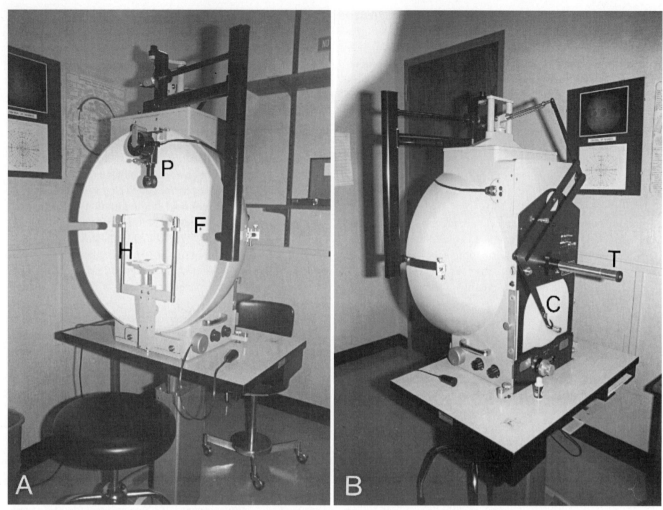

Figure 6.8. Goldmann manual perimeter. **A.** Patient's side, showing headrest *(H)*, fixation target *(F)*, and projection device for test objects *(P)*. **B.** Operator's side, showing telescope for fixation monitoring *(T)* and visual field chart *(C)* for locating and recording position of test objects.

logic sensitivity gradient (266). Other investigators have developed protocols to significantly reduce the number of test points without sacrificing sensitivity or specificity by concentrating the testing in those portions of the field where a defect is most likely to be found (267, 268).

IN-DEPTH TECHNIQUES. When a glaucomatous field defect is suspected by use of a screening technique, the physician has two choices. The patient can be asked to return another day either for a repeat screening field or an in-depth study. In many cases, however, it is more practical to proceed with the in-depth test at the time the defect is detected. The conversion from a screening to an in-depth field study is facilitated with the Armaly-Drance technique, since both are performed on a Goldmann-type perimeter with identical or similar target settings. The principle of in-depth field testing is to map out the size and shape of all scotomas, as well as complete isopters, using both the central threshold target and two or more additional targets of greater stimulus value (Fig. 6.10). Profile static perimetry is also of value in studying areas of known loss

for the depth and shape of the scotoma and for subtle evidence of progressive damage in serial fields.

Recording and Scoring Manual Visual Field Data

The complex nature of visual field data makes it difficult to reduce the information to simple descriptions or numbers. Therefore, storage of the data in its raw form, i.e., as transferred directly from the testing screen, is usually the most practical means of record-keeping. However, methods for conversion of visual fields from kinetic and static perimeter charts to computer use, for area calculations, graphic display, and storage in the patient's database, have been described (269, 270). When it is necessary to estimate the percent of functional visual field loss, a system is available (the Esterman grids), in which the field is divided into 100 blocks of varying size according to functional value with each representing 1% (271–273). The system has been adopted by the American Medical Association as a standard for rating visual field disability (274). Grids are available for scoring the tangent screen (271), perimeter (272), or the binocular field (273). In patients with severe visual loss from glaucoma, the binocular Esterman score of data generated by an automated perimeter correlated well with combined monocular visual field results (275).

Automated Perimetry

Why Automation?

The introduction of automation represents the latest step in the historic evolution of visual field technology. The first era of perimetry, which began in the mid-19th century with the work of von Graefe, was characterized by tangent screens and arc perimeters. A major limitation of these instruments was lack of standardization of the test objects and the background, as well as patient fixation. These needs were addressed in the era of standardization, which began in the middle of this century with the contributions of Goldmann. The main problem which remained, however, was the subjectivity of both the patient and perimetrist. While the former limitation is one with which we must continue to cope, the influence of the perimetrist has been eliminated to variable degrees with the advent of the era of automation, which began in the 1970s.

By reducing the influence of the perimetrist, automated perimetry improves the uniformity and reproducibility of vi-

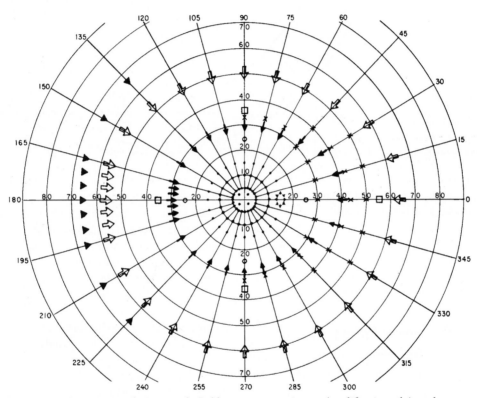

Figure 6.9. Screening technique with Goldmann-type perimeter (modification of Armaly-Drance selective perimetry). *1.* The central threshold target is determined as the smallest diameter and lowest intensity that can be visualized at any of the four threshold sites *(open circles).* *2.* The central threshold target is presented by static technique in each quadrant 5° from fixation *(solid circles)* to familiarize the patient with the testing procedure. *3.* The blind spot is outlined with kinetic checks of the central threshold target at eight cardinal points *(small arrowheads).* *4.* Isopter boundaries of the central threshold target are plotted every 5° for 15° above and below the nasal horizontal meridian and every 15° along the rest of the circumference *(solid arrows).* *5.* Spots are checked with the central threshold target along points 5, 10, and 15° from fixation *(solid circles).* *6.* The peripheral threshold target is determined at threshold site *(open squares).* *7.* Isopter boundaries of the peripheral threshold target are determined as in step 4 *(open arrows).* *8.* Spots are checked with the peripheral threshold target in the temporal periphery *(X).* *9.* The nasal peripheral isopter is plotted with the 4e target 45° above and below the horizontal meridian *(large arrowheads).* A refractive correction is used with central threshold target but not with the peripheral threshold or V_4e targets. (Reprinted with permission from de Oliveira-Rassi, M, Shields, MB: Crowding of the peripheral nasal isopters in glaucoma. *Am J Ophthalmol* 94:4, 1982.)

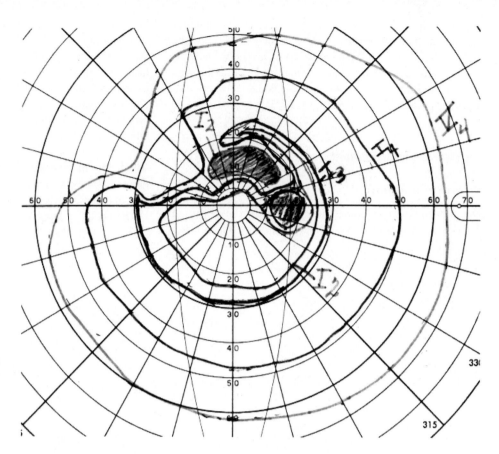

Figure 6.10. In-depth technique with Goldmann-type perimeter in which a superior arcuate scotoma and nasal step have been plotted with four targets (I₂, I₃, I₄, and V₄).

sual fields. In addition, the utilization of computers has provided new capabilities that are not possible with manual perimetry, including random presentation of targets, estimations of patient reliability, and statistical evaluation of data at many levels. It must be noted, however, that while automated perimetry is more accurate and informative, it is neither faster nor cheaper than manual perimetry.

Classification of Automated Perimeters

SEMIAUTOMATIC PERIMETERS. With these instruments, the perimetrist is still involved in a portion of the actual field testing, such as presenting the stimuli, making decisions, and recording data. These instruments are used primarily as *rapid screening devices* to aid in the detection of glaucoma.

The *Harrington-Flocks screener* utilizes the flash presentation of multiple dot patterns, and the patient is asked to indicate the number of dots seen (276). The device was found to be reliable in a study of 1500 screening tests (277). The *Friedmann visual field analyzer* is a similar instrument, which involves the static presentation of single or multiple test objects that can be varied in intensity (278, 279). Studies have also demonstrated the reliability of this device for mass screening programs (280). It was found to be at least as sensitive as careful manual perimetry with the Goldmann perimeter in detecting early glaucomatous visual field defects (281), and may even be of value in following the progression of glaucomatous damage, although it is limited by

the fact that it only measures the central 25° (282). It is also limited by the fact that normal subjects often miss stimuli in the extreme superior periphery and arcuate regions (283), although it may be possible to overcome this by comparing each field response score with scores from normal and abnormal populations (284).

Another screening device, the *Henson visual field analyzer,* presents 26 test spots on a computer monitor in a semiautomated, suprathreshold fashion (285), and was found to be useful in a vision screening study (286). Other television monitor and personal computer concepts have also been adapted for use in visual field screening (287, 288), although the value of these techniques has yet to be established.

FULLY AUTOMATIC PERIMETERS. With these instruments, the perimetrist is replaced by a computer and has no influence on the visual field results, aside from the important aspects of ensuring that the patient understands the testing procedure, is comfortably positioned at the perimeter, and complies with the requirements of the test. The remainder of this chapter deals with this class of computerized perimeters.

Instrumentation

Since the introduction of computerized perimeters in the 1970s, a wide variety of models have been designed. Many of these are no longer commercially available, while most of the others represent modifications of the originals.

Automated perimeters have two main components: the perimetric unit and the control unit. The perimetric unit in most systems utilizes a bowl-type screen, similar to that of the Goldmann manual perimeter.

STATIC TARGETS. Static targets are used in all cases, although additional kinetic targets have been evaluated in some units (144–146). The targets may either be projected onto the bowl or illuminated from light-emitting diodes (LEDs) or fiberoptics in the perimetric bowl. The former has the advantage of unlimited presentation locations on the screen, while the latter two have fixed positions in the bowl. In addition, the LEDs are recessed in dark cavities, which may allow perception by the most sensitive retinal areas of a stimulus that is of lower intensity than the background light (289, 290). This "dark hole phenomenon" is associated with increased variability in retesting the threshold (289, 290). Projected targets also have the advantage of allowing for change in size to alter the stimulus values. In practice, the size is usually kept constant, although it has been shown that larger targets may permit the measurement of visual function in areas that had been considered absolute scotomas with standard-sized stimuli (291). A larger target (size V stimulus) with a 10° test pattern was also found to be useful in patients with endstage glaucoma (292). With all target systems, the patient is provided with a device to indicate when a target is seen, which is recorded by the computer.

The standard stimulus in most automated perimeters is a white light on a white background, which tests the patient's light sense. As discussed earlier in this chapter, newer targets are being evaluated, which utilize color sense, contrast sensitivity, form sense, or motion sense.

PATIENT FIXATION. Patient fixation is monitored in a variety of ways depending on the sophistication of the instrument. Some utilize a telescope, similar to the Goldmann manual perimeter, while others allow the operator to observe the patient's eye on a television screen. Automatic fixation monitoring is also incorporated into most units either by periodically retesting the patients' response in the previously determined blind spot (the Heijl-Krakau method), or by monitoring a light reflex from this patient's cornea. With the latter, the computer can be programmed to stop the test whenever fixation is lost. Fixation is important, since eye movement has been shown to increase local short-term fluctuation and false-negative rates (293). However, maintaining fixation is difficult for many patients, and a new strategy of kinetic fixation, in which the fixation target is moved between stimuli, has been shown to improve threshold sensitivity (294).

CONTROL UNIT. The control unit provides interaction between the operator and computer through a dialog screen and either a keyboard or light pen. The computer within the control unit reads a program disc or chip, and controls and monitors instrumentation function according to that pro-

gram, evaluates patient's response, and computes data. The control unit also contains a printer, which provides a hard copy of the data in symbols or numerical values. Computers in the more sophisticated units also store data and can perform statistical analyses of the data in relation to programmed normal data or against previous fields of the same patient.

Testing Strategies

All fully automated perimeters take advantage of computer capabilities by utilizing *random presentation* of the static targets to avoid patient anticipation of the next presentation sites. In addition, an *adaptive technique* is employed, in which stimuli are presented according to the presumed normal retinal threshold contour, i.e., the relative *differential light thresholds* throughout the visual field, based on either age-corrected normal data or the patient's response to preliminary spot tests (Fig. 6.11). This approach, in comparison with the presentation of a constant stimulus value throughout a portion of the field, as with many manual techniques, improves the balance between sensitivity (the ability to detect defects) and specificity (the ability to detect normal areas). Fully automated perimeters differ at this point as to whether they are limited to suprathreshold measurements or are also capable of full thresholding.

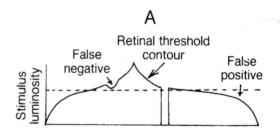

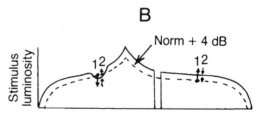

Figure 6.11. Adaptive strategy utilized in automated static perimetry. **A.** When a constant luminosity is presented throughout a portion of the visual field, true defects near fixation may be missed (false-negative), while more peripheral normal areas may be read as abnormal (false-positive). **B.** The adaptive strategy minimizes this by changing the stimulus value according to the retinal threshold contour. With full threshold programs, the retinal threshold is crossed by increasing or decreasing the stimulus value (*1*) and is then crossed a second time with smaller increments of change in luminosity (*2*).

SUPRATHRESHOLD STATIC PERIMETERS. Suprathreshold static perimeters present a stimulus value that is slightly above the anticipated normal for the corresponding retinal location. Some instruments simply indicate whether or not the target was seen, while others will present a second, high intensity target in nonseeing areas to distinguish between relative and absolute defects. In either case, however, these instruments are limited to screening functions, since they do not provide sufficient information about the depth or contour of a field defect to be used either as a baseline study or for following the patient during therapy. With the continued advances in automated perimetry, these instruments are becoming largely replaced by full threshold static perimeters.

THRESHOLD STATIC PERIMETERS. Threshold static perimeters are capable of a variety of testing strategies, in addition to suprathreshold screening. The most commonly used programs measure the retinal threshold at 70–80 points within the central 24–30°. A suprathreshold target is first presented, and the luminosity is then gradually increased or decreased until the patient's threshold is crossed, i.e., the target comes into or goes out of view, respectively. The threshold is then crossed a second time with smaller increments of change in luminosity to refine the threshold determination. Many programs will continuously adjust subsequent stimulus values according to prior measurements, e.g., the level is increased when testing near a known scotoma on the basis of optimized algorithms. Special programs have been evaluated which automatically increase the density of test locations around defective areas, although the value of this approach has yet to be established (295, 296). Other programs are designed to reduce testing time either by adjusting the initial target values according to previous fields by the same patient or by thresholding only locations that are missed with the suprathreshold target. The latter strategy, when compared to full-threshold programs, reduced the testing time by as much as two-thirds, but missed some defects that were detected with full-thresholding (297, 298).

Another thresholding strategy to reduce testing time is the FASTPAC program of the Humphrey Field Analyzer, which estimates thresholding from a single threshold crossing in 3-dB increments, in contrast to the standard double threshold crossing with 4 and 2 dB. This strategy has been evaluated by several investigative teams, most of which agree that it provides time reduction at the expense of accuracy and reliability (299–302).

VARIABILITY AND RELIABILITY. Several strategies are used to document variability and reliability of test results. With most full-thresholding programs, a percentage of random locations are retested to determine the reproducibility at those points (referred to as *short-term fluctuation* and expressed as the square root of the variance). The patient's general reliability is assessed with a series of *false-positives* (responding when no target is presented) and *false-negatives* (failing to respond to a stimulus of maximal intensity where a stimulus

was previously reported to be seen), as well as the frequency of *fixation losses* during the test, and the *number of stimuli* required to complete the test. There are several problems with this current strategy of reliability indices. With the exception of the number of stimuli, all reliability parameters add to the testing time, which may actually reduce the patient's reliability. Furthermore, since each represents a limited sampling, their usefulness is questionable. Several evaluations of the Humphrey Field Analyzer, which uses the Heijl-Krakau blind spot checking method, revealed a high percentage of tests that were considered unreliable because the patient exceeded the established criteria for fixation losses (303–305). Some suggestions for modifying reliability indices to reduce testing time have included estimating short-term fluctuation from grids of single threshold determinations (306), using intermittent monitoring for those patients who perform well during the first 1.5 minutes of testing (307), and substituting all indices with a new reliability parameter, which analyzes the inconsistency of responses to the standard thresholding algorithm (308).

TEST PATTERNS. A broad menu of test patterns are available with most instruments. The most commonly used are limited to the central 24–30° with a 6° separation between test locations. The 6° grid will miss the physiologic blind, and presumably small glaucomatous defects, in a high percentage of cases, and it has been suggested that tighter grids should be used, especially in the central 10–28° (309–311). Special programs are available to study smaller portions of the field with tighter grids. Programs are also available to study the peripheral field beyond 30° either in the nasal quadrant or for 360°. The peripheral studies can be performed alone or in conjunction with a central field program, and usually have wider target separation. Static testing of the peripheral nasal field has been shown to provide valuable additional information in detecting glaucomatous defects (312). Automated kinetic measurement of the peripheral field, especially nasally, was also found to provide useful information, in addition to that obtained from central testing, in many patients (144–146).

PRINTOUT. The computer printout records the threshold for each retinal point tested, which is theoretically the target that is just bright enough to be seen 50% of the time at that location (the *differential light threshold*). The absolute luminous intensity is measured in *apostilbs,* but is expressed in logarithmic units referred to as *decibels* (dB) which provides a more linear relationship between visual perception and a change in light intensity. A decibel is 0.1 log-unit, so that a 10-dB decrease represents a 10-fold stimulus increase, while a 20-dB decline represents a 100-fold stimulus increase. Log-units and decibels are relative and are not the same for all instruments. The printout may show the retinal threshold contour in decibels, or in a grayscale, or other symbols, with each symbol representing a decibel range (Fig. 6.12). The numerical printout may also show the difference between the test results and the age-corrected nor-

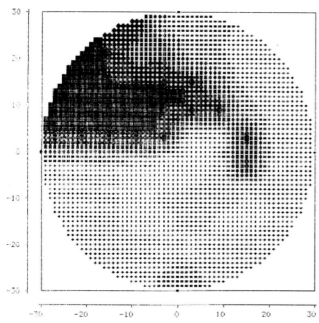

Figure 6.12. **Computer printout of visual field measured by automated static technique showing superior arcuate scotoma and nasal step. (Same patient as in Fig. 6.10.)**

mal, and a graphic method has been devised to show the development of visual field defects by superimposing two to four grayscale printouts and displaying changing areas as stripes (313).

Interpreting the Results

Computerized visual field printouts can be read by the clinician in much the same manner as with manual perimetric charts, i.e., looking primarily for nerve fiber layer defects such as paracentral and arcuate scotomas, and nasal steps. In addition, static threshold data can be analyzed mathematically, which may allow detection of more subtle visual field abnormalities. The statistical techniques used in this approach are referred to as *visual field indices.*

INDICES. An average of all threshold values is called *mean sensitivity,* while the average difference between each threshold value and the age-corrected normal is referred to as *mean defect* (or mean deviation). These indices primarily reflect diffuse changes. One way to detect localized defects is to calculate the number of threshold values that deviate significantly from the age-corrected normal, which is called *loss variance* (or pattern standard deviation). *Corrected loss variance* (or corrected pattern standard deviation) takes into account the *short-term fluctuation,* as previously discussed. These indices for localized loss are insensitive to the location of the defects. For example, three abnormal locations could either be randomly distributed or clustered. Attempts to improve the interpretation of data have led to the strategy of cluster analysis.

CLUSTER ANALYSIS. With this strategy, also referred to as *spatial correlation,* contiguous clusters of test locations, which have an increased probability of appearing together in typical glaucomatous field loss, are considered together in evaluating the visual field. They can be used in calculating local indices, which should be more sensitive than global indices, and may help to dampen long-term fluctuation. In several studies, using different cluster patterns, they have been shown to provide an enhanced probability of distinguishing normal from glaucomatous fields, as well as a stable glaucoma field from one that is deteriorating (314–317). Another strategy is to compare sums of threshold values in corresponding areas of the superior and inferior hemispheres (318, 319). In the Humphrey Field Analyzer STATPAC (discussed later), this is called the *Glaucoma Hemifield Test.* It utilizes a large normal database to calculate the significance of differences between the two hemispheres (320) and has been shown to significantly improve the ability to separate between normal and glaucoma fields (321). It has good sensitivity and specificity (322), although reproducibility is such that the use of two tests is recommended to improve specificity (323).

THRESHOLD VARIABILITY. As discussed earlier in this chapter, there is a certain degree of short-term fluctuation in the retinal threshold sensitivity profile (or hill of vision) among normal individuals, especially in the midperiphery and superior quadrant (324–326). In addition, each normal person will show some variation from test-to-test, which is referred to as *long-term fluctuation* (326). Both of these normal variations must be taken into account when attempting to interpret the significance of visual field data. Furthermore, the likelihood of increased variability in glaucomatous visual fields must also be taken into consideration. Average total long-term fluctuation in clinically stable glaucoma patients is similar to normals (327). However, long-term fluctuation can be considerable in field areas with moderate loss of sensitivity (328). In addition, short-term fluctuation is increased around both physiologic and glaucomatous scotomas (129, 329, 330). Short- and long-term fluctuations are greater among older patients (331), and short-term fluctuation is often greatest in the patients' first automated field test, indicating the influence of experience (332). In one study, a change in mean sensitivity of approximately 5–7 dB between two successive fields was needed to have 95% confidence that the trend would be confirmed by the third field (333).

TREND ANALYSIS. Statistical models are available with some automated perimeters to help the clinician determine the significance of visual field indices and variability. Those which have received the most reported investigation are the *Delta program* with the Octopus perimeter (334) and the *STATPAC* with the Humphrey Field Analyzer (335). With both systems, databases are used to calculate the probability of a measured value appearing in a given age-defined population. In the case of the Humphrey Field Analyzer, the STATPAC uses a large normal database, while STATPAC II

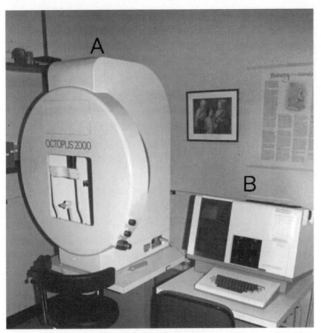

Figure 6.13. Octopus 2000R automated static perimeter, showing perimetric unit (**A**) and control unit (**B**).

200, which utilized fiberoptic light sources in a bowl perimeter, received the most reported evaluation. These models compared favorably with manual perimetry using Goldmann or Tübingen perimeters, and were felt to have great potential as quantitative visual field screening devices (341–345). The *Henson Visual Field Analyzer* has also been shown to have good predictive power (285) and was recently found to be suitable for vision screening programs (286).

THRESHOLD PERIMETERS. The first of these instruments to receive extensive study was the *Octopus 201* and subsequent models *2000* and *500* (Fig. 6.13). With each unit stimuli are projected onto a bowel and fixation is monitored by both the corneal light reflex method and a television view of the patient's eye. The models differ primarily according to computer capabilities. These automated perimeters have compared favorably to manual perimetry with Goldmann and Tübingen perimeters, and can frequently detect field loss missed with the Goldmann perimeter (346–348).

The *Humphrey Field Analyzer* also utilizes projected stimuli with strategies similar to the Octopus, except for fixation monitoring by the Heijl-Krakau periodic blind spot check method (Fig. 6.14). It is currently the most com-

uses a database of stable glaucoma patients. The STATPAC printout includes the reliability and global indices, the Glaucoma Hemifield Test, and probability maps, which display the field results in terms of the frequency with which the measured findings are seen in the defined population (336, 337). The STATPAC II also includes linear regression analysis and glaucoma change probability. A third statistical algorithm with the Humphrey Field Analyzer is the Progressor Program for analysis of serial fields downloaded to a personal computer (338).

Although most statistical models provide better agreement than experienced clinical observers with regard to significant change over time, there is no generally accepted technique for this purpose at the present time (339). One study, which compared the results of a threshold program on the Octopus perimeter to those from manual perimetry, demonstrated that indices used currently may not be clinically reliable in the assessment of changes in the visual field (340). A study evaluating the three commercially available computerized statistical algorithms with serial Humphrey fields showed a high degree of variability among the three, with none correlating well with the clinical impression (338). Until improved statistical algorithms are available, therefore, these data must be used with caution, still relying primarily on the clinical judgment of the physician.

Comparison of Specific Automated Perimeters

SUPRATHRESHOLD STATIC PERIMETERS. As previously noted, most instruments that are limited to suprathreshold measurements have now been replaced by models with full thresholding capabilities, although suprathreshold models may still have value as screening devices. The *Fieldmaster 101* and

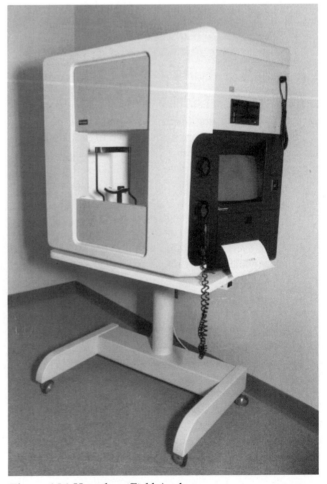

Figure 6.14. Humphrey Field Analyzer.

monly used automated perimeter. It has also compared favorably with manual perimetry on the Goldmann perimeter, often detecting defects that the latter missed (349). In one study, however, patients preferred the Goldmann perimeter, while the technician favored the Humphrey (350). The Octopus and Humphrey units have been compared in several studies. In one study, both short- and long-term fluctuations were greater with the Octopus (351). In another study, both automated perimeters identified slightly more defects by meridional threshold testing than the Tübingen manual perimeter (352).

SUMMARY

The normal visual field may be depicted as a three-dimensional contour, representing areas of relative retinal sensitivity and characterized by a peak at the point of fixation, an absolute depression corresponding to the optic nerve head (blind spot), and a sloping of the remaining areas to the boundaries of the field. Early glaucomatous damage may produce a generalized depression of this contour, which can be demonstrated with several psychophysical tests. The more specific visual field changes of glaucoma, however, are localized defects which correspond to loss of retinal nerve fiber bundles, and include paracentral and arcuate scotomas above and below fixation and step-like defects along the nasal midline (nasal step). Instruments that are used to measure the field of vision (perimeters) may have kinetic and/or static targets, which can be controlled manually or automatically. The targets are presented against a background that is either flat (tangent screen) or bowl-shaped, with the latter units providing more reliable measurements. Automated perimeters may be semiautomatic or fully automatic, and comparative studies indicate that computer-assisted static perimeters are more sensitive than manual perimeters in detecting glaucomatous visual field loss.

REFERENCES

1. Harrington, DO: The Visual Fields. A Textbook and Atlas of Clinical Perimetry. 5th ed. St. Louis, CV Mosby, 1981.
2. Hart, WM, Burde, RM: Three-dimensional topography of the central visual field. Sparing of foveal sensitivity in macular disease. Ophthalmology 90:1028, 1983.
3. Armaly, MF: The size and location of the normal blind spot. Arch Ophthalmol 81:192, 1969.
4. Jonas, JB, Gusek, GC, Fernández, MC: Correlation of the blind spot size to the area of the optic disk and parapapillary atrophy. Am J Ophthalmol 111:559, 1991.
5. Anctil, J-L, Anderson, DR: Early foveal involvement and generalized depression of the visual field in glaucoma. Arch Ophthalmol 102: 363, 1984.
6. Stamper, RL: The effect of glaucoma on central visual function. Trans Am Ophthalmol Soc 82:792, 1984.
7. Pickett, JE, Terry, SA, O'Connor, PS, O'Hara, M: Early loss of central visual acuity in glaucoma. Ophthalmology 92:891, 1985.
8. Drance, SM: Diffuse visual field loss in open-angle glaucoma. Ophthalmology 98:1533, 1991.
9. Lachenmayr, BJ, Drance, SM, Chauhan, BC, et al: Diffuse and localized field loss in light-sense, flicker and resolution perimetry. Evidence of pressure-induced damage. Fortschr Ophthalmol 88: 530, 1991.
10. Samuelson, TW, Spaeth, GL: Focal and diffuse visual field defects: their relationship to intraocular pressure. Ophthalmic Surg 24: 519, 1993.
11. Lachenmayr, BJ, Drance, SM, Airaksinen, PJ: Diffuse field loss and diffuse retinal nerve-fiber loss in glaucoma. Ger J Ophthalmol 1:22, 1992.
12. Lachenmayr, BJ, Drance, SM: Diffuse field loss and central visual function in glaucoma. Ger J Ophthalmol 1:67, 1992.
13. Åsman, P, Heijl, A: Diffuse visual field loss and glaucoma. Acta Ophthalmol 72:303, 1994.
14. Langerhorst, CT, Van den Berg, TJ, Greve EL: Is there general reduction of sensitivity in glaucoma? Int Ophthalmol 13:31, 1989.
15. Hart, WM, Yablonski, M, Kass, MA, Becker, B: Quantitative visual field and optic disc correlates early in glaucoma. Arch Ophthalmol 96:2209, 1978.
16. Flammer, J, Eppler, E, Niesel, P: Quantitative perimetry in the glaucoma patient without local visual field defects. Graefes Arch Clin Exp Ophthalmol 219:92, 1982.
17. de Oliveira-Rassi, M, Shields, MB: Crowding of the peripheral nasal isopters in glaucoma. Am J Ophthalmolal 94:4, 1982.
18. Singh, K, deFrank, MP, Shults, WT, Watzke, RC: Acute idiopathic blind spot enlargement. A spectrum of disease. Ophthalmology 98:497, 1991.
19. Drance, SM: The early field defects in glaucoma. Invest Ophthalmol 8:84, 1969.
20. Colenbrander, MC: The early diagnosis of glaucoma. Ophthalmologica 162:276, 1971.
21. Drance, SM, Lakowski, R, Schulzer, M, Douglas, GR: Acquired color vision changes in glaucoma. Use of 100-hue test and pickford anomaloscope as predictors of glaucomatous field change. Arch Ophthalmol 99:829, 1981.
22. Motolko, M, Drance, SM, Douglas, GR: The early psychophysical disturbances in chronic open-angle glaucoma. A study of visual functions with asymmetric disc cupping. Arch Ophthalmol 100: 1632, 1982.
23. Adams, AJ, Rodic, R, Husted, R, Stamper, R: Spectral sensitivity and color discrimination changes in glaucoma and glaucoma-suspect patients. Invest Ophthalmol Vis Sci 23:516, 1982.
24. Flammer, J, Drance, SM: Correlation between color vision scores and quantitative perimetry in suspected glaucoma. Arch Ophthalmol 102:38, 1984.
25. Hamill, TR, Post, RB, Johnson, CA, Keltner, JL: Correlation of color vision deficits and observable changes in the optic disc in a population of ocular hypertensives. Arch Ophthalmol 102:1637, 1984.
26. Heron, G, Adams, AJ, Husted, R: Central visual fields for short wavelength sensitive pathways in glaucoma and ocular hypertension. Invest Ophthalmol Vis Sci 29:64, 1988.
27. Adams, AJ, Heron, G, Husted, R: Clinical measures of central vision function in glaucoma and ocular hypertension. Arch Ophthalmol 105:782, 1987.
28. Yamazaki, Y, Lakowski, R, Drance, SM: A comparison of the blue color mechanism in high- and low-tension glaucoma. Ophthalmology 96:12, 1989.
29. Yamazaki, Y, Drance, SM, Lakowski, R, Schulzer, M: Correlation between color vision and highest intraocular pressure in glaucoma patients. Am J Ophthalmol 106:397, 1988.
30. Airaksinen, PJ, Lakowski, R, Drance, SM, Price, M: Color vision and retinal nerve fiber layer in early glaucoma. Am J Ophthalmol 101:208, 1986.
31. Quigley, HA, Sanchez, RM, Dunkelberg, GR, L'Hernault, NL, Baginski, TA: Chronic glaucoma selectively damages large optic nerve fibers. Invest Ophthalmol Vis Sci 28:913, 1987.
32. Breton, ME, Krupin, T: Age covariance between 100-hue color scores and quantitative perimetry in primary open angle glaucoma. Arch Ophthalmol 105:642, 1987.

33. Sample, PA, Boynton, RM, Weinreb, RN: Isolating the color vision loss in primary open-angle glaucoma. Am J Ophthalmol 106:686, 1988.

34. Gündüz, K, Arden, GB, Perry, S, et al: Color vision defects in ocular hypertension and glaucoma: quantification with a computer-driven color television system. Arch Ophthalmol 106:929, 1988.

35. Yu, TC, Falcao-Reis, F, Spileers, W, Arden, GB: Peripheral color contrast. A new screening test for preglaucomatous visual loss. Invest Ophthalmol Vis Sci 32:2779, 1991.

36. Nguyen, NX, Korth, M, Wisse, M, Junemann, A: The use of a new anomaloscope test for the diagnosis of glaucoma. Klin Monatsbl Augenheilkd 204:149, 1994.

37. Falcao-Reis, FM, O'Sullivan, F, Spileers, W, et al: Macular colour contrast sensitivity in ocular hypertension and glaucoma: evidence for two types of defect. Br J Ophthal 75:598, 1991.

38. Arden, GB, Jacobson, JJ: A simple grating test for contrast sensitivity: preliminary results indicate value in screening for glaucoma. Invest Ophthalmol Vis Sci 17:23, 1978.

39. Higgins, KE, Jaffe, MJ, Coletta, NJ, et al: Spatial contrast sensitivity. Importance of controlling the patient's visibility criterion. Arch Ophthalmol 102:1035, 1984.

40. Vaegan, Halliday, BL: A forced-choice test improves clinical contrast sensitivity testing. Br J Ophthalmol 66:477, 1982.

41. Tweten, S, Wall, M, Schwartz, BD: A comparison of three clinical methods of spatial contrast-sensitivity testing in normal subjects. Graefes Arch Clin Exp Ophthalmol 228:24, 1990.

42. Strasser, B, Haddad, R, Keibl, L: Arden test for early glaucomatous damage. Klin Monatsbl Augenheilkd 178:136, 1981.

43. Lundh, BL, Lennerstrand, G: Eccentric contrast sensitivity loss in glaucoma. Acta Ophthalmol 59:21, 1981.

44. Motolko, MA, Phelps, CD: Contrast sensitivity in asymmetric glaucoma. Int Ophthalmol 7:45, 1984.

45. Hitchings, RA, Powell, DJ, Arden, GB, Carter, RM: Contrast sensitivity gratings in glaucoma family screening. Br J Ophthalmol 65:515, 1981.

46. Stamper, RL, Hsu-Winges, C, Sopher, M: Arden contrast sensitivity testing in glaucoma. Arch Ophthalmol 100:947, 1982.

47. Ross, JE, Bron, AJ, Clarke, DD: Contrast sensitivity and visual disability in chronic simple glaucoma. Br J Ophthalmol 68:821, 1984.

48. Sample, PA, Juang, PSC, Weinreb, RN: Isolating the effects of primary open-angle glaucoma on the contrast sensitivity function. Am J Ophthalmol 112:308, 1991.

49. Zulauf, M, Flammer, J: Correlation of spatial contrast sensitivity and visual fields in glaucoma. Graefes Arch Clin Exp Ophthalmol 231:146, 1993.

50. Falcão-Reis, F, O'Donoghue, E, Buceti, R, et al: Peripheral contrast sensitivity in glaucoma and ocular hypertension. Br J Ophthalmol 74:712, 1990.

51. Sokol, S, Domar, A, Moskowitz, A: Utility of the Arden grating test in glaucoma screening: high false-positive rate in normals over 50 years of age. Invest Ophthalmol Vis Sci 19:1529, 1980.

52. Hyvarin, L, Rovamo, J, Laurinen, P, et al: Contrast sensitivity in monocular glaucoma. Acta Ophthalmol 61:742, 1983.

53. Lundh, BL: Central contrast sensitivity tests in the detection of early glaucoma. Acta Ophthalmol 63:481, 1985.

54. Sponsel, WE, DePaul, KL, Martone, JF, et al: Association of Vistech contrast sensitivity and visual field findings in glaucoma. Br J Ophthalmol 75:558, 1991.

55. Korth, M, Horn, F, Storck, B, Jonas, JB: Spatial and spatiotemporal contrast sensitivity of normal and glaucoma eyes. Graefes Arch Clin Exp Ophthalmol 227:428, 1989.

56. Owsley, C, Gardner, T, Sekuler, R, Lieberman, H: Role of the crystalline lens in the spatial vision loss of the elderly. Invest Ophthalmol Vis Sci 26:1165, 1985.

57. Pomerance, GN, Evans, DW: Test-retest reliability of the CSV-1000 contrast test and its relationship to glaucoma therapy. Invest Ophthalmol Vis Sci 35:3357, 1994.

58. Atkin, A, Bodis-Wollner, I, Wolkstein, M, et al: Abnormalities of central contrast sensitivity in glaucoma. Am J Ophthalmol 88:205, 1979.

59. Tyler, CW: Specific deficits of flicker sensitivity in glaucoma and ocular hypertension. Invest Ophthalmol Vis Sci 20:204, 1981.

60. Tyler, CW, Hardage, L, Stamper, RL: The temporal visuogram in ocular hypertension and its progression to glaucoma. J Glau 3(Suppl): S65, 1994.

61. Breton, ME, Wilson, TW, Wilson, R, et al: Temporal contrast sensitivity loss in primary open-angle glaucoma and glaucoma suspects. Invest Ophthalmol Vis Sci 32:2931, 1991.

62. Lachenmayr, BJ, Kojetinsky, S, Ostermaier, N, et al: The different effects of aging on normal sensitivity in flicker and light-sense perimetry. Invest Ophthalmol Vis Sci 35:2741, 1994.

63. Eisner, A, Cioffi, GA, Campbell, HMK, Samples, JR: Foveal flicker sensitivity abnormalities in early glaucoma: associations with high blood pressure. J Glau 3(Suppl):S19, 1994.

64. Tytla, ME, Trope, GE, Buncic, JR: Flicker sensitivity in treated ocular hypertension. Ophthalmology 97:36, 1990.

65. Regan, D, Neima, D: Balance between pattern and flicker sensitivities in the visual fields of ophthalmological patients. Br J Ophthalmol 68:310, 1984.

66. Stelmach, LB, Drance, SM, Di Lollo, V: Two-pulse temporal resolution in patients with glaucoma, suspected glaucoma, and in normal observers. Am J Ophthalmol 102:617, 1986.

67. Glovinsky, Y, Quigley, HA, Drum, B, et al: A whole-field scotopic retinal sensitivity test for the detection of early glaucoma damage. Arch Ophthalmol 110:486, 1992.

68. Quigley, HA, West, SK, Munoz, B, et al: Examination methods for glaucoma prevalence surveys. Arch Ophthalmol 111:1409, 1993.

69. Stewart, WC, Chorak, RP, Murrel, HP: Evaluation of the whole-field scotopic retinal sensitivity tester in clinical glaucoma practice. J Glau 3:280, 1994.

70. Scott, IU, Quigley, HA, Vitale, S, et al: Effect of cataract on a scotopic sensitivity screening test for glaucoma. J Glau 3: 286, 1994.

71. Bobak, P, Bodis-Wollner, I, Harnois, C, et al: Pattern electroretinograms and visual-evoked potentials in glaucoma and multiple sclerosis. Am J Ophthalmol 96:72, 1983.

72. Wanger, P, Persson, HE: Pattern-reversal electroretinograms in unilateral glaucoma. Invest Ophthalmol Vis Sci 24:749, 1983.

73. Papst, N, Bopp, M, Schnaudigel, OE: Flash and pattern electroretinograms in advanced glaucoma. Klin Monatsbl Augenheilkd 184:199, 1984.

74. Papst, N, Bopp, M, Schnaudigel, OE: Pattern of electroretinogram and visually evoked cortical potentials in glaucoma. Graefes Arch Clin Exp Ophthalmol 222:29, 1984.

75. Price, MJ, Drance, SM, Price M, et al: The pattern of electroretinogram and visual-evoked potential in glaucoma. Graefes Arch Clin Exp Ophthalmol 226:542, 1988.

76. Korth, M, Horn, F, Storck, B, Jonas, J: The pattern-evoked electroretinogram (PERG): age-related alterations and changes in glaucoma. Graefes Arch Clin Exp Ophthalmol 227:123, 1989.

77. Watanabe, I, Iijima H, Tsukahara, S: The pattern electroretinogram in glaucoma: an evaluation by relative amplitude from the Bjerrum area. Br J Ophthalmol 73:131, 1989.

78. Odom, JV, Feghali, JG, Jin, J-C, Weinstein, GW: Visual function deficits in glaucoma. Electroretinogram pattern and luminance nonlinearities. Arch Ophthalmol 108:222, 1990.

79. Wanger, P, Persson, HE: Pattern-reversal electroretinograms and high-pass resolution perimetry in suspected or early glaucoma. Ophthalmology 94:1098, 1987.

80. Weinstein, GW, Arden, GB, Hitchings, RA, et al: The pattern electroretinogram (PERG) in ocular hypertension and glaucoma. Arch Ophthalmol 106:923, 1988.

81. Trick, GL: PRRP abnormalities in glaucoma and ocular hypertension. Invest Ophthalmol Vis Sci 27:1730, 1986.

82. Trick, GL, Bickler-Bluth, M, Cooper, DG, et al: Pattern reversal electroretinogram (PRERG) abnormalities in ocular hypertension: correlation with glaucoma risk factors. Curr Eye Res 7:201, 1988.

83. Trick, GL, Nesher, R, Cooper, DG, et al: Dissociation of visual deficits in ocular hypertension. Invest Ophthalmol Vis Sci 29:1486, 1988.

84. O'Donaghue, E, Arden, GB, O'Sullivan, F, et al: The pattern electroretinogram in glaucoma and ocular hypertension. Br J Ophthalmol 76:387, 1992.

85. Pfeiffer, N, Bach, M: The pattern-electroretinogram in glaucoma and ocular hypertension. A cross-sectional and longitudinal study. Ger J Ophthalmol 1:35, 1992.

86. Pfeiffer, N, Tillmon, B, Bach, M: Predictive value of the pattern electroretinogram in high-risk ocular hypertension. Invest Ophthalmol Vis Sci 34:1710, 1993.

87. Falsini, B, Colotto, A, Porciatti, V, Porrello, G: Follow-up study with pattern ERG in ocular hypertension and glaucoma patients under timolol maleate treatment. Clin Vis Sci 7:341, 1992.

88. Bach, M, Funk, J: Pattern electroretinogram and computerized optic nerve-head analysis in glaucoma suspects. Ger J Ophthalmol 2:178, 1993.

89. Noeh, C, Kaye, SB, Brown, M, et al: Pattern electroretinogram and automated perimetry in patients with glaucoma and ocular hypertension. Br J Ophthalmol 78:359, 1994.

90. Graham, SL, Wong VAT, Drance, SM, Mikelberg, FS: Pattern electroretinograms from hemifields in normal subjects and patients with glaucoma. Invest Ophthalmol Vis Sci 35:3347, 1994.

91. Johnson, MA, Drum, BA, Quigley, HA, et al: Pattern-evoked potentials and optic nerve fiber loss in monocular laser-induced glaucoma. Invest Ophthalmol Vis Sci 30:897, 1989.

92. Siliprandi, R, Bucci, MG, Canella R, Carmignoto, G: Flash and pattern electroretinograms during and after acute intraocular pressure elevation in cats. Invest Ophthalmol Vis Sci 29:558, 1988.

93. Cappin, JM, Nissim, S: Visual evoked responses in the assessment of field defects in glaucoma. Arch Ophthalmol 93:9, 1975.

94. Towle, VL, Moskowitz, A, Sokol, S, Schwartz, B: The visual evoked potential in glaucoma and ocular hypertension: effects of check size, field size, and stimulation rate. Invest Ophthalmol Vis Sci 24:175, 1983.

95. Howe, JW, Mitchell, KW: The objective assessment of contrast sensitivity function by electrophysiological means. Br J Ophthalmol 68:626, 1984.

96. Mitchell, KW, Wood, CM, Howe, JW, et al: The visual evoked potential in acute primary angle closure glaucoma. Br J Ophthalmol 73:448, 1989.

97. Schmeisser, ET, Smith, TJ: High-frequency flicker visual-evoked potential losses in glaucoma. Ophthalmology 96:620, 1989.

98. Holopigian, K, Seiple, W, Mayron, C, et al: Electrophysiological and psychophysical flicker sensitivity in patients with primary open-angle glaucoma and ocular hypertension. Invest Ophthalmol Vis Sci 31:1863, 1990.

99. Bray, LC, Mitchell, KW, Howe, JW: Prognostic significance of the pattern visual evoked potential in ocular hypertension. Br J Ophthalmol 75:79, 1991.

100. Korth, M, Nguyen, NX, Jünemann, A, et al: VEP test of the blue-sensitive pathway in glaucoma. Invest Ophthalmol Vis Sci 35:2599, 1994.

101. Saraux, H, Grall, Y, Keller, J, et al: Electro-oculography and the glaucomatous eye. J Fr Ophthalmol 5:243, 1982.

102. Jonas, JB, Zäch, F-M, Naumann, GOH: Dark adaptation in glaucomatous and nonglaucomatous optic nerve atrophy. Graefes Arch Clin Exp Ophthalmol 228:321, 1990.

103. Goldthwaite, D, Lakowski, R, Drance, SM: A study of dark adaptation in ocular hypertensives. Can J Ophthalmol 11:55, 1976.

104. Teoh, SL, Allen, D, Dutton, GN, Foulds, WS: Brightness discrimination and contrast sensitivity in chronic glaucoma—a clinical study. Br J Ophthalmol 74:215, 1990.

105. Cummins, D, MacMillan, ES, Heron, G, Dutton, GN: Simultaneous interocular brightness sense testing in ocular hypertension and glaucoma. Arch Ophthalmol 112:1198, 1994.

106. Enoch, JM: Quantitative layer-by-layer perimetry. Invest Ophthalmol Vis Sci 17:208, 1978.

107. Bullimore, MA, Wood, JM, Swenson, K: Motion perception in glaucoma. Invest Ophthalmol Vis Sci 34:3526, 1993.

108. Fahle, M, Wehrhahn, C: Motion perception in the peripheral visual field. Graefes Arch Clin Exp Ophthalmol 229:430, 1991.

109. Ruben, S, Fitzke, F: Correlation of peripheral displacement thresholds and optic disc parameters in ocular hypertension. Br J Ophthalmol 78:291, 1994.

110. Piltz, JR, Swindale, NV, Drance, SM: Vernier thresholds and alignment bias in control, suspect, and glaucomatous eyes. J Glau 2:87, 1993.

111. Kohn, AN, Moss, AP, Podos, SM: Relative afferent pupillary defects in glaucoma without characteristic field loss. Arch Ophthalmol 97:294, 1979.

112. Thompson, HS, Montague, P, Cox, TA, Corbett, JJ: The relationship between visual acuity, pupillary defect, and visual field loss. Am J Ophthalmol 93:681, 1982.

113. Brown, RH, Zilis, JD, Lynch, MG, Sanborn, GE: The afferent pupillary defect in asymmetric glaucoma. Arch Ophthalmol 105:1540, 1987.

114. Johnson, LN, Hill, RA, Bartholomew, MJ: Correlation of afferent pupillary defect with visual field loss on automated perimetry. Ophthalmology 95:1649, 1988.

115. Browning, DJ, Buckley, EG: Reliability of brightness comparison testing in predicting afferent pupillary defects. Arch Ophthalmol 106:341, 1988.

116. Werner, EB, Drance, SM: Early visual field disturbances in glaucoma. Arch Ophthalmol 95:1173, 1977.

117. Werner, EB, Saheb, N, Thomas, D: Variability of static visual threshold responses in patients with elevated IOPs. Arch Ophthalmol 100:1627, 1982.

118. Hart, WM Jr, Becker, B: The onset and evolution of glaucomatous visual field defects. Ophthalmology 89:268, 1982.

119. Sturmer, J, Gloor, B, Tobler, HJ: How glaucomatous visual fields manifest themselves in reality. Klin Monatsbl Augenheilkd 184:390, 1984.

120. Flammer, J, Drance, SM, Zulauf, M: Differential light threshold. Short- and long-term fluctuation in patients with glaucoma, normal controls, and patients with suspected glaucoma. Arch Ophthalmol 102:704, 1984.

121. Heijl, A, Drance, SM: Changes in differential threshold in patients with glaucoma during prolonged perimetry. Br J Ophthalmol 67:512, 1983.

122. Flammer, J, Drance, SM, Fankhause, F, Augustiny, L: Differential light threshold in automated static perimetry. Factors influencing short-term fluctuation. Arch Ophthalmol 102:876, 1984.

123. Flammer, J, Drance, SM, Schulzer, M: Covariates of the long-term fluctuation of the differential light threshold. Arch Ophthalmol 102:880, 1984.

124. Harrington, DO: The Bjerrum scotoma. Am J Ophthalmol 59:646, 1965.

125. Gramer, E, Gerlach, R, Krieglstein, GK, Leydhecker, W: Topography of early visual field defects in computerized perimetry. Klin Monatsbl Augenheilkd 180:515, 1982.

126. Mikelberg, FS, Drance, SM: The mode of progression of visual field defects in glaucoma. Am J Ophthalmol 98:443, 1984.

127. Drance, SM: The glaucomatous visual field. Br J Ophthalmol 56:186, 1972.

128. Drance, SM: The glaucomatous visual field. Invest Ophthalmol 11:85, 1972.

129. Haefliger, IO, Flammer, J: Fluctuation of the differential light threshold at the border of absolute scotomas. Comparison between glaucomatous visual field defects and blind spots. Ophthalmology 98:1529, 1991.

130. Mikelberg, FS, Schulzer, M, Drance, SM, Lau, W: The rate of progression of scotomas in glaucoma. Am J Ophthalmol 101:1, 1986.

131. Harrington, DO: Differential diagnosis of the arcuate scotoma. Invest Ophthalmol 8:96, 1969.

132. LeBlanc, RP, Becker, B: Peripheral nasal field defects. Am J Ophthalmol 72:415, 1971.

133. Werner, EB, Beraskow, J: Peripheral nasal field defects in glaucoma. Ophthalmology 86:1875, 1979.

134. Lynn, JR: Correlation of pathogenesis, anatomy, and patterns of visual loss in glaucoma. In Symposium on Glaucoma. St. Louis, CV Mosby, 1975, p. 151.

135. Gilpin, LB, Stewart, WC, Shields, MB, Miller, KN: Hemianopic offsets in the visual field of patients with glaucoma. Graefes Arch Clin Exp Ophthalmol 228:450, 1990.

136. Damgaard-Jensen, L: Vertical steps in isopters at the hemiopic border in normal and glaucomatous eyes. Acta Ophthalmol 55:111, 1977.

137. Damgaard-Jensen, L: Demonstration of peripheral hemiopic border steps by static perimetry. Acta Ophthalmol 55:815, 1977.

138. Brais, P, Drance, SM: The temporal field in chronic simple glaucoma. Arch Ophthalmol 88:518, 1976.

139. Pennebaker, GE, Stewart, WC: Temporal visual field in glaucoma: a re-evaluation in the automated perimetry era. Graefes Arch Clin Exp Ophthalmol 230:111, 1992.

140. Armaly, MF: Visual field defects in early open angle glaucoma. Trans Am Ophthalmol Soc 69:147, 1971.

141. Armaly, MF: Selective perimetry for glaucomatous defects in ocular hypertension. Arch Ophthalmol 87:518, 1972.

142. Schulzer, M, Mikelberg, FS, Drance, SM: A study of the value of the central and peripheral isoptres in assessing visual field progression in the presence of paracentral scotoma measurements. Br J Ophthalmol 71:422, 1987.

143. Caprioli, J, Spaeth, GL: Static threshold examination of the peripheral nasal visual field in glaucoma. Arch Ophthalmol 103:1150, 1985.

144. Stewart, WC, Shields MB, Ollie, AR: Peripheral visual field testing by automated kinetic perimetry in glaucoma. Arch Ophthalmol 106:202, 1988.

145. Miller, KN, Shields, MB, Ollie, AR: Automated kinetic perimetry with two peripheral isopters in glaucoma. Arch Ophthalmol 107:1316, 1989.

146. Ballon, BJ, Echelman, DA, Shields, MB, Ollie, AR: Peripheral visual field testing in glaucoma by automated kinetic perimetry with the Humphrey field analyzer. Arch Ophthalmol 110:1730, 1992.

147. Lichter, RR, Ravin, JG: Risks of sudden visual loss after glaucoma surgery. Am J Ophthalmol 78:1009, 1974.

148. Caprioli, J, Sears, M, Miller, JM: Patterns of early visual field loss in open-angle glaucoma. Am J Ophthalmol 103:512, 1987.

149. Hitchings, RA, Anderton, SA: A comparative study of visual field defects seen in patients with low-tension glaucoma and chronic simple glaucoma. Br J Ophthalmol 67:818, 1983.

150. Caprioli, J, Spaeth, GL: Comparison of visual field defects in the low-tension glaucomas with those in the high-tension glaucomas. Am J Ophthalmol 97:730, 1984.

151. Drance, SM: The visual field of low tension glaucoma and shock-induced optic neuropathy. Arch Ophthalmol 95:1359, 1977.

152. Motolko, M, Drance, SM, Douglas, GR: Visual field defects in low-tension glaucoma. Comparison of defects in low-tension glaucoma and chronic open angle glaucoma. Arch Ophthalmol 100:1074, 1982.

153. Zeiter, JH, Shin, DH, Juzych, MS, et al: Visual field defects in patients with normal-tension glaucoma and patients with high-tension glaucoma. Am J Ophthalmol 114:758, 1992.

154. Radius, RL, Maumenee, AE: Visual field changes following acute elevation of intraocular pressure. Trans Am Acad Ophthalmol Otol 83:61, 1977.

155. McNaught, EI, Rennie, A, McClure, E, Chisholm, IA: Pattern of visual damage after acute angle-closure glaucoma. Trans Ophthalmol Soc UK 94:406, 1974.

156. Drance, SM: Studies in the susceptibility of the eye to raised intraocular pressure. Arch Ophthalmol 68:478, 1962.

157. Tsamparlakis, JC: Effects of transient induced elevation of the intraocular pressure on the visual field. Br J Ophthalmol 48:237, 1964.

158. Scott, AB, Morris, A: Visual field changes produced by artificially elevated intraocular pressure. Am J Ophthalmol 63:308, 1967.

159. Armaly, MF: Effect of corticosteroids on intraocular pressure and fluid dynamics. III. Changes in visual function and pupil size during topical dexamethasone application. Arch Ophthalmol 71:636, 1964.

160. Kolker, AE, Becker, B, Mills, DW: Intraocular pressure and visual fields: effects of corticosteroids. Arch Ophthalmol 72:772, 1964.

161. LeBlanc, RP, Stewart, RH, Becker, B: Corticosteriod provocative testing. Invest Ophthalmol 9:946, 1970.

162. Hart, WM Jr, Becker, B: Visual field changes in ocular hypertension. A computer-based analysis. Arch Ophthalmol 95:1176, 1977.

163. Armaly, MF: The visual field defect and ocular pressure level in open angle glaucoma. Invest Ophthalmol 8:105, 1969.

164. Heilmann, K: On the reversibility of visual field defects in glaucomas. Trans Am Acad Ophthalmol Otol 78:304, 1974.

165. Flammer, J, Drance, SM: Reversibility of a glaucomatous visual field defect after acetazolamide therapy. Can J Ophthalmol 18:139, 1983.

166. Katz, LJ, Spaeth, GL, Cantor, LB, et al: Reversible optic disk cupping and visual field improvement in adults with glaucoma. Am J Ophthalmol 107:485, 1989.

167. Tsai, CS, Shin, DH, Wan, JY, Zeiter, JH: Visual field global indices in patients with reversal of glaucomatous cupping after intraocular pressure reduction. Ophthalmology 98:1412, 1991.

168. Gandolfi, SA: Improvement of visual field indices after surgical reduction of intraocular pressure. Ophthalmic Surg 26:121, 1995.

169. Heijl, A, Bengtsson, B: The short-term effect of laser trabeculoplasty on the glaucomatous visual field. A prospective study using computerized perimetry. Acta Ophthalmol 62:705, 1984.

170. Holmin, C, Krakau, CET: Trabeculoplasty and visual field decay: a follow-up study using computerized perimetry. Cur Eye Res 3:1101, 1984.

171. Drance, SM: The disc and the field in glaucoma. Ophthalmology 85:209, 1978.

172. Zeyen, TG, Caprioli, J: Progression of disc and field damage in early glaucoma. Arch Ophthalmol 111:62, 1993.

173. Hoskins, HD Jr, Gelber, EC: Optic disk topography and visual field defects in patients with increased intraocular pressure. Am J Ophthalmol 80:284, 1975.

174. Shutt, HKR, Boyd, TAS, Salter, AB: The relationship of visual fields, optic disc appearances and age in non-glaucomatous and glaucomatous eyes. Can J Ophthalmol 2:83, 1967.

175. Drance, SM: Correlation between optic disc changes and visual field defects in chronic open-angle glaucoma. Trans Am Acad Ophthalmol Otol 81:224, 1976.

176. Holmin, C: Optic disc evaluation versus the visual field in chronic glaucoma. Acta Ophthalmol 60:275, 1982.

177. Hitchings, RA, Spaeth, GL: The optic disc in glaucoma. II: correlation of the appearance of the optic disc with the visual field. Br J Ophthalmol 61:107, 1977.

178. Quigley, HA, Addicks, EM, Green, WR: Optic nerve damage in human glaucoma. III. Quantitative correlation of nerve fiber loss and visual field defect in glaucoma, ischemic neuropathy, papilledema, and toxic neuropathy. Arch Ophthalmol 100:135, 1982.

179. Quigley, HA, Dunkelberger, GR, Green, WR: Retinal ganglion cell atrophy correlated with automated perimetry in human eyes with glaucoma. Am J Ophthalmol 107:453, 1989.

180. Read, RM, Spaeth, GL: The practical clinical appraisal of the optic disc in glaucoma: the natural history of cup progression and some specific disc-field correlations. Trans Am Acad Ophthalmol Otol 78:255, 1974.

181. Gloster, J: Quantitative relationship between cupping of the optic disc and visual field loss in chronic simple glaucoma. Br J Ophthalmol 62:665, 1978.

182. Hitchings, RA, Anderton, S: Identification of glaucomatous visual field defects from examination of monocular photographs of the optic disc. Br J Ophthalmol 67:822, 1983.

183. Nyman, K, Tomita, G, Raitta, C, Kawamura, M: Correlation of asymmetry of visual field loss with optic disc topography in normal-tension glaucoma. Arch Ophthalmol 112:349, 1994.

184. Weinreb, RN, Shakiba, S, Sample, PA, et al: Association between quantitative nerve fiber layer measurement and visual field loss in glaucoma. Am J Ophthalmol 120:732, 1995.

185. Airaksinen, JP, Drance, SM, Douglas, GR, Schulzer, M: Neuroretinal rim areas and visual field indices in glaucoma. Am J Ophthalmol 99:107, 1985.

186. Guthauser, U, Flammer, J, Niesel, P: The relationship between the visual field and the optic nerve head in glaucomas. Graefes Arch Clin Exp Ophthalmol 225:129, 1987.

187. Caprioli, J, Miller, JM: Correlation of structure and function in glaucoma: Quantitative measurements of disc and field. Ophthalmology 95:723, 1988.

188. Jonas, JB, Gusek, GC, Naumann, GOH: Optic disc morphometry in chronic primary open-angle glaucoma. II. Correlation of the intra-papillary morphometric data to visual field indices. Graefes Arch Clin Exp Ophthalmol 226:531, 1988.

189. Sommer, A, Miller, NR, Pollack, I, et al: The nerve fiber layer in the diagnosis of glaucoma. Arch Ophthalmol 95:2149, 1977.

190. Sommer, A, Pollack, I, Maumenee, AE: Optic disc parameters and onset of glaucomatous field loss. II. Static screening criteria. Arch Ophthalmol 97:1449, 1979.

191. Airaksinen, PJ, Drance, SM, Douglas, GR, et al: Visual field and retinal nerve fiber layer comparisons in glaucoma. Arch Ophthalmol 103:205, 1985.

192. Drance, SM, Airaksinen, PJ, Price, M, et al: The correlation of functional and structural measurements in glaucoma patients and normal subjects. Am J Ophthalmol 102:612, 1986.

193. Okada, K, Minato, T, Miyaji, S: A method for contrasting control visual fields in the Humphrey Field Analyzer and Monochromatic turned-over fundus photographs. Jpn J Ophthalmol 30:925, 1988.

194. Airaksinen, PJ, Heijl, A: Visual field and retinal nerve fibre layer in early glaucoma after optic disc haemorrhage. Acta Ophthalmol 61:186, 1983.

195. Katz, J, Sommer, A: Similarities between the visual fields of ocular hypertensive and normal eyes. Arch Ophthalmol 104:1648, 1986.

196. Armaly, MF: The correlation between appearance of the optic cup and visual function. Trans Am Acad Ophthalmol Otol 73:898, 1969.

197. Funk, J, Bornscheuer, C, Grehn, F: Neuroretinal rim area and visual field in glaucoma. Graefes Arch Clin Exp Ophthalmol 226:431, 1988.

198. Portney, GL, Krohn, MA: The limitations of kinetic perimetry in early scotoma detection. Ophthalmology 85:287, 1978.

199. Ourgaud, M: Static circular perimetry in open-angle glaucoma. J Fr Ophthalmol 5:387, 1982.

200. Katz, J, Tielsch, JM, Quigley, HA, Sommer, A: Automated perimetry detects visual field loss before manual Goldmann perimetry. Ophthalmology 102:21, 1995.

201. Choplin, NT, Sherwood, MB, Spaeth, GL: The effect of stimulus size on the measured threshold values in automated perimetry. Ophthalmology 97:371, 1990.

202. Hart, WM Jr, Hartz, RK, Hagen, RW, Clark, KW: Color contrast perimetry. Invest Ophthalmol Vis Sci 25:400, 1984.

203. Hart, WM Jr, Gordon, MO: Color perimetry of glaucomatous visual field defects. Ophthalmology 91:338, 1984.

204. Hart, WM Jr, Silverman, SE, Trick, GL, et al: Glaucomatous visual field damage. Luminance and color-contrast sensitivities. Invest Ophthalmol Vis Sci 31:359, 1990.

205. Logan, N, Anderson, DR: Detecting early glaucomatous visual field changes with a blue stimulus. Am J Ophthalmol 95:432, 1983.

206. Mindel, JS, Safir, A, Schare, PW: Visual field testing with red targets. Arch Ophthalmol 101:927, 1983.

207. Hart, WM Jr, Burde, RM: Color contrast perimetry: the spatial distribution of color defects in optic nerve and retinal diseases. Ophthalmology 92:768, 1985.

208. Sample, PA, Weinreb, RN: Color perimetry for assessment of primary open-angle glaucoma. Invest Ophthalmol Vis Sci 31:1869, 1990.

209. Lewis, RA, Johnson, CA, Adams, AJ: Automated perimetry and short wavelength sensitivity in patients with asymmetric intraocular pressures. Graefes Arch Clin Exp Ophthalmol 231:274, 1993.

210. Johnson, CA, Brandt, JD, Khong, AM, Adams, AJ: Short-wavelength automated perimetry in low-, medium-, and high-risk ocular hypertensive eyes. Arch Ophthalmol 113:70, 1995.

211. Sample, PA, Weinreb, RN: Progressive color visual field loss in glaucoma. Invest Ophthalmol Vis Sci 33:2068, 1992.

212. Johnson, CA, Adams, AJ, Casson, EJ, Brandt, JD: Blue-on-yellow perimetry can predict the development of glaucomatous visual field loss. Arch Ophthalmol 111:645, 1993.

213. Sample, PA, Taylor, JDN, Martinez, GA, et al: Short-wavelength color visual fields in glaucoma suspects at risk. Am J Ophthalmol 115:225, 1993.

214. Johnson, CA, Adams, AJ, Casson, EJ, Brandt, JD: Progression of early glaucomatous visual field loss as detected by blue-on-yellow and standard white-on-white automated perimetry. Arch Ophthalmol 111:651, 1993.

215. Moss, ID, Wild, JM, Whitaker, DJ: The influence of age-related cataract on blue-on-yellow perimetry. Invest Ophthalmol Vis Sci 36:764, 1995.

216. Wild, JM, Moss, ID, Whitaker, D, O'Neill, EC: The statistical interpretation of blue-on-yellow visual field loss. Invest Ophthalmol Vis Sci 36:1398, 1995.

217. Sample, PA, Martinez, GA, Weinreb, RN: Short-wavelength automated perimetry without lens density testing. Am J Ophthalmol 118:632, 1994.

218. Regan, D, Beverley, KI: Visual fields described by contrast sensitivity, by acuity, and by relative sensitivity to different orientations. Invest Ophthalmol Vis Sci 24:754, 1983.

219. Neima, D, LeBlanc, R, Regan, D: Visual field defects in ocular hypertension and glaucoma. Arch Ophthalmol 102:1042, 1984.

220. Phelps, CD: Acuity perimetry and glaucoma. Trans Am Ophthalmol Soc 82:753, 1984.

221. House, P, Schulzer, M, Drance, S, Douglas, G: Characteristics of the normal central visual field measured with resolution perimetry. Graefes Arch Clin Exp Ophthalmol 229:8, 1991.

222. Chauhan, BC, Mohandas, RN, Whelan, JH, McCormick, TA: Comparison of reliability indices in conventional and high-pass resolution perimetry. Ophthalmology 100:1089, 1993.

223. Sample, PA, Ahn, DS, Lee, PC, Weinreb, RN: High-pass resolution perimetry in eyes with ocular hypertension and primary open-angle glaucoma. Am J Ophthalmol 113:309, 1992.

224. Martinez, GA, Sample, PA, Weinreb, RN: Comparison of high-pass resolution perimetry and standard automated perimetry in glaucoma. Am J Ophthalmol 119:195, 1995.

225. Chauhan, BC, LeBlanc, RP, McCormick, TA, Rogers, JB: Comparison of high-pass resolution perimetry and pattern discrimination perimetry to conventional perimetry in glaucoma. Can J Ophthalmol 28:306, 1993.

226. Casson, EJ, Johnson, CA, Nelson-Quigg, JM: Temporal modulation perimetry: the effects of aging and eccentricity on sensitivity in normals. Invest Ophthalmol Vis Sci 34:3096, 1993.

227. Lachenmayr, BJ, Drance, SM, Douglas, GR, Mikelberg, FS: Light-sense, flicker and resolution perimetry in glaucoma: a comparative study. Graefes Arch Clin Exp Ophthalmol 229:246, 1991.

228. Lachenmayr, BJ, Gleissner, M: Flicker perimetry resists retinal image degradation. Invest Ophthalmol Vis Sci 33:3539, 1992.

229. Lachenmayr, BJ, Drance, SM: The selective effects of elevated intraocular pressure on temporal resolution. Ger J Ophthalmol 1:26, 1992.

230. Johnson, CA, Keltner, JL, Balestrery, FG: Acuity profile perimetry. Description of technique and preliminary clinical trials. Arch Ophthalmol 97:684, 1979.

231. Drum, BA, Severns, M, O'Leary, DK, et al: Selective loss of pattern discrimination in early glaucoma. Appl Optics 28:1135, 1989.

232. Stewart, WC, Kelly, DM, Hunt, HH: Long-term and short-term fluctuation in pattern discrimination perimetry. Am J Ophthalmol 114:302, 1992.

233. Wall, M, Ketoff, KM: Random dot motion perimetry in patients with glaucoma and in normal subjects. Am J Ophthalmol 120:587, 1995.

234. Johnson, CA, Keltner, JL: Optimal rates of movement for kinetic perimetry. Arch Ophthalmol 105:73, 1987.

235. Klewin, KM, Radius, RL: Background illumination and automated perimetry. Arch Ophthalmol 104:395, 1986.

236. Drum, B, Armaly, MF, Huppert, W: Scotopic sensitivity loss in glaucoma. Arch Ophthalmol 104:712, 1986.

237. Heuer, DK, Anderson, DR, Knighton, RW, et al: The influence of simulated light scattering on automated perimetric threshold measurements. Arch Ophthalmol 106:1247, 1988.

238. Bigger, JF, Becker, B: Cataracts and open-angle glaucoma. The effect of cataract extraction on visual fields. Am J Ophthalmol 71:335, 1971.

239. Wood, JM, Wild, JM, Smerdon, DL, Crews, SJ: Alterations in the shape of the automated perimetric profile arising from cataract. Graefes Arch Clin Exp Ophthalmol 227:157, 1989.

240. Guthauser, U, Flammer, J: Quantifying visual field damage caused by cataract. Am J Ophthalmol 106:480, 1988.

241. Radius, RL: Perimetry in cataract patients. Arch Ophthalmol 96:1574, 1978.

242. Ruben, JB, Lewis, RA, Johnson, CA, Adams, C: The effect of Goldmann applanation tonometry on automated static threshold perimetry. Ophthalmology 95:267, 1988.

243. Lindenmuth, KA, Skuta, GL, Rabbani, R, Musch, DC: Effects of pupillary constriction on automated perimetry in normal eyes. Ophthalmology 96:1298, 1989.

244. McCluskey, DJ, Douglas, JP, O'Connor, PS, et al: The effect of pilocarpine on the visual field in normals. Ophthalmology 93:843, 1986.

245. Heuer, DK, Anderson, DR, Feuer, WJ, Gressel, MG: The influence of decreased retinal illumination on automated perimetric threshold measurements. Am J Ophthalmol 108:643, 1989.

246. Lindenmuth, KA, Skuta, GL, Rabbani, R, et al: Effects of pupillary dilation on automated perimetry in normal patients. Ophthalmology 97:367, 1990.

247. Weinreb, RN, Perlman, JP: The effect of refractive correction on automated perimetric thresholds. Am J Ophthalmol 101:706, 1986.

248. Goldstick, BJ, Weinreb, RN: The effect of refractive error on automated global analysis program G-1. Am J Ophthalmol 104:229, 1987.

249. Heuer, DK, Anderson, DR, Feuer, WJ, Gressel, MG: The influence of refraction accuracy on automated perimetric threshold measurements. Ophthalmology 94:1550, 1987.

250. Haas, A, Flammer, J, Schneider, U: Influence of age on the visual fields of normal subjects. Am J Ophthalmol 101:199, 1986.

251. Jaffe, GJ, Alvarado, JA, Juster, RP: Age-related changes of the normal visual field. Arch Ophthalmol 104:1021, 1986.

252. Johnson, CA, Adams, AJ, Lewis, RA: Evidence for a neural basis of age-related visual field loss in normal observers. Invest Ophthalmol Vis Sci 30:2056, 1989.

253. Drance, SM, Berry, V, Hughes, A: Studies in the reproducibility of visual field areas in normal and glaucomatous subjects. Can J Ophthalmol I:14, 1966.

254. Heijl, A, Lindgren, G, Olsson, J: The effect of perimetric experience in normal subjects. Arch Ophthalmol 107:81, 1989.

255. Werner, EB, Krupin, T, Adelson, A, Feitl, ME: Effect of patient experience on the results of automated perimetry in glaucoma suspect patients. Ophthalmology 97:44, 1990.

256. Wild, JM, Dengler-Harles, M, Searle, AET, et al: The influence of the learning effect on automated perimetry in patients with suspected glaucoma. Acta Ophthalmol 67:537, 1989.

257. Zulauf, M, Flammer, J, Signer, C: The influence of alcohol on the outcome of automated static perimetry. Graefes Arch Clin Exp Ophthalmol 224:525, 1986.

258. Trobe, JD, Acosta, PC, Shuster, JJ, Krischer, JP: An evaluation of the accuracy of community-based perimetry. Am J Ophthalmol 90:654, 1980.

259. Goldmann, H: Ein selbstregistrierendes Projektionskugelperimeter. Ophthalmologica 109:71, 1945.

260. Portney, GL, Hanible, JE: A comparison of four projection perimeters. Am J Ophthalmol 81:678, 1976.

261. Harms, H: Entwicklungsmoglichkeiten der Perimetrie. Graefes Arch Clin Exp Ophthalmol 150:28, 1950.

262. Armaly, MF: Ocular pressure and visual fields. A ten-year follow-up study. Arch Ophthalmol 81:25, 1969.

263. Rock, WJ, Drance, SM, Morgan, RW: A modification of the Armaly visual field screening technique for glaucoma. Can J Ophthalmol 6:283, 1971.

264. Drance, SM, Brais, P, Fairclough, M, Bryett, J: A screening method for temporal visual defects in chronic simple glaucoma. Can J Ophthalmol 7:428, 1972.

265. Rock, WJ, Drance, SM, Morgan, RW: Visual field screening in glaucoma. An evaluation of the Armaly technique for screening glaucomatous visual fields. Arch Ophthalmol 89:287, 1973.

266. Fischer, RW: Supraliminal pattern perimetry with the Goldmann perimeter. Klin Monatsbl Augenheilkd 185:204, 1984.

267. Rabin, S, Kolesar, P, Podos, SM, Wilensky, JT: A visual field screening protocol for glaucoma. Am J Ophthalmol 92:530, 1981.

268. Stepanik, J: Diagnosis of glaucoma with the Goldmann perimeter. Klin Monatsbl Augenheilkd 183:330, 1983.

269. Hart, WM, Jr: Computer processing of visual data. II. Automated pattern analysis of glaucomatous visual fields. Arch Ophthalmol 99:133, 1981.

270. Weleber, RG, Tobler, WR: Computerized quantitative analysis of kinetic visual fields. Am J Ophthalmol 101:461, 1986.

271. Esterman, B: Grid for scoring visual fields. I. Tangent screen. Arch Ophthalmol 77:780, 1967.

272. Esterman, B: Grid for scoring visual fields. II. Perimeter. Arch Ophthalmol 79:400, 1968.

273. Esterman, B: Functional scoring of the binocular field. Ophthalmology 89:1226, 1982.

274. American Medical Association Guides to the Evaluation of Permanent Impairment. 2nd ed. Chicago: American Medical Association, 1984, p. 141.

275. Mills, RP, Drance, SM: Esterman disability rating in severe glaucoma. Ophthalmology 93:371, 1986.

276. Harrington, DO, Flocks, M: Multiple pattern method of visual field examination. JAMA 157:645, 1955.

277. Roberts, W: The multiple-pattern tachystoscopic visual field screener in glaucoma. Arch Ophthalmol 58:244, 1957.

278. Friedman, A: The assessment of the efficacy of glaucoma control by static perimetry, or "point" analysis of clinical visual thresholds. Trans Ophthalmol Soc UK 82:381, 1962.

279. Friedman, AI: Serial analysis of changes in visual field defects, employing a new instrument, to determine the activity of diseases involving the visual pathways. Ophthalmologica 152:1, 1966.

280. Greve, EL, Verduin, WM: Mass visual field investigation in 1834 persons with supposedly normal eyes. Graefes Arch Clin Exp Ophthalmol 183:286, 1972.

281. Batko, KA, Anctil, J-L, Anderson, DR: Detecting glaucomatous damage with the Friedmann analyzer compared with the Goldmann perimeter and evaluation of stereoscopic photographs of the optic disk. Am J Ophthalmol 95:435, 1983.

282. Hicks, BC, Anderson, DR: Quantitation of glaucomatous visual field defects with the Mark II Friedmann analyzer. Am J Ophthalmol 95:692, 1983.

283. Henson, DB, Dix, SM, Oborne, AC: Evaluation of the Friedmann visual field analyser Mark II. Part 1. Results from a normal population. Br J Ophthalmol 68:458, 1984.

284. Henson, DB, Dix, SM: Evaluation of the Friedmann visual field analyser Mark II. Part 2. Results from a population with induced visual field defects. Br J Ophthalmol 68:463, 1984.

285. Vernon, SA, Henry, DJ, Jones, SJ: Calculating the predictive power of the Henson field screener in a population at risk of glaucomatous field loss. Br J Ophthalmol 74:220, 1990.

286. Sponsel, WE, Ritch, R, Stamper, R, et al: Prevent blindness America visual field screening study. Am J Ophthalmol 120:699, 1995.

287. Flocks, M, Rosenthal, AR, Hopkins, JL: Mass visual screening via television. Ophthalmology 85:1141, 1978.

288. Accornero, N, Berardelli, A, Cruccu, G, Manfredi, M: Computerized video screen perimetry. Arch Ophthalmol 102:40, 1984.

289. Britt, JM, Mills, RP: The black hole effect in perimetry. Invest Ophthalmol Vis Sci 29:795, 1988.

290. Desjardins, D, Anderson, DR: Threshold variability with an automated LED perimeter. Invest Ophthalmol Vis Sci 29:915, 1988.

291. Wilensky, JT, Mermelstein, JR, Siegel, HG: The use of different-sized stimuli in automated perimetry. Am J Ophthalmol 101:710, 1986.

292. Zalta, AH: Use of a central 10° field and size V stimulus to evaluate and monitor small central islands of vision in end stage glaucoma. Br J Ophthalmol 75:151, 1991.

293. Demirel, S, Vingrys, AJ: Eye movements during perimetry and the effect that fixational instability has on perimetric outcomes. J Glau 3:28, 1994.

294. Li, Y, Mills, RP: Kinetic fixation improves threshold sensitivity in the central visual field. J Glau 1:108, 1992.

295. Fankhauser, F, Funkhouser, A, Kwasniewska, S: Evaluating the applications of the spatially adaptive program (SAPRO) in clinical perimetry: Part I. Ophthalmic Surg 17:338, 1986.

296. Asman, P, Britt, JM, Mills, RP, Heijl, A: Evaluation of adaptive spatial enhancement in suprathreshold visual field screening. Ophthalmology 95:1656, 1988.

297. Stewart, WC, Shields, MB, Ollie, AR: Full threshold versus quantification of defects for visual field testing in glaucoma. Graefes Arch Clin Exp Ophthalmol 227:51, 1989.

298. Araujo, ML, Feuer, WJ, Anderson, DR: Evaluation of baseline-related suprathreshold testing for quick determination of visual field nonprogression. Arch Ophthalmol 111:365, 1993.

299. Flanagan, JG, Wild, JM, Trope, GE: Evaluation of FASTPAC, a new strategy for threshold estimation with the Humphrey field analyzer, in a glaucomatous population. Ophthalmology 100:949, 1993.

300. Mills, RP, Barnebey, HS, Migliazzo, CV, Li, Y: Does saving time using FASTPAC or suprathreshold testing reduce quality of visual fields? Ophthalmology 101:1596, 1994.

301. O'Brien, C, Poinoosawmy, D, Wu, J, Hitchings, R: Evaluation of the Humphrey FASTPAC threshold program in glaucoma. Br J Ophthalmol 78:516, 1994.

302. Glass, E, Schaumberger, M, Lachenmayr, BJ: Simulations for FAST-PAC and the standard 4–2 dB full-threshold strategy of the Humphrey field analyzer. Invest Ophthalmol Vis Sci 36:1847, 1995.

303. Katz, J, Sommer, A: Reliability indexes of automated perimetric tests. Arch Ophthalmol 106:1252, 1988.

304. Bickler-Bluth, M, Trick, GL, Kolker, AE, Cooper, DG: Assessing the utility of reliability indices for automated visual fields: testing ocular hypertensives. Ophthalmology 96:616, 1989.

305. Nelson-Quigg, JM, Twelker, JD, Johnson, CA: Response properties of normal observers and patients during automated perimetry. Arch Ophthalmol 107:1612, 1989.

306. Schulzer, M, Mills, RP, Hopp, RH, et al: Estimation of the short-term fluctuation from a single determination of the visual field. Invest Ophthalmol Vis Sci 31:730, 1990.

307. Johnson, LN, Aminlari, A, Sassani, JW: Effect of intermittent versus continuous patient monitoring on reliability indices during automated perimetry. Ophthalmology 100:76, 1993.

308. Lee, M, Zulauf, M, Caprioli, J: A new reliability parameter for automated perimetry: inconsistent responses. J Glau 2:279, 1993.

309. King, D, Drance, SM, Douglas, GR, Wijsman K: The detection of paracentral scotomas with varying grids in computed perimetry. Arch Ophthalmol 104:524, 1986.

310. Weber, J, Dobek, K: What is the most suitable grid for computer perimetry in glaucoma patients? Ophthalmologica 192:88, 1986.

311. Gramer, E, Althaus, G, Leydhecker, W: The importance of grid density in automatic perimetry. A clinical study. Z Prakt Augenheilkd 7:197, 1986.

312. Seamone, C, LeBlanc, R, Rubillowicz, M, et al: The value of indices in the central and peripheral visual fields for the detection of glaucoma. Am J Ophthalmol 106:180, 1988.

313. Weber, J, Krieglstein, GK, Papoulis, C: Use of graphic analysis of topographical trends (GATT) for perimetric follow-up of glaucoma. Klin Monatsbl Augenheilkd 195:319, 1989.

314. Chauhan, BC, Drance, SM, Lai, C: A cluster analysis for threshold perimetry. Graefes Arch Clin Exp Ophthalmol 227:216, 1989.

315. Mandava, S, Zulauf, M, Zeyen, T, Caprioli, J: An evaluation of clusters in the glaucomatous visual field. Am J Ophthalmol 116:684, 1993.

316. Fankhauser, F I, Fankhauser F II, Giger, H: A cluster and scotoma analysis based on empiric criteria. Graefes Arch Clin Exp Ophthalmol 231:697, 1993.

317. Åsman, P, Heijl, A: Arcuate cluster analysis in glaucoma perimetry. J Glau 2:13, 1993.

318. Duggan, C, Sommer, A, Auer, C, Burkhard, K: Automated differential threshold perimetry for detecting glaucomatous visual field loss. Am J Ophthalmol 100:420, 1985.

319. Sommer, A, Enger, C, Witt, K: Screening for glaucomatous visual field loss with automated threshold perimetry. Am J Ophthalmol 103:681, 1987.

320. Åsman, P, Heijl, A: Glaucoma hemifield test. Arch Ophthalmol 110:812, 1992.

321. Åsman, P, Heijl, A: Evaluation of methods for automated hemifield analysis in perimetry. Arch Ophthalmol 110:820, 1992.

322. Susanna, R Jr, Nicolela, MT, Soriano, DS, De Carvalho, CA: Automated perimetry: a study of the glaucoma hemifield test for the detection of early glaucomatous visual field loss. J Glau 3:12, 1994.

323. Katz, J, Quigley, HA, Sommer, A: Repeatability of the glaucoma hemifield test in automated perimetry. Invest Ophthalmol Vis Sci 36:1658, 1995.

324. Jacobs, NA, Patterson, IH: Variability of the hill of vision and its significance in automated perimetry. Br J Ophthalmol 69:824, 1985.

325. Katz, J, Sommer, A: Asymmetry and variation in the normal hill of vision. Arch Ophthalmol 104:65, 1986.

326. Heijl, A, Lindgren, G, Olsson, J: Normal variability of static perimetric threshold values across the central visual field. Arch Ophthalmol 105:1544, 1987.

327. Werner, EB, Petrig, B, Krupin, T, Bishop, KI: Variability of automated visual fields in clinically stable glaucoma patients. Invest Ophthalmol Vis Sci 30:1083, 1989.

328. Heijl, A, Lindgren, A, Lindgren, G: Test-retest variability in glaucomatous visual fields. Am J Ophthalmol 108:130, 1989.

329. Haefliger, IO, Flammer, J: Increase of the short-term fluctuation of the differential light threshold around a physiologic scotoma. Am J Ophthalmol 107:417, 1989.

330. Diestelhorst, M, Kullenberg, C, Krieglstein, GK: Short-term fluctuation of retinal sensitivity at the borders of glaucomatous field defects. Klin Monatsbl Augenheilkd 191:439, 1987.

331. Katz, J, Sommer, A: A longitudinal study of the age-adjusted variability of automated visual fields. Arch Ophthalmol 105:1083, 1987.

332. Werner, EB, Adelson, A, Krupin, T: Effect of patient experience on the results of automated perimetry in clinically stable glaucoma patients. Ophthalmology 95:764, 1988.

333. Hoskins, HD, Magee, SD, Drake, MV, Kidd, MN: Confidence intervals for change in automated visual fields. Br J Ophthalmol 72: 591, 1988.

334. Hills, JF, Johnson, CA: Evaluation of the t test as a method of detecting visual field changes. Ophthalmology 95:261, 1988.

335. Enger, C, Sommer, A: Recognizing glaucomatous field loss with the Humphrey STATPAC. Arch Ophthalmol 105:1355, 1987.

336. Heijl, A, Lindgren, G, Olsson, J, Asman, P: Visual field interpretation with empiric probability maps. Arch Ophthalmol 107:204, 1989.

337. Heijl, A, Asman, P: A clinical study of perimetric probability maps. Arch Ophthalmol 107:199, 1989.

338. Birch, MK, Wishart, PK, O'Donnell, NP: Determining progressive visual field loss in serial Humphrey visual fields. Ophthalmology 102:1227, 1995.

339. Werner, EB, Bishop, KI, Koelle, J, et al: A comparison of experienced clinical observers and statistical tests in detection of progressive visual field loss in glaucoma using automated perimetry. Arch Ophthalmol 106:619, 1988.

340. Chauhan, BC, Drance, SM, Douglas, GR: The use of visual field indices in detecting changes in the visual field in glaucoma. Invest Ophthalmol Vis Sci 31:512, 1990.

341. Keltner, JL, Johnson, CA, Balestrery, FG: Suprathreshold static perimetry. Initial clinical trials with the Fieldmaster automated perimeter. Arch Ophthalmol 97:260, 1979.

342. Johnson, CA, Keltner, JL: Automated suprathreshold static perimetry. Am J Ophthalmol 89:731, 1980.

343. Bobrow, JC, Drews, RC: Clinical experience with the Fieldmaster perimeter. Am J Ophthalmol 93:238, 1982.

344. Keltner, JL, Johnson, CA: Effectiveness of automated perimetry in following glaucomatous visual field progression. Ophthalmology 89:247, 1982.

345. Krieglstein, GK, Glaab, E, Gramer, E: The Fieldmaster-200 computer perimeter: a comparative, controlled clinical study of its sensitivity and specificity in glaucomatous field defects. Klin Monatsbl Augenheilkd 179:340, 1981.

346. Li, SG, Spaeth, GL, Scimeca, HA, et al: Clinical experiences with the use of an automated perimeter (Octopus) in the diagnosis and management of patients with glaucoma and neurologic diseases. Ophthalmology 86:1302, 1979.

347. Schmied, U: Automatic (Octopus) and manual (Goldmann) perimetry in glaucoma. Graefes Arch Clin Exp Ophthalmol 213:239, 1980.

348. Wilensky, JT, Joondeph, BC: Variation in visual field measurements with an automated perimeter. Am J Ophthalmol 97:328, 1984.

349. Beck, RW, Bergstrom, TJ, Lichter, PR: A clinical comparison of visual field testing with a new automated perimeter, the Humphrey Field Analyzer, and the Goldmann perimeter. Ophthalmology 92:77, 1985.

350. Trope, GE, Britton, R: A comparison of Goldmann and Humphrey automated perimetry in patients with glaucoma. Br J Ophthalmol 71:489, 1987.

351. Brenton, RS, Argus, WA: Fluctuations on the Humphrey and Octopus perimeters. Invest Ophthalmol Vis Sci 28:767, 1987.

352. Mills, RP, Hopp, RH, Drance, SM: Comparison of quantitative testing with the Octopus, Humphrey, and Tübingen perimeters. Am J Ophthalmol 102:496, 1986.

GLAUCOMA SCREENING

The basic features of glaucoma that have been considered in this section (intraocular pressure (IOP), optic nerve head and peripapillary retina, and visual function) constitute not only the common denominators for this group of disorders, but also the main parameters by which they are detected and followed during therapy. In Section Two, we consider how these parameters relate to specific clinical forms of glaucoma. It may be helpful, however, to first take a broader look at how these basic features can be utilized in various screening programs for the early detection of glaucoma.

Since the blindness of glaucoma can only be prevented by early recognition and proper treatment of the disorder, it is essential that mechanisms for early detection be available. Some forms of glaucoma are associated with symptoms that may cause the patient to seek medical care in the early stages of the disorder. In the vast majority of cases, however, there are no early warning signs. It is for these types of glaucoma that screening mechanisms are needed. The following discussion pertains to these conditions.

PROBLEMS OF MASS SCREENING

For any screening program to be effective, it must be both sensitive and specific. *Sensitivity* is the ability to identify screenees who truly have the disease, and is expressed as the percentage screening positive of the total number of confirmed cases, i.e., a screening level with high sensitivity has few false-negatives. *Specificity* is the ability to give a negative finding when the screenee is truly free of the disease, and is expressed as the percentage screening negative of those who do not have the disorder, i.e., a screening level with high specificity has few false positives (1, 2).

In the past, most glaucoma screening programs have been limited to the use of tonometry, which has only a fair sensitivity of 50–70% and a poor specificity of 10–30% (3, 4). As a result, when the referral criterion is based on a single IOP measurement, a large percentage of the population who do not have glaucoma will be required to undergo costly followup evaluations, while a smaller, but clinically more significant, group of individuals who do have glaucoma will be told that they are free of the disease. This has led most investigators of glaucoma detection programs to feel that screening with tonometry alone is not warranted. The critical need for early detection remains, however, and continued study has shown that adding one or more additional diagnostic parameters, i.e., evaluation of the optic nerve head or visual field, as well as targeting high-risk populations, significantly improves both the sensitivity and specificity of the screening program. Other problems with mass screening for glaucoma include the location of the screening program and the mechanisms of followup. In the remainder of this chapter, we consider how the efficiency of glaucoma detection programs may be improved by directing attention to each of these areas.

SCREENING TESTS

Intraocular Pressure Measurement

Tonometer

The efficiency of a screening program is greatly influenced by the reliability of the tonometer that is used (5). For example, the Schiøtz tonometer reads significantly lower than the Goldmann applanation tonometer, which increases the chance of missing patients who actually have glaucoma. Furthermore, the effect of ocular rigidity on Schiøtz tonometry makes it difficult to simply adjust the screening level for this instrument. The Perkins applanation tonometer, because of its accuracy and portability, is a useful instrument for mass screening (6, 7), but it requires a highly skilled operator. The noncontact tonometer (NCT) can be operated with considerable accuracy by paramedical personnel with minimal training and eliminates the risk of corneal abrasion, spread of infection, and reactions to topical anesthetics (8). These advantages make the NCT particularly useful in mass screening programs, although the cost of the instrument remains a problem in many communities. Less expensive instruments that may have value in glaucoma screening include the Halberg applanation tonometer (9), the GlaucoTest (10, 11), and the Tono-Pen (12), each of which was considered in Chapter 4.

Referral Level

The main problem with IOP as a screening parameter is the overlap of the distributions in nonglaucoma and glaucoma populations, so that a simple "cutoff" pressure level between these two groups does not exist (Fig. 7.1). The optimum referral level is one that minimizes false-negatives without significantly sacrificing specificity. This level is generally set at 21 mm Hg, although some investigators have used a cutoff as high as 24 mm Hg (13). One group used a two-phase approach in which a pressure greater than 18 mm Hg with the NCT was the basis for a second measurement by a physician with applanation tonometry, in which case 21 mm Hg was the criterion for referral (14). However, since no pressure level provides a satisfactory balance between sensitivity and specificity, IOP screening may actually be counterproductive unless it is combined with one or more additional tests.

Optic Nerve Head and Peripapillary Retinal Evaluation

Relative Value of Tonometry and Ophthalmoscopy

Studies have been conducted to determine whether IOP measurement or evaluation of the optic nerve head is more useful in the early detection of glaucoma. In one trial of 11,660 subjects, 57 cases of glaucoma with field loss (0.49%) were detected, using a combination of tonometry and ophthalmoscopy (14). Of these 57 cases, tonometry alone would have detected 28 and ophthalmoscopy alone would have identified 39, but 10 cases would have been missed without the combination of both tests. In other words, IOP screening alone would have missed half of the patients with glaucoma, while disc screening alone would have overlooked nearly one-third of the cases. Most of the cases missed by ophthalmoscopy were early glaucoma with minor field change, while those overlooked by tonometry were more advanced with extensive field loss. Another study was conducted in a healthcare setting by a nonophthalmologist physician trained in the use of the NCT and the recognition of suspicious discs (13). Of 770 screenees, 2.5% were referred for elevated IOP alone, 8.7% for abnormal discs,

and 2.1% for a combination of both. These studies support the growing impression that optic nerve head screening is more practical and efficient than tonometry. However, due to the difficulty in visualizing and interpreting some discs (15), as well as those cases with high pressure prior to nerve damage, the combination of both tests is preferable to either alone in the early detection of glaucoma.

Methods of Disc Evaluation

A practical limitation of optic nerve head screening is the need for a trained physician to interpret the findings. In the office of an ophthalmologist or nonophthalmologist physician, this can be accomplished by the techniques discussed in Chapter 5. In a mass screening program, however, the use of dilatation and the need for a physician create logistic problems. One solution has been to take photographs with a nonmydriatic fundus camera and to send these to an appropriate center for detailed study (14). In one study of

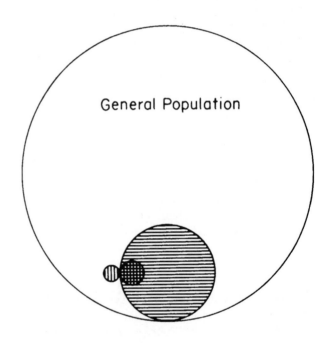

SCREENING EFFICIENCY OF TONOMETRY

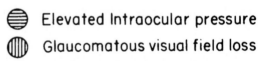

⊜ Elevated Intraocular pressure

⦀ Glaucomatous visual field loss

Figure 7.1. The problem with tonometry alone for glaucoma screening. A significant percentage of most general populations will have intraocular pressures above 21 mm Hg. Only a small percentage of the group, however, will have glaucomatous field loss, and almost an equal number of individuals with pressures below 21 mm Hg will also have glaucomatous field loss. (Reprinted with permission from Sommer A: Epidemiology and Statistics for the Ophthalmologist. New York, Oxford, Oxford University Press, 1980.)

183 first-degree relatives of glaucoma patients, photographs were taken by a technician with a nonmydriatic fundus camera and evaluated later by an ophthalmologist, which yielded six new cases of glaucoma, only one of which would have been detected by tonometry alone (16). In a 5-year followup of 26 subjects screened with nonmydriatic fundus photography, 10 of 16 subjects with initially abnormal findings showed progressive change, while all 10 with no initial abnormalities remained healthy (17). While nonmydriatic photography may, therefore, be a useful screening tool, it is not possible to obtain good quality photographs in all patients, and the technique is usually limited to two-dimensional pictures. Stereodisc photographs, obtained with a Nidek 3-DX camera through a maximally dilated pupil in 258 patients, yielded a sensitivity equivalent to screening with computerized perimetry and an accuracy significantly greater than that with tonometry (18). The risk of dilating eyes with potentially occludable angles is low (less than 1 in 333) if screenees are evaluated for shallow anterior chambers by penlight examination and checked for history of glaucoma (19).

The criteria that are considered for referral should include pallor and cup (area, asymmetry, vertical bias, and rim notching), nerve fiber bundle defect, and disc hemorrhage (13, 14). One study found that the vertical cup-to-disc ratio is the most suitable optic disc parameter for screening purposes, while the neural rim area is more valuable for followup (20). Another study found relative nerve fiber layer height to be superior to cup-to-disc ratio in discriminating between normal and glaucomatous eyes, but concluded that discriminant analysis of structural and functional measurements increases the precision of early glaucoma detection (21). With the continuing advances in technology, it may one day be possible to utilize automatic analysis of photographs of the optic nerve head and peripapillary retina to evaluate these more complex parameters in screening for glaucoma.

Visual Function Tests

Since progressive loss of visual function is the ultimate result in all forms of glaucoma, visual function screening tests may offer the most sensitive and specific method of detecting established cases. The main limitation, however, is that most standard techniques for measuring the field of vision, which is currently the most commonly used psychophysical test of visual function in glaucoma, are too time consuming to be practical for mass screening programs. Manual and automated techniques are being developed for visual field screening, which will hopefully reduce the time requirement to an acceptable level, without significantly reducing sensitivity and specificity. Many of these were considered in Chapter 6. The most promising concept is to combine automated perimetry with threshold-related testing of selected points in the field of vision that are more likely to contain early glaucomatous damage (22–24). In a population-based survey of 5341 subjects, automated suprathreshold testing with the Full Field

120 program of the Humphrey Field Analyzer was completed in 89%, required a median test time of 7.25 minutes per eye, and performed better than nonperimetric-based screening tests, but was limited by logistical weaknesses (25). In a multicenter visual acuity screening study, the Henson visual field analyzer was found to discriminate moderately to severe glaucomatous from normal fields with high sensitivity and specificity, and the authors recommended that some form of visual field measurement be added to tonometry in adult vision screening programs (26).

The discussed perimetric instruments are still limited, however, by the relatively high cost of the instruments, and less expensive, manual techniques are being developed, which may be a reasonable alternative in some parts of the world. One of these, the Damato campimeter (27), was shown in one visual field screening study to reliably detect moderate to severe visual field loss with a tolerably low false-positive rate (26). In addition, newer psychophysical tests, such as color vision and contrast sensitivity techniques, may eventually become sufficiently sophisticated to be useful as a rapid means of assessing visual function in the early detection of glaucoma (28). One such instrument is the whole-field scotopic sensitivity screener, which presents a white light, square-wave flicker that is automatically incremented until detected by the subject (29). The threshold is effected by cataracts, but it still may be of value in field-based screening for glaucoma (29).

HIGH-RISK POPULATIONS

The Public Health Service suggests that any medical screening program must detect at least 2% pathology in the general population to be considered a cost-effective measure (22). Most statistics on the overall prevalence of glaucoma indicate that this group of disorders would not meet the criterion. To become cost-effective, therefore, glaucoma screening programs must be directed at the high-risk segment of a population. With regard to chronic open-angle glaucoma, which is the most common target disorder in glaucoma screening programs, the leading risk factors are increasing age, black race, first-degree relatives with glaucoma, high myopia, and vascular disease, including diabetes mellitus (13). Since several of these factors will be more prevalent in healthcare settings than in the general population, the screening site becomes another important variable in the success of a glaucoma detection program.

SCREENING SITE

Community Programs

A commonly used site in the past has been community-based mass public screening clinics (service organization-sponsored programs, health fairs, etc.). However, studies have shown these to be the least efficient form of glaucoma screening, because they provide a low detection rate (13, 30) and an inadequate means of insuring that positive screenees follow through with a proper medical examination (31). The latter is probably due to the fact that mass screening programs are usually conducted on a periodic basis by volunteers with lack of adequate mechanisms for followup. The main value of community programs for the early detection of glaucoma appears to be the public awareness they create for the danger of glaucoma.

Healthcare Settings

The preferred alternative to community-based detection programs is the utilization of healthcare facilities, of which several options exist (1, 13, 14, 31). One approach is in-house screening in industrial settings, using *employee health clinics.* In one study, this was found to have the highest followup rate (31), and provides the potential for excellent screening if it is utilized properly with physician supervision, although it is limited to those individuals who are in a position to take advantage of it. For the remaining majority of most populations, other healthcare settings must be considered. *Public health departments* offer a logical setting for glaucoma detection programs as part of multiphasic health testing services (14). A study in North Carolina has supported the feasibility of such a program, but also indicated the need for better methods of insuring that positive screenees followup with an adequate medical examination (31). The remaining, and best, method for the early detection of glaucoma, therefore, is the *physician's office.* While some large ophthalmology groups may be able to provide effective screening programs within their clinic setting, this is not feasible in most communities. The alternative is to encourage optometrists and nonophthalmologist physicians, e.g., family physicians, internists, etc., to include glaucoma screening as part of their routine examination (1, 13). Ophthalmologists can probably be most effective in detecting glaucoma in their community by working with their colleagues in other fields of medicine with regard to recognizing suspicious discs, utilizing tonometry, and being aware of the risk factors for glaucoma.

FOLLOWUP

As noted earlier, an essential criterion for the success of any detection program is the percentage of positive screenees who follow through with an adequate medical examination. In addition, it is important to periodically evaluate the efficiency of a screening program with regard to the sensitivity and specificity of the detection methods. Both require continuing communication with the ophthalmologist to whom the positive screenees are referred, as well as periodic recall of the negative screenees. As previously discussed, the healthcare setting again provides the most effective means

for achieving this followup. However, this cannot be accomplished without careful attention to data collection, storage, and retrieval of data. With the rapid expansion of computer technology in medicine, this will undoubtedly assume an increasingly important role in this aspect of glaucoma detection.

LEGAL IMPLICATIONS

A detailed appraisal of mass screening for glaucoma (limited to tonometry) concluded that it is legally permissible since the potential benefit, i.e., detection of a sight-threatening disease, outweighs the potential hazards, such as rare ocular injury, the emotional trauma of a false-positive test, and the risk of false-negative testing (32). The same report also concluded that full disclosure to the potential screenee of all possible hazards of the test is not required.

SUMMARY

Early detection and treatment of glaucoma is necessary to prevent visual loss. The lack of early warning signs with most forms of glaucoma necessitates the use of screening programs to detect the disease in its initial stages. Tonometry is neither sufficiently sensitive nor specific to be used alone as the screening test. The use of one or more additional studies, especially the evaluation of the visual field or optic nerve head, as well as the utilization of risk factors for glaucoma, significantly improves both sensitivity and specificity. Other important factors to consider in developing a glaucoma screening program include the screening site and the methods of followup.

REFERENCES

1. Pollack, IP: The challenge of glaucoma screening. Surv Ophthalmol 13:4, 1968.
2. Packer, H, Deutsch, AR, Deweese, MW, et al: Efficiency of screening tests for glaucoma. JAMA 192:693, 1965.
3. Kahn, JA, Leibowitz, HM, Ganley, JP, et al: The Framingham eye study, outline and major prevalence finding. Am J Epidemiol 106:17, 1977.
4. Armaly, MF: Lessons to be learned from the collaborative glaucoma study. Surv Ophthalmol 25:139, 1980.
5. Schwartz, JT: Vagary in tonometric screening. Am J Ophthalmol 64:50, 1967.
6. Dunn, JS, Brubaker, RF: Perkins applanation tonometer. Clinical and laboratory evaluation. Arch Ophthalmol 89:149, 1973.
7. Krieglstein, GK, Waller, WK: Goldmann applanation versus hand-applanation and Schiøtz indentation tonometry. Graefes Arch Clin Exp Ophthalmol 194:11, 1975.
8. Shields, MB: The non-contact tonometer. Its value and limitations. Surv Ophthalmol 24:211, 1980.
9. Zimmerman, TJ, Worthen, DM: A comparison of two hand-applanation tonometers. Arch Ophthalmol 88:421, 1972.
10. Kaiden, JS, Zimmerman, TJ, Worthen, DM: An evaluation of the GlaucoTest screening tonometer. Arch Ophthalmol 92:195, 1974.

11. Krieglstein, GK: Screening tonometry by technicians. Graefes Arch Clin Exp Ophthalmol 194:221, 1975.
12. Boothe, WA, Lee, DA, Panek, WC, Pettit, TH: The Tono-Pen. A manometric and clinical study. Arch Ophthalmol 106:1214, 1988.
13. Levi, L, Schwartz, B: Glaucoma screening in the health care setting. Surv Ophthalmol 28:164, 1983.
14. Shiose, Y, Komuro, K, Itoh, T, et al: New system for mass screening of glaucoma, as part of automated multiphasic health testing services. Jpn J Ophthalmol 25:160, 1981.
15. Bechetoille, A, Aouchiche, M, Hartani, D: The study of Touggourt: a proposition for the large scale discovery of chronic glaucoma by examination of the optic disc. J Fr Ophthalmol 3:495, 1980.
16. Tuulonen, A, Airaksinen, PJ, Montagna, A, Nieminen, H: Screening for glaucoma with a non-mydriatic fundus camera. Acta Ophthalmol 68:445, 1990.
17. Komulainen, R, Tuulonen, A, Airaksinen, PJ: The follow-up of patients screened for glaucoma with non-mydriatic fundus photography. Int Ophthalmol 16:465, 1992.
18. Schultz, RO, Radius, RL, Hartz, AJ, et al: Screening for glaucoma with stereo disc photography. J Glau 4:177, 1995.
19. Patel, KH, Javitt, JC, Tielsch, JM, et al: Incidence of acute angle-closure glaucoma after pharmacologic mydriasis. Am J Ophthalmol 120:709, 1995.
20. Damms, T, Dannheim, F: Sensitivity and specificity of optic disc parameters in chronic glaucoma. Invest Ophthalmol Vis Sci 34:2246, 1993.
21. Caprioli, J: Discrimination between normal and glaucomatous eyes. Invest Ophthalmol Vis Sci 33:153, 1992.
22. Keltner, JL, Johnson, CA: Screening for visual field abnormalities with automated perimetry. Surv Ophthalmol 28:175, 1983.
23. Kosoko, O, Sommer, A, Auer, C: Screening with automated perimetry using a threshold-related three-level algorithm. Ophthalmology 93:882, 1986.
24. Henson, DB, Bryson, H: Clinical results with the Henson-Hamblin CFS 2000. Doc Ophthal Proc Series 49, 7th Internat Vis Field Symp, Amsterdam, 233, 1987.
25. Katz, J, Tielsch, JM, Quigley, HA, et al: Automated suprathreshold screening for glaucoma: the Baltimore eye survey. Invest Ophthalmol Vis Sci 34:3271, 1993.
26. Sponsel, WE, Ritch, R, Stamper, R, et al: Prevent blindness America visual field screening study. Am J Ophthalmol 120:699, 1995.
27. Damato, BE: Oculokinetic perimetry: a simple visual field test for use in the community. Br J Ophthalmol 69:927, 1985.
28. Sponsel, WE: Tonometry in question: can visual screening tests play a more decisive role in glaucoma and management? Surv Ophthalmol 33(Suppl):291, 1989.
29. Congdon, NG, Quigley, HA, Hung, PT, et al: Impact of age, various forms of cataract, and visual acuity on whole-field scotopic sensitivity screening for glaucoma in rural Taiwan. Arch Ophthalmol 113:1138, 1995.
30. Berwick, DM: Screening in health fairs. A critical review of benefits, risks, and costs. JAMA 254:1492, 1985.
31. McPherson, SD Jr: The challenge and responsibilities of a community approach to glaucoma control. Sightsaving Rev 50:15, 1980.
32. Franklin, MA: Medical mass screening programs: a legal appraisal. Cornell LQ 47:205, 1962.

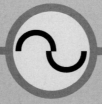

CLINICAL FORMS OF
GLAUCOMA

Chapter 8

CLASSIFICATION OF THE GLAUCOMAS

In Section One, we considered the common parameters shared by the many forms of glaucoma, which include the intraocular pressure (IOP) and the influence of elevated pressure on the optic nerve head and visual field. In Section Two, we look at the specific clinical and histopathologic features that characterize the individual glaucomas. The present chapter provides a brief introduction to the clinical forms of glaucoma within the context of classification systems for these disorders.

There are several systems by which the glaucomas may be classified. The two most commonly used are based on (a) *etiology,* i.e., the underlying disorder that leads to an alteration in aqueous humor dynamics and (b) *mechanism,* i.e., the specific alteration in the anterior chamber angle that leads to a rise in IOP.

CLASSIFICATION BASED ON ETIOLOGY

The glaucomas have traditionally been divided on the basis of primary and secondary forms. The division into "primary" and "secondary" glaucomas, however, is arbitrary and artificial, since all of the glaucomas are secondary to some abnormality. The historic basis for this division was the assumption that the initial events which lead to outflow obstruction and intraocular pressure elevation in those glaucomas called "primary" (e.g., open-angle, angle-closure, and congenital) are confined to the anterior chamber angle or conventional outflow pathway, with no apparent contribution from other ocular or systemic disorders. These conditions are typically bilateral and probably have a genetic basis. In contrast, other glaucomas have been classified as "secondary" because of a partial understanding of underlying, predisposing ocular or systemic event(s). These latter glaucomas may be unilateral or bilateral, and some may have a genetic basis, while others are acquired.

In reality, the concept of primary and secondary glaucomas is more a reflection of our incomplete understanding regarding the pathophysiologic events that ultimately lead to glaucomatous optic atrophy and visual field loss, than of any true division of the glaucomas into primary and secondary forms. As our knowledge of the mechanisms underlying the causes of the glaucomas continues to expand, the primary/secondary classification has become increasingly artificial and inadequate. Furthermore, glaucomas due to developmental anomalies of the anterior chamber angle do not fit neatly into either category. It is time, therefore, to rethink our classification of the glaucomas and to replace traditional concepts with a new scheme that provides a better working foundation for the new concepts of mechanism, diagnosis, and therapy that will shape management the of glaucomas in the 21st century.

Stages of Glaucoma

One way to think of the glaucomas is in five stages:

stage 1–initiating events;
stage 2–structural alterations;
stage 3–functional alterations;
stage 4–optic nerve damage; and
stage 5–visual loss.

The initiating events (stage 1) include the condition or series of conditions that set in motion the chain of events that may eventually lead to optic nerve damage and visual loss, but which precede any pathologic or physiologic alterations related to aqueous humor dynamics or optic nerve function. Structural alterations (stage 2) are those tissue changes which precede, but may eventually lead to, alterations of aqueous humor dynamics and/or optic nerve function. Functional alterations (stage 3) are those physiologic abnormalities that may lead indirectly and/or directly to optic nerve damage. Optic nerve damage (stage 4) represents the loss of axons as a result of the events in stage 3, which will eventually lead to progressive loss of vision (stage 5). The first three stages could be further subdivided into events related to elevated IOP and those that are at least partially pressure-independent (Table 8.1).

In the pressure-related subdivision, the initiating events (stage 1) are the conditions that may lead to structural alterations in the aqueous outflow system. In some glaucomas, this could be a genetic defect with an associated protein abnormality, while other glaucomas might have acquired events such as trauma, inflammation, or a retinal vascular disorder, some of which may also have a genetic predisposition or may be indirectly influenced by genetic disorders. The structural alternations (stage 2) are tissue changes in the outflow system, which may lead to increased resistance to aqueous outflow and subsequent elevation of the IOP. Such changes might be subtle alterations in the endothelial cells or extracellular matrix of the trabecular meshwork or more obvious obstructive mechanisms, such as membranes over the anterior chamber angle, scar tissue within the meshwork, intertrabecular debris or developmental anomalies. These changes can sometimes, but not always, be detected by gonioscopy. The functional alterations (stage 3) include obstruction to aqueous outflow and subsequent elevation of IOP, which (in pressure-related glaucoma mechanisms) may lead to the glaucomatous optic neuropathy (stage 4) and eventual, progressive loss of visual field (stage 5).

The specific events in the pressure-independent subdivision are less well understood and are, in large part, only speculative at this time. It is quite likely, however, that the initiating events (stage 1) have a genetic basis with alterations in proteins that may lead to structural changes directly related to the optic nerve head. The structural alterations (stage 2) may be subtle tissue changes in blood vessels supplying the optic nerve head or in supportive elements of the lamina cribrosa or quite likely in additional ways that have yet to be disclosed. The functional alterations (stage 3) may be reduced vascular perfusion to the optic nerve head or a progressive deformity of the lamina cribrosa that may lead (either alone or in conjunction with a relative IOP elevation) to the optic neuropathy (stage 4) and subsequent loss of visual field (stage 5).

Although our knowledge regarding the events leading to optic nerve damage, as well as our ability to detect and treat these events, is incomplete for most of the glaucomas, there are some glaucomas for which we have not only a partial knowledge of the events in each stage, but also treatments for early intervention at stage 1. In neovascular glaucoma, for example, we know that an initiating event (stage 1) may be a central retinal vein occlusion, which may lead to a structural alteration (stage 2) in the form of a fibrovascular membrane over the anterior chamber angle, which may eventually cause a functional alteration (stage 3) by obstructing aqueous outflow with a rise in IOP, which usually leads to optic nerve damage (stage 4) and eventual loss of visual field (stage 5). An understanding of this sequence of stages provides a rational basis for early intervention with panretinal photocoagulation at stage 1 in selected patients. Such an approach to diagnosis and management should be the ultimate goal for all forms of glaucoma. As knowledge of the initial events becomes available for an ever increasing number of the glaucomas, we may eventually be able to develop a complete classification scheme, based on these initial events. Until continued research provides the answers to these gaps in our knowledge, however, the following classification scheme can only be partially developed (Table 8.2).

Chronic (Idiopathic) Open-Angle Glaucomas

This category of glaucomas constitutes at least half of all the glaucomas and has been referred to by a variety of names, including primary open-angle glaucoma, chronic open-angle glaucoma, and chronic simple glaucoma. To deemphasize use of the "primary/secondary" terminology in glaucoma, the term chronic open-angle glaucoma is used in this text. A more appropriate term, however, might be idiopathic open-angle glaucoma, since our failure to provide more precise terminology stems from our lack of knowledge regarding the related mechanisms.

Table 8.1.
A STAGING SYSTEM FOR GLAUCOMA

Stages	Definitions	Pressure-Related	Pressure-Independent
1. Initiating events	The series of events that may lead to . . .	Genetic; acquired	Genetic? (less well understood
2. Structural alterations	Tissue changes that may lead to . . .	Alterations in aqueous outflow system	Alterations related to optic nerve head (e.g., vascular, structural, etc.?)
3. Functional alterations	Physiologic changes that may lead to . . .	Elevated intraocular pressure	Reduced vascular perfusion, laminar deformity, etc.?
4. Optic nerve damage	Axonal loss that leads to . . .	Glaucomatous optic neuropathy	
5. Visual loss	Progressive loss of visual field . . .	Glaucomatous visual field loss	

Table 8.2.

CLASSIFICATION OF THE GLAUCOMAS BASED ON INITIAL EVENTS

A. Open-angle glaucomas
   1. Chronic open-angle glaucoma
   2. Normal-tension glaucoma
B. Angle-closure glaucomas
   1. Pupillary block glaucoma
   2. Plateau iris syndrome (see also D2c)
   3. Combined mechanism glaucoma
C. Developmental glaucomas
   1. Congenital glaucoma
   2. Juvenile glaucoma
   3. Axenfeld-Rieger syndrome
   4. Peters' anomaly
   5. Aniridia
   6. Other developmental anomalies
D. Glaucomas associated with other ocular and systemic disorders
   1. Glaucomas associated with disorders of the corneal endothelium
      a. Iridocorneal endothelial syndrome
      b. Posterior polymorphous dystrophy
      c. Fuchs' endothelial dystrophy
   2. Glaucomas associated with disorders of the iris and ciliary body
      a. Pigmentary glaucoma
      b. Iridoschisis
      c. Plateau iris
      d. Iris and ciliary body cysts
   3. Glaucoma associated with disorders of the lens
      a. Exfoliation syndrome
      b. Glaucomas associated with cataracts
      c. Glaucomas associated with lens dislocation
   4. Glaucomas associated with disorders of the retina, choroid, and vitreous
      a. Neovascular glaucoma
      b. Glaucomas associated with retinal detachment and vitreoretinal abnormalities
   5. Glaucomas associated with intraocular tumors
      a. Malignant melanoma
      b. Retinoblastoma
      c. Metastatic carcinoma
      d. Leukemias and lymphomas
      e. Benign tumors
   6. Glaucomas associated with elevated episcleral venous pressure
   7. Glaucomas associated with inflammation
      a. Glaucomas associated with uveitis
      b. Glaucomas associated with keratitis, episcleritis, and scleritis
   8. Steroid-induced glaucoma
   9. Glaucomas associated with ocular trauma
   10. Glaucomas associated with hemorrhage
   11. Glaucomas following intraocular surgery
      a. Ciliary block (malignant) glaucoma
      b. Glaucomas in aphakia and pseudophakia
      c. Epithelial, fibrous, and endothelial proliferation
      d. Glaucomas associated with corneal surgery
      e. Glaucomas associated with vitreoretinal surgery

Although the initial events have not been determined, it is likely that genetic defects initiate the series of events that eventually lead to increased resistance to aqueous outflow, as well as increased vulnerability of the optic nerve head to a particular IOP level. There is also growing evidence that this category of glaucomas represents several different entities. For example, one group of investigators have described two conditions: "senile sclerotic glaucoma," which is seen in the elderly, with relatively low IOPs and normal appearing anterior chamber angles, and "high tension glaucoma," which occurs in a younger population, with high pressures and signs of developmental abnormalities of the angle (1). A third variation may be "normal-tension glaucoma" in which the IOP never exceeds the statistical norm. It is in the latter patients that the pressure-independent causative factors, such as vascular or structural defects of the optic nerve head, most likely play their biggest role. However, even in this condition a relative IOP elevation appears to be an important factor in many cases (2).

Pupillary Block Glaucoma

This is the most common variation of the glaucomas that have been called primary angle-closure glaucomas. However, there is a considerable amount of information available regarding the initial events and mechanisms of outflow obstruction in pupillary block glaucoma. Therefore, there is no basis for distinguishing this condition as a primary glaucoma from other disorders such as pigmentary glaucoma that were previously called secondary glaucomas. Pupillary block glaucoma may be divided into "acute" and "subacute" forms, although these only represent different clinical manifestations, which can both occur at different times in the same patient. A third form is called "chronic angle closure glaucoma," which is characterized by the presence of peripheral anterior synechiae. A subset of chronic angle-closure glaucoma has been called "creeping angle-closure glaucoma," in which peripheral anterior synechiae slowly advance forward circumferentially, giving the appearance that the iris insertion is becoming more and more anterior. Another form has been called "combined mechanism glaucoma" in which elevated IOP persists after peripheral iridotomy for the angle-closure component, despite an open, normal-appearing anterior chamber angle. Some classification schemes have included the "plateau iris syndrome" with primary angle-closure glaucomas, although recent studies of the mechanism suggest that it might more appropriately be included with glaucomas associated with disorders of the iris and ciliary body (3).

Developmental Anomalies of the Anterior Chamber Angle

Numerous developmental disorders associated with anomalies of the anterior chamber angle can lead to IOP elevation. The initial event is probably a genetic defect in most cases, although some may have an acquired, intrauterine insult. The developmental anomaly may be a high insertion of the anterior uvea into the trabecular meshwork, incomplete development of the meshwork or Schlemm's canal, or broad iridocorneal adhesions. One group of developmental glaucomas has previously been classified among the primary glaucomas because there is no apparent consistent association with other ocular or systemic anomalies. This group includes "congenital or infantile glaucoma" and "juvenile glaucoma," which differ primarily according to the age of onset. Other conditions within this category have a wide range of associated ocular and systemic developmental abnormalities. In addition, there are other developmental disorders, such as those associated with the vitreous and retina, which may lead to glaucoma usually by an angle-closure mechanism. In the present scheme, the latter disorders are classified under glaucomas associated with abnormalities of a particular ocular structure, e.g., persistent hyperplastic primary vitreous.

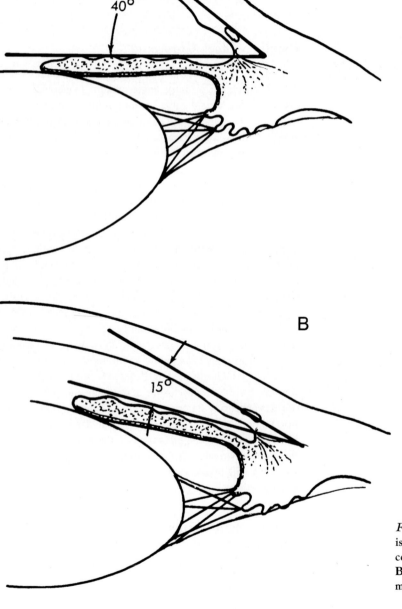

Figure 8.1. The angle of the anterior chamber is formed by the cornea and iris. **A.** The typical configuration in open-angle forms of glaucoma. **B.** The narrow angle that typically precedes most forms of angle-closure glaucoma.

Glaucomas Associated with Other Ocular Disorders

It is this large group of glaucomas that was previously classified as "secondary glaucomas." In some cases, the initial events involve an abnormality of a specific ocular structure such as the corneal endothelium, iris, ciliary body, lens, retina, choroid, or vitreous. In other cases, the initial events may involve a tumor, inflammation, hemorrhage, or accidental or surgical trauma. Many of these initial events most likely begin with a genetic defect, while others are acquired. For each of these broad categories of glaucoma, there are usually subdivisions based on different series of events that eventually lead to outflow obstruction.

CLASSIFICATION BASED ON MECHANISM

As previously discussed, an understanding of the initial events in each form of glaucoma will eventually allow an improved classification, as well as a rationale for early glaucoma intervention. Until that information becomes available, however, most treatment strategies will continue to focus on IOP and will depend on an understanding of the mechanisms of aqueous outflow obstruction.

One disadvantage of a classification based on the mechanism of aqueous outflow obstruction is that it ignores the pressure-independent causative factors. In addition, many of the glaucomas have more than one mechanism of outflow obstruction at different times in the course of the disease. As a result, it is necessary to classify some glaucomas under more than one mechanistic heading. It is for this reason that a classification based on initial events, rather than mechanisms of outflow obstruction, is used for organizing the chapters on clinical forms of glaucoma in this text.

On the other hand, there are distinct advantages to the mechanistic classification. First, our understanding of the mechanisms of aqueous outflow obstruction is more complete than our knowledge of the initial events. Second, since most of our current treatment strategies are directed at lowering IOP, an understanding of the precise mechanism that leads to aqueous outflow obstruction is important in developing a rationale for controlling the pressure in each form of glaucoma.

Barkan (4) first recognized the distinction between open-angle and closed-angle forms of glaucoma, which led to the basis for the mechanistic classification of the glaucomas (Fig. 8.1). A third group of glaucomas that do not fit well into either the open- or closed-angle mechanisms are the developmental glaucomas. The mechanistic classification, therefore, can be divided into three categories: (a) open-angle glaucoma mechanisms, (b) angle-closure glaucoma mechanisms, and (c) developmental anomalies of the anterior chamber angle (Table 8.3; Fig. 8.2).

Open-Angle Glaucoma Mechanisms

The open-angle mechanisms are those in which the anterior chamber angle structures, i.e., trabecular meshwork, scleral spur, and ciliary body band, are visible by gonioscopy. The elements obstructing aqueous outflow may be located on the anterior chamber-side of the trabecular meshwork (pretrabecular mechanisms), within the trabeculum (trabecular mechanisms), or distal to the meshwork, in Schlemm's canal, or further along the aqueous drainage system (posttrabecular mechanisms).

In the *pretrabecular mechanisms,* a translucent membrane extends across the open iridocorneal angle, leading to the obstruction of aqueous outflow. This obstructive element may be a fibrovascular membrane, an endothelial layer with a Descemet-like membrane, an epithelial membrane, a connective tissue membrane, or an inflammatory-related membrane.

In the *trabecular mechanisms,* the obstruction to aqueous outflow is located within the trabecular meshwork. The chronic open-angle glaucomas are included in this category, although the precise mechanisms of the obstruction are not known. As previously noted, this category of the glaucomas may represent several distinct entities with differing mechanisms of outflow obstruction. In other glaucomas with a trabecular mechanism there may be a "clogging" of the meshwork with red blood cells, macrophages, neoplastic cells, pigment particles, protein, lens zonules, viscoelastic agents, or vitreous. In still other cases, obstruction to outflow may result from acquired alterations of the trabecular meshwork tissue such as edema associated with inflammatory conditions, trauma with subsequent scarring, and toxic reactions associated with intraocular foreign bodies. Steroid-induced glaucoma and certain glaucomas associated with systemic diseases may also have obstruction to aqueous outflow in the trabecular meshwork.

In the *posttrabecular mechanisms,* obstruction to aqueous outflow may result from increased resistance in Schlemm's canal due to collapse or absence of the canal, or a clogging of the canal, as with sickled red blood cells. Most of the posttrabecular cases, however, are due to elevated episcleral venous pressure.

Angle-Closure Glaucoma Mechanisms

The angle-closure mechanisms include situations in which the peripheral iris is in apposition to the trabecular meshwork or peripheral cornea. The peripheral iris may either be "pulled" (anterior mechanisms) or "pushed" (posterior mechanisms) into this position.

In the *anterior mechanisms* of angle-closure glaucoma, an abnormal tissue bridges the anterior chamber angle and subsequently undergoes contraction, pulling the peripheral iris into the iridocorneal angle. Examples of the contracting tissue include a fibrovascular membrane, an endothelial

Table 8.3

CLASSIFICATION OF THE GLAUCOMAS BASED ON MECHANISMS
OF OUTFLOW OBSTRUCTION*

I. Open-angle glaucoma mechanisms
   A. Pretrabecular (membrane overgrowth)
      1. Fibrovascular membrane (neovascular glaucoma)
      2. Endothelial layer, often with Descemet-like membrane
         a. Iridocorneal endothelial syndrome
         b. Posterior polymorphous dystrophy
         c. Penetrating and nonpenetrating trauma
      3. Epithelial downgrowth
      4. Fibrous ingrowth
      5. Inflammatory membrane
         a. Fuchs' heterochromic iridocyclitis
         b. Luetic interstitial keratitis
   B. Trabecular
      1. Idiopathic
         a. Chronic open-angle glaucomas
         b. Steroid-induced glaucoma
      2. "Clogging" of the trabecular meshwork
         a. Red blood cells
            1) Hemorrhagic glaucoma
            2) Ghost cell glaucoma
         b. Macrophages
            1) Hemolytic glaucoma
            2) Phacolytic glaucoma
            3) Melanomalytic glaucoma
         c. Neoplastic cells
            1) Malignant tumors
            2) Neurofibromatosis
            3) Nevus of Ota
            4) Juvenile xanthogranuloma
         d. Pigment particles
            1) Pigmentary glaucoma
            2) Exfolilation syndrome (glaucoma capsulare)
            3) Uveitis
            4) Malignant melanoma
         e. Protein
            1) Uveitis
            2) Lens-induced glaucoma
         f. Viscoelastic agents
         g. α-chymotrypsin-induced glaucoma
         h. Vitreous
      3. Alterations of the trabecular meshwork
         a. Edema
            1) Uveitis (trabeculitis)
            2) Scleritis and episcleritis
            3) Alkali burns
          b. Trauma (angle recession)
         c. Intraocular foreign bodies (hemosiderosis, chalcosis)
   C. Posttrabecular
      1. Obstruction of Schlemm's canal
         a. Collapse of canal
         b. Clogging of canal (e.g., sickled red blood cells)
      2. Elevated episcleral venous pressure
         a. Carotid-cavernous fistula
         b. Cavernous sinus thrombosis
         c. Retrobulbar tumors

         d. Thyrotropic exophthalmos
         e. Superior vena cava obstruction
         f. Mediastinal tumors
         g. Sturge-Weber syndrome
         h. Familial episcleral venous pressure elevation
II. Angle-closure glaucoma mechanisms
   A. Anterior ("pulling" mechanism)
      1. Contracture of membranes
         a. Neovascular glaucoma
         b. Iridocorneal endothelial syndrome
         c. Posterior polymorphous dystrophy
         d. Penetrating and nonpenetrating trauma
      2. Contracture of inflammatory precipitates
   B. Posterior ("pushing" mechanism)
      1. With pupillary block
         a. Pupillary block glaucoma
         b. Lens-induced mechanisms
            1) Intumescent lens
            2) Subluxation of lens
            3) Mobile lens syndrome
         c. Posterior synechiae
            1) Iris-vitreous block in aphakia
            2) Pseudophakia
            3) Uveitis
      2. Without pupillary block
         a. Plateau iris syndrome
         b. Ciliary block (malignant) glaucoma
         c. Lens-induced mechanisms
            1) Intumescent lens
            2) Subluxation of lens
            3) Mobile lens syndrome
         d. Following lens extraction (forward vitreous shift)
         e. Following scleral buckling
         f. Following panretinal photocoagulation
         g. Central retinal vein occlusion
         h. Intraocular tumors
            1) Malignant melanoma
            2) Retinoblastoma
         i. Cysts of the iris and ciliary body
         j. Retrolenticular tissue contracture
            1) Retinopathy of prematurity (retrolental fibroplasia)
            2) Persistent hyperplastic primary vitreous
III. Developmental anomalies of the anterior chamber angle
   A. High insertion of anterior uvea
      1. Congenital (infantile) glaucoma
      2. Juvenile glaucoma
      3. Glaucomas associated with other developmental anomalies
   B. Incomplete development of trabecular
      meshwork/Schlemm's canal
      1. Axenfeld-Rieger syndrome
      2. Peters' anomaly
      3. Glaumomas associated with other developmental anomalies
   C. Iridocorneal adhesions
      1. Broad strands (Axenfeld-Rieger syndrome)
      2. Fine strands which contract to close angle (Aniridia)

Clinical examples cited in this table do not represent an inclusive list of the glaucomas.

layer with a Descemet-like membrane, and inflammatory precipitates.

In the *posterior mechanisms,* pressure behind the iris, lens, or vitreous causes the peripheral iris to be pushed into the anterior chamber angle. This may occur with or without pupillary block.

Posterior mechanisms *with pupillary block* include pupillary block glaucoma, as previously discussed. Functional apposition between the peripupillary iris and lens in this condition increases resistance of aqueous humor flow into the anterior chamber, resulting in a relative increase in posterior chamber pressure and forward bowing of the peripheral iris. The functional apposition in these patients is due to a genetically-determined configuration of the anterior ocular segment. In other conditions, the same functional apposition may result from an acquired forward shift of the lens (e.g., intumescent cataract or subluxed lens). In still other cases, a pupillary block may be due to posterior synechia associated with inflammation of the anterior ocular segment. In each of these conditions, apposition between the iris and the lens, in-

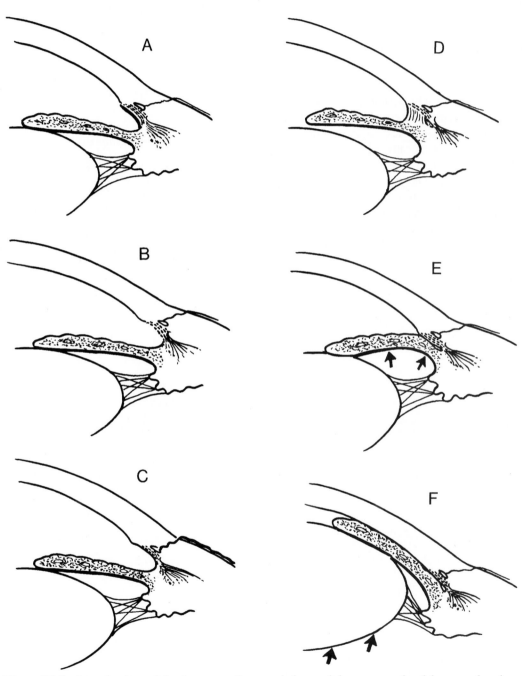

Figure 8.2. Basic mechanisms of the glaucomas. Open-angle forms of glaucoma may be of the pre-trabecular (**A**), trabecular (**B**), or posttrabecular type (**C**). Angle-closure forms of glaucoma may be of the anterior "pulling" type (**D**) or of the posterior "pushing" type. The latter may occur with (**E**) or without (**F**) pupillary block *(arrows* indicate location of force pushing the iris or lens-iris diaphragm forward).

traocular lens or vitreous obstructs the flow of aqueous humor into the anterior chamber, resulting in increased pressure in the posterior chamber and forward bowing of the peripheral iris into the anterior chamber angle.

In the posterior mechanisms of angle-closure glaucoma *without pupillary block,* increased pressure in the posterior portion of the eye pushes the lens-iris or vitreous-iris diaphragm forward. Examples include malignant (ciliary block) glaucoma, plateau iris syndrome, intraocular tumors, cysts of the iris and ciliary body, or contracture of retrolenticular tissue.

Developmental Anomalies of the Anterior Chamber Angle

These glaucomas are not readily separated into open-angle and angle-closure mechanisms, but typically represent incomplete development of structures in the conventional aqueous outflow pathway. Clinically recognized developmental defects include a high insertion of the anterior uvea, as in congenital (infantile) and juvenile glaucoma and many of the glaucomas associated with other developmental abnormalities. In other cases, the defect may manifest as an incomplete development of the trabecular meshwork and/or Schlemm's canal (e.g., Peters' anomaly) or as iridocorneal adhesions (e.g., Axenfeld-Rieger syndrome).

SUMMARY

Two methods of classifying the many clinical forms of glaucoma are (a) etiologic and (b) mechanical. The former is based on the underlying disorder that leads through a five-stage pathway to alterations in aqueous humor dynamics and/or optic neuropathy. The mechanical classification is based on alterations in the anterior chamber angle, which may result from the underlying abnormality and lead to the elevated IOP. The latter classification is first divided into open-angle and angle-closure mechanisms and developmental anomalies of the anterior chamber angle, which are then subdivided according to the underlying etiology and specific structural alterations.

REFERENCES

1. Geijssen HC, Greve, EL: The spectrum of open angle glaucoma. I: senile sclerotic glaucoma versus high tension glaucoma. Ophthalmic Surg 18:207, 1987.
2. Cartwright, MJ, Anderson, DR: Correlation of asymmetric damage with asymmetric intraocular pressure in normal-tension glaucoma (low-tension glaucoma). Arch Ophthalmol 106:898, 1988.
3. Pavlin, CJ, Ritch, R, Foster, FS: Ultrasound biomicroscopy in plateau iris syndrome. Am J Ophthalmol 113:390, 1992.
4. Barkan, O: Glaucoma: classification, causes, and surgical control. Results of microgonioscopic research. Am J Ophthalmol 21: 1099, 1938.

OPEN-ANGLE GLAUCOMAS

TERMINOLOGY

Chronic Open-Angle Glaucoma

As discussed in Chapter 8, it has been traditional to classify the glaucomas according to primary and secondary forms. Within the former group, and indeed among all the glaucomas, by far the most prevalent condition has been commonly referred to as *primary open-angle glaucoma.* Continued research, however, has shown the concept of primary and secondary glaucomas to be arbitrary and one that should probably be abandoned. Research has also suggested that the view of primary open-angle glaucoma as a single entity is no longer valid. Within this large group of glaucomas, the most common form (or forms) is typically defined by the following three criteria: (a) an intraocular pressure (IOP) consistently above 21 mm Hg in at least one eye; (b) an open, normal appearing anterior chamber angle with no apparent ocular or systemic abnormality that might account for the elevated IOP; and (c) typical glaucomatous visual field and/or optic nerve head damage, as described in Chapters 6 and 5, respectively. Alternative terms that may be more appropriate for this condition(s)

are *open-angle glaucoma, chronic open-angle glaucoma* (COAG), or *idiopathic open-angle glaucoma.* Other synonymous terms that may also appear in the literature include *chronic simple glaucoma,* and *open-angle glaucoma with damage.*

It is likely that COAG represents a spectrum of disorders in which several causative factors, of which IOP is one, have varying degrees of influence. For example, one group of investigators has described two subgroups of COAG (1). The first of these, which they refer to as *senile sclerotic glaucoma,* is seen in the elderly, with relatively low IOP and normal anterior chamber angles, while the second, *high tension glaucoma,* occurs in a younger age group with high IOP and signs of developmental abnormalities of the angle. The two groups are also distinguished by the nature of the optic atrophy, and the appearance of the peripapillary retina and the choroid. In another study, a population of COAG patients revealed two statistically distinct groups: a smaller group with evidence of vasospastic abnormalities and a high correlation between mean deviation index of visual field severity and the highest IOP, and a larger group with evidence of coagulation and biochemical abnormalities, but no correlation between the field index and highest IOP (2).

Significance of Intraocular Pressure

The commonly used IOP level of 21 mm Hg is based on the concept that 2 standard deviations above the mean within a Gaussian distribution represents the upper limit of "normal" for that biologic parameter. However, since the distribution of IOP in the general population is skewed to the right or higher pressures, this principle provides only a rough approximation of the normal limits. What is even more important, many eyes will not develop glaucomatous optic atrophy or visual field loss, at least not for long periods of time, despite IOP well above 21 mm Hg, while others will suffer progressive glaucomatous damage at pressures that are never recorded to exceed this level. These latter observations have brought into question the role of IOP in the mechanism of COAG. While many studies have confirmed a correlation between the level of IOP and the rate of visual field loss in some groups of patients with COAG, this correlation is not seen in all cases (3–5). Other causative factors figure into the formula for glaucomatous damage (6), which appears to explain the lack of absolute correlation between IOP and the development of COAG. In any case, this discrepancy between IOP level and glaucomatous damage has led to the use of additional terms (and confusion) within the general category of COAG.

Ocular Hypertension

Patients who have the first two criteria for COAG, i.e., an IOP above 21 mm Hg for which there is no apparent cause, but who have normal optic nerve heads and visual fields, are commonly said to have *ocular hypertension* (7, 8). Some investigators, however, have pointed out disadvantages of this term, suggesting that it does not connote the potential seriousness of the situation, i.e., that a certain percentage of these patients eventually will develop glaucomatous damage, and may lead to a false sense of security on the part of both patient and physician. Furthermore, it is hard to know whether the terminology should arbitrarily be changed to "glaucoma" when the IOP reaches a level at which treatment for pressure alone is felt to be indicated. Chandler and Grant (9) suggested the term *early open-angle glaucoma without damage* for this condition, while Shaffer (10) preferred *glaucoma suspect*. The latter term may also include other risk factors for glaucoma such as suspicious optic nerve heads. Whatever term one chooses to use for this condition, the most important point is that both physician and patient must be fully aware of its potential consequences. Later in this chapter, we consider the management of such patients.

Normal-Tension Glaucoma

At the other end of the spectrum with regard to susceptibility to IOP are those patients with open, normal appearing anterior chamber angles, who have glaucomatous optic nerve head and visual field damage despite pressures that have never been documented above 21 mm Hg. These patients are said to have *normal-tension glaucoma* (or *low-tension glaucoma*). The former term is becoming more popular, since the IOP in these individuals is usually "normal" or "high normal" and rarely "low normal." Some investigators feel that normal-tension glaucoma is a variant of COAG (11–13), while others believe that the mechanism of optic atrophy in the two conditions is different (14, 15). Although a number of differences between the two disorders has been described, which are considered later in this chapter, an overlap of findings makes it difficult to clearly separate all of these patients into one category or the other.

Open-Angle Glaucomas with Associated Abnormalities

There are some forms of open-angle glaucoma, such as pigmentary glaucoma and the exfoliation syndrome, that have been identified as distinct entities because of a partial understanding of associated, causative abnormalities and mechanisms of aqueous outflow obstruction. These conditions are considered in subsequent chapters in Section Two. In the present chapter, we focus on those open-angle glaucomas for which laboratory and clinical findings have yet to clarify the glaucoma mechanisms and in which IOP plays a variable role. As the search continues into the causes and mechanisms of the open-angle glaucomas, especially in the field of molecular biology, it is quite likely that an ever increasing number of separate entities will be recognized within this spectrum of disorders.

EPIDEMIOLOGY

Frequency Among the Glaucomas

Chronic open-angle glaucoma is clearly the most common single form of glaucoma, although it is difficult to precisely establish the ratio of individuals with this disorder to the total number of patients with all forms of glaucoma. In a British survey of 4231 individuals between the ages of 40 and 75 years, 39 glaucoma patients were detected, of whom 13 (i.e., one-third of the glaucoma population or 0.28% of the general population) had COAG (16). However, in a study of 8126 subjects, 40 years of age or older, in Japan, open-angle glaucomas accounted for 73% of the glaucomas detected (exclusive of ocular hypertensives), of which the majority were diagnosed with normal-tension glaucoma (17). These epidemiologic surveys will obviously be influenced by the population being studied, as well as the methods and criteria used to identify patients with glaucoma.

Prevalence Within General Populations

Several large surveys have been conducted to determine the number of patients with ocular hypertension and COAG (or glaucoma in general) within a population at a given time (16–21). The prevalence of glaucoma is between 1% and 2% in most studies, although reports again vary considerably according to the population being studied, the diagnostic criteria, and the screening techniques. However, most surveys show that the prevalence of ocular hypertension is considerably higher than that of glaucoma, even when all forms of glaucoma are included, which some investigators take as evidence that elevated IOP does not invariably lead to glaucoma (22).

Incidence Among Ocular Hypertensives

Numerous studies have been conducted to determine the rate of occurrence of COAG within populations of untreated ocular hypertensives (Table 9.1) (23–33). Most studies spanned an observation period of 5–10 years, during which time the incidence of patients developing glaucomatous field loss was roughly 1% per year. However, there are large differences in the results of these studies, which suggest variable degrees of susceptibility among populations of ocular hypertensives. It should also be kept in mind that "normotensive" individuals may develop glaucoma. Some of these patients may have normal-tension glaucoma, while others may initially or on one examination have IOPs below 21 mm Hg, but later be found to have elevated pressures and subsequently develop COAG (32, 33).

Natural History of Field Loss in Chronic Open-Angle Glaucoma

Leydhecker (34) studied the distribution of IOP and glaucomatous visual field loss in a large population survey. When persons with pressures higher than 20 mm Hg and those with definite glaucomatous field defects were plotted against their age, the two slopes were parallel and separated horizontally by 18 years, which led to the notion that 10–20 years may elapse between the onset of ocular hypertension and the development of visual field loss. Lichter and Shaffer (35), however, found that field loss in a population of 378 ocular hypertensives, observed for a period averaging 12¾ years, occurred earlier than Leydhecker suggested, despite the fact that most were being treated during this time. The level of IOP appears to influence the rate of visual field loss. In one study of 177 untreated COAG patients, comparing the mean age of presentation with the degree of field loss, it was estimated that untreated disease is likely to progress from early to end stage visual field loss in 14.4 years at pressures of 21–25 mmHg, in 6.5 years at 25–30 mmHg, and in 2.9 years at pressures over 30 mmHg (36). Furthermore, once field loss has occurred, further damage tends to progress more rapidly than in the fellow undamaged eye exposed to the same IOP, which appears to reflect the increased susceptibility of the damaged eye (37–39).

RISK FACTORS

Chronic open-angle glaucoma has no associated symptoms or other warning signs prior to the development of advanced visual field loss. It is for this reason that glaucoma screening

Table 9.1.

INCIDENCE OF CHRONIC OPEN-ANGLE GLAUCOMA AMONG OCULAR HYPERTENSIVES

Investigator(s)	No. Ocular Hypertensives (Patients)	Observation Period (Years)	No. Developed Open-Angle Glaucoma (Patients)
Perkins (23, 33)	124	5–7	4 (3.2%)
Walker (24)	109	11	11 (11%)
Wilensky, et al. (25)	50	avg. 6	3 (6%)
Norskov (26)	68	5	0
Linner (27)	92	10	0
Kitazawa, et al. (28)	75	avg. 9.5	7 (9.3%)
David, et al. (29)	61	avg. 3.3 range 1–11	10 (16.4%)
Hart, et al. (30	92	5	33 (35%)
Armaly, et al. (32)	5886	13	(1.7%)
Lundberg, et al. (31)	41	20	14 (34%)

programs, as discussed in Chapter 7, are needed for the early detection of this disorder. Such programs must utilize the following risk factors, that are commonly associated with the disease, to identify those segments of the population requiring the closest attention. In addition, once a patient has been found to have persistent IOP elevation (the most significant risk factor), but no apparent optic nerve head or visual field damage, the additional risk factors must be considered by the physician in trying to decide which of these individuals require closer observation or the initiation of therapy before definite damage. These risk factors can be considered in two categories: (a) the general features of patients with COAG and (b) the clinical features that are detected during the basic glaucoma examination.

General Features of Patients

Age

All studies agree that the prevalence of chronic open-angle glaucoma increases with the age of the population being considered (40–44). It is unusual for the disorder to reach the clinical stage before the age of 40, and most cases are seen after age 65. For example, in one general population survey of 3000 individuals, the prevalence of COAG and normal-tension glaucoma by age group was 0.22% among 40–49-year-olds, 0.10% for 50–59-year-olds, 0.57% for 60–69-year-olds, 2.81% for 70–79-year-olds, and 14.29% for patients 80+ years of age (40). Age, therefore, becomes an increasingly significant risk factor with each decade.

It is important to emphasize, however, that COAG is by no means limited to those over 40 years of age. In one study, 25% of glaucoma patients 10–35 years old had this form of glaucoma (45). Another study of 13 COAG patients under 40 years of age, four of whom were in their teens, emphasized the unusual severity of the disease in younger patients and stressed the need for applanation tonometry in all individuals old enough to permit the study (46).

Race

Several studies have shown that COAG is more prevalent, develops at an earlier age, and is more severe in black individuals as compared to whites (47–53). In a population-based study of 5308 individuals (2395 blacks and 2913 whites) in Baltimore, the prevalence of COAG for age groups between 40 and 80 years or older was from 1.23% to 11.26% among blacks and 0.92% to 2.16% among whites (53). In another study, 25 black and 47 white ocular hypertensives were followed 1–12 years, during which time glaucomatous damage developed in 18.1% of the former and 5.4% of the latter group (49). Furthermore, nonwhites are said to have seven- to eight-times more blindness from glaucoma than whites (51). One possible explanation for the increased susceptibility of black patients with COAG to progressive glaucomatous damage is the larger physiologic cup-disc ratios as compared to whites (54). In one study of 40 blacks undergoing filtering surgery for COAG, sickle cell anemia did not appear to explain the increased susceptibility, with only two patients having sickle trait (55).

Sex

The prognostic significance of sex is less clear than that of age and race, although some studies suggest a higher prevalence among men (18, 44, 56, 57).

Diabetes Mellitus

The prevalence of COAG and ocular hypertension is several times higher in the diabetic population than in the general population according to most surveys (57–61). One survey failed to support the association of diabetes and COAG, although the diagnosis of diabetes was limited to the patient's history (62). The prevalence of diabetes or a positive glucose tolerance test has also been shown to be higher in patients with COAG (59, 63) or a high IOP response to topical steroids (59, 64). Diabetes also appears to influence the nature of visual field loss in patients with COAG, with a prevalence of inferior field loss of 64.4% versus 36.4% in diabetics versus nondiabetics, respectively (65), and a 32% prevalence of diabetes among COAG patients with primarily inferior loss, compared to 13% in those without such a defect (66).

Other Endocrine Disorders

An increased prevalence of various thyroid disorders among COAG patients was suggested over 30 years ago (67), and a more recent study revealed *hypothyroidism* in 23.4% of COAG patients, compared to 4.7% of controls (68). Treating hypothyroidism was also shown to improve IOP and the facility of aqueous outflow (69). Low normal protein bound iodine and radioactive iodine uptake have also been noted in patients with COAG (70), although baseline thyroxine, thyrotropin (TSH), and triiodothyronine (T$_3$) resin uptake levels did not differ from normal values (71).

Other endocrine disorders have not been found to be associated with COAG, but may influence the IOP and, therefore, should be considered in the diagnosis and management of glaucoma. For example, elevated IOP has occurred in patients with Cushing's syndrome, with normalization of pressure after treatment of the systemic disease (72, 73). One study showed that relatives of such patients were often positive topical steroid responders (discussed later in this chapter), suggesting increased steroid sensitivity as the mechanism of the pressure rise (73). Pituitary dysfunction may be associated with instability of IOP (74) and aqueous humor dynamics (75), and elevated estrogen or progesterone may lower the pressure (76), while male hormones may raise it (77).

Cardiovascular and Hematologic Abnormalities

Cardiovascular and hematologic abnormalities are particularly common among patients with normal-tension glaucoma, which is discussed later in this chapter. The association of these abnormalities is less clear among patients with the high pressure form of COAG. Some investigators have found an association with hemodynamic crisis and low diastolic ophthalmic artery pressure or diastolic blood pressure (57, 78, 79). However, other studies showed an association with increased systemic blood pressure (52, 80–82), and yet others revealed no significant deviation in blood pressure from the general population (83, 84). A more meaningful measure may be the perfusion pressure (blood pressure minus intraocular pressure), a reduction of which was shown to have a strong association with an increased prevalence of COAG (85). Visual field progression, despite well-controlled IOP, was significantly associated with lower systolic blood pressure during both day and night (86), and nocturnal reductions in blood pressure have been associated with progressive visual field loss (87) and with a focal ischemic type of glaucomatous damage (88). While most patients do not suffer optic nerve damage following a sudden loss in blood pressure, there is evidence that this may increase the risk of further nerve damage among glaucoma patients (89). These individuals should be followed closely for evidence of changes in their optic nerve head or visual field during situations such as the adjustment of medication for systemic hypertension and general surgery.

Family History

A family history of COAG is generally considered to be a significant prognostic indicator. Chronic open-angle glaucoma is believed to have a genetic basis. Although the exact hereditary mode is unknown, indirect evidence suggests that it is most likely polygenetic or multifactorial (the genetic basis of COAG is discussed later in this chapter). One survey revealed a family history of glaucoma in 50% of patients with open-angle glaucoma (90). The prevalence of COAG among close relatives of glaucoma patients ranges between 5% and 19% according to two reports (91, 92). In a 10–12-year followup of 101 patients with a family history of COAG, 3% developed glaucoma and another 6% became glaucoma suspects (93). The age-adjusted association between COAG and a family history of glaucoma, in one population-based survey, was higher when the relative was a sibling rather than a parent or child, with odds ratios of 3.69, 2.17, and 1.12, respectively (94).

Clinical Features

Intraocular Pressure

As previously noted, an elevated IOP is only one of several risk factors for the development of COAG, although it is a causative risk factor and most studies agree that it is the most important single prognostic risk factor. The degree of risk for developing glaucomatous damage is related to the level of IOP. One study of 307 patients revealed the following association of optic nerve head damage with the presenting IOP (95):

IOP(mm Hg)	Percent with Nerve Damage
25–29	7
30–34	14
35–39	52
40–44	61
45–49	73
50–54	83
55–59	83
>60	70

Another study revealed the probability of glaucoma to be near zero at IOP less than 18 mm Hg, while it reaches 0.5 at 27–28 mm Hg, and approaches 1 (i.e., certainty) at approximately 35 mm Hg (96). As previously noted, the level of IOP also influences the rate of visual field loss in patients with established glaucomatous damage (36).

A fluctuation in the IOP is also important and may have more prognostic value than an individual pressure reading (81). In one study, ocular hypertensives whose pressures increased with time had a greater risk of developing glaucomatous damage (97). In another study, 15% of ocular hypertensive patients had an IOP rise of 5 to 9 mm Hg when going from the sitting to supine position, suggesting the value of measuring the supine pressure when evaluating these individuals (98).

Despite the importance of IOP as a risk factor in most forms of glaucoma, it must be emphasized, as discussed in Chapter 7, that this parameter will not always be abnormal, especially with single measurements. In one population survey, 8 of 15 newly diagnosed cases had pressures below 20.5 mm Hg (99), while another revealed screening pressures below 21 mm Hg in more than half of all glaucomatous eyes (100).

Optic Nerve Head

The second most significant risk factor for the development of COAG is the size of the physiologic cup before glaucomatous damage occurs. Chandler and Grant (101) observed that a wide, deep physiologic cup tolerates increased IOP poorly, and the tendency is to enlargement and total cupping. This concept was supported by a study in which 27 of 102 ocular hypertensives who developed field loss during a 5-year observation period had significantly larger vertical cup/disc ratios than those who did not develop field loss (102). In that study, eyes with the combination of IOP consistently above 28 mm Hg and cup/disc ratios of 0.5 or greater were at such a high risk of developing glaucomatous damage that therapy should probably be initiated in these patients.

The greatest diagnostic value of observing the optic nerve head comes when the first definite evidence of progressive glaucomatous damage is detected (103). A helpful early finding is defects in the retinal nerve fiber layer, which may be a sign of glaucomatous optic atrophy before apparent changes are seen in the nerve head (104). Other early findings include thinning or saucerizing of the neural rim, disc hemorrhages, and parapapillary atrophy. These features were considered in detail in Chapter 5. The importance of close observation for these changes in glaucoma suspects is reemphasized.

Myopia

There is an increased prevalence of COAG among myopes (105), as well as an increased frequency of myopia among patients who have COAG, ocular hypertension, and normal-tension glaucoma (106). Of particular clinical significance is the observation that myopic eyes are more susceptible to the effects of elevated IOP. Of 10 ocular hypertensive patients who developed glaucomatous field defects during observation, six were myopic (less than −1.00 diopter), three were emmetropic (+1.00 to −1.00 diopters), and one was hyperopic (more than +1.00 diopter) (106). Conversely, once IOP has been lowered by therapy, the visual fields of myopic eyes more often improve and less often worsen than those of nonmyopic eyes, which may relate to the increased susceptibility of the latter group to risk factors that are independent of IOP, such as low ophthalmic artery pressure (107).

Cornea

The cornea is typically normal in COAG. In one study, patients with cornea guttata were reported to frequently have abnormal tonographic values (108), and preliminary specular microscopic studies of patients with chronic glaucoma suggested abnormal corneal endothelium (109). However, a subsequent study, comparing individuals with normal IOP, untreated ocular hypertension, treated ocular hypertension, or COAG, revealed no significant difference in the central corneal endothelial density or central corneal thickness (110). Yet, another study suggested that patients diagnosed with ocular hypertension have a higher incidence of increased corneal thickness than glaucoma or control subjects, which may cause an artifactual elevation of the IOP measurements (111).

Gonioscopy

By traditional definition, the anterior chamber angle in eyes with COAG is open and grossly normal, as described in Chapter 3. Preliminary studies, however, suggest that these patients may have more iris processes, a higher insertion of the iris root, more trabecular meshwork pigmentation (112), and a greater than normal degree of segmentation in the pigmentation of the meshwork (113).

Visual Abnormalities

Central visual acuity, as measured by standard clinical tests, typically remains normal until peripheral visual field loss is advanced and is, therefore, of no value in the early detection of COAG. Preliminary evidence, however, suggests that more subtle measures of vision dysfunction, such as contrast sensitivity, color vision, and motion perception (discussed in Chapter 6), may one day be useful as prognostic indicators in diagnosing COAG prior to the development of typical visual field loss. Once typical glaucomatous damage to the visual field has been documented in one eye, the diagnosis of glaucoma is usually established, and there is a high incidence of subsequent field loss in the fellow eye. The latter was reported to be 29% in 31 patients followed 3–7 years (114), and 25% of 104 individuals after 5 years of followup in another series (115).

NORMAL-TENSION GLAUCOMA

As noted earlier in this chapter, some investigators consider normal-tension glaucoma to be clearly distinguishable from the high tension form of COAG. There is, in fact, considerable evidence, considered in this section, that the two entities differ in several ways beyond just the IOP levels. However, reports are conflicting and it is difficult to draw a clear division between the two conditions. It may be that COAG is a spectrum of disorders in which elevated IOP is the most influential causative factor at one end, while other factors that influence glaucomatous optic atrophy predominate at the other end. In any case, we now consider some of the clinical differences between normal-tension glaucoma and the high tension form of COAG and the mechanisms that might be responsible for these differences.

Clinical Differences from High-Tension Chronic Open-Angle Glaucoma

Optic Nerve Head

The neural rim has been found by some investigators to be significantly thinner in normal-tension patients, especially inferiorly and inferotemporally, than in high-tension patients with comparable total visual field loss (116–118). Other studies, however, have revealed less striking differences. In one study, the discs were similar, although cupping in the normal-tension glaucoma was broadly sloping, resulting in less disc volume alteration (119). In another study, the only significant difference in disc appearance was an increased prevalence in the high-tension group of an "hourglass pattern" to the lamina cribrosa, in which thick connective tissue bundles crossed horizontally between 3 o'clock and 9 o'clock, with thinner bundles and larger pores above and below (120). While this finding was not so striking as to allow segregation of the two forms of open-angle glaucoma on that basis alone, it was felt to suggest that the architecture of the lamina may be a causative factor in normal-tension glaucoma. Studies comparing disc area between eyes with normal-tension and high-tension open-angle glaucoma have also been conflicting, with one showing significantly larger discs in the former group (121), and another showing no significant difference (118).

One study found that optic disc hemorrhages were more prevalent in the normal-tension group, raising the possibility of vascular disease as another causative factor in these patients (122). In that study, the normal-tension eyes could be divided into those which frequently develop recurrent disc hemorrhages and those which rarely bleed, providing more evidence for multiple causative factors in normal-tension glaucoma. Another study looked at normal-tension glaucoma patients with unilateral cilioretinal arteries, which revealed no association between this vascular finding and the degree of disc or field damage (123). The retinal nerve fiber layer has also been compared between normal-tension and high-tension open-angle glaucoma patients, with the former having more localized and the latter more diffuse defects (124).

Visual Fields

Differences have also been reported in the nature of visual field loss between normal-tension and high-tension open-angle glaucoma patients with comparable optic nerve damage. In general, normal-tension glaucoma patients appear to have deeper, more localized scotomas (117, 125–127), although one study found this to be true only for the inferior hemifield (128), and another found no significant difference in the depth or slopes of the scotomas (129). There are also conflicting reports regarding the proximity of scotomas to fixation between the two groups, which may relate to the testing methods (129, 130). One study found a significantly greater rate of progressive visual field loss in normal-tension glaucoma (131), and another revealed a difference in the pattern of the progression, with the high-tension patients initially increasing mainly in area and later in depth, while the increases in area and depth remained in constant proportion in normal-tension glaucoma patients (132).

Possible Mechanisms of Normal-Tension Glaucoma

Influence of Intraocular Pressure

Although normal-tension glaucoma, by definition, is distinguished from the high-tension form of open-angle glaucoma by an IOP that is never recorded to exceed 21 mm Hg, the pressures do tend to be higher than those in the normal population (133). One study revealed a significant influence of

IOP on the progression of visual field damage in normal-tension glaucoma (134), although another study showed no significant difference in IOP between those patients with and without field progression (135). In two studies of normal-tension patients with asymmetric IOP, the visual field loss was typically worse in the eye with the higher pressure (136, 137). The bulk of the evidence, therefore, suggests that slightly elevated IOP is a causative factor in normal-tension glaucoma, although other factors are also involved. In making the diagnosis of normal-tension glaucoma and in the management of these patients it is important to know the diurnal variation in IOP in order to confirm that their pressures are consistently below 21 mm Hg before therapy and are staying within the target level while on treatment. One study suggested that patients with normal-tension glaucoma have wider diurnal fluctuations than the normal population (133), although other investigators found no significant difference in diurnal variation of IOP (138, 139) or of aqueous humor flow or resistance to outflow (139). A multiple regression analysis showed that the peak diurnal IOP could be predicted by the mean of six clinic IOPs, with no peak exceeding 21 mm Hg when using a cutoff for clinic IOPs of 16 mm Hg (140).

Other Causative Factors

As noted earlier in this section, additional causative factors may relate to the architecture of the lamina cribrosa (120) and the vascular perfusion of the optic nerve head (122). Drance and coworkers (11, 12) described two forms of normal-tension glaucoma: (a) a *nonprogressive form,* which is usually associated with a transient episode of vascular shock, and (b) a *progressive form,* which is believed to result from chronic vascular insufficiency of the optic nerve head. A variety of cardiovascular and hematologic abnormalities have been described, which might account for both forms (141). Hayreh (142) has suggested that normal-tension glaucoma differs from anterior ischemic optic neuropathy only in that the latter is a more acute process. Reported associated findings include hemodynamic crises (11, 12) reduced diastolic ophthalmodynamometry levels (11, 141) and ocular pulse amplitudes (143, 144), and increased vascular resistance of the ophthalmic artery by color Doppler analysis (145, 146). Reports of alterations in systemic blood pressure are conflicting (11, 14, 80, 141). Visual-evoked responses during stepwise artificially-increased IOP were significantly different between patients with normal-tension and high-tension open-angle glaucoma, suggesting a greater lack of autoregulation of optic nerve head circulation in the former group (147).

Patients with normal-tension glaucoma were noted to have an increased frequency of headaches with or without migraine features (148). Another study failed to confirm this association (149), while a third investigation found that normal-tension glaucoma patients with headaches had significantly lower IOP than normal-tension glaucoma patients without headaches, suggesting a subset within this group of patients (150). An abnormally reduced blood flow in the fingers, especially in response to exposure to cold, has also been reported (151, 152), although one study failed to confirm this finding (153). Other investigators again found two subsets of open-angle glaucoma: a smaller one with vasospastic finger blood flow measurements and a highly positive correlation between visual field loss and IOP and a larger group with disturbed coagulation and biochemical measurement, suggestive of vascular disease, with no correlation between field and highest IOP (154). The bulk of the observations, therefore, suggests that vasospastic events are involved in the mechanism of at least some forms of normal-tension glaucoma. The therapeutic implications of this is discussed at the end of this chapter.

Hematologic abnormalities that have been reported to be associated with normal-tension glaucoma include increased blood and plasma viscosity (155) and hypercoagulability (e.g., increased platelet adhesiveness and euglobulin lysis time) (11, 137). Other studies, however, have revealed no statistically significant abnormalities in coagulation tests (156, 157), or in vascular or rheological profiles (157). Hypercholesterolemia has also been reported to be higher among patients with normal-tension glaucoma (158). Magnetic resonance imaging in patients with normal-tension glaucoma have revealed an increased incidence of diffuse cerebral ischemia, which may be further evidence for a vascular etiology (159, 160).

There is also some evidence that immune mechanisms may play a role in the mechanism of normal-tension glaucoma. In one study, 30% of the patients had one or more immune-related diseases, compared to 8% in a matched group of ocular hypertensives (161). Additional support for an immune mechanism includes the increased incidence of paraproteinemia and autoantibodies (162) and antirhodopsin antibodies (163) in patients with normal-tension glaucoma.

Whatever factors may have a causative role in normal-tension glaucoma, it is likely that they have a genetic basis, with one reported family having an autosomal dominant mode (164).

Differential Diagnosis of Normal-Tension Glaucoma

The differential diagnosis of normal-tension glaucoma should include wide diurnal IOP fluctuations in which high pressures are occurring at times when they are not being recorded. Other patients may have once had high pressures that caused damage, but which have since spontaneously normalized. One example of this is pigmentary glaucoma, in which the IOP often improves with increasing age (165). Another situation to distinguish from normal-tension glaucoma is the individual with advanced optic atrophy and visual field loss, in which even high normal pressures often cause further progressive damage. It is also important to rule out nonglaucomatous causes of disc and field changes as discussed in Chapters 5 and 6.

ADJUNCTIVE TESTS

Numerous tests have been studied in an attempt to find additional prognostic indicators of COAG. Although none of these have yet been clearly proven to be of clinical value, the physician should be familiar with some of the more frequently discussed adjunctive tests.

Tonography

The details of this procedure and its limitations as a clinical tool in the diagnosis of COAG were discussed in Chapter 3.

Provocative Tests

Water Provocative Test

Drinking a large quantity of water in a short period of time will generally lead to a rise in the IOP. Based on the theory that glaucomatous eyes have a greater pressure response to water drinking, a "provocative" test was developed for the early detection of COAG.

PROCEDURE. After an 8-hour fast, the test begins with baseline applanation tonometric readings. Indentation tonometry is unsatisfactory, since water drinking reduces ocular rigidity (166). The patient is then instructed to drink approximately 1 liter of tap water, following which applanation tonometry is performed every 15 minutes for 1 hour. The maximum IOP rise usually occurs in 15–30 minutes and returns to the initial level after approximately 60 minutes in both normal and glaucomatous eyes (167). A rise of 8 mm Hg is generally felt to be a significant response. It has also been suggested that performing tonography after a water drinking test has additional diagnostic value (168, 169).

MECHANISM. The mechanism of IOP rise after water drinking is uncertain. One theory is that reduced serum osmolality might cause increased aqueous inflow, although studies have revealed an inconsistent correlation between the IOP and serum osmolality (170, 171). Tonographic studies have shown reduced aqueous outflow facility in human (172–174) and rabbit (175) eyes, and a suggestion of increased aqueous production has been observed in monkeys (176).

CLINICAL VALUE. Kronfeld (174) found that the combined water drinking test and tonography gave statistically significant lowering of aqueous outflow facility in 35 ocular hypertensives. However, the response was too small to be clinically significant for the individual patient. He concluded that the two tests in this situation added little to the information provided by tonometry. Two additional studies suggest that the water provocative test has no diagnostic value, since 22% false-positives and 48% false-negatives were found in one series (177), while the other group had 24% false-negatives (178).

Dilatation Provocative Tests

These tests are used primarily in eyes suspected of having potentially occludable anterior chamber angles, which are discussed in the next chapter. However, cycloplegics and mydriatics have also been studied with regard to their influence on open-angle forms of glaucoma. Although these studies have not yet provided clinically useful diagnostic tests for COAG, it is important to understand how different eyes respond to these drugs, especially when interpreting a mydriatic provocative test for angle-closure glaucoma.

CYCLOPLEGIC EFFECT. *Strong topical cycloplegics* such as 1% cyclopentolate, 1% atropine, 5% homatropine, or 0.25% scopolamine, have been shown to cause a significant IOP rise (greater than 6 mm Hg) in many eyes with COAG (179). Oral atropine did not influence IOP with short-term administration in COAG patients (180), although some had a pressure rise after 1 week of medication (181). A pressure response to topical cycloplegics may also occur in eyes with angle-closure glaucoma when an uncontrolled pressure persists despite a patent iridectomy (182), and in nonglaucomatous eyes after several weeks of topical dexamethasone (183). Chronic open-angle glaucoma patients are more likely to have this pressure rise if they are being treated with miotics (184), and the mechanism of the pressure response to strong cycloplegics is felt to include inhibition of the miotic effect and direct inhibitory action on the ciliary muscle (184, 185).

A *weak cycloplegic* such as 1% tropicamide may also cause a pressure rise in some patients with open-angle glaucoma, especially when on miotic therapy, suggesting the mechanism is competition with the miotic (186, 187). In one study, this did not correlate with the early IOP response after argon laser trabeculoplasty (187).

MYDRIATIC EFFECT. The mydriatic action of cycloplegic-mydriatic agents, or a mydriatic such as phenylephrine, is also felt to be a cause of elevated IOP in some eyes with open anterior chamber angles (188–192). This occurs only when there is an associated shower of pigment in the anterior chamber. The mechanism is felt to be temporary obstruction of the trabecular meshwork by pigment granules. This occurs predominantly in eyes with the exfoliation syndrome or pigmentary glaucoma, but may also occur in some cases of COAG with heavy pigmentation in the anterior chamber angle (188–192). In one case of COAG, the postdilatation pressure rise was permanent, and histopathogy of the trabeculectomy specimens suggested that this

was due to a breakdown of the endothelium covering the trabecular beams (192).

Therapeutic Trials

Based on a theory that eyes with COAG respond to antiglaucoma drugs with a greater IOP response than is the case with nonglaucomatous eyes, these attempts have been made to develop prognostic tests.

Epinephrine Test

There is evidence that patients with COAG may be particularly sensitive to epinephrine (193). Such individuals reportedly have a greater IOP drop and more frequent cardiac arrhythmias in response to topical epinephrine than patients with other forms of glaucoma (193). It has been theorized that the mechanism of this increased responsiveness is an epinephrine-stimulated rise in intraocular cyclic adenosine monophosphate to which the COAG patient may be unusually sensitive (194, 195). Based on this apparent sensitivity to epinephrine, a test was devised in which 1–2% epinephrine twice daily was administered, and a pressure drop of more than 5 mm Hg over a 1–7 day period was considered a "response" (196). (A subsequent study indicated that the pressure drop 4 hours after a single dose could also be used as the indicator of response (197).) In a 5–10-year followup of 80 ocular hypertensives, 85% of those who developed field loss were positive responders, while only 28% without field loss had shown the positive response (196). However, in another study the positive response was found in 53% of 32 ocular hypertensives and 56% of 18 open-angle glaucoma patients with field loss (198). Further study is needed, therefore, to confirm the prognostic value of this test.

Other Therapeutic Trials

Other therapeutic trials that have been suggested include the *pilocarpine test,* in which an IOP drop of more than 4 mm Hg at the peak of the diurnal curve, in response to pilocarpine therapy, is felt to suggest glaucoma (199). The *acetazolamide test* is used to estimate the coefficient of aqueous outflow facility based on applanation IOP measurements after the drug is given intravenously (200). Neither of these tests, however, have confirmed clinical value.

UNIOCULAR THERAPEUTIC TRIAL. While the value of the therapeutic trials discussed above awaits further study, there is an entirely different concept of therapeutic trials which has clinical value today. Administration of a topical antiglaucoma drug to one eye (using the other as a control) is a valuable clinical adjunct in helping to decide whether or not to institute medical therapy in ocular hypertensives, as well as in establishing the efficacy of a particular medical regimen. The purpose of this trial is simply to determine the effectiveness in reducing IOP and the side effects that can be expected from that medication (201). It has been suggested that this information can be obtained, at least in part, during a 4-hour office trial with 2% pilocarpine (202), although a 1-month trial is preferable for most drugs, since this allows time to better determine the long-term IOP-lowering efficacy of the drug as well as the patient's tolerance of any side effects.

Topical Steroid Response

In the next section, we consider the influence of corticosteroids in the mechanism of COAG. The tendency of these patients, as well as a certain percentage of the general population, to respond to topical steroid therapy with an IOP rise has also been evaluated as a predictive test for COAG. Of 788 normotensives or ocular hypertensives treated with 0.1% dexamethasone four times daily for 6 weeks and followed for a minimum of 5 years, glaucomatous visual field loss developed in 31% of high responders (IOP greater than 31 mm Hg during the steroid administration), 3.4% of intermediate responders (20–30 mm Hg), and in no low responders (less than 20 mm Hg) (203). However, another study of 134 patients, followed for 5–15 years, showed no correlation between corticosteroid response and the development of glaucoma (204), and the predictive value of this test is not as good as a multivariate analysis of the risk factors discussed earlier in this chapter.

Intraocular Pressure Effect on Visual Function

The influence of transient, artificially-induced IOP elevation on the visual field helps to identify which eyes are more susceptible to raised pressure (205), and may provide a possible approach to the early identification of COAG patients (206). Using the reverse approach, a reduction in the vertical diameter of the blind spot has been correlated with declining IOP following oral antiglaucoma medication to establish the pressure level which the eye can tolerate (207). However, long-term investigations are needed to establish the value of these tests as prognostic indicators.

Other Reported Tests

It was once suggested that populations of COAG patients have significantly more nontasters of phenylthiourea (208) or phenylthiocarbamide, although this was not confirmed in a subsequent study (209). It was also reported that patients with COAG have a higher prevalence of the histocompatibility (HLA) antigens, HLA-B12 and HLA-B7 (210), although numerous studies have subsequently shown no significant correlation between HLA antigens and glaucoma (211–220).

THEORIES OF MECHANISM

As with virtually all forms of glaucoma, elevation of the IOP in COAG is due to obstruction of aqueous outflow. However, the precise mechanism(s) of outflow obstruction in this condition has not been fully explained, despite the fact that it has been studied more than in any other type of glaucoma. The data from these studies provide only suggestions of what the final answer may hold.

Histopathologic Observations

The most likely source for the eventual explanation of aqueous outflow obstruction in COAG lies in the study of histopathologic material. However, the interpretation of these findings must take into consideration additional influences, such as age, the secondary effects of prolonged IOP elevation, the alterations that medical and surgical treatment of the glaucoma might have induced, and artifacts created by tissue processing.

Alterations of the Trabecular Meshwork

Grant (221) demonstrated that the largest proportion of resistance to aqueous outflow in enucleated human eyes could be eliminated by incising the trabecular meshwork. Whether this tissue is the actual site of abnormal resistance in COAG has not been determined, but the following observations have been reported.

Collagen of the trabecular beams is fragmented, with thickening of the glass membrane, increased curly collagen, diffuse nodular proliferation of extracellular long-spacing collagen, coiling of fiber bundles, and changes in orientation and osmophilia of the fibers (222–225). However, similar changes are seen in association with aging, and one study found the changes correlated more closely with age than with reduction in outflow facility (226), while another revealed no statistical difference in mean collagen levels of the meshwork between eyes with COAG and age matched normal eyes (227). It has been suggested that the changes in COAG may represent an exaggeration of the normal aging process (228).

Endothelial cells lining the trabeculae appear to be more active than in normotensive eyes (223–225), and are reported to show proliferation with foamy degeneration and basement membrane thickening (222, 224). The cellularity of the trabecular meshwork in eyes with COAG is lower than in nonglaucomatous eyes, but the rate of decline with age is similar in the two groups (229). A reduced frequency of actin filaments (contractile proteins) in trabecular endothelium has also been demonstrated in eyes with COAG (230). Cross-linked actin networks, which alter the function of trabecular cells, was found in higher levels and to increase more in response to dexamethasone in glaucoma eyes than in normal controls in tissue culture (231).

Intertrabecular spaces, as might be anticipated from the general thickening of the trabeculae, are narrowed (225, 227). In addition, they may contain red blood cells, pigment, and dense amorphous material (224). It has also been reported that glycosaminoglycans are more abundant in the meshwork of human eyes with COAG (225, 232). However, hyaluronic acid has been shown to be decreased in the trabecular meshwork of eyes with COAG, and the loss of its surface-active properties may influence aqueous outflow resistance (233). A scanning electron microscopic study of 10 trabeculectomy specimens revealed an unknown substance coating the meshwork, which was felt to be sufficient to obstruct aqueous outflow (234), although this finding has not been confirmed by other investigators (235–237).

Perfusion of cationized ferritin in enucleated eyes of COAG patients suggests that the outflow obstruction is segmental (255).

Juxtacanalicular connective tissue just beneath the inner wall endothelium of Schlemm's canal has been noted by several observers to contain a layer of amorphous, osmophilic material (225, 226, 238–241). This has been described as moderately electron-dense, nonfibrillar material (226) with characteristics of basement membrane and curly collagen (240) and cytochemical properties of chondroitin sulfate protein complex (226). However, the concentration of electron-dense materials, while significantly higher than that of normal controls, is not felt to be enough to account for the outflow reduction characteristic of COAG (241). Matrix vesicles, representing extracellular lysosomes (242), a sheath material from subendothelial elastic-like fibers (243), the extracellular glycoprotein, fibronectin (244), and elastin (245) have also been found in abnormal amounts in the juxtacanalicular tissue of eyes with COAG. These patients also differ from the normal population in collagen binding of plasma fibronectin (246). In a small sample of COAG eyes, pigment in the juxtacanalicular tissue did not appear sufficient to contribute to resistance to aqueous outflow (247). Pores and giant vacuoles, as described in Chapter 2, are found in the inner wall endothelium of Schlemm's canal in normal eyes and are felt to be related to aqueous transport. In eyes with COAG, the giant vacuoles have been found in most studies to be decreased or absent (210, 211, 224, 225, 240, 248, 249). Pore density has also been shown to be reduced and more unevenly distributed in COAG than in normal eyes (250). In addition, cul-de-sacs, which are described as terminations of aqueous channels, are markedly reduced in eyes with COAG (251).

Collapse of Schlemm's Canal

Collapse of Schlemm's canal will also increase resistance to aqueous outflow and has been proposed as the mechanism of outflow obstruction in COAG (252, 253). The collapse represents a bulge of trabecular meshwork into the canal, which might result from alterations in the meshwork and/or relaxation of the ciliary muscle. In support of this theory, some histopathologic studies have revealed a narrowed Schlemm's canal with adhesions between the inner and outer walls (224, 225, 252). A mathematical model of Schlemm's canal, however, tentatively suggests that resistance to aqueous outflow is in the inner wall of the canal and is not caused by a weakening of the trabecular meshwork with a resultant collapse of Schlemm's canal alone (254).

In interpreting the histologic findings in the juxtacanalicular tissue and Schlemm's canal, it is advisable to take into account a certain amount of segmental variability (255, 256), and to examine at least three quadrants per eye (256).

Alterations of the Intrascleral Channels

Alterations of the intrascleral channels could also be a mechanism of increased resistance to aqueous outflow in COAG. Histopathologic observations have revealed attenuation of the channels, which may be due to a swelling of glycosaminoglycans in the adjacent sclera (222). Krasnov (257) has suggested that intrascleral blockage may be the mechanism of outflow obstruction in approximately half of the eyes with COAG. However, this theory was not supported by a study in which removal of tissue overlying Schlemm's canal did not improve outflow facility until the canal was actually entered (252).

Influence of Aqueous Humor

There is also growing evidence that abnormal constituents of the aqueous humor may adversely effect the outflow structures to increase resistance to outflow. In one study, the relative concentration of a protein doublet was significantly different in the aqueous of COAG patients as compared to controls (258). Transforming growth factors (TGF) are a family of multifunctional polypeptides with several cellular regulatory properties, including inhibition of epithelial cell proliferation, induction of extracellular matrix protein synthesis, and stimulation of mesenchymal cell growth. Porcine trabecular cells have been shown to express the messenger RNA for TFG-β1 (259) and the aqueous humor of patients with COAG was found to have a significantly greater amount of TGF-β2 than normal subjects (260). These authors postulate that abnormal levels of TGF in the aqueous of patients with COAG may decrease the cellularity of the trabecular meshwork and promote a buildup of excessive amounts of extracellular matrix materials with subsequent increased resistance to aqueous outflow. Another study revealed a significant decrease of functional collagenase activity, a higher concentration of tissue inhibitor of metalloproteinase-1, and increased collagen synthesis activity in the aqueous of patients with COAG, as compared to a control group with cataracts, and these authors suggested that an increase of collagen synthesis and a decrease of collagen degradation may contribute to an excess deposition of collagen with loss of trabecular cells during the development of COAG (261).

Corticosteroid Sensitivity

As previously noted, there is evidence that patients with COAG are unusually sensitive to corticosteroids and that this steroid sensitivity may be related to the abnormal resistance to aqueous outflow. We consider first the evidence for the increased sensitivity and then look at theories of how this may influence outflow.

Topical Corticosteroid Response

It has been well-documented that chronic corticosteroid therapy, especially with topical administration, leads to elevated IOP in many individuals. In a small percentage of the general population, the magnitude of this pressure rise is sufficient to cause a severe form of glaucoma, which is considered in Chapter 20. The present discussion is limited to prospective studies of topical steroid response in various populations.

General population studies have been performed in which a potent topical corticosteroid such as 0.1% betamethasone or 0.1% dexamethasone was given three to four times daily for 3–6 weeks. These studies all agree that a significant number of individuals will respond with variable degrees of IOP elevation. The studies differ considerably, however, with regard to many important aspects of this pressure response. For example, the distribution of pressure responses in the general population was found in some studies to be trimodal, with approximately two-thirds having a low response (usually defined as a rise of less than 5 mm Hg), one-third showing an intermediate response (6–15 mm Hg rise), and 4–5% having a rise greater than 15 mm Hg (262–264). Another study, however, could not confirm the trimodal concept (265), and when the topical corticosteroid test was repeated in the same population, individuals did not always give the same response each time (266).

Chronic open-angle glaucoma populations have been shown to have a greater number of individuals with a high IOP response to topical corticosteroids. The actual reported percentage of high responders, however, varies according to the criteria used to define this group (262–264). Reports also differ as to whether ocular hypertensives do (267) or do not (268) have a greater incidence of high responders than the general population. In one study, a significant number of ocular hypertensives with high responses were reported to have reversible glaucomatous field defects (269). Another study suggested that high corticosteroid responders, whether ocular normotensive or hypertensive at the time of testing, have an increased chance of developing glaucomatous damage (270). As previously discussed, however, the topical corticosteroid response has not been found to be a useful prognostic indicator for COAG (203, 204).

Eyes that have sustained an attack of *angle-closure glaucoma* also have a high percentage of topical steroids responders (271), although those at risk of angle closure (271), or that have undergone prophylactic peripheral iridectomies (272), do not differ from the general population. It has also been shown that topical corticosteroid responsiveness among insulin-dependent diabetics does not correlate with the rate of development of diabetic retinopathy (273).

Inheritance of the topical corticosteroid response and how this may relate to COAG have been matters of particular controversy. Becker (262, 274) postulated an autosomal recessive mode for the corticosteroid response and suggested that the gene is either closely related or identical to that for COAG, which he felt had an autosomal recessive inheritance. Armaly (264) agreed that the two conditions might be genetically related, but proposed a polygenetic inheritance for COAG with the gene for the topical corticosteroid response being one of the genes involved. Results of additional studies were consistent with a genetic basis for the topical corticosteroid response, but could confirm neither the recessive mode (275) nor even a relationship to glaucoma (268). Still other investigators could not even substantiate that the corticosteroid response was entirely genetic. A twin-heritability study of monozygotic and like-sex dizygotic twins revealed a low estimate of heritability that did not support a predominant role of inheritance in the response to corticosteroids, and suggested that nongenetic factors play the major role (265, 276–278). In further support of the nongenetic concept of topical corticosteroid response, eyes with unilateral angle-closure glaucoma (279) or angle-recession (280) responded to topical corticosteroids with a higher pressure rise in the involved eye than the fellow eye, which had not suffered angle closure or trauma. These observations suggest that topical corticosteroid responsiveness, at least in some individuals, may be acquired.

Plasma Cortisol Studies

Plasma cortisol studies have been felt by some investigators to provide additional evidence that patients with COAG may be unusually sensitive to corticosteroids. The results of these studies, however, are again conflicting. Higher than normal plasma cortisol levels (281), as well as percent plasma free cortisol (not bound to plasma proteins) of total plasma cortisol (282), have been demonstrated in COAG patients. Other investigators, however, were unable to confirm the association of elevated plasma cortisol and COAG (283, 284). One study suggested that an elevated plasma cortisol level is closely related to the IOP at the time of cortisol sampling (285). Noncortisol glucocorticoid activity has been shown to be increased in the plasma of patients with COAG, and the authors suggest that these may be responsible for elevating biologic plasma glucocorticoid activity (286).

Plasma cortisol suppression has also been suggested to be abnormal in patients with COAG. This test consists of measuring plasma cortisol before and after the oral administration of dexamethasone. The normal response is a reduction in plasma cortisol of 35% or more approximately 9 hours after administration of the corticosteroid, due to suppression of trophic hormones. The reported results of plasma cortisol suppression in COAG patients are conflicting, in that some investigators have found less than normal suppression (281, 287), which did not appear to be genetically determined (288), while other investigators found no significant difference from nonglaucomatous individuals (283, 289). Pretreatment with diphenylhydantoin (Dilantin) normally prevents plasma cortisol suppression, presumably by enhancing liver enzyme degradation of the dexamethasone before it suppresses the release of trophic hormones from the pituitary. However, in 89% of COAG patients, diphenylhydantoin did not prevent the plasma cortisol suppression (283). This observation did not appear to be due to an alteration in liver enzyme degradation of dexamethasone (290), but rather to an increased sensitivity to lower levels of circulating steroids (291). The corticosteroid sensitivity in COAG patients appears to be relatively specific, since oral dexamethasone does not have an abnormal effect on baseline thyroid function tests or thyroid stimulating hormone suppression in these individuals (292). However, a study of cultured skin fibroblast sensitivity to corticosteroids suggested that a generalized cellular hypersensitivity to glucocorticoids is not intrinsic to COAG (293). These authors postulated that environmental alterations and/or endogenous factors may influence steroid responses.

The relationship of topical corticosteroid response to plasma cortisol suppression has also been investigated, and a correlation between high topical corticosteroid responders and reduced plasma cortisol suppression has been reported (289, 294, 295). In addition, approximately half of the high topical corticosteroid responders from a general population study had plasma cortisol suppression despite pretreatment with diphenylhydantoin (283). The latter individuals also more closely resembled COAG patients on the basis of other parameters, such as a larger cup/disc ratio and an abnormal glucose tolerance test (283). However, a 5-year prospective study failed to show that plasma cortisol suppression can predict the development of COAG among high topical steroid responders (296).

Lymphocyte Transformation Inhibition

Lymphocyte transformation inhibition studies may offer yet another source of evidence for increased corticosteroid sensitivity in patients with COAG, although reports continue to be conflicting. Lymphocytes from peripheral blood can be transformed from the usual state of relative metabolic inactivity to a metabolically active state by mitogenic agents such as phytohemagglutinin. The degree of transformation can be measured by the uptake of tritiated thymidine into DNA. Corticosteroids inhibit the lymphocyte transformation and the degree of inhibition can be taken as a measure of sensitivity to corticosteroids. Using this model, some studies have revealed increased corticosteroid sensitivity among patients with COAG (297, 298), while other investigators have been unable to confirm these findings (299–301). The

effect of ouabain on lymphocyte transformation is normal in COAG patients and high topical corticosteroid responders, suggesting that steroid sensitivity, if it exists, is specific and not the general vulnerability of "sick cells" (302).

Relationship of Intraocular Pressure to Corticosteroid Sensitivity

If patients with COAG are unusually sensitive to corticosteroids, by what mechanism(s) might this lead to elevated IOP? Furthermore, does this mechanism(s) only function in response to exogenously administered corticosteroids, or do normal circulating corticosteroids also adversely influence the IOP in COAG patients? Attempts to answer these question include these theories.

HYPOTHALAMIC-PITUITARY-ADRENAL AXIS THEORY. It has been suggested that an abnormal response of the hypothalamic-pituitary-adrenal axis in COAG patients, and possibly in other forms of glaucoma, may be related to alterations in aqueous humor dynamics in response to corticosteroids (295, 303).

CYCLIC-ADENOSINE MONOPHOSPHATE THEORY. It may be that corticosteroids influence the IOP by altering cyclic-adenosine monophosphate (cyclic-AMP). Corticosteroids have a permissive effect on the β-adrenergic stimulation of adenyl cyclase, the enzyme responsible for the synthesis of cyclic-AMP (304). How this relates to aqueous humor dynamics is uncertain, although COAG patients and high topical steroid responders appear to be unusually sensitive to cyclic-AMP. Evidence for this increased sensitivity has been observed in studies of lymphocyte transformation, as previously described, which is normally inhibited by cyclic-AMP. Theophylline inhibits the enzyme, phosphodiesterase, which destroys cyclic-AMP, and COAG patients reportedly require less theophylline than control subjects to stimulate inhibition of lymphocyte transformation (305).

GLYCOSAMINOGLYCANS THEORY. It has also been proposed that IOP elevation associated with corticosteroid sensitivity may be related to glycosaminoglycans in the trabecular meshwork (306). When polymerized, glycosaminoglycans become hydrated, swell, and obstruct aqueous outflow. Catabolic enzymes, released from lysosomes in the trabecular cells depolymerize the glycosaminoglycans. Corticosteroids stabilize the lysosome membrane preventing release of these enzymes, thereby increasing the polymerized form of glycosaminoglycans and the resistance to aqueous outflow.

PHAGOCYTOSIS THEORY. Yet another possible effect of steroids on IOP may be related to the phagocytic activity of endothelial cells lining the trabecular meshwork. As discussed in Chapter 2, these cells are normally phagocytic, and it may be that they function to "clean" the aqueous of debris before it reaches the inner wall endothelium of Schlemm's canal. Failure to do so might result in a buildup of material that could account for the amorphous layer in the juxtacanalicular connective tissue, as previously described. Corticosteroids suppress phagocytosis, and it may be that the trabecular endothelium in COAG patients is unusually sensitive even to endogenous corticosteroids (307).

Cells cultured from trabecular meshwork of patients with COAG have been found to have abnormal metabolism of cortisol (308).

Immunologic Studies

Increased γ-globulin (309) and plasma cells (310) in the trabecular meshwork of eyes with COAG have been reported, and a high percentage of patients with this disease were found in one study to have positive antinuclear antibodies reactions (311). These reports suggested a possible immunologic mechanism in the pathogenesis of COAG. However, subsequent assays for specific immunoglobulins in the trabecular meshwork of eyes with COAG revealed no difference from nonglaucomatous eyes (312–314). In addition, further evaluation of antinuclear antibodies in patients with COAG (315, 316), as well as C1q binding immune complexes, collagen antibodies, anti-nDNA-antibodies (316), and cell-mediated immunity, as indicated by leukocyte migration inhibition in vitro (317), have all failed to show any significant difference from the nonglaucoma population. The absence of a correlation between HLA antigens and COAG was discussed earlier in this chapter. At the present time, therefore, the bulk of the evidence is against an immunogenic mechanism in COAG.

Genetic Basis of Open-Angle Glaucomas

The next major breakthrough in our understanding of the etiology and mechanisms of the open-angle glaucomas will quite likely come through studies of genetic linkage. Two families with autosomal dominantly inherited open-angle glaucomas of juvenile onset have shown genetic linkage to the long arm of chromosome 1 (318–320). The eventual identification of the gene responsible for this and other forms of glaucomas will not only provide a means of classifying and detecting the various conditions, but also of identifying the protein defect, which may lead to the mechanism of the glaucomas and ultimately to the appropriate therapy.

MANAGEMENT

The present discussion will be limited to the principles of deciding when to begin treatment and what basic type of therapy to use. The details of the drugs and surgical procedures are considered in Section Three.

When to Treat

In the typical case of COAG with established visual field and/or optic nerve head damage, treatment to reduce the IOP is clearly indicated whatever the pressure may be. The importance of elevated IOP as a causative factor of COAG and the importance of reducing the pressure in the management of the disease has been clinically established (321, 322). However, in the case of ocular hypertension with normal optic nerve heads and visual fields, the appropriate course is less clear. As discussed earlier in this chapter, not all such patients appear destined to develop glaucomatous damage and there is no way of predicting with certainty which ones will go on to manifest the full picture of COAG. Prospective studies have indicated that elevated IOP, abnormalities of the optic nerve head, black race, advancing age, myopia, a family history of glaucoma, and cardiovascular disorders are significant risk factors for the development of this disorder (25, 323, 324). However, no single risk factor or group of factors has yet been shown to predict the future development of glaucomatous damage with reasonable accuracy (325).

For lack of a precise indicator of future glaucomatous damage, it has been customary practice that patients with moderate IOP elevations be followed without treatment, but with periodic visual field and optic nerve head examinations. However, the concept of treating elevated IOP prior to established glaucomatous damage has received considerable attention. In two randomized, prospective studies of ocular hypertension, one randomizing patients (326) and the other randomizing right and left eyes (327) between timolol therapy and no treatment, the treated eyes had a more favorable course with regard to glaucomatous damage. In a third study, however, randomizing patients between timolol treatment and no treatment, no significant differences in outcomes were found (328). A national Ocular Hypertension Treatment Study is currently underway to shed more light on this important issue.

Most ophthalmologists will initiate therapy at a certain IOP level despite normal discs and fields based on the belief that, beyond that particular pressure, the increased risk of developing glaucomatous damage is sufficient to justify therapeutic intervention. Goldmann (329) began medical therapy at 25 mm Hg, while Chandler and Grant (101) suggested 30 mm Hg as a guideline for initiating treatment in the absence of apparent damage. Clearly, any arbitrary pressure level should be adjusted for each patient on the basis of that individual's risk factors. In addition to the risk factors for COAG, other situations for which the initiation of therapy at lower pressure levels might be considered include the risk of central retinal vein occlusion, as well as individuals who are one-eyed, who are more likely to return for followup if they are being treated, who desire treatment, or in whom visual fields or disc evaluation is not possible. In doubtful cases, a uniocular trial of therapy, as discussed earlier in this chapter, may be helpful, since a good pressure reduction with minimal side effects might argue in favor of continuing the therapy in both eyes.

How to Treat

Once the decision has been made to begin treatment, the next questions are what form of therapy should be used and what should be the guidelines for successful therapy?

Medical Therapy

Chronic open-angle glaucoma has traditionally been thought of as a medical disease, in that laser and incisional surgery are usually reserved for cases that cannot be controlled with medication. Although the question of earlier or initial surgical intervention is being revisited, as discussed below, an initial trial of medical therapy is still the standard of practice for most patients with COAG. The basic principle of medical therapy is to use the least amount of medicine that will control the glaucoma with the fewest side effects. To this end, it is customary to begin with a low dose of topical medication and to increase the concentration and/or advance to combinations of drugs until the desired pressure level is reached. It is good practice to treat only one eye initially in symmetric cases, so the fellow eye can be used as a control in determining the efficacy of therapy. The question of which drug to use first depends on the ocular and systemic status of each individual patient, as well as the physician's personal preference. The relative advantages and disadvantages of the various antiglaucoma drugs are considered in Section Three.

A common tendency, which should be resisted, is to add more and more, stronger and stronger medicines in an effort to control the IOP. This often leads only to additional side effects without significant additional IOP-lowering efficacy. One study showed that a significant IOP reduction is usually associated with any initial medication, whereas the pressure does not decline significantly more with a change to a stronger medication or combined medical therapy (330). It is important, therefore, to carefully document the efficacy and patient tolerance of any new medication that is added and to move on to surgical intervention if the target pressure is not reached with a reasonable regimen of well tolerated medication.

Although IOP reduction has been shown to be important in preventing visual loss in glaucoma (321, 322), it is not possible to predict what pressure level will be adequate to prevent progressive glaucomatous damage in each individual case. Traditionally, a pressure below 20 mm Hg was felt to be adequate for eyes with early damage, while a pressure below 18 mm Hg was felt to be desirable for advanced cases (331). Those figures, however, may be too high (332), especially for patients with advanced glaucoma. Patients with marked visual field loss tend to experience further loss at a greatly accelerated rate (333) and these individuals may re-

quire pressures in the mid- to low-teens (334). However, at least one study has shown a poor correlation between IOP reduction and progressive visual field loss (335), and the main guide to therapy should be the appearance of the optic nerve heads and visual fields. Progressive change in the latter parameters demands further pressure reduction regardless of what the pressure level may be. In fact, it has been shown that the appearance of the disc and field may improve with IOP reduction (336–338), and it has suggested that improvement in these parameters, rather than just arrested progression, is necessary to establish with certainty that the glaucoma is controlled (336, 337).

If the IOP begins to rise after long-term treatment with a particular medical regimen, the explanation may either be progression of the disease or a loss of responsiveness to the medication. Before increasing the concentration or adding other drugs, therefore, it is best to first test the second possibility by temporarily discontinuing the current medication in one eye (one drug at a time). If the pressure does not go up significantly with this uniocular trial of discontinuation, it suggests that the drug has lost part or all of its effectiveness, and it is probably best to change to a different medication or consider surgical intervention. In some cases, it is possible to return to the first drug after several months or years with renewed effectiveness of that medication.

TOLERANCE AND COMPLIANCE WITH MEDICAL THERAPY. Surgical intervention is usually indicated whenever there is progressive glaucomatous damage despite "maximum tolerable medical therapy." In some cases, this may mean that all available forms of effective antiglaucoma drugs in their highest effective concentrations are being used. Other cases of medical failure may result from inability to use one or more medications due to drug intolerances, while others may be related to poor compliance with the recommended therapy. In one study, 11 of 40 randomly selected COAG patients failed to comply with their medical therapy (339), while 42% of patients in another study missed at least some of their medications (340). Patients more often miss doses during the middle of the day and are more compliant with twice daily medication than when the drug is prescribed three or four times each day (340). Reported factors related to poor compliance include males, no other medical disease, glaucoma not ranked most troubling when other disorders were present, side effects with medication, and failure to relate glaucoma to blindness (339).

Surgical Intervention

When the glaucoma is uncontrolled medically, laser trabeculoplasty is usually the first surgical procedure of choice, followed by incisional surgical intervention when necessary. Trabeculectomy is usually the preferred incisional surgical technique for COAG.

In advanced cases with total cupping of the disc and a small, central field, it is no longer possible to use progressive disc and field change as a guide to laser or incisional surgical intervention, and reliance must be placed on the IOP. As noted earlier, these eyes probably require pressures in the mid- to low-teens.

Loss of central vision may occur after glaucoma surgery as well as during medical therapy. Kolker (331) found this to occur with equal frequency with these two modalities of treatment, and the potential risk of central field loss after filtering surgery should not constitute a contraindication to proceeding with the surgery if the glaucoma cannot be adequately controlled with medication and laser trabeculoplasty.

EARLY SURGERY Although the present standard of practice for most ophthalmologists is to consider medical therapy, laser surgery, and then incisional surgery in the sequence of treating patients with COAG, a trend to earlier surgical intervention is receiving considerable attention. The Glaucoma Laser Trial (discussed in Section Three) provided some support for laser trabeculoplasty as initial therapy. However, most of these patients eventually require the addition of medical therapy, and other investigators are looking at trabeculectomy as early or initial treatment for COAG. At question is the balance between the risk of inadequate IOP control and side effects with medical therapy versus the potential complications of filtering surgery. In one study of 52 COAG patients assigned to either medial therapy or filtering surgery and followed for up to 17.5 years, the early surgery group had less visual field loss but more rapid deterioration of visual acuity due to cataracts (341). In another study of 99 COAG patients in whom one eye was randomly assigned either to medial therapy or a trabeculectomy as the initial therapy, early surgery was associated with a lower mean IOP (15 mm Hg vs. 20.8 mm Hg, respectively) and better protection of the visual field (342). These authors concluded that the risk of delaying surgery is significantly greater than that of performing trabeculectomy as primary treatment. Yet, a third study of 168 COAG patients compared medical therapy, laser trabeculoplasty, and filtering surgery, and found that the latter gave the greatest IOP reduction, with no further deterioration of the visual fields, while medical therapy provided the least protection against progressive damage (343, 344). Clearly, there is a need for further evaluation of early surgery in the management of COAG.

Treatment of Normal-Tension Glaucoma

Damage to the optic nerve head and visual field may progress even at low normal pressures in this condition. Indeed, there is no firm evidence that treating the IOP improves the prognosis. Nevertheless, most clinicians try to keep the pressure as low as possible with medication or with laser or incisional surgery. Medical therapy may be adequate in some cases. In the Normal Tension Glaucoma Study,

57% of the patients achieved a stable 30% IOP reduction with topical medication and/or laser trabeculoplasty (345). The remaining 43% underwent filtering surgery. Although filtering surgery did not help in one reported series (346), other surgeons have found that it may prevent progressive damage (347–349).

The most important aspect of managing the patient with normal-tension glaucoma may be the treatment of any cardiovascular abnormality, e.g., gastrointestinal lesions, anemia, congestive heart failure, transient ischemic attacks, and cardiac arrhythmias, to ensure maximum perfusion of the optic nerve head (14). Ultimately, the treatment of choice may prove to be therapy which directly improves the function of the optic nerve head. A pilot study of 25 normal-tension glaucoma patients suggested that long-term oral therapy with nifedipine, a calcium channel blocker, may protect the visual field in these patients, possibly by relieving the effect of vasospasm on the nerve head (350). Although another study suggested that nifedipine therapy provided no difference in the rate of neuroretinal rim change, as compared to treatment with acetazolamide or no therapy (351), two other calcium channel blockers, verapamil and nimodipine, were shown to reduce IOP and vascular resistance in the central retinal artery (352), and improve contrast sensitivity (353), respectively. In another study, normal-tension glaucoma patients who were receiving concurrent calcium channel blocker therapy had a significant reduction in the rate of disc and field progression, as compared to similar normal-tension glaucoma group who were not receiving the concomitant therapy (354).

SUMMARY

Open-angle glaucomas are the most common form of glaucoma. The most prevalent of these, chronic open-angle glaucoma, has a familial tendency and is more prevalent with increasing age, black race, myopia, and certain systemic diseases, such as diabetes and cardiovascular abnormalities. It is typically asymptomatic until advanced visual field loss occurs and is characterized by an open, normal appearing anterior chamber angle. By definition, the IOP is consistently above 21 mm Hg, although there is a clinical variation, normal-tension glaucoma, in which disc and field changes develop despite pressures that never reach this level. Other patients have pressure elevation without glaucomatous damage, and no test has yet been developed to predict which of these individuals will develop glaucomatous damage. The precise mechanism of increased resistance to aqueous outflow remains unclear, although it is most likely related to subtle alterations in the trabecular meshwork and/or Schlemm's canal. Initial treatment in nearly all cases is topical and oral medication. When progressive damage continues, despite maximum tolerable medical therapy, laser trabeculoplasty is usually indicated, followed by glaucoma filtering surgery if necessary.

REFERENCES

1. Geijssen, HC, Greve, EL: The spectrum of primary open angle glaucoma. I: senile sclerotic glaucoma versus high tension glaucoma. Ophthalmic Surg 18:207, 1987.
2. Schulzer, M, Drance, SM, Carter, CJ, et al: Biostatistical evidence for two distinct chronic open angle glaucoma populations. Br J Ophthalmol 74:196, 1990.
3. O'Brien, C, Schwartz, B, Takamoto, T, Wu DC: Intraocular pressure and the rate of visual field loss in chronic open-angle glaucoma. Am J Ophthalmol 111:491, 1991.
4. Weber, J, Koll, W, Krieglstein, GK: Intraocular pressure and visual field decay in chronic glaucoma. Ger J Ophthalmol 2: 165, 1993.
5. Chauhan, BC, Drance, SM: The relationship between intraocular pressure and visual field progression in glaucoma. Graefes Arch Clin Exp Ophthalmol 230:521, 1992.
6. Anderson, DR: Glaucoma: The damage caused by pressure. Am J Ophthalmol 108:485, 1989.
7. Kolker, AE, Becker, B: "Ocular hypertension" vs. open-angle glaucoma: a different view. Arch Ophthalmol 95:586, 1977.
8. Phelps, CD: Ocular hypertension: to treat or not to treat? Arch Ophthalmol 95:588, 1977.
9. Chandler, PA, Grant, WM: "Ocular hypertension" vs. open-angle glaucoma. Arch Ophthalmol 95:585, 1977.
10. Shaffer, R: "Glaucoma suspect" or "ocular hypertension"? Arch Ophthalmol 95:588, 1977.
11. Drance, SM, Sweeney, VP, Morgan, RW, Feldman, F: Studies of factors involved in the production of low tension glaucoma. Arch Ophthalmol 89:457, 1973.
12. Drance, SM, Morgan, RW, Sweeney, VP: Shock-induced optic neuropathy. A cause of nonprogressive glaucoma. N Engl J Med 288:392, 1973.
13. Lewis, RA, Hayreh, SS, Phelps, CD: Optic disk and visual field correlations in primary open-angle and low-tension glaucoma. Am J Ophthalmol 96:148, 1983.
14. Chumbley, LC, Brubaker, RF: Low-tension glaucoma. Am J Ophthalmol 81:761, 1976.
15. Caprioli, J, Spaeth, GL: Comparison of visual field defects in the low-tension glaucomas with those in the high-tension glaucomas. Am J Ophthalmol 97:730, 1984.
16. Hollows, FC, Graham, PA: Intra-ocular pressure, glaucoma, and glaucoma suspects in a defined population. Br J Ophthalmol 50:570, 1966.
17. Shiose, Y, Kitazawa, Y, Tsukahara, S, et al: Epidemiology of glaucoma in Japan. A nationwide glaucoma survey. Jpn J Ophthalmol 35:133, 1991.
18. Kahn, HA, Leibowitz, HM, Ganley, JP, et al: The Framingham eye study. I. Outline and major prevalence findings. Am J Epidemiol 106:17, 1977.
19. Leske, MC, Rosenthal, J: Epidemiologic aspects of open-angle glaucoma. Am J Epidemiol 109:250, 1979.
20. Klein, BEK, Klein, R, Sponsel, WE, et al: Prevalence of glaucoma. The Beaver Dam eye study. Ophthalmology 99:1499, 1992.
21. Dielemans, I, Vingerling, JR, Wolfs, RCW et al: The prevalence of primary open-angle glaucoma in a population-based study in the Netherlands. The Rotterdam study. Ophthalmology 101: 1851, 1994.
22. Graham, PA: Epidemiology of simple glaucoma and ocular hypertension. Br J Ophthalmol 56:223, 1972.
23. Perkins, ES: The Bedford glaucoma survey. I. Long-term follow-up of borderline cases. Br J Ophthalmol 57:179, 1973.
24. Walker, WM: Ocular hypertension. Follow-up of 109 cases from 1963 to 1974. Trans Ophthalmol Soc UK 94:525, 1974.
25. Wilensky, JT, Podos, SM, Becker, B: Prognostic indicators in ocular hypertension. Arch Ophthalmol 91:200, 1974.
26. Norskov, K: Routine tonometry in ophthalmic practice. II. Five-year follow-up. Acta Ophthalmol 48:873, 1970.
27. Linner, E: Ocular hypertension. I. The clinical course during ten years without therapy. Aqueous humour dynamics. Acta Ophthalmol 54:707, 1976.
28. Kitazawa, Y, Horie, T, Aoki, S, et al: Untreated ocular hypertension. A long-term prospective study. Arch Ophthalmol 95:1180, 1977.
29. David, R, Livingston, DG, Luntz, MH: Ocular hypertension—a long-term follow-up of treated and untreated patients. Br J Ophthalmol 61:668, 1977.
30. Hart, WM Jr, Yablonski, M, Kass, MA, Becker, B: Multivariate analysis of the risk of glaucomatous visual field loss. Arch Ophthalmol 97:1455, 1979.
31. Lundberg, L, Wettrell, K, Linner, E: Ocular hypertension. A prospective twenty-year follow-up study. Acta Ophthalmol 65:705, 1987.
32. Armaly, MF: Ocular pressure and visual fields. A ten-year follow-up study. Arch Ophthalmol 81:25, 1969.
33. Perkins, ES: The Bedford glaucoma survey. II. Rescreening of normal population. Br J Ophthalmol 57:186, 1973.
34. Leydhecker, W: Zur verbreitung des glaucoma simplex in der scheinbar gesunden, augenarztlich nicht behandelten bevolkerung. Doc Ophthalmol 13:359, 1959.
35. Lichter, PR, Shaffer, RN: Ocular hypertension and glaucoma. Trans Pacific Coast Oto-Ophthalmol Soc 54:63, 1973.
36. Jay, JL, Murdoch, JR: The rate of visual field loss in untreated primary open angle glaucoma. Br J Ophthalmol 77:176, 1993.
37. Harbin, TS Jr, Podos, SM, Kolker, AE, Becker, B: Visual field progression in open-angle glaucoma patients presenting with monocular field loss. Trans Am Acad Ophthalmol Otol 81:253, 1976.
38. Grant, WM, Burke, JF Jr: Why do some people go blind from glaucoma? Ophthalmology 89:991, 1982.
39. Ekstrom C, Haglund B: Chronic open-angle glaucoma and advanced visual field defects in a defined population. Acta Ophthalmol 69: 574, 1991.
40. Wright, JE: The Bedford glaucoma survey. In: Glaucoma Symposium. Hunt, ed. Edinburgh, E&S Livingston, Ltd., 1966, p. 12.
41. Martinez, GS, Campbell, AJ, Reinken, J, Allan, BC: Prevalence of ocular disease in a population study of subjects 65 years old and older. Am J Ophthalmol 94:181, 1982.
42. Podgor, MJ, Leske, MC, Ederer, F: Incidence estimates for lens changes, macular changes, open-angle glaucoma and diabetic retinopathy. Am J Epidemiol 118:206, 1983.
43. Quigley, HA, Enger, C, Katz, J, et al: Risk factors for the development of glaucomatous visual field loss in ocular hypertension. Arch Ophthalmol 112:644, 1994.
44. Leske, MC, Connell, AMS, Wu, S-Y, et al: Risk factors for open-angle glaucoma. Arch Ophthalmol 113:918, 1995.
45. Goldwyn, R, Waltman, SR, Becker, B: Primary open-angle glaucoma in adolescents and young adults. Arch Ophthalmol 84:579, 1970.
46. Mandell, AI, Elfervig, J: Open-angle glaucoma in patients under forty years of age. Perspect Ophthalmol 1:215, 1977.
47. Wilensky, JT, Gandhi, N, Pan, T: Racial influences in open-angle glaucoma. Ann Ophthalmol 10:1398, 1978.
48. David, R, Livingston, D, Luntz, MH: Ocular hypertension: A comparative follow-up of black and white patients. Br J Ophthalmol 62:676, 1978.
49. Wallace, J, Lovell, HG: Glaucoma and intraocular pressure in Jamaica. Am J Ophthalmol 67:93, 1969.
50. Martin, MJ, Sommer, A, Gold, EB, Diamond, EL: Race and primary open-angle glaucoma. Am J Ophthalmol 99:383, 1985.
51. Hiller, R, Kahn, HA: Blindness from glaucoma. Am J Ophthalmol 80:62, 1975.
52. Wilson, MR, Hertzmark, E, Walker, AM, et al: A case-control study of risk factors in open angle glaucoma. Arch Ophthalmol 105: 1066, 1987.
53. Tielsch, JM, Sommer, A, Katz, J, et al: Racial variations in the prevalence of primary open-angle glaucoma. JAMA 266:369, 1991.

54. Beck, RW, Messner, DK, Musch, DC, et al: Is there a racial difference in physiologic cup size? Ophthalmology 92:873, 1985.

55. Schwartz, AL, Helfgott, MA: The incidence of sickle trait in blacks requiring filtering surgery. Ann Ophthalmol 9:957, 1977.

56. Kahn, HA, Milton, RC: Alternative definitions of open-angle glaucoma. Effect on prevalence and associations in the Framingham eye study. Arch Ophthalmol 98:2172, 1980.

57. Richler, M, Werner, EB, Thomas, D: Risk factors for progression of visual field defects in medically treated patients with glaucoma. Can J Ophthalmol 17:245, 1982.

58. Armstrong, JR, Daily, RK, Dobson, HL, Girard, LJ: The incidence of glaucoma in diabetes mellitus. A comparison with the incidence of glaucoma in the general population. Am J Ophthalmol 50: 55, 1960.

59. Becker, B: Diabetes mellitus and primary open-angle glaucoma. Am J Ophthalmol 71:1, 1971.

60. Vesti, N: The prevalence of glaucoma and ocular hypertension in type 1 and 2 diabetes mellitus. An epidemiological study of diabetes mellitus on the island of Falster, Denmark. Acta Ophthalmol 61: 662, 1983.

61. Klein, BEK, Klein, R, Jensen, SC: Open-angle glaucoma and older-onset diabetes. The Beaver Dam eye study. Ophthalmology 101:1173, 1994.

62. Tielsch, JM, Katz, J, Quigley, HA, et al: Diabetes, intraocular pressure, and primary open-angle glaucoma in the Baltimore eye survey. Ophthalmology 102:48, 1995.

63. Marre, E, Marre, M: A contribution to glaucoma in the presence of diabetes mellitus. Klin Monatsbl Augenheilkd 153:396, 1968.

64. Armaly, MF: Dexamethasone ocular hypertension and eosinopenia, and glucose tolerance test. Arch Ophthalmol 78:193, 1967.

65. Zeiter, JH, Shin, DH, Baek, NH: Visual field defects in diabetic patients with primary open-angle glaucoma. Am J Ophthalmol 111:581, 1991.

66. Zeiter, JH, Shin, DH: Diabetes in primary open-angle glaucoma patients with inferior visual field defects. Graefes Arch Clin Exp Ophthalmol 232:205, 1994.

67. McLenachan, J, Davies, DM: Glaucoma and the thyroid. Br J Ophthalmol 49:441, 1965.

68. Smith, KD, Arthurs, BP, Saheb, N: An association between hypothyroidism and primary open-angle glaucoma. Ophthalmology 100:1580, 1993.

69. Smith, KD, Tevaarwerk, GJM, Allen, LH: An ocular dynamic study supporting the hypothesis that hypothyroidism is a treatable cause of secondary open-angle glaucoma. Can J Ophthalmol 27: 341, 1992.

70. Becker, B, Kolker, AE, Ballin, N: Thyroid function and glaucoma. Am J Ophthalmol 61:997, 1966.

71. Krupin, T, Jacobs, LS, Podos, SM, Becker, B: Thyroid function and the intraocular pressure response to topical corticosteroids. Am J Ophthalmol 83:643, 1977.

72. Neuner, HP, Dardenne, U: Ocular changes in the Cushing syndrome. Klin Monatsbl Augenheilkd 152:570, 1968.

73. Haas, JS, Nootens, RH: Glaucoma secondary to benign adrenal adenoma. Am J Ophthalmol 78:497, 1974.

74. Abdel-Aziz, M, Labib, MA: The relationship of the intraocular pressure and the hormonal disturbance. Part II: the pituitary gland. Bull Ophthalmol Soc Egypt 62:61, 1969.

75. Caygill, WM: Aqueous humor dynamics following pituitary irradiation in diabetic patients with retinopathy. Am J Ophthalmol 71: 826, 1971.

76. Treister, G, Mannor, S: Intraocular pressure and outflow facility. Effect of estrogen and combined estrogen-progestin treatment in normal human eyes. Arch Ophthalmol 83:311, 1970.

77. Abdel-Aziz, M, Labib, MA: The relationship of the intra-ocular pressure to hormonal disturbance. Part IV. The gonads. Bull Ophthalmol Soc Egypt 62:83, 1969.

78. Morgan, RW, Drance, SM: Chronic open-angle glaucoma and ocular hypertension. An epidemiological study. Br J Ophthalmol 59: 211, 1975.

79. Drance, SM, Schulzer, M, Thomas, B, Douglas, GR: Multivariate analysis in glaucoma. Use of discriminant analysis in predicting glaucomatous visual field damage. Arch Ophthalmol 99:1019, 1981.

80. Leighton, DA, Phillips, CI: Systemic blood pressure in open-angle glaucoma, low tension glaucoma, and the normal eye. Br J Ophthalmol 56:447, 1972.

81. Nagin, P, Schwartz, B: Detection of increased pallor over time. Computerized image analysis in untreated ocular hypertension. Ophthalmology 91:252, 1984.

82. Dielemans, I, Vingerling, JR, Algra, D, et al: Primary open-angle glaucoma, intraocular pressure, and systemic blood pressure in the general elderly population. The Rotterdam study. Ophthalmology 102:54, 1995.

83. Kahn, HA, Leibowitz, HM, Ganley, JP, et al: The Framingham eye study. II. Association of ophthalmic pathology with single variables previously measured in the Framingham heart study. Am J Epidemiol 106:33, 1977.

84. Bengtsson, B: Findings associated with glaucomatous visual field defects. Acta Ophthalmol 58:20, 1980.

85. Tielsch, JM, Katz, J, Sommer, A, et al: Hypertension, perfusion pressure, and primary open-angle glaucoma. Arch Ophthalmol 113: 216, 1995.

86. Kaiser, HJ, Flammer, J, Graf, T, Stümpfig, D: Systemic blood pressure in glaucoma patients. Graefes Arch Clin Exp Ophthalmol 231:677, 1993.

87. Graham, SL, Drance, SM, Wijsman, K, et al: Ambulatory blood pressure monitoring in glaucoma. The nocturnal dip. Ophthalmology 102:61, 1995.

88. Béchetoille, A, Bresson-Dumont, H: Diurnal and nocturnal blood pressure drops in patients with focal ischemic glaucoma. Graefes Arch Clin Exp Ophthalmol 232:675, 1994.

89. Said, A, Labib, MAM, Abboud, I, Hegazi, A: The relationship between systemic hypertension and chronic simple glaucoma. Bull Ophthalmol Soc Egypt 60:71, 1967.

90. Shin, DH, Becker, B, Kolker, AE: Family history in primary open-angle glaucoma. Arch Ophthalmol 95:598, 1977.

91. Perkins, ES: Family studies in glaucoma. Br J Ophthalmol 58:529, 1974.

92. Kolker, AE: Glaucoma family study. Ten-year follow-up (preliminary report). Israel J Med Sci 8:1357, 1972.

93. Rosenthal, AR, Perkins, ES: Family studies in glaucoma. Br J Ophthalmol 69:664, 1985.

94. Tielsch, JM, Katz, J, Sommer, A, et al: Family history and risk of primary open angle glaucoma. The Baltimore eye survey. Arch Ophthalmol 112:69, 1994.

95. Pohjanpelto, PEJ, Plava, J: Ocular hypertension and glaucomatous optic nerve damage. Acta Ophthalmol 52:194, 1974.

96. Davanger, M, Ringvold, A, Bilka, S: The probability of having glaucoma at different IOP levels. Acta Ophthalmol 69:565, 1991.

97. Schwartz, B, Talusan, AG: Spontaneous trends in ocular pressure in untreated ocular hypertension. Arch Ophthalmol 98:105, 1980.

98. Leonard, TJK, Kerr-Muir, MG, Kirkby, GR, Hitchings, RA: Ocular hypertension and posture. Br J Ophthalmol 67:362, 1983.

99. Bengtsson, B: The prevalence of glaucoma. Br J Ophthalmol 65: 46, 1981.

100. Sommer, A, Tielsch, JM, Katz, J, et al: Relationship between intraocular pressure and primary open angle glaucoma among white and black Americans. The Baltimore eye survey. Arch Ophthalmol 109:1090, 1991.

101. Chandler, PA, Grant, WM: Lectures on Glaucoma. Philadelphia, Lea & Febiger, 1965, p. 13.

102. Yablonski, ME, Zimmerman, TJ, Kass, MA, Becker, B: Prognostic significance of optic disk cupping in ocular hypertensive patients. Am J Ophthalmol 89:585, 1980.

103. Hitchings, RA, Wheeler, CA: The optic disc in glaucoma. IV: optic disc evaluation in the ocular hypertensive patient. Br J Ophthalmol 64:232, 1980.

104. Sommer, A, Miller, NR, Pollack, I, et al: The nerve fiber layer in the diagnosis of glaucoma. Arch Ophthalmol 95:2149, 1977.

105. Daubs, JG, Crick, RP: Effect of refractive error on the risk of ocular hypertension and open angle glaucoma. Trans Ophthalmol Soc UK 101:121, 1981.

106. Perkins, ES, Phelps, CD: Open angle glaucoma, ocular hypertension, low-tension glaucoma, and refraction. Arch Ophthalmol 100: 1464, 1982.

107. Phelps, CD: Effect of myopia on prognosis in treated primary open-angle glaucoma. Am J Ophthalmol 93:622, 1982.

108. Buxton, JN, Preston, RW, Riechers, R, Guilbault, N: Tonography in cornea guttata. A preliminary report. Arch Ophthalmol 77:602, 1967.

109. Hiles, DA, Biglan, AW, Fetherolf, EC: Central corneal endothelial cell counts in children. Am Intra-Ocular Implant Soc J V:292, 1979.

110. Korey, M, Gieser, D, Kass, MA, et al: Central corneal endothelial cell density and central corneal thickness in ocular hypertension and primary open-angle glaucoma. Am J Ophthalmol 94:610, 1982.

111. Argus, WA: Ocular hypertension and central corneal thickness. Ophthalmology 102:1810, 1995.

112. Kimura, R, Levene, RZ: Gonioscopic differences between primary open-angle glaucoma and normal subjects over 40 years of age. Am J Ophthalmol 80:56, 1975.

113. Campbell, DG, Boys-Smith, JW, Woods, WD: Variation of pigmentation and segmentation of pigmentation in primary open angle glaucoma. Invest Ophthalmol Vis Sci 25(Suppl):122, 1984.

114. Kass, MA, Kolker, AE, Becker, B: Prognostic factors in glaucomatous visual field loss. Arch Ophthalmol 94:1274, 1976.

115. Susanna, R, Drance, SM, Douglas, GR: The visual prognosis of the fellow eye in uniocular chronic open-angle glaucoma. Br J Ophthalmol 62:327, 1978.

116. Caprioli, J, Spaeth, GL: Comparison of the optic nerve head in high- and low-tension glaucoma. Arch Ophthalmol 103:1145, 1985.

117. Gramer, E, Althaus, G, Leydhecker, W: Localization and depth of glaucomatous visual field defects in relation to the size of the neuroretinal rim area of the disk in low-tension glaucoma, glaucoma simplex, and pigmentary glaucoma. Clinical study with the octopus 201 perimeter and the optic nerve head analyzer. Klin Monatsbl Augenheilkd 189:190, 1986.

118. Yamagami, J, Araie, M, Shirato, S: A comparative study of optic nerve head in low- and high-tension glaucomas. Graefes Arch Clin Exp Ophthalmol 230:446, 1992.

119. Fazio, P, Krupin, T, Feitl, ME, et al: Optic disc topography in patients with low-tension and primary open angle glaucoma. Arch Ophthalmol 108:705, 1990.

120. Miller, KM, Quigley, HA: Comparison of optic disc features in low-tension and typical open-angle glaucoma. Ophthalmic Surg 18: 882, 1987.

121. Tuulonen, A, Airaksinen, PJ: Optic disc size in exfoliative, primary open angle, and low-tension glaucoma. Arch Ophthalmol 110: 211, 1992.

122. Kitazawa, Y, Shirato, S, Yamamoto, T: Optic disc hemorrhage in low-tension glaucoma. Ophthalmology 93:853, 1986.

123. Mikelberg, FS, Drance, SM, Schulzer, M, Wijsman, K: Possible significance of cilioretinal arteries in low-tension glaucoma. Can J Ophthalmol 25:298, 1990.

124. Yamazaki, Y, Koide, C, Miyazawa, T, et al: Comparison of retinal nerve-fiber layer in high- and normal-tension glaucoma. Graefes Arch Clin Exp Ophthalmol 229:517, 1991.

125. Drance, SM, Douglas, GR, Airaksinen, PJ, et al: Diffuse visual field loss in chronic open-angle and low-tension glaucoma. Am J Ophthalmol 104:577, 1987.

126. Chauhan, BC, Drance, SM, Douglas, GR, Johnson, CA: Visual field damage in normal-tension and high-tension glaucoma. Am J Ophthalmol 108:636, 1989.

127. Gramer, E, Althaus, G: The impact of intraocular pressure on visual field loss in primary open angle glaucoma. Klin Monatsbl Augenheilkd 197:218, 1990.

128. Zeiter, JH, Shin, DH, Juzych, MS, et al: Visual field defects in patients with normal-tension glaucoma and patients with high-tension glaucoma. Am J Ophthalmol 114:758, 1992.

129. King, D, Drance, SM, Douglas, G, et al: Comparison of visual field defects in normal-tension glaucoma and high-tension glaucoma. Am J Ophthalmol 101:204, 1986.

130. Caprioli, J, Spaeth GL: Comparison of visual field defects in the low-tension glaucomas with those in the high-tension glaucomas. Am J Ophthalmol 97:730, 1984.

131. Gliklich, RE, Steinmann, WC, Spaeth, GL: Visual field change in low-tension glaucoma over a five-year follow-up. Ophthalmology 96:316, 1989.

132. Gramer, E, Althaus, G: Quantification and progression of visual field damage in low-tension, primary open angle, and pigmentary glaucoma. Klin Monatsbl Augenheilkd 191:184, 1987.

133. Gramer, E, Leydhecker, W: Glaucoma without elevated IOP: A clinical study. Klin Monatsbl Augenheilkd 186:262, 1985.

134. Araie, M, Sekine, M, Suzuki, Y, Koseki, N: Factors contributing to the progression of visual field damage in eyes with normal-tension glaucoma. Ophthalmology 101:1440, 1994.

135. Noureddin, BN, Poinoosawmy, D, Fietzke, FW, Hitchings, RA: Regression analysis of visual field progression in low tension glaucoma. Br J Ophthalmol 75:493, 1991.

136. Cartwright, MJ, Anderson, DR: Correlation of asymmetric damage with asymmetric intraocular pressure in normal-tension glaucoma (low-tension glaucoma). Arch Ophthalmol 106:898, 1988.

137. Crichton, A, Drance, SM, Douglas, GR, Schulzer, M: Unequal intraocular pressure and its relation to asymmetric visual field defects in low-tension glaucoma. Ophthalmology 96:1312, 1989.

138. Tadayoshi, I, Tomita, G, Kitazawa, Y: Diurnal variation of intraocular pressure of normal-tension glaucoma. Influence of sleep and arousal. Ophthalmology 98:296, 1991.

139. Larsson, L-I, Rettig, ES, Sheridan, PT, Brubaker, RF: Aqueous humor dynamics in low-tension glaucoma. Am J Ophthalmol 116:590, 1993.

140. Yamagami, J, Araie, M, Aihara, M, Yamamoto, S: Diurnal variation in intraocular pressure of normal-tension glaucoma eyes. Ophthalmology 100:643, 1993.

141. Goldberg, I, Hollows, FC, Kass, MA, Becker, B: Systemic factors in patients with low-tension glaucoma. Br J Ophthalmol 65:56, 1981.

142. Hayreh, SS: Anterior Ischemic Optic Neuropathy. New York, Springer-Verlag, 1975, p. 22.

143. Perkins, ES, Phelps, CD: Ocular pulse amplitudes in low-tension glaucoma. Klin Monatsbl Augenheilkd 184:303, 1984.

144. James, CB, Smith, SE: Pulsatile ocular blood flow in patients with low tension glaucoma. Br J Ophthalmol 75:466, 1991.

145. Harris, A, Sergott, RC, Spaeth, GL, et al: Color Doppler analysis of ocular vessel blood velocity in normal-tension glaucoma. Am J Ophthalmol 118:642, 1994.

146. Yamazaki, Y, Hayamizu, F: Comparison of flow velocity of ophthalmic artery between primary open angle glaucoma and normal tension glaucoma. Br J Ophthalmol 79:732, 1995.

147. Pillunat, LE, Stodtmeister, R, Wilmanns, I: Pressure compliance of the optic nerve head in low tension glaucoma. Br J Ophthalmol 71:181, 1987.

148. Phelps, CD, Corbett, JJ: Migraine and low-tension glaucoma: A case-control study. Invest Ophthalmol Vis Sci 26:1105, 1985.

149. Usui, T, Iwata, K, Shirakashi, M, Abe, H: Prevalence of migraine in low-tension glaucoma and primary open-angle glaucoma in Japanese. Br J Ophthalmol 75:224, 1991.

150. Orgül, S, Flammer, J: Headache in normal-tension glaucoma patients. J Glau 3:292, 1994.

151. Drance, SM, Douglas, GR, Wijsman, K, et al: Response of blood flow to warm and cold in normal and low-tension glaucoma patients. Am J Ophthalmol 105:35, 1988.

152. Gasser, P, Flammer, J: Blood-cell velocity in the nailfold capillaries of patients with normal-tension and high-tension glaucoma. Am J Ophthalmol 111:585, 1991.

153. Usui, T, Iwata, K: Finger blood flow in patients with low tension glaucoma and primry open-angle glaucoma. Br J Ophthalmol 76:2, 1992.

154. Schulzer, M, Drance, SM, Carter, CJ, et al: Biostatistical evidence for two distinct chronic open angle glaucoma populations. Br J Ophthalmol 74:196, 1990.

155. Klaver, JHJ, Greve, EL, Goslinga, H, et al: Blood and plasma viscosity measurements in patients with glaucoma. Br J Ophthalmol 69:765, 1985.

156. Joist, JH, Lichtenfeld, P, Mandell, AI, Kolker, AE: Platelet function, blood coagulability, and fibrinolysis in patients with low tension glaucoma. Arch Ophthalmol 94:1893, 1976.

157. Carter, CJ, Brooks, DE, Doyle, DL, Drance, SM: Investigations into a vascular etiology for low-tension glaucoma. Ophthalmology 97:49, 1990.

158. Winder, AF: Circulating lipoprotein and blood glucose levels in association with low-tension and chronic simple glaucoma. Br J Ophthalmol 61:641, 1977.

159. Stroman, GA, Stewart, WC, Golnik, KC, et al: Magnetic resonance imaging in patients with low-tension glaucoma. Arch Ophthalmol 113:168, 1995.

160. Ong, K, Farinelli, A, Billson, F, et al: Comparative study of brain magnetic resonance imaging findings in patients with low-tension glaucoma and control subjects. Ophthalmology 102:1632, 1995.

161. Cartwright, MJ, Grajewski, AL, Friedberg, ML, et al: Immune-related disease and normal-tension glaucoma. A case-control study. Arch Ophthalmol 110:500, 1992.

162. Wax, MB, Barrett, DA, Pestronk, A: Increased incidence of paraproteinemia and autoantibodies in patients with normal-pressure glaucoma. Am J Ophthalmol 117:561, 1994.

163. Romano, C, Barrett, DA, Li, Z, et al: Anti-rhodopsin antibodies in sera from patients with normal-pressure glaucoma. Invest Ophthalmol Vis Sci 36:1968, 1995.

164. Bennett, SR, Alward, WLM, Folberg, R: An autosomal dominant form of low-tension glaucoma. Am J Ophthalmol 108:238, 1989.

165. Ritch, R: Nonprogressive low-tension glaucoma with pigmentary dispersion. Am J Ophthalmol 94:190, 1982.

166. Vucicevic, ZM, Ralston, J, Burns, WP, Gaffney, HP: Influence of the water drinking test on scleral rigidity. Arch Ophthalmol 82:761, 1969.

167. Armaly, MF: Water-drinking test. I. Characteristics of the ocular pressure response and the effect of age. Arch Ophthalmol 83:169, 1970.

168. Becker, B, Christensen, RE: Water-drinking and tonography in the diagnosis of glaucoma. Arch Ophthalmol 56:321, 1956.

169. Becker, B: Tonography in the diagnosis of simple (open angle) glaucoma. Trans Am Acad Ophthalmol Otol 65:156, 1961.

170. Spaeth, GL: The water drinking test. Indications that factors other than osmotic considerations are involved. Arch Ophthalmol 77:50, 1967.

171. Kimura, R: Clinical studies on glaucoma. Report III. The diagnostic significance of the water-drinking test. Acta Soc Ophthalmol Jpn 71:2133, 1967.

172. Ballin, N, Becker, B: Provocative testing for primary open-angle glaucoma in "senior citizens." Invest Ophthalmol 6:126, 1967.

173. Armaly, MF, Sayegh, RE: Water-drinking test. II. The effect of age on tonometric and tonographic measures. Arch Ophthalmol 83:176, 1970.

174. Kronfeld, PC: Water drinking and outflow facility. Invest Ophthalmol 14:49, 1975.

175. Thorpe, RM, Kolker, AE: A tonographic study of water loading in rabbits. Arch Ophthalmol 77:238, 1967.

176. Casey, WJ: Intraocular pressure and facility in monkeys after water drinking. A study in the Cynomolgus monkey, Macaca irus. Arch Ophthalmol 74:841, 1965.

177. Roth, JA: Inadequate diagnostic value of the water-drinking test. Br J Ophthalmol 58:55, 1974.

178. Rasmussen, KE, Jørgensen, HA: Diagnostic value of the water-drinking test in early detection of simple glaucoma. Acta Ophthalmol 54:160, 1976.

179. Harris, LS: Cycloplegic-induced intraocular pressure elevations. A study of normal and open-angle glaucomatous eyes. Arch Ophthalmol 79:242, 1968.

180. Lazenby, GW, Reed, JW, Grant, WM: Short-term tests of anticholinergic medication in open-angle glaucoma. Arch Ophthalmol 80:443, 1968.

181. Lazenby, GW, Reed, JW, Grant, WM: Anticholinergic medication in open-angle glaucoma. Long-term tests. Arch Ophthalmol 84:719, 1970.

182. Harris, LS, Galin, MA: Cycloplegic provocative testing. Arch Ophthalmol 81:356, 1969.

183. Harris, LS, Galin, MA, Mittag, TW: Cycloplegic provocative testing after topical administration of steroids. Arch Ophthalmol 86:12, 1971.

184. Harris, LS, Galin, MA: Cycloplegic provocative testing. Effect of miotic therapy. Arch Ophthalmol 81:544, 1969.

185. Båråny, E, Christensen, RE: Cycloplegia and outflow resistance in normal human and monkey eyes and in primary open-angle glaucoma. Arch Ophthalmol 77:757, 1967.

186. Portney, GL, Purcell, TW: The influence of tropicamide on intraocular pressure. Ann Ophthalmol 7:31, 1975.

187. Shaw, BR, Lewis, RA: Intraocular pressure elevation after pupillary dilation in open angle glaucoma. Arch Ophthalmol 104:1185, 1986.

188. Kristensen, P: Mydriasis-induced pigment liberation in the anterior chamber associated with acute rise in intraocular pressure in open-angle glaucoma. Acta Ophthalmol 43:714, 1965.

189. Kristensen, P: Pigment liberation test in open-angle glaucoma. Acta Ophthalmol 46:586, 1968.

190. Valle, O: The cyclopentolate provocative test in suspected or untreated open-angle glaucoma. III. The significance of pigment for the result of the cyclopentolate provocative test in suspected or untreated open-angle glaucoma. Acta Ophthalmol 54:654, 1976.

191. Mapstone, R: Pigment release. Br J Ophthalmol 65:258, 1981.

192. Haddad, R, Strasser, G, Heilig, P, Jurecka, W: Decompensation of chronic open-angle glaucoma following mydriasis-induced pigmentary dispersion into the aqueous humour: a light and electron microscopic study. Br J Ophthalmol 65:252, 1981.

193. Becker, B, Montgomery, SW, Kass, MA, Shin, DH: Increased ocular and systemic responsiveness to epinephrine in primary open-angle glaucoma. Arch Ophthalmol 95:789, 1977.

194. Shin, DH, Kass, MA, Becker, B: Intraocular pressure response to topical epinephrine and HLA-B12. Arch Ophthalmol 96:1012, 1978.

195. Palmberg, PF, Hajek, S, Cooper, D, Becker, B: Increased cellular responsiveness to epinephrine in primary open-angle glaucoma. Arch Ophthalmol 95:855, 1977.

196. Becker, B, Shin, DH: Response to topical epinephrine. A practical prognostic test in patients with ocular hypertension. Arch Ophthalmol 94:2057, 1976.

197. Kass, MA, Becker, B: A simplified test of epinephrine responsiveness. Arch Ophthalmol 96:999, 1978.

198. Drance, SM, Saheb, NE, Schulzer, M: Response to topical epinephrine in chronic open-angle glaucoma. Arch Ophthalmol 96:1001, 1978.

199. Hollwich, F: The pilocarpine-test for the early diagnosis of glaucoma. Klin Monatsbl Augenheilkd 163:115, 1973.

200. Nissen, OI, Kjer, P, Olsen, L: A comparison between an acetazolamide test and weight tonography in pathological and apathological circulation of the aqueous humor. Invest Ophthalmol 15:844, 1976.

201. Drance, SM: The uniocular therapeutic trial in the management of elevated intraocular pressure. Surv Ophthalmol 25:203, 1980.

202. Rothkoff, L, Biedner, B, Biger, Y, Blumenthal, M: A proposed pilocarpine therapeutic test. Arch Ophthalmol 96:1380, 1978.

203. Lewis, JM, Priddy, T, Judd, J, et al: Intraocular pressure response to topical dexamethasone as a predictor for the development of primary open-angle glaucoma. Am J Ophthalmol 106:607, 1988.

204. Klemetti, A: The dexamethasone provocative test: A predictive tool for glaucoma? Acta Ophthalmol 68:29, 1990.

205. Drance, SM: Studies in the susceptibility of the eye to raised intraocular pressure. Arch Ophthalmol 68:478, 1962.

206. Goldmann, H: Open-angle glaucoma. Br J Ophthalmol 56:242, 1972.

207. Wodowosow, AM, Boriskina, MG, Kotjeljnikowa, OF: Further observations concerning the campimetric method of measuring individually tolerated intraocular pressure in glaucoma. Klin Monatsbl Augenheilkd 180:135, 1982.

208. Becker, B, Morton, WR: Phenylthiourea taste testing and glaucoma. Arch Ophthalmol 72:323, 1964.

209. Kalmus, H, Lewkonia, I: Relation between some forms of glaucoma and phenylthiocarbamide tasting. Br J Ophthalmol 57:503, 1973.

210. Shin, DH, Becker, B, Waltman, SR, et al: The prevalence of HLA-B12 and HLA-B7 antigens in primary open-angle glaucoma. Arch Ophthalmol 95:224, 1977.

211. Ritch, R, Podos, SM, Henley, W, et al: Lack of association of histocompatibility antigens with primary open-angle glaucoma. Arch Ophthalmol 96:2204, 1978.

212. Shaw, JF, Levene, RZ, Sowell, JG: The incidence of HLA antigens in black primary open-angle glaucoma patients. Am J Ophthalmol 86:501, 1978.

213. Damgaard-Jensen, L, Kissmeyer-Nielsen, F: HLA histocompatibility antigens in open-angle glaucoma. Acta Ophthalmol 56:384, 1978.

214. Scharf, J, Gideoni, O, Zonis, S, Barzilai, A: Histocompatibility antigens (HLA) and open-angle glaucoma. Ann Ophthalmol 10:914, 1978.

215. David, R, Maier, G, Baumgarten, I, Abrahams, C: HLA antigens in glaucoma and ocular hypertension. Br J Ophthalmol 63:293, 1979.

216. Rosenthal, AR, Payne, R: Association of HLA antigens and primary open-angle glaucoma. Am J Ophthalmol 88:479, 1979.

217. Ticho, U, Cohen, T, Brautbar, C: Absence of association betwen HLA antigens and primary open-angle glaucoma in Israel. Israel J Med Sci 15:124, 1979.

218. Kass, MA, Palmberg, P, Becker, B, Miller, JP: Histocompatibility antigens and primary open-angle glaucoma. A reassessment. Arch Ophthalmol 96:2207, 1978.

219. Olivius, E, Polland, W: Histocompatibility (HLA) antigens in capsular glaucoma and simplex glaucoma. Acta Ophthalmol 58:406, 1980.

220. Slagsvold, JE, Nordhagen, R: The HLA system in primary open-angle glaucoma and in patients with pseudoexfoliation of the lens capsule (exfoliation or fibrillopathia epitheliocapsularis). Acta Ophthalmol 58:188, 1980.

221. Grant, WM: Further studies on facility of flow through the trabecular meshwork. Arch Ophthalmol 60:523, 1958.

222. Ashton, N: The exit pathway of the aqueous. Trans Ophthalmol Soc UK 80:397, 1960.

223. Speakman, JS, Leeson, TS: Site of obstruction to aqueous outflow in chronic simple glaucoma. Br J Ophthalmol 46:321, 1962.

224. Zatulina, NI: Electron-microscopy of trabecular tissue in far-advanced stage of simple open-angle glaucoma. Oftal Z 28:117, 1973.

225. Li, Y, Yi, Y: Histochemical and electron microscopic studies of the trabecular meshwork in primary open-angle glaucoma. Eye Sci 1:17, 1985.

226. Segawa, K: Electron microscopic changes of the trabecular tissue in primary open-angle glaucoma. Ann Ophthalmol 11:49, 1979.

227. Finkelstein, I, Trope, GE, Basu, PK, et al: Quantitative analysis of collagen content and amino acids in trabecular meshwork. Br J Ophthalmol 74:280, 1990.

228. Fine, BS, Yanoff, M, Stone, RA: A clinicopathologic study of four cases of primary open-angle glaucoma compared to normal eyes. Am J Ophthalmol 91:88, 1981.

229. Alvarado, J, Murphy, C, Juster, R: Trabecular meshwork cellularity in primary open-angle glaucoma and nonglaucomatous normals. Ophthalmology 91:564, 1984.

230. Tripathi, RC, Tripathi, BJ: Contractile protein alteration in trabecular endothelium in primary open-angle glaucoma. Exp Eye Res 31:721, 1981.

231. Clark, AF, Miggans, ST, Wilson, K, et al: Cytoskeletal changes in cultured human glaucoma trabecular meshwork cells. J Glau 4:183, 1995.

232. Armaly, MF, Wang, Y: Demonstration of acid mucopolysaccharides in the trabecular meshwork of the Rhesus monkey. Invest Ophthalmol 14:507, 1975.

233. Knepper, PA, Covici, S, Fadel, JR, et al: Surface-tension properties of hyaluronic acid. J Glau 4:194, 1995.

234. Chaudhry, HA, Dueker, DK, Simmons, RJ, et al: Scanning electron microscopy of trabeculectomy specimens in open-angle glaucoma. Am J Ophthalmol 88:78, 1979.

235. Maglio, M, McMahon, C, Hoskins, D, Alvarado, J: Potential artifacts in scanning electron microscopy of the trabecular meshwork in glaucoma. Am J Ophthalmol 90:645, 1980.

236. Quigley, HA, Addicks, EM: Scanning electron microscopy of trabeculectomy specimens from eyes with open-angle glaucoma. Am J Ophthalmol 90:854, 1980.

237. Gieser, DK, Tanenbaum, M, Smith, ME, et al: Amorphous coating in open-angle glaucoma. Am J Ophthalmol 92:130, 1981.

238. Rohen, JW: Fine structural changes in the trabecular meshwork of the human eye in different forms of glaucoma. Klin Monatsbl Augenheilkd 163:401, 1973.

239. Zimmerman, LE: The outflow problem in normal and pathologic eyes. Trans Am Acad Ophthalmol Otol 70:767, 1966.

240. Rodrigues, MM, Spaeth, GL, Sivalingam, E, Weinreb, S: Value of trabeculectomy specimens in glaucoma. Ophthalmic Surg 9:29, 1978.

241. Alvarado, JA, Yun, AJ, Murphy, CG: Juxtacanalicular tissue in primary open angle glaucoma and in nonglaucomatous normals. Arch Ophthalmol 104:1517, 1986.

242. Rohen, JW: Presence of matrix vesicles in the trabecular meshwork of glaucomatous eyes. Graefes Arch Clin Exp Ophthalmol 218:171, 1982.

243. Rohen, JW: Why is intraocular pressure elevated in chronic simple glaucoma? Ophthalmology 90:758, 1983.

244. Babizhayev, MA, Brodskaya, MW: Fibronectin detection in drainage outflow system of human eyes in ageing and progression of open-angle glaucoma. Mech Ageing Dev 47:145, 1989.

245. Umihira, J, Nagata, S, Nohara, M, et al: Localization of elastin in the normal and glaucomatous human trabecular meshwork. Invest Ophthalmol Vis Sci 35:486, 1994.

246. Worthen, DM, Cleveland, PH, Slight, JR, Abare, J: Selective binding affinity of human plasma fibronectin for the collagens I-IV. Invest Ophthalmol Vis Sci 26:1740, 1985.

247. Murphy, CG, Johnson, M, Alvarado, JA: Juxtacanalicular tissue in pigmentary and primary open angle glaucoma. The hydrodynamic role of pigment and other constituents. Arch Ophthalmol 110:1779, 1992.

248. Tripathi, RC: Ultrastructure of the trabecular wall of Schlemm's canal. (A study of normotensive and chronic simple glaucomatous eyes.) Trans Ophthalmol Soc UK 89:449, 1969.

249. Tripathi, RC: Ultrastructure of Schlemm's canal in relation to aqueous outflow. Exp Eye Res 7:335, 1968.

250. Allingham, RR, de Kater, AW, Ethier, CR, et al: The relationship between pore density and outflow facility in human eyes. Invest Ophthalmol Vis Sci 33:1661, 1992.

251. Alvarado, JA, Murphy, CG: Outflow obstruction in pigmentary and primary open angle glaucoma. Arch Ophthalmol 110:1769, 1992.

252. Nesterov, AP, Batmanov, YE: Trabecular wall of Schlemm's canal in the early stage of primary open-angle glaucoma. Am J Ophthalmol 78:639, 1974.

253. Moses, RA, Grodski, WJ Jr, Etheridge, EL, Wilson, CD: Schlemm's canal: the effect of intraocular pressure. Invest Ophthalmol Vis Sci 20:61, 1981.

254. Johnson, MC, Kamm, RD: The role of Schlemm's canal in aqueous outflow from the human eye. Invest Ophthalmol Vis Sci 24:320, 1983.

255. de Kater, AW, Melamed, S, Epstein, DL: Patterns of aqueous human outflow in glaucomatous and nonglaucomatous human eyes. A tracer study using cationized ferritin. Arch Ophthalmol 107:572, 1989.

256. Buller, C, Johnson, D: Segmental variability of the trabecular meshwork in normal and glaucomatous eyes. Invest Ophthalmol Vis Sci 35:3841, 1994.

257. Krasnov, MM: Sinusotomy. Foundations, results, prospects. Trans Am Acad Ophthalmol Otol 76:368, 1972.

258. Herschler, J, Litin, BS: Biochemical abnormalities in the aqueous in chronic open-angle glaucoma. Ophthalmic Surg 18:792, 1987.

259. Tripathi, RC, Li, J, Borisuth, NSC, Tripathi, BJ: Trabecular cells of the eye express messenger RNA for transforming growth factor-β1 and secrete this cytokine. Invest Ophthalmol Vis Sci 34:2562, 1993.

260. Tripathi, RC, Li, J, Chan, WFA, Tripathi, BJ: Aqueous humor in glaucomatous eyes contains an increased level of TGF-β2. Exp Eye Res 59:723, 1994.

261. Gonzalez-Avila, G, Ginebra, M, Hayakawa, T, et al: Collagen metabolism in human aqueous humor from primary open-angle glaucoma. Decreased degradation and increased biosynthesis play a role in its pathogenesis. Arch Ophthalmol 113:1319, 1995.

262. Becker, B, Hahn, KA: Topical corticosteroids and heredity in primary open-angle glaucoma. Am J Ophthalmol 57:543, 1964.

263. Armaly, MF: The heritable nature of dexamethasone-induced ocular hypertension. Arch Ophthalmol 75:32, 1966.

264. Armaly, MF: Inheritance of dexamethasone hypertension and glaucoma. Arch Ophthalmol 77:747, 1967.

265. Schwartz, JT, Reuling, FH, Feinleib, M, et al: Twin study on ocular pressure after topical dexamethasone. 1. Frequency distribution of pressure response. Am J Ophthalmol 76:126, 1973.

266. Palmberg, PF, Mandell, A, Wilensky, JT, et al: The reproducibility of the intraocular pressure response to dexamethasone. Am J Ophthalmol 80:844, 1975.

267. Dean, GO Jr, Deutsch, AR, Hiatt, RL: The effect of dexamethasone on borderline ocular hypertension. Ann Ophthalmol 7:193, 1975.

268. Levene, R, Wigdor, A, Edelstein, A, Baum, J: Topical corticosteroid in normal patients and glaucoma suspects. Arch Ophthalmol 77:593, 1967.

269. LeBlanc, RP, Stewart, RH, Becker, B: Corticosteroid provocative testing. Invest Ophthalmol 9:946, 1970.

270. Kitazawa, Y, Horie, T: The prognosis of corticosteroid-responsive individuals. Arch Ophthalmol 99:819, 1981.

271. Akingbehin, AO: Corticosteroid-induced ocular hypertension. I. Prevalence in closed-angle glaucoma. Br J Ophthalmol 66:536, 1982.

272. Kitazawa, Y: Primary angle-closure glaucoma. Corticosteroid responsiveness. Arch Ophthalmol 84:724, 1970.

273. Krupin, T, Schoch, LH, Cooper, D, Becker, B: Lack of correlation between ocular hypertensive response to topical corticosteroids and progression of retinopathy in insulin-dependent diabetes mellitus. Am J Ophthalmol 96:52, 1983.

274. Becker, B: The genetic problem of chronic simple glaucoma. Ann Ophthalmol 3:351, 1971.

275. Francois, J, Heintz-De Bree, C, Tripathi, RC: The cortisone test and the heredity of primary open-angle glaucoma. Am J Ophthalmol 62:844, 1966.

276. Schwartz, JT, Reuling, FH, Feinleib, M, et al: Twin heritability study of the effect of corticosteroids on intraocular pressure. J Med Genet 9:137, 1972.

277. Schwartz, JT, Reuling, FH Jr, Feinleib, M, et al: Twin heritability study of the corticosteroid response. Trans Am Acad Ophthalmol Otol 77:126, 1973.

278. Schwartz, JT, Reuling, FH, Feinleib, M, et al: Twin study on ocular pressure following topically applied dexamethasone. II. Inheritance of variation in pressure response. Arch Ophthalmol 90:281, 1973.

279. Akingbehin, AO: Corticosteroid-induced ocular hypertension. II. An acquired form. Br J Ophthalmol 66:541, 1982.

280. Spaeth, GL: Traumatic hyphema, angle recession, dexamethasone hypertension, and glaucoma. Arch Ophthalmol 78:714, 1967.

281. Schwartz, B, Levene, RZ: Plasma cortisol differences between normal and glaucomatous patients. Before and after dexamethasone suppression. Arch Ophthalmol 87:369, 1972.

282. Schwartz B, McCarty, G, Rosner, B: Increased plasma free cortisol in ocular hypertension and open angle glaucoma. Arch Ophthalmol 105:1060, 1987.

283. Krupin, T, Podos, SM, Becker, B: Effect of diphenylhydantoin on dexamethasone suppression of plasma cortisol in primary open-angle glaucoma. Am J Ophthalmol 71:997, 1971.

284. Meredig, WE, Puelhorn, G, Jentzen, F, Hartmann, F: The plasmacortisol-level in patients suffering from glaucoma. Graefes Arch Clin Exp Ophthalmol 213:215, 1980.

285. Schwartz, B, Seddon, JM: Increased plasma cortisol levels in ocular hypertension. Arch Ophthalmol 99:1791, 1981.

286. McCarty, GR, Schwartz, B: Increased plasma noncortisol glucocorticoid activity in open-angle glaucoma. Invest Ophthalmol Vis Sci 32:1600, 1991.

287. Rosenberg, S, Levene, R: Suppression of plasma cortisol in normal and glaucomatous patients. Arch Ophthalmol 92:6, 1974.

288. Levene, RZ, Schwartz, B, Workman, PL: Heritability of plasma cortisol. Arch Ophthalmol 87:389, 1972.

289. Becker, B, Ramsey, CK: Plasma cortisol and the intraocular pressure response to topical corticosteroids. Am J Ophthalmol 69:999, 1970.

290. Podos, SM, Becker, B, Beaty, C, Cooper, DG: Diphenylhydantoin and cortisol metabolism in glaucoma. Am J Ophthalmol 74:498, 1972.

291. Becker, B, Podos, SM, Asseff, CF, Cooper, DG: Plasma cortisol suppression in glaucoma. Am J Ophthalmol 75:73, 1973.

292. Krupin, T, Jacobs, LS, Podos, SM, Becker, B: Thyroid function and the intraocular pressure response to topical corticosteroids. Am J Ophthalmol 83:643, 1977.

293. Polansky, J, Palmberg, P, Matulich, D, et al: Cellular sensitivity to glucocorticoids in patients with POAG. Steroid receptors and responses in cultured skin fibroblasts. Invest Ophthalmol Vis Sci 26:805, 1985.

294. Levene, RZ, Schwartz, B: Depression of plasma cortisol and the steroid ocular pressure response. Arch Ophthalmol 80:461, 1968.

295. Schwartz, B: Hypothalamic-pituitary-adrenal axis and steroid glaucoma. Klin Monatsbl Augenheilkd 161:280, 1972.

296. Kass, MA, Krupin, T, Becker, B: Plasma cortisol suppression test used to predict the development of primary open-angle glaucoma. Am J Ophthalmol 82:496, 1976.

297. Bigger, JF, Palmberg, PF, Becker, B: Increased cellular sensitivity to glucocorticoids in primary open-angle glaucoma. Invest Ophthalmol 11:832, 1972.

298. Foon, KA, Yuen, K, Ballintine, EF, Rosenstreich, DL: Analysis of the systemic corticosteroid sensitivity of patients with primary open-angle glaucoma. Am J Ophthalmol 83:167, 1977.

299. BenEzra, D, Ticho, U, Sachs, U: Lymphocyte sensitivity to glucocorticoids. Am J Ophthalmol 82:866, 1976.

300. Sowell, JC, Levene, RZ, Bloom, J, Bernstein, M: Primary open-angle glaucoma and sensitivity to corticosteroids in vitro. Am J Ophthalmol 84:715, 1977.

301. McCarty, G, Schwartz, B, Miller, K: Absence of lymphocyte glucocorticoid hypersensitivity in primary open-angle glaucoma. Arch Ophthalmol 99:1258, 1981.

302. Palmberg, PF, Rachlin, D, Becker, B: Differential sensitivity at the cellular level in primary open-angle glaucoma: prednisolone and ouabain. Invest Ophthalmol 15:403, 1976.

303. Schwartz, B, Golden, MA, Wiznia, RA, Miller, SA: Differences of adrenal stress control mechanisms in subjects with glaucoma and normal subjects. Effect of vasopressin and pyrogen. Arch Ophthalmol 99:1770, 1981.

304. Kass, MA, Shin, DH, Becker, B: The ocular hypotensive effect of epinephrine in high and low corticosteroid responders. Invest Ophthalmol 16:530, 1977.

305. Zink, HA, Palmberg, PF, Bigger, JF: Increased sensitivity to theophylline associated with primary open-angle glaucoma. Invest Ophthalmol 12:603, 1973.

306. Francois, J, Victoria-Troncoso, V: Mucopolysaccharides and pathogenesis of cortisone glaucoma. Klin Monatsbl Augenheilkd 165:5, 1974.

307. Bill, A: The drainage of aqueous humor. Invest Ophthalmol 14:1, 1975.

308. Southren, AL, Gordon, GG, Munnangi, PR, et al: Altered cortisol metabolism in cells cultured from trabecular meshwork specimens obtained from patients with primary open-angle glaucoma. Invest Ophthalmol Vis Sci 24:1413, 1983.

309. Becker, B, Keates, EU, Coleman, SL: Gamma-globulin in the trabecular meshwork of glaucomatous eyes. Arch Ophthalmol 68:643, 1962.

310. Becker, B, Unger, H-H, Coleman, SL, Keates, EU: Plasma cells and gamma-globulin in trabecular meshwork of eyes with primary open-angle glaucoma. Arch Ophthalmol 70:38, 1963.

311. Waltman, SR, Yarian, D: Antinuclear antibodies in open-angle glaucoma. Invest Ophthalmol 13:695, 1974.

312. Shields, MB, McCoy, RC, Shelburne, JD: Immunofluorescent studies on the trabecular meshwork in open-angle glaucoma. Invest Ophthalmol 15:1014, 1976.

313. Rodrigues, MM, Katz, SI, Foidart, JM, Spaeth, GL: Collagen, Factor VIII antigen, and immunoglobulins in the human aqueous drainage channels. Ophthalmology 87:337, 1980.

314. Radda, TM, Gnad, HC, Aberer, W: The questionable immunopathogenesis of primary open-angle glaucoma. Klin Monatsbl Augenheilkd 181:388, 1982.

315. Felberg, NT, Leon, SA, Gasparini, J, Spaeth, GL: A comparison of antinuclear antibodies and DNA-binding antibodies in chronic open-angle glaucoma. Invest Ophthalmol Vis Sci 16:757, 1977.

316. Radda, TM, Menzel, J, Drobec, P, Aberer, W: Immunological investigation in primary open angle glaucoma. Graefes Arch Clin Exp Ophthalmol 218:55, 1982.

317. Henley, WL, Okas, S, Leopold, IH: Cellular immunity in chronic ophthalmic disorders. 4. Leukocyte migration inhibition in diseases associated with glaucoma. Am J Ophthalmol 76:60, 1973.

318. Johnson, AT, Drack, AV, Kwitek, AE, et al: Clinical features and linkage analysis of a family with autosomal dominant juvenile glaucoma. Ophthalmology 100:524, 1993.

319. Richards, JE, Lichter, PR, Boehnke, M, et al: Mapping of a gene for autosomal dominant juvenile-onset open-angle glaucoma to chromosome 1q. Am J Hum Gen 54:62, 1994.

320. Lichter, PR: Genetic clues to glaucoma's secrets. The L. Edward Jackson Memorial Lecture. Part 2. Am J Ophthalmol 117:706, 1994.

321. Quigley, HA, Maumenee, AE: Long-term follow-up of treated open-angle glaucoma. Am J Ophthalmol 87:519, 1979.

322. Vogel, R, Crick, RP, Newson, RB, et al: Association between intraocular pressure and loss of visual field in chronic simple glaucoma. Br J Ophthalmol 74:3, 1990.

323. Drance, SM, Schulzer, M, Douglas, GR, Sweeney, VP: Use of discriminant analysis. II. Identification of persons with glaucomatous visual field defects. Arch Ophthalmol 96:1571, 1978.

324. Kass, MA, Hart, WM Jr, Gordon, M, Miller, JP: Risk factors favoring the development of glaucomatous visual field loss in ocular hypertension. Surv Ophthalmol 25:155, 1980.

325. Armaly, MF, Krueger, DE, Maunder, L, et al: Biostatistical analysis of the collaborative glaucoma study. I. Summary report of the risk factors for glaucomatous visual-field defects. Arch Ophthalmol 98:2163, 1980.

326. Epstein, DL, Krug, JH, Jr, Hertzmark, E, et al: A long-term clinical trial of timolol therapy versus no treatment in the management of glaucoma suspects. Ophthalmology 96:1460, 1989.

327. Kass, MA, Gordon, MO, Hoff, MR, et al: Topical timolol administration reduces the incidence of glaucomatous damage in ocular hypertensive individuals. Arch Ophthalmol 107:1590, 1989.

328. Schulzer, M, Drance, SM, Douglas, GR: A comparison of treated and untreated glaucoma suspects. Ophthalmology 98:301, 1991.

329. Goldmann, H: An analysis of some concepts concerning chronic simple glaucoma. Am J Ophthalmol 80:409, 1975.

330. Begg, IS, Cottle, RW, Collaborative Glaucoma Study Group: Epidemological approach to open-angle glaucoma: 1. Control of intraocular pressure. Report of the Canadian Ocular Adverse Drug Reaction Registry Program. Can J Ophthalmol 23:273, 1988.

331. Kolker, AE: Visual prognosis in advanced glaucoma: a comparison of medical and surgical therapy for retention of vision in 101 eyes with advanced glaucoma. Trans Am Ophthalmol Soc 75:539, 1977.

332. Mao, LK, Stewart, WC, Shields, MB: Correlation between intraocular pressure control and progressive glaucomatous damage in primary open-angle glaucoma. Am J Ophthalmol 111:51, 1991.

333. Wilson, R, Walker, AM, Dueker, DK, Crick, RP: Risk factors for rate of progression of glaucomatous visual field loss. A computer-based analysis. Arch Ophthalmol 100:737, 1982.

334. Odberg, T: Visual field prognosis in advanced glaucoma. Acta Ophthalmol 65(Suppl) 182:27, 1987.

335. Schulzer, M, Mikelberg, FS, Drance, SM: Some observations on the relation between intraocular pressure reduction and the progression of glaucomatous visual loss. Br J Ophthalmol 71:486, 1987.

336. Spaeth, GL: Control of glaucoma: a new definition. Ophthalmic Surg 14:303, 1983.

337. Spaeth, GL, Fellman, RL, Starita, RL, et al: A new management system for glaucoma based on improvement of the appearance of the optic disc or visual field. Trans Am Ophthalmol Soc 83:268, 1985.

338. Shin, DH, Bielik, M, Hong, YJ, et al: Reversal of glaucomatous optic disc cupping in adult patients. Arch Ophthalmol 115:1599, 1989.

339. Bloch, S, Rosenthal, AR, Friedman, L, Caldarolla, P: Patient compliance in glaucoma. Br J Ophthalmol 61:531, 1977.

340. MacKean, JM, Elkington, AR: Compliance with treatment of patients with chronic open-angle glaucoma. Br J Ophthalmol 67:46, 1983.

341. Smith, RJH: The enigma of primary open angle glaucoma. Trans Ophthalmol Soc UK 105:618, 1986.

342. Jay, JL, Murray, SB: Early trabeculectomy versus conventional management in primary open angle glaucoma. Br J Ophthalmol 72:881, 1988.

343. Migdal, C, Hitchings, R: Control of chronic simple glaucoma with primary medical, surgical and laser treatment. Trans Ophthalmol Soc UK 105:653, 1986.

344. Migdal, C, Gregory, W, Hitchings, R: Long-term functional outcome after early surgery compared with laser and medicine in open-angle glaucoma. Ophthalmology 101:1651, 1994.

345. Schulzer, M, The Normal Tension Glaucoma Study Group: Intraocular pressure reduction in normal-tension glaucoma patients. Ophthalmology 99:1468, 1992.

346. Bloomfield, S: The results of surgery for low-tension glaucoma. Am J Ophthalmol 36:1067, 1953.

347. Sugar, HS: Low tension glaucoma: a practical approach. Ann Ophthalmol 11:1155, 1979.

348. Abedin, S, Simmons, RJ, Grant, WM: Progressive low-tension glaucoma. Treatment to stop glaucomatous cupping and field loss when these progress despite normal intraocular pressure. Ophthalmology 89:1, 1982.

349. Yamamoto, T, Ichien, M, Suemori-Matsushita, H, Kitazawa, Y: Trabeculectomy with mitomycin C for normal-tension glaucoma. J Glau 4:158, 1995.

350. Kitazawa, Y, Shirai, H, Go, FJ: The effect of Ca^{2+}-antagonist on visual field in low-tension glaucoma. Graefes Arch Clin Exp Ophthalmol 227:408, 1989.

351. Lumme, P, Tuulonen, A, Airaksinen, PJ, Alanko, HI: Neuroretinal rim area in low tension glaucoma: Effect of nifedipine and acetazolamide compared to no treatment. Acta Ophthalmol 69: 293, 1991.

352. Netland, PA, Grosskreutz, CL, Feke, GT, Hart, LJ: Color doppler ultrasound analysis of ocular circulation after topical calcium channel blocker. Am J Ophthalmol 119:694, 1995.

353. Bose, S, Piltz, JR, Breton, ME: Nimodipine, a centrally active calcium antagonist, exerts a beneficial effect on contrast sensitivity in patients with normal-tension glaucoma and in control subjects. Ophthalmology 102:1236, 1995.

354. Netland, PA, Chaturvedi, N, Dreyer, EB: Calcium channel blockers in the management of low-tension and open-angle glaucoma. Am J Ophthalmol 115:608, 1993.

Chapter 10

PUPILLARY-BLOCK GLAUCOMAS[a]

TERMINOLOGY

"Primary" versus "Secondary" Angle-Closure Glaucomas

As discussed in Chapter 8, angle-closure glaucomas are characterized by apposition of peripheral iris against trabecular meshwork, resulting in obstruction of aqueous outflow. Traditionally, some forms of angle-closure glaucoma have been referred to as *primary angle-closure glaucoma,* either because the mechanisms of angle closure were not felt to be associated with other ocular or systemic abnormalities or because the mechanisms were not well-understood. Conditions that have been included in this group are *pupillary block glaucoma, plateau iris,* and *combined mechanism glaucoma.* Other forms of angle-closure glaucoma have been called *secondary angle-closure glaucoma,* either because of associated ocular or systemic abnormalities or because of more apparent mechanisms of angle closure, such as contracting membranes or inflammatory precipitates that pull the angle closed, or space occupying lesions that push it closed. As continued research has expanded our knowledge concerning the associ-

ated abnormalities and mechanisms of "primary" angle-closure glaucomas, however, a distinction between the "primary" and "secondary" forms has become increasingly artificial, and the concept should probably be abandoned.

One example of how continued expansion of our knowledge has progressively blurred the distinction between "primary" and "secondary" glaucomas is seen in the condition called plateau iris (1–3). As noted above, this condition has traditionally been included with the "primary angle-closure glaucomas." However, as a result of new information regarding the mechanism of plateau iris, it is considered with the glaucomas associated with disorders of the iris and ciliary body in Chapter 14.

In this chapter, we consider several forms of glaucoma which share the common mechanism of pupillary block and that have traditionally been grouped as "primary angle-closure glaucomas." Those conditions that have been called "secondary angle-closure glaucomas" are considered in subsequent chapters in Section Two.

Pupillary-Block Glaucoma

This category of angle-closure glaucoma is the most common form within these conditions. The initiating event is felt

[a]Refer to Shields, MB: Color Atlas of Glaucoma. Baltimore, Williams & Wilkins, 1998, Plates II2–3.

to be a functional block between the pupillary portion of the iris and the anterior lens surface (4), which is associated with mid-dilatation of the pupil (5). The functional block causes a buildup of aqueous in the posterior chamber, leading to a forward shift of the peripheral iris and closure of the anterior chamber angle (Fig. 10.1) (4–6). Four forms of pupillary block glaucoma may be distinguished on the basis of symptoms and clinical findings.

Acute Angle-Closure Glaucoma

In this form of pupillary block glaucoma, the symptoms are sudden and severe, with marked pain, blurred vision, and a red eye. The condition was once referred to as congestive glaucoma (7).

Subacute Angle-Closure Glaucoma

This clinical entity is felt to have the same pupillary block mechanism as the acute form, but symptoms are either mild or absent (8). The condition has also been called intermittent, prodromal, or subclinical (9), and was probably once lumped with the "noncongestive" glaucomas (7). However, the latter term also included open-angle glaucoma and has been largely abandoned since Barkan (7) classified the glaucomas on the basis of an open or closed anterior chamber angle. Patients with subacute angle-closure glaucoma may have repeated subacute or subclinical attacks before finally having an acute attack or developing peripheral anterior synechiae with chronic pressure elevation (8).

Chronic Angle-Closure Glaucoma

In this condition, portions of the anterior chamber angle are permanently closed by peripheral anterior synechiae, and the intraocular pressure (IOP) is chronically elevated (9, 10). The synechial closure may result from a prolonged acute attack or repeated subacute attacks of angle-closure glaucoma. A vari-

ation of this condition has been called shortening of the angle (11), or creeping angle-closure glaucoma (12).

Combined Mechanism Glaucoma

In some eyes there appears to be both an open-angle and an angle-closure mechanism to the glaucoma. The diagnosis is usually made after an acute angle-closure glaucoma attack in which the IOP remains elevated after a peripheral iridotomy, despite an open, normal appearing angle. In one study, this was seen in 6 of 267 (2.2%) eyes that underwent peripheral iridectomy for presumed angle-closure glaucoma (13).

EPIDEMIOLOGY

In most populations, pupillary block glaucoma is considerably less common than chronic open-angle glaucoma, although a precise ratio between the two conditions has not been clearly established. However, there is a reversal in the ratio of angle-closure and open-angle glaucoma among Canadian (14), Alaskan (15), and Greenland (16, 17) Eskimos, with the former disorder occurring in approximately 0.5% of the general population and in 2–3% of those over 40 years of age, with a predilection for women. A similar observation was made in a mixed ethnic group in South Africa, in which the prevalence of angle-closure glaucoma was 2.3%, compared to 1.5% for open-angle glaucoma, with the former showing a four-fold predilection for women (18). This prevalence of angle-closure glaucoma may be due to a smaller corneal diameter and anterior chamber depth, and a thicker, more anteriorly placed lens among effected individuals (19–21). A study among Alaskan Eskimos also showed a rapid increase in hyperopia after age 50 years, reaching 71.5% in persons above 80 years of age (22).

Studies of the anterior chamber angle in general populations provide an impression of the prevalence of those at risk of developing pupillary block glaucoma. In two large stud-

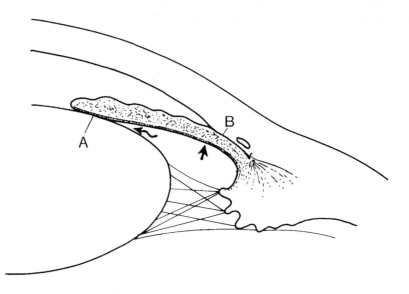

Figure 10.1. Pupillary-block glaucoma. A functional block between the lens and iris (A) leads to increased pressure in the posterior chamber *(arrows)* with forward shift of the peripheral iris and closure of the anterior chamber angle (B).

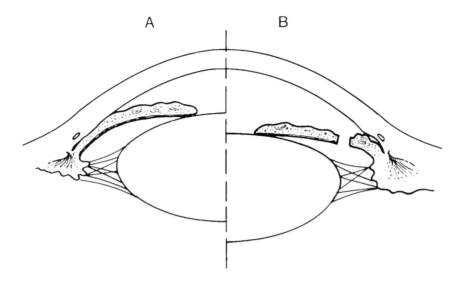

Figure 10.2. Pupillary-block glaucoma (**A**) contrasted with the plateau iris syndrome (**B**). In the latter situation, note the relatively deeper central anterior chamber, the flat iris plane, patent iridectomy, and bunching up of peripheral iris in the anterior chamber angle.

ies, 5–6% of those screened had suspicious anterior chamber angles, but only 0.64–1.1% were considered to have critically narrow angles (23, 24).

CLINICAL FEATURES

The diagnosis of pupillary-block glaucoma has several facets. During the course of every ocular examination, the physician must consider general risk factors in the medical history and look for anatomic features that might predispose to angle-closure. When suspicious findings are noted, provocative tests are sometimes used to determine the potential for angle-closure glaucoma. In other situations, the patient may present with signs and symptoms suggestive of angle-closure glaucoma, and the correct diagnosis will depend on an understanding of the symptoms, predisposing circumstances, and physical findings of the disease, as well as the differential diagnosis (Fig. 10.2). These various aspects of diagnosing potential or manifest pupillary-block glaucoma will now be considered.

Risk Factors

General Features of Patients

These factors influence the configuration of the anterior chamber angle and the risk of developing pupillary-block glaucoma.

AGE. The depth and volume of the anterior chamber diminish with age (25), which may result from a thickening and forward displacement of the lens (26, 27). Consequently, the percent of individuals with critically narrow angles is higher in older age groups. The prevalence of pupillary-block glaucoma also increases with age, although it may peak earlier

in life than with chronic open-angle glaucoma. One study found a bimodal peak, with the first at ages 53–58 years and the second at 63–70 years (26). However, it can occur at any age, including rare cases in childhood (28).

RACE. Angle-closure glaucoma is less common among blacks, and is more often of the chronic form when it does occur in that race (29–31). The explanation for this difference is uncertain. One study suggested it might be due to a thinner average lens thickness (30), although another investigation revealed the anterior chamber depth in Nigerian blacks to be equivalent to that of whites (32). It has also been suggested that the weaker response to mydriatics observed among African blacks could indicate that darker irides are less able to exert the force which may lead to pupillary block (33). Angle-closure glaucoma also has a reduced prevalence among American Indians and is often secondary to a swollen lens when it did occur in this group (31). As previously noted, the relative prevalence of pupillary-block glaucoma among all the glaucomas is increased in various populations of Eskimos (14–17).

SEX. There is a statistically significant predominance of *females* in populations with pupillary-block glaucoma, which is felt to be due to the shallower anterior chamber among women in general (14–16, 25, 32, 34).

REFRACTIVE ERROR. The depth and volume of the anterior chamber are also related to the degree of ametropia, with smaller dimensions in *hyperopes* (25). However, the presence of myopia does not eliminate the possibility of angle-closure glaucoma since rare cases have been reported in such patients (35), possibly related to a spherical or anteriorly displaced lens or an increase in corneal curvature (36).

FAMILY HISTORY. The potential for pupillary-block glaucoma is generally believed to be inherited. In one study,

A

B

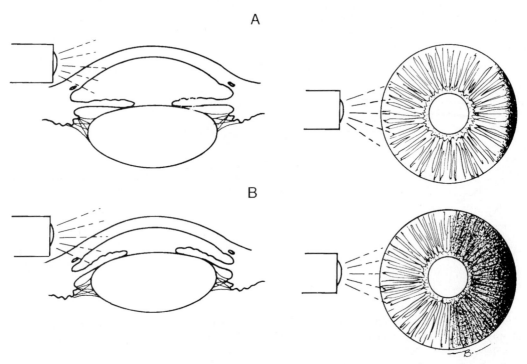

Figure 10.3. Oblique flashlight illumination as a screening measure for estimating the anterior chamber depth. **A.** With a deep chamber, nearly the entire iris is illuminated. **B.** When the iris is bowed forward, only the proximal portion is illuminated, and a shadow is seen in the distal half.

20% of 95 relatives of angle-closure glaucoma patients were felt to have potentially occludable angles (37). However, aside from a few reported families in which many members developed angle-closure glaucoma, the family history is not very useful in predicting a future angle-closure attack (38).

HLA antigens were studied in 35 angle-closure glaucoma patients, and no correlation was found (39).

SYSTEMIC DISORDERS. One study has shown an inverse correlation between type 2 diabetes or an abnormal glucose-tolerance test and the anterior chamber depth (40). The same authors have suggested an increased prevalence of denervation supersensitivity to autonomic agonists in angle closure glaucoma (41).

Findings During Routine Examination

These observations during the course of a routine ocular examination will help to establish the potential for angle closure.

INTRAOCULAR PRESSURE. Unless the patient has angle closure at the time of the examination, the IOP will usually be normal. One study, however, found a larger-than-normal amplitude in the diurnal IOP curve, which the authors felt might have prognostic value (42). Tonography also characteristically reveals normal outflow facility before or between attacks, unless peripheral anterior synechiae have begun to develop (5).

EVALUATION OF PERIPHERAL ANTERIOR CHAMBER. Photogrammetric studies of all forms of angle-closure glaucoma have revealed anterior chamber depths, volumes, and diameters that are smaller than matched controls (43). Anterior chamber depth and volume have also been shown to have diurnal variation, with lower values in the evening (44), although a correlation between diurnal variations of chamber depth and IOP is not clear. In any case, the most important step in the diagnosis of either potential or manifest angle-closure glaucoma is to evaluate the anterior chamber depth and especially the configuration of the anterior chamber angle. While this is best accomplished by gonioscopy, there are preliminary screening measures that may be useful in some situations, as well as techniques of quantifying the anterior chamber depth.

PENLIGHT EXAMINATION. For situations in which a slitlamp and goniolens are not available, the anterior chamber depth can be estimated with oblique penlight illumination across the surface of the iris. With the light coming from the temporal side of the eye, a relatively flat iris will be illuminated on both the temporal and nasal side of the pupil, while an iris that is bowed forward will have a shadow on the nasal side (Fig. 10.3) (45).

SLITLAMP EXAMINATION. The *central anterior chamber depth* may be estimated during examination with the slitlamp, and several techniques for quantitating this parameter have been proposed (46–48). However, the central anterior chamber depth has been shown to have a weak correlation with the angle width (49), and the parameter of greater diagnostic value within the context of angle-closure glaucoma is the *peripheral anterior chamber depth.* van Herick and coworkers (50) developed a technique for making this estimation with the slitlamp by comparing the peripheral anterior chamber depth to the thickness of the adjacent cornea (Figs. 10.4 and 10.5). This is commonly referred to as the *van Herick technique.* When the peripheral anterior chamber depth is less than 1/4-corneal thickness, the anterior chamber angle may be dangerously narrow (50).

GONIOSCOPY. Whenever the peripheral anterior chamber depth is felt to be shallow (van Herick slitlamp Grade 1 or 2), careful gonioscopic examination of the angle is required. Numerous grading systems have been suggested in an attempt to correlate gonioscopic appearance with the potential for angle-closure. Scheie (51) proposed a system based on the extent of the *anterior chamber angle structures* that can be visualized (Fig. 10.6). He noted a high risk of angle closure in eyes with Grade III or IV angles. Shaffer (52) suggested using the *angular width* of the angle recess as the criterion for grading the angle and attempted to correlate this with the potential for angle-closure (Fig. 10.7).

Other authors feel that any single criterion does not fully describe the anterior chamber angle. Becker (53) proposed combining an estimation of the anterior chamber angle width and the height of the iris insertion, while Spaeth (24) suggested an evaluation of three variables: (a) angular width of the angle recess; (b) configuration of the peripheral iris; and (c) apparent insertion of the iris root (Fig. 10.8). Whatever system the clinician prefers to use to document the appearance of the anterior chamber angle, it is important to pay close attention to these three aspects of the angle. Additional features of the angle should also be studied and documented, such as peripheral anterior synechiae and degrees or abnormalities in pigmentation. It was noted in one study that patients with narrow angles may have a predominance of trabecular meshwork pigmentation in the superior quadrant, rather than the more common inferior location, which the authors felt might be due to a rubbing between the peripheral iris and the meshwork (54).

NEWER TECHNIQUES. Several newer forms of technology are being applied to evaluation of the anterior segment of the eye to more accurately quantify the anterior chamber depth

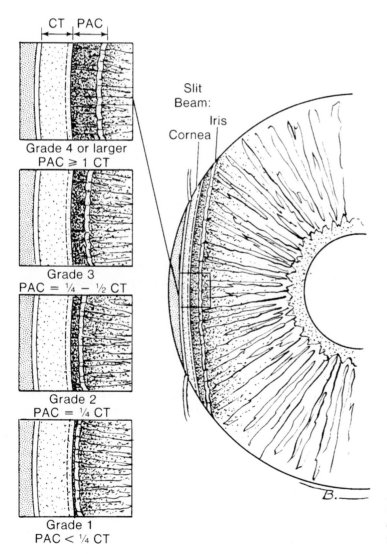

Figure 10.4. Slitlamp technique of van Herick, et al. (50), for estimating the depth of the peripheral anterior chamber (PAC) by comparing it to the adjacent corneal thickness (CT).

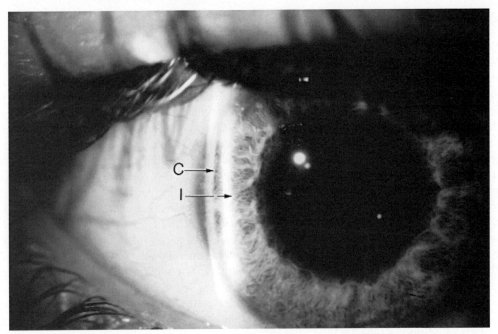

Figure 10.5. Slitlamp photograph of van Herick technique for estimation of peripheral anterior chamber depth showing slit beam on cornea (C) and iris *(I)*.

and related dimensions. The use of high frequency ultrasound, referred to as *ultrasound biomicroscopy,* allows definition of the relationship between the iris, posterior chamber, lens, zonules, and ciliary body. This technique has potential value in understanding the mechanisms of glaucoma (55), as well as aiding in the diagnosis of pupillary block glaucoma, especially when the media is not clear (56). It may also be of value in identifying eyes with potentially occludable anterior chamber angles. It has been suggested that the biometric calculation of the lens thickness/axial length ratio can be used as a prognostic indicator of pupillary block glaucoma (57, 58). Ultrasound biomicroscopy has also been used to image the dynamic changes in anterior ocular structures during darkroom provocative testing (59) (discussed later).

Specialized photographic techniques are also being used to gain better understanding of the anterior segment structures in angle-closure glaucomas (43, 44, 61–62). With one of these techniques, *Scheimpflug video imaging,* the iridocorneal angle can be quantitatively assessed and observed longitudinally (62).

Yet another new technology that may prove to be useful in assessing the relationship of the anterior segment structures is *optical coherence tomography* (63). (The principles of this technology were reviewed in Chapter 5 in relation to image analyses of the optic nerve head and peripapillary retina.)

Provocative Tests

Having decided that a patient has suspiciously narrow anterior chamber angles, the physician is now faced with a difficult decision. If it could be predicted that the patient would one day have an attack of angle-closure glaucoma, the ap-propriate course in most cases would be prophylactic peripheral iridotomies. The results of one study suggest that optic nerve damage occurs in the early time period after IOP rise, supporting the value of detecting potentially occludable angles and performing prophylactic surgery prior to an attack (64). However, it is not usually possible to predict with certainty, on the basis of the anterior chamber angle appearance, which eyes will eventually suffer an angle-closure attack.

Some surgeons utilize provocative tests when attempting to identify those patients for whom treatment should be recommended. A variety of such tests have been designed to precipitate an angle-closure attack, with the rationale that it is better for this to occur in the physician's office, where it can be treated promptly, than in a situation where it might go unrecognized or where medical attention might not be readily available. It is important that a provocative test be as physiologic as possible in an effort to create a situation that might occur under natural circumstances.

Mydriatic Provocative Tests

A short-acting topical mydriatic (e.g., 0.5% tropicamide) is instilled and a rise in IOP of 8 mm Hg or more is considered to be a positive test. However, gonioscopic confirmation of angle closure is essential, since mydriatics and cycloplegics can also cause pressure rises in eyes with open anterior chamber angles, as discussed in Chapter 9.

Dark Room Provocative Test

Mydriasis is induced by placing the patient in a dark room for 60–90 minutes. It is important that the patient remain awake during this time to avoid the miosis of sleep. A positive test

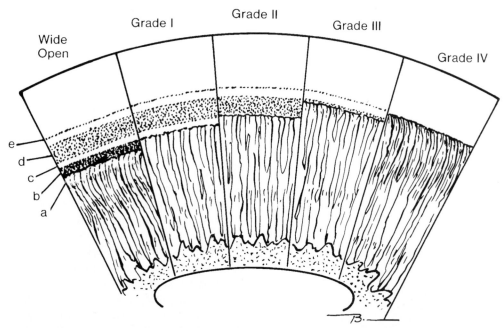

Figure 10.6. Scheie's (51) gonioscopic classification of the anterior chamber angle, based on the extent of visible angle structures: *a,* Root of the iris; *b,* Ciliary body band; *c,* Scleral spur; *d,* Trabecular meshwork; and *e,* Schwalbe's line.

Classification	Gonioscopic Appearance
Wide open	All structures visible
Grade I narrow	Hard to see over iris root into recess
Grade II narrow	Ciliary body band obscured
Grade III narrow	Posterior trabeculum obscured
Grade IV narrow (closed)	Only Schwalbe's line visible

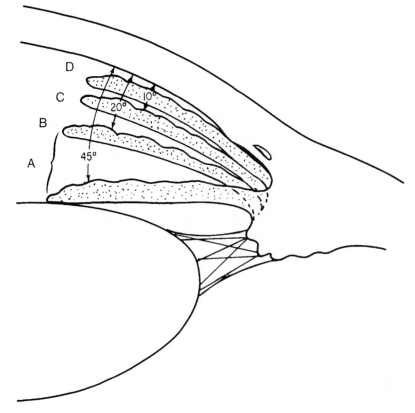

Figure 10.7. Shaffer's (52) gonioscopic classification of the anterior chamber angle, based on the angular width of the angle recess:

Angular Width	Clinical Interpretation
A. Wide open (20–45°)	Closure improbable
B. Moderately narrow (10–20°)	Closure possible
C. Extremely narrow	Closure possible
D. Partially or totally closed	Closure present

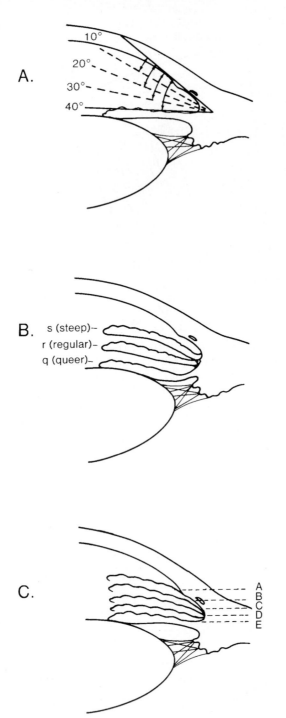

Figure 10.8. Spaeth's (24) gonioscopic classification of the anterior chamber angle, based on three variables: **A.** Angular width of the angle recess; **B.** Configuration of the peripheral iris; and **C.** Apparent insertion of the iris root.

again is taken with a pressure rise of 8 mm Hg or more and gonioscopic confirmation of angle closure. Exposure to light should be kept to a minimum during the post-dark room studies to avoid reversing the pressure-inducing mechanism (65). It has been reported that using a 30% decrease in the tonographic facility of outflow as an additional parameter in-

creased the positive yield from 30% to 67% (66). As noted earlier, ultrasound biomicroscopy has also been suggested as an adjunct to dark room provocative testing (59).

Prone Provocative Test

The patient is placed in a prone position for 60 minutes and a pressure rise of 8 mm Hg or more is taken as a positive response (67). The mechanism of angle closure with this test is uncertain, but it is apparently not related to mydriasis (68). One theory holds that angle closure during prone provocative testing is due to pupillary block associated with a slight forward shift of the lens, although in one study no significant shallowing of the anterior chamber could be demonstrated in patients with positive prone provocative tests (69).

The prone provocative test was compared to the mydriatic and dark room tests in 76 angle-closure glaucoma eyes and was found to yield 71% positive responses before peripheral iridectomy and 6.5% after surgery, in contrast to 58% and 1.4%, respectively, for the mydriatic test, and 48% and 6.5% with the dark room test (70). In another study of 19 patients with a diagnosis of narrow angle glaucoma, the percentage of positive provocative tests was approximately 50% with either the prone or dark room test alone, compared to 11% and 16% with phenylephrine or cyclopentolate mydriatic provocative testing, respectively (68). When a combined prone and a dark room test was performed on the same patient, the yield was almost 90% positive (68).

Pilocarpine/Phenylephrine Test

Two percent pilocarpine and 10% phenylephrine are instilled simultaneously every minute for three applications to achieve a mid-dilated pupil. If this does not achieve a positive response (IOP rise greater than 8 mm Hg) in 2 hours, the test is repeated. If the second test is also negative after 90 minutes, it is terminated with 0.5% thymoxamine, and a mydriatic provocative test with 0.5% tropicamide is performed on another day (71–74). In a study of 119 high-risk patients, 74 had positive responses with the initial pilocarpine/phenylephrine test, while nine more had positive responses to tropicamide, and only one of the remaining 36 developed angle-closure glaucoma during a followup that averaged 3 years (71). However, in another study with a 10-year followup, the pilocarpine/phenylephrine test showed both poor sensitivity (40% of fellow eyes and 60% of eyes with a history of subacute attacks that eventually developed angle closure glaucoma had negative pilocarpine/phenylephrine tests) (75) and poor specificity (only 1 of 13 untreated fellow eyes of patients with a positive pilocarpine/phenylephrine test developed angle-closure glaucoma) (76).

Value of Provocative Tests

Most ophthalmologists today question the clinical value of any provocative test for angle-closure glaucoma. In one study of 129 angle-closure glaucoma suspects who underwent gonioscopy, refraction, anterior chamber pachymetry, ultrasound biomicroscopy, and an angle-closure provocative test, it was concluded that none of the test factors studied showed a high sensitivity or positive predictive accuracy in detecting eyes that later developed angle closure (77). It has been suggested that an accurate history and physical examination provides the best guide to management of angle-closure glaucoma suspects (78).

Precipitating Factors

In an eye that is anatomically predisposed to develop angle-closure, these factors may precipitate an attack.

Factors Which Produce Mydriasis

DIM ILLUMINATION. A common history for the development of pupillary-block glaucoma is the onset of an acute attack when the patient is in a dark room, such as a theater or restaurant. It has been reported that the incidence of angle closure increases in the winter and autumn (34, 79). In one study, however, there was a direct association with hours of sunshine and an inverse association with cloud amount, which the authors thought might be related to the contrast between day and evening levels of illumination (79).

EMOTIONAL STRESS. Occasionally, an acute angle-closure attack will follow severe emotional stress. It may be that this is related to the mydriasis of increased sympathetic tone, although the exact mechanism is not fully understood.

DRUGS. Mydriatics may also precipitate an angle-closure attack in an anatomically predisposed eye.

Anticholinergics (e.g., atropine, cyclopentolate, tropicamide, etc.) create a particularly high risk when administered topically (80). In one study, 0.5% cyclopentolate precipitated attacks in 9 of 21 (43%) high-risk eyes, while 0.5% tropicamide did the same in 19 of 58 (33%) eyes (81). However, in a population-based screening study of 4870 subjects whose eyes were dilated with 1% tropicamide and 2.5% phenylephrine after penlight examination of the anterior chamber depth, none developed an acute angle-closure attack (82). Systemic atropine and other mydriatics can also create a hazard, especially when large doses are used along with spinal or general anesthesia during surgery (83). It has been suggested that high-risk eyes should be protected with topical pilocarpine before, during, and after surgery (84). However, miosis can also precipitate angle-closure attacks, and an alternative approach to managing the high-risk eye is close observation during the postoperative period, or prophylactic peripheral iridotomy, depending on the degree of risk. Other systemic drugs with weaker anticholinergic properties (e.g., antihistaminic, anti-Parkinsonism, antipsychotic, and gastrointestinal spasmolytic drugs) also present a

risk proportional to the pupillary effect (81, 85, 86). The tricyclic antidepressants have the greatest anticholinergic properties of the various psychoactive drugs, and four cases have been reported in which imipramine was believed to trigger pupillary-block glaucoma (85). Botulinum toxin, used in the treatment of strabismus and blepharospasm, inhibits acetylcholine release with subsequent mydriasis, and has been reported to cause acute angle-closure glaucoma (87).

Adrenergics, such as topical epinephrine, may precipitate an angle-closure attack in the predisposed eye. Phenylephrine can also precipitate an attack, although it was found to be safer than cyclopentolate or tropicamide for dilating high risk eyes (83). In addition, systemic drugs with adrenergic properties (e.g., vasoconstrictors, central nervous system stimulants, appetite depressants, bronchodilators, and hallucinogenic agents) may present a risk in the predisposed eye (80).

Factors Which Produce Miosis

As previously noted, miotic therapy may occasionally lead to an acute attack of pupillary-block glaucoma. This has also been observed following the miosis induced by reading or bright lights. Possible mechanisms include (a) an increase in the relative pupillary block due to a wider zone of contact between iris and lens, and (b) relaxation of the lens zonules, allowing a forward shift of the iris-lens diaphragm. With strong miotics, such as the cholinesterase inhibitors (e.g., diisopropyl fluorophosphate and echothiophate iodide), the mechanism of angle-closure may be either the miosis or congestion of the uveal tract. Chandler (5) favored the former theory, since he noted that an acute rise in IOP following the use of a miotic did not occur in an eye with a peripheral iridectomy.

Sulfa-based compounds may cause transient myopia, presumably due to lens swelling and a forward movement of the lens-iris diaphragm associated with choroidal detachments and ciliary body swelling. Oral hydrochlorothiazide was reported to precipitate bilateral angle-closure glaucoma, presumably by this mechanism (88).

Vasodilators were also once felt to create a risk of precipitating angle-closure attacks, but this was subsequently disproved (80).

Symptoms of Angle-Closure Attack

Angle-closure glaucoma, in marked contrast to chronic open-angle glaucoma, is characterized by profound symptoms, although the severity of these symptoms varies considerably in different forms of the disorder.

Subacute Angle-Closure Glaucoma

This form of pupillary-block glaucoma may have no recognizable symptoms. In other cases, the patient may notice a dull ache behind the eye and/or slight blurring of vision. A symptom that is especially typical of the subacute attack is colored halos around lights. This is felt to result from an alteration in the cornea, which causes it to act as a diffraction grating, producing a blue-green central and yellow-red peripheral halo. These symptoms, which more often occur at night after the patient has been in a dark room, will often spontaneously clear by the following morning, presumably due to the miosis of sleep.

Acute Angle-Closure Glaucoma

This condition is characterized by pain, redness, and blurred vision. The pain is typically a severe, deep ache, which follows the trigeminal distribution and may be associated with nausea, vomiting, bradycardia, and profuse sweating. The conjunctival hyperemia is marked and usually consists of both a ciliary flush and peripheral conjunctival congestion. The blurred vision, which is also typically marked, may be due to stretching of the corneal lamellae initially and later to edema of the cornea, as well as a direct effect of the IOP on the optic nerve head. Rarely, the corneal decompensation may persist, requiring penetrating keratoplasty (89).

Chronic Angle-Closure Glaucoma

This form of pupillary-block glaucoma is typically asymptomatic until advanced visual field loss develops, although the patient may give a history suggestive of one or more episodes of subacute or acute angle-closure glaucoma.

Clinical Findings During an Acute Attack

The patient who presents during an acute angle-closure attack will typically have marked IOP elevation in the range of 40–60 mm Hg or more, with a profound reduction in central visual acuity. The following additional findings help to confirm the diagnosis.

External Examination

Characteristic findings include the previously noted conjunctival hyperemia, as well as a cloudy cornea and an irregular (usually vertically oval), mid-dilated, fixed pupil (Fig. 10.9). The pupillary change is thought to result from paralysis of the sphincter, which is apparently due to a reduction in circulation induced by the elevated IOP (90–92), and possibly to degeneration of the ciliary ganglion (93).

Slitlamp Examination

This step of the evaluation confirms the presence of the corneal edema, which frequently must be cleared by topical application of glycerin before the anterior chamber can be studied. The corneal edema usually clears after the pressure is normalized, although, as previously noted, this is not always the case (89). Specular microscopic examination has revealed significant corneal endothelial cell loss in these cases, which correlates with the duration of IOP elevation (94), the degree of visual field loss, a large cup-disc ratio, and previous intraocular surgery (95).

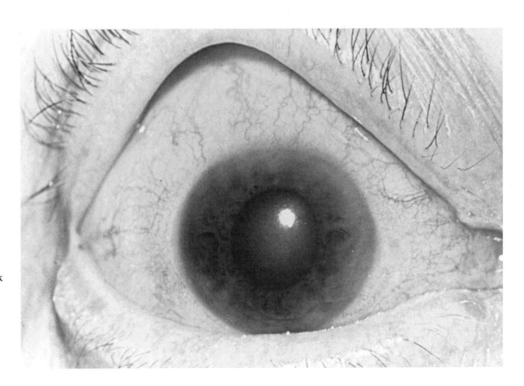

Figure 10.9. External appearance of eye during attack of acute angle-closure glaucoma, showing diffuse conjunctival hyperemia, cloudy cornea, and irregular, mid-dilated pupil. (Courtesy of H. Saul Sugar, M.D.)

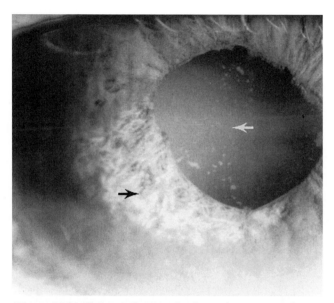

Figure 10.10. Slitlamp photograph of eye after acute angle-closure glaucoma attack, showing glaukomflecken (*white arrow*) and sector iris atrophy (*black arrow*).

The anterior chamber is shallow, but typically is formed centrally with anterior bowing of the mid-peripheral iris, often making contact with peripheral cornea. Aqueous flare may be present. Other findings may include *pigment dispersion, sector atrophy* of the iris, and *glaukomflecken,* which are irregular white opacities in the anterior portion of the lens (Fig. 10.10).

Gonioscopy

It is essential to confirm the diagnosis of angle-closure glaucoma by demonstrating a closed anterior chamber angle. If gonioscopy is not possible due to persistent corneal edema, gonioscopy of the fellow eye may provide useful information if it reveals an extremely narrow angle. In a study of 10 eyes with angle-closure glaucoma, the Koeppe lens was felt to be more reliable than the Goldmann three-mirror or Zeiss four-mirror lenses in determining whether the angle was open or closed, because it caused no artifactual widening of the angle and allowed the best view over a convex iris (96).

Peripheral anterior synechiae may also be present, and documenting the presence and extent of the synechiae is important in establishing the nature of the angle-closure glaucoma and in selecting the appropriate treatment (discussed later in this chapter). Forbes (97, 98) described an office procedure *(compressive gonioscopy)* in which the degree of synechial closure is determined by indenting the central cornea with a Zeiss four-mirror gonioprism. This forces aqueous into the peripheral portion of the anterior chamber, which deepens it and facilitates visualization of the angle (Fig. 10.11).

Fundus Examination

The optic nerve head may be hyperemic and edematous in the early stages of the attack. Monkeys exposed to high IOPs usually developed congestion of the optic nerve head within 12–15 hours, which persisted for 4–5 days (99). The disc then became pale, and glaucomatous cupping was observed after 9–10 days. In a study of human eyes with a history of angle-closure glaucoma, pallor without cupping was seen in eyes following acute attacks, while both pallor and cupping occurred in chronic cases (100). Central retinal vein occlusion may also occur during acute angle-closure glaucoma (101). Conversely, central retinal vein occlusion may cause a form of angle-closure glaucoma, which is discussed in Chapter 16.

Visual Fields

As discussed in Chapter 6, visual field changes associated with acute elevation of IOP most often show nonspecific constriction. In one study of 25 patients with acute angle-closure glaucoma that had been surgically corrected, the most common field defect was constriction of the upper field (102), while another revealed nerve fiber bundle defects in 7 of 18 acute and 9 of 11 chronic cases (100).

THEORIES OF MECHANISM

Relative Pupillary Block

As noted earlier in this chapter, the most common mechanism leading to angle-closure glaucoma appears to be

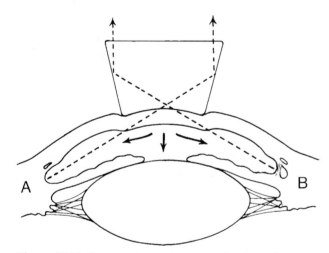

Figure 10.11. Compressive gonioscopy with a Zeiss four-mirror gonioprism deepens the peripheral anterior chamber by displacing aqueous from the central portion of the chamber (*arrows*). This facilitates gonioscopic examination of the anterior chamber angle before surgery by helping to distinguish between appositional (**A**) and synechial (**B**) closure of the angle (97, 98).

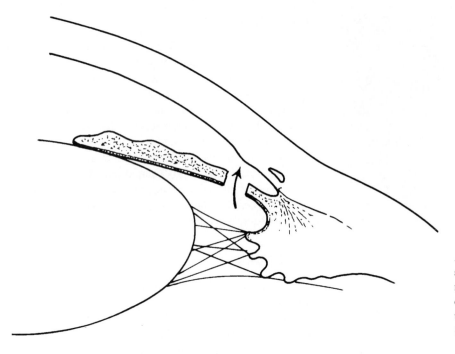

Figure 10.12. The strongest evidence in support of the pupillary block mechanism of angle-closure glaucoma is the excellent response to peripheral iridotomy, which circumvents the block *(arrow).*

increased resistance to aqueous flow from the posterior to the anterior chamber between the iris and lens. This concept was suggested by Curran (4) and Banziger (6) in the early 1920s, and advanced by the teachings of Chandler (5), who noted that an eye with a shallow anterior chamber has a wider zone of contact between the surfaces of the iris and lens. He postulated that the musculature of the iris exerts a backward pressure against the lens which increases the resistance to flow of aqueous into the anterior chamber. This increases the pressure in the posterior chamber, causing the thin peripheral iris to bulge into the anterior chamber angle. It has been suggested on the basis of gonioscopic studies that the angle closure occurs in two stages, with the first being iridocorneal contact anterior to the trabecular meshwork, followed by apposition of the iris to the meshwork as the pressure rises (103, 104). There is considerable clinical evidence which strongly favors the basic concept of pupillary block, the most convincing of which is the excellent response to peripheral iridotomy, which presumably works by circumventing the block (Fig. 10.12) (5).

Anatomic Factors Predisposing to Pupillary Block

Several anatomic aspects of the eye combine to produce a shallow anterior chamber. These include a thicker, more anteriorly placed lens, a smaller diameter and shorter posterior curvature of the cornea, and a shorter axial length of the globe (105–111). A study of chronic angle-closure glaucoma patients of Oriental or African ethnic background revealed an abnormal anterior lens position without an increase in lens thickness, suggesting an ethnic influence on these biometric parameters (112). As previously noted, the lens thickness/axial length ratio appears to correlate best

with the predisposition to angle closure (57, 58). It has also been shown that the anterior chamber depth is not a static dimension, but can undergo rapid, transient change (113).

Relatives of patients with pupillary block glaucoma have been noted to have a more anterior insertion of the iris into the ciliary body, a narrower angular approach to the recess of the anterior chamber angle, and a more anterior peripheral convexity of the iris as compared to average eyes in the general population (24). All of these parameters are variably influenced by hyperopia, increasing age, and genetics.

Another factor predisposing to a pupillary block mechanism may be a forward displacement to the lens due to loose zonules, which is made worse by miotic therapy and relieved with cycloplegia (David G. Campbell, M.D., personal communication).

Significance of Pupillary Dilatation

Chandler (2) emphasized that a mid-dilated pupil of 3.5–6 mm is the critical degree of dilatation that seems to bring on the acute attack. He felt this might be due to continued pupillary block combined with sufficient relaxation of peripheral iris to allow its forward displacement into the anterior chamber. Mapstone (114) proposed a mathematical model to explain the influence of a mid-dilated pupil, in which the combined pupil-blocking forces of the dilator and sphincter muscles and the stretching force of the iris were greatest with the iris in the mid-dilated position. Tiedeman (115), however, using basic physical principles, noted that Mapstone's model involved incorrect usage of the physical concepts of force and tension. He developed a model that can predict the profile of the iris by using the radii of the pupil and iris root and the anterior displacement of the pupil from the iris root. If the latter measurement were constant, the angle between the peripheral iris and trabecular meshwork would progressively narrow as the pupillary radius increased. However, due to the contour of the lens, the anterior displacement of the pupil decreases as the pupil dilates, resulting in the narrowest angle when the pupil is mid-dilated (115). Biometric photographs of subjects with narrow anterior chamber angles supported the validity of the Tiedeman model (116).

Chronic Angle-Closure Glaucoma

Peripheral anterior synechiae may eventually develop with prolonged or recurrent acute or subacute attacks, leading to chronic angle-closure glaucoma. The peripheral anterior synechiae in patients after acute angle-closure attacks tend to be broad based, are most commonly seen in the superior quadrant, and correlate with the duration of the acute attacks (120). In addition, a more insidious form has been recognized in which the angle slowly closes from the periphery toward Schwalbe's line (9–12). The synechial closure usually begins superiorly, where the angle is normally narrowest, and progresses inferiorly (10). This condition has been referred to as *shortening of the angle* (11) or *creeping angle closure* (12). These cases are frequently cured by peripheral iridotomy if detected early enough, but occasionally require filtering surgery.

Plateau Iris

As noted at the outset of this chapter, plateau iris has traditionally been included among the "primary" angle-closure glaucomas largely because of an incomplete understanding of the mechanism of angle closure (1–3). More recent evidence suggests that an anterior position of the ciliary body may cause the angle closure (117–119). This condition is considered in more detail in Chapter 14.

DIFFERENTIAL DIAGNOSIS

The sudden onset of pain, redness, and blurred vision, which characterizes the acute angle-closure attack, may also be seen with other forms of glaucoma, creating a differential diagnostic problem.

Open-Angle Glaucomas

Open-angle glaucomas may occasionally present as an acute attack, especially when associated with events such as inflammation, hemorrhage, or rubeosis iridis. These cases are usually readily distinguished from acute angle-closure glaucoma on the basis of the gonioscopic appearance and associated findings. However, in the eye with an elevated IOP and a narrow anterior chamber angle, it may be difficult to distinguish between pupillary-block glaucoma and open-angle

glaucoma with narrow angles. A *thymoxamine test* has been suggested for this situation (121). Unlike cholinergic miotics, which can lower IOP by either opening a closed angle or by reducing resistance to trabecular outflow, thymoxamine, an α-adrenergic blocker, produces miosis by relaxation of the dilator muscle without effecting outflow through cyclotropia. As a result, topical thymoxamine 0.5% can often open a narrow or appositionally-closed angle and lower the IOP in angle-closure glaucoma, but will not alter the pressure in an eye with open-angle glaucoma. An alternative approach to distinguishing between these two conditions is to perform a laser iridotomy, which will relieve the pressure elevation in a pure angle-closure case, while additional measures will be required if an open-angle component is present.

Angle-Closure Glaucomas with Associated Abnormalities

There are many forms of angle-closure glaucoma with associated abnormalities, which may present even more difficult diagnostic problems, especially when the initiating event is posterior to the lens-iris diaphragm, where early detection can be difficult. The following are some of the ocular disorders that may lead to these forms of angle closure (the details of these conditions are considered in subsequent chapters):

1. Plateau iris (Chapter 14).
2. Central retinal vein occlusion (Chapter 16).
3. Ciliary body swelling, inflammation, or cysts (Chapters 18, 19).
4. Ciliary block (malignant) glaucoma (Chapter 23).
5. Posterior segment tumors (Chapter 18).
6. Contracting retrolental tissue (Chapter 16).
7. Scleral buckling procedures and panretinal photocoagulation (Chapter 23).
8. Nanophthalmos (Chapter 16).
9. Corneal thickening (Chapter 13).

MANAGEMENT

The details regarding drugs and surgical procedures used in the treatment of pupillary-block glaucoma are considered in Section Three. The present discussion is limited to the general approach and basic concepts of the management.

Medical Therapy

Although the vast majority of eyes with pupillary-block glaucoma are managed surgically, it is desirable to first bring the glaucoma under medical control. In the case of an acute attack, this constitutes a medical emergency and should be approached in two stages: (a) reduce the IOP and (b) relieve the angle closure.

Reduction of Intraocular Pressure

Miotic therapy is frequently ineffective when the IOP is high, presumably due to pressure-induced ischemia of the iris, which leads to paralysis of the sphincter muscle (90–92). For this reason, the first line of defense is to administer drugs that will promptly lower the IOP. Oral or topical *carbonic anhydrase inhibitors,* topical β-*adrenergic blockers,* and/or α2-*adrenergic agonists* will, in many cases, lower the pressure sufficiently to allow effective miotic therapy to open the angle (122, 123). In especially difficult cases, *hyperosmotics* may also be used to help in the initial pressure reduction. They may be given orally as glycerol or isosorbide or, if the patient is too nauseated to tolerate oral medication, they may be given intravenously as mannitol or urea.

Relief of Angle-Closure

Once the IOP has been reduced, a miotic is instilled to break the pupillary block and open the anterior chamber angle. A single drop of *pilocarpine* approximately 3 hours after administration of acetazolamide or timolol has been reported to effectively break the angle-closure attack (122, 123). This is also safer than copious use of pilocarpine, since it reduces the chances of drug toxicity. The concentration of pilocarpine does not appear to be important in this situation, and a low dosage of 1–2% is preferable. α-Adrenergic antagonists, such as thymoxamine, have theoretic advantages over pilocarpine, since the mechanism of miosis, as previously noted, is relaxation of the dilator muscle, which may allow effective pupillary constriction even when the IOP is elevated (124, 125). However, other investigators have not found thymoxamine alone to be effective in the treatment of angle-closure glaucoma (126). Strong miotics, such as eserine and echothiophate iodide, are generally contraindicated in acute angle-closure glaucoma, since they may aggravate the situation by producing vascular congestion or increasing the pupillary block.

Surgical Management

Once the IOP has been brought under control medically (or all efforts at medical control have been exhausted), the surgeon is then faced with two decisions: (a) when to operate and (b) what procedure to use. These considerations have been significantly influenced by the replacement, in most cases, of incisional iridectomy with laser iridotomy.

When to Operate

In the days of incisional iridectomy when the elevated pressure could not be controlled medically, Chandler and Grant (127) advised considering surgery within the next few hours, especially if the vision was failing. However, the risks of incisional surgery are considerably higher under these circumstances, and mechanical techniques to lower the IOP before surgery may prove helpful. For example, indentation of the central cornea for several 30-second intervals, using a blunt instrument such as a cotton-tipped applicator, may lower the pressure and occasionally break the attack by forcing aqueous from the central to the peripheral anterior chamber (Fig. 10.13) (128). Even with a laser iridotomy, it may be helpful to lower the IOP first to allow clearing of corneal edema. In any case, the safest approach to medically-unresponsive cases is to proceed with the iridotomy. When an iridotomy cannot be achieved due to corneal edema, laser pupilloplasty or peripheral iridoplasty may break the attack (129, 130). Once the attack is broken and the cornea has cleared, a laser iridotomy should then be formed.

If the IOP does respond to medical therapy, the eye should be reexamined gonioscopically to determine the mechanism of the pressure reduction. An open anterior chamber angle without compressive gonioscopy suggests that the angle-closure attack has been broken. In this situation, there is less urgency as to when surgical intervention should be performed. In the days of incisional surgical iridectomy, some surgeons preferred to wait a day or two until inflammation had subsided. With laser iridotomy, however, there is no advantage in waiting unless marked iritis or corneal edema are present. In one long-term study of 116 cases, delay in treatment had a detrimental effect on the final outcome (131). If the gonioscopy reveals that the angle is still closed, despite medical lowering of the IOP, it may be that the pressure reduction is due to the drug-induced reduction of aqueous production and/or vitreous volume and that the angle-closure has not actually been relieved. Since the high pressure may recur as the effects of these medications begin to wear off, there is all the more urgency in proceeding promptly with the laser iridotomy.

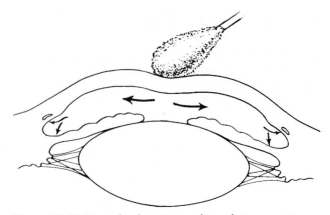

Figure 10.13. Corneal indentation with a soft instrument, such as a cotton-tipped applicator, may lower the intraocular pressure during an acute angle-closure attack by forcing aqueous from the central to the peripheral anterior chamber (*arrows*), thereby temporarily opening the chamber angle and reestablishing aqueous outflow (128).

What Operation to Use

The eye with pupillary-block glaucoma typically responds well to a peripheral iridotomy, and the initial procedure of choice in nearly every case is a laser iridotomy. One study compared 50 eyes treated with incisional iridectomy or laser iridotomy to 64 treated medically and found that the former group had a greater number of improved anterior chamber configurations, a lower incidence of peripheral anterior synechiae, and a greater reduction in the need for glaucoma medications (132). Studies of anterior ocular segment configuration before and after iridotomy, using the Scheimpflug imaging technique, revealed a significant widening of the anterior chamber angle (133) and a straightening of the iris contour (134), but no significant change in the position of the anterior lens surface (133, 134).

Followup studies, however, indicate that many eyes treated with an iridotomy alone will eventually require medication to control chronic pressure elevation and some will need filtering surgery (13, 135–139). Factors associated with the need for additional treatment include the duration of the angle-closure attack and a history of intermittent, spontaneously resolved angle closure episodes (138, 139). These factors relate to the amount of permanent damage to the anterior chamber angle, which sometimes correlates with the extent of gonioscopically visible peripheral anterior synechiae.

Chamber deepening procedures have been devised in an attempt to quantitate the degree of synechial closure in eyes with angle-closure glaucoma. Compressive gonioscopy as an office procedure was discussed earlier in this chapter. Similar approaches have been used at the time of incisional surgery. Chandler and Simmons (140) suggested deepening the anterior chamber with saline to study the angle with a Koeppe goniolens before proceeding with the surgery, while Shaffer (141) performed the same maneuver after making an iridectomy. The purpose of these maneuvers was to help decide whether an incisional iridectomy alone or a filtering procedure should be performed, based on the extent of synechial angle closure. Other factors that are said to be helpful in this decision making process are a poor tonographic facility of outflow (142) and visual field loss (143).

The advent of laser iridotomy has provided an alternative approach for the determination of which eyes may require filtering surgery. Even if compressive gonioscopy reveals partial synechial closure of the anterior chamber angle, it is best to proceed first with the laser iridotomy, since this has been shown to control the pressure in many cases of chronic angle-closure glaucoma (144). If the iridotomy does not restore a normal IOP, the eye is then treated with medication or filtering surgery if required. Caution must be taken when performing filtering surgery (as well as an incisional surgical iridectomy) on eyes with angle-closure glaucoma, due to the increased risk of malignant (ciliary block) glaucoma (discussed in Chapter 23) (145).

Care must also be taken with the prolonged use of topical corticosteroids following laser or incisional surgery in these patients, since a high percentage will have steroid-induced IOP elevation after an attack of angle-closure glaucoma (146, 147).

A prophylactic peripheral iridotomy is generally recommended for the fellow eye following an attack of pupillary-block glaucoma. Several large studies have shown that approximately 50–75% of the patients who develop angle closure in one eye will have an attack in the fellow, unoperated eye within 5–10 years despite miotic prophylaxis (148–153), whereas such an attack is rare after an iridectomy (151, 154, 155). Since the attack in the fellow eye usually occurs in the first year after the initial event (156, 157), the prophylactic procedure should be done promptly. Rare exceptions include a deeper anterior chamber in the fellow eye due to anisometropia, pseudophakia, aphakia, or a dislocated lens. Some surgeons have suggested that fellow eyes with negative provocative tests might be followed closely without surgery (156, 158). However, with the relative safety of laser iridotomy, a prophylactic procedure in all high risk fellow eyes appears to be prudent.

Extracapsular cataract extraction with posterior chamber intraocular lens implantation has also been shown to be effective surgical therapy for pupillary-block glaucoma (159, 160). This, of course, should be limited to eyes with a significant cataract, should include an iridectomy, and is best suited for chronic cases, in which case the lysis of peripheral anterior synechiae has also been shown to be beneficial (161).

SUMMARY

Pupillary-block glaucomas are much less common than open-angle glaucomas in most populations. A predisposing factor to angle closure is a narrow anterior chamber angle, which has a familial tendency and is associated with increasing age and hyperopia. An angle-closure attack may be precipitated in a predisposed individual by factors which induce mydriasis, such as dim illumination, emotional stress, and drugs. The basic mechanism of pupillary-block glaucoma is a functional block between the lens and iris, which obstructs aqueous flow from the posterior to the anterior chamber, resulting in increased pressure in the posterior chamber, forward bowing of the peripheral iris, and closure of the anterior chamber angle. The clinical presentation may be that of an acute attack with severe pain, marked conjunctival hyperemia, a cloudy cornea, and profound visual loss, or as a subacute attack with a dull ache, slight blurring of vision, and colored halos around lights. Still other cases may be chronic and typically asymptomatic. Treatment usually begins with medical therapy to lower the IOP and relieve the angle closure, followed by a peripheral iridotomy to prevent future attacks.

REFERENCES

1. Tornquist, R: Angle-closure glaucoma in an eye with a plateau type of iris. Acta Ophthalmol 36:413, 1958.

2. Shaffer, RN: Gonioscopy, ophthalmoscopy, and perimetry. Trans Am Acad Ophthalmol Otol 64:112, 1960.

3. Wand, M, Grant, WM, Simmons, RJ, Hutchinson, BT: Plateau iris syndrome. Trans Am Acad Ophthalmol Otol 83:122, 1977.

4. Curran, EJ: A new operation for glaucoma involving a new principle in the aetiology and treatment of chronic primary glaucoma. Arch Ophthalmol 49:131, 1920.

5. Chandler, PA: Narrow-angle glaucoma. Arch Ophthalmol 47:695, 1952.

6. Banziger, TH: The mechanism of acute glaucoma and the explanation for the effectiveness of iridectomy for the same. Ber Deutsch Ophthalmol Ges 43:43, 1922.

7. Barkan, O: Glaucoma: classification, causes, and surgical control. Results of microgonioscopic research. Am J Ophthalmol 21:1099, 1938.

8. Chandler, PA, Trotter, RR: Angle-closure glaucoma. Subacute types. Arch Ophthalmol 53:305, 1955.

9. Pollack, IP: Chronic angle-closure glaucoma. Diagnosis and treatment in patients with angles that appear open. Arch Ophthalmol 85:676, 1971.

10. Bhargava, SK, Leighton, DA, Phillips, CI: Early angle-closure glaucoma. Distribution of iridotrabecular contact and response to pilocarpine. Arch Ophthalmol 89:369, 1973.

11. Gorin, G: Shortening of the angle of the anterior chamber in angle-closure glaucoma. Am J Ophthalmol 49:141, 1960.

12. Lowe, RF: Primary creeping angle-closure glaucoma. Br J Ophthalmol 48:544, 1964.

13. Hyams, SW, Keroub, C, Pokotilo, E: Mixed glaucoma. Br J Ophthalmol 61:105, 1977.

14. Drance, SM: Angle closure glaucoma among Canadian Eskimos. Can J Ophthalmol 8:252, 1973.

15. Arkell, SM, Lightman, DA, Sommer, A, et al: The prevalence of glaucoma among Eskimos of Northwest Alaska. Arch Ophthalmol 105:482, 1987.

16. Clemmesen, V, Alsbirk, PH: Primary angle-closure glaucoma (a.c.g.) in Greenland. Acta Ophthalmol 49:47, 1971.

17. Alsbirk, PH: Early detection of primary angle-closure glaucoma. Limbal and axial chamber depth screening in a high risk population (Greenland Eskimos). Acta Ophthalmol 49:47, 1971.

18. Salmon, JF, Mermoud, A, Ivey, A, et al: The prevalence of primary angle closure glaucoma and open angle glaucoma in Mamre, Western Cape, South Africa. Arch Ophthalmol 111:1263, 1993.

19. Drance, SM, Morgan, RW, Bryett, J, et al: Anterior chamber depth and gonioscopic findings among the Eskimos and Indians of the Canadian artic. Can J Ophthalmol 8:255, 1973.

20. Alsbirk, PH: Corneal diameter in Greenland Eskimos. Acta Ophthalmol 53:635, 1975.

21. Alsbirk, PH: Anterior chamber depth, genes and environment. A population study among long-term Greenland Eskimo immigrants in Copenhagen. Acta Ophthalmol 60:223, 1982.

22. Van Rens, GHMB, Arkell, SM: Refractive errors and axial length among Alaskan Eskimos. Acta Ophthalmol 69:27, 1991.

23. Kolker, A, Hetherington, J Jr: Becker-Shaffer's Diagnosis and Therapy of the Glaucomas. 4th ed. St. Louis, CV Mosby, 1976, p. 183.

24. Spaeth, GL: The normal development of the human anterior chamber angle: a new system of descriptive grading. Trans Ophthalmol Soc UK XCI:709, 1971.

25. Fontana, ST, Brubaker, RF: Volume and depth of the anterior chamber in the normal aging human eye. Arch Ophthalmol 98:1803, 1980.

26. Markowitz, SN, Morin, JD: Angle-closure glaucoma: relation between lens thickness, anterior chamber depth and age. Can J Ophthalmol 19:300, 1984.

27. Okabe, I, Taniguchi, T, Yamamoto, T, Kitazawa, Y: Age-related changes of the anterior chamber width. J Glau 1:100, 1992.

28. Appleby, RS Jr, Kinder, RSL: Bilateral angle-closure glaucoma in a 14-year-old boy. Arch Ophthalmol 86:449, 1971.

29. Alper, MG, Laubach, JL: Primary angle-closure glaucoma in the American Negro. Arch Ophthalmol 79:663, 1968.

30. Clemmesen, V, Luntz, MH: Lens thickness and angle-closure glaucoma. A comparative oculometric study in South African Negroes and Danes. Acta Ophthalmol 54:193, 1976.

31. Wilensky, J: Racial influences in glaucoma. Ann Ophthalmol 9:1545, 1977.

32. Olurin, O: Anterior chamber depths of Nigerians. Ann Ophthalmol 9:315, 1977.

33. Emiru, VP: Response to mydriatics in the African. Br J Ophthalmol 55:538, 1971.

34. Teikari, J, Raivio, I, Nurminen, M: Incidence of acute glaucoma in Finland from 1973 to 1982. Graefes Arch Clin Exp Ophthalmol 225:357, 1987.

35. Hagan, JC III, Lederer, CM Jr: Primary angle closure glaucoma in a myopic kinship. Arch Ophthalmol 103:363, 1985.

36. Cherny, M, Brooks, AMV, Gillies, WE: Progressive myopia in early onset chronic angle closure glaucoma. Br J Ophthalmol 76:758, 1992.

37. Spaeth, GL: Gonioscopy: uses old and new. The inheritance of occludable angles. Ophthalmology 85:222, 1978.

38. Lichter, PR, Anderson, DR, ed: Discussions on Glaucoma. New York, Grune & Stratton, 1977, p. 139.

39. Gieser, DK, Wilensky, JT: HLA antigens and acute angle-closure glaucoma. Am J Ophthalmol 88:232, 1979.

40. Mapstone, R, Clark, CV: Prevalence of diabetes in glaucoma. Br Med J 291:93, 1985.

41. Mapstone, R, Clark, CV: The prevalence of autonomic neuropathy in glaucoma. Trans Ophthalmol Soc UK 104:265, 1985.

42. Shapiro, A, Zauberman, H: Diurnal changes of the intraocular pressure of patients with angle-closure glaucoma. Br J Ophthalmol 63:225, 1979.

43. Lee, DA, Brubaker, RF, Ilstrup, DM: Anterior chamber dimensions in patients with narrow angles and angle-closure glaucoma. Arch Ophthalmol 102:46, 1984.

44. Mapstone, R, Clark, CV: Diurnal variation in the dimensions of the anterior chamber. Arch Ophthalmol 103:1485, 1985.

45. Vargas, E, Drance, SM: Anterior chamber depth in angle-closure glaucoma. Clinical methods of depth determination in people with and without the disease. Arch Ophthalmol 90:438, 1973.

46. Smith, RJH: A new method of estimating the depth of the anterior chamber. Br J Ophthalmol 63:215, 1979.

47. Jacobs, IH: Anterior chamber depth measurement using the slit-lamp microscope. Am J Ophthalmol 88:236, 1979.

48. Douthwaite, WA, Spence, D: Slit-lamp measurement of the anterior chamber depth. Br J Ophthalmol 70:205, 1986.

49. Makabe, R: Comparative studies of the anterior chamber angle width by ultrasonography and gonioscopy. Klin Monatsbl Augenheilkd 194:6, 1989.

50. van Herick, W, Shaffer, RN, Schwartz, A: Estimation of width of angle of anterior chamber. Incidence and significance of the narrow angle. Am J Ophthalmol 68:626, 1969.

51. Scheie, HG: Width and pigmentation of the angle of the anterior chamber. A system of grading by gonioscopy. Arch Ophthalmol 58:510, 1957.

52. Shaffer, RN: Symposium: Primary Glaucomas. III. Gonioscopy, ophthalmoscopy and perimetry. Trans Am Acad Ophthalmol Otol 62:112, 1960.

53. Becker, S: Clinical Gonioscopy—A Test and Stereoscopic Atlas. St. Louis, CV Mosby, 1972.

54. Desjardins, D, Parrish, RK II: Inversion of anterior chamber pigment as a possible prognostic sign in narrow angles. Am J Ophthalmol 100:480, 1985.

55. Pavlin, CJ, Harasiewicz, K, Foster, FS: Ultrasound biomicroscopy of anterior segment structures in normal and glaucomatous eyes. Am J Ophthalmol 113:381, 1992.

56. Aslanides, IM, Libre, PE, Silverman, RH, et al: High frequency ultrasound imaging in pupillary block glaucoma. Br J Ophthalmol 79:972, 1995.

57. Markowitz, SN, Morin, JD: The clinical course in primary angle-closure glaucoma: a reassessment. Can J Ophthalmol 21:130, 1986.

58. Panek, WC, Christensen, RE, Lee, DA, et al: Biometric variables in patients with occludable anterior chamber angles. Am J Ophthalmol 110:185, 1990.

59. Pavlin, CJ, Harasiewicz, K, Foster, FS: An ultrasound biomicroscopic dark-room provocative test. Ophthalmic Surg 26:253, 1995.

60. Richards, DW, Russell, SR, Anderson, DR: A method for improved biometry of the anterior chamber with a Scheimpflug technique. Invest Ophthalmol Vis Sci 29:1826, 1988.

61. Kondo, T, Miura, M: A method of measuring pupil-blocking force in the human eye. Graefes Arch Clin Exp Ophthalmol 225:361, 1987.

62. Bosem, ME, Morsman, D, Lusky, M, Weinreb, RN: Reproducibility of quantitative anterior chamber angle measurements with Scheimpflug video imaging. J Glau 1:254, 1992.

63. Izatt, JA, Hee, MR, Swanson, EA, et al: Micrometer-scale resolution imaging of the anterior eye in vivo with optical coherence tomography. Arch Ophthalmol 112:1584, 1994.

64. Hillman, JS: Acute closed-angle glaucoma: an investigation into the effect of delay in treatment. Br J Ophthalmol 63:817, 1979.

65. Gloster, J, Poinoosawmy, D: Changes in intraocular pressure during and after the dark-room test. Br J Ophthalmol 57:170, 1973.

66. Foulds, WS: Observations on the facility of aqueous outflow in closed-angle glaucoma. Br J Ophthalmol 43:613, 1959.

67. Hyams, SW, Friedman, BZ, Neumann, E: Elevated intraocular pressure in the prone position. A new provocative test for angle-closure glaucoma. Am J Ophthalmol 66:661, 1968.

68. Harris, LS, Galin, MA: Prone provocative testing for narrow angle glaucoma. Arch Ophthalmol 87:493, 1972.

69. Neumann, E, Hyams, SW: Gonioscopy and anterior chamber depth in the prone-position provocative test for angle-closure glaucoma. Ophthalmologica 167:9, 1973.

70. Friedman, Z, Neumann, E: Comparison of prone-position, darkroom, and mydriatic tests for angle-closure glaucoma before and after peripheral iridectomy. Am J Ophthalmol 74:24, 1972.

71. Mapstone, R: Provocative tests in closed-angle glaucoma. Br J Ophthalmol 60:115, 1976.

72. Mapstone, R: Normal response to pilocarpine and phenylephrine. Br J Ophthalmol 61:510, 1977.

73. Mapstone, R: Outflow changes in positive provocative tests. Br J Ophthalmol 61:634, 1977.

74. Mapstone, R: Partial angle closure. Br J Ophthalmol 61:525, 1977.

75. Wishart, PK: Does the pilocarpine phenylephrine provocative test help in the management of acute and subacute angle closure glaucoma? Br J Ophthalmol 75:284, 1991.

76. Wishart, PK: Can the pilocarpine phenylephrine provocative test be used to detect covert angle closure? Br J Ophthalmol 75:615, 1991.

77. Wilensky, JT, Kaufman, PL, Frohlichstein, D, et al: Follow-up of angle-closure glaucoma suspects. Am J Ophthalmol 115:338, 1993.

78. Lowe, RF: Primary angle-closure glaucoma. A review of provocative tests. Br J Ophthalmol 51:727, 1967.

79. Hillman, JS, Turner, JDC: Association between acute glaucoma and the weather and sunspot activity. Br J Ophthalmol 61:512, 1977.

80. Grant, WM: Ocular complications of drugs. Glaucoma. JAMA 207:2089, 1969.

81. Mapstone, R: Dilating dangerous pupils. Br J Ophthalmol 61:517, 1977.

82. Patel, KH, Javitt, JC, Tielsch, JM, et al: Incidence of acute angle-closure glaucoma after pharmacologic mydriasis. Am J Ophthalmol 120:709, 1995.

83. Fazio, DT, Bateman, JB, Christensen, RE: Acute angle-closure glaucoma associated with surgical anesthesia. Arch Ophthalmol 103:360, 1985.

84. Schwartz, H, Apt, L: Mydriatic effect of anticholinergic drugs used during reversal of nondepolarizing muscle relaxants. Am J Ophthalmol 88:609, 1979.

85. Ritch, R, Krupin, T, Henry, C, Kurata, F: Oral imipramine and acute angle closure glaucoma. Arch Ophthalmol 112:67, 1994.

86. Potash, SD, Ritch, R: Acute angle-closure glaucoma secondary to chlortrimeton. J Glau 1:258, 1992.

87. Corridan, P, Nightingale, S, Mashoudi, N, Williams AC: Acute angle-closure glaucoma following botulinum toxin injection for blepharospasm. Br J Ophthalmol 74:309, 1990.

88. Geanon, JD, Perkins, TW: Bilateral acute angle-closure glaucoma associated with drug sensitivity to hydrochlorothiazide. Arch Ophthalmol 113:1231, 1995.

89. Krontz, DP, Wood, TO: Corneal decompensation following acute angle-closure glaucoma. Ophthalmic Surg 19:334, 1988.

90. Charles, ST, Hamasaki, DI: The effect of intraocular pressure on the pupil size. Arch Ophthalmol 83:729, 1970.

91. Rutkowski, PC, Thompson, HS: Mydriasis and increased intraocular pressure. I. Pupillographic studies. Arch Ophthalmol 87:21, 1972.

92. Anderson, DR, Davis, EB: Sensitivities of ocular tissues to acute pressure-induced ischemia. Arch Ophthalmol 93:267, 1975.

93. Kapoor, S, Sood, M: Glaucoma-induced changes in the ciliary ganglion. Br J Ophthalmol 59:573, 1975.

94. Bigar, F, Witmer, R: Corneal endothelial changes in primary acute angle-closure glaucoma. Ophthalmology 89:596, 1982.

95. Markowitz, SN, Morin, JD: The endothelium in primary angle-closure glaucoma. Am J Ophthalmol 98:103, 1984.

96. Campbell, DG: A comparison of diagnostic techniques in angle-closure glaucoma. Am J Ophthalmol 88:197, 1979.

97. Forbes, M: Gonioscopy with corneal indentation. A method for distinguishing between appositional closure and synechial closure. Arch Ophthalmol 76:488, 1966.

98. Forbes, M: Indentation gonioscopy and efficacy of iridectomy in angle-closure glaucoma. Trans Am Ophthalmol Soc LXXII:488, 1974.

99. Zimmerman, LE, de Venecia, G, Hamasaki, DI: Pathology of the optic nerve in experimetnal acute glaucoma. Invest Ophthalmol 6:109, 1967.

100. Douglas, GR, Drance, SM, Schulzer, M: The visual field and nerve head in angle-closure glaucoma. A comparison of the effects of acute and chronic angle closure. Arch Ophthalmol 93:409, 1975.

101. Sonty, S, Schwartz, B: Vascular accidents in acute angle closure glaucoma. Ophthalmology 88:225, 1981.

102. McNaught, EI, Rennie, A, McClure, E, Chisholm, IA: Pattern of visual damage after acute angle-closure glaucoma. Trans Ophthalmol Soc UK 94:406, 1974.

103. Mapstone, R: One gonioscopic fallacy. Br J Ophthalmol 63:221, 1979.

104. Mapstone, R: The mechanism and clinical significance of angle closure. Glaucoma 2:249, 1980.

105. Tornquist, R: Corneal radius in primary acute glaucoma. Br J Ophthalmol 41:421, 1957.

106. Lowe, RF: Causes of shallow anterior chamber in primary angle-closure glaucoma. Ultrasonic biometry of normal and angle-closure glaucoma eyes. Am J Ophthalmol 67:87, 1969.

107. Phillips, CI: Aetiology of angle-closure glaucoma. Br J Ophthalmol 56:248, 1972.

108. Lowe, RF, Clark, BAJ: Posterior corneal curvature. Correlations in normal eyes and in eyes involved with primary angle-closure glaucoma. Br J Ophthalmol 57:464, 1973.

109. Tomlinson, A, Leighton, DA: Ocular dimensions in the heredity of angle-closure glaucoma. Br J Ophthalmol 57:475, 1973.

110. Kerman, BM, Christensen, RE, Foos, RY: Angle-closure glaucoma: a clinicopathologic correlation. Am J Ophthalmol 76:887, 1973.

111. Markowitz, SN, Morin, JD: The ratio of lens thickness to axial length for biometric standardization in angle-closure glaucoma. Am J Ophthalmol 99:400, 1985.

112. Salmon, JF, Swanevelder, SA, Donald, MA: The dimensions of eyes with chronic angle-closure glaucoma. J Glau 3:237, 1994.

113. Mapstone, R: Acute shallowing of the anterior chamber. Br J Ophthalmol 65:446, 1981.

114. Mapstone, R: Mechanics of pupil block. Br J Ophthalmol 52:19, 1968.

115. Tiedeman, JS: A physical analysis of the factors that determine the contour of the iris. Am J Ophthalmol 111:338, 1991.

116. Anderson, DR, Jin, JC, Wright, MM: The physiologic characteristics of relative pupillary block. Am J Ophthalmol 111:344, 1991.

117. Pavlin, CJ, Ritch, R, Foster, FS: Ultrasound biomicroscopy in plateau iris syndrome. Am J Ophthalmol 113:390, 1992.

118. Ritch, R: Plateau iris is caused by abnormally positioned ciliary processes. J Glau 1:23, 1992.

119. Wand, M, Pavlin, CJ, Foster, FS: Plateau iris syndrome: ultrasound biomicroscopic and histologic study. Ophthalmic Surg 24:129, 1993.

120. Inoue, T, Yamamoto, T, Kitazawa, Y: Distribution and morphology of peripheral anterior synechiae in primary angle-closure glaucoma. J Glau 2:171, 1993.

121. Wand, M, Grant, WM: Thymoxamine test. Differentiating angle-closure glaucoma from open-angle glaucoma with narrow angles. Arch Ophthalmol 96:1009, 1978.

122. Ganias, F, Mapstone, R: Miotics in closed-angle glaucoma. Br J Ophthalmol 59:205, 1975.

123. Airaksinen, PJ, Saari, KM, Tiainen, TJ, Jaanio, E-AT: Management of acute closed-angle glaucoma with miotics and timolol. Br J Ophthalmol 63:822, 1979.

124. Rutkowski, PC, Fernandez, JL, Galin, MA, Halasa, AH: Alpha-adrenergic receptor blockade in the treatment of angle-closure glaucoma. Trans Am Acad Ophthalmol Otol 77:137, 1973.

125. Halasa, AH, Rutkowski, PC: Thymoxamine therapy for angle-closure glaucoma. Arch Ophthalmol 90:177, 1973.

126. Wand, M, Grant, WM: Thymoxamine hydrochloride: an alpha-adrenergic blocker. Surv Ophthalmol 25:75, 1980.

127. Chandler, PA, Grant, WM: Glaucoma. 2nd ed. Philadelphia, Lea & Febiger, 1979, p. 140.

128. Anderson, DR: Corneal indentation to relieve acute angle-closure glaucoma. Am J Ophthalmol 88:1091, 1979.

129. Ritch, R: Argon laser treatment for medically unresponsive attacks of angle-closure glaucoma. Am J Ophthalmol 94:197, 1982.

130. Shin, DH: Argon Laser treatment for relief of medically unresponsive angle-closure glaucoma attacks. Am J Ophthalmol 94:821, 1982.

131. David, R, Tessler, Z, Yassur, Y: Long-term outcome of primary acute angle-closure glaucoma. Br J Ophthalmol 69:261, 1985.

132. Schwartz, GF, Steinmann, WC, Spaeth, GL, Wilson, RP: Surgical and medical management of patients with narrow anterior chamber angles: comparative results. Ophthalmic Surg 23:108, 1992.

133. Morsman, CD, Lusky, M, Bosem, ME, Weinreb, RN: Anterior chamber angle configuration before and after iridotomy measured by Scheimpflug video imaging. J Glau 13:114, 1994.

134. Jin, JC, Anderson, DR: The effect of iridotomy on iris contour. Am J Ophthalmol 110:260, 1990.

135. Krupin, T, Mitchell, KB, Johnson, MF, Becker, B: The long-term effects of iridectomy for primary acute angle-closure glaucoma. Am J Ophthalmol 86:506, 1978.

136. Playfair, TJ, Watson, PG: Management of acute primary angle-closure glaucoma: a long-term follow-up of the results of peripheral iridectomy used as an initial procedure. Br J Ophthalmol 63:17, 1979.

137. Romano, JH, Hitchings, RA, Pooinasawmy, D: Role of Nd: YAG peripheral iridectomy in the management of ocular hypertension with a narrow angle. Ophthalmic Surg 19:814, 1988.

138. Saunders, DC: Acute closed-angle glaucoma and Nd-YAG laser iridotomy. Br J Ophthalmol 74:523, 1990.

139. Buckley, SA, Reeves, B, Burdon, M, et al: Acute angle closure glaucoma: relative failure of YAG iridotomy in affected eyes and factors influencing outcome. Br J Ophthalmol 78:529, 1994.

140. Chandler, PA, Simmons, RJ: Anterior chamber deepening for gonioscopy at time of surgery. Arch Ophthalmol 74:177, 1965.

141. Shaffer, RN: Operating room gonioscopy in angle closure glaucoma surgery. Trans Am Ophthalmol Soc 55:59, 1957.

142. Williams, DJ, Gills, JP Jr, Hall, GA: Results of 233 peripheral iridectomies for narrow-angle glaucoma. Am J Ophthalmol 65:548, 1968.

143. Playfair, TJ, Watson, PG: Management of chronic or intermittent primary angle-closure glaucoma: a long-term follow-up of the results of peripheral iridectomy used as an initial procedure. Br J Ophthalmol 63:23, 1979.

144. Gieser, DK, Wilensky, JT: Laser iridectomy in the management of chronic angle-closure glaucoma. Am J Ophthalmol 98:446, 1984.

145. Eltz, H, Gloor, B: Trabeculectomy in cases of angle closure glaucoma—successes and failures. Klin Monatsbl Augenheilkd 177:556, 1980.

146. Akingbehin, AO: Corticosteroid-induced ocular hypertension. I. Prevalence in closed-angle glaucoma. Br J Ophthalmol 66:536, 1982.

147. Akingbehin, AO: Corticosteroid-induced ocular hypertension. II. An acquired form. Br J Ophthalmol 66:541, 1982.

148. Lowe, RF: Acute angle-closure glaucoma. The second eye: an analysis of 200 cases. Br J Ophthalmol 46:641, 1962.

149. Benedikt, O: Prophylactic iridectomy in the partner eye after angle closure glaucoma. Klin Monatsbl Augenheilkd 156:80, 1970.

150. Ritzinger, I, Benedikt, O, Dirisamer, F: Surgical or conservative prophylaxis of the partner eye after primary acute angle bloc glaucoma. Klin Monatsbl Augenheilkd 164:645, 1974.

151. Wollensak, J, Ehrhorn, J: Angle block glaucoma and prophylactic iridectomy in the eye without symptoms. Klin Monatsbl Augenheilkd 167:791, 1975.

152. Imre, Gy, Bogi, J: The fellow eye in acute angle-closure glaucoma. Klin Monatsbl Augenheilkd 169:264, 1976.

153. Snow, JT: Value of prophylactic peripheral iridectomy on the second eye in angle-closure glaucoma. Trans Ophthalmol Soc UK 97:189, 1977.

154. Lowe, RF: Primary angle-closure glaucoma. A review 5 years after bilateral surgery. Br J Ophthalmol 57:457, 1973.

155. Imre, G, Bogi, J: Results of prophylactic iridectomy. Klin Monatsbl Augenheilkd 181:409, 1982.

156. Mapstone, R: The fellow eye. Br J Ophthalmol 65:410, 1981.

157. Edwards, RS: Behaviour of the fellow eye in acute angle-closure glaucoma. Br J Ophthalmol 66:576, 1982.

158. Hyams, SW, Friedman, Z, Keroub, C: Fellow eye in angle-closure glaucoma. Br J Ophthalmol 59:207, 1975.

159. Greve, EL: Primary angle closure glaucoma: Extracapsular extraction or filtering procedure? Int Ophthalmol 12:157, 1988.

160. Reibaldi, A, Uva, MG, Ott, JP, Russo, V: A new surgical approach to the closed angle glaucoma. Klin Monatsbl Augenheilkd 200:658, 1992.

161. Matsumura, M, Ido, W, Shirakami, Y, Koizumi, K: Treatment of primary closed angle glaucoma with cataract by lysis of peripheral anterior synechiae and intraocular lens implantation. Jpn J Clin Ophthalmol 45:1567, 1991.

CONGENITAL GLAUCOMAS[a]

TERMINOLOGY

Classification of Childhood Glaucomas

As noted in Chapter 8, the glaucomas of childhood may be classified into three groups: (a) *congenital glaucomas,* in which a developmental abnormality of the anterior chamber angle leads to obstruction of aqueous outflow without a consistent association with other ocular or systemic developmental anomalies; (b) *developmental glaucomas with associated anomalies,* in which a developmental abnormality is responsible for the glaucoma, but in which additional ocular and systemic anomalies are typically present; and (c) *glaucomas in childhood with associated abnormalities,* in which the mechanism of obstruction to outflow is acquired from other events, such as inflammation or neoplasia, rather than a developmental anomaly of the angle. In one study of 63 cases of glaucoma in childhood, the relative proportions of these three groups were 22.2%, 46%, and 31.8%, respectively (1).

Congenital glaucomas are the subject of this chapter, while developmental glaucomas with associated anomalies are considered in Chapter 12. Since children are subject to many of the same glaucomas with associated abnormalities as adults, these will be discussed together in subsequent chapters of Section Two, with special attention being given to those situations that are unique to children.

Classification of Congenital Glaucomas

Because these glaucomas tend to occur without a consistent association with other ocular or systemic anomalies, they have traditionally been called *primary congenital glaucoma* or *primary congenital open-angle glaucoma* (2). They appear to represent a group of disorders, and other terms that have been used for this group refer primarily to the age of onset or clinical appearance. *Infantile glaucoma* is a term that is often applied to those cases which appear during the first few years of life (3). This form of congenital glaucoma has also been called "buphthalmos" (cow's eye) or "hydrophthalmia," referring to the enlargement of the eye that may occur with this condition. However, the latter names should not be used as synonyms for infantile glaucoma since enlargement of the globe may also be seen with other childhood glaucomas if they occur early enough in life. When congenital glaucoma appears later in childhood or early adulthood, it is sometimes referred to as *juvenile glaucoma* (4). Three years of age is generally taken as the division between infantile and juvenile glaucoma, because it is at approximately this age that the eye no longer expands in response to elevated intraocular pressure (IOP) (2, 4). Others prefer a broader definition for juvenile glaucoma, which includes all forms of open-angle glaucoma diagnosed between the ages of 10 and 35 years (5).

GENERAL FEATURES

Frequency

As noted above, congenital glaucomas were found to occur in 22.2% of all childhood glaucomas in one study (1).

[a]Refer to Shields, MB: Color Atlas of Glaucoma. Baltimore, Williams & Wilkins, 1998, Plates II4–7.

However, it occurs much less frequently than the open-angle and angle-closure glaucomas that are seen in adults, and it was once estimated that the average ophthalmic practice will have only one case of congenital glaucoma every 5 years (3).

Age of Onset

Infantile glaucoma is usually diagnosed at birth or shortly thereafter, and most cases are recognized in the first year of life. Juvenile glaucoma may become apparent at any time throughout childhood or even in young adults.

Heredity

Although it is generally believed that the congenital glaucomas have a genetic basis, reports vary as to the precise mode of inheritance. An autosomal recessive mode with incomplete or variable penetrance has been suspected (3), although more recent studies suggest that most cases are caused by multifactorial inheritance (6, 7). In studies of identical twins, congenital glaucoma was usually present in both siblings (6, 8), although only one member was afflicted in one pair of monozygotic twins (9), suggesting that nongenetic factors may also be involved. An incomplete form of the disease has also been observed in a child whose sibling had the typical findings of congenital glaucoma (10).

Chromosomal abnormalities have been reported with various congenital glaucomas, although most of these patients have not had the typical clinical findings of congenital glaucoma (11). More recently, an autosomal dominant juvenile glaucoma was identified in several pedigrees in which the disease-causing gene was mapped to chromosome 1q21–q31 (12). These individuals are typically myopic with open, normal appearing angles except for a possible increase in iris processes (13, 14). The average age of onset is 18, and the IOP tends to be high, in the range of 30–50 mm Hg or more, with a high percentage of patients requiring surgery. In addition, the gene for an infantile glaucoma, characterized by bilateral involvement and diagnosis within the first 6 months of life, has been linked to the 2p21 region of chromosome 2 (15). In both of these glaucomas, however, not all pedigrees linked to chromosomes 1q21–q31 or 2p21, supporting the genetic heterogeneity for this group of glaucomas.

Reports are conflicting as to whether parents of children with congenital glaucoma have an increased prevalence of abnormal anterior chamber angles or topical corticosteroid responses (16, 17). No statistically significant differences in HLA histocompatibility antigens were found in one study of patients with congenital glaucoma as compared to controls (18).

Race

In one study of juvenile glaucoma, which used the liberal definition of all open-angle glaucomas diagnosed between the ages of 10 and 35 years, blacks tended to present at younger ages than whites, and had a higher proportion with glaucomatous damage (5).

CLINICAL FEATURES

Congenital glaucoma is typically bilateral, although a significant IOP elevation may occur in only one eye in 25–30% of the cases. The following ocular features, with the possible exception of gonioscopic findings, are not unique to the congenital glaucomas, but may be a part of any childhood glaucoma during the first few years of life.

History

There is a classic triad of manifestations, any one of which should arouse suspicion of glaucoma in an infant or young child: (a) *epiphora* (excessive tearing); (b) *photophobia* (hypersensitivity to light), which is due to corneal edema and is manifested by the child hiding his face in bright lighting, or even in ordinary lighting in severe cases; and (c) *blepharospasm* (squeezing the eyelids), which may be another manifestation of the photophobia.

External Examination

Corneal Diameter

The average horizontal corneal diameter at birth is normally 10.5 mm (3, 19). In a study of premature infants, the mean corneal diameter was 8.2 mm (20). Both the corneal diameter and axial length are positively correlated with gestational age and birth weight in premature infants, with horizontal corneal diameters ranging from 6.2 to 10 mm for gestational ages ranging from 23 to 36 weeks, respectively (21, 22). Distention of the globe in response to elevated IOP (*buphthalmos*) leads to enlargement of the cornea, especially at the corneoscleral junction, and a diameter over 12 mm in the first year of life is highly suspicious. Grossly, this is more obvious in asymmetric cases (Fig. 11.1). In one study, corneal diameter was found to be a more reliable guide than axial length in the assessment of congenital glaucoma (19).

Corneal Edema

Initially, this may be a direct result of the elevated IOP, producing a corneal haze that clears with normalization of the pressure. In more advanced cases, a dense opacification of

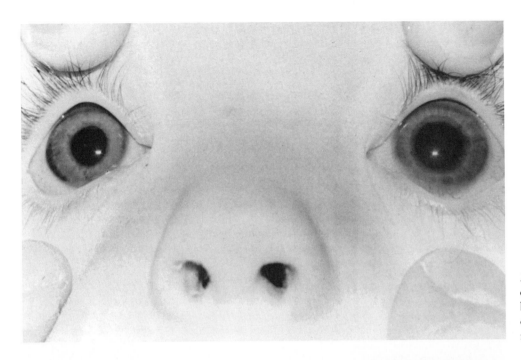

Figure 11.1. Infant with congenital glaucoma showing buphthalmos and corneal clouding, both of which are more marked in the left eye.

the corneal stroma may persist despite reduction of the IOP (Fig. 11.2). One study suggests that the latter may result from reduced aqueous production with poor corneal nutrition (23).

Refractive Error

The enlargement of the globe with elevated IOP during the first 3 years of life creates a *myopic shift* in the refractive error, which may lead to amblyopia if significantly asymmetric. As previously noted, myopia is also commonly associated with forms of juvenile glaucoma (5), although it is not clear as to how often the glaucoma or the myopia was the primary event. It has also been noted that an excessive loss of hyperopia in an aphakic child should alert the clinician to the possible diagnosis of juvenile glaucoma (24).

Tonometry

Any one of the aforementioned findings demands a thorough examination to rule out congenital glaucoma. Since the pressure is often measured during general anesthesia, the possible influence of the anesthesia on IOP (see Chapter 4) must be considered. The normal pressure in an infant under halothane anesthesia is said to be approximately 9–10 mm Hg (25, 26), and a pressure of 20 mm Hg or more should arouse suspicion (25). It has also been reported that children can be successfully examined under chloral hydrate sedation and, using this approach, the pressures by Mackay-Marg tonometry in 17 nonglaucomatous eyes ranged from 11 to 17 mm Hg (27). However, the most reliable method of measuring the IOP is probably with the child awake, if cooperation permits. The Perkins tonome-

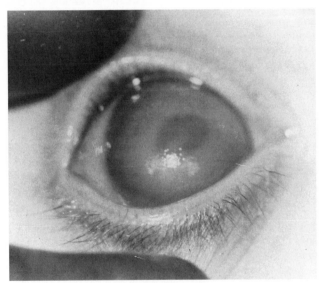

Figure 11.2. Dense corneal opacity of newborn with congenital glaucoma.

ter has been found to be particularly suitable in this situation (28). In one study, the mean IOP in unanesthetized newborns was 11.4 ± 2.4 mm Hg (29). Studies of premature infants are conflicting, with a mean pressure of 18 mm Hg when measured with a Perkins tonometer without anesthesia (20), but 10.3 ± 3.5 mm Hg when measured with a Tonopen II (21).

Slitlamp Examination

This portion of the examination is best performed with a portable slitlamp, with or without general anesthesia. A

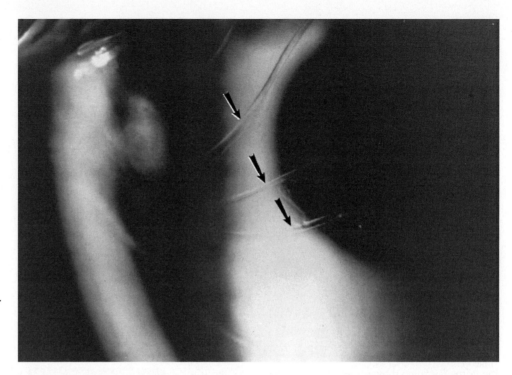

Figure 11.3. Slitlamp appearance of tears in Descemet's membrane, or Haab's striae *(arrows),* in patient with congenital glaucoma.

common finding in the cornea is tears in Descemet's membrane *(Haab's striae),* which may be single or multiple and are characteristically oriented horizontally or concentric to the limbus (Fig. 11.3). They are typically associated with corneal edema in the early phases of the glaucoma. However, as the IOP is normalized and the tears are repaired by endothelial overgrowth, the edema may clear but the linear opacities will persist. Specular microscopy has shown that these patients also have a significantly reduced corneal endothelial cell count (30).

The anterior chamber is characteristically deep, especially when distention of the globe is present. The iris is typically normal, although it may have stromal hypoplasia with loss of the crypts.

Gonioscopy

Evaluation of the anterior chamber angle is essential for the accurate diagnosis of congenital glaucoma. The instruments and techniques of gonioscopy were discussed in Chapter 3. In performing gonioscopy on infants and children under anesthesia, an infant Koeppe goniolens is recommended.

The normal anterior chamber angle in childhood differs significantly from that of adults, and the ophthalmologist must be familiar with these differences in order to recognize the abnormal state. The most characteristic feature of the child's anterior chamber angle is the trabecular meshwork, which has the appearance of a smooth, homogeneous membrane, extending from peripheral iris to Schwalbe's line, during the first year of life. It becomes coarser and more pigmented with the passing years. In addition, the peripheral iris in the young child tends to be thinner and flatter (2).

In congenital glaucoma, the typical gonioscopic appearance is an open angle, with a high insertion of the iris root, which forms a scalloped line (Fig. 11.4). Abnormal tissue, with a shagreened, glistening appearance, may be seen in the angle, and appears to pull the peripheral iris anteriorly. Although the angle is usually avascular, loops of vessels from the major arterial circle may be seen above the iris root, which has been called the "Loch Ness monster phenomenon" (31). In addition, the peripheral iris may be covered by a fine, fluffy tissue that has been referred to as "Lister's morning mist" (31).

The clinical features of congenital glaucoma seem to merge with other forms of developmental glaucoma. A gonioscopic assessment of over 100 eyes with developmental glaucoma revealed a spectrum ranging from the common form described above, through a more cicatrized, vascularized condition, to the gross anomalies of the Axenfeld-Rieger syndrome (32), which is discussed in Chapter 12.

Funduscopy

Evaluation of the optic nerve head is one of the most important methods for diagnosing congenital glaucoma, as well as for following the response to therapy. This is usually done with the child anesthetized or sedated, often with an undilated pupil, in which case visualization of the disc may be facilitated by using a direct ophthalmoscope with a Koeppe lens on the cornea (Fig. 11.5) or a lens designed for vitrectomy surgery (33).

The optic nerve head in normal newborns is typically pink but may have slight pallor, and a small physiologic cup is usually present (34). The morphology of glaucomatous optic atrophy in childhood resembles that seen in adult eyes, with a preferential loss of neural tissue in the vertical poles (35). A child's eye does differ from that of the adult, however, in that the scleral canal in children enlarges in response to elevated IOP, especially in the horizontal meridian, causing further enlargement of the cup in addition to that resulting from the actual loss of neural tissue (35).

Cupping of the optic nerve head proceeds more rapidly in infants than in adults, and is more likely to be reversible if the pressure is lowered early enough (36–39). This appears to be due to incomplete development of connective tissue in the lamina cribrosa, which allows compression or posterior movement of the optic disc tissue in response to elevated IOP, with an elastic return to normal when the pressure is lowered (37).

Visual Fields

When tested after the child becomes old enough for a reliable study, the visual fields are identical to those in adult-onset glaucoma, with an initial predilection for the arcuate areas (35).

Visual Acuity

Good vision may be achieved if the IOP is controlled before optic atrophy occurs. Occasionally, however, the acuity is poor despite adequate pressure control. In some cases this is due to optic nerve damage, corneal clouding, or irregular astigmatism (35, 40). Other children, may have normal appearing optic nerve heads and clear media, but develop amblyopia from an-

isometropia or strabismus (41). Retinal detachment is also an occasional cause of poor visual results (42).

Ultrasonography

It has been suggested that ultrasonography may be helpful in documenting progression of infantile glaucoma by recording changes in the axial length of the globe (43, 44). It has also been reported that the axial length may decrease up to 0.8 mm following surgical reduction of the IOP (44). As previously noted, axial length in the premature infant correlates with gestational age and birth weight, with a range of 12.6 mm to 16.2 mm for gestational ages of 25–37 weeks, respectively (21).

ETIOLOGY

Normal Development of the Anterior Ocular Segment

A basic understanding of the normal development of the anterior ocular segment is necessary before considering the theories of mechanism for congenital glaucoma or for any of the developmental glaucomas with associated anomalies.

General Development

The lens vesicle begins to develop as an invagination of surface ectoderm during the third week of gestation and separates from the latter structure by the sixth week (45). A study

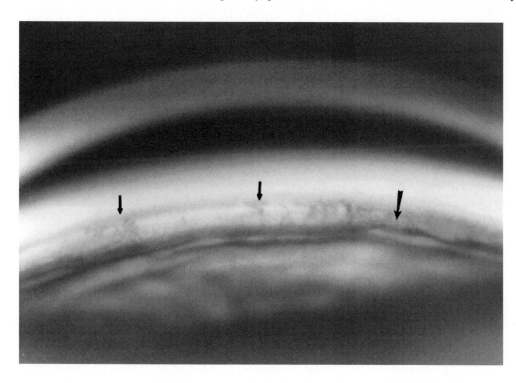

Figure 11.4. Gonioscopic appearance of patient with juvenile glaucoma showing high insertion of iris *(large arrow)* and numerous iris processes *(small arrows)*.

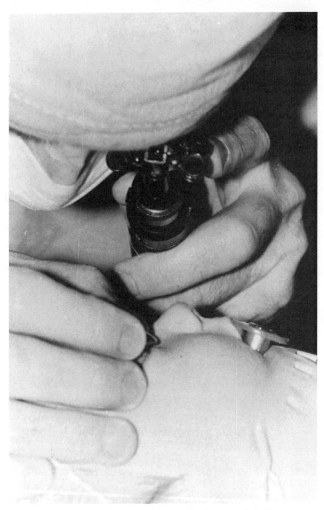

Figure 11.5. Fundus examination with direct ophthalmoscope through infant Koeppe lens during examination under anesthesia of infant with suspected glaucoma.

dicate that the tissue is of cranial neural crest cell origin. Johnston and coworkers (47) studied orofacial development in chick embryos by transplanting labeled neural crest or mesodermal cells into unlabeled host embryos. The donor tissue was either labeled with tritiated thymidine or was material from the Japanese quail. Cells from the latter bird are characterized by condensed chromatin in the center of the nucleus, in contrast to a more diffuse chromatin pattern in chick cells. Using these models, it was determined that corneal endothelium and stroma, iris, ciliary body, and sclera are of neural crest origin, except for the associated vascular endothelium, which is derived from mesodermal mesenchyme. Immunohistochemical studies have provided support for the concept that cells of human trabecular meshwork are also of neural crest origin by showing evidence of neuronal-specific enolase, an enzyme that is normally confined to neurons and cells of the neuroendocrine system (48, 49). These cells were found in the anterior region of the meshwork and in the inner uveal beams (48, 49), while the cells lining Schlemm's canal were found to share many immunophenotypical features with vascular endothelial cells (49).

Development of Cornea and Iris

From the mass of undifferentiated cells, three waves of tissue come forward between the surface ectoderm and lens. The first of these layers differentiates into the primordial corneal endothelium by the eighth week and subsequently produces Descemet's membrane, while the second wave grows between the corneal endothelium and epithelium to produce the stroma of the cornea (50, 51). The third wave insinuates between the primordia of the cornea and the lens and gives rise to the pupillary membrane and the stroma of the iris. In later months, the pigment epithelial layer of the iris develops from neural ectoderm.

Development of Anterior Chamber Angle

The aqueous outflow structures in the anterior chamber angle appear to arise from the same mesenchymal mass of neural crest cell origin. The precise details of this development, however, are not fully understood. Theories have included atrophy (45) or resorption (52) (progressive disappearance of portions of fetal tissue), cleavage (53) (separation of two preexisting tissue layers due to differential growth rates), and rarefaction (54) (mechanical distention due to growth of the anterior ocular segment). More recent work, however, suggests that none of these concepts are completely correct.

Anderson (55) studied 40 normal fetal and infant eyes by light and electron microscopy and found that the anterior surface of the iris at 5 months gestation inserts at the edge of the corneal endothelium, covering the cells that are destined to become trabecular meshwork. This appears to be what Worst (31) called the fetal pectinate ligament, separating the

of 53 human embryos showed that the adhesion between the lens vesicle and presumptive corneal epithelium at the 8-mm stage is replaced by a "clear zone" at the 12.5-mm stage (46). The same study suggested that the formation of the eye is influenced by signals from neural and pigmented layers, and that the lens, with its relatively large size and high mitosis, participates in the early embryogenesis of the rudimentary anterior chamber, most likely by its active metabolic flow.

At the same time that the lens vesicle is separating from surface ectoderm, the optic cup, which arises from neural ectoderm, has reached the periphery of the lens, and a triangular mass of undifferentiated cells overrides the rim of the cup and surrounds the anterior periphery of the lens. From this tissue mass will arise portions of the cornea, iris, and the anterior chamber angle structures.

Neural Crest Cell Contribution

It was traditionally taught that the undifferentiated cell mass is derived from mesoderm. Subsequent studies, however, in-

corneoscleral meshwork primordium from the anterior chamber angle. Anderson noted a posterior repositioning of the anterior uveal structures in relation to the cornea and sclera in progressively older tissue specimens, presumably due to the differential growth rates. At birth, the insertion of the iris and ciliary body is near the level of the scleral spur, and the posterior migration of these structures continues for about the first year of life.

There is some difference of interpretation regarding the innermost layer of the trabecular meshwork primordium as it is uncovered by the posteriorly receding iris. Anderson (55) felt that the smooth surface represents multilayered mesenchymal tissue, which begins to cavitate by the seventh fetal month. Others have suggested, however, that a true endothelial layer covers the meshwork during gestation. Hansson and Jerndal (56) studied human fetal eyes by scanning electron microscopy and described a single layer of endothelium, continuous with that of the cornea, extending over the primitive anterior chamber angle and iridopupillary structures, creating a closed cavity at the beginning of the fifth fetal month. Worst (31) observed a similar sheet of flat endothelial cells on the pupillary membrane and felt that the disappearance of this layer progresses centrifugally toward the anterior chamber angle.

Hansson and Jerndal (56) noted that the anterior chamber angle portion of the endothelial layer begins to flatten, with loss of clear-cut cell borders, by the seventh fetal month. During the final weeks of gestation and the first weeks after birth, the endothelial layer undergoes fenestration with migration of cells into the underlying uveal meshwork. Van Buskirk (57) also observed intact endothelium completely lining the anterior chamber angle by the second gestational trimester in macaque monkey eyes studied by scanning electron microscopy. He noted that fenestration and gradual retraction of this tissue occurs in the third trimester and progresses in a posterior-to-anterior direction. McMenamin (58), however, in a scanning electron microscopic study of 32 human fetal eyes, found that the endothelial layer in the iridocorneal angle was perforated by discrete intercellular gaps by 12–14 weeks and that the gaps between the inner uveal trabecular endothelial cells was sufficiently developed by 18–20 weeks to allow a route of communication between the fetal anterior chamber and primitive trabecular tissue.

McMenamin (59) also showed, in light and electron microscopic studies of human fetal eyes between 12 and 22 weeks gestation, that the trabecular anlage doubles in cross-sectional area, cell density decreases but the absolute number of cells increases two- to three-fold, extracellular matrix increases in a predictable fashion by 360%, and the intertrabecular spaces increase in a more variable manner by 200%. Thus it appears that the trabecular meshwork develops by a simple process of growth and differentiation. These observations have been combined into a concept of anterior chamber angle development, depicted in Figure 11.6**A–D** (60).

Theories of Abnormal Development in Congenital Glaucoma

Although it is generally agreed that the IOP elevation in congenital glaucoma is due to an abnormal development of the anterior chamber angle which leads to obstruction of aqueous outflow, there is no universal agreement as to the nature of the developmental alteration. Theories of pathogenesis parallel the basic concepts regarding the normal development of the anterior chamber angle, as discussed above, most of which are no longer accepted as being entirely correct. We will first review the major theories that have been proposed in the past and then consider how they fit with our current understanding of the developmental abnormality of congenital glaucoma.

In 1928, Mann (61) postulated that incomplete atrophy of anterior chamber mesoderm resulted in retention of abnormal tissue that blocked aqueous outflow. In 1955, Barkan (52) suggested that incomplete resorption of the mesodermal cells by adjacent tissue led to the formation of a membrane across the anterior chamber angle. This "membrane" became known as *Barkan's membrane*, although its existence has not been proved histologically. Electron microscopic studies by Anderson (55, 62) revealed no membrane, despite the appearance of such a structure by gonioscopy and the dissecting microscope. In 1955, Allen, Burian, and Braley (53) postulated that incomplete cleavage of mesoderm in the anterior chamber angle resulted in the congenital defect. Worst (31), in 1966, proposed a combined theory, which included elements of the atrophy and resorption concepts, but rejected the cleavage theory. However, all of the theories for normal development of the anterior chamber angle, on which each of the above theories of pathogenesis were based, are no longer felt to be correct.

In 1959, Maumenee (63, 64) observed an abnormal anterior insertion of the ciliary musculature into the trabecular meshwork, and reasoned that this might compress the scleral spur forward and externally, thus narrowing Schlemm's canal. Anderson (55) and others (65) provided further histopathologic support for the high insertion of the anterior uvea into the trabecular meshwork, suggesting that this is due to a developmental arrest in the normal migration of the uvea across the meshwork in the third trimester of gestation. Maumenee (64) also noted the absence of Schlemm's canal in some histopathologic specimens and suggested that this might be a cause of aqueous outflow obstruction in congenital glaucoma, although Anderson (62) feels this may be a secondary change.

In 1971, Smelser and Ozanics (54) explained congenital glaucoma as a failure of anterior chamber angle anlage to become properly rearranged into the normal trabecular meshwork. Subsequent light and electron microscopic studies favor this theory by showing structural changes of the uveal meshwork (62, 66–70) and, in some cases of both in-

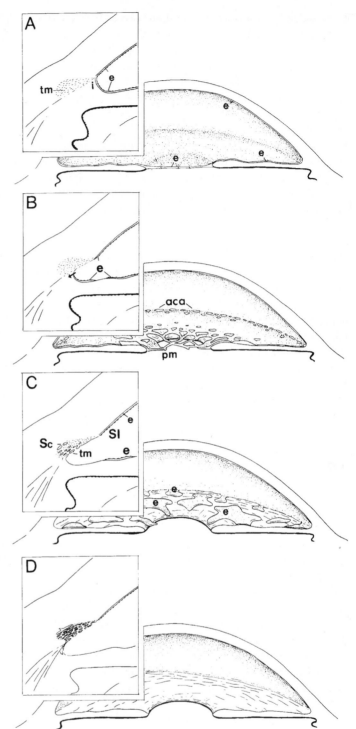

Figure 11.6. A concept of anterior chamber angle development (insets show cross-sectional views of chamber angle). **A.** At 5 months gestation, a continuous layer of endothelium *(e)* creates a closed cavity of the anterior chamber (according to most, but not all, studies), and the anterior surface of the iris *(i)* inserts in front of the primordial trabecular meshwork *(tm)*. **B.** During the third trimester, the endothelial layer progressively disappears from the pupillary membrane *(pm)* and iris and cavitates over the anterior chamber angle *(aca)*, possibly becoming incorporated in the trabecular meshwork. At the same time, the peripheral uveal tissue begins to slide posteriorly in relation to the chamber angle structures *(arrow)*. **C.** Development of the trabecular lamellae and intertrabecular spaces begins in the inner, posterior aspect of the primordial tissue and progresses toward Schlemm's canal *(Sc)* and Schwalbe's line *(S1)*. **D.** The normal anterior chamber angle is not fully developed until one year of life. (Reprinted with permission from Shields, MB: Axenfeld-Rieger Syndrome. A theory of mechanism and distinctions from the iridocorneal endothelial syndrome. Trans Am Ophthalmol Soc 81:736, 1983.)

fantile and juvenile glaucoma, a thick layer of amorphous material beneath the internal endothelium of Schlemm's canal (68–70). Kupfer and associates (71, 72) emphasized the contribution of the cranial neural crest cells in the development of the anterior chamber angle and suggested that abnormal development of structures derived from these cells may result in the defects of the various forms of congenital glaucoma.

In summary, most forms of congenital glaucoma appear to result from a developmental arrest of anterior chamber angle tissue derived from neural crest cells, leading to aqueous outflow obstruction by one or more of several mechanisms. The high insertion of ciliary body and iris into the posterior portion of the trabecular meshwork may compress the trabecular beams. In addition, there may be primary developmental defects at various levels of the meshwork and, in some cases, of Schlemm's canal. However, a true membrane over the meshwork does not appear to be a feature of this disorder.

DIFFERENTIAL DIAGNOSIS

Some of the clinical features of congenital glaucoma are also found in other conditions, and these must be considered in the differential diagnosis.

Excessive Tearing

In the infant, excessive tearing is most commonly caused by obstruction of the lacrimal drainage system. The epiphora of nasolacrimal duct obstruction is distinguished from that of infantile-onset glaucoma in that the former condition is usually associated with fullness of the lacrimal sac and often has purulent discharge. In addition, the epiphora of infantile glaucoma is frequently associated with photophobia and blepharospasm, although these three findings can also result from a variety of external ocular disorders.

Corneal Disorders

Large Corneas

Large corneas may represent congenital megalocornea without glaucoma or an enlarged globe due to high myopia. However, infantile-onset glaucoma also typically causes progressive myopia secondary to enlargement of the globe. In addition, a pedigree has been described with autosomal dominant megalocornea and congenital glaucoma, in which the inheritance is felt to represent germ-line mosaicism (73).

Tears in Descemet's Membrane

Tears in Descemet's membrane may result from birth trauma (74). These tears are usually vertical or oblique in contrast to those of congenital glaucoma (Haab's striae), which tend to be horizontal or concentric with the limbus. The tears in Descemet's membrane may also be confused with band-like structures in posterior polymorphous dystrophy (75) and posterior corneal vesicles (76). Haab's striae may be distinguished from these disorders by thin, smooth areas between thickened, curled edges in contrast to central thickening in the latter conditions (75).

Corneal Opacification

Corneal opacification in infancy may be associated with a variety of disorders (77): (a) developmental anomalies (Peters' anomaly and sclerocornea); (b) dystrophies (congenital hereditary corneal dystrophy and posterior polymorphous dystrophy); (c) choristomas (dermoid and dermis-like choristoma); (d) edema due to birth trauma; (e) intrauterine inflammation (congenital syphilis and rubella): and (f) inborn errors of metabolism (mucopolysaccharidoses and cystinosis). Three children have been described with the association of congenital hereditary endothelial dystrophy and congenital glaucoma, and the authors suggest that this combination should be suspected when total corneal opacification fails to resolve after normalization of IOP (78).

Other Glaucomas of Childhood

The differential diagnosis of congenital glaucoma should also include developmental glaucomas with associated anomalies, as well as the childhood glaucomas associated with other ocular and systemic disorders, all of which are discussed in subsequent chapters.

MANAGEMENT

Medical Therapy

Congenital glaucoma is almost always managed surgically with medical therapy being used only as a temporizing measure before surgery or when surgical intervention has repeatedly failed. In general, the same basic principles of medical therapy apply to the treatment of congenital glaucoma as to the adult glaucomas. One possible exception is the use of miotics, which, paradoxically, may raise the IOP by collapse of the trabecular meshwork due to the high insertion of uveal tissue into the posterior meshwork. Dosages for children and special precautions are discussed in Section Three.

Surgery

The primary surgical techniques are designed to eliminate the resistance to aqueous outflow created by the structural abnormalities in the anterior chamber angle. This is presently accomplished with incisional surgery, using either an internal (goniotomy) or external (trabeculotomy) approach, although pulsed lasers may one day become effective for this purpose. The present discussion is limited to the concepts of management, while details of the operative procedures are considered in Section Three.

Goniotomy

Barkan (79, 80) described a technique in which abnormal tissue (originally felt to be Barkan's membrane) is incised under direct visualization with the aid of a goniolens. It is now believed that the incision is not through a membrane, but rather through the inner portion of the trabecular meshwork. This presumably relieves the compressive traction of the anterior uvea on the meshwork, and eliminates any resistance imposed by incompletely developed inner meshwork.

Trabeculotomy

Harms and Dannheim (81) described a technique in which Schlemm's canal is identified by external dissection, and the trabecular meshwork is incised by passing a probe into the canal and then rotating it into the anterior chamber. One advantage of this procedure is that it can be performed in eyes with cloudy corneas, which is not the case with goniotomy. While some surgeons employ the technique only in cases with corneal opacification or when multiple goniotomies have failed, others prefer it as the initial procedure in congenital glaucoma.

Both goniotomy and trabeculotomy have their advocates, and reported success rates vary considerably, with neither procedure having clear-cut superiority. A more detailed comparison of the two operations is presented in Section Three. With both procedures, success is related to the severity and duration of the glaucoma. The worst prognosis occurs in infants with elevated pressures and cloudy corneas at birth. The most favorable outcome is seen in infants operated between the second and eighth month of life, and the surgery then becomes less effective with increasing age (82). One study of long-term surgical outcome after trabeculotomy, divided 71 children into congenital glaucoma (existing before age 2 months), infantile glaucoma (occurring between 2 months and 2 years), and juvenile glaucoma (after 2 years), and reported success rates with one or more trabeculotomies of 60.3 ± 15.9%, 96.3 ± 3.6%, and 76.4 ± 7.5%, respectively (83).

Other Glaucoma Procedures

When multiple goniotomies and/or trabeculotomies have failed, the surgeon usually resorts to a filtering procedure, such as a trabeculectomy. One study showed that trabeculectomy was the most successful procedure for congenital glaucoma in the hands of general ophthalmologists (84). Some surgeons prefer a full-thickness technique, such as thermal sclerostomy (85), which may have a better chance of pressure control, but may also be associated with a higher risk of postoperative complications. With the advent of adjunctive antimetabolites, especially mitomycin C, a trabeculectomy is probably a better choice for filtering surgery in children. A combined trabeculectomy/trabeculotomy may also be used when repeated surgery is required. Drainage implant devices may also have a role in the more difficult cases. A study of Molteno implants in 27 eyes of 20 children with a variety of developmental glaucomas revealed IOP control without medication in nine eyes, while 12 eyes required additional surgery (86). In some desperate situations, in which all else has failed, a cyclodestructive procedure may be useful. In one small series of cases with marked buphthalmos and congenitally opaque corneas, cyclocryotherapy led to both normalization of IOP and a reduction in corneal diameter, allowing subsequent successful penetrating keratoplasty (87).

Penetrating Keratoplasty

Corneal cloudiness may persist following normalization of the IOP, leading to the need for penetrating keratoplasty. These patients typically do not do well, with only 25% of eyes achieving 20/40 or better vision in one series (88). The most common postoperative complications are IOP elevation and graft failure. While significant visual improvement can be achieved with penetrating keratoplasty (87), it is suggested that it be reserved for patients with severe visual disability whose glaucoma is well-controlled (88).

Postoperative Care

The followup care of patients with congenital glaucoma has several important facets. In the early postoperative period, close observation is required regarding success of the glaucoma procedure. Corneal edema may persist for weeks after successful reduction of IOP and is, therefore, an unreliable indicator of early success, while changes in the optic nerve head provide the most important indicator of the course of the disease (41). The IOP is also a significant factor in postoperative visual capacity, with substantially better vision among those whose pressures remain no higher than 19 mm Hg (82), although for many children with advanced nerve damage, even this is often too high.

Even when the pressure is well-controlled, a significant number of children never achieve good vision. In two large studies, approximately half of the patients had visual acuities of less than 20/50 (82, 89). As previously noted, this reduction may result from persistent corneal changes, occasionally requiring penetrating keratoplasty. A high percentage of patients, however, suffer amblyopia from the induced anisometropia, and it is critical that this be diagnosed early and managed appropriately.

Finally, the patient and family must understand that pressure elevation can recur at any age in individuals with congenital glaucoma, and these patients must be followed throughout their life.

SUMMARY

Congenital glaucomas represent one group of glaucomas in childhood, and are characterized by a developmental abnormality of the anterior chamber angle without consistently associated systemic or other ocular anomalies. The conditions are believed to have a genetic basis, are often diagnosed during the first year of life, and are usually bilateral. Characteristic clinical features include epiphora, photophobia, blepharospasm, and an enlarged, cloudy cornea. The normal development of the anterior chamber angle primarily involves tissues of cranial neural crest cell origin, and incomplete development of these tissues is believed to be the pathogenesis of the congenital glaucomas. The differential diagnosis must include other causes of epiphora and corneal abnormalities, as well as the additional forms of glaucoma in childhood. Congenital glaucoma is usually managed surgically, with either a goniotomy or trabeculotomy, although attention must also be given to the amblyopia, which is common sequelae of these disorders.

REFERENCES

1. Barsoum-Homsy, M, Chevrette, L: Incidence and prognosis of childhood glaucoma. A study of 63 cases. Opthalmology 93:1323, 1986.
2. Walton, DS: Primary Congenital Open-Angle Glaucoma. In: Glaucoma. Chandler, PA, Grant, WM, eds. Philadelphia, Lea and Febiger, 1979, p. 329.
3. Shaffer, RN, Weiss, DI: Congenital and Pediatric Glaucomas. St. Louis, CV Mosby, 1970, p. 37.
4. Kwitko, ML: Glaucomas in Infants and Children. New York, Appleton-Century-Crofts, 1973, p. 185.
5. Lotufo, D, Ritch, R, Szmyd, L, Burris, JE: Juvenile glaucoma, race, and refraction. JAMA 261:249, 1989.
6. Merin, S, Morin, D: Heredity of congenital glaucoma. Br J Ophthalmol 56:414, 1972.
7. Demenais, F, Elston, RC, Bonaiti, C, et al: Segregation analysis of congenital glaucoma. Approach by two different models. Am J Hum Genet 33:300, 1981.
8. Rasussen, DH, Ellis, PP: Congenital glaucoma in identical twins. Arch Ophthalmol 84:827, 1970.
9. Fried, K, Sachs, R, Krakowsky, D: Congenital glaucoma in only one of identical twins. Ophthalmologica 174:185, 1977.
10. Pollack, A, Oliver, M: Congenital glaucoma and incomplete congenital glaucoma in two siblings. Acta Ophthalmol 62:359, 1984.
11. Katsushima, H, Kii, T, Soma, K, et al: Primary congenital glaucoma in a patient with trisomy 2q (q33→qter)and monosomy 9p (p24→pter). Arch Ophthalmol 105:323, 1987.
12. Sheffield, VC, Stone, EM, Alward, WLM, et al: Genetic linkage of familial open angle glaucoma to chromosome 1q21–q31. Nat Genet 4:47, 1993.
13. Johnson, AT, Drack, AV, Kwitek, AE, et al: Clinical features and linkage analysis of a family with autosomal dominant juvenile glaucoma. Ophthalmology 100:524, 1993.
14. Wiggs, JL, Del Bono, EA, Schuman, JS, et al: Clinical features of five pedigrees genetically linked to the juvenile glaucoma locus on chromosome 1q21–q31. Ophthalmology 102:1782, 1995.
15. Sarfarazi, M, Akarsu, AN, Hossain, A, et al: Assignment of a locus (GLC3A) for primary congenital glaucoma (buphthalmos) to 2q21 and evidence for genetic heterogeneity. Genomics 30:171, 1995.
16. Kaufman, PL, Kolker, AE: Ocular findings and corticosteroid responsiveness in parents of children with primary infantile glaucoma. Invest Ophthalmol 14:46, 1975.
17. Jerndal, T, Munkby, M: Corticosteroid response in dominant congenital glaucoma. Acta Ophthalmol 56:373, 1978.
18. Hvidberg, A, Kessing, SVV, Svejgaard, A: HLA histocompatibility antigens in primary congenital glaucoma. Glaucoma 1:134, 1979.
19. Kiskis, AA, Markowitz, SN, Morin, JD: Corneal diameter and axial length in congenital glaucoma. Can J Ophthalmol 20:93, 1985.
20. Musarella, MA, Morin, JD: Anterior segment and intraocular pressure measurements of the unanesthetized premature infant. Metab Pediatr Syst Ophthalmol 8:53, 1985.
21. Tucker, SM, Enzenauer, RW, Levin, AV, et al: Corneal diameter, axial length, and intraocular pressure in premature infants. Ophthalmology 99:1296, 1992.
22. Al-Umran, KU, Pandolfi, MF: Corneal diameter in premature infants. Br J Ophthalmol 76:292, 1992.
23. Imre, G, Bogi, J: Corneal edema in young glaucoma patients. Klin Monatsbl Augenheilkd 179:465, 1981.
24. Egbert, JE, Kushner, BJ: Excessive loss of hyperopia. A presenting sign of juvenile aphakic glaucoma. Arch Ophthalmol 108:1257, 1990.
25. Dominquez, A, Banos, MS, Alvarez, MG, et al: Intraocular pressure measurement in infants under general anesthesia. Am J Ophthalmol 78:110, 1974.
26. Grote, P: Augeninnendruckmessungen bei Kleinkindern ohne Glaukam in Halothanmaskennarkose. Ophthalmologica 171:202, 1975.
27. Judisch, GF, Anderson, S, Bell, WE: Chloral hydrate sedation as a substitute for examination under anesthesia in pediatric ophthalmology. Am J Ophthalmol 89:560, 1980.
28. Van Buskirk, EM, Plamer, EA: Office assessment of young children for glaucoma. Ann Ophthalmol 11:1749, 1979.
29. Radtke, ND, Cohen, BF: Intraocular pressure measurement in the newborn. Am J Ophthalmol 78:501, 1974.
30. Wenzel, M, Krippendorff, U, Hunold, W, Reim, M: Endothelial cell damage in congenital and juvenile glaucoma. Klin Monatasbl Augenheilkd 195:344, 1989.
31. Worst, JGF: The Pathogenesis of Congenital Glaucoma. An Embryological and Goniosurgical Study. Springfield, IL, Charles C Thomas, 1966.
32. Luntz, MH: Congenital, infantile, and juvenile glaucoma. Ophthalmology 86:793, 1979.
33. Budenz, DL, Hodapp, E: Vitrectomy lens for examination of the optic disk in young children with glaucoma. Am J Ophthalmol 119:523, 1995.
34. Khodadoust, AA, Ziai, M, Biggs, SL: Optic disc in normal newborns. Am J Ophthalmol 66:502, 1968.
35. Robin, AL, Quigley, HA, Pollack, IP, et al: An analysis of visual acuity, visual fields, and disk cupping in childhood glaucoma. Am J Ophthalmol 88:847, 1979.
36. Shaffer, RN, Hetherington, J Jr: The glaucomatous disc in infants. A suggested hypothesis for disc cupping. Trans Am Acad Ophthalmol Otol 73:929, 1969.
37. Quigley, HA: The pathogenesis of reversible cupping in congenital glaucoma. Am J Ophthalmol 84:358, 1977.
38. Robin, AL, Quigley, HA: Transient reversible cupping in juvenile-onset glaucoma. Am J Ophthalmol 88:580, 1979.
39. Quigley, HA: Childhood glaucoma. Results with trabeculotomy and study of reversible cupping. Ophthalmology 89:219, 1982.
40. Morin, JD, Bryars, JH: Causes of loss of vision in congenital glaucoma. Arch Ophthalmol 93:1575, 1980.
41. Rice, NSC: Management of infantile glaucoma. Br J Ophthalmol 56:294, 1972.
42. Cooling, RJ, Rice, NSC, McLeod, D: Retinal detachment in congenital glaucoma. Br J Ophthalmol 64:417, 1980.
43. Sampaolesi, R, Caruso, R: Ocular echometry in the diagnosis of congenital glaucoma. Arch Ophthalmol 100:574, 1982.
44. Tarkkanen, A, Uusitalo, R, Mianowicz, J: Ultrasonographic biometry in congenital glaucoma. Acta Ophthalmol 61:618, 1983.
45. Mann, IC: The Development of the Human Eye. 3rd ed. New York, Grune & Stratton, 1964.
46. Kashani, AA: Early formation of the anterior chamber of the eye in the human embryo. Ital J Ophthalmol 3:65, 1989.
47. Johnston, MC, Noden, DM, Hazelton, RD, et al: Origins of avian ocular and periocular tissues. Exp Eye Res 29:27, 1979.
48. Tripathi, BJ, Tripathi, RC: Neural crest origin of human trabecular meshwork and its implications for the pathogenesis of glaucoma. Am J Ophthalmol 107:583, 1989.
49. Foets, B, van den Oord, J, Engelmann, K, Missotten, L: A comparative immunohistochemical study of human corneotrabecular tissue. Graefes Arch Clin Exp Ophthalmol 230:269, 1992.

50. Wulle, KG: Electron microscopy of the fetal development of the corneal endothelium and Descemet's membrane of the human eye. Invest Ophthalmol 11:397, 1972.

51. Hay, ED: Development of the vertebrate cornea. Int Rev Cytol 63:263, 1980.

52. Barkan, O: Pathogenesis of congenital glaucoma. Gonioscopic and anatomic observation of the angle of the anterior chamber in the normal eye and in congenital glaucoma. Am J Ophthalmol 40:1, 1955.

53. Allen, L, Burian, HM, Braley, AE: A new concept of the development of the anterior chamber angle. Its relationship to developmental glaucoma and other structural anomalies. Arch Ophthalmol 53:783, 1955.

54. Smelser, GK, Ozanics, V: The development of the trabecular meshwork in primate eyes. Am J Ophthalmol 71:366, 1971.

55. Anderson, DR: The development of the trabecular meshwork and its abnormality in primary infantile glaucoma. Trans Am Ophthalmol Soc 79:458, 1981.

56. Hansson, H-A, Jerndal, T: Scanning electron microscopic studies on the development of the iridocorneal angle in human eyes. Invest Ophthalmol 10:252, 1971.

57. Van Buskirk, EM: Clinical implications of iridocorneal angle development. Ophthalmology 88:361, 1981.

58. McMenamin, PG: Human fetal iridocorneal angle: A light and scanning electron microscopic study. Br J Ophthalmol 73:871, 1989

59. McMenamin, PG: A quantitative study of the prenatal development of the aqueous outflow system in the human eye. Exp Eye Res 53:507, 1991.

60. Shields, MB: Axenfeld-Rieger Syndrome. A theory of mechanism and distinctions from the iridocorneal endothelial syndrome. Trans Am Ophthalmol Soc 81:736, 1983.

61. Mann, IC: Development of the Human Eye. Cambridge, England, Cambridge University Press, 1928.

62. Anderson, Dr: Pathology of the glaucomas. Br J Ophthalmol 56:146, 1972.

63. Maumenee, AE: The pathogenesis of congenital glaucoma. A new theory. Am J Ophthalmol 47:827, 1959.

64. Maumenee, AE: Further observations on the pathogenesis of congenital glaucoma. Am J Ophthalmol 55:1163, 1963.

65. Wright, JD Jr, Robb, RM, Dueker, DK, Boger, WP III: Congenital glaucoma unresponsive to conventional therapy: a clinicopathological case presentation. J Pediatr Ophthalmol Strabismus 20:172, 1983.

66. Sampaolesi, R, Argento, C: Scanning electron microscopy of the trabecular meshwork in normal and glaucuomatous eyes. Invest Ophthalmol Vis Sci 16:302, 1977.

67. Maul, E, Strozzi, L, Munoz, C, Reyes, C: The outflow pathway in congenital glaucoma. Am J Ophthalmol 89:667, 1980.

68. Rodrigues, MM, Spaeth, GL, Weinreb, S: Juvenile glaucoma associated with goniodysgenesis. Am J Ophthalmol 81:786, 1976.

69. Tawara, A, Inomata, H: Developmental immaturity of the trabecular meshwork in congenital glaucoma. Am J Ophthalmol 92:508, 1981.

70. Tawara, A, Inomata, H: Developmental immaturity of the trabecular meshwork in juvenile glaucoma. Am J Ophthalmol 98:82, 1984.

71. Kupfer, C, Ross, K: The development of outflow facility in human eyes. Invest Ophthalmol 10:513, 1971.

72. Kupfer, C, Kaiser-Kupfer, MI: Observations on the development of the anterior chamber angle with reference to the pathogenesis of congenital glaucomas. Am J Ophthalmol 88:424, 1979.

73. Pearce, WG: Autosomal dominant megalocornea with congenital glaucoma: evidence for germ-line mosaicism. Can J Ophthalmol 26:21, 1991.

74. Angell, LK, Robb, RM, Berson, FG: Visual prognosis in patients with ruptures in Descemet's membrane due to forceps injuries. Arch Ophthalmol 99:2137, 1981.

75. Cibis, GW, Tripathi, RC: The differential diagnosis of Decemet's tears (Haab's Striae) and posterior polymorphous dystrophy bands. A clinicopathologic study. Ophthalmology 89:614, 1982.

76. Pardos, GJ, Krachmer, JH, Mannis, MJ: Posterior corneal vesicles. Arch Ophthalmol 99:1573, 1981.

77. Ching, FC: Corneal opacification in infancy. Med Coll Va Quart 8:230, 1972.

78. Mullaney, PB, Risco, JM, Teichmann, K, Millar, L: Congenital hereditary endothelial dystrophy associated with glaucoma. Ophthalmology 102:186, 1995.

79. Barkan, O: Operation for congenital glaucoma. Am J Ophthalmol 25:552, 1942.

80. Barkan, O: Goniotomy for the relief of congenital glaucoma. Br J Ophthalmol 32:701, 1948.

81. Harms, H, Dannheim, R: Trabeculotomy results and problems. In Microsurgery in Glaucoma. Mackenson, G, ed. Basel, S. Karger, 1970, p. 121.

82. Dannheim, R, Haas, H: Visual acuity and intraocular pressure after surgery in congenital glaucoma. Klin Monatsbl Augenheilkd 177:296, 1980.

83. Akimoto, M, Tanihara, H, Negi, A, Nagata, M: Surgical results of trabeculotomy ab externo for developmental glaucoma. Arch Ophthalmol 112:1540, 1994.

84. Elder, MJ: Congenital glaucoma in the West Bank and Gaza Strip. Br J Ophthalmol 77:413, 1993.

85. Cadera, W, Pachtman, MA, Cantor, LB, et al: Congenital glaucoma with corneal cloudiness treated by thermal sclerostomy. Can J Ophthalmol 20:98, 1985.

86. Nesher, R, Sherwood, MB, Kass, MA, et al: Molteno implants in children. J Glau 1:228, 1992.

87. Frucht-Pery, J, Feldman, ST, Brown, SI: Transplantation of congenitally opaque corneas from eyes with exaggerated buphthalmos. Am J Ophthalmol 107:655, 1989.

88. Huang, SCM, Soong, HK, Benz, RM, et al: Problems associated with penetrating keratoplasty for corneal edema in congenital glaucoma. Ophthalmic Surg 20:399, 1989.

89. Morgan, KS, Black, B, Ellis, FD, Helveston, EM: Treatment of congenital glaucoma. Am J Ophthalmol 92:799, 1981.

Chapter 12

DEVELOPMENTAL GLAUCOMAS WITH ASSOCIATED ANOMALIES

The glaucomas considered in this chapter all have a developmental abnormality of the anterior chamber angle as the mechanism of aqueous outflow obstruction. Unlike the congenital glaucomas discussed in the previous chapter, however, these conditions are consistently associated with additional ocular and systemic anomalies, which help to characterize each clinical entity.

GENERAL TERMINOLOGY

There has been considerable discussion and confusion regarding the lumping, splitting, and classifying of this large number of disorders. Based on the observation that most of the ocular and facial structures involved in these developmental disorders are of neural crest origin (1, 2), the term *neurocristopathies* has been used as a unifying concept for

diseases arising from neural crest maldevelopment (3, 4). Hoskins and associates (5) advocated a shift away from eponyms and syndrome names for individual disorders toward an emphasis on descriptive terminology. Noting that the trabecular meshwork, iris, and cornea are the three major structures involved in these conditions, they suggested the terms "trabeculodysgenesis," "iridodysgenesis," and "corneodysgenesis," or combinations thereof, as a system of classifying the developmental defects.

While there is value in categorizing disorders on the basis of anatomic descriptions and mechanisms, the overlapping of manifestations and limited understanding of disease mechanisms make it difficult to apply such a system in all cases of developmental glaucomas with associated anomalies. For this reason, traditional eponyms and syndrome names are retained, with some suggested modifications, for purpose of discussion in this chapter.

AXENFELD-RIEGER SYNDROME[a]

Terminology

In 1920, Axenfeld (6) described a patient with a white line in the posterior aspect of the cornea, near the limbus, and tissue strands extending from peripheral iris to this prominent line. Beginning in the mid-1930s, Rieger (7–9) reported cases with similar anterior segment anomalies, but with additional changes in the iris, including corectopia, atrophy, and hole formation. It was also discovered that some of these patients had associated systemic developmental defects, especially of the teeth and facial bones (10, 11). Axenfeld (6) referred to his case as "posterior embryotoxon of the cornea," while Rieger (9) used the term, "mesodermal dysgenesis of the cornea and iris." Traditionally, these conditions have been designated by three eponyms: (a) *Axenfeld's anomaly* (limited to peripheral anterior segment defects); (b) *Rieger's anomaly* (peripheral abnormalities with additional changes in the iris); and (c) *Rieger's syndrome* (ocular anomalies plus systemic developmental defects).

The similarity of anterior chamber angle abnormalities in Axenfeld's anomaly and Rieger's anomaly and syndrome has led most investigators to agree that these three arbitrary categories represent a spectrum of developmental disorders (12–15). Furthermore, the overlap of ocular and systemic anomalies is such that the traditional classification is difficult to apply in all cases. Various collective terms have been applied to this spectrum of disorders, such as "anterior chamber cleavage syndrome"(13) and "mesodermal dysgenesis of the cornea and iris" (9). As noted in Chapter 11, however, the theories of normal development on which these names are based are no longer felt to be correct. In addition, the former collective term included the central ocular defects of Peters' anomaly, which is discussed later in this chapter. While some patients may have the combined defects of Axenfeld's or Rieger's anomaly and Peters' anomaly, the association is rare and the mechanisms of the two disorders, in most cases, are different.

The alternative term, *Axenfeld-Rieger* (A-R) *syndrome,* was proposed for all clinical variations within this spectrum of developmental disorders (15, 16), and is now commonly used in the literature. This name retains reference to the original eponyms, and is not dependent on any theory of normal development, understanding of which is still incomplete, nor does it require arbitrary subclassification of the clinical variations.

General Features

All patients with the A-R syndrome, irrespective of ocular manifestations, share the same general features: (a) a bilat-

eral, developmental disorder of the eyes; (b) a frequent family history of the disorder, with an autosomal dominant mode of inheritance; (c) no sex predilection; (d) frequent systemic developmental defects; and (e) a high incidence of associated glaucoma. The age at which the A-R syndrome is diagnosed ranges from birth to adulthood, with most cases becoming recognized during infancy or childhood. The diagnosis may result from discovery of an abnormal iris or other ocular anomaly, signs of congenital glaucoma, reduced vision in older patients, or systemic anomalies. Other cases are diagnosed during a routine examination, which may have been prompted by a family history of the disorder.

Ocular Features

Ocular defects in the A-R syndrome are typically bilateral. The structures most commonly involved are the peripheral cornea, anterior chamber angle, and iris.

Cornea

The characteristic abnormality of the cornea is a *prominent, anteriorly displaced Schwalbe's line.* This appears on slit-lamp examination as a white line on the posterior cornea near the limbus. The prominent line may be incomplete, usually limited to the temporal quadrant (Fig. 12.1), while in other patients it may be seen for 360° (Fig. 12.2). In some cases, the line can only be seen by gonioscopy, while rare cases with other ocular and systemic features of the syndrome may have grossly normal Schwalbe's lines (17).

It is not uncommon for an individual to have a prominent Schwalbe's line with no other evidence of the A-R syndrome. This isolated defect is often referred to as *posterior embryotoxon,* the term originally used by Axenfeld (6), and reportedly occurs in 8% (12) to 15% (18) of the general population. It may represent a forme fruste of the A-R syndrome, but is not included in this spectrum of anomalies, since it is neither associated with an increased incidence of glaucoma nor with systemic anomalies. A prominent Schwalbe's line may rarely be associated with other disorders, including congenital glaucoma (Chapter 11) (19) and the iridocorneal endothelial syndrome (Chapter 13) (20).

The cornea is otherwise normal in the typical case of the A-R syndrome, with the exception of occasional patients with variation in the overall size (megalocornea or, less often, microcornea) or shape of the cornea (12). Congenital opacities of the central cornea have also been observed in a few cases. The corneal endothelium is typically normal. By specular microscopy, the cells have distinct margins, although mild-to-moderate variation in the size and shape is commonly observed, especially in older patients and in those with long-standing glaucoma or previous intraocular surgery (15).

[a]Refer to Shields, MB: Color Atlas of Glaucoma. Baltimore, Williams & Wilkins, 1998, Plates II8–10.

Anterior Chamber Angle

Gonioscopic examination typically reveals a prominent Schwalbe's line, although there is considerable variation among patients in the extent to which Schwalbe's line is enlarged and anteriorly displaced. In occasional cases, the line is suspended from the cornea in some areas by a thin membrane (15, 21). Tissue strands bridge the anterior chamber angle from the peripheral iris to the prominent ridge (Fig. 12.3). These *iridocorneal adhesions* are typically similar in color and texture to the adjacent iris. The strands range in size from threadlike structures to broad bands extending for nearly 15% of the circumference. In some eyes, only one to two tissue strands are seen, while others have several per quadrant. Beyond the tissue strands, the anterior chamber angle is open and the trabecular meshwork is visible, but the scleral spur is typically obscured by peripheral iris, which inserts into the posterior portion of the meshwork (12, 15, 18).

Iris

Aside from the peripheral abnormalities, the iris may be normal in some eyes with the A-R syndrome. In other cases, defects of the iris range from mild stromal thinning to marked atrophy with hole formation, corectopia and ectropion uveae (Fig. 12.4). When corectopia is present, the pupil is usually displaced toward a prominent peripheral tissue strand, which is often visible by slitlamp biomicroscopy. The atrophy and hole formation typically occur in the quadrant away from the direction of the corectopia.

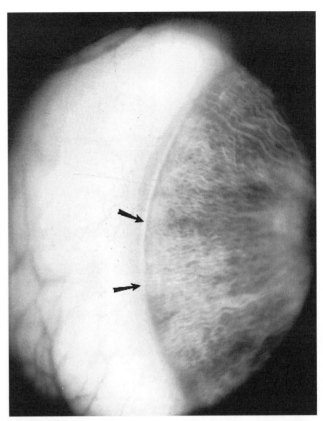

Figure 12.1. Prominent, anteriorly displaced Schwalbe's line (posterior embryotoxon) in temporal quadrant *(arrows)*. (Reprinted with permission from Ritch R, Shields MB, eds: The Secondary Glaucomas, Chapter 2. St. Louis, CV Mosby, 1982.)

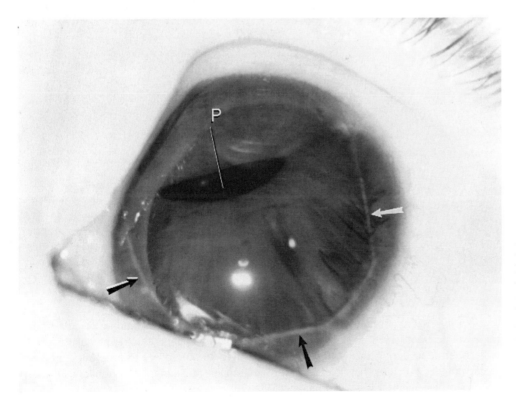

Figure 12.2. Prominent, anteriorly displaced Schwalbe's line in all quadrants *(arrows)* with pupillary distortion (P) in patient with Axenfeld-Rieger syndrome. (Reprinted with permission from Ritch R, Shields MB, eds: The Secondary Glaucomas, Chapter 2. St. Louis, CV Mosby, 1982.)

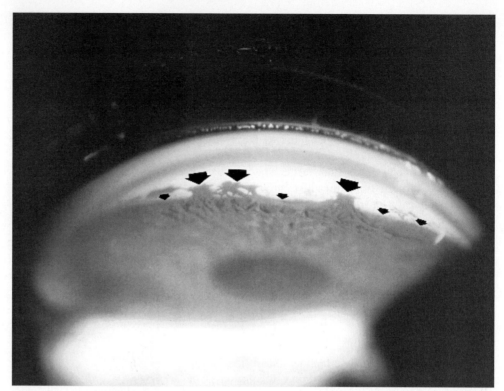

Figure 12.3. Gonioscopic appearance of patient with Axenfeld-Rieger syndrome showing tissue strands extending from peripheral iris to prominent Schwalbe's line *(large arrows)* and high insertion of iris into trabecular meshwork *(small arrows)*. (Reprinted with permission from Shields, MB: Axenfeld-Rieger syndrome. A theory of mechanism and distinctions from the iridocorneal endothelial syndrome. Trans Am Ophthalmol Soc 81:736, 1983.)

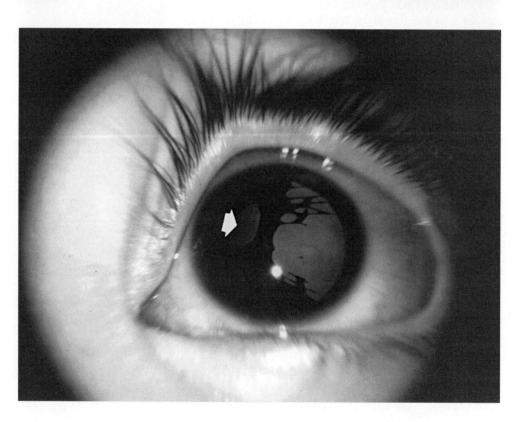

Figure 12.4. Advanced iris changes in patient with Axenfeld-Rieger syndrome showing small, markedly displaced pupil *(arrow)* and large iris hole in opposite quadrants. (Reprinted with permission from Shields, MB: Axenfeld-Rieger syndrome. A theory of mechanism and distinctions from the iridocorneal endothelial syndrome. Trans Am Ophthalmol Soc 81:736, 1983.)

In a small number of patients with the A-R syndrome, abnormalities of the central iris have been observed to progress (15, 22–24). This is more often seen during the first years of life, but may also occur in older patients. The progressive changes usually consist of displacement or distortion of the pupil and occasional thinning or hole formation of the iris. Abnormalities of the peripheral iris or anterior chamber angle do not appear to progress after birth, except for occasional thickening of iridocorneal tissue strands (15).

Additional Ocular Abnormalities

Many additional ocular abnormalities have been reported in one or more cases or pedigrees. While none of these occur with sufficient frequency to be included as a typical feature of the A-R syndrome, and may actually represent separate entities, there is the impression that these patients are subject to a wide range of ocular anomalies (12, 15). Reported abnormalities include strabismus, limbal dermoids, corneal pannus (25), cataracts (26), congenital ectropion uveae (27), congenital pupillary-iris-lens membrane (28), peripheral spoke-like transillumination defects of the iris, retinal detachment (29), macular degeneration, chorioretinal colobomas, choroidal hypoplasia, and hypoplasia of the optic nerve heads (12, 15).

Glaucoma

Slightly more than half of the patients with the A-R syndrome develop glaucoma. This may become manifest during infancy, although it more commonly appears in childhood or young adulthood. The extent of the iris defects and iridocorneal strands does not correlate precisely with the presence or severity of the glaucoma. On the other hand, the high insertion of peripheral iris into the trabecular meshwork, which is present to some degree in all cases, appears to be more pronounced in those eyes with glaucoma (15).

Systemic Features

The systemic anomalies most commonly associated with the A-R syndrome are developmental defects of the teeth and facial bones. The dental abnormalities include a reduction in crown size (microdontia), a decreased but evenly spaced number of teeth (hypodontia), and a focal absence of teeth (oligodontia or anodontia) (Fig. 12.5) (10, 11, 30). The teeth most commonly missing are anterior maxillary primary and permanent central incisors. Facial anomalies include maxillary hypoplasia with flattening of the midface and a receding upper lip and prominent lower lip, especially in association with dental hypoplasia (Fig. 12.6). Hypertelorism, telecanthus, a broad flat nose, micrognathia and mandibular prognathism have also been described (12, 25).

Anomalies in the region of the pituitary gland are a less common but more serious finding associated with the A-R syndrome. A primary empty sella syndrome has been documented in several patients (15, 31), and one case of congenital parasellar arachnoid cyst has been reported (15). Growth hormone deficiency and short stature have also been described in association with the entity (32, 33). Other abnormalities reported in association with the A-R syndrome include redundant periumbilical skin and hypospadias (34), oculocutaneous albinism (35), heart defects, middle ear deafness, mental deficiency, and a variety of neurologic, dermatologic (12) and skeletal (36) disorders.

Histopathologic Features

The central cornea is typically normal, while the peripheral cornea has the characteristic prominent, anteriorly displaced Schwalbe's line. The latter structure is composed of dense collagen and ground substance covered by a monolayer of spindle-shaped cells with a basement membrane (Fig. 12.7) (15, 18, 21). The peripheral iris is attached in some areas to

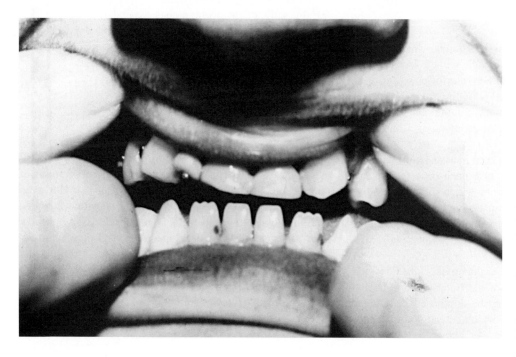

Figure 12.5. Patient with Axenfeld-Rieger syndrome demonstrating typical dental anomaly of microdontia (reduction in crown size of teeth). (Reprinted with permission from Ritch R, Shields MB, eds: The Secondary Glaucomas, Chapter 2. St. Louis, CV Mosby, 1982.)

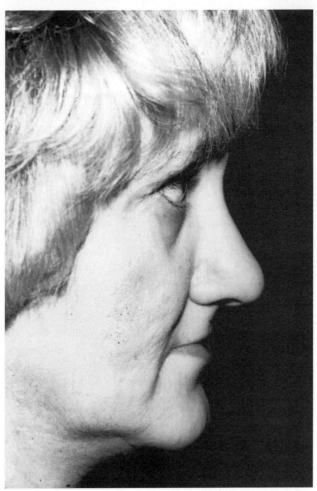

Figure 12.6. Patient with Axenfeld-Rieger syndrome demonstrating characteristic facial configuration of midface flattening (upper lip and cheek) and protruding lower lip. (Reprinted with permission from Ritch R, Shields MB, eds: The Secondary Glaucomas, Chapter 2. St. Louis, CV Mosby, 1982.)

the corneoscleral junction by tissue strands, which usually connect with the prominent Schwalbe's line. Occasionally, however, the adhesions insert either anterior or posterior to Schwalbe's line or on both sides of the ridge (15). The strands consist of either iris stroma, a membrane composed of a monolayer of spindle-shaped cells and/or a basement membrane-like layer, or both.

A membrane, similar to that seen in association with the iridocorneal tissue strands, has also been observed on the iris, usually on the portion toward which the pupil is distorted (12, 15, 37). In the quadrants away from the direction of pupillary displacement, the stroma of the iris is often thin or absent, exposing pigment epithelium which may also contain holes.

The iris peripheral to the iridocorneal adhesions inserts into the posterior aspect of the trabecular meshwork (Fig. 12.8). The meshwork may be composed of a scant number of attenuated lamellae, which extend from beneath the

peripheral iris to the prominent Schwalbe's line and are often compressed, especially in the outer layers. Transmission electron microscopic study suggests that the apparent compression may be due to incomplete development of the trabecular meshwork (15). Schlemm's canal is either rudimentary or absent.

Theories of Mechanism

Based on clinical and histopathologic observations and the current concepts of normal anterior segment development, as discussed in Chapter 11, a developmental arrest, late in gestation, of certain anterior segment structures derived from neural crest cells, has been postulated as the mechanism of the A-R syndrome (15). This leads to the abnormal retention of the primordial endothelial layer on portions of the iris and anterior chamber angle, and alterations in the aqueous outflow structures (Fig. 12.9). The retained endothelium with associated basement membrane is believed to create the iridocorneal strands, while contraction of this tissue layer on the iris leads to the iris changes, which sometimes continues to progress after birth. The developmental arrest also accounts for the high insertion of anterior uvea into the posterior trabecular meshwork, similar to the alterations seen in congenital glaucoma, and results in the incomplete maturation of the trabecular meshwork and Schlemm's canal. The latter defects are felt to be responsible for the associated glaucoma.

The neural crest cells also give rise to most of the mesenchyme related to the forebrain and pituitary gland, bones and cartilages of the upper face, and dental papillae (3, 4). This could explain the developmental anomalies involving the pituitary gland, the facial bones, and the teeth. Neural crest cells also contribute to many other structures, including the walls of the aortic arches, genitalia, spinal ganglia, long bones (36), and melanocytes (35), which appears to explain the wide range of systemic anomalies that may be seen in some patients with the A-R syndrome.

Genetic Linkage

As previously noted, the A-R syndrome is felt to have a genetic basis with an autosomal dominant pattern of inheritance. Cases have been reported with various aberrations of chromosomes 4, 6, 10, 13, 16, and 22 (38–44). However, chromosome 4 anomalies were the only ones that included both the ocular and systemic features of the A-R syndrome. Four patients with fully developed A-R syndrome had deletions in the region of chromosome 4q23–26 (45–48). Using a group of highly polymorphic short tandem repeat polymorphisms, including a new tetranucleotide repeat for epidermal growth factor, significant linkage of the A-R syndrome to chromosome band 4q25 was identified (49).

Epidermal growth factor appeared to be an excellent candidate gene because of its effects on dental development and corneal endothelial cell activity. However, single strand conformation polymorphism analysis of all 24 axons of the epidermal growth factor gene in five pedigrees, as well as two unrelated patients with balanced translocations of chromosome 4q26, suggest that mutations in epidermal growth factor are unlikely to cause the A-R syndrome (50).

Differential Diagnosis

Iridocorneal Endothelial Syndrome

The iris and anterior chamber angle abnormalities in this spectrum of disease (Chapter 13) resemble those of A-R syndrome both clinically and histopathologically. This has led some investigators to suggest that the two syndromes are parts

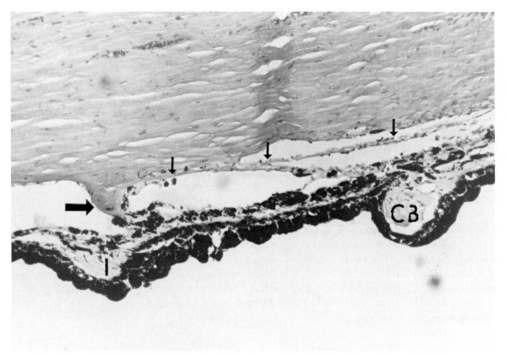

Figure 12.7. Light microscopic view of eye with Axenfeld-Rieger syndrome showing prominent, anteriorly displaced Schwalbe's line *(large arrow)* attached to iris (I) by tissue strand. Scant, attenuated trabecular lamellae *(small arrows)* extend to Schwalbe's line and attach to peripheral iris; anterior portion of ciliary body (CB). (Hematoxylin & eosin, ×150). (Reprinted with permission from Shields, MB: Axenfeld-Rieger syndrome. A theory of mechanism and distinctions from the iridocorneal endothelial syndrome. Trans Am Ophthalmol Soc 81:736, 1983.)

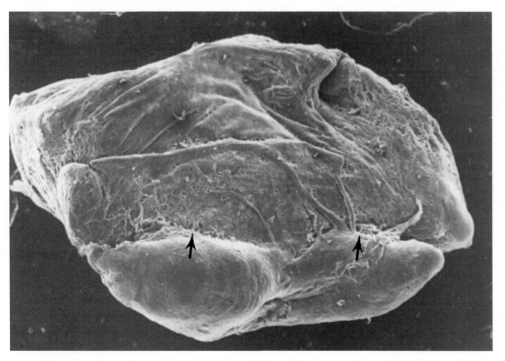

Figure 12.8. Scanning electron microscopic view of trabeculectomy specimen from patient with Axenfeld-Rieger syndrome showing high insertion of iris into trabecular meshwork (arrows). (Reprinted with permission from Shields, MB, Buckley, E, Klintworth, GK, Thresher, R: Axenfeld-Rieger syndrome. A spectrum of developmental disorders. Surv Ophthalmol 29:387, 1985.)

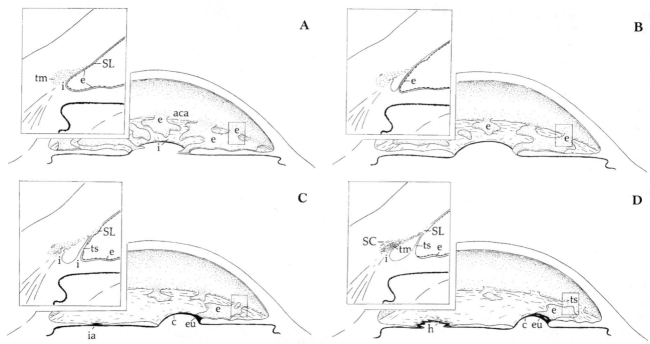

Figure 12.9. Theory of mechanism for ocular abnormalities of Axenfeld-Rieger syndrome (*insets* show cross-sectional views of anterior chamber angle corresponding to area within rectangle): **A.** Partial retention of primordial endothelium *(e)* on iris *(i)* and anterior chamber angle *(aca)*; incomplete posterior recession of peripheral uvea from trabecular meshwork *(tm)*; abnormal differentiation between corneal and chamber angle endothelium with prominent, anteriorly displaced Schwalbe's line *(SL)*. **B.** Development of tissue strands from retained endothelium crossing anterior chamber angle. **C.** Contraction of retained endothelium with iris changes of corectopia *(c)*, ectropion uvea *(eu)*, and iris atrophy *(ia)*, which may continue after birth; tissue strand *(ts)*. **D.** Incomplete development of trabecular meshwork and Schlemm's canal *(SC)*; continued traction on iris, with possible secondary ischemia leads to hole formation *(h)*. (Reprinted with permission from Shields, MB: Axenfeld-Rieger syndrome. A theory of mechanism and distinctions from the iridocorneal endothelial syndrome. Trans Am Ophthalmol Soc 81:736, 1983.)

of a common spectrum of disorders (37, 51). However, clinical features which distinguish the iridocorneal endothelial (ICE) syndrome include corneal endothelial abnormalities, unilaterality, absence of family history, and onset in young adulthood. Both conditions are characterized histopathologically by a membrane over the angle and iris, which is associated with many of the alterations in each disorder. However, while the membrane in the A-R syndrome represents a primordial remnant, that of the ICE syndrome is due to a proliferation from the abnormal corneal endothelium.

Posterior Polymorphous Dystrophy

One variation of this developmental disorder of the corneal endothelium (Chapter 13) has changes of the iris and anterior chamber angle similar to those of the A-R syndrome. However, the differentiation can be made on the basis of the typical corneal endothelial abnormality.

Peters' Anomaly

This spectrum of disorders, which is discussed next in this chapter, involves the central portion of the cornea, iris, and lens. Similar changes have been reported in association with

the peripheral defects of the A-R syndrome, and the two conditions were once included in a single category of developmental disorders (13, 14). However, this association is rare, and the mechanisms for the two groups of disorders are distinctly different.

Aniridia

The rudimentary iris and anterior chamber abnormalities with associated glaucoma in this developmental disorder, which is discussed later in this chapter, may lead to confusion with the A-R syndrome in some cases.

Congenital Iris Hypoplasia

Patients may have congenital hypoplasia of the iris without the anterior chamber angle defects of the A-R syndrome or any other ocular abnormality (52). Iris hypoplasia has also been reported in association with juvenile-onset glaucoma with autosomal dominant inheritance (53).

Oculodentodigital Dysplasia

The dental anomalies in this condition are similar to those seen in the A-R syndrome. In addition, these patients may occasionally have mild stromal hypoplasia of the iris (12), anterior chamber angle defects, microphthalmia, and glaucoma (54).

Ectopia Lentis et Pupillae

This autosomal recessive condition is characterized by bilateral displacement of the lens and pupil (55), with the two typically displaced in opposite directions. The corectopia in this disorder may resemble that of the A-R syndrome, but the absence of anterior chamber angle defects is a differential feature.

Congenital Ectropion Uveae

This condition has been described as a rare, nonprogressive anomaly characterized by the presence of pigment epithelium on the stroma of the iris (56, 57). It may be an isolated finding, or appear in association with systemic anomalies, including neurofibromatosis, facial hemiatrophy, and the Prader-Willi syndrome (56). Glaucoma is present in a high percentage of cases and the ectropion uvea may be confused with that found in some patients with the A-R syndrome.

As previously discussed, patients with the A-R syndrome may have a wide variety of associated ocular and systemic developmental abnormalities, and it has not yet been established in many of these cases whether the patient has a variation of the A-R syndrome or whether the findings should be considered as a separate entity.

Management

The primary concern regarding the management of ocular defects in a patient with the A-R syndrome is detection and control of the associated glaucoma. Intraocular pressure (IOP) elevation most often develops between childhood and early adulthood, but may appear in infancy or, in rare cases, not until the elderly years (15). Therefore, patients with the A-R syndrome must be followed for suspicion of glaucoma throughout their life.

With the exception of infantile cases, medical therapy should usually be tried before surgical intervention is recommended. Pilocarpine and other miotics are often ineffective, and drugs which reduce aqueous production, such as β-adrenergic blockers, carbonic anhydrase inhibitors and α₂-adrenergic agonists, are most likely to be beneficial. Surgical options include goniotomy, trabeculotomy, and trabeculectomy. The former two have been utilized in infantile cases with limited success. Trabeculectomy is the surgical procedure of choice for most patients with glaucoma associated with the A-R syndrome.

While laser surgery has not been found effective in managing the glaucoma in the A-R syndrome, it has been reported that the Nd:YAG laser can be used to lyse irido-corneal adhesions to minimize corectopia when it is impairing vision (58).

PETERS' ANOMALY[b]

In 1897, von Hippel (59) reported a case of buphthalmos with bilateral central corneal opacities and adhesions from these defects to the iris. Peters, beginning in 1906 (60), described similar patients with what has become generally known as Peters' anomaly.

General Features

The condition is present at birth and is usually bilateral. Most cases are sporadic, although there are reported cases of autosomal recessive inheritance and, less commonly, autosomal dominant transmission (61, 62). Chromosomal defects have also been described (63–65). It typically occurs in the absence of additional abnormalities, although associations with a wide range of systemic and other ocular anomalies have been reported, including defects of the ear and auditory system, orofacial system, heart, genitourinary system, spine, and musculoskeletal system (66–69). Because of the varied genetic and nongenetic patterns and the spectrum of ocular and systemic abnormalities, it is likely that Peters' anomaly is a morphologic finding rather than a distinct entity (66).

Clinicopathologic Features

The hallmark of Peters' anomaly is a central defect in Descemet's membrane and corneal endothelium with thinning and opacification of the corresponding area of corneal stroma (Fig. 12.10) (70–73). Iris adhesions may extend to the borders of this corneal defect. Bowman's layer may also be absent centrally (72, 73). Immunohistochemical studies of the cornea suggest that extracellular matrix elements such as fibronectin may be important in the pathogenesis of Peters' anomaly (74).

The disorder has been subdivided into the following three groups (Fig. 12.11), each of which may have more than one pathogenic mechanism (71).

Not Associated with Keratolenticular Contact or Cataract

In these cases, the defect in Descemet's membrane may represent primary failure of corneal endothelial development (72). However, rare cases may be secondary to intrauterine

---

[b]Refer to Shields, MB: *Color Atlas of Glaucoma*. Baltimore, Williams & Wilkins, 1998, Plate II11.

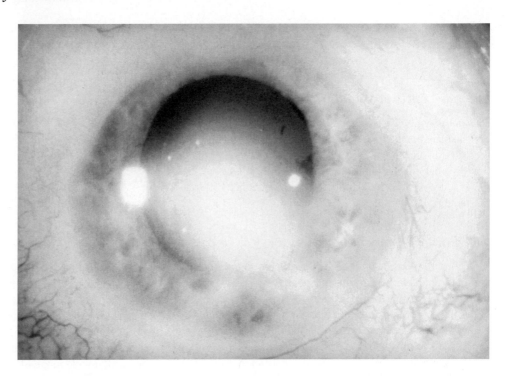

Figure 12.10. External appearance of patient with Peters' anomaly showing central corneal opacity. (Courtesy George O. Waring, M.D.)

inflammation (75), which was originally postulated by von Hippel (59) and gave rise to the term "von Hippel's internal corneal ulcer."

Associated with Keratolenticular Contact or Cataract

Most histopathologic studies of this variation suggest that the lens developed normally and was then secondarily pushed forward against the cornea by one of several mechanisms, causing the loss of Descemet's membrane (Fig. 12.12) (71, 72, 76). It is also possible that some cases may result from incomplete separation of the lens vesicle from surface ectoderm.

Associated with Axenfeld-Rieger Syndrome

This rare association was discussed earlier in this chapter.

Associated Glaucoma

Approximately half of the patients with Peters' anomaly will develop glaucoma, which is frequently present at birth. The mechanism of the glaucoma is uncertain, since the anterior chamber angle is usually grossly normal by clinical examination. Histopathologic studies have revealed peripheral anterior synechiae in some cases (71), while ultrastructural studies of two young patients with Peters' anomaly and open angles revealed changes in the trabecular meshwork that are characteristic of aging (77, 78). In cases of Peters' anomaly associated with the anterior chamber angle abnormalities of the Axenfeld-Rieger syndrome, the mechanism of glaucoma

is presumably the same as in the latter condition as discussed earlier in this chapter.

Differential Diagnosis

Other Causes of Central Corneal Opacities in Infants

The corneal clouding of Peters' anomaly must be distinguished from that of congenital glaucoma, birth trauma, the mucopolysaccharidoses, and congenital hereditary endothelial dystrophy. Several of the mucopolysaccharidoses have been associated with glaucoma, which are discussed later in this chapter, and one case of congenital glaucoma and iris hypoplasia has been reported in association with congenital hereditary endothelial dystrophy (79).

Posterior Keratoconus

This rare disorder is characterized by a thinning of the central corneal stroma, with excessive curvature of the posterior corneal surface and variable overlying stromal haze (14, 80). An ultrastructural study revealed a multilaminar Descemet's membrane with abnormal anterior banding and localized posterior excrescences (81). Glaucoma is rarely associated with posterior keratoconus (14).

Congenital Corneal Leukomas and Staphylomas

These cases represent the more severe forms of central dysgenesis of the anterior ocular segment and are frequently associated with glaucoma (12).

Management

All infants and children with cloudy corneas must be examined carefully for the possibility of associated glaucoma. The glaucoma usually requires surgical intervention, and a trabeculotomy or trabeculectomy may offer the best chance of success. In refractory cases, a drainage implant device or cyclodestructive surgery may be required. Penetrating keratoplasty is also frequently necessary, although the results are typically poor, which is probably due, at least in part, to the associated glaucoma. In one series of 16 eyes in 10 patients, five eyes had glaucoma before keratoplasty and 10 more developed it postoperatively (82). Of those 15 eyes with glaucoma, 14 required cyclodestructive surgery or a

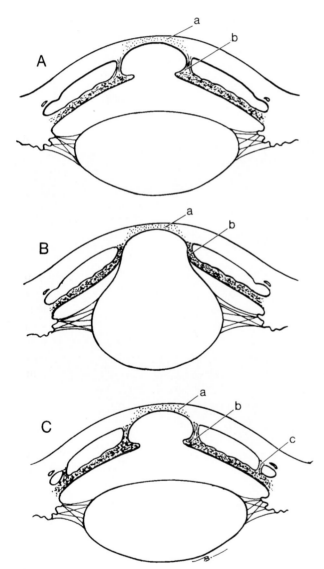

Figure 12.11. Peters' anomaly with central corneal defect *(a)* and adhesions *(b)* from corneal defect to central iris, showing three forms according to Townsend, et al. (71). **A.** Without keratolenticular contact or cataract; **(B)** with keratolenticular contact or cataract; or **(C)** with peripheral defects of Axenfeld-Rieger syndrome *(c)*.

Molteno implant or both, and of the 10 receiving cyclodestructive surgery, nine developed graft failure shortly after the procedure.

ANIRIDIA[c]

General Features

Aniridia is a bilateral developmental disorder, characterized by the congenital absence of a normal iris. The name "aniridia," however, is a misnomer, since the iris is only partially absent, with a rudimentary stump of variable width. Aniridia is associated with multiple ocular defects, some of which are present at birth, while others may become manifest later in childhood or early adulthood. In addition, some forms of aniridia may have associated systemic abnormalities.

Four phenotypes of aniridia have been identified on the basis of associated ocular and systemic abnormalities (83): (a) associated with foveal hypoplasia, nystagmus, corneal pannus, glaucoma, and reduced vision; (b) predominant iris changes and normal visual acuity; (c) associated with Wilms' tumor (the *aniridia–Wilms' tumor syndrome)* or other genitourinary anomalies; and (d) associated with mental retardation.

Most cases are inherited by autosomal dominant transmission, although sporadic cases also occur. The latter patients frequently have the associated Wilms' tumor, and a deletion of the short arm of the eleventh chromosome 11p13 has been identified in some of these cases (84–89). It has been reported that approximately 68% of patients with a deletion of chromosome 11 and aniridia will develop Wilms' tumor before age 3 years (88). However, the deletion has also been seen in an autosomal dominant pedigree of five generations without Wilms' tumor (90). Patients with the 11p13 deletion, aniridia, and Wilms' tumor also have a wide range of other ocular and nonocular development disorders (89). Other patients, especially those with mental retardation, have an autosomal recessive mode of inheritance (91).

Clinicopathologic Features

Iris

In some cases, the iris is so rudimentary that it can only be seen by gonioscopy (Fig. 12.13), while other eyes may have enough peripheral iris to be visible by external and slitlamp examination (Fig. 12.14). In some cases, the iris involvement is so minimal that other features of the disorder, as discussed below, must be used to make the diagnosis (92). Iris and retinal fluorescein angiography have also been shown to

[c]Refer to Shields, MB: Color Atlas of Glaucoma. Baltimore, Williams & Wilkins, 1998, Plate II12.

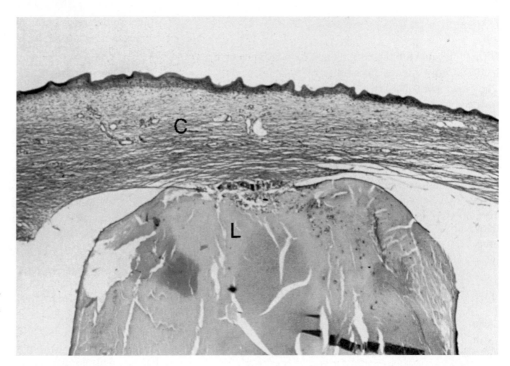

Figure 12.12. Light microscopic view of eye with Peters' anomaly showing central defect of posterior cornea *(C)* in contact with lens *(L)*. (Courtesy of George O. Waring, M.D.)

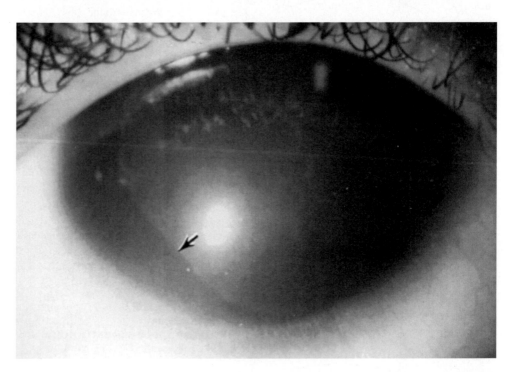

Figure 12.13. Slitlamp view of patient with aniridia in which no iris is visible, revealing equator of lens *(arrow)*.

help in identifying these patients by showing abnormal iris vascular remodeling that resulted in incomplete iris collarettes and decreased retinal foveal avascular zones (90).

Cornea

In a high percent of cases, a corneal pannus and opacity begins in the peripheral cornea in early life and advances toward the center of the cornea with increasing age. A study of ocular surface abnormalities in nine patients with nearly total aniridia and superficial corneal opacification and vas-

cularization of either the peripheral or entire cornea revealed a complete absence of the palisades of Vogt and an increase in goblet cell density, suggesting that the conjunctival epithelium had invaded the cornea (93). Microcornea (94, 95) and iridocorneal (89) and keratolenticular (96) adhesions have also been reported.

Lens

Localized congenital opacities of the lens are common but usually insignificant. However, progressive cataracts may lead to significant visual impairment by approximately the third decade of life. The lens may also be subluxed (94), or congenitally absent or reabsorbed (95, 97).

Foveal Hypoplasia

Poor visual acuity and nystagmus are typical findings in patients with aniridia. It was once thought that the absence of a pupillary effect caused the visual impairment, although some aniridic patients have reasonably good vision and no nystagmus despite significant hypoplasia of the iris (83). Foveal hypoplasia is a frequent finding in aniridia and presumably accounts for the poor visual acuity and nystagmus. However, in three infants with sporadic aniridia and nystagmus, normal ERGs suggested that the poor visual function was not due to gross retinal anomalies (98).

Other Ocular and Systemic Defects

As noted previously, aniridia has been reported in association with a wide range of other ocular and nonocular developmental anomalies. These reports include choroidal colobomas, persistent pupillary membranes (99), sclerocornea and the Hallermann-Streiff syndrome (85), small optic nerve heads, strabismus, ptosis (97, 100), Marfan's syndrome with cervical ribs and dental anomalies (101), tracheomalacia and delayed closure of the anterior fontanelle (89), and retinoblastoma (102).

Associated Glaucoma

Glaucoma occurs in 50–75% of patients with aniridia, but usually does not appear before late childhood or adolescence (103). The development of the glaucoma appears to correlate with the gonioscopic appearance of the anterior chamber angle. In infancy, the angle is usually open and unobstructed, although some eyes may have strands of tissue with occasional fine blood vessels extending from the iris root to the trabecular meshwork or higher (103). Some patients have congenital anomalies in the filtration angle, which appears to be more common in patients with chromosomal defects and may lead to glaucoma early in life (86).

During the first 5–15 years of life, many eyes with aniridia will undergo progressive change in the anterior chamber angle as the rudimentary stump of iris comes to lie over the trabecular meshwork (Fig. 12.15). The progressive obstruction of the anterior chamber angle may be due to contracture of the tissue strands between the peripheral iris and angle wall (Fig. 12.16) (103). In eyes with mild IOP elevation, the obstruction to aqueous outflow may be limited to the superior quadrant, while in eyes with more advanced glaucoma, the iris stroma covers most of the trabecular meshwork.

Management

Glaucoma

Conventional medical therapy, especially with agents to reduce aqueous production, may control the IOP initially, but eventually proves to be inadequate in most cases. A filtering procedure is usually the first surgical intervention to be attempted, although it is often unsuccessful, especially in children. Drainage implant devices may offer a reasonable alternative, while cyclocryotherapy or cyclophotocoagulation may have lasting benefit in some cases. In one surgical

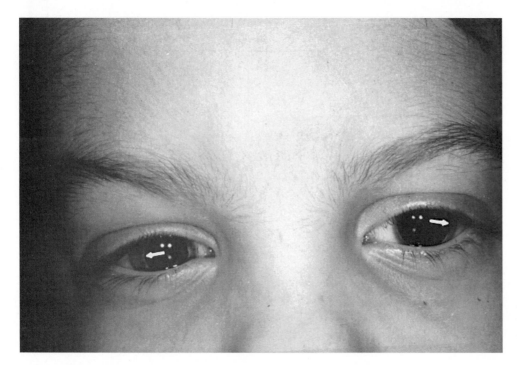

Figure 12.14. External view of patient with aniridia in which rudimentary, peripheral iris is visible in both eyes *(arrows).*

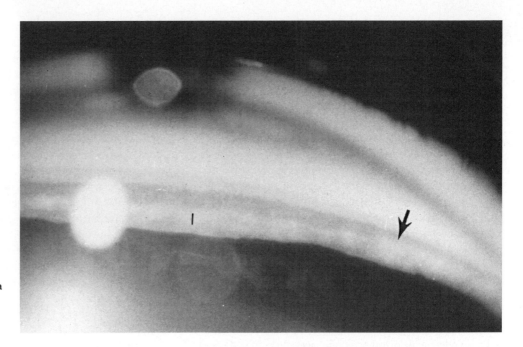

Figure 12.15. Gonioscopic view of patient with aniridia and glaucoma showing rudimentary, peripheral iris *(I)*, a portion of which has been drawn up toward the trabecular meshwork *(arrow)*.

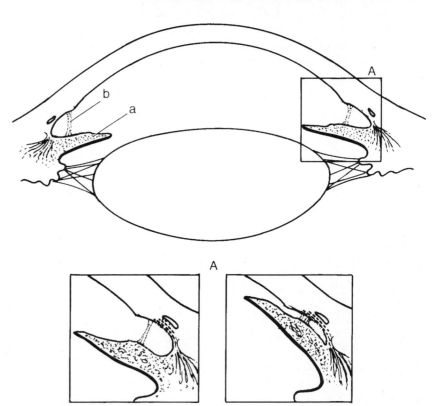

Figure 12.16. Aniridia with rudimentary iris *(a)* and fine tissue strands *(b)* extending across the anterior chamber angle. Insets *(A)* show theory of progressive angle closure by contracture of tissue strands.

series, trabeculectomy was successful in only 9% of the cases in which it was performed (1 of 11), while cyclocryotherapy was successful in 25% (5 of 20) and a Molteno implant was successful in 83% (5 of 6) (104). Goniotomy is of no value in advanced cases, but preliminary experience suggests that early goniotomy to separate the strands between the iris and the trabecular meshwork may prevent the development of glaucoma (103, 105).

Cataracts and Corneal Opacities

Cataract surgery is often difficult in the aniridic eye due to reduced corneal clarity, limited iris support, and poor zonular integrity. Nevertheless, successful extracapsular cataract extraction with capsular fixation of a posterior chamber intraocular lens was reported in four patients (106). Presumably, phacoemulsification with a small capsulorhexis might be a better option in eyes with good zonular support. The remaining anterior capsule often opacifies, which might create a "pseudo iris." Other attempts to compensate for the missing iris include intraocular lens with a peripheral black diaphragm (107) or frosted surface (108).

Penetrating keratoplasty is also difficult in these patients, presumably because of the high incidence of corneal vascularization. In one series of eight patients who underwent keratoplasty in 11 eyes, graft rejection occurred in seven (64%), and the glaucoma became more difficult to control in 5 of 9 eyes (56%) (109).

OTHER SYNDROMES WITH ASSOCIATED GLAUCOMA[d]

In addition to the disorders already considered in this chapter, glaucoma may be a feature of many other congenital syndromes. The present discussion is limited to those syndromes that represent multiple-system, developmental anomalies, and undoubtedly represents only a partial list of this extensive group of developmental disorders.

Lowe's (Oculocerebrorenal) Syndrome

Lowe's syndrome is a sex-linked disorder characterized by mental retardation, renal rickets, aminoaciduria, hypotonia, acidemia, and irritability. The two principal ocular abnormalities are cataracts, which are usually bilateral and occur in nearly all cases, and glaucoma, which is seen in approximately two-thirds of the patients. Other ocular findings include microphthalmia, strabismus, nystagmus, miosis, and iris atrophy. Female carriers may be identified by cortical lens opacities and genetic studies (110).

The mechanism of the glaucoma is related to faulty development of the filtration angle. Gonioscopy reveals only minor anatomic defects, including poor visualization of the scleral spur and a narrow ciliary body band. Goniotomy may be beneficial in some cases.

Chromosomal Anomalies

Trisomy 21 (Down's Syndrome)

This condition is characterized by mental retardation and a typical facies. Ocular findings include epicanthus, blepharitis, nystagmus, strabismus, light-colored and spotted irides, keratoconus, cataracts, and congenital glaucoma (111). The glaucoma usually appears in infancy, with the typical findings of infantile glaucoma (112).

[d]Refer to Shields, MB: *Color Atlas of Glaucoma*. Baltimore, Williams & Wilkins, 1998, Plate II13.

Trisomy D (Trisomy 13–15) Syndrome

The principal systemic features include mental retardation, deafness, heart disease, and motor seizures. The condition is usually not compatible with life, although milder forms have been reported (113). Ocular findings include microphthalmia, coloboma with cartilage, congenital cataracts, retinal dysplasia, hyperplastic primary vitreous, and dysembryogeneses of the anterior chamber angle (114). Glaucoma may be present as a result of several of these developmental defects.

Trisomy 18 (Edwards' Syndrome)

The ocular histopathologic findings in one infant included an anterior position of the iris obstructing the anterior chamber angle (115).

Turner's Syndrome (XO)

These patients are typically short-stature, postadolescent females with sexual infantilism and multiple systemic anomalies. Ocular findings include ptosis, epicanthus, cataract, strabismus, blue sclera, corneal nebulae, and color blindness (116). Developmental glaucoma is rarely associated.

Stickler's Syndrome

Stickler's syndrome, or hereditary progressive arthro-ophthalmopathy, is an autosomal dominant connective tissue dysplasia, characterized by ocular, orofacial, and generalized skeletal abnormalities (117). The *Pierre-Robin anomaly* of mandibular hypoplasia, glossoptosis, and cleft palate may be seen in some patients. The most common ocular manifestations are high myopia, open-angle glaucoma, cataracts, vitreoretinal degeneration, and retinal detachment (118, 119). In one study of 39 patients from 12 families, 10% had ocular hypertension, which may be associated with numerous iris processes, suggestive of a developmental abnormality of the angle (119). Neovascular glaucoma has also been reported in association with Stickler's syndrome (120). The open-angle glaucoma can usually be controlled medically, although miotics should be avoided if possible, due to the potential for retinal detachment.

Zellweger Syndrome

Zellweger syndrome, or the cerebrohepatorenal syndrome, is a multisystem congenital disorder characterized by central nervous system abnormalities, hepatic interstitial fibrosis, and renal cysts. Ocular findings include nystagmus, corneal clouding, cataracts, retinal vascular and pigmentary abnormalities, optic nerve head lesions, and congenital glaucoma (121). Iridocorneal adhesions may be the mechanism of the glaucoma (122).

Hallermann-Streiff Syndrome

Micrognathia and dwarfism in this condition may be associated with ocular findings, including cataracts and microphthalmos. Glaucoma may also be present due to absorption of lens material or associated aniridia (85).

Rubinstein-Taybi (Broad Thumb) Syndrome

These individuals have mental and motor retardation and typical congenital skeletal deformities with characteristically large thumbs and first toes. Ocular findings include bushy brows, hypertelorism, epicanthus, antimongoloid slant of eyelids, and hyperopia. Infantile or juvenile glaucoma has also been observed in several patients (123–125).

Oculodentodigital Dysplasia

The systemic features of this disorder are hypoplastic dental enamel, microdontia, bilateral syndactyly and a characteristic thin nose. Multiple ocular anomalies have been described, including glaucoma. There are probably several mechanisms of glaucoma in this syndrome, with reported cases of mild developmental abnormalities of the anterior chamber angle (54), gonioscopic changes resembling infantile glaucoma (126), and one case of chronic angle closure glaucoma associated with bilateral microcornea (127).

Mucopolysaccharidoses

The prototype, *Hurler's syndrome,* is an autosomal recessive disease with central nervous system, skeletal, and visceral abnormalities. The typical ocular finding is corneal clouding. Glaucoma has also been reported in Hurler's syndrome and was felt to result from mucopolysaccharide-containing cells in the aqueous outflow system (128). In a 3-year-old child with Hurler's syndrome and open-angle glaucoma, the IOP returned to normal after bone marrow transplantation (129). Patients with mucopolysaccharidosis type VI, the *Maroteaux-Lamy syndrome,* may have acute or chronic angle-closure glaucoma, which appears to be associated more with increased thickness of the peripheral cornea than with pupillary block (130). Glaucoma, apparently with open angles, was also described in two siblings with mucopolysaccharidosis type IV, the *Morquio syndrome* (131).

Cystinosis

This is a rare autosomal recessive metabolic disorder characterized by widespread accumulation of cystine crystals in ocular and nonocular tissues. A case of pupillary-block glaucoma was reported in one patient, which was felt to be due to the cystine accumulation in the iris stroma (132).

Prader-Willi Syndrome

This condition is characterized by muscular hypotonia, hypogonadism, obesity, and mental retardation, and is frequently caused by an abnormality of chromosome 15. Ocular findings include oculocutaneous albinism (133) and congenital ectropion uveae, which may be associated with open-angle glaucoma (56). One patient with Prader-Willi syndrome, congenital ectropion uvea, and glaucoma had factor XI deficiency and the suggestion of a primary hypothalamic defect (134).

Waardenburg Syndrome

This autosomal dominant disorder is characterized by lateral displacement of the medial canthi, hyperplasia of the medial brows, a prominent, broad root of the nose, sectoral or complete iris heterochromia, congenital deafness, and a white forelock (135, 136). It is felt to represent a defect of neural crest-derived tissues. Open-angle glaucoma is an uncommon finding, although was present in one of Waardenburg's original cases, and may be due to a developmental abnormality of neural crest-derived tissues in the angle (136).

Cockayne's Syndrome

This autosomal recessive disorder is characterized by dwarfism and a "bird-like" facies. Ocular manifestations include "salt-and-pepper" retinopathy, cataracts, corneal ulcers or opacities, nystagmus, hypoplastic irides, and irregular pupils. While glaucoma has not been associated, the histopathologic examination of one case revealed a high insertion of the anterior uvea into the posterior aspect of the trabecular meshwork (137) similar to that seen in congenital glaucoma and the Axenfeld-Rieger syndrome.

Fetal Alcohol Syndrome

This condition presumably results from a teratogenic effect of alcohol during a critical period of gestation, possibly influenced by a genetic background. The anterior ocular segment may be involved, with developmental abnormalities resembling those of the Axenfeld-Rieger syndrome and Peters' anomaly (138). Mouse studies suggest that the ocular abnormalities result from an acute insult to the optic primordia during a specific period that corresponds to the third week after fertilization in the human (139).

Michel's Syndrome

This condition is characterized by congenital anomalies of the anterior ocular segment, eyelids, and skeletal system with an apparent autosomal recessive transmission (141, 142). Ocular findings include corneal opacities, conjunctival telangiectasia, and iridocorneal adhesions, with blepharoptosis, blepharophimosis and telecanthus, while systemic findings include oromandibular anomalies, short stature, clinodactyly, subnormal intelligence, and hearing loss. Glaucoma may occur in eyes with extensive anterior segment anomalies (142).

SUMMARY

Several conditions are characterized by glaucoma due to developmental defects of the anterior chamber angle with additional ocular and systemic abnormalities. These disorders are typically bilateral, are usually diagnosed at birth or in early childhood, and most are felt to have a genetic basis. One such condition, the Axenfeld-Rieger syndrome, is a spectrum of disorders in which the ocular anomalies include a prominent Schwalbe's line, tissue strands across the anterior chamber angle, and variable degrees of iris distortion, while systemic defects most often involve the teeth and facial bones. Peters' anomaly also has variable clinical manifestations with alterations primarily of the central cornea, iris, and lens. In aniridia, the hallmark is a rudimentary stump of peripheral iris, although there may be additional ocular abnormalities of the cornea, lens, or fovea, as well as systemic disorders including Wilms' tumor and mental retardation. A large number of other syndromes with ocular and systemic abnormalities may occasionally have developmental glaucoma.

REFERENCES

1. LeDourain, N: The neural crest in the neck and other parts of the body. Birth Defects 11:19, 1975.
2. Johnston, MC, Norden, DM, Hazelton, RD, et al: Origins of avian ocular and periocular tissues. Exp Eye Res 29:27, 1979.
3. Bolande, RP: The neurocristopathies: a unifying concept of disease arising in neural crest maldevelopment. Hum Pathol 5:279, 1974.
4. Beauchamp, GR, Knepper, PA: Role of the neural crest in anterior segment development and disease. J Pediatr Ophthalmol Strabismus 21:209, 1984.
5. Hoskins, HD, Shaffer, RN, Hetherington, J: Anatomical classification of the developmental glaucomas. Arch Ophthalmol 102:1331, 1984.
6. Axenfeld, TH: Embryotoxon corneae posterius. Ber Deutsch Ophthalmol Ges 42:301, 1920.
7. Rieger, H: Demonstration von zwei: Fallen von Verlagerung und Schlitzform der Pupille mit Hypoplasie des Irisvorderblattes an beiden Augen einer 10-und 25-jahrigen Patientin. Z Augenheilk 84:98, 1934.
8. Rieger, H: Beitrage zur Kenntnis seltener Missbildungen der Iris. II. Uber Hypoplasie des Irisvorderblattes mit Verlagerung und Entrundung der Pupille. Graefes Arch Clin Exp Ophthalmol 133:602, 1935.
9. Rieger, H: Dysgenesis mesodermalis Corneae et Iridis. Z Augenheilk 86:333, 1935.
10. Mathis, H: Zahnunterzahl und Missbildungen der Iris. Z Stomatol 34:895, 1936.
11. Rieger, H: Erbfragen in der Augenheilkunde. Graefes Arch Clin Exp Ophthalmol 143:277, 1941.
12. Alkemade, PPH: Dysgenesis Mesodermalis of the Iris and the Cornea. Assen, Netherlands, Charles C Thomas, 1969.
13. Reese, AB, Ellsworth, RM: The anterior chamber cleavage syndrome. Arch Ophthalmol 75:307, 1966.
14. Waring, GO III, Rodrigues, MM, Laibson, PR: Anterior chamber cleavage syndrome. A stepladder classification. Surv Ophthalmol 20:3, 1975.
15. Shields, MB: Axenfeld-Rieger syndrome. A theory of mechanism and distinctions from the iridocorneal endothelial syndrome. Trans Am Ophthalmol Soc 81:736, 1983.
16. Shields, MB, Buckley, E, Klintworth, GK, Thresher, R: Axenfeld-Rieger syndrome. A spectrum of developmental disorders. Surv Ophthalmol 29:387, 1985.
17. Chisholm, IA, Chudley, AE: Autosomal dominant iridogoniodysgenesis with associated somatic anomalies: four-generation family with Rieger's syndrome. Br J Ophthalmol 67:529, 1983.
18. Burian, HM, Braley, AE, Allen, L: External and gonioscopic visibility of the ring of Schwalbe and the trabecular zone. An interpretation of the posterior corneal embryotoxon and the so-called congenital hyaline membranes on the posterior corneal surface. Trans Am Ophthalmol Soc 51:389, 1955.
19. Maumenee, AE: Further observations on the pathogenesis of congenital glaucoma. Am J Ophthalmol 55:1163, 1963.
20. Shields, MB, Campbell, DG, Simmons, RF: The essential iris atrophies. Am J Ophthalmol 85:749, 1978.
21. Wolter, JR, Sandall, GS, Fralick, FB: Mesodermal dysgenesis of anterior eye with a partially separated posterior embryotoxon. J Pediatr Ophthalmol Strabismus 4:41, 1967.
22. Cross, HE, Maumenee, AE: Progressive spontaneous dissolution of the iris. Surv Ophthalmol 18:186, 1973.
23. Judisch, GF, Phelps, CD, Hanson, J: Rieger's syndrome. A case report with a 15-year follow-up. Arch Ophthalmol 97:2120, 1979.
24. Gregor, Z, Hitchings, RA: Rieger's anomaly: a 42-year follow-up. Br J Ophthalmol 64:56, 1980.
25. Piper, HF, Schwinger, E, Von Domarus, H: Dysplasia of the limbus corneae, the mesodermal iris layer, and the facial skeleton in one family. Klin Monastsbl Augenheilkd 186:287, 1985.
26. Henkind, P, Friedman, AH: Iridogoniodysgenesis with cataract. Am J Ophthalmol 72:949, 1971.
27. Dowling, JL, Albert, DM, Nelson, LB, Walton, DS: Primary glaucoma associated with iridotrabecular dysgenesis and ectropion uveae. Ophthalmology 92:912, 1985.
28. Cibis, GW, Waeltermann, JM, Hurst, E, et al: Congenital pupillary-iris-lens membrane with goniodysgenesis (a new entity). Ophthalmology 93:847, 1986.
29. Spallone, A: Retinal detachment in Axenfeld-Rieger syndrome. Br J Ophthalmol 73:559, 1989.
30. Wesley, RK, Baker, JD, Golnick, AL: Rieger's syndrome (oligodontia and primary mesodermal dysgenesis of the iris): clinical features and report of an isolated case. J Pediatr Ophthalmol Strabismus 15:67, 1978.
31. Kleinman, RE, Kazarian, EL, Raptopoulos, V, Braverman, LE: Primary empty sella and Rieger's anomaly of the anterior chamber of the eye: a familial syndrome. N Engl J Med 304:90, 1981.
32. Feingold, M, Shiere, F, Fogels, HR, Donaldson, D: Rieger's syndrome. Pediatrics 44:564, 1969.
33. Sadeghi-Nejad, A, Senior, B: Autosomal dominant transmission of isolated growth hormone deficiency in iris-dental dysplasia (Rieger's syndrome). J Pediatr 85:644, 1974.
34. Jorgenson, RJ, Levin, LS, Cross, HE, et al: The Rieger syndrome. Am J Med Genet 2:307, 1978.
35. Lubin, JR: Oculocutaneous albinism associated with corneal mesodermal dysgenesis. Am J Ophthalmol 91:347, 1981.

36. Steinsapir, KD, Lehman, E, Ernest, JT, Tripathi, RC: Systemic neurocristopathy associated with Rieger's syndrome. Am J Ophthalmol 110:437, 1990.

37. Troeber, R, Rochels, R: Histological findings in dysgenesis mesodermalis iridis et corneae Rieger. Graefes Arch Clin Exp Ophthalmol 213:169, 1980.

38. Tabbara, KF, Khouri, FP, der Kaloustian VM: Rieger's syndrome with chromosomal anomaly (report of a case). Can J Ophthalmol 8:488, 1973.

39. Wilcox, LM, Bercovitch, L, Howard, RO: Ophthalmic features of chromosome deletion 4p (Wolf-Hirschhorn syndrome). Am J Ophthalmol 86:834, 1978.

40. Heinemann, M, Breg, R, Cotlier, E: Rieger's syndrome with pericentric inversion of chromosome 6. Br J Ophthalmol 63:40, 1979.

41. Akazawa, K, et al: A case of retinoblastoma associated with Rieger's anomaly and 13q deletion. Jpn J Ophthalmol 25:321, 1981.

42. Herve, J, Warnet, JF, Jeanu-Bellego, E, et al: Monosomie partielle du bras court d'un chromosome 10, associee a un syndrome de Rieger et a un deficit immunitaire partiel, type Di George. Ann Pediatr 31:77, 1984.

43. Ferguson, JG, Jr, Hicks, EL: Rieger's anomaly and glaucoma associated with partial trisomy 16q. Arch Ophthalmol 105:323, 1987.

44. Stathacopoulos, RA, Bateman, JB, Sparkes, RS, Hepler, RS: The Reiger syndrome and a chromosome 13 deletion: J Pediatr Ophthalmol Strabismus 24:198, 1987.

45. Ligutic, I, Brecevic, L, Petkovic, I, Kalogjera, T, Rajic, Z: Interstitial deletion 4q and Rieger syndrome. Clin Genet 20:323, 1981.

46. Serville, F, Broustet, A: Pericentric inversion and partial monosomy 4q associated with congenital anomalies. Hum Genet 39:239, 1977.

47. Mitchell, JA, Packman, S, Loughman, WD, et al: Deletions of different segments of the long arm of chromosome 4. Am J Med Genet 8:73, 1981.

48. Vaux, C, Sheffield, L, Keith, CG, Voullaire, L: Evidence that Rieger syndrome maps to 4q25 or 4q27. J Med Genet 29:256, 1992.

49. Murray, JC, Bennett, SR, Kwitek, AE, et al: Linkage of Rieger syndrome to the region of the epidermal growth factor gene on chromosome 4. Nat Genet 2:46, 1992.

50. Alward, WLM, Murray, JC: Axenfeld-Rieger syndrome. In: Wiggs, JL: Molecular Genetics of Ocular Disease. New York, Wiley-Liss, 1994, pp. 31–50.

51. Kupfer, C, Kaiser-Kupfer, MI, Datiles, M, McCain, L: The contralateral eye in the iridocorneal endothelial (ICE) syndrome. Ophthalmology 90:1343, 1983.

52. Rubel, E: Angeborene Hypoplasie bzw. Aplasie des Irisvorderblattes. Klin Monatsbl Augenheilkd 51:174, 1913.

53. Jerndal, T: Goniodysgenesis and hereditary juvenile glaucoma. Acta Ophthalmol Suppl 107:1, 1970.

54. Judisch, GF, Martin-Casals, A, Hanson, JW, Olin, WH: Oculodentodigital dysplasia. Four new reports and a literature review. Arch Ophthalmol 97:878, 1979.

55. Cross, He: Ectopia lentis et pupillae. Am J Ophthalmol 88:381, 1979.

56. Ritch, R, Forbes, M, Hetherington, J Jr, et al: Congenital ectropion uveae with glaucoma. Ophthalmology 91:326, 1984.

57. Gramer, E, Krieglstein, GK: Infantile glaucoma in unilateral uveal ectropion. Graefes Arch Clin Exp Ophthalmol 211:215, 1979.

58. Chang, JSM Jr, Lee, DA, Christensen, RE: Neodymium:YAG laser lysis of iridocorneal adhesions in mesodermal dysgenesis. Am J Ophthalmol 108:598, 1989.

59. von Hippel, E: Ueber Hydrophthalmus congenitus nebst Bemerkungen uber die Verfarbung der Cornea durch Blutfarbstoff. Pathologisch-anatomische Untersuchung. Graefes Arch Clin Exp Ophthalmol 44:539, 1897.

60. Peters, A: Ueber angeborene Defektbildung der Descemetschen Membran. Klin Monatsbl Augenheilkd 44:27, 1906.

61. DeRespinis, PA, Wagner, RS: Peters' anomaly in a father and son: Am J Ophthalmol 104:545, 1987.

62. Holmström, GE, Reardon, WP, Baraitser, M, et al: Heterogeneity in dominant anterior segment malformations. Br J Ophthalmol 75: 591, 1991.

63. Bateman, JB, Maumenee, IH, Sparkes, RS: Peters' anomaly associated with partial deletion of the long arm of chromosome 11. Am J Ophthalmol 97:11, 1984.

64. Cibis, GW, Waeltermann, J, Harris, DJ: Peters' anomaly in association with ring 21 chromosomal abnormality. Am J Ophthalmol 100:733, 1985.

65. Azuma, I: Peters' anomaly associated with glaucoma and chromosomal abnormality. Folia Ophthalmol Jpn 35:1869, 1984.

66. Kivlin, JD, Fineman, RM, Crandall, AS, Olson, RJ: Peters' anomaly as a consequence of genetic and nongenetic syndromes. Arch Ophthalmol 104:61, 1986.

67. Van Schooneveld, MJ, Delleman, JW, Beemer, FA, Bleeker-Wagemakers, EM: Peters'- plus: a new syndrome: Ophthalmol Pediatr Genet 4:141, 1984.

68. Traboulsi, EI, Maumenee, IH: Peters' anomaly and associated congenital malformations. Arch Ophthalmol 110:1739, 1992.

69. Sullivan, TJ, Clarke, MP, Heathcote, JG, et al: Multiple congenital contractures (arthrogryposis) in association with Peters' anomaly and chorioretinal colobomata. J Pediatr Ophthalmol Strabismus 29:370, 1992.

70. Townsend, WM: Congenital corneal leukomas. 1. Central defect in Descemet's membrane. Am J Ophthalmol 77:80, 1974.

71. Townsend, WM, Font, RL, Zimmerman, LE: Congenital corneal leukomas. 2. Histopathologic findings in 19 eyes with central defect in Descemet's membrane. Am J Ophthalmol 77:192, 1974.

72. Stone, DL, Kenyon, KR, Green, WR, Ryan, SJ: Congenital central corneal leukoma (Peters' anomaly). Am J Ophthalmol 81:173, 1976.

73. Nakanishi, I, Brown, SI: The histopathology and ultrastructure of congenital, central corneal opacity (Peters' anomaly). Am J Ophthalmol 72:801, 1971.

74. Lee, C-F, Yue, BYJT, Robin, J, et al: Immunohistochemical studies of Peters' anomaly. Ophthalmology 96:958, 1989.

75. Polack, FM, Graue, EL: Scanning electron microscopy of congenital corneal leukomas (Peters' anomaly). Am J Ophthalmol 88:169, 1979.

76. Myles, WM, Flanders, ME, Chitayat, D, Brownstein, S: Peters' anomaly: a clinicopathologic study. J Pediatr Ophthalmol Strabismus 29:374, 1992.

77. Kupfer, C, Kuwabara, T, Stark, WJ: The histopathology of Peters' anomaly. Am J Ophthalmol 80:653, 1975.

78. Heath, DH, Shields, MB: Glaucoma and Peters' anomaly. A clinicopathologic case report. Graefes Arch Clin Exp Ophthalmol 229: 277, 1991.

79. Pedersen, OO, Rushood, A, Olsen EG: Anterior mesenchymal dysgenesis of the eye. Congenital hereditary endothelial dystrophy and congenital glaucoma. Acta Ophthalmol 67:470, 1989.

80. Wolter, JR, Haney, WP: Histopathology of keratoconus posticus circumscriptus. Arch Ophthalmol 69:357, 1963.

81. Krachmer, JH, Rodrigues, MM: Posterior keratoconus. Arch Ophthalmol 96:1867, 1978.

82. Parmley, VC, Stonecipher, KG, Rowsey, JJ: Peters' anomaly: a review of 26 penetrating keratoplasties in infants. Ophthalmic Surg 24:31, 1993.

83. Elsas, FJ, Maumenee, IH, Kenyon, KR, Yoder, F: Familial aniridia with preserved ocular function. Am J Ophthalmol 83:718, 1977.

84. Hittner, HM, Riccardi, VM, Franke, U: Anirida caused by a heritable chromosome 11 deletion. Ophthalmology. 86:1173, 1979.

85. Schanzlin, DJ, Goldberg, DB, Brown, SI: Hallermann-Streiff syndrome associated with sclerocornea, aniridia, and a chromosomal abnormality. Am J Ophthalmol 90:411, 1980.

86. Margo, CE: Congenital anirida: a histopathologic study of the anterior segment in children. J Pediatr Ophthalmol Strabismus 20: 192, 1983.

87. Bateman, JB, Sparkes, MC, Sparkes, RS: Aniridia: enzyme studies in an 11p-chromosomal deletion. Invest Ophthalmol Vis Sci 25: 612, 1984.

88. Turleau, C, DeGrouchy, J, Tournade, M-F, et al: Del 11p/aniridia complex. Report of three patients and review of 37 observations from the literature. Clin Genet 26:356, 1984.

89. Jotterand, V, Boisjoly, HM, Harnois, C, et al: 11p13 deletion, Wilms' tumour, and aniridia: unusual genetic, non-ocular and ocular features of three cases. Br J Ophthalmol 74:568, 1990.
90. Mintz-Hittner, HA, Ferrell, RE, Lyons, LA, Kretzer, FL: Criteria to detect minimal expressivity within families with autosomal dominant aniridia. Am J Ophthalmol 114:700, 1992.
91. Gillespie, FD: Aniridia, cerebellar ataxia, and oligophrenia in siblings. Arch Ophthalmol 73:338, 1965.
92. Pearce, WG: Variability of iris defects in autosomal dominant aniridia. Can J Ophthalmol 29:25, 1994.
93. Nishida, K, Kinoshita, S, Ohashi, Y, et al: Ocular surface abnormalities in aniridia. Am J Ophthalmol 120:368, 1995.
94. David, R, MacBeath, L, Jeenkins, T: Aniridia associated with microcornea and subluxated lenses. Br J Ophthalmol 62:118, 1978.
95. Yamamoto, Y, Hayasaka, S, Setogawa, T: Family with aniridia, microcornea, and spontaneously reabsorbed cataract. Arch Ophthalmol 106:502, 1988.
96. Beauchamp, GR: Anterior segment dysgenesis keratolenticular adhesion and aniridia. J Pediatr Ophthalmol Strabismus 17:55, 1980.
97. Shields, MB, Reed, JW: Aniridia and congenital ptosis. Ann Ophthal 7:203, 1975.
98. Harnois, C, Boisjoly, HM, Jotterand, V: Sporadic aniridia and Wilms' tumor: visual function evaluation of three cases. Graefes Clin Exp Ophthalmol 227:244, 1989.
99. Hamming, N, Wilensky, J: Persistent pupillary membrane associated with with aniridia. Am J Ophthalmol 86:118, 1978.
100. Bergamini, L, Ferraris, F, Gandiglio, G, Inghirami, L: Su di una singolare sindrome neuro-oftalmologica congenita e familiare (ptosi palpebrale, aniridia, cataratta, nistagomo, subatrofia ottica). Riv Oto-Neuro-Oftalmologica 41:81, 1966.
101. Sachdev, MS, Sood, NN, Kumar, H, Ghose, S: Bilateral aniridia with Marfan's syndrome and dental anomalies—a new association. Jpn J Ophthalmol 30:360, 1986.
102. To, KW, Mukai, S, Friedman, AH: Association and chance occurrence of aniridia and retinoblastoma. Am J Ophthalmol 118:820, 1994.
103. Grant, WM, Walton, DS: Progressive changes in the angle in congenital aniridia with development of glaucoma. Am J Ophthalmol 78:842, 1974.
104. Wiggins, RE, Tomey, KF: The results of glaucoma surgery in aniridia. Arch Ophthalmol 110:503, 1992.
105. Walton, DS: Aniridic glaucoma: the results of gonio-surgery to prevent and treat this problem. Tr Am Ophthalmol Soc 84:59, 1986.
106. Johns, KJ, O'Day, DM: Posterior chamber intraocular lenses after extracapsular cataract extraction in patients with aniridia. Ophthalmology 98:1698, 1991.
107. Sundmacher, R, Reinhard, T, Althaus, C: Black-diaphragm intraocular lens for correction of aniridia. Ophthalmic Surg 25:180, 1994.
108. Vajpayee, RB, Majji, AB, Taherian, K, Honavar, SG: Frosted-iris, intraocular lens for traumatic aniridia with cataract. Ophthalmic Surg 25:730, 1994.
109. Kremer, I, Rajpal, RK, Rapuano, CJ, et al: Results of penetrating keratoplasty in aniridia. Am J Ophthalmol 115:317, 1993.
110. Wadelius, C, Fagerholm, P, Pettersson, U, Anneren, G: Lowe oculocerebrorenal syndrome. DNA-based linkage of the gene to Xq24-q26, using tightly linked flanking markers and the correlation to lens examination in carrier diagnosis. Am J Hum Genet 44:241, 1989.
111. Shapiro, MB, France, TD: The ocular features of Down's syndrome. Am J Ophthalmol 99:659, 1985.
112. Traboulsi, EI, Levine, E, Mets, MB, et al: Infantile glaucoma in Down's syndrome (trisomy 21). Am J Ophthalmol 105:389, 1988.
113. Lichter, PR, Schmickel, RD: Posterior vortex vein and congenital glaucoma in a patient with trisomy 13 syndrome. Am J Ophthalmol 80:939, 1975.
114. Hoepner, J, Yanoff, M: Ocular anomalies in trisomy 13–15: an analysis of 13 eyes with two new findings. Am J Ophthalmol 74:729, 1972.
115. Mayer, UM, Grosse, KP, Schwanitz, G: Ophthalmologic findings in trisomy 18. Graefes Arch Clin Exp Ophthalmol 218:46, 1982.
116. Lessell, S, Forbes, AP: Eye signs in Turner's syndrome. Arch Ophthalmol 76:211, 1966.
117. Stickler, GB, Belau, PG, Farrell, FJ, et al: Hereditary progressive arthro-opthalmopathy. Mayo Clin Proc 40:433, 1965.
118. Blair, NP, Albert, DM, Liberfarb, RM, Hirose, T: Hereditary progressive arthro-ophthalmopathy of Stickler. Am J Ophthalmol 88:876, 1979.
119. Spallone, A: Stickler's syndrome: a study of 12 families. Br J Ophthalmol 71:504, 1987.
120. Young, NJA, Hitchings, RA, Sehmi, K, Bird, AC: Stickler's syndrome and neovascular glaucoma. Br J Ophthalmol 63:826, 1979.
121. Cohen, SM, Brown, FR III, Martyn, L, et al: Ocular histopathologic and biochemical studies of the cerebrohepatorenal syndrome (Zellweger's syndrome) and its relationship to neonatal adrenoleukodystrophy. Am J Ophthalmol 96:488, 1983.
122. Haddad, R, Font, RL, Friendly, DS: Cerebro-hepato-renal syndrome of Zellweger. Ocular histopathologic findings. Arch Ophthalmol 94:1927, 1976.
123. Mangitti, E, Lavin, JR: Le Glaucoma congenital dans le syndrome de Rubinstein-Taybi. Ann Oculist 205:1005, 1972.
124. Weber, U, Bernsmeier, H: Rubinstein-Taybi syndrome and juvenile glaucoma. Klin Monatsbl Augenheilkd 183:47, 1983.
125. Shihab, ZM: Pediatric glaucoma in Rubinstein-Taybi syndrome. Glaucoma 3:288, 1984.
126. Traboulsi, EI, Parks, MM: Glaucoma in oculo-dento-osseous dysplasia. Am J Ophthalmol 109:310, 1990.
127. Sugar, HS: Oculodentodigital dysplasia syndrome with angle-closure glaucoma. Am J Ophthalmol 86:36, 1978.
128. Spellacy, E, Bankes, JLK, Crow, J, et al: Glaucoma in a case of Hurler disease. Br J Ophthalmol 64:773, 1980.
129. Christiansen, SP, Smith, TJ, Henslee-Downey, PJ: Normal intraocular pressure after a bone marrow transplant in glaucoma associated with mucopolysaccharidosis type I-H. Am J Ophthalmol 109:230, 1990.
130. Cantor, LB, Disseler, JA, Wilson FM, II: Glaucoma in the Maroteaux-Lamy syndrome. Am J Ophthalmol 108:426, 1989.
131. Cahane, M, Treister, G, Abraham, FA, Melamed, S: Glaucoma in siblings with Morquio syndrome. Br J Ophthalmol 74:382, 1990.
132. Wan, WL, Minckler, DS, Rao, NA: Pupillary-block glaucoma associated with childhood cystinosis. Am J Ophthalmol 101:700, 1986.
133. Hittner, HM, King, RA: Oculocutaneous albinoidism as a manifestation of reduced neural crest derivatives in the Prader-Willi syndrome. Am J Ophthalmol 94:328, 1982.
134. Futterweit, W, Ritch, R, Teekhasaenee, C, Nelson, ES: Coexistence of Prader-Willi syndrome, congenital ectropion uveae with glaucoma, and factor XI deficiency. JAMA 255:3280, 1986.
135. Enright, KA, Neelon, FA: The eyes have it: Waardenburg's syndrome. N C Med J 47:592, 1986.
136. Nork, TM, Shihab, ZM, Young, RSL, Price, J: Pigment distribution in Waardenburg's syndrome: a new hypothesis. Graefes Arch Clin Exp Ophthalmol 224:487, 1986.
137. Levin, PS, Green, WR, Victor, DI, MacLean, AL: Histopathology of the eye in Cockayne's syndrome. Arch Ophthalmol 101:1093, 1983.
138. Miller, MT, Gammon, JA, Epstein, RJ, et al: Anterior segment anomalies associated with the fetal alcohol syndrome. J Pediatr Ophthalmol Strabismus 21:8, 1984.
139. Cook, CS, Nowotny, AZ, Sulik, KK: Fetal Alcohol syndrome. Eye malformations in a mouse model. Arch Ophthalmol 105:1576, 1987.
140. Michels, VV, Hittner, HM, Beaudet, AL: A clefting syndrome with ocular anterior chamber defect and lid anomalies. J Pediatr 93:444, 1978.
141. De La Paz, MA, Lewis, RA, Patrinely, JR, et al: A sibship with unusual anomalies of the eye and skeleton (Michels' syndrome). Am J Ophthalmol 112:572, 1991.

Chapter 13

GLAUCOMAS ASSOCIATED WITH DISORDERS OF THE CORNEAL ENDOTHELIUM

GLAUCOMA AND CORNEAL DISORDERS

Glaucoma and disorders of the cornea may be associated in one of three ways (1). In one set of conditions, the concomitant findings may be due to *common anterior segment abnormalities*. These situations include developmental disorders such as Peters' anomaly, sclerocornea, aniridia, and the Axenfeld-Rieger syndrome, as well as acquired conditions such as anterior uveitis and trauma. A second set of conditions includes *corneal abnormalities secondary to the glaucoma*. These include pressure-induced changes, such as epithelial and stromal edema with acute or especially high elevations of intraocular pressure (IOP), endothelial changes with chronic pressure elevation, and Haab's striae in childhood glaucomas. Corneal changes may also be secondary to the use of topical anti-glaucoma medications.

In the third set of conditions, a *corneal disorder leads to IOP elevation*. These situations include corneal inflammation with associated glaucoma either due to the inflammation or treatment of the inflammation, i.e., steroid-induced glaucoma, and glaucomas following penetrating keratoplasty. In addition, certain primary disorders of the corneal endothelium may have associated glaucoma. Two of these situations, the iridocorneal endothelial syndrome and posterior polymorphous dystrophy, represent spectra of clinical and histopathologic abnormalities, with strong evidence for an association between the glaucoma and the corneal disease. In a third condition, Fuchs' endothelial dystrophy, an association with glaucoma has also been suggested. This group of primary corneal endothelial disorders is the subject of the present chapter, while the other conditions noted above are considered in other chapters (Table 13.1).

Table 13.1.

GLAUCOMA AND CORNEAL DISORDERS

I. Common anterior segment abnormalities
  A. Developmental disorders   (Chapter 12)
    1. Peters' anomaly
    2. Sclerocornea
    3. Aniridia
    4. Axenfeld-Rieger syndrome
  B. Acquired conditions
    1. Anterior uveitis   (Chapter 19)
    2. Trauma   (Chapter 21)
II. Glaucoma with secondary corneal
   abnormalities
  A. Pressure-induced corneal changes
    1. Epithelial and stromal edema   (Chapter 10)
      (acute or marked IOP elevation)
    2. Endothelial changes (chronic   (Present
      IOP elevation)   chapter)
    3. Haab's striae (childhood glaucoma)   (Chapter 11)
  B. Drug-induced ocular surface changes
    1. Miotics   (Chapter 25)
    2. Epinephrine compounds   (Chapter 26)
    3. β-blockers   (Chapter 27)
III. Corneal disorders with associated glaucoma
  A. Keratitis
    1. Glaucoma due to inflammation   (Chapter 19)
    2. Steroid-induced glaucoma   (Chapter 20)
  B. Glaucoma following penetrating   (Chapter 23)
    keratoplasty
  C. Glaucomas associated with primary   (Present
    disorders of the corneal endothelium   chapter)
    1. Iridocorneal endothelial syndrome
    2. Posterior polymorphous dystrophy
    3. Fuchs' endothelial dystrophy

(Modified from Miller, KN, Carlson, AN, Foulks, GN, Shields, MB: Associated glaucoma and corneal disorders. Focal Points, Am Acad Ophthal, Vol. 7, Module 4, 1989.)

IRIDOCORNEAL ENDOTHELIAL SYNDROME

Terminology[a]

The term "iridocorneal endothelial (ICE) syndrome" was suggested by Eagle and Yanoff (2–4) to denote a spectrum of disease that is characterized by a primary corneal endothelial abnormality. The endothelial disease is variably associated with corneal edema, anterior chamber angle changes, alterations in the iris, and glaucoma. The following three clinical variations within the ICE syndrome have been distinguished primarily on the basis of changes in the iris (Table 13.2).

[a]Refer to Shields, MB: Color Atlas of Glaucoma. Baltimore, Williams & Wilkins, 1998, Plates II14–16.

Progressive Iris Atrophy

In 1903, Harms (5) described a condition that is characterized by extreme atrophy of the iris with hole formation. This variation has been called "essential iris atrophy" or "progressive essential iris atrophy." However, subsequent observations, which are discussed later in this chapter, indicate that iris atrophy is not the "essential" or primary feature in this disease.

Chandler's Syndrome

This variation was described by Chandler (6) in 1956 and differs from progressive iris atrophy in that changes in the iris are limited to slight corectopia and mild stromal atrophy, or may be absent altogether. In one study of 37 consecutive cases of the ICE syndrome, Chandler's syndrome was the most common clinical variation, accounting for 21 cases (56%), and was characterized by more severe corneal edema despite less severe glaucoma than in the rest of the group (7). Intermediate variations between progressive iris atrophy and Chandler's syndrome are also seen, in which changes in the iris are more extensive than in the latter condition, but lack the hole formation of the former variation.

Cogan-Reese Syndrome

In 1969, Cogan and Reese (8) reported two cases with pigmented nodules of the iris, associated with some features of the ICE syndrome. Subsequent studies have revealed that these nodules may occur on the surface of the iris throughout the complete spectrum of this syndrome (9, 10). Similar cases have been described with diffuse nevi, rather than nod-

Table 13.2.

IRIDOCORNEAL ENDOTHELIAL (ICE) SYNDROME

Major Clinical Variations	Characteristic Features
1. Progressive Iris Atrophy	Iris features predominate with marked corectopia, atrophy, and hole formation.
2. Chandler's Syndrome	Changes in the iris are mild-to-absent, while corneal edema, often at normal intraocular pressures, is typical.
3. Cogan-Reese Syndrome	Nodular, pigmented lesions of the iris are the hallmark, and may be seen with the entire spectrum of corneal and other iris defects.

ules, on the surface of iris, which has been called *iris nevus syndrome* (9). There has been a tendency to lump the Cogan-Reese and iris nevus syndromes together as variants of the ICE syndrome. However, the iris lesions of the two conditions are clinically and histologically different, and there is insufficient evidence at this time to include the iris nevus syndrome as a clinical variation of the ICE syndrome.

General Features (7, 11, 12)

The ICE syndrome is nearly always clinically unilateral, although subclinical abnormalities of the corneal endothelium in the fellow eye are common. The condition is usually recognized in early to middle adulthood, with a predilection for women. Familial cases are rare, and there is no consistent association with systemic diseases. The most common presenting manifestations are abnormalities of the iris, reduced visual acuity, or pain. The latter two symptoms are usually due to corneal edema, but also may result from the elevated IOP.

Clinicopathologic Features

Corneal Alterations

A common feature throughout the ICE syndrome is a corneal endothelial abnormality, which may be seen by slitlamp biomicroscopy as a fine hammered silver appearance of the posterior cornea, similar to that of Fuchs' dystrophy (Fig. 13.1). This defect may occur by itself without symptoms, or may cause corneal edema with variable degrees of reduced vision and pain (13). In some cases, the corneal edema may occur at IOP levels that are normal or only slightly elevated. Specular microscopy reveals a characteristic, diffuse abnormality of the corneal endothelial cells, with variable degrees of pleomorphism in size and shape, dark areas within the cells, and loss of the clear hexagonal margins (Fig. 13.2) (14–18). The similarity of these findings among the three main clinical variations of the ICE syndrome is further evidence that they represent a spectrum of disease. Some studies have revealed focal areas of normal and abnormal cells separated by a distinct border (16, 17), with gradual disappearance of the normal areas with time (17). Decreased endothelial cell counts and cellular pleomorphism have also been observed in fellow, asymptomatic eyes of patients with the ICE syndrome (19). Endothelial permeability, studied by fluorophotometry, was markedly decreased in the eye with the clinically apparent disorder, but normal in the fellow eye (20).

The appearance of the corneal endothelium by specular microscopy is virtually pathognomonic of the ICE syndrome. So typical are certain cells in this condition that they have been called *ICE cells* (21). These endothelial cells appear dark by specular microscopy except for a light central spot and a light peripheral zone. When clustered as continuous cells, which has been called ICE tissue, they give the ap-

pearance of a negative of the normal endothelium. These cells are said to form four basic variations with the remaining corneal endothelium: (a) *disseminated ICE,* characterized by ICE cells that are scattered among large endothelial cells with vague margins; is always associated with elevated IOP and progresses rapidly to the second variation; (b) *total ICE,* in which the whole posterior corneal surface is ICE tissue; (c) *subtotal ICE (+),* characterized by clearly defined ICE tissue with the remaining endothelium composed of distinct small cells; is associated with normal IOP and slowly progresses to the fourth variation; and (d) *subtotal ICE (–),* which occurs relatively late in the disease process and consists of ICE tissue and larger than normal remaining endothelial cells (21).

The course of the abnormal corneal endothelium may not be as predictable as described above. In three patients, followed for more than 10 years, partial corneal involvement spread to cover the entire posterior corneal surface in two patients, while in the third it disappeared to be completely replaced by normal corneal endothelium (22).

Electron microscopic studies of the posterior cornea in advanced cases have revealed varied and complex alterations of cells, lining multilayered collagenous tissue poste-

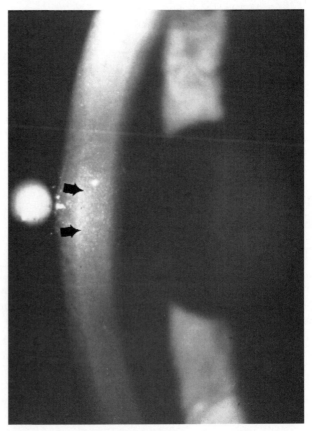

Figure 13.1. Slitlamp view showing fine beaten silver appearance of corneal endothelial abnormality *(arrows)* in the ICE syndrome. (Reprinted with permission from Shields, MB, Campbell, DG, Simmons, RJ: The essential iris atrophies. Am J Ophthalmol 85:749, 1978.)

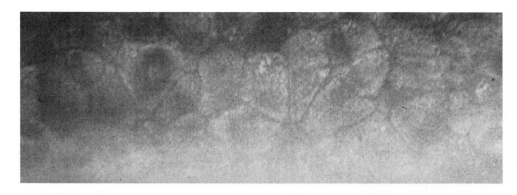

Figure 13.2. Specular microscopic appearance of corneal endothelial cells in the ICE syndrome showing pleomorphism in size and shape, dark areas within the cells, and loss of clear hexagonal margins.

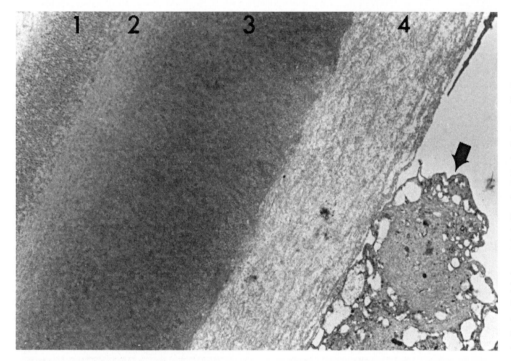

Figure 13.3. Transmission electron microscopic view of inner corneal surface in ICE syndrome showing part of an abnormal cell (*arrow*) on a four-layered membrane, composed of the anterior nonbanded (1) and posterior banded (2) portions of Descemet's membrane with abnormal compact collagenous (3) and loose collagenous (4) layers (×6875). (Reprinted with permission from Shields, MB, McCracken, JS, Klintworth, GK, Campbell, DG: Corneal edema in essential iris atrophy. Ophthalmology 86:1533, 1979.)

rior to Descemet's membrane (Fig. 13.3) (13, 23–30). Most studies are in agreement with regard to the collagenous structures, which consist of the normal prenatal and postnatal layers of Descemet's membrane, lined posteriorly by abnormal collagen zones of variable thickness. Descriptions of the cellular layer differ among reports, however, which may relate to the varied response of the corneal endothelium in this syndrome, even within different areas of the same eye. Some cells have evidence of metabolic activity or have undergone division. Filopodial processes and cytoplasmic actin filaments suggest that they are migrating cells (26, 28, 30). Groups of blebs are found in some cells, which may be the explanation for the dark spots seen by specular microscopy (26). Other cells are disrupted and necrotic.

One histologic study described the ICE cells as rounded and hexagonal with numerous microvilli on the apical surface, tonofilaments in the cytoplasm, and indentations on the basal surface containing clumps of fibrillar collagenous material (31). The ICE cells have also been described as being morphologically similar to epithelial cells (32), although studies differ on the question of whether the endothelial cells in this syndrome truly have characteristics of epithelium (25, 26, 28–35). In favor of an association with epithelial cells are immunohistochemical studies showing cytokeratins (33, 34), although cross-reaction with vimentin suggests that these cells retain or derive some endothelial staining characteristics (34). Cell density varies, with some specimens revealing multiple endothelial layers, suggesting loss of contact inhibition (26). The typical finding, however, is a monolayer of reduced cell density with occasional acellular zones. Chronic inflammatory cells have also been observed in some cases (26, 28, 30, 31), with one study describing mononuclear inflammatory cells between the ICE cells in the monolayer (31).

Anterior Chamber Angle Alterations

Peripheral anterior synechia, usually extending to or beyond Schwalbe's line, is another clinical feature common to all variations of the ICE syndrome (Fig. 13.4). Histologic studies reveal a cellular membrane, consisting of a single layer of endothelial cells and a Descemet's-like membrane, extending down from the peripheral cornea. The membrane may cover an open anterior chamber angle in some areas and may be associated with synechial closure of the angle elsewhere in the same eye (2, 29, 36–38).

Elevated IOP usually begins as the synechiae progressively close the anterior chamber angle. However, the glaucoma does not correlate precisely with the degree of synechial closure (11), and has been reported to occur when

the entire angle was open, but apparently covered by the cellular membrane (39, 40). Presumably, obstruction to aqueous outflow may result from either the membrane covering the trabecular meshwork or synechial closure of the anterior chamber angle.

Alterations of the Iris

The abnormalities of the iris constitute the primary basis for distinguishing clinical variations within the ICE syndrome.

PROGRESSIVE IRIS ATROPHY. This variation is characterized by marked atrophy of the iris, associated with variable degrees of corectopia and ectropion uvea. The latter two features are usually directed toward the quadrant with the most prominent area of peripheral anterior synechia (11, 31). The hallmark of progressive iris atrophy is hole formation of the iris, which occurs in two forms (11). With *stretch holes,* the iris is markedly thinned in the quadrant away from the direction of pupillary distortion, and the holes develop within the area that is being stretched (Fig. 13.5). In other eyes, *melting holes* develop without associated corectopia or thinning of the iris. Fluorescein angiographic studies suggest that this is associated with ischemia of the iris (10).

Histopathology of the iris in this and all variations of the ICE syndrome includes a cellular membrane on portions of the anterior surface of the iris (Fig. 13.6), which is similar to and continuous with that seen over the anterior chamber angle (2, 36). The membrane is most often found in the quadrant toward which the pupil is distorted (36).

CHANDLER'S SYNDROME. In this clinical form, there is minimal corectopia and mild atrophy of the stroma of the iris

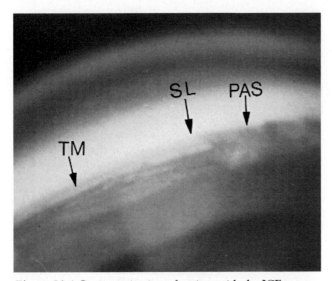

Figure 13.4. Gonioscopic view of patient with the ICE syndrome showing peripheral anterior synechia *(PAS)* extending beyond trabecular meshwork *(TM)* to Schwalbe's line *(SL).* (Reprinted with permission from Shields, MB, Campbell, DG, Simmons, RJ: The essential iris atrophies. Am J Ophthalmol 85:749, 1978.)

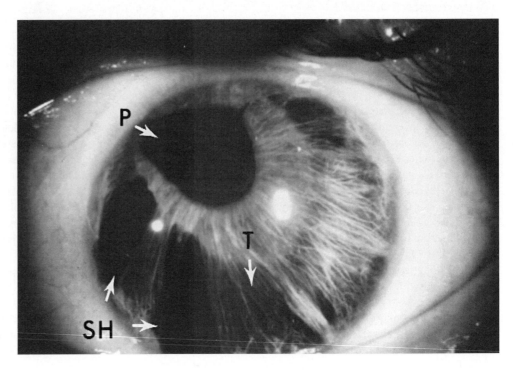

Figure 13.5. Progressive iris atrophy, a variation of the ICE syndrome, with pupillary distortion *(P)*, thinning of the iris *(T)*, and stretch holes *(SH)*. (Reprinted with permission from Shields, MB, Campbell, DG, Simmons, RJ: The essential iris atrophies. Am J Ophthalmol 85:749, 1978.)

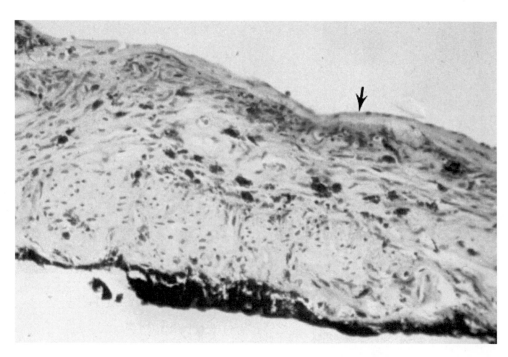

Figure 13.6. Light microscopic view of iris specimen from eye with the ICE syndrome showing Descemet-like membrane and scant monolayer of cells *(arrow)* extending across the stroma (Hematoxylin & eosin, ×250). (Reprinted with permission from Shields, MB, McCracken, JS, Klintworth, GK, Campbell, DG: Corneal edema in essential iris atrophy. Ophthalmology 86:1533, 1979.)

(Fig. 13.7) (6). In some cases, there may be no detectable change in the iris.

COGAN-REESE SYNDROME. The eyes in this variation of the ICE syndrome may have any degree of iris atrophy, but are distinguished by the presence of pigmented, pedunculated nodules on the surface of the iris (Fig. 13.8) (8–10). In some cases, other features of the ICE syndrome may be present for many years before the nodules appear (10, 41). One case has been reported in which the pigmented nodules appeared on the iris 20 years after the initial diagnosis of the ICE syndrome (42). The nodular lesions have an ultrastructure similar to that of the underlying stroma of the iris and are always surrounded by the previously described cellular membrane (Fig. 13.9) (2, 36, 41–44).

Theories of Mechanism

Campbell and associates (36) proposed a "membrane theory" which holds that the abnormality of the corneal endothelium is the primary defect in the ICE syndrome (Fig. 13.10). The endothelial defect causes the corneal edema and also leads to the proliferation of the cellular membrane across the anterior chamber angle and onto the surface of the iris. The observation of filopodial processes, cytoplasmic actin filaments, and apparent loss of contact inhibition are consistent with the concept of migrating cells (26, 28–30). Contracture of the cellular membrane causes the formation of peripheral anterior synechiae, the corectopia, and the ectropion uvea. Stretching of the iris in the direction away from the corectopia, especially when the iris is anchored by peripheral anterior synechiae on both sides, un-

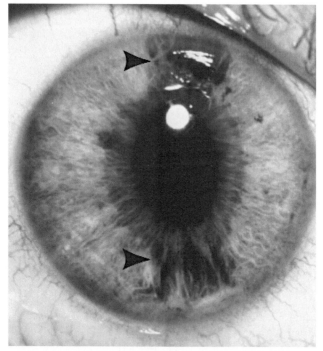

Figure 13.7. Chandler's syndrome, a variation of the ICE syndrome, with slight pupillary distortion and thinning of iris stroma at the vertical poles *(arrows)*. (Reprinted with permission from Shields, MB, Campbell, DG, Simmons, RJ: The essential iris atrophies. Am J Ophthalmol 85:749, 1978.)

doubtedly contributes to the atrophy and hole formation, although additional factors, such as ischemia, may also be involved (12). The cellular membrane is also believed to be responsible for the development of the nodular lesions of the iris in the Cogan-Reese syndrome, possibly by encircling

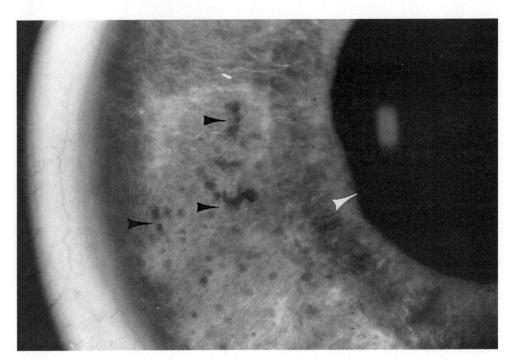

Figure 13.8. Cogan-Reese syndrome, a variation of the ICE syndrome, showing ectropion uvea *(white arrow)* and numerous dark nodules *(black arrows)* on area of flattened iris stroma. (Reprinted with permission from Shields, MB, Campbell, DG, Simmons, RJ, Hutchinson, BT: Iris nodules in essential iris atrophy. Arch Ophthalmol 94:406, 1976.)

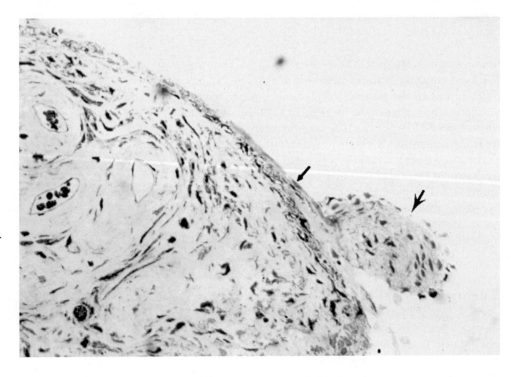

Figure 13.9. Light microscopic view of iridectomy specimen from eye with Cogan-Reese syndrome showing nodule composed of cells resembling the iris stroma *(large arrow)* and portion of a monolayer of spindle-shaped cells *(small arrow)* (Toluidine blue & basic fuchsin, ×200). (Reprinted with permission from Shields, MB, Campbell, DG, Simmons, RJ, Hutchinson, BT: Iris nodules in essential iris atrophy. Arch Ophthalmol 94:406, 1976.)

and pinching off portions of the iris stroma to form the nodules (36, 43). As previously noted, the associated glaucoma may be due to obstruction of the trabecular meshwork by either the cellular membrane or, more commonly, the peripheral anterior synechiae.

Each clinical variation is believed to have the same basic mechanism described above. In some cases, the difference in clinical features may simply be due to the time at which the patient is seen. For example, a patient with the ini-

tial findings of Chandler's syndrome may later develop iris hole formation and/or nodules, changing the diagnosis to progressive iris atrophy or the Cogan-Reese syndrome, respectively. In other cases, however, patients do not progress and, as previously noted, Chandler's syndrome appears to be the most common variant of the ICE syndrome (7). It may be that the endothelial cells in these patients are more disrupted and/or less able to migrate, which could explain the more severe corneal edema, as well as the less severe

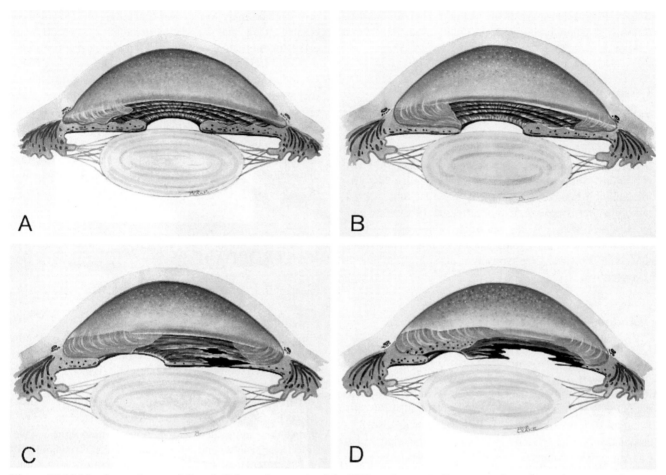

Figure 13.10. Membrane theory of Campbell for pathogenesis of the ICE syndrome. **A.** Extension of membrane from corneal endothelium over anterior chamber angle and onto iris. **B.** Contraction of membrane, creating peripheral anterior synechiae and corectopia. **C.** Thinning and atrophy of iris in quadrants away from corectopia. **D.** Hole formation in area of atrophy (in progressive iris atrophy), ectropion uvea in direction of corectopia, and nodules in area of membrane (in Cogan-Reese syndrome). (Reprinted with permission from Shields, MB: Progressive essential iris atrophy, Chandler's syndrome, and the iris nevus (Cogan-Reese) syndrome: a spectrum of disease. Surv Ophthalmol 24:3, 1979.)

glaucoma and iris changes, as compared to the other variants in this spectrum of disease (7, 26).

The underlying condition that leads to the corneal endothelial changes is unknown. The absence of a positive family history and the presence of the postnatal layer of Descemet's membrane suggest an acquired disorder. The observation of chronic inflammatory cells has raised the possibility of a viral etiology (26). An early suspect for the viral etiology was the Epstein-Barr virus, based on serologic profiles of 13 patients with the ICE syndrome (45), although this was never substantiated. More recently, using primer pairs and polymerase chain reaction methods, 16 of 25 corneas from ICE patients and four of six from patients with herpetic keratitis were positive for *herpes simplex virus* DNA, but negative for herpes zoster and Epstein-Barr viruses (46). All control corneas were negative for herpes simplex virus. These observations provide strong support for a viral etiology of the ICE syndrome and could eventually lead to more cause-specific therapeutic interventions.

Differential Diagnosis

There are several disorders of the cornea or iris, many of which have associated glaucoma, that could be confused with the various forms of the ICE syndrome. It is helpful to think of these in the following three categories: corneal endothelial disorders, dissolution of the iris, and nodular lesions of the iris.

Corneal Endothelial Disorders

Posterior polymorphous dystrophy may have associated glaucoma, as well as changes of the anterior chamber angle and iris that resemble the ICE syndrome. However, the corneal abnormalities, as well as other clinical features, clearly distinguish these two spectra of disease. Specular microscopy has been shown to be especially helpful in distinguishing the ICE syndrome and posterior polymorphous dystrophy (47). *Fuchs' endothelial dystrophy* has corneal changes that are clinically very similar to those of the

ICE syndrome, but none of the chamber angle or iris features of the latter condition. Both conditions are considered later in this chapter.

Dissolution of the Iris

The *Axenfeld-Rieger syndrome* has striking clinical and histopathologic similarities to the ICE syndrome, but the congenital nature and bilaterality, as well as the other features described in Chapter 12, help to separate the two conditions. Some advanced cases of progressive iris atrophy might resemble *aniridia*, but the bilaterality of the latter disorder is again a helpful differential feature (Chapter 12). *Iridoschisis* is characterized by separation of superficial layers of iris stroma and may be associated with glaucoma. However, it is typically a disease of the elderly (Chapter 14).

Nodular Lesions of the Iris

Patients with the Cogan-Reese syndrome have had enucleation for presumed *melanomas* of the iris (8). Patients with *iris melanosis* may also have pedunculated nodules, strikingly similar to those of the Cogan-Reese syndrome, but this condition is typically bilateral and may be familial (48, 49). Bilateral diffuse iris nodular nevi have been described in association with a variety of conditions, including bilateral congenital cataracts, neurofibromatosis, oculodermal melanocytosis, congenital ptosis, morning glory anomaly, the Axenfeld-Reiger syndrome, and Peters' anomaly (50). In addition, differentiation must be made from nodular *inflammatory disorders* such as sarcoidosis.

Management

Patients with the ICE syndrome may require treatment for corneal edema, the associated glaucoma, or both. The glaucoma can often be controlled medically in the early stages, especially with drugs that reduce aqueous production. When the IOP can no longer be controlled medically, surgical intervention is indicated, and a high percentage of patients with the ICE syndrome eventually require surgery. In one study of 66 patients, glaucoma occurred in 33 (50%), and 22 (66%) of these underwent surgery (51). Laser trabeculoplasty is usually not effective in these cases. Filtering surgery is reasonably successful (11, 52), although late failures have occurred due to endothelialization of the filtering bleb (41, 52). In the series noted above, 45% of the patients undergoing a trabeculectomy required more than one procedure (51). Adjunctive use of 5-fluorouracil was not found to improve these results (53).

Lowering the IOP may also control the corneal edema, although the additional use of hypertonic saline solutions and soft contact lenses may be required. In some cases,

even an extremely low pressure may not reverse advanced corneal edema, and penetrating keratoplasty is usually indicated for this situation after the glaucoma has been controlled (13, 54).

In the future, it may be that therapy can be directed more specifically at the underlying disease process. For example, as noted earlier, if the viral theory of etiology proves to be correct, it may allow treatment with antiviral agents (46). Another approach might be to prevent the growth of the endothelial membrane. An immunotoxin has been described that inhibits the proliferation of human corneal endothelium in tissue culture (55).

POSTERIOR POLYMORPHOUS DYSTROPHY[b]

General Features

Posterior polymorphous dystrophy is a bilateral, familial disorder of the corneal endothelium. Inheritance is usually autosomal dominant and there is no race or sex predilection. Although it is probably congenital, it typically remains asymptomatic until adulthood. As with the ICE syndrome, posterior polymorphous dystrophy represents a spectrum of disorders (56–58). In one form, the characteristic corneal changes are associated with peripheral iridocorneal adhesions, iris atrophy, and corectopia (56, 58). Glaucoma occurs in approximately 15% of patients with posterior polymorphous dystrophy, both with and without the iridocorneal adhesions.

Clinicopathologic Features

Corneal Alterations

By slitlamp biomicroscopy, the posterior cornea has the appearance of blisters or vesicles at the level of Descemet's membrane (Fig. 13.11). The vesicles may be linear or in groups and surrounded by an aureole of gray haze (57, 58). Band-like thickenings may also be seen at the level of Descemet's membrane (59). Two patterns of endothelial abnormality have been identified by slitlamp biomicroscopy and specular microscopy (60, 61). One is characterized by localized vesicular and band patterns resembling craters, or doughnut-like lesions, and snail tracks, with retention of corneal clarity. The second type has a geographic pattern with associated haze of Descemet's membrane and deep corneal stroma. The latter variety may be associated with iridocorneal adhesions and glaucoma.

Ultrastructural studies reveal an unusually thin Descemet's membrane covered by multiple layers of coll-

[b]Refer to Shields, MB: Color Atlas of Glaucoma. Baltimore, Williams & Wilkins, 1998, Plate II17.

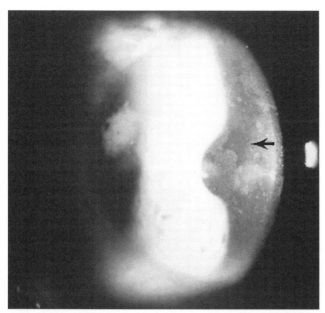

Figure 13.11. Slitlamp view of patient with posterior polymorphous dystrophy showing typical, irregular lesions *(arrow)* of the posterior corneal surface. (Reprinted with permission from Bourgeois, J, Shields, MB, Thresher, R: Open-angle glaucoma associated with posterior polymorphous dystrophy. A clinicopathologic study. Ophthalmology 91:420, 1984.)

agen (62–66), and lined by cells that have been variably described as having features of abnormal endothelium (66, 67), fibroblasts (63, 65), or epithelium (62, 64, 65, 68, 69). These differences in cellular morphology may represent an evolving process of metaplasia (63). The ultrastructural study of the corneal button from a 5-month-old baby revealed a thinned, incomplete anterior banded zone of Descemet's membrane, suggesting an onset of the disorder before the twelfth week of gestation (66). A mosaic of preserved and dystrophic endothelial cells is believed to be responsible for depositing the irregular Descemet's membrane and additional collagen layers (66). Clinically, the cornea may remain clear and produce no symptoms, although corneal edema may develop in some cases.

Anterior Chamber Angle and Iris Alterations

A small number of patients may have broad peripheral anterior synechiae extending to or beyond Schwalbe's line, which may be associated with corectopia, ectropion uvea, and atrophy of the iris (56–58, 70). Histopathologic studies of such cases have revealed a membrane composed of endothelial- (71) or epithelial-like (38, 58) cells and a Descemet's-like membrane extending over the anterior chamber angle and onto the iris (Fig. 13.12). Three types of peripheral anterior synechiae have been described: (a) without an associated membrane; (b) with iridotrabecular and iridocorneal apposition; and (c) bridging open trabecular meshwork (71). The abnormal membrane is associated with the latter two configurations.

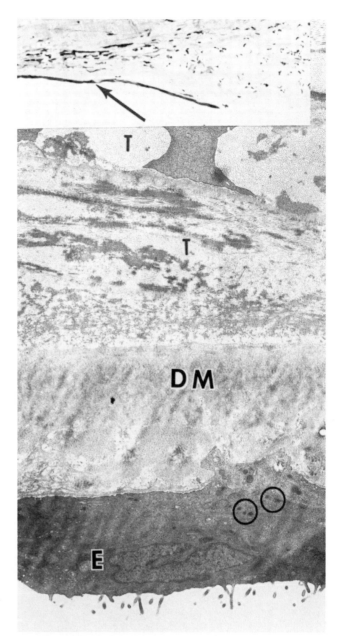

Figure 13.12. Transmission electron microscopic view of trabeculectomy specimen from eye with posterior polymorphous dystrophy showing trabecular beams *(T)* covered by Descemet-like membrane *(DM)* and transformed endothelial cells *(E)* with numerous microvillous projections and desmosomal attachments *(circles)* (×8200). Inset shows light microscopic appearance of membrane on trabecular meshwork *(arrow)* (Toluidine blue, ×130). (Reprinted with permission from Rodrigues, MM, Phelps, CD, Krachmer, JH, et al: Glaucoma due to endothelialization of the anterior chamber angle. A comparison of posterior polymorphous dystrophy of the cornea and Chandler's syndrome. Arch Ophthalmol 98:688, 1980.)

Glaucoma may be present in some of the cases with peripheral anterior synechiae, but has also been observed in eyes with open angles (57, 58, 70, 72). In the latter situation, gonioscopy may reveal a high insertion of the iris into the posterior aspect of the trabecular meshwork (72). An ultrastructural evaluation of such an eye confirmed the high insertion of anterior uvea into the meshwork with collapse of the trabecular beams (Fig. 13.13) (72).

Theories of Mechanism

A membrane theory, similar to that for the ICE syndrome, has been proposed for those cases of posterior polymorphous dystrophy with iridocorneal adhesions. It is postulated that a dystrophic endothelium (or epithelium), producing a basement membrane-like material, extends across the anterior chamber angle and onto the iris, and subsequently causes the synechia formation and changes in the iris (57, 58, 71). The glaucoma may be due to the iridocorneal adhesions in these cases. However, the extent of the iridocorneal adhesions does not correlate with the presence or severity of glaucoma, since those adhesions which bridge an otherwise open trabecular meshwork may not obstruct aqueous outflow (71). In the eyes with open angles, the high insertion of the anterior uvea may represent a developmental anomaly of the anterior chamber angle similar to that seen in several of the developmental glaucomas, and may be responsible for the subsequent collapse of the trabecular meshwork and the secondary glaucoma (72). In other cases with associated glaucoma and an open angle by gonioscopy, the mechanism of aqueous outflow obstruction may be the abnormal membrane covering the trabecular meshwork (38, 58, 71).

Differential Diagnosis

Conditions that may be confused with posterior polymorphous dystrophy include other forms of posterior corneal dystrophy, such as Fuchs' endothelial dystrophy, congenital hereditary corneal dystrophy, and posterior amorphous corneal dystrophy. The latter is characterized by diffuse gray-white, sheet-like opacities of the posterior stroma, with occasional fine iris processes extending to Schwalbe's line for 360° and various abnormalities of the iris, but no glaucoma (73). When iridocorneal adhesions are present, the Axenfeld-Rieger syndrome and the ICE syndrome should also be considered. The band-like thickenings of posterior polymorphous dystrophy may be confused with the Haab's striae of congenital glaucoma, although the latter are distinguished by the characteristic thinned areas with thickened edges (59).

Management

Most cases of posterior polymorphous dystrophy are asymptomatic and do not require treatment. However, corneal edema may require conservative management or penetrating keratoplasty. In one series of 21 keratoplasties for posterior polymorphous dystrophy, nine grafts failed, six of which had iridocorneal adhesions and glaucoma, and it has been suggested that keratoplasty should be avoided in these patients until absolutely necessary (58). Recurrence of posterior polymorphous dystrophy has been reported following penetrating keratoplasty (74). The glaucoma, when present, may respond to drugs that lower aqueous production. Laser trabeculoplasty is not likely to be successful in these cases, and filtering surgery generally is indicated when medical therapy is no longer adequate. It has also been noted that posterior polymorphous dystrophy is a common feature of Alport syndrome (a basement membrane disorder with hereditary

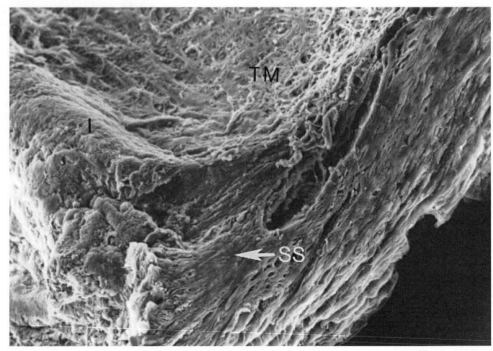

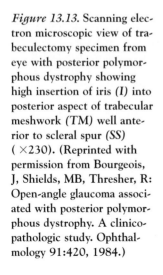

Figure 13.13. Scanning electron microscopic view of trabeculectomy specimen from eye with posterior polymorphous dystrophy showing high insertion of iris *(I)* into posterior aspect of trabecular meshwork *(TM)* well anterior to scleral spur *(SS)* (×230). (Reprinted with permission from Bourgeois, J, Shields, MB, Thresher, R: Open-angle glaucoma associated with posterior polymorphous dystrophy. A clinicopathologic study. Ophthalmology 91:420, 1984.)

nephritis, sensorineural hearing loss, anterior lenticonus, and retinal flecks) and the management of patients with posterior polymorphous dystrophy should include an examination for renal abnormalities and hearing loss (75).

FUCHS' ENDOTHELIAL DYSTROPHY

Terminology and Clinicopathologic Features

Cornea Guttata

Cornea guttata is a common condition, the incidence of which increases significantly with age (76). Slitlamp biomicroscopy reveals a beaten silver appearance of the central posterior cornea, similar to that seen in the ICE syndrome. However, by specular microscopic study a more characteristic pattern is seen, consisting of enlarged endothelial cells with dark areas that overlap the cell borders (77). The primary pathology is an alteration in the corneal endothelium which leads to a deposition of collagen on the posterior surface of Descemet's membrane. Histologically, this may appear as warts or excrescences in the pure form of cornea guttata. In other cases, focal accumulations may be covered by additional basement membrane or there may be a uniform thickening of the posterior collagen layers (78, 79).

Fuchs' Endothelial Dystrophy

The vast majority of individuals with cornea guttata have otherwise normal corneas with no visual impairment. A small number of patients with the same posterior corneal changes as described above, however, will develop edema of the corneal stroma and endothelium. The clinical entity was described by Fuchs (80) in 1910, and the association with a dystrophy of the corneal endothelium was subsequently recognized. The disorder is bilateral with a predilection for women and an onset usually between the ages of 40 and 70 years. There is a strong familial tendency, and an autosomal dominant inheritance has been described (78). Viral particles have been found in the corneal endothelium of one eye, suggesting the possibility of an acquired etiology in some cases (81). Aqueous humor composition is normal, consistent with the theory that Fuchs' dystrophy is a primary disorder of the corneal endothelium (82). The condition may lead to severe visual reduction, often requiring penetrating keratoplasty.

Association with Glaucoma

Influence of Intraocular Pressure on Corneal Endothelium

Reports are conflicting regarding the association of glaucoma with cornea guttata and Fuchs' endothelial dystrophy.

This may be due, at least in part, to the fact that elevated IOP often induces secondary changes in the corneal endothelium. Reduced cell densities have been reported in association with open-angle glaucoma (83), angle-closure glaucoma (84–86), and other forms of glaucomas (86–88). However, the degree of endothelial alteration does not always correlate with the height of IOP elevation, suggesting that other factors may also influence the association between glaucoma and corneal endothelial changes (83). It has been shown, for example, that the morphology of corneal endothelium is altered by increasing age (89) and anterior uveitis, including glaucomatocyclitic crises (86, 88, 90). These observations must be taken into consideration with any reported association between glaucoma and an alteration of the corneal endothelium.

Cornea Guttata and Aqueous Outflow

It has been reported that patients with cornea guttata have a high incidence of abnormal tonographic facilities of outflow (91). However, in a subsequent study using wide-field specular microscopy, the mean value for facility of outflow in patients with cornea guttata was not statistically different from the normal population and there was no correlation between the extent of guttata and facility of outflow (92). Another study of patients with cornea guttata showed a lower mean IOP in this group as compared to a matched population without guttata (93).

Fuchs' Endothelial Dystrophy and Glaucoma

Patients with shallow anterior chambers and Fuchs' dystrophy may develop *angle-closure glaucoma*. This was once thought to be due to a gradual thickening of the cornea with eventual closure of the anterior chamber angle (94). More recent studies, however, indicate that Fuchs' corneal endothelial dystrophy patients have a high incidence of angle-closure glaucoma due to the high incidence of axial hypermetropia and shallow anterior chambers (95, 96).

It was once estimated that 10–15% of patients with Fuchs' endothelial dystrophy have open-angle glaucoma (97). However, a study of 64 families with the Fuchs' endothelial dystrophy revealed only one case of open-angle glaucoma (98). In another study, no genetic overlap between Fuchs' endothelial dystrophy and open-angle glaucoma was found on the basis of in vitro lymphocyte responsiveness to corticosteroids (99).

MANAGEMENT

Although glaucoma is usually not present in eyes with Fuchs' endothelial dystrophy, medical efforts to further reduce the normal IOP may sometimes help to minimize the corneal edema. When glaucoma is present, the open-angle form is managed the same as chronic open-angle glaucoma, while the angle-closure form requires an iridotomy or filtering procedure.

SUMMARY

The iridocorneal endothelial (ICE) syndrome is a primary disorder of the corneal endothelium, which presents in young adulthood as a unilateral abnormality of the cornea, anterior chamber angle, and iris. It appears to be an acquired condition, possibly with a viral etiology. The abnormal endothelium often causes corneal edema and proliferates over the angle and iris with subsequent contraction, leading to glaucoma and variable degrees of iris distortion. The latter changes are the basis for clinical variations including Chandler's syndrome, progressive iris atrophy, and the Cogan-Reese syndrome. Posterior polymorphous dystrophy is another spectrum of disease in which an endothelial abnormality is the fundamental disorder. Glaucoma is present in a small percentage of these cases and, in some patients, a proliferation of the abnormal endothelium causes changes of the anterior chamber angle and iris, resembling those in the ICE syndrome. The condition differs from the latter syndrome, however, in that it is inherited and bilateral and has a different clinical appearance of the posterior cornea. A third primary disorder of the corneal endothelium, Fuchs' endothelial dystrophy, occasionally has associated glaucoma, usually with an angle-closure mechanism.

REFERENCES

1. Miller, KN, Carlson, AN, Foulks, GN, Shields, MB: Associated glaucoma and corneal disorders. Focal Points, Am Acad Ophthalmol, Vol. 7, Module 4, 1989.
2. Eagle, RC Jr, Font, RL, Yanoff, M, Fine, BS: Proliferative endotheliopathy with iris abnormalities. The iridocorneal endothelial syndrome. Arch Ophthalmol 97:2104, 1979.
3. Yanoff, M: In discussion of Shields, MB, McCracken, JS, Klintworth, GK, Campbell, DG: Corneal edema in essential iris atrophy. Ophthalmology 86:1549, 1979.
4. Yanoff, M: Iridocorneal endothelial syndrome. Unification of a disease spectrum. Surv Ophthalmol 24:1, 1979.
5. Harms, C: Einseitige spontane Luckenbildung der Iris durch Atrophie ohne mechanische Zerrung. Klin Monatsbl Augenheilkd 41:522, 1903.
6. Chandler, PA: Atrophy of the stroma of the iris. Endothelial dystrophy, corneal edema, and glaucoma. Am J Ophthalmol 41:607, 1956.
7. Wilson, MC, Shields, MB: A comparison of the clinical variations of the iridocorneal endothelial syndrome. Arch Ophthalmol 107:1465, 1989.
8. Cogan, DG, Reese, AB: A syndrome of iris nodules, ectopic Descemet's membrane, and unilateral glaucoma. Doc Ophthalmol 26:424, 1969.
9. Scheie, HG, Yanoff, M: Iris nevus (Cogan-Reese) syndrome. A cause of unilateral glaucoma. Arch Ophthalmol 93:963, 1975.
10. Shields, MB, Campbell, DG, Simmons, RJ, Hutchinson, BT: Iris nodules in essential iris atrophy. Arch Ophthalmol 94:406, 1976.
11. Shields, MB, Campbell, DG, Simmons, RJ: The essential iris atrophies. Am J Ophthalmol 85:749, 1978.
12. Shields, MB: Progressive essential iris atrophy, Chandler's syndrome, and the iris nevus (Cogan-Reese) syndrome: a spectrum of disease. Surv Ophthalmol 24:3, 1979.
13. Shields, MB, McCracken, JS, Klintworth, GK, Campbell, DG: Corneal edema in essential iris atrophy. Ophthalmology 86:1533, 1979.
14. Setala, K, Vannas, A: Corneal endothelial cells in essential iris atrophy. A specular microscopic study. Acta Ophthalmol 57:1020, 1979.
15. Hirst, LW, Quigley, HA, Stark, WJ, Shields, MB: Specular microscopy of iridocorneal endothelia syndrome. Am J Ophthalmol 89:11, 1980.
16. Neubauer, L, Lund, O-E, Leibowitz, HM: Specular microscopic appearance of the corneal endothelium in iridocorneal endothelial syndrome. Arch Ophthalmol 101:916, 1983.
17. Bourne, WM: Partial corneal involvement in the iridocorneal endothelial syndrome. Am J Ophthalmol 94:774, 1982.
18. Wang, Y: Specular microscopic studies of the corneal endothelium in iridocorneal endothelial (ICE) syndrome. Eye Sci 1:53, 1985.
19. Kupfer, C, Kaiser-Kupfer, MI, Datiles, M, McCain, L: The contralateral eye in the iridocorneal endothelial (ICE) syndrome. Ophthalmology 90:1343, 1983.
20. Bourne, WM, Brubaker, RF: Decreased endothelial permeability in the iridocorneal endothelial syndrome. Ophthalmology: 89:591, 1982.
21. Sherrard, ES, Frangoulis, MA, Kerr Muir, MG, Buckley, RJ: The posterior surface of the cornea in the irido-corneal endothelial syndrome: a specular microscopical study. Trans Ophthalmol Soc UK 104:766, 1985.
22. Bourne, WM, Brubaker, RF: Progression and regression of partial corneal involvement in the iridocorneal endothelial syndrome. Am J Ophthalmol 114:171, 1992.
23. Quigley, HA, Forster, RF: Histopathology of cornea and iris in Chandler's syndrome. Arch Ophthalmol 96:1878, 1978.
24. Richardson, RM: Corneal decompensation in Chandler's syndrome. A scanning and transmission electron microscopic study. Arch Ophthalmol 97:2112, 1979.
25. Portis, JM, Stamper, RL, Spencer, WH, Webster, RG, Jr: The corneal endothelium and Descemet's membrane in the iridocorneal endothelial syndrome. Trans Am Ophthalmol Soc 83:316, 1985.
26. Alvarado, JA, Murphy, CG, Maglio, M, Hetherington, J: Pathogenesis of Chandler's syndrome, essential iris atrophy and the Cogan-Reese syndrome. I. Alterations of the corneal endothelium. Invest Ophthalmol Vis Sci 27:853, 1986.
27. Alvarado, JA, Murphy, CG, Juster, RP, Hetherington, J: Pathogenesis of Changler's syndrome, essential iris atrophy and the Cogan-Reese syndrome. II. Estimated age at disease onset. Invest Ophthalmol Vis Sci 27:873, 1986.
28. Rodrigues, MM, Stulting, RD, Waring, GO, III: Clinical, electron microscopic, and immunohistochemical study of the corneal endothelium and Descemet's membrane in the iridocorneal endothelial syndrome. Am J Ophthalmol 101:16, 1986.
29. Eagle, RC Jr, Shields, JA: Iridocorneal endothelial syndrome with contralateral guttate endothelial dystrophy. A light and electron microscopic study. Ophthalmology 94:862, 1987.
30. Rodrigues, MM, Jester, JV, Richards, R, et al: Essential iris atrophy. A clinical, immunohistologic, and electron microscopic study in an enucleated eye. Ophthalmology 95:69, 1988.
31. Lee, WR, Marshall, GE, Kirkness, CM: Corneal endothelial cell abnormalities in an early stage of the iridocorneal endothelial syndrome. Br J Ophthalmol 78:624, 1994.
32. Levy, SG, McCartney, ACE, Baghai, MH, et al: Pathology of the iridocorneal-endothelial syndrome. The ICE-cell. Invest Ophthalmol Vis Sci 36:2592, 1995.
33. Kramer, TR, Grossniklaus, HE, Vigneswaran, N, et al: Cytokeratin expression in corneal endothelium in the iridocorneal endothelial syndrome. Invest Ophthalmol Vis Sci 33:3581, 1992.
34. Hirst, LW, Bancroft, J, Yamauchi, K, Green, WR: Immunohistochemical pathology of the corneal endothelium in iridocorneal endothelial syndrome. Invest Ophthalmol Vis Sci 36:820, 1995.

35. Hirst, LW, Green, WR, Luckenbvach, M, et al: Epithelial characteristics of the endothelium in Chandler's syndrome. Invest Ophthalmol Vis Sci 24:603, 1983.
36. Campbell, DG, Shields, MB, Smith, TR: The corneal endothelium and the spectrum of essential iris atrophy. Am J Ophthalmol 86:317, 1978.
37. Rodrigues, MM, Streeten, BW, Spaeth, GL: Chandler's syndrome as a variant of essential iris atrophy. A clinicopathologic study. Arch Ophthalmol 96:643, 1978.
38. Rodrigues, MM, Phelps, CD, Krachmer, JH, et al: Glaucoma due to endothelialization of the anterior chamber angle. A comparison of posterior polymorphous dystrophy of the cornea and Chandler's syndrome. Arch Ophthalmol 98:688, 1980.
39. Benedikt, O, Roll, P: Open-angle glaucoma through endothelialization of the anterior chamber angle. Glaucoma 2:368, 1980.
40. Weber, PA, Gibb, G: Iridocorneal endothelial syndrome: glaucoma without peripheral anterior synechias. Glaucoma 6:128, 1984.
41. Daicker, B, Sturrock, G, Guggenheim, R: Clinicopathological correlation in Cogan-Reese syndrome. Klin Monatsbl Augenheilkd 180:531, 1982.
42. Daus, W, Volcker, HE, Steinbruck, M, Rentsch, F: Clinicopathological correlation in a case of Cogan-Reese syndrome. Klin Monatsbl Augenheilkd 197:150, 1990.
43. Eagle, RC Jr, Font, RL, Yanoff, M, Fine, BS: The iris naevus (Cogan-Reese) syndrome: light and electron microscopic observations. Br J Ophthalmol 64:446, 1980.
44. Radius, RL, Herschler, J: Histopathology in the iris-nevus (Cogan-Reese) syndrome. Am J Ophthalmol 89:780, 1980.
45. Tsai, CS, Ritch, R, Straus, SE, et al: Antibodies to Epstein-Barr virus in iridocorneal endothelial syndrome. Arch Ophthalmol 108:1572, 1990.
46. Alvarado, JA, Underwood, JL, Green, WR, et al: Detection of herpes simplex viral DNA in the iridocorneal endothelial syndrome. Arch Ophthalmol 112:1601, 1994.
47. Laganowski, HC, Sherrard, ES, Kerr Muir, MG, Buckley, RJ: Distinguishing features of the iridocorneal endothelial syndrome and posterior polymorphous dystrophy: value of endothelial specular microscopy. Br J Ophthalmol 75:212, 1991.
48. Traboulsi, EI, Maumenee, IH: Bilateral melanosis of the iris. Am J Ophthalmol 103:115, 1987.
49. Joondeph, BC, Goldberg, MF: Familial iris melanosis—a misnomer? Br J Ophthalmol 73:289, 1989.
50. Ticho, BH, Rosner, M, Mets, MB, Tso, MOM: Bilateral diffuse iris nodular nevi. Clinical and histopathologic characterization. Ophthalmology 102:419, 1995.
51. Laganowski, HC, Kerr Muir, MG, Hitchings, RA: Glaucoma and the iridocorneal endothelial syndrome. Arch Ophthalmol 110:346, 1992.
52. Kidd, M, Hetherington, J, Magee, S: Surgical results in iridocorneal endothelial syndrome. Arch Ophthalmol 106:199, 1988.
53. Wright, MM, Grajewski, AL, Cristol, SM, Parrish, RK: 5-fluorouracil after trabeculectomy and the iridocorneal endothelial syndrome. Ophthalmology 98:314, 1991.
54. Buxton, JN, Lash, RS: Results of penetrating keratoplasty in the iridocorneal endothelial syndrome. Am J Ophthalmol 98:297, 1984.
55. Fulcher, S, Lui, G, Houston, LL, et al: Use of immunotoxin to inhibit proliferating human corneal endothelium. Invest Ophthalmol Vis Sci 29:755, 1988.
56. Grayson, M: The nature of hereditary deep polymorphous dystrophy of the cornea: its association with iris and anterior chamber dygenesis. Trans Am Ophthalmol Soc 72:516, 1974.
57. Cibis, GW, Krachmer, JA, Phelps, CD, Weingeist, TA: The clinical spectrum of posterior polymorphous dystrophy. Arch Ophthalmol 95:1529, 1977.
58. Krachmer, JH: Posterior polymorphous corneal dystrophy: a disease characterized by epithelial-like endothelial cells which influence management and prognosis. Trans Am Ophthalmol Soc 83:413, 1985.
59. Cibis, GW, Tripathi, RC: The differential diagnosis of Descemet's Tears (Haab's Striae) and posterior polymorphous dystrophy bands. A clinicopathologic study. Ophthalmology 89:614, 1982.
60. Hirst, LW, Waring, GO III: Clinical specular microscopy of posterior polymorphous endothelial dystrophy. Am J Ophthalmol 95:143, 1983.
61. Brooks, AMV, Grant, G, Gillies, WE: Differentiation of posterior polymorphous dystrophy from other posterior corneal opacities by specular microscopy. Ophthalmology 96:1639, 1989.
62. Boruchoff, SA, Kuwabara, T: Electron microscopy of posterior polymorphous degeneration. Am J Ophthalmol 72:879, 1971.
63. Johnson, BL, Brown, SI: Posterior polymorphous dystrophy: a light and electron microscopic study. Br J Ophthalmol 62:89, 1978.
64. Rodrigues, MM, Sun, T-T, Krachmer, J, Newsome, D: Epithelialization of the corneal endothelium in posterior polymorphous dystrophy. Invest Ophthalmol Vis Sci 19:832, 1980.
65. Henriquez, AS, Kenyon, KR, Dohlman, CH, et al: Morphologic characteristics of posterior polymorphous dystrophy. A study of nine corneas and review of the literature. Surv Ophthalmol 29:139, 1984.
66. Sekundo, W, Lee, WR, Kirkness, CM, et al: An ultrastructural investigation of an early manifestation of the posterior polymorphous dystrophy of the cornea. Ophthalmology 101:1422, 1994.
67. Polack, FM, Bourne, WM, Forstot, SL, Yamaguchi, T: Scanning electron microscopy of posterior polymorphous corneal dystrophy. Am J Ophthalmol 89:575, 1980.
68. Richardson, WP, Hettinger, ME: Endothelial and epithelial-like cell formations in a case of posterior polymorphous dystrophy. Arch Ophthalmol 103:1520, 1985.
69. de Felice, GP, Braidotti, P, Viale, G, et al: Posterior polymorphous dystrophy of the cornea. An ultrastructural study. Graefes Arch Clin Exp Ophthalmol 223:265, 1985.
70. Cibis, GW, Krachmer, JH, Phelps, CD, Weingeist, TA: Iridocorneal adhesions in posterior polymorphous dystrophy. Trans Am Acad Ophthalmol Otol 81:770, 1976.
71. Threlkeld, AB, Green, WR, Quigley, HA, et al: A clinicopathologic study of posterior polymorphous dystrophy: implications for pathogenetic mechanism of the associated glaucoma. Tr Am Ophthalmol Soc 92:133, 1994.
72. Bourgeois, J, Shields, MB, Thresher, R: Open-angle glaucoma associated with posterior polymorphous dystrophy. A clinicopathologic study. Ophthalmology 91:420, 1984.
73. Dunn, SP, Krachmer, JH, Ching, SST: New findings in posterior amorphous corneal dystrophy. Arch Ophthalmol 102:236, 1984.
74. Boruchoff, SA, Weiner, MJ, Albert, DM: Recurrence of posterior polymorphous corneal dystrophy after penetrating keratoplasty. Am J Ophthalmol 109:323, 1990.
75. Teekhasaenee, C, Nimmanit, S, Wutthiphan, S, et al: Posterior polymorphous dystrophy and Alport syndrome. Ophthalmology 98:1207, 1991.
76. Lorenzetti, DWC, Uotila, MH, Parikh, N, Kaufman, HE: Central cornea guttata. Incidence in the general population. Am J Ophthalmol 64:1155, 1967.
77. Laing, RA, Leibowitz, HM, Oak, SS, et al: Endothelial mosaic in Fuch's dystrophy. A qualitative evaluation with the specular microscope. Arch Ophthalmol 99:80, 1981.
78. Magovern, M, Beauchamp, GR, McTigue, JW, et al: Inheritance of Fuchs' combined dystrophy. Ophthalmology 86:1897, 1979.
79. Rodrigues, MM, Krachmer, JH, Hackett, J, et al: Fuchs' corneal dystrophy. A clinicopathologic study of the variation in corneal edema. Ophthalmology 93:789, 1986.
80. Fuchs, E: Dystrophis epithelialis corneae. Arch Ophthalmol 76:478, 1910.
81. Roth, SI, Stock, EL, Jutabha, R: Endothelial viral inclusions in Fuchs' corneal dystrophy. Hum Pathol 18:338, 1987.
82. Wilson, SE, Bourne, WM, Maguire, LJ, et al: Aqueous humor composition in Fuchs' dystrophy. Invest Ophthalmol Vis Sci 30:449, 1989.
83. Hong, C, Kandori, T, Kitazawa, Y, Tanishima, T: Corneal endothelial cells in ocular hypertension. Jpn J Ophthalmol 26:183, 1982.
84. Bigar, F, Witmer, R: Corneal endothelial changes in primary acute angle-closure glaucoma. Ophthalmology 89:596, 1982.

85. Olsen, T: The endothelial cell damage in acute glaucoma. On the corneal thickness response to intraocular pressure. Acta Ophthalmol 58:257, 1980.

86. Setala, K: Response of human corneal endothelial cells to increased intraocular pressure. A specular microscopic study. Acta Ophthalmol 144(Suppl):547, 1980.

87. Vannas, A, Setala, K, Ruusuvaara, P: Endothelial cells in capsular glaucoma. Acta Ophthalmol 55:951, 1977.

88. Setala, K, Vannas, A: Endothelial cells in the glaucomato-cyclitic crisis. Adv Ophthalmol 36:218, 1978.

89. Kaufman, HE, Capella, JA, Robbins, JE: The human corneal endothelium. Am J Ophthalmol 61:835, 1966.

90. Olsen, T: Changes in the corneal endothelium after acute anterior uveitis as seen with the specular microscope. Acta Ophthalmol 58:250, 1980.

91. Buxton, JN, Preston, RW, Riechers, R, Guilbault, N: Tonography in cornea guttata. A preliminary report. Arch Ophthalmol 77:602, 1967.

92. Roberts, CW, Steinert, RF, Thomas, JV, Boruchoff, SA: Endothelial guttata and facility of aqueous outflow. Cornea 3:5, 1984.

93. Burns, RR, Bourne, WM, Brubaker, RF: Endothelial function in patients with cornea guttata. Invest Ophthalmol Vis Sci 20:77, 1981.

94. Stocker, FW: The Endothelium of the Cornea and Its Clinical Implications. 2nd ed. Springfield, IL, Charles C Thomas, 1971, p. 79.

95. Pitts, JF, Jay, JL: The association of Fuchs's corneal endothelial dystrophy with axial hypermetropia, shallow anterior chamber, and angle closure glaucoma. Br J Ophthalmol 74:601, 1990.

96. Loewenstein, A, Hourvitz, D, Goldstein, M, et al: Association of Fuchs' corneal endothelial dystrophy with angle-closure glaucoma. J Glau 3:201, 1994.

97. Kolker, AE, Hetherington, J Jr: Becker, Shaffer's Diagnosis and Therapy of the Glaucomas. 4th ed. St. Louis, CV Mosby, 1976, pp. 265–266.

98. Krachmer, JH, Purcell, JJ Jr, Yound, CW, Bucher, KD: Corneal endothelial dystrophy. A study of 64 families. Arch Ophthalmol 96:2036, 1978.

99. Waltman, SR, Palmberg, PF, Becker, B: In vitro corticosteroid sensitivity in patients with Fuchs' dystrophy. Doc Ophthalmol Proc Series 18:321, 1979.

Chapter 14

GLAUCOMAS ASSOCIATED WITH DISORDERS OF THE IRIS AND CILIARY BODY

CONDITIONS WITH IRIS OR CILIARY BODY DISORDERS AND ASSOCIATED GLAUCOMA

There are several conditions in which a disorder of the iris and/or ciliary body is believed to be involved in the initial events that eventually lead to various forms of glaucoma (Table 14.1). Most of these, such as developmental disorders, inflammatory conditions, and intraocular tumors, are considered in other chapters in Section Two. In the present chapter, we will consider three additional conditions (pigmentary glaucoma, iridoschisis, and the plateau iris), which do not fit precisely into any one of these general systems of disease.

PIGMENTARY GLAUCOMA[a]

Terminology

As a normal feature of maturation and aging, a variable amount of uveal pigment is chronically released and dispersed into the anterior ocular segment. This is best appreciated by observing the trabecular meshwork, which is non-

pigmented in the infant eye, but becomes progressively pigmented to variable degrees with the passage of years, due to the accumulation of the dispersed pigment in the aqueous outflow system. There is, therefore, a spectrum of ocular pigment dispersion within the general population. As might be anticipated, this spectrum of pigment dispersion is also found among individuals with various forms of glaucoma, although the pigment in most of these cases is not believed to be a major factor in the mechanism of the glaucoma. There are several ocular conditions, however, that are associated with an unusually heavy dispersion of pigment, which may be significantly involved in the increased resistance to aqueous outflow. In 1940, Sugar (1) briefly described one such case with marked pigment dispersion and glaucoma. Subsequently, in 1949, Sugar and Barbour (2) reported the details of this entity, which differed from other forms of pigment dispersion by typical clinical and histopathologic features. They referred to the condition as *pigmentary glaucoma* (2). When the typical findings are encountered without associated glaucoma, the term *pigment dispersion syndrome* has been advocated (3).

---

[a]Refer to Shields, MB: Color Atlas of Glaucoma. Baltimore, Williams & Wilkins, 1998, Plates II18–19.

Table 14.1.

CONDITIONS WITH IRIS OR CILIARY BODY DISORDERS AND ASSOCIATED GLAUCOMA

1. Developmental defects   (Chapter 12)
   a. Axenfeld-Rieger syndrome
   b. Peters' anomaly
   c. Aniridia
2. Iris atrophy with corneal disease   (Chapter 13)
   a. Iridocorneal endothelial syndrome
   b. Posterior polymorphous dystrophy
3. Pigmentary glaucoma   (Present Chapter)
4. Iridoschisis   (Present Chapter)
5. Plateau iris   (Present Chapter)
6. Exfoliation syndrome   (Chapter 15)
7. Neovascular glaucoma   (Chapter 16)
8. Iris tumors   (Chapter 18)
9. Anterior uveitis   (Chapter 19)
10. Trauma   (Chapter 22)
11. Complications of intraocular surgery   (Chapter 23)

General Features

The typical patient is a young, myopic male. The disorder appears most frequently in the third decade, and there is a tendency for it to decrease in severity or disappear in later life (4–5). Most studies agree that the pigment dispersion syndrome is more common among men, with a male/female ratio of approximately 2:1, although studies differ as to the ratio of those converting to pigmentary glaucoma (3–11). The reason for the male predilection appears to be the gender difference in anterior chamber depth, which one study showed to be 3.22 ± 0.42 mm in men and 2.88 ± 0.38 mm in women (12). The significance of chamber depth in the mechanism of pigment dispersion is discussed later in this chapter.

Pigmentary glaucoma is seen predominantly in Caucasians (3–11). In one report, 20 black patients were felt to have pigmentary glaucoma on the basis of heavy pigment deposition on the corneal endothelium and trabecular meshwork, but they differed from the typical patient population in having a mean age of 73 years, a preponderance of hyperopia and women, and no iris transillumination defects (13). An hereditary basis has been suggested (3, 7), but this has not been clearly established.

Clinical Features

Slitlamp Biomicroscopic Findings

CORNEAL FINDINGS

PIGMENT DISPERSION. Pigment dispersion occurs throughout the anterior ocular segment, but is seen by slitlamp examination primarily on the cornea and iris. *Krukenberg's spindle* is an accumulation of pigment on the posterior surface of the central cornea in a vertical spindle-shaped pattern (Fig. 14.1). Dispersed pigment is deposited on the cornea in this pattern due to aqueous convection currents and is then phagocytosed by adjacent endothelial cells (3). This feature is commonly seen in eyes with pigmentary glaucoma, but is neither invariable nor pathognomonic of the disorder. In one study of 43 patients with Krukenberg's spindles, only two developed field loss during a followup that averaged 5.8 years (14). Krukenberg's spindle is actually more common in women (14) and may have a hormonal relationship (15). Specular microscopy of the corneal endothelium reveals distinct pleomorphism and polymegathism (abnormality in shape and size of cells) (16), but normal cell counts (16, 17) and central corneal thickness (17).

IRIS FINDINGS

IRIS TRANSILLUMINATION. Iris transillumination is the most diagnostic clinical feature of pigmentary glaucoma since it represents the source of the dispersed pigment. The characteristic appearance is a radial spoke-like pattern in the midperiphery of the iris (Fig. 14.2) (18, 19). This feature can

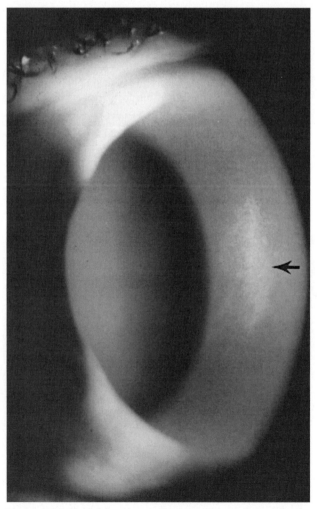

Figure 14.1. Krukenberg's spindle *(arrow)* in patient with pigmentary glaucoma.

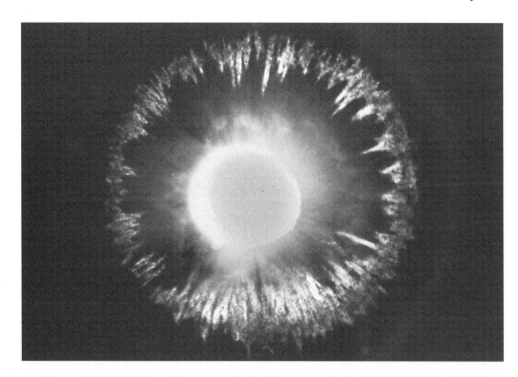

Figure 14.2. Transillumination of the iris in patient with pigmentary glaucoma showing typical midperipheral spoke-like defects.

be seen during slitlamp biomicroscopy by directing the light beam through the pupil perpendicular to the plane of the iris, or by using scleral transillumination, and observing the retinal light reflex through the defects in the iris. In some patients, however, a dark, thick iris stroma may prevent transillumination of the defects, so that the absence of this finding does not rule out the diagnosis of pigmentary glaucoma. This could explain the absence of iris transillumination in black patients with pigmentary glaucoma (13). An infrared videographic technique has been developed which allows visualization of discrete iris transillumination defects that were not visible by slitlamp examination (20).

Pigment granules are also frequently dispersed on the stroma of the iris, which may give the iris a progressively darker appearance or create heterochromia in asymmetric cases (Fig. 14.3) (9). Asymmetric pigment dispersion has also been reported in association with unilateral cataract formation or extraction (21) and unilateral angle recession (22). Patients with the pigment dispersion syndrome may also have anisocoria, in which the eye with the larger pupil is on the side with the greater iris transillumination (23, 24). The iris heterochromia and anisocoria of the pigment dispersion syndrome may mimic Horner's syndrome (25).

OTHER ANTERIOR SEGMENT FINDINGS. Other locations where pigment dispersion may be seen by slitlamp examination include the posterior lens capsule, lens zonules, and the interior of a glaucoma filtering bleb (9).

Gonioscopic Findings

The principal gonioscopic feature of pigmentary glaucoma is a dense, homogeneous band of dark brown pigment in the full circumference of the trabecular meshwork (Fig. 14.4). The dispersed pigment may also accumulate along Schwalbe's line, especially inferiorly, creating a thin, dark band. Abundant iris processes inserting anterior to the scleral spur were also observed in one small series of patients with pigmentary glaucoma (26), but do not appear to be a consistent finding in this condition.

Fundus Findings

Retinal detachments are more common in patients with the pigment dispersion syndrome or pigmentary glaucoma (27), occurring in 6.4% of one study (11). A study of 60 pigment dispersion or pigmentary glaucoma patients revealed lattice degeneration in 12 (20%) and full-thickness retinal breaks in seven patients (11.7%) (28). Retinal pigment epithelial dystrophy has also been reported in two brothers with pigmentary glaucoma (29).

Clinical Course of the Glaucoma

Patients with the pigment dispersion syndrome may go for years before developing pigmentary glaucoma or may never have a rise in intraocular pressure (IOP). In one study of 97 eyes with pigment dispersion throughout the anterior ocular segment, glaucoma was present in 42 (18), while in another study of 407 patients with the dispersion syndrome, only one-fourth had glaucoma (11). In a long-term study that spanned 5–35 years, 13 of 37 patients (35%) with the pigment dispersion syndrome converted to pigmentary glaucoma (6). The glaucoma usually develops within 15 years of the presentation of the pigment dispersion syndrome, although some may take more than 20 years (6). In another

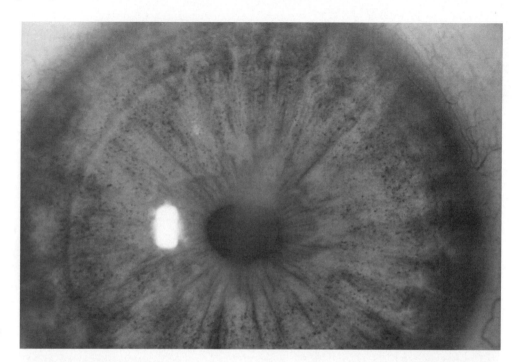

Figure 14.3. Pigment granules on iris stroma in patient with pigmentary glaucoma.

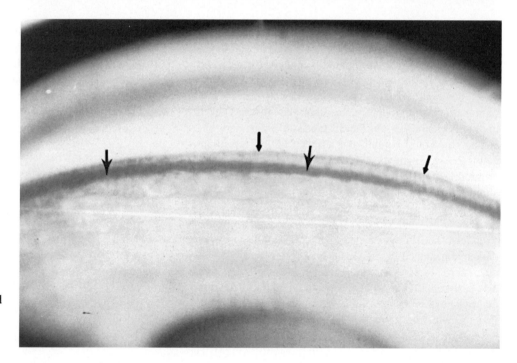

Figure 14.4. Gonioscopic view of patient with pigmentary glaucoma showing typical features of wide-open angle with dense, homogenous pigmentation of trabecular meshwork *(large arrows)* and heavy pigment accumulation on Schwalbe's line *(small arrows)*.

followup study averaging 27 months, progression of the iris transillumination defects and pigment dispersion could be documented in 31 of 55 patients and correlated with worsening of the glaucoma in most of these (30). A study of 111 patients with the pigment dispersion syndrome or pigmentary glaucoma identified male gender, black race, high myopia, and Krukenberg spindles as risk factors for the development and severity of glaucoma within this population (10). However, another study found that sex did not influence the development or severity of the glaucoma among patients with the pigment dispersion syndrome (6).

In some patients, strenuous exercise, such as jogging, or spontaneous changes in the pupillary diameter may cause an increased liberation of pigment into the anterior chamber (31), although this does not appear to cause significant IOP elevation in most cases (32, 33). In those patients in whom exercise-induced pigment dispersion does cause a significant IOP rise, pilocarpine has been effective in inhibiting this phenomenon (33, 34). Phenylephrine-induced mydriasis will also cause a significant shower of pigment into the anterior chamber in some patients with pigmentary glaucoma or the pigment dispersion syndrome, although this transient liberation of pigment is not consistently associated with IOP elevations (35).

Once pigmentary glaucoma becomes established, it may be somewhat more difficult to control than chronic open-angle glaucoma. In one long-term followup of 38 patients (75 eyes), 39 eyes were controlled medically, 15 required laser trabeculoplasty, and 20 underwent a trabeculectomy (36). However, 89% of the eyes in that study retained normal vision during the mean followup of 10 years. With increasing age there is a tendency for the glaucoma to become less severe, but the condition must be treated aggressively during the active years to avoid irreversible loss of vision in later life.

Theories of Mechanism

Two fundamental questions must be considered regarding the pathogenesis of the pigment dispersion syndrome and the mechanism of pigmentary glaucoma: (a) What are the factors leading to the pigment dispersion? and (b) How does the dispersed pigment and/or additional features cause the glaucoma?

Mechanism of Pigment Dispersion

Histopathologic observations of the iris in eyes with the pigment dispersion syndrome or pigmentary glaucoma have revealed changes in the iris pigment epithelium, which include focal atrophy and hypopigmentation, an apparent delay in melanogenesis, and a hyperplasia of the dilator muscle (37–39). In contrast, eyes with chronic open-angle glaucoma and varying degrees of pigment dispersion had minimal hypopigmentation of the iris epithelium with normal dilator muscle and melanogenesis (39). These observations have led some observers to feel that a developmental abnormality of the iris pigment epithelium is the fundamental defect in the pigment dispersion syndrome (37–39). The additional observation of retinal pigment epithelial dystrophy in two brothers with pigmentary glaucoma raises the possibility of an inherited defect of pigment epithelium in both the anterior and posterior ocular segments (29). Fluorescein angiography of the iris also suggests that hypovascularity of the iris may play a role in the pigment dispersion syndrome (40, 41).

Campbell (42) proposed an alternative theory for the mechanism of pigment liberation from the iris. He noted that the peripheral radial defects of the iris correspond in location and number to anterior packets of lens zonules and suggested that a background bowing of the peripheral iris leads to the mechanical rubbing of the lens zonules against the iris pigment epithelium with the subsequent dispersion of pigment. This hypothesis was supported by histologic studies showing a correlation between packets of zonules and deep groves in the iris pigment epithelium and posterior stroma (Fig. 14.5) (42, 43). Sugar (7) suggested that the radial folds of iris pigment epithelium rubbing against the lens capsule itself may be an additional mechanism of pigment release.

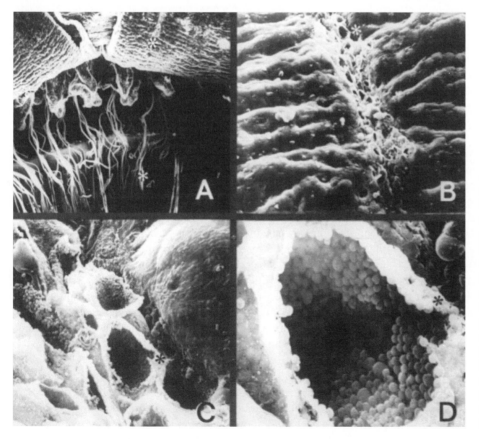

Figure 14.5. Scanning electron microscopic view of peripheral iris from patient with pigment dispersion syndrome showing: **A.** Incomplete radial defect in pigment epithelial layer of iris *(upper asterisk)* and underlying lens zonular packet *(lower asterisk)* at ×30; **B.** Radial defect *(asterisk)* with many pigment cells (×260); **C.** Ruptured pigment epithelial cell *(asterisk)* in radial defect (×1300); **D.** Pigment granules lining ruptured cell (×4500). (Reprinted with permission from Campbell, DG: Pigmentary dispersion and glaucoma. A new theory. Arch Ophthalmol 97:1667, 1979.)

The mechanical theory of Campbell is also supported by biometric (44) and photogrammetric (45) studies of anterior chamber dimensions, which revealed deeper anterior chambers and flatter lenses in the involved eyes of unilateral cases (44), and a deeper than normal midperipheral chamber depth with corresponding concavity of the iris in eyes with the pigment dispersion syndrome (45). In addition, the mechanical theory is consistent with clinical observations and helps to explain certain features of the disease. For example, the low incidence of the condition in the nonwhite population may be due to the heavy pigmentation and compactness of the iris stroma in these individuals, which prevents posterior sagging of the midperipheral iris (46). Furthermore, the tendency for the disease to ameliorate with increasing age may be due to increasing axial length of the lens, which pulls the peripheral iris away from the zonules (5, 42). A case has also been reported in which subluxation of the lens apparently caused remission of pigmentary glaucoma (47).

The mechanical theory must include an explanation of the mechanism by which the peripheral iris is bowed backwards. This missing piece of the puzzle came with the observation that a laser iridotomy relieves the posterior bowing, which led to the concept of *reverse pupillary block* (48). This concept suggests that aqueous is "pumped" into the anterior chamber against the normal pressure gradient, possibly by the movement of the peripheral iris in response to movement of the eye. Once in the anterior chamber, the aqueous is prevented from returning to the posterior chamber by a one-way valve effect between the iris and lens, resulting in a relatively greater pressure in the anterior chamber and subsequent backward bowing of the peripheral iris. The theory of reverse pupillary block has been supported by studies with ultrasound biomicroscopy (49, 50) and Scheimpflug photography (51), both of which demonstrate the posterior bowing of the iris in patients with the pigment dispersion syndrome and pigmentary glaucoma. The posterior bowing is eliminated by a peripheral iridotomy (49, 50), miotic therapy (50), or prevention of blinking (51, 52). Exercise, on the other hand, increases the iris concavity (53). The latter two observations appear to support the concept that eye movement is responsible for the pumping of aqueous into the anterior chamber. It has also been observed that accommodation in patients with the pigment dispersion syndrome leads to increased posterior bowing of the iris, which the authors explain by the forward movement of the lens, which reduces the volume, thereby increasing the pressure in the anterior chamber (54).

The mechanical theory, however, does not fully explain why all eyes with myopia are not subject to the pigment dispersion syndrome, and it may be that additional iris defects, as previously discussed, are necessary for development of the pigment dispersion syndrome.

Mechanism of Intraocular Pressure Elevation

In 1963, Grant (55) demonstrated that pigment granules perfused in human autopsy eyes caused a significant obstruction to aqueous outflow. Clinical studies have also shown that pigment release due to pharmacologically-induced movement of the iris causes a transient pressure rise in some eyes (35, 56). However, perfusion of living monkey eyes with uveal pigment particles caused only a transient obstruction to aqueous outflow (57), and histologic studies of human eyes with pigmentary glaucoma showed that only 3.5% of the pigment in the trabecular meshwork was in the juxtacanalicular tissue, which was not felt to be sufficient to account for the outflow obstruction (58). It would appear, therefore, that other or additional factors must be involved in the mechanism of pigmentary glaucoma.

While many histopathologic studies of eyes with pigmentary glaucoma have revealed excessive amounts of pigment granules and cell debris in the trabecular meshwork (39, 59–61), it is the associated changes in the trabecular endothelial cells and collagen beams that is believed to lead to the glaucoma (Fig. 14.6) (60–62). Based on these observations, the following pathophysiologic sequence of events has been proposed for the development of pigmentary glaucoma (62). Trabecular cells engulf melanin, which eventually leads to cell injury and death due to a phagocytic overload. Since melanoprotein is only partially digested, it is retained within intracellular storage vacuoles where it generates deleterious oxygen free radicals. Macrophages migrate to the necrotic trabecular cells, possibly in response to cytokines released by the injured cells, and carry off the pigment and debris through Schlemm's canal and into the circulation. The trabecular cell loss leaves the collagen beams denuded and vulnerable to fusion, with obliteration of the aqueous channels. Histologic studies reveal that the cul-de-sacs, in which aqueous channels normally terminate, are markedly reduced in pigmentary glaucoma, accounting for a major portion of the increased resistance to aqueous outflow (62).

An alternative theory suggests that a primary developmental anomaly of the anterior chamber angle may lead to aqueous outflow obstruction (9). This is based on the previously described abundant iris processes that have been seen in some cases (26, 39). However, this is not a consistent finding and probably plays little, if any, role in the mechanism of pigmentary glaucoma.

A third hypothesis that has been proposed for pigmentary glaucoma is that it represents a variation of chronic open-angle glaucoma. This theory was derived from observations that both chronic open-angle glaucoma and pigmentary glaucoma may be seen in the same family (26, 63). In one study, individuals with Krukenberg's spindles had topical corticosteroid responses that were similar to those seen among close relatives of patients with chronic open-angle glaucoma (63). However, patients with pigmentary glaucoma were not found to have the same corticosteroid sensitivity to in vitro inhibition of lymphocyte transformation as do chronic open-angle glaucoma patients (64). HLA-antigen testing revealed differences between the pigment dispersion syndrome, pigmentary glaucoma, and chronic open-angle glaucoma (65), but another study showed no significant difference among patients with pigmentary glaucoma, the pigment dispersion syndrome, and normal controls (66). The bulk of the current evidence suggests that pigmentary glaucoma and chronic open-angle glaucoma are separate entities.

Differential Diagnosis

As noted at the outset of this chapter, there are several disorders in which an excessive dispersion of pigment may be associated with glaucoma either with or without a cause-and-effect relationship. These conditions constitute the differential diagnosis for pigmentary glaucoma. One such condition is the exfoliation syndrome (Chapter 15), in which rubbing between the midperipheral lens and peripupillary iris leads to the pigment dispersion. This condition is usually distinguished from pigmentary glaucoma by the typical lens appearance and older age of the patients, although the two conditions have been reported to occur together (67). Other conditions associated with increased anterior segment pigmentation and glaucoma include some forms of uveitis (Chapter 19), trauma (Chapter 22), ocular melanosis and melanoma (Chapter 18), complications of intraocular surgery (Chapter 23), and chronic open-angle glaucoma with excessive pigment dispersion (Chapter 9).

Management

Medical Therapy

The mechanical theory of Campbell (42) suggests that measures to eliminate contact between the iris and lens zonules would be the most appropriate measure to prevent the progressive development of pigmentary glaucoma. Pilocarpine has the theoretic advantage of relieving this mechanism of pigment dispersion by creating miosis, while at the same time lowering the IOP by the direct effect on aqueous outflow. However, it is usually not tolerated by the young myope due to further induced myopia. Pilocarpine in an ocular insert delivery system (Ocusert) may provide the desired miosis and improved facility of outflow without excessive induced myopia in some pigmentary glaucoma patients. When using cholinergic agonists in patients with pigmentary glaucoma, special attention must be given to the risk of retinal detachment, which is more common in this population (27). The α-adrenergic antagonist *thymoxamine* may be useful since it produces miosis without cyclotropia (42), but it is not available in most parts of the world. An alternative α-blocker, *dapiprazole,* is commercially available in the United States for the reversal of pupillary dilatation after eye examinations, but was not as effective as 1.6% pilocarpine in constricting the pupil or relieving posterior iris bowing in patients with the pigment dispersion syndrome (68).

Alternative medications to miotic therapy include β-adrenergic antagonists, epinephrine compounds, and carbonic anhydrase inhibitors. In one study of 35 patients with pigmentary glaucoma, timolol was well-tolerated by the majority (69). With all of these nonmiotic drugs, however, the IOP may be reduced, but the mechanism of continued pigment dispersion is not eliminated.

Laser Surgery

In 1991, Campbell reported to the American Glaucoma Society, in a lecture honoring Dr. Saul Sugar, that a laser iridotomy

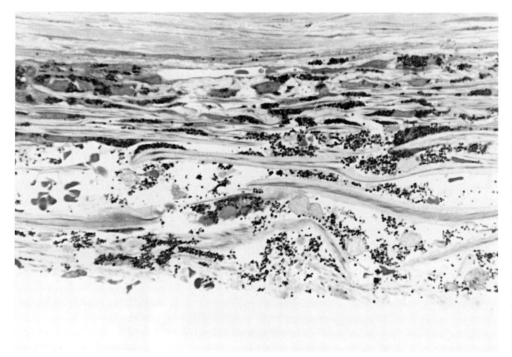

Figure 14.6. Light microscopic view of trabecular meshwork from patient with pigmentary glaucoma showing free pigment granules primarily in the uveal meshwork and in the inner portion of the corneoscleral meshwork, with intracellular pigment in the deeper portions of the meshwork. (Reprinted with permission from Richardson TM: Pigmentary glaucoma. In The Secondary Glaucomas. Ritch R, Shields MB, eds. St. Louis, CV Mosby, 1982.)

was effective in relieving the posterior iris bowing in pigmentary glaucoma. This was confirmed by Karickhoff (48) the following year in a report of six patients. This effect, however, has not been observed in all cases (70), and an iridotomy did not completely eliminate exercise-induced pigment dispersion in a patient with the pigment dispersion syndrome (71). Whether a prophylactic laser iridotomy can prevent the development of glaucoma in pigment dispersion patients or prevent the progression in patients with pigmentary glaucoma awaits the results of long-term, multicenter trials.

When the glaucoma can no longer be controlled medically, laser trabeculoplasty is usually indicated. Patients with pigmentary glaucoma respond well initially to the laser treatment, although the IOP control tends to decline with time and the surgery is less effective in patients who are older (e.g., patients in their 50s as compared to in their 30s) or who have had the glaucoma for a longer period of time (10 years as compared to 2–3 years) (72–74). In one study of 32 eyes of 32 patients with a mean age of 45.1 ± 13.1 years and a mean followup of 33.0 ± 5.0 months, lifetable analysis indicated a cumulative success of 80% at 1 year, 62% at 2 years, and 45% at 6 years (74).

Incisional Surgery

When both medical therapy and laser trabeculoplasty have failed, glaucoma-filtering surgery is usually indicated. A higher percentage of patients with pigmentary glaucoma require surgery, as compared to those with chronic open-angle glaucoma, and men appear to require it at an earlier age than women (10, 11). Success rates are similar to other forms of open-angle glaucoma at comparable age levels.

Activity

As previously noted, exercise may induce increased pigment dispersion and IOP elevation, which can be a concern in this population of young, active individuals (31–34). One approach to dealing with this question is to measure the IOP (and observe the amount of pigment in the anterior chamber) before and 30 minutes after the patient's typical exercise. If a significant pressure rise is observed, the use of 0.5% pilocarpine during exercise may be beneficial (33, 34).

IRIDOSCHISIS[b]

General Features

Iridoschisis is an uncommon condition and, in contrast to the young age of onset in pigmentary glaucoma, it usually appears in the sixth or seventh decade of life, although it

---

[b]Refer to Shields, MB: Color Atlas of Glaucoma. Baltimore, Williams & Wilkins, 1998, Plate II20.

may be seen in younger individuals. A case has been reported in a child with associated microphthalmos (75) and in a 30-year-old with keratoconus (76). The hallmark is a bilateral separation of the layers of iris stroma, typically in the inferior quadrants. The disorder is complicated by glaucoma in approximately half the cases. Corneal edema is also an occasional sequelae. Most cases are not associated with other ocular disorders, although concomitant conditions may be seen, including, in addition to those noted earlier, angle-closure glaucoma (77), angle-recession glaucoma (78), and syphilitic interstitial keratitis (79).

Clinicopathologic Features

Slitlamp biomicroscopic examination typically reveals sheets or strands of iris stroma that have partially separated from the rest of the iris, especially in the inferior quadrants (Fig. 14.7). In some cases, the loose tissue may touch the corneal endothelium with adjacent edema of the cornea. By gonioscopy, the strands of iris tissue may obscure visualization of the anterior chamber angle.

Histopathologic studies of involved iris revealed marked atrophy of the iris stroma with scant or absent collagen fibrils in the area of separation, although there was no evidence of vascular or neural alterations (80). Specular microscopy of the corneal endothelium has revealed a marked decrease in cell density and a high degree of polymegathism in the area directly over the iridoschisis (81). Histopathology of a corneal button, removed due to bullous keratopathy, showed degeneration and focal loss of endothelial cells, patchy posterior banding (110 nm) of Descemet's membrane with irregular connective tissue, and stromal and epithelial edema (80).

Mechanisms of Glaucoma

Some patients with iridoschisis and glaucoma have angle closure (77, 80), and it is presumed that a pupillary block mechanism is present, since an iridectomy results in deepening of the anterior chamber (80). It has been suggested that iridoschisis may be an unusual manifestation of iris stromal atrophy resulting from the intermittent or acute IOP evaluation of pupillary-block glaucoma (77). In other patients, the angle is open, in which case the meshwork is apparently obstructed either by release of pigment from the iris or by the shredded iris stroma (80).

Differential Diagnosis

The main conditions that must be distinguished from iridoschisis are other causes of iris stromal dissolution such as the iridocorneal endothelial syndrome and Axenfeld-Rieger syndrome, both of which differ from iridoschisis by a much younger age of onset. It should also be noted that trauma can lead to disruption of the iris creating clinical findings that resemble iridoschisis, which may explain the relationship to angle-recession glaucoma (78). In one patient with iridoschisis, strands of iris floating in the anterior chamber after a trabeculectomy was mistaken for a fungal infection (82).

Management

Cases with an angle-closure mechanism of glaucoma should be treated with a laser iridotomy, or with conventional surgical iridectomy if corneal edema prevents laser surgery. The open-angle form of glaucoma can be controlled medically in some cases, using an approach similar to that for chronic open-angle glaucoma, while other patients require glaucoma filtering surgery.

PLATEAU IRIS

One mechanism leading to angle-closure glaucoma appears to result from an abnormal anatomic configuration of the anterior chamber angle without pupillary block (83, 84). It is far less common than pupillary-block glaucoma and is usually only recognized after a peripheral iridotomy for a presumed pupillary-block mechanism has failed. Consequently, two variations of plateau iris have been described (85).

Plateau Iris Configuration

This diagnosis is made preoperatively based on the gonioscopic findings of a closed anterior chamber angle, but a flat iris plane (as opposed to the forward bowing of peripheral iris with the pupillary block mechanism) and a more normal central anterior chamber depth. Relative pupillary block plays a significant role in this situation, and most of these cases are cured by peripheral iridotomy.

Plateau Iris Syndrome

This constitutes a small percent of eyes with the plateau iris configuration and represents the true plateau iris mechanism. The peripheral iris appears to bunch up in the anterior chamber angle when the pupil is dilated, despite a patent iridotomy. This was traditionally felt to be due, at least in part, to an anterior insertion of the iris, although studies with ultrasound biomicroscopy now suggest that an anterior position of the ciliary processes prevents the peripheral iris from falling posteriorly after an iridotomy (86–88). These cases are usually treated with pilocarpine.

SUMMARY

Pigmentary glaucoma is typically seen in young adult myopes, with a predilection for males. The ocular configuration in these individuals apparently leads to rubbing between the iris and lens zonules which causes liberation of pigment granules. This can be seen clinically as transillumination defects in the peripheral iris and as deposition of the dispersed pigment on the corneal endothelium, iris stroma and other anterior ocular structures. It is in the trabecular meshwork, however, where the accumulation of pigment and subsequent alteration of the trabecular beams leads to a severe

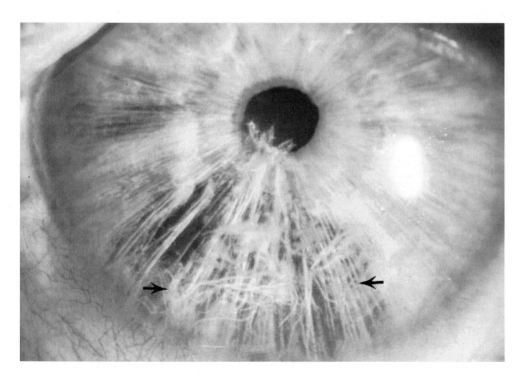

Figure 14.7. Slitlamp view of patient with iridoschisis showing characteristic strands of iris stroma (*arrows*) that have partially separated from the rest of the iris in the inferior quadrant.

form of open-angle glaucoma. Iridoschisis, is an uncommon affliction of the elderly, characterized by a separation of layers of iris stroma with occasional associated glaucoma. Plateau iris is a form of angle-closure glaucoma, in which an anterior position of the ciliary processes appears to be responsible for the angle closure.

REFERENCES

1. Sugar, HS: Concerning the chamber angle. I. Gonioscopy. Am J Ophthalmol 23:853, 1940.
2. Sugar, HS, Barbour, FA: Pigmentary glaucoma. A rare clinical entity. Am J Ophthalmol 32:90, 1949.
3. Sugar, HS: Pigmentary glaucoma. A 25-year review. Am J Ophthalmol 62:499, 1966.
4. Speakman, JS: Pigmentary dispersion. Br J Ophthalmol 65:249, 1981.
5. Ritch, R: Nonprogressive low-tension glaucoma with pigmentary dispersion. Am J Ophthalmol 94:190, 1982.
6. Migliazzo, CV, Shaffer, RN, Nykin, R, Magee, S: Long-term analysis of pigmentary dispersion syndrome and pigmentary glaucoma. Ophthalmology 93:1528, 1986.
7. Sugar, S: Pigmentary glaucoma and the glaucoma associated with the exfoliation-pseudoexfoliation syndrome: update. Ophthalmology 91:307, 1984.
8. Lichter, PR, Shaffer, RN: Diagnostic and prognostic signs in pigmentary glaucoma. Trans Am Acad Ophthalmol Otol 74:984, 1970.
9. Lichter, PR: Pigmentary glaucoma—current concepts. Trans Am Acad Ophthalmol Otol 78:309, 1974.
10. Farrar, SM, Shields, MB, Miller, KN, Stoup, CM: Risk factors for the development and severity of glaucoma in the pigment dispersion syndrome. Am J Ophthalmol 108:223, 1989.
11. Scheie, HG, Cameron, JD: Pigment dispersion syndrome: a clinical study. Br J Ophthalmol 65:264, 1981.
12. Orgul, S, Hendrickson, P, Flammer, J: Anterior chamber depth and pigment dispersion syndrome. Am J Ophthalmol 117:575, 1994.
13. Semple, HC, Ball, SF: Pigmentary glaucoma in the black population. Am J Ophthalmol 109:518, 1990.
14. Wilensky, JT, Buerk, KM, Podos, SM: Krukenberg's spindles. Am J Ophthalmol 79:220, 1975.
15. Duncan, TE: Krukenberg spindles in pregnancy. Arch Ophthalmol 91:355, 1974.
16. Lehto, I, Ruusuvaara, P, Setala, K: Corneal endothelium in pigmentary glaucoma and pigment dispersion syndrome. Acta Ophthalmol 68:703, 1990.
17. Murrell, WJ, Shihab, Z, Lamberts, DW, Avera, B: The corneal endothelium and central corneal thickness in pigmentary dispersion syndrome. Arch Ophthalmol 104:845, 1986.
18. Scheie, HG, Fleischhauer, HW: Idiopathic atrophy of the epithelial layers of the iris and ciliary body. A clinical study. Arch Ophthalmol 59:216, 1958.
19. Donaldson, DD: Transillumination of the iris. Trans Am Ophthal Soc LXXII:89, 1974.
20. Alward, WLM, Munden, PM, Verdick, RE, et al: Use of infrared videography to detect and record iris transillumination defects. Arch Ophthalmol 108:748, 1990.
21. Ritch, R, Chaiwat, T, Harbin, TS Jr: Asymmetric pigmentary glaucoma resulting from cataract formation. Am J Ophthalmol 114:484, 1992.
22. Ritch, R, Alward, WLM: Asymmetric pigmentary glaucoma caused by unilateral angle recession. Am J Ophthalmol 115:765, 1993.
23. Feibel, RM, Perlmutter, JC: Anisocoria in the pigmentary dispersion syndrome. Am J Ophthalmol 110:657, 1990.
24. Haynes, WL, Alward, WLM, Thompson, HS: Distortion of the pupil in patients with the pigment dispersion syndrome. J Glau 3:329, 1994.
25. Haynes, WL, Thompson, HS, Kardon, RH, Alward, WLM: Asymmetric pigmentary dispersion syndrome mimicking Horner's syndrome. Am J Ophthalmol 112:463, 1991.
26. Lichter, PR, Shaffer, RN: Iris processes and glaucoma. Am J Ophthalmol 70:905, 1970.
27. Delaney, WV Jr: Equatorial lens pigmentation, myopia, and retinal detachment. Am J Ophthalmol 79:194, 1975.
28. Weseley, P, Liebmann, J, Walsh, JB, Ritch, R: Lattice degeneration of the retina and the pigment dispersion syndrome. Am J Ophthalmol 114:539, 1992.
29. Piccolino, FC, Calabria, G, Polizzi, A, Fioretto, M: Pigmentary retinal dystrophy associated with pigmentary glaucoma. Graefes Arch Clin Exp Ophthalmol 227:335, 1989.
30. Richter, CU, Richardson, TM, Grant, WM: Pigmentary dispersion syndrome and pigmentary glaucoma. A prospective study of the natural history. Arch Ophthalmol 104:211, 1986.
31. Schenker, HI, Luntz, MH, Kels, B, Podos, SM: Exercise-induced increase of intraocular pressure in the pigmentary dispersion syndrome. Am J Ophthalmol 89:598, 1980.
32. Smith, DL, Kao, SF, Rabbani, R, Musch, DC: The effects of exercise on intraocular pressure in pigmentary glaucoma patients. Ophthalmic Surg 20:561, 1989.
33. Haynes, WL, Johnson, AT, Alward, WLM: Effects of jogging exercise on patients with the pigmentary dispersion syndrome and pigmentary glaucoma. Ophthalmology 99:1096, 1992.
34. Haynes, WL, Johnson, AT, Alward, WL: Inhibition of exercise-induced pigment dispersion in a patient with the pigmentary dispersion syndrome. Am J Ophthalmol 109:601, 1990.
35. Epstein, DL, Boger, WP III, Grant, WM: Phenylephrine provocative testing in the pigmentary dispersion syndrome. Am J Ophthalmol 85:43, 1978.
36. Lehto, I: Long-term prognosis of pigmentary glaucoma. Acta Ophthalmol 69:437, 1991.
37. Fine, BS, Yanoff, M, Scheie, HG: Pigmentary "glaucoma." A histologic study. Trans Am Acad Ophthalmol Otol 78:314, 1974.
38. Kupfer, C, Kuwabara, T, Kaiser-Kupfer, M: The histopathology of pigmentary dispersion syndrome with glaucoma. Am J Ophthalmol 80:857, 1975.
39. Rodrigues, MM, Spaeth, GL, Weinreb, S, Sivalingam, E: Spectrum of trabecular pigmentation in open-angle glaucoma: a clinicopathologic study. Trans Am Acad Ophthalmol Otol 81:258, 1976.
40. Gillies, WE, Tangas, C: Fluorescein angiography of the iris in anterior segment pigment dispersal syndrome. Br J Ophthalmol 70:284, 1986.
41. Brooks, AMV, Gillies, WE: Hypoperfusion of the iris and its consequences in anterior segment pigment dispersal syndrome. Ophthalmic Surg 25:307, 1994.
42. Campbell, DG: Pigmentary dispersion and glaucoma. A new theory. Arch Ophthalmol 97:1667, 1979.
43. Kampik, A, Green, WR, Quigley, HA, Pierce, LH: Scanning and transmission electron microscopic studies of two cases of pigment dispersion syndrome. Am J Ophthalmol 91:573, 1981.
44. Strasser, G, Hauff, W: Pigmentary dispersion syndrome. A biometric study. Acta Ophthalmol 63:721, 1985.
45. Davidson, JA, Brubaker, RF, Ilstrup, DM: Dimensions of the anterior chamber in pigment dispersion syndrome. Arch Ophthalmol 101:81, 1983.
46. Richardson, TM: Pigmentary glaucoma. In: The Secondary Glaucomas. Ritch, R, Shields, MB, eds. St. Louis, CV Mosby, 1982.
47. Ritch, R, Manusow, D, Podos, SM: Remission of pigmentary glaucoma in a patient with subluxed lenses. Am J Ophthalmol 94:812, 1982.
48. Karickhoff, JR: Pigmentary dispersion syndrome and pigmentary glaucoma: a new mechanism concept, a new treatment, and a new technique. Ophthalmic Surg 23:269, 1992.
49. Pavlin, CJ, Macken, P, Trope, G, et al: Ultrasound biomicroscopic features of pigmentary glaucoma. Can J Ophthalmol 29:187, 1994.

50. Potash, SD, Tello, C, Liebmann, J, Ritch, R: Ultrasound biomicroscopy in pigment dispersion syndrome. Ophthalmology 101: 332, 1994.

51. Doyle, JW, Hansen, JE, Smith, MF, et al: Use of Scheimpflug photography to study iris configuration in patients with pigment dispersion syndrome and pigmentary glaucoma. J Glau 4:398, 1995.

52. Liebmann, JM, Tello, C, Chew, S-J, et al: Prevention of blinking alters iris configuration in pigment dispersion syndrome and in normal eyes. Ophthalmology 102:446, 1995.

53. Jensen, PK, Nissen, O, Kessing, SV: Exercise and reversed pupillary block in pigmentary glaucoma. Am J Ophthalmol 120:110, 1995.

54. Pavlin, CJ, Harasiewicz, Foster, FS: Posterior iris bowing in pigmentary dispersion syndrome caused by accomodation. Am J Ophthalmol 118:114, 1994.

55. Grant, WM: Experimental aqueous perfusion in enucleated human eyes. Arch Ophthalmol 69:783, 1963.

56. Mapstone, R: Pigment release. Br J Ophthalmol 65:258, 1981.

57. Epstein, DL, Freddo, TF, Anderson, PJ, et al: Experimental obstruction to aqueous outflow by pigment particles in living monkeys. Invest Ophthalmol Vis Sci 27:387, 1986.

58. Murphy, CG, Johnson, M, Alvarado, JA: Juxtacanalicular tissue in pigmentary and primary open angle glaucoma. Arch Ophthalmol 110:1779, 1992.

59. Rodrigues, MM, Spaeth, GL, Sivalingam, E, Weinreb, S: Value of trabeculectomy specimens in glaucoma. Ophthalmic Surg 9:29, 1978.

60. Richardson, TM, Hutchinson, BT, Grant, WM: The outflow tract in pigmentary glaucoma. A light and electron microscopic study. Arch Ophthalmol 95:1015, 1977.

61. Shimizu, T, Hara, K, Futa, R: Fine structure of trabecular meshwork and iris in pigmentary glaucoma. Graefes Arch Clin Exp Ophthalmol 215: 171, 1981.

62. Alvarado, JA, Murphy, CG: Outflow obstruction in pigmentary and primary open angle glaucoma. Arch Ophthalmol 110:1769, 1992.

63. Becker, B, Podos, SM: Krukenberg's spindles and primary open-angle glaucoma. Arch Ophthalmol 76:635, 1966.

64. Zink, HA, Palmberg, PF, Sugar, A, et al: Comparison of in vitro corticosteriod response in pigmentary glaucoma and primary open-angle glaucoma. Am J Ophthalmol 80:478, 1975.

65. Becker, B, Shin, DH, Cooper, DG, Kass, MA: The pigment dispersion syndrome. Am J Ophthalmol 83:161, 1977.

66. Kaiser-Kupfer, MI, Mittal, KK: The HLA and ABO antigens in pigment dispersion syndrome. Am J Ophthalmol 85:368, 1978.

67. Layden, WE, Ritch, R, King, DG, Teekhasaenee, C: Combined exfoliation and pigment dispersion syndrome. Am J Ophthalmol 109: 530, 1990.

68. Haynes, WL, Thompson, HS, Johnson, AT, Alward, WLM: Comparison of the miotic effects of dapiprazole and dilute pilocarpine in patients with the pigment dispersion syndrome. J Glau 4:379, 1995.

69. Lehto, I: Side effects of topical treatment in pigmentary glaucoma. Acta Ophthalmol 70:225, 1992.

70. Jampel, HD: Lack of effect of peripheral laser iridotomy in pigment dispersion syndrome. Arch Ophthalmol 111:1606, 1993.

71. Haynes, WL, Alward, WLM, Tello, C, et al: Incomplete elimination of exercise-induced pigment dispersion by laser iridotomy in pigment dispersion syndrome. Ophthalmic Surg Lasers 26:484, 1995.

72. Lunde, MW: Argon laser trabeculoplasty in pigmentary dispersion syndrome with glaucoma. Am J Ophthalmol 96:721, 1983.

73. Lehto, I: Long-term follow-up of argon laser trabeculoplasty in pigmentary glaucoma. Ophthalmic Surg 23:614, 1992.

74. Ritch, R, Liebmann, J, Robin, A, et al: Argon laser trabeculoplasty in pigmentary glaucoma. Ophthalmology 100:909, 1993.

75. Summers, CG, Doughman, DJ, Letson, RD, Lufkin, M: Juvenile iridoschisis and microphthalmos. Am J Ophthalmol 100:437, 1985.

76. Eiferman, RA, Law, M, Lane, L: Iridoschisis and keratoconus. Cornea 13:78, 1994.

77. Salmon, JF, Murray, AND: The association of iridoschisis and primary angle-closure glaucoma. Eye 6:267, 1992.

78. Salmon, JF: The association of iridoschisis and angle-recession glaucoma. Am J Ophthalmol 114:766, 1992.

79. Pearson, PA, Amrien, JM, Baldwin, LB, Smith, TJ: Iridoschisis associated with syphilitic interstitial keratitis. Am J Ophthalmol 107:88, 1989.

80. Rodrigues, MC, Spaeth, GL, Krachmer, JH, Laibson, PR: Iridoschisis associated with glaucoma and bullous keratopathy. Am J Ophthalmol 95:73, 1983.

81. Weseley, AC, Freeman, WR: Iridoschisis and the corneal endothelium. Ann Ophthalmol 15:955, 1983.

82. Zimmerman, TJ, Dabezies, OH Jr, Kaufman, HE: Iridoschisis: a case report. Ann Ophthalmol 13:297, 1981.

83. Tornquist, R: Angle-closure glaucoma in an eye with a plateau type of iris. Acta Ophthalmol 36:413, 1958.

84. Shaffer, RN: Gonioscopy, ophthalmoscopy, and perimetry. Trans Am Acad Ophthalmol Otol 64:112, 1960.

85. Wand, M, Grant, WM, Simmons, RJ, Hutchinson, BT: Plateau iris syndrome. Trans Am Acad Ophthalmol Otol 83:122, 1977.

86. Pavlin, CJ, Ritch, R, Foster, FS: Ultrasound biomicroscopy in plateau iris syndrome. Am J Ophthalmol 113:390, 1992.

87. Ritch, R: Plateau iris is caused by abnormally positioned ciliary processes. J Glau 1:23, 1992.

88. Wand, M, Pavlin, CJ, Foster, FS: Plateau iris syndrome: Ultrasound biomicroscopic and histologic study. Ophthalmic Surg 24:129, 1993.

Chapter 15

GLAUCOMAS ASSOCIATED WITH DISORDERS OF THE LENS

Several disorders of the crystalline lens are associated with various forms of glaucoma. In some cases, such as the exfoliation syndrome, a cause-and-effect relationship between the lenticular abnormality and the glaucoma is uncertain. In other situations, including some forms of dislocated lenses and cataracts, the glaucoma is more clearly a result of the alteration in the lens.

EXFOLIATION SYNDROME[a]

Terminology

In 1917, Lindberg (1) described cases of chronic glaucoma in which flakes of whitish material adhered to the pupillary

border of the iris. Subsequent study revealed that this material is derived, at least in part, from exfoliation of the anterior lens capsule. Two types of exfoliation have now been distinguished, which has led to confusion with the nomenclature.

Capsular Delamination

In this condition, superficial layers of lens capsule separate from the deeper capsular layers to form scroll-like margins and occasionally to float in the anterior chamber as thin, clear membranes (Fig. 15.1). Elschnig (2) first described this condition in glassblowers, leading to the term "glassblower's cataracts," and it was subsequently found that extended exposure to infrared radiation in a variety of occupations was the responsible element. The condition is uncommon since the widespread use of protective goggles by exposed workers, although clinically similar cases may be seen in association with trauma (3), intraocular inflam-

[a]Refer to Shields, MB: Color Atlas of Glaucoma. Baltimore, Williams & Wilkins, 1998, Plates II21–22.

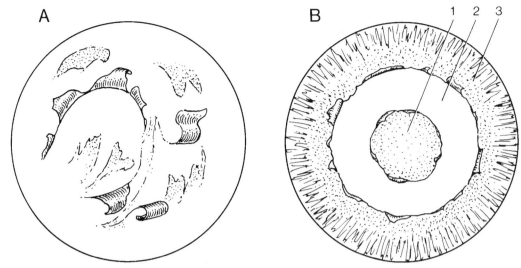

Figure 15.1. Two types of exfoliation of the anterior lens capsule. **A.** Capsular delamination, characterized by thin, clear membranes separating from the anterior lens capsule and often curling at the margins. **B.** The exfoliation syndrome, with three distinct zones: *(1)* central, translucent disc; *(2)* clear zone; *(3)* peripheral granular zone, often with radial striations.

mation (4), and idiopathically, usually with advanced age (5–7). Glaucoma is not a common feature of this disorder. The condition has been called *capsular delamination* or *exfoliation of the lens capsule,* and Dvorak-Theobald (8) suggested the term *true exfoliation of the lens capsule* to distinguish it from the condition to be discussed next.

Exfoliation Syndrome

Vogt (9), in 1925, described what he felt to be a senile form of capsular delamination, which he called "senile exfoliation." In addition to occurring in an older patient population, this condition differs from the other forms of exfoliation of the lens capsule in clinical appearance (Fig. 15.1), as well as in a frequent association with glaucoma (9, 10). Dvorak-Theobald (8) felt that this disorder is not a true exfoliation of the lens capsule, but rather represents precipitates of an unknown substance that are deposited on the anterior lens capsule and other structures in the anterior ocular segment. She recommended the term "pseudo-exfoliation of the lens capsule," to distinguish the condition from capsular delamination or "true" exfoliation, and the term *pseudoexfoliation syndrome* is commonly used in modern literature. However, more recent ultrastructural studies have suggested that the exfoliative material on the lens capsule is derived, at least in part, from the lens, and it has been proposed that this entity be called the *exfoliation syndrome* (11–13). Both terms, pseudoexfoliation syndrome and exfoliation syndrome, are still commonly used in current literature. Glaucoma is not always present in eyes with this disorder, but when it does occur in association with the exfoliation syndrome, the condition has been called glaucoma capsulare or *capsular glaucoma.*

Epidemiology

Reports vary considerably regarding the prevalence of the exfoliation syndrome, apparently due to differences within the populations that have been studied. Geographic and ethnic differences appear to be important factors, with high prevalences in Scandinavian countries (14–17) and among people of Mediterranean origin (18). Considerable geographic variation, however, exists even within countries; e.g., three municipalities in middle-Norway had prevalences ranging from 10% to 21% among persons over 64 years (17). In the United States, the exfoliation syndrome is less common, with one study revealing a prevalence of 1.6% for a population over 30 years of age and 3.2% for those over 60 years (19), and another showing 0.67% for ages 52–64, 2.6% for 65–74, and 5.0% for 75 to 85 years (20).

The reported prevalence of exfoliation syndrome among patients with open-angle glaucoma also shows considerable geographic variation, with 26% in Denmark (14), 75% in Sweden (15), 60% in Norway (21), 46.9% in the Eastern Mediterranean area of Turkey (22), and 44.5% in the Northwest of Spain (23), compared to reports of 1% (24), 3% (12), 6% (19), and 12% (25) in the United States.

General Features

As noted earlier, the exfoliation syndrome is more common in older age groups, with most cases occurring in the late 60s and early 70s. The influence of race differs among geographic populations. In South Africa, the exfoliation syndrome was found in 20% of black patients with open-angle glaucoma, compared to 1.4% of the whites in that country (26), whereas a study in southern Louisiana revealed a prevalence of 0.3% in blacks and 2.0% in whites (24). The reported influence of sex is also conflicting, with one study showing a preponderance of women (27) and two others of men (28, 29), while most suggest no sex predilection. One study suggested that men may have higher intraocular pressures (IOP) than women with capsular glaucoma (30). No hereditary pattern has been clearly established for the exfoliation syndrome, and two studies gave conflicting results with regard to a positive correlation with HLA typing (31, 32). A study of married couples showed a higher than expected prevalence among both spouses, suggesting a possible environmental influence (33). The condition may be unilateral or bilateral, and some unilateral cases will become bilateral with time (25, 27, 34).

Clinical Features

Lens Changes

The characteristic appearance of exfoliation material on the anterior lens capsule has three distinct zones (Fig. 15.2): (a) a translucent, central disc with occasional curled edges, (b) a clear zone, probably corresponding to contact with the moving iris, and (c) a peripheral granular zone, which may have radial striations (12). The central zone is not always apparent, but the peripheral defect is a consistent finding, and the pupil must be dilated before the lens changes can be seen in some cases. Cataracts occur frequently in

eyes with the exfoliation syndrome (20, 25, 28, 30). While this may be, at least in part, a function of the age of the patient population, cataracts in eyes with the exfoliation syndrome have been observed to differ from those without associated diseases by a higher percentage of nuclear and fewer cortical and supranuclear cataracts in the former group (35). Phacodonesis and subluxation of the lens may also be seen in some patients (36, 37), which is apparently due to degenerative changes in the zonular fibers of these individuals (36).

Iris Changes

Exfoliation material may also be seen as white flecks on the pupillary margin of the iris, with loss of pigment at the pupillary ruff (38). Iris transillumination typically reveals a "moth-eaten" pattern near the pupillary sphincter (12, 38), and a significant percentage of patients also have diffuse mid-peripheral transillumination defects (39) (Fig. 15.3). Fluorescein angiographic studies of the iris have revealed hypoperfusion, peripupillary leakage, and neovascularization (40, 41). These findings are more pronounced with increasing age of the patient, longer duration of the disease, and the presence of glaucoma, and may represent a secondary feature of the disease (41). Ultrastructural studies suggests that vascular abnormalities or abnormal extracellular matrix production causes tissue hypoxia (42, 43). Conversely, it has been noted that eyes with transient ischemic

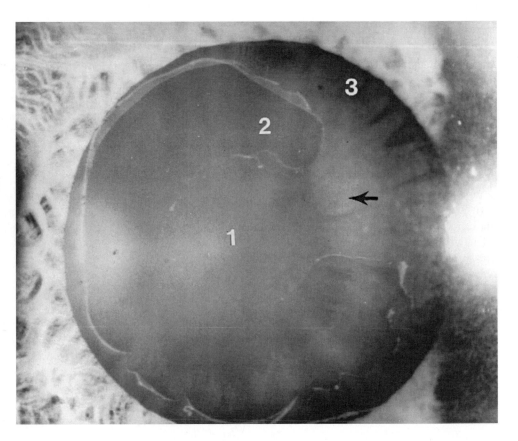

Figure 15.2. Slitlamp view of lens in patient with the exfoliation syndrome showing three zones on the anterior lens capsule: *(1)* central, translucent disc; *(2)* middle clear zone except for bridge between central and peripheral zones *(arrow)*; *(3)* peripheral granular zone with radial striations. (Reprinted with permission from Layden WE: Exfoliation syndrome. In: The Secondary Glaucomas. Ritch R, Shields MB, eds. St. Louis, CV Mosby, 1982.)

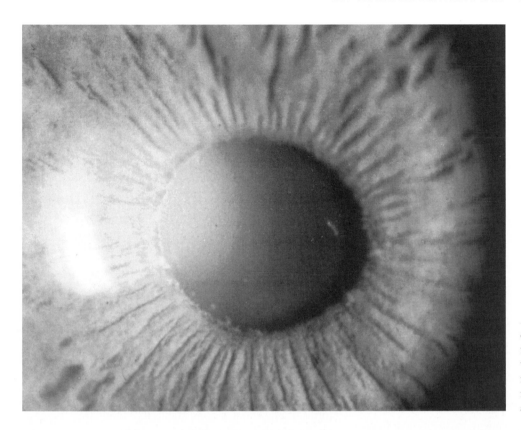

Figure 15.3. Slitlamp view of iris in patient with the exfoliation syndrome showing white flecks of exfoliative material on the pupillary margin and loss of pigment at the pupillary ruff.

attacks have an increased incidence of abnormal iris transillumination and exfoliation material, suggesting that hypoperfusion may be a contributory factor in the development of the exfoliation syndrome (44, 45).

Whether a primary or secondary feature, the iris hypoxia is associated with atrophy of the iris pigment epithelium, stroma, and muscle cells (43). Atrophy of the pigment epithelium may be associated with anterior chamber melanin dispersion, which may be seen as a whorl-like pattern of pigment particles on the iris sphincter and pigment deposition on the peripheral iris (38), while atrophy of the muscle cells may account for the poor mydriasis, which is also a typical finding in the exfoliation syndrome (43).

Other Slitlamp Findings

Exfoliation material may also be seen on lens zonules, on the anterior hyaloid in aphakic eyes (46), and on a posterior chamber intraocular lens in pseudophakic eyes (47). Specular microscopy of the corneal endothelium has revealed a significantly lower than normal cell density in eyes with the exfoliation syndrome, as well as morphologic changes in cell size and shape (48, 49). These findings have also been observed in the unaffected eye of unilateral cases, leading the authors to suggest that these corneal endothelial changes might serve as an early sign of the disorder (48). Ultrastructural studies have revealed clumps of exfoliation material adhering to the corneal endothelium and incorporated into the posterior Descemet's membrane, which the authors believe indicate that the exfoliation ma-

terial was formed by degenerative endothelial cells (50). Eyes with the exfoliation syndrome may also have increased aqueous flare and cells as quantitated by a laser flare-cell meter (51).

Gonioscopic Findings

The exfoliation syndrome is associated with excessive pigment dispersion, which leads to increased trabecular meshwork pigmentation. The pigmentation of the meshwork has a more uneven distribution than that seen in pigmentary glaucoma and may be associated with flecks of exfoliation material (Fig. 15.4). An accumulation of pigment may also be seen along Schwalbe's line *(Sampaolesi's line)*. In eyes with marked asymmetry of meshwork pigmentation, glaucoma is more common in the more pigmented eye (52). However, increased pigmentation of the trabecular meshwork has also been observed in the fellow eye without exfoliation, and it has been suggested that this may be the earliest detectable sign of the exfoliation syndrome (52). Although the anterior chamber depth is normal in most eyes with the exfoliation syndrome (53), the anterior chamber angle is occludable in a high percentage of cases (54). In studies of patients with the exfoliation syndrome, 9–18% had angles that were considered to be occludable (52, 55) and 14% had evidence of angle closure on the basis of peripheral anterior synechiae (52). When the ciliary processes can be visualized by a special gonioscopic technique (cycloscopy), the exfoliation material may be seen on these structures (56).

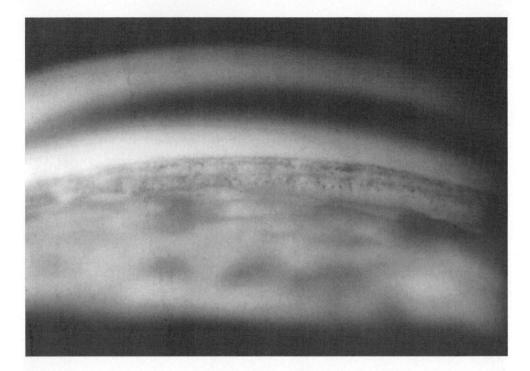

Figure 15.4. Gonioscopic view of eye with exfoliation syndrome showing irregular pigmentation of trabecular meshwork and white flecks of exfoliative material.

Course of the Glaucoma

As previously noted, not all patients with the exfoliation syndrome develop glaucoma, and reports vary considerably regarding the frequency of glaucoma in eyes with this condition. Sugar (57) found elevated IOP in 55% of 643 cases in the literature and in 81.8% of his own series. A study of 100 consecutive patients with the exfoliation syndrome revealed 22% with pressure elevations, only one-third of whom had glaucomatous damage (27), while in another series of 518 patients, more than half had glaucoma (58). In one study of patients with the exfoliation syndrome but without glaucoma on the initial examination, one-third developed glaucoma during a 1.5-year followup (59). Some patients with bilateral exfoliation syndrome will have glaucoma in both eyes, while others will have a pressure rise in only one of the eyes with exfoliation. Less commonly, a patient with unilateral exfoliation may have open-angle glaucoma in both eyes (15).

Most eyes with capsular glaucoma have an open-angle mechanism, although acute angle-closure glaucoma also occurs in a small number of cases (12, 25, 58, 60). It is not uncommon for a patient with the exfoliation syndrome to present with an acute onset of high IOP, although the majority of these will have open angles. In one series of 139 exfoliation syndrome patients presenting with acute glaucoma, 86 had open angles, 18 had angle closure, 21 had neovascular glaucoma, and 14 had absolute glaucoma (60). Once open-angle glaucoma has developed in an eye with exfoliation, the IOP tends to run higher (61, 62) and may be more difficult to control than cases of chronic open-angle glaucoma (62, 63). It has also been observed that the probability of developing glaucomatous optic neuropathy is higher in eyes with exfoliation syndrome than in other forms of glaucoma at comparable IOP levels (60), suggesting an intrinsic vulnerability in the optic nerve in the former group. Although disc area and other morphometric features of the nerve head do not differ in nonglaucomatous eyes with and without exfoliation (65), glaucomatous neuroretinal rim damage tends to be more diffuse with capsular glaucoma, as opposed to the sectorial preference in chronic open-angle glaucoma (66). Immunoelectron microscopic studies of the lamina cribrosa have shown elastosis, suggesting abnormal regulation of elastin synthesis and/or degradation in the optic nerve head of patients with the exfoliation syndrome (67).

Histopathologic Features and Theories of Mechanism

Questions that must be considered regarding the pathogenesis of the exfoliation syndrome include: (a) the nature and source of the exfoliation material, and (b) how this material contributes to elevation of the IOP.

Exfoliation Material

NATURE. The ultrastructural appearance of the exfoliation material is that of a fibrillar protein (68), arranged in an irregular meshwork and occasionally coiled as spirals (69). The material has staining characteristics of oxytalan, a microtubular component of connective and elastic tissues (70–72). Immunoelectron microscopy has revealed elastin and tropoelastin (73). These observations led to the theory that the exfoliation syndrome is a type of elastosis, with elastic microfibrils being abnormally secreted by local ocular cells (72, 73). Other studies indicate that the exfoliation material may be a basement membrane proteoglycan (74–77). Immunohistochemical studies have shown heparan sulfate and chondroitin sulfate proteoglycans, laminin, entactin/nidogen, fibronectin, and amyloid P protein to be integral components of exfoliation material (77, 78). It has been suggested that the material is a multicomponent expression of a disordered extracellular matrix synthesis, including the incorporation of principal noncollagenous basement membrane components (77). The presence of glycosaminoglycans in anterior ocular structures and the aqueous humor has also been demonstrated in eyes with the exfoliation syndrome (69, 79, 80), and the possibility has been raised that this disease may involve abnormal metabolism of glycosaminoglycans in the iris (80). Still other studies have suggested that the protein of the exfoliation material may be of the amyloid group (68, 81), and there are clinical similarities between the exfoliation syndrome and primary amyloidosis (82, 83). However, immunohistochemical staining demonstrated amyloid P protein, a minor serum component, on the periphery of the exfoliation fibers, suggesting that it is not an intrinsic fiber component, but binds to sites similar to those on normal elastic fibers (84).

SOURCE. The exfoliation material occurs on and in the *lens* capsule, and adjacent to the lens epithelium (85–87). The source of the material on the outer surface of the lens capsule has been controversial. Some investigators felt it to be unlikely that this material could be derived from the lens epithelium since early ultrastructural studies showed no continuity between the capsular and epithelial exfoliation material (85), and studies with horseradish peroxidase suggested that this material could not pass through the capsule (79). These observations led to the theory that the exfoliation material on the lens capsule must have been deposited there from other ocular structures. However, small amounts of fibrillar protein have been seen in the otherwise normal aging lens capsule (88), and discoid plaques of exfoliation material near the epithelium correspond in location and appearance to material on the capsular surface with connections between the material at the two levels, suggesting that the lens epithelium does contribute, at least in part, to the exfoliation material on the anterior lens capsule (86, 87, 89).

A precapsular film has been noted on the anterior lens capsule of many older individuals, which has a ground glass appearance and has been shown by ultrastructural studies as a fibrillar layer similar to exfoliation material (90, 91). It has been suggested that the precapsular layer may be a precursor of the exfoliation syndrome (90, 91).

The exfoliation material is also found in the *iris* in the anterior limiting layer, on the posterior aspect of the pigment epithelium, in the vessel walls (92), and in the perivascular matrix (93). The material is attached in irregular areas to the iris

vessels (94) and is located in indentations of the cell membrane of the pigment epithelium, but not in the cytoplasm of those cells (95). It has been suggested that the iris may be a source of the exfoliation material on the lens capsule (46, 57), which may explain the presence of the material on the anterior hyaloid in aphakic eyes (46, 96, 97) and on a posterior chamber lens in pseudophakia (47). The material has also been demonstrated in the ciliary epithelium (98) and on lens zonules, although it is not clear as to whether these represent additional primary sources or secondary deposition.

Exfoliation material has also been found in extrabulbar tissue including the *conjunctiva* (72, 99–103), which appears to be another independent source of the material (104). This has been demonstrated in conjunctival biopsies of eyes that did not have the typical clinical appearance of exfoliation material on the anterior lens capsule but were suspected on the basis of other signs, such as pigment dispersion and iris transillumination defects (101). Other extrabulbar sites where exfoliation material has been identified include extraocular muscles, orbital septa, posterior ciliary arteries, vortex veins, and central retinal vessels passing through the optic nerve sheaths (102, 103).

The exfoliation material has also been demonstrated in tissues throughout the body of patients with the exfoliation syndrome, including lung, heart, liver, gallbladder, skin, kidney, and cerebral meninges (105, 106), suggesting a systemic process involving generalized abnormal connective-tissue metabolism.

Mechanism of the Pigment Dispersion

It has been generally held that the obstruction to aqueous outflow which leads to elevated IOP in glaucoma capsulare is due to blockage of the outflow channels by the exfoliation material, melanin granules from the iris pigment epithelium, or both. Whether the exfoliation material is derived locally from trabecular cells or accumulates by dispersion from distant sites is not fully understood. It may be that both the exfoliation material and pigment are liberated from the lens and iris as a result of the rubbing of iris pigment epithelium against the rough lens capsule. Sugar (57), however, felt the pigment dispersion may result from a fundamental defect of the iris.

Ultrastructural studies of eyes with the exfoliation syndrome have revealed both fibrillar material and pigment granules in the trabecular meshwork (107–110), which may lead to the obstruction of aqueous outflow. In one morphometric, ultrastructural study, comparing five eyes with glaucoma capsulare, 10 with the exfoliation syndrome without evidence of glaucomas, and six age-matched control eyes, large deposits of exfoliation material were seen in the juxtacanalicular tissue and uveal meshwork of the first two groups, with a significant correlation between the presence of glaucoma and the amount of exfoliation material (110). There was evidence that the material in the juxtacanalicular tissue was produced locally by endothelial and connective tissue cells, while that in the uveal meshwork was derived partly from the aqueous. Other features that correlated with the presence of glaucoma included increased thickness of the juxtacanalicular tissue and reduced area of Schlemm's canal, both of which appeared to result from the accumulation of locally produced exfoliation material, dysfunction of endothelial cells and disorganization of the juxtacanalicular tissue and Schlemm's canal. However, the glaucoma status did not correlate with the concentration of melanin granules.

Mechanism of the Glaucoma

The observation that glaucoma does not develop in all eyes with the exfoliation syndrome, and yet may develop in both eyes of a patient with unilateral exfoliation (12, 25, 107, 111), has led to the theory that capsular glaucoma and chronic open-angle glaucoma may share the same mechanism of outflow obstruction. However, the increased incidence of glaucoma in eyes with the exfoliation syndrome is felt to indicate a causal relationship between the abnormal material and the elevated IOP (112). Furthermore, patients with the exfoliation syndrome do not have the same response to topical corticosteroids as do chronic open-angle glaucoma patients (113, 114). It appears, therefore, that glaucoma capsulare represents a distinct form of glaucoma, but may be superimposed on chronic open-angle glaucoma in some patients.

As previously noted, a less common mechanism of glaucoma in patients with the exfoliation syndrome is angle-closure glaucoma (12, 25, 52, 58, 60).

Differential Diagnosis

The exfoliation syndrome must be distinguished from other forms of lens exfoliation as well as other causes of pigment dispersion.

Capsular Delamination

As noted earlier in this chapter, there is another group of disorders that involve exfoliation of the anterior lens capsule and have been referred to as "true" exfoliation of the lens capsule (5, 7, 8), or capsular delamination (6). These cases differ from the exfoliation syndrome in that an underlying precipitating factor, such as trauma (3, 4), exposure to intense heat (2), or severe uveitis (4), is often, but not always (5–7), present. The nature of the lens exfoliation also differs, with thin, clear membrane-like material separating from the anterior lens capsule and often curling at the margins (5–7). Glaucoma is infrequent with capsular delamination.

Primary Amyloidosis

This generalized, systemic disease, which may be familial (82) or nonfamilial (83), has numerous ocular manifesta-

tions, including glaucoma. The amyloid may be deposited as a white, flaky substance throughout the eye, including the pupillary margin of the iris, the anterior lens capsule, and the anterior chamber angle, creating a clinical picture that resembles the exfoliation syndrome (82, 83). In the autosomal dominant condition, familial amyloidotic polyneuropathy, glaucoma is the most common ocular manifestation, and an ultrastructural study revealed accumulations of amyloid fibrils and multilayered plaques of basement membrane-like material in the intertrabecular spaces (115).

Pigment Dispersion

A variety of conditions, in addition to the exfoliation syndrome, are characterized by increased pigmentation of the trabecular meshwork. These include the pigment dispersion syndrome and pigmentary glaucoma (Chapter 14), some forms of anterior uveitis (Chapter 19), melanosis and melanomas (Chapter 18), and chronic open-angle glaucoma, or otherwise normal eyes with unusually heavy pigment dispersion. These conditions can usually be distinguished from the exfoliation syndrome by observing the characteristic appearance of the anterior lens capsule and iris in the latter disorder. However, the exfoliation syndrome has been observed to develop in patients with the pigment dispersion syndrome (116).

Management

Glaucoma

The glaucoma associated with the exfoliation syndrome is basically treated the same as chronic open-angle glaucoma, although it has been emphasized that the former glaucoma is typically more difficult to control (62, 63). When medical therapy is no longer adequate, laser trabeculoplasty is usually indicated and has a high success rate with this form of glaucoma. When conventional surgical intervention becomes necessary, filtering surgery is generally advocated. One study suggested that while capsular glaucoma has a poorer response to medical therapy than chronic open-angle glaucoma, it has a better response to trabeculectomy (117). The influence of lens removal on the course of the glaucoma is unclear. It has been reported that the exfoliation material diminishes and regresses after intracapsular cataract extraction (118), although others have observed the development of the exfoliation syndrome years after intracapsular lens removal (46, 47, 96, 97). A new surgical modality that is being evaluated for treatment of glaucoma capsulare attempts to remove intertrabecular and pretrabecular debris by trabecular aspiration (119).

Cataract

Although lens extraction is not advocated for the management of glaucoma in the exfoliation syndrome, cataract extraction for improvement of visual acuity is frequently indicated and requires special consideration in these patients. With extracapsular cataract surgery, patients with the exfoliation syndrome have a higher than average risk of zonular and capsular breaks (120–124). This is most likely due to degeneration of the zonular fibrils (36, 125), but may also be associated with a thin posterior lens capsule (126). Other factors that may complicate cataract surgery in these patients are poor pupillary dilatation (121, 123, 124, 127) and occasional synechiae between the iris pigment epithelium and the peripheral anterior lens capsule (128). Preoperatively, the surgeon should look for evidence of zonular dialysis, such as phacodonesis and asymmetric anterior chamber depth (36, 118), and care must be taken during surgery to avoid excessive stress on the zonules or posterior capsule (120–126). When a successful extracapsular cataract extraction or phacoemulsification has been performed, the implantation of a posterior chamber intraocular lens appears to be well tolerated in patients with the exfoliation syndrome (121). However, there is an increased incidence of fibrinoid iritis in the early postoperative period following cataract extraction with intraocular lens implantation in patients with the exfoliation syndrome (123, 129), and it has been reported that this complication can be reduced by the use of heparin surface modified intraocular lenses (130).

GLAUCOMAS ASSOCIATED WITH DISLOCATION OF THE LENS[b]

Terminology

Several terms have been applied to the clinical situation in which the crystalline lens is displaced from its normal, central position behind the iris. *Subluxation* of the lens implies an incomplete dislocation in which the lens is still at least partially behind the iris, but is tilted or displaced slightly in either an anterior or posterior direction or perpendicular to the optical axis. With *complete dislocation,* the entire lens may be in the anterior chamber or may have fallen posteriorly into the vitreous cavity. The term ectopia of the lens, or *ectopia lentis,* is also applied to cases of lens dislocation, but is nonspecific with regard to the degree of lens displacement.

Subluxation or complete dislocation of the lens may be associated with a number of clinical conditions, all of which can lead to glaucoma by a variety of mechanisms. We will first review the more common clinical forms of ectopia lentis and then consider the mechanisms by which these conditions may lead to IOP elevation and how these glaucomas are managed.

[b]Refer to Shields, MB: Color Atlas of Glaucoma. Baltimore, Williams & Wilkins, 1998, Plate II23.

Clinical Forms of Ectopia Lentis

Traumatic Dislocation

Trauma is the most common cause of a displaced lens (131, 132). In one series of 166 cases, injury was reported to account for 53% of the total group (132). The patient population with traumatic dislocation of the lens has a higher than normal incidence of serologic evidence for syphilis (132), although a direct cause-and-effect relationship between this disease and ectopia lentis has not been established. It may simply be that the patient who is likely to acquire syphilis is also more prone to place himself in situations that lead to trauma (132).

Simple Ectopia Lentis

Dislocation of the lens may occur without associated ocular or systemic abnormalities either as a congenital anomaly or as a spontaneous disorder later in life (133, 134). Both forms are typically inherited by an autosomal dominant mode (134). The condition is usually bilateral and symmetric, with lens dislocation generally upward and outward and occasionally into the anterior chamber. Associated problems include glaucoma and retinal detachment.

Ectopia Lentis et Pupillae

This is a rare, autosomal recessive condition characterized by small, subluxed lenses, and oval or slit-shaped pupils that are displaced usually in the opposite direction from that of the lens (Fig. 15.5) (133–136). The condition is associated with a wide variety of other ocular abnormalities, including severe axial myopia with related fundus changes, enlarged corneal diameters, iris transillumination defects, poor pupillary dilation, persistent pupillary membranes, iridohyaloid adhesions, prominent iris processes, cataracts, retinal detachment, and glaucoma (136). The condition is usually bilateral, although marked variation may be seen between eyes of the same patient (136).

It has been suggested that simple ectopia lentis may be an incomplete expression of ectopia lentis et pupillae since both may occur in the same family and have peripheral iris transillumination (136). In addition, some patients with ectopia lentis et pupillae may have mild systemic changes suggestive of Marfan's syndrome (133).

Marfan's Syndrome

This autosomal dominant disorder is characterized by a tall, slender individual with long, slender fingers and toes (arachnodactyly) and frequent cardiovascular disease (134, 137). Marfan's syndrome and ectopia lentis have been linked to a single fibrillin gene on chromosome 15, while arachnodactyly was linked to the fibrillin gene on chromosome 5 (138). In a review of 160 consecutive patients, the

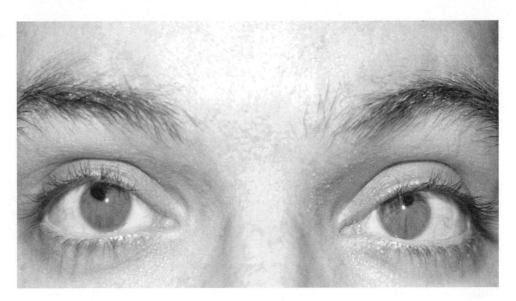

Figure 15.5. Patient with ectopia lentis et pupillae showing typical displacement of pupils.

most striking ocular abnormality was enlargement of the globe, presumably due to scleral stretching (139). The lens was dislocated in 193 of the eyes, and this correlated with increased ocular axial length, suggesting that stretching and rupture of the zonular fibers leads to the dislocation. The ectopia lentis typically appears in the fourth to fifth decade of life and is rarely complete, but is usually seen as an upward subluxation. Glaucoma may result from the lens dislocation, but also occurs in association with surgical aphakia, or as an anomaly of the anterior chamber angle. In one review of 573 patients, 29 (5%) had glaucoma, with the most common mechanisms being chronic open-angle, postlens extraction, and postscleral buckling procedure (140). Retinal detachment is also a common finding in either the phakic or aphakic eye of a patient with Marfan's syndrome.

Homocystinuria

These patients may resemble those with Marfan's syndrome in habitus and ocular problems, but differ by an autosomal recessive inheritance and frequent mental retardation (134, 137). Homocystinuria may result from one of several enzyme deficiencies in homocysteine metabolism. The diagnosis can be confirmed by the demonstration of homocysteine in the urine. The differentiation between Marfan's syndrome and homocystinuria is important since the homocystinuric patient is subject to thromboembolic episodes, which can lead to death in early adulthood and creates a significant surgical risk. In addition, if the condition is diagnosed in the newborn, appropriate dietary treatment and vitamin supplementation can substantially reduce the risk of ocular complications (141). The lens dislocation occurs earlier in life than in Marfan's syndrome, is more often in a downward direction, and there is frequently complete dislocation into the vitreous or anterior chamber. Glaucoma is more commonly related to the lens disloca-

tion than in Marfan's syndrome. Retinal detachment is also a frequent problem.

Weill-Marchesani Syndrome

Weill-Marchesani syndrome is the antithesis of the aforementioned conditions with respect to habitus in that the patients are short and stocky. The principal features of the syndrome are short fingers (brachydactyly) and small, round lenses (microspherophakia). Lens dislocation occurs with equal frequency as compared to Marfan's syndrome and homocystinuria, and glaucoma is more common than in either of the latter two conditions (142). An ultrastructural study of the lens from a patient with Weill-Marchesani syndrome revealed degeneration and necrosis of the epithelial cells and destruction of cortical fibers, which was felt to be due, at least in part, to the trauma and irritation of a highly mobile lens in close contact with the iris (143). The small, round lens in this condition also has loose zonules, and the glaucoma may be related to either lens dislocation (142) or a forward shift of the lens, causing pupillary-block glaucoma (144, 145), which can be precipitated or aggravated by miotic therapy. Bilateral angle-closure glaucoma has also been reported following mid-dilatation with cyclopentolate in a child with the Weill-Marchesani Syndrome but without lens subluxation (146). Angle-closure glaucoma may be treated with either laser iridotomy or peripheral iridoplasty depending on the relative proportion of pupillary block as the mechanism of the angle closure (147).

Spontaneous Dislocation

In some middle-aged or older individuals, dislocation of the lens may occur spontaneously, usually in association with cataract formation (131). Spontaneous dislocation has also been reported in eyes with high myopia, uveitis, buphthalmos, or megalocornea (131).

Other Conditions with Associated Ectopia Lentis

Other rare congenital disorders associated with lens dislocation include Ehlers-Danlos syndrome, hyperlysemia (148), sulfite oxidase deficiency (149), and aniridia (150). Additional conditions associated with ectopia lentis are included in Table 15.1.

Mechanisms of Associated Glaucoma

Subluxation or complete dislocation of the lens in any of the aforementioned clinical conditions may lead to glaucoma by a variety of mechanisms. In general, these mechanisms of glaucoma apply to all forms of ectopia lentis.

Pupillary Block

The lens may block aqueous flow through the pupil if it is dislocated into the pupil or anterior chamber, or if it is subluxed or tilted forward against the iris without entering the anterior chamber (131, 145, 151). This mechanism is partic-

Table 15.1.

CONDITIONS ASSOCIATED WITH ECTOPIA LENTIS

Trauma
Simple ectopia lentis
Ectopia lentis et pupillae
Marfan's syndrome
Homocystinuria
Weill-Marchesani syndrome
High myopia
Uveitis
Buphthalmos
Megalocornea
Ehlers-Danlos syndrome
Hyperlysemia
Sulfite oxidase deficiency
Aniridia
Scleroderma
Alport's syndrome
Mandibulofacial dysostosis
Klinefelter's syndrome
Retinitis pigmentosa
Persistent pupillary membrane
Axenfeld-Rieger syndrome
Dominantly inherited blepharoptosis and high myopia
Marfan-like syndrome with hyaloretinal degeneration
Sturge-Weber syndrome
Syphilis
Crouzon's disease
Refsum's syndrome

Modified from Nelson, LB, Maumenee, IH: Ectopia lentis. Surv Ophthal 27:143, 1982 and Ritch, R, Wand, M: Treatment of the Weill-Marchesani syndrome. Ann Ophthal 13:665, 1981.

ularly common with microspherophakia, as in the Weill-Marchesani syndrome, due to loose zonules of the lens. Pupillary block in the latter condition is often made worse by miotic therapy, which allows further relaxation of zonular support, while cycloplegics may help by pulling the lens posteriorly. Pupillary block may also occur in association with a dislocated lens due to herniation of vitreous into the pupil. Peripheral anterior synechiae may develop from a long-standing pupillary block and produce chronic IOP elevation.

Phacolytic Glaucoma

In other cases, the lens may dislocate completely into the vitreous cavity and later undergo degenerative changes with release of material that obstructs aqueous outflow (152). In one reported case, this condition was associated with retinal perivasculitis, which cleared along with the glaucoma after removal of the lens (153). Phacolytic glaucoma without dislocation is discussed later in this chapter.

Concomitant Trauma

In cases of traumatic dislocation of the lens, concomitant trauma to the anterior chamber angle from the initial injury may be the cause of the associated glaucoma (131, 134). In addition, a transient pressure elevation of uncertain etiology may persist for days or weeks after traumatic dislocation of the lens. The mechanisms of glaucoma associated with trauma are considered in more detail in Chapter 22.

Management

Pupillary Block

If the lens is displaced anteriorly, either in the anterior chamber or partially through the pupil, it may be possible to relieve the condition by dilating the pupil and allowing the lens to reposit back into the posterior chamber (154). A miotic may then be used to keep the lens behind the iris. As previously noted, however, miotic therapy should be avoided when the pupillary block is due to loose zonules, since contraction of the ciliary muscle further relaxes the zonular support, making the pupillary block worse (145). In addition, if the lens is totally dislocated in the anterior chamber, it is probably better to constrict the pupil and surgically remove the lens, rather than letting it fall back into the vitreous. Cycloplegics may help to break the attack by pulling the lens posteriorly. Hyperosmotic agents, carbonic anhydrase inhibitors, or topical β-blockers may also be useful in breaking the attack. The definitive treatment, however, is a laser iridotomy (or incisional iridectomy if necessary). The iridotomy should be placed peripherally to avoid subsequent obstruction by the lens. Prophylactic iridotomy in cases of microspherophakia, to avoid pupillary block glaucoma, has also been advocated (145, 155). As previously noted, laser peripheral iridoplasty may also be helpful in some cases of angle-closure glaucoma without a significant pupillary block component (147). The extraction of a subluxed lens is associated with increased surgical risk, and should usually be avoided unless the lens in the anterior chamber or lens extraction is needed to relieve the glaucoma or improve vision.

Phacolytic Glaucoma

This is the only situation in cases of lens dislocation in which cataract extraction is the procedure of choice (156). It has been shown that subluxed lenses can be successfully removed through a pars plana approach with vitreous instruments (153,157).

Chronic Glaucomas

Chronic glaucoma due to peripheral anterior synechiae or concomitant trauma in eyes with dislocated lenses is generally managed by standard medical measures. Laser trabeculoplasty has a low success rate in eyes with open-angle glaucoma associated with trauma, although it is often reasonable to try this approach when medical therapy is no longer adequate before recommending incisional surgical intervention.

GLAUCOMAS ASSOCIATED WITH CATARACT FORMATION[c]

It has long been recognized clinically that several forms of glaucoma may occur in association with the formation of cataracts. However, an incomplete understanding of the various mechanisms for these glaucomas has led to a plethora of terms, accompanied by considerable controversy and confusion. More recent observations have provided new explanations and terminology for several of the glaucomas that are associated with cataract formation.

Phacolytic (Lens Protein) Glaucoma[c]

Terminology

In 1900, Gifford (158) described a form of open-angle glaucoma associated with a hypermature cataract. Among the terms subsequently suggested for this condition were "phacogenetic glaucoma" (159) and "lens-induced uveitis" (160). Flocks and coworkers (161) reported histologic findings which suggested that the glaucoma-inducing mechanism was a macrophagic response to lens material. They proposed that this condition be called *phacolytic glaucoma,* which is the term most often used today. However, Epstein and associates (162, 163) have provided evidence that lens

[c]Refer to Shields, MB: Color Atlas of Glaucoma. Baltimore, Williams & Wilkins, 1998, Plate II24.

protein may be primarily responsible for the obstruction to aqueous outflow in this disorder, and the term *lens protein glaucoma* has been suggested (164).

Clinical Features

The typical patient presents with the acute onset of monocular pain and redness. There is usually a history of gradual reduction in visual acuity over the preceding months or years, and vision at the time of presentation may be reduced to only inaccurate light perception. The examination reveals a high IOP, conjunctival hyperemia, and diffuse corneal edema. It is important to note that the anterior chamber angle is open and usually grossly normal. A heavy flare is typically seen in the anterior chamber, often associated with iridescent or hyperrefringent particles. The latter have been variably reported to represent calcium oxalate (165) or cholesterol (166, 167) crystals, and are a helpful diagnostic sign in phacolytic glaucoma. Chunks of white material may also be seen in the aqueous and on the anterior lens capsule and corneal endothelium. In five cases, specular microscopy revealed regular, round cells, about three times the size of an erythrocyte, which were found by histologic study of aqueous aspirates to represent macrophages (166). The cataract is typically mature (totally opaque) or hypermature (liquid cortex), but may rarely be immature. A less common variation of phacolytic glaucoma is the previously discussed situation in which the lens has dislocated into the vitreous and undergone phacolysis. The latter cases differ clinically in that the glaucoma tends to be more subacute.

Theories of Mechanism

It is generally accepted that part of the pathogenesis in phacolytic glaucoma is the release of soluble lens protein into the aqueous through microscopic defects in the lens capsule. However, theories vary as to how this protein leads to the elevated IOP.

As previously noted, it has been postulated that macrophages, laden with phagocytosed lens material, block the trabecular meshwork to produce the acute glaucoma (161). This theory has been supported by the demonstration of macrophages in the aqueous (168) and trabecular meshwork (169) of eyes with phacolytic glaucoma. By electron microscopic study, these macrophages were found to have phagocytized degenerated lens material (170). Electron microscopy has also demonstrated free-floating degenerated lens material in the aqueous and trabecular meshwork of an eye with phacolytic glaucoma (170). Against the macrophage theory is the observation that lens-laden macrophages in the anterior chamber do not invariably lead to elevated IOP. For example, a macrophagic cellular reaction has been found in the anterior chamber aspirate following needling and aspiration of a cataract, but did not appear to obstruct aqueous outflow (171). However, the number of macrophages in the aqueous may be greater in phacolytic glaucoma.

An alternative theory is that heavy molecular weight (HMW) soluble protein from the lens directly obstructs the outflow of aqueous (162–164). Such protein has been shown to cause a significant decrease in outflow when perfused in enucleated human eyes (162). HMW soluble protein is known to increase in the cataractous lens (172) and has been demonstrated in the aqueous of eyes with phacolytic glaucoma in quantities sufficient to obstruct aqueous outflow (163). HMW protein is rare in childhood lenses (173, 174), which may explain why phacolytic glaucoma rarely, if ever, occurs in children.

Differential Diagnosis

Several forms of glaucoma may present with the sudden onset of pain and redness, creating diagnostic confusion with phacolytic glaucoma. *Acute angle-closure glaucoma* must be ruled out on the basis of the gonioscopic examination. *Open-angle glaucoma associated with uveitis* may be more difficult to distinguish. In some cases, a paracentesis and microscopic examination of the aqueous may be helpful by demonstrating amorphous protein-like fluid and occasional macrophages in eyes with phacolytic glaucoma (164). A therapeutic trial of topical steroids will produce only temporary remission when phacolysis is the underlying problem, which may help to distinguish it from a primary uveitis. Other conditions, such as neovascular glaucoma and trauma, may also cause a sudden IOP rise, but can usually be distinguished on the basis of history and/or clinical findings.

Management

Phacolytic glaucoma should be handled as an emergency, ultimately by removal of the lens (175, 176). It is desirable, however, to first bring the IOP under medical control with hyperosmotics, carbonic anhydrase inhibitors and topical β-blockers and/or α$_2$-agonists, and possibly to minimize associated inflammation with topical steroid therapy (164). When the pressure cannot be lowered medically, it may be necessary to accomplish this at the time of surgery by gradual release of aqueous through a paracentesis incision. Extracapsular cataract extraction with posterior chamber intraocular lens implantation was performed in five patients with phacolytic glaucoma with uniformly good results (177). The anterior chamber should be thoroughly irrigated and all lens material removed to avoid postoperative IOP rise. Following uncomplicated cataract surgery, the glaucoma usually clears and there is often a return of good vision, despite a significant preoperative reduction.

Lens Particle Glaucoma

Terminology

It was once felt that a primary toxicity of cataractous lens material caused an inflammatory reaction called "phaco-

toxic uveitis," and led to glaucoma in some cases. Subsequent studies, however, have not supported the concept that liberated lens material is toxic (178). It appears that cases incorrectly given this diagnosis are actually due to liberation of lens particles and debris following disruption of the lens capsule, and the term *lens particle glaucoma* has been proposed for this entity (164).

Clinical Features

This condition is typically associated with disruption of the lens capsule either by cataract extraction or a penetrating injury. The onset of IOP elevation is usually soon after the primary event and is generally proportional to the amount of "fluffed up" lens cortical material in the anterior chamber. Uncommon clinical variations include an onset of glaucoma many years after capsular disruption or following a spontaneous rupture in the lens capsule. The latter condition may be hard to distinguish from phacolytic glaucoma, although cases of lens particle glaucoma tend to have a greater inflammatory component, often associated with posterior and anterior synechiae and inflammatory pupillary membranes (164).

Theories of Mechanism

It has been demonstrated by perfusion studies with enucleated human eyes that small amounts of free particulate lens material significantly reduce outflow (162). This is presumed to be the principal mechanism of trabecular meshwork obstruction in cases of lens particle glaucoma. However, it is possible that the associated inflammation, whether in response to the surgery, trauma, or retained lens material, may also contribute to the glaucoma in this condition.

Differential Diagnosis

In its typical form, the diagnosis of lens particle glaucoma is usually easy to make on the basis of history and physical findings. In atypical forms, such as delayed onset or spontaneous capsule rupture, the diagnosis might be confused with phacoanaphylaxis, phacolytic glaucoma, or uveitic conditions with associated open-angle glaucoma. When doubt exists, microscopic examination of aqueous from an anterior chamber tap may help to establish the diagnosis of lens particle glaucoma by demonstrating leukocytes and macrophages along with lens cortical material (164).

Management

In some cases, it is possible to control the IOP medically with drugs that reduce aqueous production. Because inflammation is also present, the pupil should be dilated and topical steroids used, although it may be advisable to use the latter only in moderate amounts since steroid therapy may delay absorption of the lens material (164). The IOP will usually return to normal after the lens material has been absorbed. When the pressure cannot be adequately controlled medically, the residual lens material should be surgically removed either by irrigation if the material is loose or with vitrectomy instruments when it is adherent to ocular structures.

Phacoanaphylaxis

Terminology

In 1922, Verhoeff and Lemoine (179) reported that a small percent of individuals are hypersensitive to lens protein, and that rupture of the lens capsule in these cases leads to an intraocular inflammation, which they called "endophthalmitis phacoanaphylactica." Although such cases are apparently rare, there is evidence that a true *phacoanaphylaxis* does occur in response to lens protein antigen (180), with subsequent inflammation and occasional open-angle glaucoma.

Clinical Features

As in the case of lens particle glaucoma, there is usually a preceding disruption of the lens capsule by extracapsular cataract surgery or penetrating injury (181). The distinguishing feature, however, is a latent period during which sensitization to lens protein occurs. A particularly likely setting for the development of phacoanaphylaxis is when lens material, especially the nucleus, is retained in the vitreous. The typical physical finding is a chronic, relentless "granulomatous-type" of inflammation, which is centered around lens material either in the primarily involved eye or in the fellow eye after it has undergone extracapsular cataract surgery or phacoemulsification. Associated glaucoma is only rarely a feature of phacoanaphylaxis.

Theories of Mechanism

It has been demonstrated in rabbits that autologous lens protein is antigenic (180), and it was assumed that the lens capsule isolates the lenticular antigens from the immune response, with sensitization occurring only when the capsule is violated. This concept was not supported, however, by human studies which failed to demonstrate lens antibodies after injury to the lens and which showed an equal incidence of antibody in cataract patients and controls (182). The same study did show a higher prevalence of antibodies in a small group with hypermature cataracts and more frequent postoperative uveitis in patients with antibodies in preoperative blood specimens, although the latter observation was not statistically significant. In the rabbit study cited above, there was considerable variation in the response to autologous lens antigen (180) which may explain the infrequency with which phacoanaphylaxis is seen clinically. The cellular appearance of the immune response is characterized by polymorphonuclear leukocytes and lymphoid, epithelioid, and

giant cells, usually around a nidus of lens material. It may be that the occasional glaucoma in phacoanaphylaxis is related to the accumulation of these cells in the trabecular meshwork, although lens protein or particles may also be present and could account for the glaucoma.

Differential Diagnosis

Other chronic forms of uveitis, especially sympathetic ophthalmia, may occur in association with phacoanaphylaxis. Phacolytic and lens particle glaucomas must also be considered. Microscopic examination of the aqueous may be helpful, although variations in cytology have not been fully studied in this condition, and the diagnosis may require histologic examination of the surgically removed lens material.

Management

Steroid therapy should be used to control the uveitis, with antiglaucoma medication as required. When medical measures are inadequate, the retained lens material should be surgically removed.

Intumescent Lens

In some eyes with advanced cataract formation, the lens may become swollen or intumescent, with progressive reduction in the anterior chamber angle, eventually leading to a form of angle-closure glaucoma. This has been referred to as "phacomorphic glaucoma" (183). The angle closure may be either secondary to an enhanced pupillary block mechanism or to forward displacement of the lens-iris diaphragm. In either case, the diagnosis is usually made by observing a mature, intumescent cataract associated with a central anterior chamber depth that is significantly shallower than that of the fellow eye. The treatment is initial medical reduction of the IOP with hyperosmotics, carbonic anhydrase inhibitors, and topical β-blockers and/or α_2-agonists, followed by extraction of the cataract. However, in 10 patients with phacomorphic glaucoma, the acute angle-closure glaucoma attack was relieved in all cases by laser iridotomy (184), which may be helpful to bring the pressure under control before proceeding with cataract surgery.

SUMMARY

The exfoliation syndrome, a relatively common disorder among older individuals and within certain ethnic populations, is characterized by a protein-like material of the lens, iris, and various other ocular and extraocular structures. It is recognized clinically by the typical appearance of the exfoliative material on the anterior lens capsule. The condition may be unilateral or bilateral, and some cases have associated glaucoma due to the accumulation of the exfoliation material and possibly iris pigment granules in the trabecular meshwork.

The lens may also be associated with glaucoma when it is dislocated, which may occur with trauma or certain inherited disorders, such as Marfan's syndrome, homocystinuria, and the Weill-Marchesani syndrome. Mechanisms by which a dislocated lens may be associated with glaucoma include pupillary block, degenerative changes of the lens, and concomitant damage of the anterior chamber angle.

A cataractous lens may also lead to glaucoma by obstruction of the trabecular meshwork with lens protein and macrophages (phacolytic glaucoma), lens particles and debris (lens particle glaucoma), or inflammatory cells as part of an immune response (phacoanaphylaxis). In addition, an intumescent lens may lead to angle-closure glaucoma.

REFERENCES

1. Lindberg, JG: Clinical investigations on depigmentation of the pupillary border and translucency of the iris. In cases of senile cataract and in normal eyes in elderly persons. Academic Dissertation, Helsinki, 1917. English translation by Tarkkanen, A, Forsius, H. Acta Ophthalmol 66(Suppl 190), Helsinki, University Press, 1989.
2. Elschnig, A: Ablosung der Zonulalamelle bei Glasblasern. Klin Monatsbl Augenheilkd 69:732, 1922.
3. Kraupa, E: Linsenkapselrisse ohne Wundstar. Zeitschrift fur Augenheilkunde 48:93, 1922.
4. Butler, TH: Capsular glaucoma. Trans Ophthalmol Soc UK 68: 575, 1938.
5. Radda, TM, Klemen, UM: Idiopathic true exfoliation. Klin Monatsbl Augenheilkd 181:276, 1982.
6. Brodrick, JD, Tate, GW Jr: Capsular delamination (true exfoliation) of the lens. Report of a case. Arch Ophthalmol 97:1693, 1979.
7. Cashwell, LF Jr, Holleman, IL, Weaver, RG, van Rens GH: Idiopathic true exofoliation of the lens capsule. Ophthalmology 96: 348, 1989.
8. Dvorak-Theobald, G: Pseudo-exfoliation of the lens capsule. Relation to "true" exfoliation of the lens capsule as reported in the literature and role in the production of glaucoma capsulocuticulare. Am J Ophthalmol 37:1, 1954.
9. Vogt, A: Ein neues Spaltlampenbild des Pupillengebietes: Hellblauer Pupillensaumfilz mit Hautchenbildung auf der Linsenvorderkapsel. Klin Monatsbl Augenheilkd 75:1, 1925.
10. Vogt, A: Vergleichende Uebersicht uber Klinik und Histologie der Alters- und Feuerlamelle der Linsenvorderkapsel. Klin Monatsbl Augenheilkd 89:587, 1932.
11. Sunde, OA: Senile exfoliation of the anterior lens capsule. Acta Ophthalmol 45(Suppl):27, 1956.
12. Layden, WE, Shaffer, RN: Exfoliation syndrome. Am J Ophthalmol 78:835, 1974.
13. Tarkkanen, A, Forsius, H, eds: Exfoliation syndrome. Acta Ophthalmol 66(Suppl 184), Copenhagen, Scriptor, 1988.
14. Ohrt, V, Nehen, JH: The incidence of glaucoma capsulare based on a Danish hospital material. Acta Ophthalmol 59:888, 1981.
15. Lindblom, B, Thorburn, W: Observed incidence of glaucoma in Halsingland, Sweden. Acta Ophthalmol 62:217, 1984.
16. Lindblom, B, Thorburn, W: Prevalence of visual field defects due to capsular and simple glaucoma in Halsingland, Sweden. Acta Ophthalmol 60:353, 1982.
17. Ringvold, A, Blika, S, Elsas, T, et al: The prevalence of pseudoexfoliation in three separate municipalities of Middle-Norway. A preliminary report. Acta Ophthalmol 65(Suppl 182):17, 1987.
18. Meyer, E, Haim, T, Zonis, S, et al: Pseudoexfoliation: epidemiology, clinical and scanning electrom microscopic study. Ophthalmologica 188:141, 1984.
19. Cashwell, LF, Shields, MB: Exfoliation syndrome. Prevalence in a southeastern United States population. Arch Ophthalmol 106:335, 1988.
20. Hiller, R, Sperduto, RD, Krueger, DE: Pseudoexfoliation, intraocular pressure, and senile lens changes in a population-based survey. Arch Ophthalmol 100:1080, 1982.
21. Blika, S, Ringvold, A: The occurrence of simple and capsular glaucoma in Middle-Norway. Acta Ophthalmol 65(Suppl 182):11, 1987.
22. Yalaz, M, Othman, I, Nas, K, et al: The frequency of pseudoexfoliation syndrome in the Eastern Mediterranean area of Turkey. Acta Ophthalmol 70:209, 1992.
23. Moreno-Montanes, J, Alvarez Serna, A, Alcolea Paredes, A: Pseudoexfoliative glaucoma in patients with open-angle glaucoma in the Northwest of Spain. Acta Ophthalmol 68:695, 1990.
24. Ball, SF, Graham, S, Thompson, H: The racial prevalence and biomicroscopic signs of exfoliation syndrome in the glaucoma population of southern Louisiana. Glaucoma 11:169, 1989
25. Roth, M, Epstein, DL: Exfoliation syndrome. Am J Ophthalmol 89:477, 1980.
26. Luntz, MH: Prevalence of pseudo-exfoliation syndrome in an urban South African clinic population. Am J Ophthalmol 74:581, 1972.
27. Kozart, DM, Yanoff, M: Intraocular pressure status in 100 consecutive patients with exfoliation syndrome. Ophthalmology 89:214, 1982.
28. Taylor, HR: The environment and the lens. Br J Ophthalmol 64: 303, 1980.
29. Khanzada, AM: Exfoliation syndrome in Pakistan. Pak J Ophthalmol 2:7, 1986.
30. Madden, JG, Crowley, MJ: Factors in the exfoliation syndrome. Br J Ophthalmol 66:432, 1982.
31. Olivius, E, Polland, WP: Histocompatibility (HLA) antigens in capsular glaucoma and simplex glaucoma. Acta Ophthalmol 58:406, 1980.
32. Slagsvold, JE, Nordhagen, R: The HLA system in primary open-angle glaucoma and in patients with pseudoexfoliation of the lens capsule (exfoliation or fibrillopathia epitheliocapsularis). Acta Ophthalmol 58:188, 1980.
33. Ringvold, A, Blika, S, Elsas, T, et al: The Middle-Norway eye-screening study. I. Epidemiology of the pseudo-exfoliation syndrome. Acta Ophthalmol 66:652, 1988.
34. Crittendon, JJ, Shields, MB: Exfoliation syndrome in the southeastern United States. II. Characteristics of patient population and clinical courses. Acta Ophthalmol 66(Suppl 184):103, 1988.
35. Seland, JH, Chylack, LT Jr: Cataracts in the exfoliation syndrome (fibrillopathia epitheliocapsularis). Trans Ophthalmol Soc UK 102:375, 1982.
36. Futa, R, Furoyoshi, N: Phakodonesis in capsular glaucoma: a clinical and electron microscopic study. Jpn J Ophthalmol 33:311, 1989.
37. Freissler, K, Küchle, M, Naumann, GOH: Spontaneous dislocation of the lens in pseudoexfoliation syndrome. Arch Ophthalmol 113:1095, 1995.
38. Prince, AM, Ritch, R: Clinical signs of the pseudoexfoliation syndrome. Ophthalmology 93:803, 1986.
39. Repo, LP, Teräsvirta, ME, Tuovinen, EJ: Generalized peripheral iris transluminance in the pseudoexfoliation syndrome. Ophthalmology 97:1027, 1990.
40. Sakai, K, Kojima, K: Fluorescein angiography and electron microscopic study of the iris with exfoliation syndrome. Folia Ophthalmol Jpn 33:72, 1982.
41. Brooks, AMV, Gillies, WE: The development of microneovascular changes in the iris in pseudoexfoliation of the lens capsule. Ophthalmology 94:1090, 1987.
42. Ringvold, A, Davanger, M: Iris neovascularisation in eyes with pseudoexfoliation syndrome. Br J Ophthalmol 65:138, 1981.
43. Asano, N, Schlötzer-Schrehardt, U, Naumann, GOH: A histopathologic study of iris changes in pseudoexfoliation syndrome. Ophthalmology 102:1279, 1995.

44. Repo, LP, Teräsvirta, ME, Koivisto, KJ: Generalized transluminance of the iris and the frequency of the pseudoexfoliation syndrome in the eyes of transient ischemic attack patients. Ophthalmology 100:352, 1993.

45. Repo, LP, Suhonen, MT, Teräsvirta, ME, Koivisto, KJ: Color doppler imaging of the ophthalmic artery blood flow spectra of patients who have had a transient ischemic attack. Ophthalmology 102:1199, 1995.

46. Sugar, HS: Onset of the exfoliation syndrome after intracapsular lens extraction. Am J Ophthalmol 89:601, 1980.

47. Ringvold, A, Bore J: Pseudo-exfoliation pattern on posterior IOL. Acta Ophthalmol 68:353, 1990.

48. Miyake, K, Matsuda, M, Inaba, M: Corneal endothelial changes in pseudoexfoliation syndrome. Am J Ophthalmol 108:49, 1989.

49. Knorr, HLJ, Jünemann, A, Händel, A, Naumann, GOH: Morphometric and qualitative changes of the corneal endothelium in pseudoexfoliation syndrome. Fortschr Ophthalmol 88:786, 1991.

50. Schlötzer-Schrehardt, UM, Dörfler, S, Naumann, GOH: Corneal endothelial involvement in pseudoexfoliation syndrome. Arch Ophthalmol 111:666, 1993.

51. Kuchle, M, Nguyen, NX, Horn, F, Naumann, GOH: Quantitative assessment of aqueous flare and aqueous "cells" in pseudoexfoliation syndrome. Acta Ophthalmol 70:201, 1992.

52. Wishart, PK, Spaeth, GL, Poryzees, EM: Anterior chamber angle in the exfoliation syndrome. Br J Ophthalmol 69:103, 1985.

53. Bartholomew, RS: Anterior chamber depth in eyes with pseudoexfoliation. Br J Ophthalmol 64:322, 1980.

54. Ritch, R: Exfoliation syndrome and occludable angles. Trans Am Ophthalmol Soc 92:845, 1994.

55. Gross, FJ, Tingey, D, Epstein, DL: Increased prevalence of occludable angles and angle-closure glaucoma in patients with pseudoexfoliation. Am J Ophthalmol 117:333, 1994.

56. Mizuno, K, Muroi, S: Cycloscopy of pseudoexfoliation. Am J Ophthalmol 87:513, 1979.

57. Sugar, S: Pigmentary glaucoma and the glaucoma associated with the exfoliation-pseudoexfoliation syndrome: update. Ophthalmology 91:307, 1984.

58. Brooks, AMV, Gillies, WE: The presentation and prognosis of glaucoma in pseudoexfoliation of the lens capsule. Ophthalmology 95:271, 1988.

59. Slagsvold, JE: The follow-up in patients with pseudoexfoliation of the lens capsule with and without glaucoma. 2. The development of glaucoma in persons with pseudoexfoliation. Acta Ophthalmol 64:241, 1986.

60. Gillies, WE, Brooks, AMV: The presentation of acute glaucoma in pseudoexfoliation of the lens capsule. Aust NZ J Ophthalmol 16:101, 1988.

61. Lindblom, B, Thorburn, W: Functional damage at diagnosis of primary open-angle glaucoma. Acta Ophthalmol 62:223, 1984.

62. Futa, R, Shimizu, T, Furuyoshi, N, et al: Clinical features of capsular glaucoma in comparison with primary open-angle glaucoma in Japan. Acta Ophthalmol 70:214, 1992.

63. Olivius, E, Thorburn, W: Prognosis of glaucoma simplex and glaucoma capsulare. A comparative study Acta Ophthalmol 56:921, 1978.

64. Davanger, M, Ringvold, A, Blika, S: Pseudo-exfoliation, IOP and glaucoma. Acta Ophthalmol 69:569, 1991.

65. Puska, P, Raitta, C: Exfoliation syndrome as a risk factor for optic disc changes in nonglaucomatous eyes. Graefes Arch Clin Exp Ophthalmol 230:501, 1992.

66. Tezel, G, Tezel, TH: The comparative analysis of optic disc damage in exfoliative glaucoma. Acta Ophthalmol 71:744, 1993.

67. Netland, PA, Ye, H, Streeten, BW, Hernandez, MR: Elastosis of the lamina cribrosa in pseudoexfoliation syndrome with glaucoma. Ophthalmology 102:878, 1995.

68. Dark, AJ, Streeten, BW, Cornwall, CC: Pseudoexfoliative disease of the lens: a study in electron microscopy and histochemistry. Br J Ophthalmol 61:462, 1977.

69. Davanger, M: The pseudo-exfoliation syndrome. A scanning electron microscopic study. I. The anterior lens surface. Acta Ophthalmol 53:809, 1975.

70. Garner, A, Alexander, RA: Pseudoexfoliative disease: histochemical evidence of an affinity with zonular fibres. Br J Ophthalmol 68:574, 1984.

71. Streeten, BW, Dark, AJ, Barnes, CW: Pseudoexfoliative material and oxytalan fibers. Exp Eye Res 38:523, 1984.

72. Streeten, BW, Bookman, L, Ritch, R, et al: Pseudoexfoliative fibrillopathy in the conjunctiva. A relation to elastic fibers and elastosis. Ophthalmology 94:1439, 1987.

73. Li, Z-Y, Streeten, BW, Wallace, RN: Association of elastin with pseudoexfoliative material: an immunoelectron microscopic study. Cur Eye Res 7:1163, 1988.

74. Eagle, RC Jr, Font, RL, Fine, BS: The basement membrane exfoliation syndrome. Arch Ophthalmol 97:510, 1979.

75. Bertelsen, TI, Drablos, PA, Flood, PR: The so-called senile exfoliation (pseudoexfoliation) of the anterior lens capsule. A product of the lens epithelium. Fibrillopathia epitheliocapsularis. A microscopic, histochemical and electron microscopic investigation. Acta Ophthalmol 42:1096, 1964.

76. Harnisch, JP, Barrach, HJ, Hassell, JR, Sinha, PK: Identification of a basement membrane proteoglycan in exfoliation material. Graefes Arch Clin Exp Ophthalmol 215:273, 1981.

77. Schlötzer-Schrehardt, UM, Dörfler, S, Naumann, GOH: Immunohistochemical localization of basement membrane components in pseudoexfoliation material of the lens capsule. Curr Eye Res 11:343, 1992.

78. Konstas, AG, Marshall, GE, Lee, WR: Immunogold localisation of laminin in normal and exfoliative iris. Br J Ophthalmol 74:450, 1990.

79. Davanger, M, Pedersen, OO: Pseudo-exfoliation material on the anterior lens surface. Demonstration and examination of an interfibrillar ground substance. Acta Ophthalmol 53:3, 1975.

80. Baba, H: Histochemical and polarization optical investigation for glycosaminoglycans in exfoliation syndrome. Graefes Arch Clin Exp Ophthalmol 221:106, 1983.

81. Ringvold, A, Husby, G: Pseudo-exfoliation material—an amyloid-like substance. Exp Eye Res 17:289, 1973.

82. Tsukahara, S, Matsuo, T: Secondary glaucoma accompanied with primary familial amyloidosis. Ophthalmologica 175:250, 1977.

83. Schwartz, MF, Green, RW, Michels, RG, et al: An unusual case of ocular involvement in primary systemic nonfamilial amyloidosis. Ophthalmology 89:394, 1982.

84. Li, Z-Y, Streeten, BW, Yohai, N: Amyloid P protein in pseudoexfoliative fibrillopathy. Cur Eye Res. 8:217, 1989.

85. Benedikt, O, Aubock, L, Gottinger, W, Waltinger, H: Comparative transmission and scanning electronmicroscopical studies on lenses in so-called exfoliation syndrome. Graefes Arch Clin Exp Ophthalmol 187:249, 1973.

86. Seland, JH: The ultrastructure of the deep layer of the lens capsule in fibrillopathia epitheliocapsularis (FEC), so-called senile exfoliation or pseudoexfoliation. A scanning electron microscopic study. Acta Ophthalmol 56:335, 1978.

87. Seland, JH: Histopathology of the lens capsule in fibrillopathia epitheliocapsularis (FEC) or so-called senile exfoliation or pseudoexfoliation. An electron microscopic study. Acta Ophthalmol 57:477, 1979.

88. Dark, AJ, Streeten, BW, Jones, D: Accumulation of fibrillar protein in the aging human lens capsule. With special reference to the pathogenesis of pseudoexfoliative disease of the lens. Arch Ophthalmol 82:815, 1969.

89. Bergmanson, JPG, Jones, WL, Chu, LW-F: Ultrastructural observations on (pseudo-) exfoliation of the lens capsule: a re-examination of the involvement of the lens epithelium. Br J Ophthalmol 68:118, 1984.

90. Dark, AJ, Streeten, BW: Precapsular film on the aging human lens: precursor of pseudoexfoliation? Br J Ophthalmol 74:717, 1990.

91. Tetsumoto, K, Schlötzer-Schrehardt, U, Küchle, M, et al: Precapsular layer of the anterior lens capsule in early pseudoexfoliation syndrome. Graefes Arch Clin Exp Ophthalmolmol 230:252, 1992.

92. Ghosh, M, Speakman, JS: The iris in senile exfoliation of the lens. Can J Ophthalmol 9:289, 1974.

93. Konstas, AGP, Marshall, GE, Cameron, SA, Lee, WR: Morphology of iris vasculopathy in exfoliation glaucoma. Acta Ophthalmol 71:751, 1993.

94. Shimizu, T: Changes of iris vessels in capsular glaucoma: three-dimensional and electron microscopic studies. Jpn J Ophthalmol 29:434, 1985.

95. Shimizu, T, Futa, R: The fine structure of pigment epithelium of the iris in capsular glaucoma. Graefes Arch Clin Exp Ophthalmol 223:77, 1985.

96. Radian, AB, Radian, AL: Senile pseudoexfoliation in aphakic eyes. Br J Ophthalmol 59:577, 1975.

97. Caccamise, WC: The exfoliation syndrome in the aphakic eye. Am J Ophthalmol 91:111, 1981.

98. Ghosh, M, Speakman, JS: The ciliary body in senile exfoliation of the lens. Can J Ophthalmol 8:394, 1973.

99. Speakman, JS, Ghosh, M: The conjunctiva in senile lens exfoliation. Arch Ophthalmol 94:1757, 1976.

100. Roh, YB, Ishibashi, T, Ito, N, Inomata, H: Alteration of microfibrils in the conjunctiva of patients with exfoliation syndrome. Arch Ophthalmol 105:978, 1987.

101. Prince, AM, Streeten, BW, Ritch, R, et al: Preclinical diagnosis of pseudoexfoliation syndrome. Arch Ophthalmol 105:1076, 1987.

102. Küchle, M, Schlötzer-Schrehardt, U, Naumann, GOH: Occurrence of pseudoexfoliative material in parabulbar structures in pseudoexfoliation syndrome. Acta Ophthalmol 69:124, 1991.

103. Schlötzer-Schrehardt, U, Küchle, M, Naumann, GOH: Electron-microscopic identification of pseudoexfoliation material in extrabulbar tissue. Arch Ophthalmol 109:565, 1991.

104. Ringvold, A, Davanger, M: Notes on the distribution of pseudoexfoliation material with particular reference to the uveoscleral route of aqueous humour. Acta Ophthalmol 55:807, 1977.

105. Schlötzer-Schrehardt, Koca, MR, M, Naumann, GOH, Volkholz, H: Pseudoexfoliation syndrome. Ocular manifestation of a systemic disorder? Arch Ophthalmol 110:1752, 1992.

106. Streeten, BW, Li, Z-Y, Wallace, RN, et al: Pseudoexfoliative fibrillopathy in visceral organs of a patient with pseudoexfoliation syndrome. Arch Ophthalmol 110:1757, 1992.

107. Sampaolesi, R, Argento, C: Scanning electron microscopy of the trabecular meshwork in normal and glaucomatous eyes. Invest Ophthalmol Vis Sci 16:302, 1977.

108. Rodrigues, MM, Spaeth, GL, Sivalingam, E, Weinreb, S: Value of trabeculectomy specimens in glaucoma. Ophthalmic Surg 9:29, 1978.

109. Benedikt, O, Roll, P: The trabecular meshwork of a non-glaucomatous eye with the exfoliation syndrome. Electronmicroscopic study. Virchows Arch A Path Anat Histol 384:347, 1979.

110. Schlötzer-Schrehardt, M, Naumann, GOH: Trabecular meshwork in pseudoexfoliation syndrome with and without open-angle glaucoma. A morphometric, ultrastructural study. Invest Ophthalmol Vis Sci 36:1750, 1995.

111. Cebon, L, Smith, RJH: Pseudoexfoliation of lens capsule and glaucoma. Case report. Br J Ophthalmol 60:279, 1976.

112. Aasved, H: Intraocular pressure in eyes with and without fibrillopathia epitheliocapsularis (so-called senile exfoliation or pseudoexfoliation). Acta Ophthalmol 49:601, 1971.

113. Pohjola, S, Horsmanheimo, A: Topically applied corticosteroids in glaucoma capsulare. Arch Ophthalmol 85:150, 1971.

114. Gillies, WE: Corticosteroid-induced ocular hypertension in pseudoexfoliation of lens capsule. Am J Ophthalmol 70:90, 1970.

115. Silva-Araújo, AC, Tavares, MA, Cotta, JS, Castro-Correia, JF: Aqueous outflow system in familial amyloidotic polyneuropathy, Portuguese type. Graefes Arch Clin Exp Ophthalmol 231:131, 1993.

116. Layden, WE, Ritch, R, King, DG, Teekhasaenee, C: Combined exfoliation and pigment dispersion syndrome. Am J Ophthalmol 109:530, 1990.

117. Konstas, AGP, Jay, JL, Marshall, GE, Lee, WR: Prevalence, diagnostic features, and response to trabeculectomy in exfoliation glaucoma. Ophthalmology 100:619, 1993.

118. Gillies, WE: Effect of lens extraction in pseudoexfoliation of the lens capsule. Br J Ophthalmol 57:46, 1973.

119. Jacobi, PC, Kreiglstein, GK: Trabecular aspiration. A new mode to treat pseudoexfoliation glaucoma. Invest Ophthalmol Vis Sci 36:2270, 1995.

120. Skuta, GL, Parrish, RK II, Hodapp, E, et al: Zonular dialysis during extracapsular cataract extraction in pseudoexfoliation syndrome. Arch Ophthalmol 105:632, 1987.

121. Raitta, C, Tarkkanen, A: Posterior chamber lens implantation in capsular glaucoma. Acta Ophthalmol 65(Suppl 182):24, 1987.

122. Hovding, G: The association between fibrillopathy and posterior capsular/zonular breaks during extracapsular cataract extraction and posterior chamber IOL implantation. Acta Ophthalmol 66:662, 1988.

123. Zetterström, C, Olivestedt, G, Lundvall, A: Exfoliation syndrome and extracapsular cataract extraction with implantation of posterior chamber lens. Acta Ophthalmol 70:85, 1992.

124. Lumme, P, Laatikainen, L: Exfoliation syndrome and cataract extraction. Am J Ophthalmol 116:51, 1993.

125. Chijiiwa, T, Araki, H, Ishibashi, T, Inomata, H: Degeneration of zonular fibrils in a case of exfoliation glaucoma. Ophthalmologica 199:16, 1989.

126. Ruotsalainen, J, Tarkkanen, A: Capsule thickness of cataractous lenses with and without exfoliation syndrome. Acta Ophthalmol 65:444, 1987.

127. Carpel, EF: Pupillary dilation in eyes with pseudoexfoliation syndrome. Am J Ophthalmol 105:692, 1988.

128. Dark, AJ: Cataract extraction complicated by capsular glaucoma. Br J Ophthalmol 63:465, 1979.

129. Drolsum, L, Haaskjold, E, Davanger, M: Results and complications after extracapsular cataract extraction in eyes with pseudoexfoliation syndrome. Acta Ophthalmol 71:771, 1993.

130. Zetterström, C, Lundvall, A, Olivestedt, G: Exfoliation syndrome and heparin surface modified intraocular lenses. Acta Ophthalmol 70:91, 1992.

131. Chandler, PA: Choice of treatment in dislocation of the lens. Arch Ophthalmol 71:765, 1964.

132. Jarrett, WH: Dislocation of the lens. A study of 166 hospitalized cases. Arch Ophthalmol 78:289, 1967.

133. Luebbers, JA, Goldberg, MF, Herbst, R, et al: Iris transillumination and variable expression in ectopia lentis et pupillae. Am J Ophthalmol 83:647, 1977.

134. Nelson, LB, Maumenee, IH: Ectopia lentis. Surv Ophthalmol 27:143, 1982.

135. Townes, PL: Ectopia lentis et pupillae. Arch Ophthalmol 94:1126, 1976.

136. Goldberg, MF: Clinical manifestations of ectopia lentis et pupillae in 16 patients. Ophthalmology 95:1080, 1988.

137. Cross, HE, Jensen, AD: Ocular manifestations in the Marfan syndrome and homocystinuria. Am J Ophthalmol 75:405, 1973.

138. Tsipouras, P, Del Mastro, R, Sarfarazi, M, et al: Genetic linkage of the Marfan syndrome, ectopia lentis, and congenital contractural arachnodactyly to the fibrillin genes on chromosomes 15 and 5. N Engl J Med 326:905, 1992.

139. Maumenee, IH: The eye in the Marfan syndrome. Trans Am Ophthalmol Soc 79:684, 1981.

140. Izquierdo, NJ, Traboulsi, EI, Enger, C, Maumenee, IH: Glaucoma in the Marfan syndrome. Trans Am Ophthalmol Soc 90:111, 1992.

141. Burke, JP, O'Keefe, M, Bowell, R, Naughten, ER: Ocular complications in homocystinuria—early and late treated. Br J Ophthalmol 73:427, 1989.

142. Jensen, AD, Cross, HE, Patton, D: Ocular complications in the Weill-Marchesani syndrome. Am J Ophthalmol 77:261, 1974.

143. Fujiwara, H, Takigawa, Y, Ueno, S, Okuda, K: Histology of the lens in the Weill-Marchesani syndrome. Br J Ophthalmol 74:631, 1990.

144. Willi, M, Kut, L, Cotlier, E: Pupillary-block glaucoma in the Marchesani syndrome. Arch Ophthalmol 90:504, 1973.

145. Ritch, R, Wand, M: Treatment of the Weill-Marchesani Syndrome. Ann Ophthalmol 13:665, 1981.

146. Wright, KW, Chrousos, GA: Weill-Marchesani syndrome with bilateral angle-closure glaucoma. J Ped Ophthalmol Strabismus 22:129, 1985.

147. Ritch, R, Solomon, LD: Argon laser peripheral iridoplasty for angle-closure glaucoma in siblings with Weill-Marchesani syndrome. J Glau 1:243, 1992.

148. Smith, TH, Holland, MG, Woody, NC: Ocular manifestations of familial hyperlysinemia. Trans Am Acad Ophthalmol Otol 75:355, 1971.

149. Shih, VE, Abroms, IF, Johnson, JL, et al: Sulfite oxidase deficiency. Biochemical and clinical investigations of a hereditary metabolic disorder in sulfur metabolism. N Engl J Med 297:1022, 1977.

150. David, R, MacBeath, L, Jenkins, T: Aniridia associated with microcornea and subluxated lenses. Br J Ophthalmol 62:118, 1978.

151. Hein, HF, Maltzman, B: Long-standing anterior dislocation of the crystalline lens. Ann Ophthalmol 7:66, 1975.

152. Pollard, ZF: Phacolytic glaucoma secondary to ectopia lentis. Ann Ophthalmol 7:999, 1975.

153. Friberg, TR: Retinal perivasculitis in phacolytic glaucoma. Am J Ophthalmol 91:761, 1981.

154. Jay, B: Glaucoma associated with spontaneous displacement of the lens. Br J Ophthalmol 56:258, 1972.

155. Johnson, GJ, Bosanquet, RC: Spherophakia in a Newfoundland family: 8 years experience. Can J Ophthalmol 18:159, 1983.

156. Chandler, PA: Completely dislocated hypermature cataract and glaucoma. Trans Am Ophthalmol Soc 57:242, 1959.

157. Treister, G, Machemer, R: Pars plana surgical approach for various anterior segment problems. Arch Ophthalmol 97:909, 1979.

158. Gifford, H: Danger of the spontaneous cure of senile cataracts. Am J Ophthalmol 17:289, 1900.

159. Zeeman, WPC: Zwei Falle von Glaucoma phacogeneticum mit anatomischem Befund. Ophthalmologica 106:136, 1943.

160. Irvine, SR, Irvine, AR Jr: Lens-induced uveitis and glaucoma. Part III. "Phacogenetic glaucoma": lens-induced glaucoma; mature or hypermature cataract; open iridocorneal angle. Am J Ophthalmol 35:489, 1952.

161. Flocks, M, Littwin, CS, Zimmerman, LE: Phacolytic glaucoma. A clinicopathologic study of one hundred thirty-eight cases of glaucoma associated with hypermature cataract. Arch Ophthalmol 54:37, 1955.

162. Epstein, DL, Jedziniak, JA, Grant, WM: Obstruction of aqueous outflow by lens particles and by heavy-molecular-weight soluble lens proteins. Invest Ophthalmol Vis Sci 17:272, 1978.

163. Epstein, DL, Jedziniak, JA, Grant, WM: Identification of heavy-molecular-weight soluble protein in aqueous humor in human phacolytic glaucoma. Invest Ophthalmol Vis Sci 17:398, 1978.

164. Epstein, DL: Diagnosis and management of lens-induced glaucoma. Ophthalmology 89:227, 1982.

165. Bartholomew, RS, Rebello, PF: Calcium oxalate crystals in the aqueous. Am J Ophthalmol 88:1026, 1979.

166. Brooks, AMV, Grant, G, Gillies, WE: Comparison of specular microscopy and examination of aspirate in phacolytic glaucoma. Ophthalmology 97:85, 1990.

167. Brooks, AMV, Drewe, RH, Grant, GB, et al: Crystalline nature of the iridescent particles in hypermature cataracts. Br J Ophthalmol 78:581, 1994.

168. Goldberg, MF: Cytological diagnosis of phacolytic glaucoma utilizing Millipore filtration of the aqueous. Br J Ophthalmol 51:847, 1967.

169. Tomita, G, Watanabe, K, Funahashi, M, et al: Lens induced glaucoma—histopathological study of the filtrating angle. Folia Ophthalmol Jpn 35:1345, 1984.

170. Ueno, H, Tamai, A, Iyota, K, Moriki, T: Electron microscopic observation of the cells floating in the anterior chamber in a case of phacolytic glaucoma. Jpn J Ophthalmol 33:103, 1989.

171. Yanoff, M, Scheie, HG: Cytology of human lens aspirate. Its relationship to phacolytic glaucoma and phacoanaphylactic endophthalmitis. Arch Ophthalmol 80:166, 1968.

172. Jedziniak, JA, Kinoshita, JH, Yates, EM, et al: On the presence and mechanism of formation of heavy molecular weight aggregates in human normal and cataractous lenses. Exp Eye Res 15:185, 1973.

173. Spector, A, Li, S, Sigelman, J: Age-dependent changes in the molecular size of human lens proteins and their relationship to light scatter. Invest Ophthalmol 13:795, 1974.

174. Jedzinisk, JA, Nicoli, DF, Baram, H, Benedek, GB: Quantitative verification of the existence of high molecular weight protein aggregates in the intact normal human lens by light-scattering spectroscopy. Invest Ophthalmol Vis Sci 17:51, 1978.

175. Chandler, PA: Problems in the diagnosis and treatment of lens-induced uveitis and glaucoma. Arch Ophthalmol 60:828, 1958.

176. Volcker, HE, Naumann, G: Clinical findings in phakolytic glaucoma. Klin Monatsbl Augenheilkd 166:613, 1975.

177. Lane, SS, Kopietz, LA, Lindquist, TD, Leavenworth, N: Treatment of phacolytic glaucoma with extracapsular cataract extraction. Ophthalmology 95:749, 1988.

178. Muller, H: Phacolytic glaucoma and phacogenic ophthalmia (lens-induced uveitis). Trans Ophthalmol Soc UK 83:689, 1963.

179. Verhoeff, FH, Lemoine, AN: Endophthalmitis phacoanaphylactica. Trans Int Cong Ophthal, Wash, DC. Philadelphia, William F Fell, 1922, p. 234.

180. Rahi, AHS, Misra, RN, Morgan, G: Immunopathology of the lens. III. Humoral and cellular immune responses to autologous lens antigens and their roles in ocular inflammation. Br J Ophthalmol 61:371, 1977.

181. Perlman, EM, Albert, DM: Clinically unsuspected phacoanaphylaxis after ocular trauma. Arch Ophthalmol 95:244, 1977.

182. Nissen, SH, Andersen, P, Andersen, HMK: Antibodies to lens antigens in cataract and after cataract surgery. Br J Ophthalmol 65:63, 1981.

183. Duke-Elder, S: System of Ophthalmology. Vol II. London, Henry Kimpton Publishers, 1969, p. 662.

184. Tomey, KF, Al-Rajhi, AA: Neodymium:YAG laser iridotomy in the initial management of phacomorphic glaucoma. Ophthalmology 99:660, 1992.

Chapter 16

GLAUCOMAS ASSOCIATED WITH DISORDERS OF THE RETINA, VITREOUS, AND CHOROID

Several types of glaucoma are associated with diseases of the retina. The most common of these is neovascular glaucoma, which is usually associated with one of several retinal disorders, although some cases are associated with other ocular or extraocular conditions. In addition, retinal detachments and a variety of less common disorders of the retina, vitreous, or choroid may cause or occur in association with various forms of glaucoma.

NEOVASCULAR GLAUCOMA[a]

Terminology

In 1906, Coats (1) described new vessel formation on the iris in eyes with central retinal vein occlusion. This neovascu-

larization of the iris is commonly known as *rubeosis iridis* and is now recognized as a complication of many diseases of the retina and other ocular and extraocular disorders. Rubeosis iridis is frequently associated with a severe form of glaucoma, which has been given several different names on the basis of various clinical features: "hemorrhagic glaucoma," referring to the hyphema that is present in some cases, "congestive glaucoma," describing the frequently acute nature of the condition, and "thrombotic glaucoma," implying an underlying vascular thrombotic etiology. However, none of these terms accurately describes the glaucoma in all cases and more nonspecific names are preferable, such as *rubeotic glaucoma* (2), or *neovascular glaucoma* (which

[a]Refer to Shields, MB: Color Atlas of Glaucoma. Baltimore, Williams & Wilkins, 1998, Plates II25–26.

was proposed by Weiss and coworkers (3) and is found most often in current literature).

Factors Predisposing to Rubeosis Iridis

Most cases of rubeosis iridis are preceded by an hypoxic disease of the retina. Diabetic retinopathy and occlusion of major retinal vessels account for over half of these with the former possibly being slightly more common (4, 5). However, many additional retinal diseases, as well as certain other ocular or extraocular disorders, have now been recognized, resulting in a long list of conditions which may predispose to the development of rubeosis iridis (Table 16.1).

Diabetic Retinopathy

Approximately one-third of the patients with rubeosis iridis have diabetic retinopathy (4, 5). The frequency with which this condition occurs in association with diabetic retino-

Table 16.1.
FACTORS PREDISPOSING TO RUBEOSIS IRIDIS AND NEOVASCULAR GLAUCOMA

Diabetic retinopathy
Retinal vascular occlusive disorders
    Central retinal vein occlusion
    Central retinal artery occlusion (32, 33)
    Branch retinal vein occlusion (36)
    Branch retinal artery occlusion (32, 37)
Other retinal disorders
    Retinal detachment
    Choroidal melanoma
    Retinoblastoma (42)
    Hemorrhagic retinal disorders
    Coat's exudative retinopathy
    Retinopathy of prematurity
    Sickle cell retinopathy (40, 41)
    Syphilitic retinal vasculitis (43)
    Retinoschisis (44)
    Stickler's syndrome (inherited vitreoretinal degeneration) (45)
    Optic nerve glioma with subsequent venous stasis retinopathy (46)
    Photoradiation (47) and helium ion irradiation (48) for uveal melanoma
Other ocular disorders
    Uveitis
    Intraocular lens implantation (49)
    Iris melanoma (50)
Extraocular vascular disorders
    Carotid artery obstructive disease (51)
    Carotid-cavernous fistula (52, 53)
    Internal carotid artery occlusion (54)

Modified from Hoskins, HD Jr: Neovascular glaucoma: current concepts. Trans Am Acad Ophthal Otol 78:330, 1974, and Brown, GC, Magargal, LE, Schachat, A, Shah, H: Neovascular glaucoma: etiologic considerations. Ophthalmology 91:315, 1984.

pathy is greatly influenced by surgical interventions. Following pars plana vitrectomy for diabetic retinopathy, the reported incidence of rubeosis iridis ranges from 25% to 42%, while neovascular glaucoma ranges from 10% to 23% (6–10) with most of these developing during the first 6 months after surgery (11). In these cases, the occurrence of rubeosis iridis and neovascular glaucoma are much higher in aphakic eyes (9, 10, 12–16). In one series, vitreous cavity lavage of hemorrhage following pars plana vitrectomy for diabetic retinopathy was associated with rubeosis iridis in 76% of aphakic eyes and 14% of phakic eyes (16). Postoperative neovascular glaucoma is also more common when rubeosis iridis is present before the vitrectomy (17).

An unrepaired retinal detachment following vitrectomy for diabetic retinopathy is also a risk factor for postoperative rubeosis iridis. The acute onset or exacerbation of rubeosis iridis after diabetic vitrectomy can indicate the presence of a peripheral traction retinal detachment (18). Successful surgical reattachment of the retina during vitrectomy for diabetic retinopathy often leads to regression of preoperative rubeosis iridis, especially when the lens is retained (19). A completely attached retina and aggressive anterior/peripheral coagulation therapy have been shown to be the most important factors in controlling (18) or preventing (20) neovascular glaucoma after vitrectomy for proliferative diabetic retinopathy. Intraocular silicone oil also reduces the incidence of anterior segment neovascularization, possibly by acting as a diffusion/convection barrier to the posterior movement of oxygen from the anterior chamber (21), or the anterior movement of an angiogenesis factor.

Intracapsular cataract surgery alone in eyes with diabetic retinopathy was also associated with an increased incidence of postoperative rubeosis iridis and neovascular glaucoma (22). The incidence is similar with extracapsular extraction and a primary capsulotomy (23). Leaving the posterior capsule intact appears to prevent this complication (23), although a subsequent laser capsulotomy in diabetic patients may lead to neovascular glaucoma (24).

Retinal Vascular Occlusive Disorders

Central retinal vein occlusion accounted for 28% of all rubeosis iridis in one series (4). Elevated intraocular pressure (IOP), with or without glaucomatous damage, is felt by most (25–27), but not all (28), investigators to be a predisposing factor for the development of retinal vein occlusion. Other risk factors for central or branch retinal vein occlusion include systemic hypertension, diabetes, and male gender (27–30). Retinal vein occlusion may occur in a wide range of ages (14–92 years in one large study, although 51% of these patients were 65 years or older (31)).

Rubeosis iridis and neovascular glaucoma may also be associated with *central retinal artery occlusion,* although less commonly than with central vein occlusion (32). In two series of patients with central retinal artery occlusion, the incidence of rubeosis iridis was 16.67% (33) and 18.2% (34).

Patients who develop neovascular glaucoma in association with central retinal artery occlusion are usually elderly with severe carotid artery disease and atherosclerosis, which may be predisposing factors for development of the retinal artery occlusion (35), as well as, in some cases, the ocular neovascularization (32). *Branch retinal vein occlusion* may rarely cause rubeosis iridis (4) and neovascular glaucoma (36). *Branch retinal artery occlusion* has also been reported as a rare cause of rubeosis iridis (32, 37), although the association with neovascular glaucoma is uncertain.

Other Retinal Disorders

Rubeosis iridis may be associated with a *rhegmatogenous retinal detachment* (38), especially when complicated by proliferative vitreoretinopathy (39). In some cases, the detachment may overlie a *choroidal melanoma,* and a chronic retinal detachment with glaucoma should always raise the suspicion of melanoma. Neovascular glaucoma may also be associated with sickle-cell retinopathy (40, 41) and many other retinal disorders which are listed in Table 16.1 (42–48).

Other Ocular Disorders

Uveitis was present in 11% of rubeotic eyes in one series (4) and in 1.5% of another study (5). One case has been reported in which neovascular glaucoma followed implantation of a posterior chamber intraocular lens (49). An iris melanoma has also been associated with neovascular glaucoma, which resolved after the tumor was excised (50). End stage glaucoma (open-angle or angle-closure) has been said to give rise to rubeosis iridis (4), which may be related to associated central retinal vein occlusion.

Extraocular Vascular Disorders

Carotid artery obstructive disease is probably the third most common cause of neovascular glaucoma, accounting for 13% of all cases in one series (5). These eyes may initially be normotensive or even hypotensive due to decreased perfusion of the ciliary body with reduced aqueous production, and fluorescein angiography may reveal an increased arm-to-retina time and leakage from the major retinal arterioles (51). A *carotid-cavernous fistula* may also cause rubeosis iridis and neovascular glaucoma as a result of decreased arterial flow and subsequent reduction in the ocular perfusion pressure, which may occur either before or after treatment of the fistula (52, 53). It has also been reported that internal carotid artery occlusion may create an "ophthalmic artery steal phenomenon" with associated rubeosis iridis (54).

Theories of Neovasculogenesis

The mechanism(s) by which the aforementioned clinical situations lead to the development of rubeosis iridis is not

fully understood, although the following theories have been proposed.

Retinal Hypoxia

Since most, but not all, of the conditions associated with rubeosis iridis involve diminished perfusion of the retina, it may be that retinal hypoxia is at least one factor in the formation of new vessels on the iris and anterior chamber angle, as well as on the retina and optic nerve head (55). This concept is supported by the clinical observation that rubeosis iridis in association with either proliferative diabetic retinopathy (56) or central retinal vein occlusion (57) is more likely to occur when significant capillary nonperfusion is present.

Angiogenesis Factors

It has been demonstrated that tumors possess a diffusible factor, "tumor angiogenesis factor," that is capable of eliciting new vessel growth toward the tumor (58). Subsequent studies have suggested that human and animal retina, as well as other vascular ocular tissues, have similar angiogenic activity, which may explain why ocular neovascularization can occur in areas remote from the site of retinal capillary nonperfusion (59–61). Tissue culture studies have revealed vasoproliferative activity in the aqueous and vitreous of human eyes with neovascular glaucoma or proliferative diabetic retinopathy, and in animal models of neovascularization, but not in fluids from normal eyes (62). The exact nature of this angiogenic factor is unknown. It was characterized in one study as diffusible, heat-labile, and noninflammatory (60), and possibilities that have been considered regarding the identity of this substance include lactic acid (63), biogenic amines (64), and prostaglandins (65). More recently it has been suggested that the angiogenic peptide, vascular endothelial growth factor (VEGF), mediates retinal ischemia-associated ocular neovascularization, and neutralizing anti-VEGF antibodies prevented iris neovascularization in a nonhuman primate model of retinal vein occlusion (66).

Chronic Dilatation of Ocular Vessels

It has also been proposed that dilatation of vessels is the stimulus that leads to new vessel growth in response to hypoxia, or any other factor that causes a vessel to dilate (67, 68). According to this theory, rubeosis iridis results from local hypoxia of the iris, which causes dilatation of iris vessels and subsequent new vessel formation.

Vasoinhibitory Factors

It has also been postulated that ocular tissues may produce substances that inhibit neovascularization. The vitreous (69) and lens (70) have been suggested as possible sources of these vasoinhibitory factors, which could explain why vitrectomy or lensectomy increases the risk of rubeosis iridis in eyes with diabetic retinopathy. More recently, retinal pigment epithelial cells have been shown to release an inhibitor of neovascularization (71).

Clinicopathologic Course

The clinical and histologic events that lead from a predisposing factor, through rubeosis iridis, to advanced neovascular glaucoma may be thought of in these four stages (Fig. 16.1):

Prerubeosis Stage

In patients with a predisposing factor such as diabetic retinopathy or central retinal vein occlusion, it is helpful to understand what the likelihood is for developing rubeosis iridis and what the chances are that this may progress to neovascular glaucoma. There are additional circumstances, especially with the two noted predisposing factors, that may increase the risk of neovascular glaucoma to the extent that treatment may be indicated even before rubeosis is detected.

DIABETIC RETINOPATHY. The prevalence of rubeosis iridis among patients with diabetes mellitus ranges from 0.25% to 20% according to various reports (72). The diabetes will generally have been present for many years before rubeosis develops and concomitant proliferative diabetic retinopathy is usually found. In populations of patients with proliferative diabetic retinopathy, rubeosis iridis is reported to occur in approximately half of the cases (72, 73). Rubeosis iridis may also rarely occur in an eye with nonproliferative retinopathy (72), although other predisposing factors, such as carotid artery disease, should be considered in these cases.

As previously discussed, the risk of rubeosis iridis and neovascular glaucoma in patients with diabetic retinopathy is greatly increased when arteriolar or capillary nonperfusion is present (56) or following vitrectomy or lensectomy (6–16). There is also a highly significant correlation between rubeosis iridis and optic disc neovascularization (74), as well as a rhegmatogenous retinal detachment (19, 20). The demonstration of peripupillary leakage by iris fluorescein angiography correlates with the presence of abnormal iris vessels and the risk of developing rubeosis iridis following vitrectomy for diabetic retinopathy (Fig. 16.2) (75–78). Slitlamp biomicroscopy was shown to be less reliable than angiography in detecting the presence of diabetic iris lesions (78). In looking for the earliest biomicroscopic evidence of anterior segment rubeosis, it is important to pay close attention to the pupillary margin of the iris, where neovascularization is typically seen first (79). However, gonioscopy is also important, since angle neovascularization may occasionally precede that of the iris (80).

CENTRAL RETINAL VEIN OCCLUSION. During the early months after a central retinal vein occlusion, hypotony may develop (81, 82). The explanation for this is unclear, although the possible influences of anterior segment ischemia, or an angiogenic factor have been considered (81, 82).

As in diabetic retinopathy, the incidence of rubeosis iridis and neovascular glaucoma in eyes with central retinal vein occlusion is significantly correlated with the extent of retinal capillary nonperfusion (57, 83–86). In one study, the incidence of rubeosis iridis following central retinal vein occlusion was 60% when retinal ischemia was demonstrated by fluorescein angiography, compared to 1% in those eyes with good capillary perfusion (84).

Fluorescein angiography is the most direct method of evaluating capillary nonperfusion, but is not always feasible, due to obstruction of visualization by the blood or other media opacities. The ophthalmoscopic findings may be helpful in determining the risk of neovascular glaucoma, which has been reported in 14% (87) to 27% (88) of eyes with hemorrhagic retinopathy (complete venous occlusion), but in no cases of venous stasis retinopathy (incomplete occlusion) (87–89). Several other techniques have also been shown to have predictive value. Fluorescein angiography of the iris reveals abnormal, leaking vessels in virtually all eyes with extensive retinal capillary closure following central retinal vein occlusion (90). Aqueous protein and cell concentrations, as indicated by a laser flare-cell meter, have been shown to correlate with fluorescein angiographic findings and the severity of retinal vein occlusion (91). A relative afferent pupillary defect also indicates an increased risk of rubeosis iridis following central retinal vein occlusion (92), and infrared pupillometry has been shown to be an objective method of documenting this finding (93). Electroretinography also has useful predictive value (94–100). The most diagnostic findings include a b-wave-implicit time delay and a reduced b-wave/a-wave amplitude ratio (94–98). The flicker electroretinogram is also reported to have diagnostic value (99, 100). Blood flow velocities of the central retinal vein and artery can be measured with color Doppler imaging and are reported to provide a high degree of predictability regarding the risk of iris neovascularization (101).

Despite evidence of good perfusion and a low risk of iris neovascularization by any of the noted techniques, it is important to follow all patients with central retinal vein occlusion for the possibility of rubeosis iridis and neovascular glaucoma. A certain number of patients with perfused retinas will progress to nonperfusion. In one study this was seen in 15% of cases (102). Time and age appear to influence this percentage. In one study, the cumulative probability of converting from nonischemic to ischemic central retinal vein occlusion in 6 and 18 months was 13.2% and 18.6%, respectively, in persons 65 years or older, and 6.7% and 8.1%, respectively, in individuals 45–64 years of age (31). It was also found that 83% of patients with indeterminate perfusion eventually developed nonperfusion or neovascularization of the iris or anterior chamber angle (103).

Preglaucoma Stage (Rubeosis Iridis)

CLINICAL FEATURES. This stage is characterized by a normal IOP, unless preexisting chronic open-angle glaucoma is present. Slitlamp biomicroscopy early in the disease process

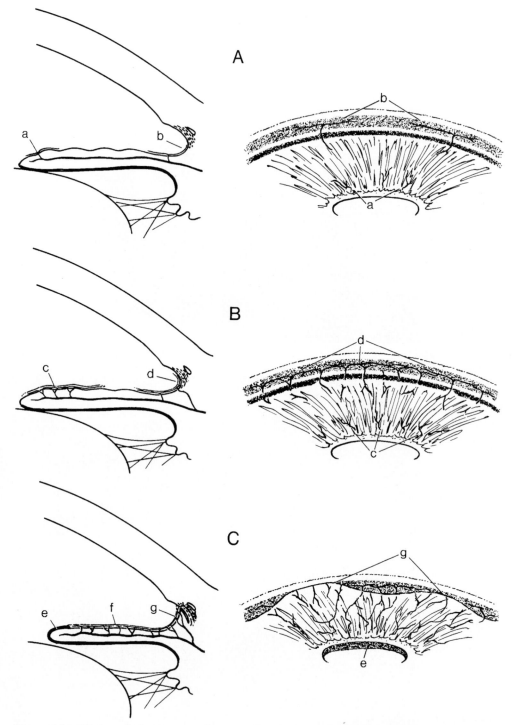

Figure 16.1. Clinicopathologic stages of neovascular glaucoma. **A.** Preglaucoma stage (rubeosis iridis), characterized by new vessels on the surface of the iris (*a*) and in the anterior chamber angle (*b*). **B.** Open-angle glaucoma stage, characterized by an increase in neovascularization and a fibrovascular membrane on the iris (*c*) and in the anterior chamber angle (*d*). **C.** Angle-closure glaucoma stage, characterized by contracture of the fibrovascular membrane, causing corectopia, ectropion uvea (*e*), flattening of the iris (*f*), and peripheral anterior synechiae (*g*).

typically reveals dilated tufts of preexisting capillaries and fine, randomly oriented vessels on the surface of the iris near the pupillary margin (104) (Fig. 16.3). The new vessels are also characterized by leakage of fluorescein (104, 105). As previously noted, neovascularization in the majority of cases is first seen on the peripupillary iris (79, 104), although it may be first seen in the anterior chamber angle (80, 106). Gonioscopy, therefore, may reveal a normal anterior chamber angle, or may show a variable amount of angle neovascularization. The latter is characterized by single vascular

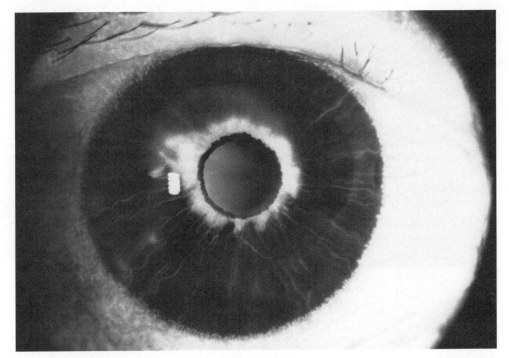

Figure 16.2. Fluorescein angiographic view of the iris in patient with proliferative diabetic retinopathy showing peripupillary microvascular leakage despite absence of clinically apparent rubeosis. (Reprinted with permission from Ehrenberg M, McCuen BW, Schindler RH, Machemer R: Rubeosis iridis: preoperative iris fluorescein angiography and periocular steroids. Ophthalmology 91:321, 1984.)

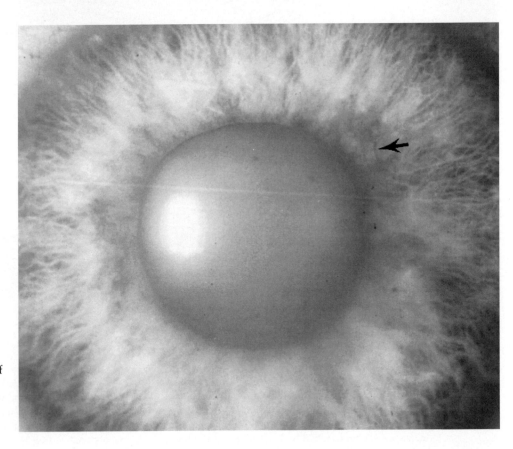

Figure 16.3. Slitlamp view of iris in patient with rubeosis iridis showing fine, tortuous vessels on surface of peripupillary iris *(arrow)*.

trunks crossing the ciliary body band and scleral spur and arborizing on the trabecular meshwork.

HISTOPATHOLOGIC FEATURES. The rubeosis iridis begins intrastromally and then develops on the surface of the iris (69,

107). Experimental retinal vein occlusion in monkey eyes indicates that the rubeosis iridis begins with dilatation of normal iris vessels and marked increase in metabolism of vascular endothelial cells followed by new vessel formation (108). Silicone injection studies indicate that the new vessels on the iris arise from normal iris arteries and drain primarily into iris and ciliary body veins, while new vessels in the angle arise from arteries of the iris and ciliary body and connect with the peripheral neovascular network on the iris (109). Although the clinical appearance of rubeosis iridis is said to be the same in cases of diabetes and central retinal vein occlusion (105), the silicone injections show tighter and more evenly distributed neovascularization in the diabetic eye (109). The silicone injection studies also show that new vessels in the angle run circumferentially in the trabecular meshwork, with branches coursing into the fibrosed Schlemm's canal and occasionally into collector channels (109). The new vessels are characterized histologically as having thin fenestrated walls (107, 110, 111) and are arranged in irregular patterns (107). The ultrastructure of iris neovascularization associated with sickle cell retinopathy is said to be similar to that in diabetes and retinal occlusive disease with open interendothelial cell junctions, attenuated intraendothelial cytoplasm, and pericyte formation (112).

Open-Angle Glaucoma Stage

CLINICAL FEATURES. Neovascular glaucoma does not invariably follow the development of rubeosis iridis (72, 73, 81, 104), and the latter condition may rarely resolve spontaneously, especially that associated with diabetic retinopathy (72). The reported incidence of neovascular glaucoma in diabetic patients with rubeosis iridis ranges from 13% to 22% (72, 73, 104), while that associated with central retinal vein occlusion is probably significantly higher. The latter condition typically occurs 8–15 weeks after the vascular oc-

clusive event (81). It has been called "90-day glaucoma" because the average time interval was felt to be 3 months. It is important to note, however, that the glaucoma can develop during the first month or any time after a central retinal vein occlusion.

The rubeosis iridis is typically more florid in this stage and biomicroscopic examination of the aqueous often reveals an inflammatory reaction (Fig. 16.4). By gonioscopy, the anterior chamber angle is still open, but the neovascularization is intense (Fig. 16.5). The IOP is now elevated and may rise suddenly, causing the patient to present with acute onset glaucoma. Hyphema may also be present in this stage.

HISTOPATHOLOGIC FEATURES. The hallmark of this stage is a fibrovascular membrane which covers the anterior chamber angle and anterior surface of the iris (107, 110), and may even extend onto the posterior iris (110). Chronic inflammatory changes are also typically seen on histologic examination (107, 110). The glaucoma in this stage probably results from obstruction of the trabecular meshwork by the fibrovascular membrane, with variable contribution from the inflammation and hemorrhage.

Angle-Closure Glaucoma Stage

CLINICAL FEATURES. In this stage, the stroma of the iris has become flattened, with a smooth, glistening appearance. Ectropion uvea is frequently present, and the iris is often dilated and pulled anteriorly from the lens (Fig. 16.6). In the anterior chamber angle, the contracture leads to peripheral anterior synechia formation, with eventual total synechial

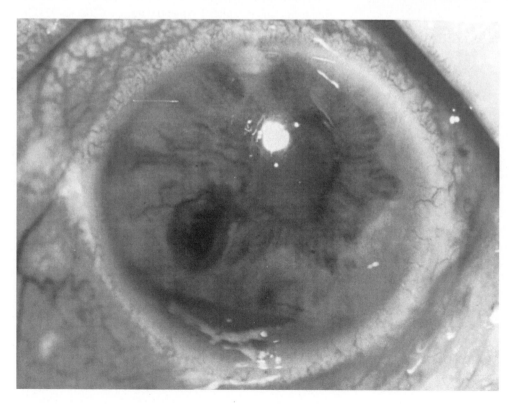

Figure 16.4. Slitlamp appearance of iris in patient with neovascular glaucoma showing marked rubeosis and hyphema.

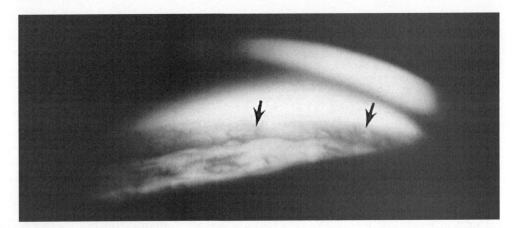

Figure 16.5. Gonioscopic view of patient with open-angle stage of neovascular glaucoma showing intense neovascularization (*arrows*) in an open anterior chamber angle. (Courtesy of Brooks W. McCuen, II, M.D.)

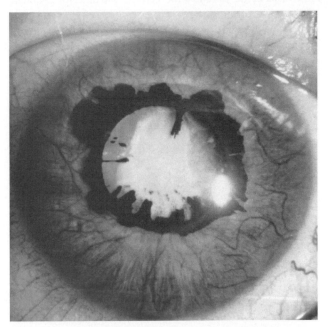

Figure 16.6. Slitlamp view of patient with angle-closure stage of neovascular glaucoma showing numerous new vessels on iris, with pupillary dilatation and ectropion uvea due to contracture of the fibrovascular membrane.

closure of the angle. The glaucoma in this stage is typically severe and usually requires surgical intervention.

HISTOPATHOLOGIC FEATURES. The clinically observed alterations of the iris and anterior chamber angle in this stage result from contracture of tissue overlying these structures. Histopathologic studies reveal peripheral anterior synechiae and flattening of the anterior iris surface by a confluent fibrovascular membrane (113, 114). Overlying the new vessels is a clinically inapparent, superficial layer of myofibroblasts (fibroblastic cells with smooth muscle differentiation), which may be responsible for the tissue contraction (113). A layer of endothelium, continuous with the corneal endothelium at the pseudoangle, is also seen in some cases (114–116) and has been observed to possess features of myoblastic differentiation (116), which may explain the origin of these cells.

Differential Diagnosis

In the open-angle stage, neovascular glaucoma must be distinguished from other glaucomas with acute onset such as angle-closure glaucoma and glaucoma associated with anterior uveitis. This differentiation can usually be made on the basis of new vessels on the iris and in the anterior chamber angle with neovascular glaucoma, although eyes with uveitis often have dilatation of normal iris vessels that may be confused with neovascularization, especially with blue irides. Patients with Fuchs' heterochromic iridocyclitis also typically have new vessels in the anterior chamber angle (Chapter 19). In the angle-closure stage of neovascular glaucoma, the new vessels may be less apparent, and the differential diagnosis must include other causes of iris distortion and peripheral anterior synechiae, such as the iridocorneal endothelial syndrome (Chapter 13) and old trauma (Chapter 22).

Management

Panretinal Photocoagulation

Ablation of peripheral retina with laser (usually argon) photocoagulation is the first line of therapy for most cases of neovascular glaucoma. This procedure has been shown to significantly reduce or eliminate anterior segment neovascularization in many cases (117–122), and to reduce the chances of developing rubeosis iridis in eyes with diabetic retinopathy or central retinal vein occlusion (84, 104, 123–126). The mechanism by which panretinal photocoagulation influences neovascularization is uncertain, although it may be related to decreasing the retinal oxygen demand, which is consistent with the reported observation that the photoreceptor-retinal pigment epithelial complex accounts for two-thirds of the total retinal oxygen consumption (127). This, in turn, may reduce the stimulus for release of an angiogenesis factor and/or may reduce the hypoxia in the anterior ocular segment. However, in 27 eyes with ischemic central retinal vein occlusion treated with panretinal photocoagulation, five eyes developed posterior neovascarization, which had not been present preoperatively, suggesting that the photocoagulation does not always eliminate retinal ischemia (128).

PROPHYLACTIC THERAPY. Panretinal photocoagulation is most effective as prophylaxis against the development of neovascular glaucoma. It was once felt by some surgeons that photocoagulation should be performed during the pre-rubeosis stage in central retinal vein occlusion, if the risk of developing rubeosis iridis was sufficiently high. However, a multicenter, randomized clinical trial revealed that prophylactic photocoagulation does not totally prevent iris and angle neovascularization, and that prompt regression of the rubeosis is more likely to occur in response to photocoagulation in eyes that have not been treated previously (129). With regard to central retinal vein occlusion, therefore, it is apparently better to follow the patients closely and intervene promptly with panretinal photocoagulation at the early signs of rubeosis.

The risk of rubeosis iridis in eyes with diabetic retinopathy is more difficult to predict than those with central retinal vein occlusion, but vitrectomy or lensectomy, especially in association with peripupillary fluorescein leakage, may be indications for prophylactic therapy. The latter is often performed as endophotocoagulation in conjunction with pars plana vitrectomy for diabetic retinopathy. By the time rubeosis iridis appears *(preglaucoma stage),* panretinal photocoagulation is indicated in all cases, including those due to central retinal artery occlusion (130) and carotid artery insufficiency. Even though neovascular glaucoma does not invariably follow rubeosis iridis, it does so with sufficient frequency that prophylactic laser therapy is justified in nearly all of these cases.

TREATMENT OF GLAUCOMA. It is reported that panretinal photocoagulation may reverse IOP elevation in the open-angle glaucoma stage (117, 118, 131), and in some cases of early angle-closure neovascular glaucoma, provided the synechial closure has not exceeded 270° (120). Even in the latter situation, panretinal photocoagulation may be useful in reducing anterior segment neovascularization prior to intraocular surgery (132). However, one study showed that panretinal photocoagulation prior to vitrectomy for diabetic retinopathy did not prevent postoperative rubeosis iridis (133). In these cases, intraocular panretinal photocoagulation at the time of vitrectomy may be the procedure of choice (134).

Panretinal Cryotherapy

When cloudy media precludes panretinal photocoagulation, it has been reported that transscleral panretinal cryotherapy, often combined with cyclocryotherapy, in eyes with neovascular glaucoma will control the IOP and reduce or abolish the neovascularization (135, 136).

Goniophotocoagulation

This technique involves the direct application of argon laser therapy to new vessels in the anterior chamber angle (137). It is most effective when used in the early stages of the disease to prevent the progressive angle changes and eventual intractable neovascular glaucoma (138). Although no longer commonly used, it may be beneficial in patients with a high risk of developing neovascular glaucoma, when panretinal photocoagulation has not been successful, or is not possible or advisable, and prior to intraocular surgery (138).

Medical Management

Once the IOP begins to rise, medical therapy is usually required and is frequently sufficient to control the pressure during the *open-angle glaucoma stage.* The mainstay of the therapy at this stage is drugs that reduce aqueous production such as carbonic anhydrase inhibitors, topical β-blockers and α₂-agonists. Miotics are rarely helpful and should usually be avoided since they may increase the inflammation and discomfort. Topical corticosteroids may be useful in minimizing the inflammation and pain (139). In addition, intravitreal triamcinolone has been shown to reduce retinal neovascularization in rabbit eyes (140), raising the question of a possible direct benefit of topical steroids on rubeotic vessels. In far advanced or blind eyes, atropine is helpful for relief of pain. Hyperosmotic agents may also be required for temporary control of cases with marked IOP elevation.

Glaucoma Surgical Procedures

CYCLODESTRUCTIVE PROCEDURES. If the disease follows its natural course to the *angle-closure glaucoma stage,* medical therapy nearly always becomes ineffective and surgical intervention is required. Even at this stage, panretinal photocoagulation may be beneficial by reducing the anterior segment neovascularization to allow filtration surgery. With active rubeosis, however, standard filtering surgery has a low chance of success, and a cyclodestructive procedure may be preferable.

While good results have been reported by some surgeons with the use of *cyclocryotherapy* for neovascular glaucoma (141, 142), other reports have been less encouraging (143–145). In one 2-year followup of 50 eyes, one-third were uncontrolled and one-third developed phthisis (143). An alternative cyclodestructive procedure is *transscleral Nd:YAG cyclophotocoagulation.* Preliminary experience suggests that this may become the surgical procedure of choice for neovascular glaucoma when filtering surgery is not felt to be indicated (146).

FILTERING SURGERY. It has been a general belief that standard filtering procedures in eyes with neovascular glaucoma are rarely successful, primarily due to the high risk of intraoperative bleeding and postoperative progression of the fibrovascular membrane. As noted earlier, however, a successful panretinal photocoagulation, possibly combined with goniophotocoagulation, will often reduce the neovascularization sufficiently to make it possible to perform a standard filtering operation such as trabeculectomy or a full-thickness filtering procedure (147). The adjunctive use of 5-fluorouracil provided success rates of 71% and 67% in the first and second postoperative years, respectively, although this fell to 41% and 28% by the fourth and fifth years, respectively (148). Other techniques of filtering surgery for neovascular glaucoma that have been described include a modified trabeculectomy with intraocular bipolar cautery of peripheral iris and ciliary processes (149, 150), and creation of a limbal fistula with a carbon dioxide laser (151). Encouraging preliminary experience has also been reported with the implantation of drainage tubes (152–157) or valves (158) into the anterior chamber in eyes with neovascular glaucoma. Details regarding the techniques and reported results of these procedures are considered in Section Three.

OTHER SURGICAL PROCEDURES. Several new techniques have been evaluated for the treatment of neovascular glaucoma. Silicone oil injection during revision of vitrectomy after unsuccessful diabetic vitreous surgery achieved stabilization or regression of anterior ocular neovascular changes in 83% of eyes in one study (159). Vascular occlusion has been created in experimental models following photosensitization of vessels with intravenous hematoporphyrin and exposure to red light (160) or intravenous injection of rose bengal and exposure to filtered light with a wavelength of 550 nm (the absorption maximum of rose bengal) (161). Exposure to 100% oxygen under hyperbaric conditions has been shown to significantly increase the partial pressure of oxygen in the aqueous humor of animal eyes which may have an application in treating hypoxic diseases of the anterior segment, including rubeosis iridis (162).

FUTURE TREATMENTS. The ultimate treatment for neovascular glaucoma would be to prevent the initiating event, such as diabetic retinopathy or central retinal vein occlusion, or at least to prevent that event from progressing to aqueous outflow obstruction. While the latter goal has been achieved, at least in part, with panretinal photocoagulation, this involves destruction of functional tissue and is not uniformly successful. As previously noted, neutralizing anti-VEGF antibodies have been shown to prevent iris neovascularization in a nonhuman primate model of retinal vein occlusion (66). In another study, systemic α-interferon, a polypeptide that inhibits proliferation and migration of endothelial cells and neovascularization, caused regression of iris neovascularization in a monkey model (163). Troxerutin, a semisynthetic, flavonoid derivative of rutin that improves microvascular flow by inhibiting platelet and red cell aggregation, increasing erythrocyte deformability, and reducing blood viscosity, was shown to improve retinal circulation and diminish progression of ischemia in patients with retinal vein occlusion (164). Such therapeutic approaches may eventually become the mainstay in preventing neovascular glaucoma.

ALTERATIONS OF INTRAOCULAR PRESSURE ASSOCIATED WITH RETINAL DETACHMENT

Reduced Intraocular Pressure and Retinal Detachment

An eye with a rhegmatogenous retinal detachment typically has a reduced IOP. Experimental studies with retinal detachments in monkeys suggest that an early, transient pressure drop may result from inflammation and reduced aqueous production (165), while a more prolonged hypotony may be due to posterior flow of aqueous through the retinal hole (166). A study with kinetic vitreous fluorophotometry indicated a posterior flow, presumably through a break in the retinal pigment epithelium, in patients with vitreous and rhegmatogenous retinal detachments (167). Campbell (168) has described a condition, the *iris retraction syndrome,* in which a patient presents with a rhegmatogenous retinal detachment, a secluded pupil, and angle closure with iris bombé. Pharmacologic suppression of aqueous production in these individuals leads to hypotony and a posterior retraction of the iris, presumably due to a shift in the predominant direction of aqueous flow toward the subretinal space.

Glaucomas Associated with Retinal Detachment

The coexistence of glaucoma and a retinal detachment in the same eye occurs under three circumstances: (a) glaucomas associated with retinal detachment, in which a cause-and-effect relationship is uncertain; (b) glaucoma directly related to retinal detachment; and (c) glaucomas following treatment for retinal detachment. The first two situations are discussed in this chapter, and the third is considered in Chapter 23.

Chronic Open-Angle Glaucoma and Retinal Detachment

EPIDEMIOLOGY. Chronic open-angle glaucoma is more common in eyes with a rhegmatogenous retinal detachment than in the general population. In one study of 817 cases of retinal detachment, open-angle glaucoma was present in 4%, and an additional 6.5% had elevated IOP without glaucomatous damage (169).

THEORIES OF MECHANISM. It is not known why chronic open-angle glaucoma and rhegmatogenous retinal detachment occur in the same eye more frequently than would be anticipated on the basis of chance occurrence. Neither myopia nor the use of miotics have been found to be the common denominator (169). In 30 cases of spontaneous rhegmatogenous retinal detachment, 53% had a cup/disc ratio greater than 0.3 and 20% were high topical steroid responders (170). These values are significantly higher than in the general population and resemble the findings in groups of patients with chronic open-angle glaucoma, which led the authors to suggest that the two diseases may be related genetically by multifactorial inheritance.

MANAGEMENT. When chronic open-angle glaucoma and retinal detachment coexist, one disorder may mask the presence of the other, necessitating careful attention to certain details during the management of either condition. When following a patient with open-angle glaucoma, the peripheral retina should be examined before initiating therapy and at least annually, or whenever warning signs such as floaters, flashing lights, loss of peripheral vision, or a sudden decrease in the IOP appear. Although the role of miotics in the pathogenesis of rhegmatogenous retinal detachment has not been clearly established, circumstantial evidence indicates that particular caution is warranted when these drugs are used (171).

In an eye with a rhegmatogenous retinal detachment, the reduced IOP may mask a preexisting glaucoma. In addition, retinal detachment surgery lowers ocular rigidity, which will cause a Schiøtz tonometer to read falsely low (172). In one study of 115 eyes, the mean disparity between applanation and Schiøtz pressure measurements averaged 8.6 mm Hg 1 month after retinal detachment surgery and 5.8 mm Hg 6 months postoperatively (172). An applanation tonometer, therefore, should be used following retinal detachment surgery, and the optic nerve head should be carefully inspected during the fundus examination to avoid missing coexisting glaucoma.

The success of retinal detachment surgery is not adversely affected by the presence of glaucoma (169), although the visual outcome may be worse due to the concomitant glaucomatous optic atrophy (169, 173). Following retinal detachment surgery, special caution should be given to the use of topical steroids, due to the increased incidence of high topical steroid responders (170), and miotics should be used with caution in either eye.

Pigmentary Glaucoma and Retinal Detachment

Patients with the pigment dispersion syndrome, with or without glaucoma, may have an increased incidence of retinal detachment. In addition, patients with retinal detachment are reported to have varying degrees of pigment dispersion in the anterior chamber angle in a significant number of cases (174). As in the case of chronic open-angle glaucoma, no definite cause-and-effect relationship has been established, but the same considerations as mentioned earlier must be employed in the management of coexisting pigmentary glaucoma and retinal detachment.

Schwartz Syndrome

As previously noted, a rhegmatogenous retinal detachment is typically associated with a slight reduction in the IOP. However, Schwartz described a rare condition in which the patient presents with unilateral pressure elevation, a retinal detachment, and an open anterior chamber angle with aqueous cells and flare (175). The condition has become known as the *Schwartz syndrome.*

THEORIES OF MECHANISM. Photoreceptor outer segments with few inflammatory cells have been demonstrated in the aqueous of patients with the Schwartz syndrome (176, 177), and the injection of rod outer segments into human autopsy and living cat eyes has been shown to significantly reduce outflow facility by obstructing the trabecular meshwork (178). Other mechanisms that have been considered include ocular trauma with concomitant damage to the trabecular meshwork (167, 175), anterior uveitis secondary to the retinal detachment (175) and obstruction of the trabecular meshwork by pigment from the retinal pigment epithelium (179) or glycosaminoglycans from the visual cells (180).

MANAGEMENT. The treatment of both the rhegmatogenous retinal detachment and the associated glaucoma is repair of the detachment, which typically results in resolution of the glaucoma within a few days (175, 177). In the differential diagnosis, it is important to remember that an eye with a retinal detachment and glaucoma may harbor a malignant melanoma (181).

Glaucoma Associated with Other Forms of Retinal Detachment

In addition to rhegmatogenous retinal detachment, there are several other forms of retinal detachment which may be associated with glaucoma. These include traction detachments, as with proliferative diabetic retinopathy and retinopathy of prematurity (discussed in this chapter), exudative retinal detachments (Chapter 19) and detachments associated with neoplasia, such as melanomas and retinoblastoma (Chapter 18). Each of these conditions may lead to either a neovascular or angle-closure mechanism of glaucoma.

ANGLE-CLOSURE GLAUCOMAS ASSOCIATED WITH DISORDERS OF THE RETINA, VITREOUS, AND CHOROID

Central Retinal Vein Occlusion

The neovascular glaucoma following retinal vascular occlusive disease was discussed earlier in this chapter. In addition, a small number of cases have been described in which shallowing of the anterior chamber after a central retinal vein occlusion led to transient angle-closure glaucoma (182–185).

Examination typically reveals a forward shift of the lens-iris diaphragm in the involved eye and a normal anterior chamber depth in the fellow eye. The mechanism of the angle-closure is uncertain, although it has been postulated that transudation of fluid from the retinal vessels into the vitreous leads to forward displacement of the lens with a subsequent pupillary block (182). The differential diagnosis should include pupillary-block glaucoma, which may lead to occlusion of the central retinal vein, and neovascular glaucoma, which can cause synechial closure of the anterior chamber angle. The former situation might be recognized by a potentially occludable angle in the fellow eye, while the latter can usually be identified by the presence of rubeosis iridis.

Treatment should usually be medical, since the angle returns to normal depth over a several-week period. Carbonic anhydrase inhibitors, topical β-blockers, and α₂-agonists may be helpful, and success has been reported with both pilocarpine (182, 183) and cycloplegics (184).

Hemorrhagic Retinal or Choroidal Detachment

Acute angle-closure glaucoma may follow a spontaneous massive hemorrhagic retinal or choroidal detachment (186). The hemorrhagic detachment is typically due to a disciform macular lesion, and associated conditions include systemic hypertension, primary clotting disorders, and the systemic use of anticoagulants and thrombolytic agents (186, 187). The mechanism of the angle closure is felt to be the abrupt forward displacement of the lens-iris diaphragm by the massively detached retina and choroid (186). Visual prognosis is poor in these eyes, and the management is directed primarily at relief of pain through IOP control with antiglaucoma medications or cyclodestructive surgery.

Hemorrhagic choroidal detachment may also occur during or after intraocular surgery, especially filtering surgery, with associated IOP elevation and flattening of the anterior chamber. This is discussed in Section Three as a complication of trabeculectomy.

Ciliochoroidal Effusion

In the following conditions, uveal effusion with ciliochoroidal detachment may lead to a forward rotation of the lens-iris diaphragm and angle-closure glaucoma.

Nanophthalmos

This rare ocular anomaly is characterized by a small eye with a small cornea, shallow anterior chamber, narrow angle, and high lens/eye volume ratio (188–190). The eyes are highly hyperopic due to the short axial length (< 20 mm by most definitions) and frequently develop angle-closure glaucoma in the fourth to sixth decades of life. Additional reported retinal disorders include pigmentary retinal dystrophy (191) and a family with pigmentary retinal degeneration and cystic macular degeneration in an autosomal-recessive syndrome (192). Uveal effusion and nonrhegmatogenous retinal detachment may follow intraocular surgery in these cases (188–190, 193). There is also evidence that, in some patients, the uveal effusion and retinal detachment may precede the surgery and actually cause the angle-closure glaucoma by producing a forward shift of the lens-iris diaphragm, leading to a pupillary block mechanism (194).

Histopathologic studies reveal an unusually thick sclera with irregular interlacing collagen bundles (195, 196), fraying of collagen fibrils (197), reduced glycosaminoglycans (196) and elevated fibronectin (198). Altered metabolism of glycosaminoglycans and fibronectin may be related to the development of abnormal sclera in nanophthalmos (195, 196, 198). Tissue culture studies of sclerocytes from a patient with nanophthalmos revealed modified glycosaminoglycan metabolism, which may contribute to the abnormal packing of collagen bundles and thickening of the sclera (199). It has been proposed that the uveal effusion may be due to reduced scleral permeability to proteins by the thickened sclera (200), or compression of venous drainage channels by the dense collagen around the vortex veins (201). However, no collagen abnormality was seen in three patients of one study, leading the authors to suggest that nanophthalmos may result from several distinct defects (197).

This form of glaucoma responds poorly to conventional surgical therapy, with a high complication rate, associated primarily with the uveal effusion (189, 193). Medical therapy may be effective, although miotics may increase the pupillary block (189). Laser iridotomy and laser gonioplasty (retraction of the peripheral iris) appear to have the highest success rate and are the procedures of choice (189, 194), although these are not uniformly successful. One suggested approach to managing the uveal effusion is to decompress the vortex veins by making large scleral flaps over the veins and, in some cases, drainage of choroidal and/or subretinal fluid with air injection into the vitreous cavity (201). It has also been reported that lamellar sclerectomy, by dissecting areas of sclera to two-thirds thickness, relieved both the IOP elevation and the shallow anterior chamber (202).

Uveal Effusion Syndrome

This condition has similarities to nanophthalmos with the main exception being an eye of normal size. It occurs more frequently in males and is characterized by dilated episcleral vessels, thickened or detached choroid and ciliary body, and nonrhegmatogenous retinal detachment (200). As with nanophthalmos, the sclera may be thickened and impermeable, although one ultrastructural study revealed increased glycosaminoglycan-like deposits between the scleral fibers and dilated rough endoplasmic reticulum and large intracellular glycogen-like granules in scleral cells (203). The IOP may be normal, unless angle-closure glaucoma is present, which reportedly responds to cycloplegics, aqueous suppressants, and corticosteroids (204).

Other Causes of Ciliochoroidal Effusion

Several additional causes of ciliochoroidal effusion are considered in subsequent chapters: arteriovenous malformation (Chapter 17), tumors (Chapter 18), inflammatory conditions (Chapter 19), trauma (Chapter 22), and surgery (Chapter 23).

Retinopathy of Prematurity (Retrolental Fibroplasia)

Contracture of the retrolental mass in retinopathy of prematurity can cause progressive shallowing of the anterior chamber with eventual angle-closure glaucoma. This complication coincides with the cicatricial phase of the disease, which usually has its onset at 3–6 months of age. However, the angle-closure glaucoma may occur later in childhood (205, 206), or even young adulthood (206, 207), and there is a need for continued observation. Although the typical mechanism of glaucoma is angle closure due to the retrolental mass, anterior chamber angle abnormalities, including hypopigmentation of the iris root, a translucent material in the angle, and a prominent Schwalbe's line, suggest a developmental origin in some cases (208).

The glaucoma usually does not respond well to medical therapy, although some success has been reported with the use of cycloplegics (209) and topical corticosteroids (210). Iridectomy or trabeculectomy may be effective in some cases (206). Lens aspiration, with anterior vitrectomy, has been successful in other patients in controlling the IOP, although the procedure is usually only to relieve pain and avoid enucleation since useful vision is often lost by this stage (205, 211, 212). Vitrectomy techniques to reattach the retina are resulting in improved vision in some cases (213, 214), although patients with concomitant glaucoma usually have a poor visual outcome despite reattachment of the retina (215). In one case, however, an infant regained vision after treatment of the glaucoma with antihypertensive medication (216).

Persistent Hyperplastic Primary Vitreous

Retention and hyperplasia of the primary vitreous is usually unilateral and often associated with microphthalmia and elongated ciliary processes (217). Small pupillary notches, due to anastomotic vessels between the anterior and posterior tunica vasculosa lentis, may be a helpful sign of persistent hyperplastic primary vitreous, especially when the diagnosis is obscured by an opaque lens (218). The appearance of persistent hyperplastic primary vitreous by computed tomography is sufficiently characteristic as to also make this a useful diagnostic modality (219).

Glaucoma is usually a late finding with persistent hyperplastic primary vitreous. Angle-closure mechanisms are most common, resulting from anterior displacement of the lens-iris diaphragm due to contracture of the fibrous retrolenticular mass or a swollen lens. Other cases of angle-closure glaucoma may have extensive peripheral anterior synechiae. Open-angle mechanisms may include chronic uveitis, intraocular hemorrhage, and abnormal development of the anterior chamber angle. A case was reported of a 4-day-old newborn with bilateral glaucoma, which was felt to be related to the latter mechanism (220).

If left untreated, the vast majority of these eyes will show progressive deterioration (221). The recommended treatment is aspiration of the lens and removal of the fibrovascular mass with scissors (222) or vitrectomy instruments (221, 222–226). Since the retina in these cases often extends as far anteriorly as the pars plicata, a pars plana incision is felt to be contraindicated (226), and success with a limbal incision has been reported (221). This treatment may prevent or eliminate the angle-closure glaucoma, although postoperative visual rehabilitation is difficult and treatment to avoid amblyopia is usually required (222, 223).

Attention should also be given to the fellow eye in these cases, since two adult patients with uncomplicated unilateral persistent hyperplastic primary vitreous were found to have open-angle glaucoma in the contralateral eye, associated with anomalous blood vessels in the entire circumference of the anterior chamber angle, band keratopathy, and heterochromia iridis (227).

Retinal Dysplasia

This condition is usually bilateral and associated with multiple congenital anomalies, especially in trisomy 13–15 (228). The dysplastic retina may be pulled up behind the lens, and glaucoma may result from angle-closure or an associated dysgenesis of the anterior chamber angle.

RETINITIS PIGMENTOSA

Retinitis pigmentosa has been described in association with glaucoma, which appears most often to be of the open-angle type (229). However, the association is infrequent, and a true cause-and-effect relationship has not been established.

SUMMARY

Neovascular glaucoma is a relatively common and serious complication of several retinal disorders, especially diabetic retinopathy and central retinal vein occlusion, as well as certain other ocular and extraocular conditions. By mechanisms that are not fully understood, a fibrovascular membrane develops on the iris and in the anterior chamber angle, which initially obstructs aqueous outflow in an open angle and then contracts to produce an angle-closure form of glaucoma. The most effective treatment is panretinal photocoagulation in the early stages of the disease to reduce the stimulus for anterior segment neovascularization.

Retinal detachments are usually associated with a reduction in IOP, although some patients may have concomitant retinal detachment and glaucoma, which may or may not have a cause-and-effect relationship. There are also a group of conditions in which angle-closure glaucoma may be associated with a retinal, choroidal, or vitreous disorder, including central retinal vein occlusion, nanophthalmos, retinopathy of prematurity, persistent hyperplastic primary vitreous, and retinal dysplasia.

REFERENCES

1. Coats, G: Further cases of thrombosis of the central vein. Roy Lond Ophthal Hosp Rep 16:516, 1906.
2. Smith, RJH: Rubeotic glaucoma. Br J Ophthmol 65:606, 1981.
3. Weiss, DI, Shaffer, RN, Nehrenberg, TR: Neovascular glaucoma complicating carotid-cavernous fistula. Arch Ophthalmol 69:304, 1963.
4. Hoskins, HD Jr: Neovascular glaucoma: current concepts. Trans Am Acad Ophthalmol Otol 78:330, 1974.
5. Brown, GC, Magargal, LE, Schachat, A, Shah, H: Neovascular glaucoma: etiologic considerations. Ophthalmology 91:315, 1984.
6. Mandelcorn, MS, Blankenship, G, Machemer, R: Pars plana vitrectomy for the management of severe diabetic retinopathy. Am J Ophthal 81:561, 1976.
7. Aaberg, TM, Van Horn, DL: Late complications of pars plana vitreous surgery. Ophthalmology 85:126, 1978.
8. Michels, RG: Vitrectomy for complications of diabetic retinopathy. Arch Ophthalmol 96:237, 1978.
9. Blankenship, G, Cortez, R, Machemer, R: The lens and pars plana vitrectomy for diabetic retinopathy complications. Arch Ophthalmol 97:1263, 1979.
10. Machemer, R, Blankenship, G: Vitrectomy for proliferative diabetic retinopathy associated with vitreous hemorrhage. Ophthalmology 88:643, 1981.
11. Blankenship, GW, Machemer, R: Long-term diabetic vitrectomy results. Report of 10 year follow-up. Ophthalmology 92:503, 1985.
12. Schachat, AP, Oyakawa, RT, Michels, RG, Rice, TA: Complications of vitreous surgery for diabetic retinopathy. II. Postoperative complications. Ophthalmology 90:522, 1983.
13. Blankenship, GW: The lens influence on diabetic vitrectomy results. Report of a prospective randomized study. Arch Ophthalmol 98:2196, 1980.
14. Aaberg, TM: Pars plana vitrectomy for diabetic traction retinal detachment. Ophthalmology 88:639, 1981.
15. Rice, TA, Michels, RG, Maguire, MG, Rice, EF: The effect of lensectomy on the incidence of iris neovascularization and neovascular glaucoma after vitrectomy for diabetic retinopathy. Am J Ophthalmol 95:1, 1983.
16. Blankenship, GW: Management of vitreous cavity hemorrhage following pars plana vitrectomy for diabetic retinopathy. Ophthalmology 93:39, 1986.
17. Blankenship, GW: Preoperative iris rubeosis and diabetic vitrectomy results. Ophthalmology 87:176, 1980.
18. Bopp, S, Lucke, K, Laqua, H: Acute onset of rubeosis iridis after diabetic vitrectomy can indicate peripheral traction retinal detachment. Ger J Ophthmol 1:375, 1992.
19. Scuderi, JJ, Blumenkranz, MS, Blankenship, GW: Regression of diabetic rubeosis iridis following successful surgical reattachment of the retina by vitrectomy. Retina 2:193, 1982.
20. Wand, M, Madigan, JC, Gaudio, AR, Sorokanich, S: Neovascular glaucoma following pars plana vitrectomy for complications of diabetic retinopathy. Ophthalmic Surg 21:113, 1990.
21. de Juan, E Jr, Hardy, M, Hatchell, DL, Hatchell, MC: The effect of intraocular silicone oil on anterior chamber oxygen pressure in cats. Arch Ophthalmolmol 104:1063, 1986.
22. Aiello, LM, Wand, M, Liang, G: Neovascular glaucoma and vitreous hemorrhage following cataract surgery in patients with diabetes mellitus. Ophthalmology 90:814, 1983.
23. Poliner, LS, Christianson, DJ, Escoffery, RF, et al: Neovascular glaucoma after intracapsular and extracapsular cataract extraction in diabetic patients. Am J Ophthalmol 100:637, 1985.
24. Weinreb, RN, Wasserstrom, JP, Parker, W: Neovascular glaucoma following Neodymium-YAG laser posterior capsulotomy. Arch Ophthalmol 104:730, 1986.
25. Gartner, S, Henkind, P: Neovascularization of the iris (rubeosis iridis). Surg Ophthal 22: 291, 1978.
26. David, R, Zangwill, L, Badarna, M, Yassur, Y: Epidemiology of retinal vein occlusion and its association with glaucoma and increased intraocular pressure. Ophthalmologica 197:69, 1988.
27. Rath, EZ, Frank, RN, Shin, DH, Kim, C: Risk factors for retinal vein occlusions. A case-control study. Ophthalmology 99:509, 1992.
28. Cole, MD, Dodson, PM, Hendeles, S: Medical conditions underlying retinal vein occlusion in patients with glaucoma or ocular hypertension. Br J Ophthalmol 73:693, 1989
29. Elman, MJ, Bhatt, AK, Quinlan, PM, Enger, C: The risk for systemic vascular diseases and mortality in patients with central retinal vein occlusion. Ophthalmology 97:1543, 1990.
30. The Eye Disease Case-control Study Group: Risk factors for branch retinal vein occlusion. Am J Ophthalmol 116:286, 1993.
31. Hayreh, SS, Zimmerman, MB, Podhajsky, P: Incidence of various types of retinal vein occlusion and their recurrence and demographic characteristics. Am J Ophthalmol 117:429, 1994.
32. Hayreh, SS, Podhajsky, P: Ocular neovascularization with retinal vascular occlusion. II. Occurrence in central and branch retinal artery occlusion. Arch Ophthalmol 100:1585, 1982.
33. Duker, JS, Brown, GC: Iris neovascularization associated with obstruction of the central retinal artery. Ophthalmology 95:1244, 1988.
34. Duker, JS, Sivalingam, A, Brown, GC, Reber, R: A prospective study of acute central retinal artery obstruction. The incidence of secondary ocular neovascularization. Arch Ophthalmol 109:339, 1991.
35. Peternel, P, Keber, D, Videcnik, V: Carotid arteries in central retinal vessel occlusion as assessed by Doppler ultrasound. Br J Ophthmol 73:880, 1989.
36. Magargal, LE, Brown, GC, Augsburger, JJ, Parrish, RK: Neovascular glaucoma following branch retinal vein obstruction. Glaucoma 3:333, 1981.
37. Bresnick, GH, Gay, AJ: Rubeosis iridis associated with branch retinal arteriolar occlusions. Arch Ophthalmol 77:176, 1967.
38. Tanaka, S, Ideta, H, Yonemoto, J, et al: Neovascularization of the iris in rhegmatogenous retinal detachment. Am J Ophthalmol 112:632, 1991.
39. Comaratta, MR, Chang, S, Sparrow, J: Iris neovascularization in proliferative vitreoretinopathy. Ophthalmology 99:898, 1992.
40. Goldberg, MF, Tso, MOM: Rubeosis iridis and glaucoma associated with sickle cell retinopathy: A light and electron microscopic study. Ophthalmology 85:1028, 1978.
41. Bergren, RL, Brown, GC: Neovascular glaucoma secondary to sickle-cell retinopathy. Am J Ophthalmol 113:718, 1992.
42. Walton, DS, Grant, WM: Retinoblastoma and iris neovascularization. Am J Ophthalmol 65:598, 1968.

43. Savir, H, Kurz, O: Fluorescein angiography in syphilitic retinal vasculitis. Ann Ophthal 8:713, 1976.

44. Hung, JY, Hilton, GF: Neovascular glaucoma in a patient with X-linked juvenile retinoschisis. Ann Ophthalmol 12:1054, 1980.

45. Young, NJA, Hitchings, RA, Sehmi, K, Bird, AC: Stickler's syndrome and neovascular glaucoma. Br J Ophthmol 63:826, 1979.

46. Buchanan, TAS, Hoyt, WF: Optic nerve glioma and neovascular glaucoma: report of a case. Br J Ophthmol 66:96, 1982.

47. Lewis, RA, Tse, DT, Phelps, CD, Weingeist, TA: Neovascular glaucoma after photoradiation therapy for uveal melanoma. Arch Ophthalmol 102:839, 1984.

48. Kim, MK, Char, DH, Castro, JL, et al: Neovascular glaucoma after helium ion irradiation for uveal melanoma. Ophthalmology 93:189, 1986.

49. Apple, DJ, Craythorn, JM, Olson, RJ, et al: Anterior segment complications and neovascular glaucoma following implantation of a posterior chamber intraocular lens. Ophthalmology 91:403, 1984.

50. Shields, MB, Proia, AD: Neovascular glaucoma associated with an iris melanoma. A clinicopathologic report. Arch Ophthalmol 105:672, 1987.

51. Coppeto, JR, Wand, M, Bear, L, Sciarra, R: Neovascular glaucoma and carotid artery obstructive disease. Am J Ophthalmol 99:567, 1985.

52. Sugar, HS: Neovascular glaucoma after cartoid-cavernous fistula formation. Ann Ophthalmol 11:667, 1979.

53. Harris, GJ, Rice, PR: Angle closure in carotid-cavernous fistula. Ophthalmology 86:1521, 1979.

54. Huckman, MS, Haas, J: Reversed flow through the ophthalmic artery as a cause of rubeosis iridis. Am J Ophthalmol 74:1094, 1972.

55. Wise, GN: Retinal neovascularization. Trans Am Ophthalmol Soc 54:729, 1956.

56. Bresnick, GH, De Venecia, G, Myers, FL, et al: Retinal ischemia in diabetic retinopathy. Arch Ophthalmol 93:1300, 1975.

57. Laatikainen, L, Kohner, EM: Fluorescein angiography and its prognostic significance in central retinal vein occlusion. Br J Ophthmol 60:411, 1976.

58. Folkman, J, Merler, E, Abernathy, C, Williams, G: Isolation of a tumor factor responsible for angiogenesis. J Exp Med 133:275, 1971.

59. Glaser, BM, D'Amore, PA, Michels, RG, et al: The demonstration of angiogenic activity from ocular tissues. Preliminary report. Ophthalmology 87:440, 1980.

60. Federman, JL, Brown, GC, Felberg, NT, Felton, SM: Experimental ocular angiogenesis. Am J Ophthalmol 89:231, 1980.

61. Patz, A: Studies on retinal neovascularization. Invest Ophthalmol Vis Sci 19:1133, 1980.

62. Gu, XQ, Fry, GL, Lata, GF, et al: Ocular neovascularization. Tissue culture studies. Arch Ophthalmol 103:111, 1985.

63. Imre, G: Studies on the mechanism of retinal neovascularization. Role of lactic acid. Br J Ophthmol 48:75, 1964.

64. Zauberman, H, Michaelson, IC, Bergmann, F, Maurice, DM: Stimulation of neovascularization of the cornea by biogenic amines. Exp Eye Res 8:77, 1969.

65. Ben Ezra, D: Neovasculogenesis. Triggering factors and possible mechanisms. Surv Ophthalmol 24:167, 1979.

66. Adamis, AP, Shima, DT, Tolentino, MJ, et al: Inhibition of vascular endothelial growth factor prevents retinal ischemia-associated iris neovascularization in a nonhuman primate. Arch Ophthalmol 114:66, 1996.

67. Wolbarsht, ML, Landers, MB III, Stefansson, E: Vasodilation and the etiology of diabetic retinopathy: a new model. Ophthalmic Surg 12:104, 1981.

68. Stefansson, E, Landers, MB III, Wolbarsht, ML: Oxygenation and vasodilatation in relation to diabetic and other proliferative retinopathies. Ophthalmic Surg 14:209, 1983.

69. Henkind, P: Ocular neovascularization. Am J Ophthalmol 85:287, 1978.

70. Williams, GA, Eisenstein, R, Schumacher, B, et al: Inhibitor of vascular endothelial cell growth in the lens. Am J Ophthalmol 97:366, 1984.

71. Glaser, BM, Campochiaro, PA, Davis, JL Jr, Jerdan, JA: Retinal pigment epithelial cells release inhibitors of neovascularization. Ophthalmology 94:780, 1987.

72. Ohrt, V: The frequency of rubeosis iridis in diabetic patients. Acta Ophthalmol 49:301, 1971.

73. Madsen, PH: Rubeosis of the iris and haemorrhagic glaucoma in patients with proliferative diabetic retinopathy. Br J Ophthmol 55:368, 1971.

74. Bonnet, M, Jourdain, M, Francoz-Taillanter, N: Clinical correlation between rubeosis iridis and optic disc neovascularization. J Fr Ophthalmol 4:405, 1981.

75. Kluxen, G, Friedburg, D, Ruppert, A: Circular neovascularization of the circulus arteriosus iridis minor. Klin Monatsbl Augenheilkd 176:160, 1980.

76. Laqua, H: Rubeosis iridis following pars plana vitrectomy. Klin Monatsbl Augenheilkd 177:24, 1980.

77. Ehrenberg, M, McCuen, BW II, Schindler, RH, Machemer, R: Rubeosis iridis: preoperative iris fluorescein angiography and periocular steroids. Ophthalmology 91:321, 1984.

78. Bandello, F, Brancato, R, Lattanzio, R, et al: Biomicroscopy versus fluorescein angiography of the iris in the detection of diabetic iridopathy. Graefes Arch Clin Exp Ophthalmol 231:444, 1993.

79. Browning, DJ: Risk of missing angle neovascularization by omitting screening gonioscopy in patients with diabetes mellitus. Am J Ophthalmol 112:212, 1991.

80. Blinder, KJ, Friedman, SM, Mames, RN: Diabetic iris neovascularization. Am J Ophthalmolmol 120:393, 1995.

81. Cappin, JM, Whitelocke, R: The iris in central retinal vein thrombosis. Proc Roy Soc Med 67:1048, 1974.

82. Hayreh, S, March, W, Phelps, CD: Ocular hypotony following retinal vein occlusion. Arch Ophthalmol 96:827, 1978.

83. Sinclair, SH, Gragoudas, ES: Prognosis for rubeosis iridis following central retinal vein occlusion. Br J Ophthmol 63:735, 1979.

84. Tasman, W, Magargal, LE, Augsburger, JJ: Effects of argon laser photocoagulation on rubeosis iridis and angle neovascularization. Ophthalmology 87:400, 1980.

85. Magargal, LE, Donoso, LA, Sanborn, GE: Retinal ischemia and risk of neovascularization following central retinal vein obstruction. Ophthalmology 89:1241, 1982.

86. Hayreh, SS, Rojas, P, Podhajsky, P, et al: Ocular neovascularization with retinal vascular occlusion—III. Incidence of ocular neovascularization with retinal vein occlusion. Ophthalmology 90:488, 1983.

87. Priluck, IA, Robertson, DM, Hollenhorst, RW: Long-term follow-up of occlusion of the central retinal vein in young adults. Am J Ophthalmol 90:190, 1980.

88. Zegarra, H, Gutman, FA, Conforto, J: The natural course of central retinal vein occlusion. Ophthalmology 86:1931, 1979.

89. Zegarra, H, Gutman, FA, Zakov, N, Carim, M: Partial occlusion of the central retinal vein. Am J Ophthalmol 96:330, 1983.

90. Laatikainen, L, Blach, RK: Behavior of the iris vasculature in central retinal vein occlusion: a fluorescein angiographic study of the vascular response of the retina and the iris. Br J Ophthmol 61:272, 1977.

91. Nguyen, NX, Küchle, M: Aqueous flare and cells in eyes with retinal vein occlusion—correlation with retinal fluorescein angiographic findings. Br J Ophthmol 77:280, 1993.

92. Servais, GE, Thompson, HS, Hayreh, SS: Relative afferent pupillary defect in central retinal vein occlusion. Ophthalmology 93:301, 1986.

93. Bloom, PA, Papakostopoulos, D, Gogolitsyn, Y, et al: Clinical and infrared pupillometry in central retinal vein occlusion. Br J Ophthmol 77:75, 1993.

94. Sabates, R, Hirose, T, McMeel, JW: Electroretinography in the prognosis and classification of central retinal vein occlusion. Arch Ophthalmol 101:232, 1983.

95. Kaye, SB, Harding, SP: Early electroretinography in unilateral central retinal vein occlusion as a predictor of rubeosis iridis. Arch Ophthalmol 106:353, 1988.

96. Johnson, MA, Marcus, S, Elman, MJ, McPhee, TJ: Neovascularization in central retinal vein occlusion: electroretinographic findings. Arch Ophthalmol 106:348, 1988.

97. Breton, ME, Montzka, DP, Brucker, AJ, Quinn, GE: Electroretinogram intrepretation in central retinal vein occlusion. Ophthalmology 98:1837, 1991.

98. Breton, ME, Schueller, AW, Montzka, DP: Electroretinogram b-wave implicit time and b/a wave ratio as a function of intensity in central retinal vein occlusion. Ophthalmology 98:1845, 1991.

99. Severns, ML, Johnson, MA: Predicting outcome in central retinal vein occlusion using the flicker electroretinogram. Arch Ophthalmol 111:1123, 1993.

100. Johnson, MA, McPhee, TJ: Electroretinographic findings in iris neovascularization due to acute central retinal vein occlusion. Arch Ophthalmol 111:806, 1993.

101. Williamson, TH, Baxter, GM: Central retinal vein occlusion, an investigation by color Doppler imaging. Blood velocity characteristics and prediction of iris neovascularization. Ophthalmology 101:1362, 1994.

102. Chen, JC, Klein, ML, Watzke, RC, et al: Natural course of perfused central retinal vein occlusion. Can J Ophthalmol 30:21, 1995.

103. Central Vein Occlusion Study Group. Baseline and early natural history report. The Central Vein Occlusion Study. Arch Ophthalmol 111:1087, 1993.

104. Wand, M, Dueker, DK, Aiello, LM, Grant, WM: Effects of panretinal photocoagulation on rubeosis iridis, angle neovascularization, and neovascular glaucoma. Am J Ophthalmol 86:332, 1978.

105. Madsen, PH: Haemorrhagic glaucoma. Comparative study in diabetic and nondiabetic patients. Br J Ophthmol 55:444, 1971.

106. Laatikainen, L: Development and classification of rubeosis iridis in diabetic eye disease. Br J Ophthmol 63:150, 1979.

107. Schulze, RR: Rubeosis iridis. Am J Ophthalmol 63:487, 1967.

108. Nork, TM, Tso, MOM, Duvall, J, Hayreh, SS: Cellular mechanisms of iris neovascularization secondary to retinal vein occlusion. Arch Ophthalmol 107:581, 1989.

109. Jocson, VL: Microvascular injection studies in rubeosis iridis and neovascular glaucoma. Am J Ophthalmol 83:508, 1977.

110. Anderson, DM, Morin, JD, Hunter, WS: Rubeosis iridis. Can J Ophthalmol 6:183, 1971.

111. Peyman, GA, Raichand, M, Juarez, CP, et al: Hypotony and experimental rubeosis iridis in primate eyes. A clinicopathologic study. Graefes Arch Clin Exp Ophthalmol 224:435, 1986.

112. Goldberg, MF, Tso, MOM: Rubeosis iridis and glaucoma associated with sickle cell retinopathy: a light and electron microscopic study. Ophthalmology 85:1028, 1978.

113. John, T, Sassani, JW, Eagle, RC Jr: The myofibroblastic component of rubeosis iridis. Ophthalmology 90:721, 1983.

114. Nomura, T: Pathology of anterior chamber angle in diabetic neovascular glaucoma: Extension of corneal endothelium onto iris surface. Jpn J Ophthalmol 27:193, 1983.

115. Gartner, S, Taffet, S, Friedman, AH: The association of rubeosis iridis with endothelialisation of the anterior chamber: report of a clinical case with histopathological review of 16 additional cases. Br J Ophthmol 61:267, 1977.

116. Harris, M, Tso, AY, Kaba, FW, et al: Corneal endothelial overgrowth of angle and iris. Evidence of myoblastic differentiation in three cases. Ophthalmology 91:1154, 1984.

117. Little, HL, Rosenthal, AR, Dellaporta, A, Jacobson, DR: The effect of pan-retinal photocoagulation on rubeosis iridis. Am J Ophthalmol 81:804, 1976.

118. Laatikainen, L: Preliminary report on effect of retinal panphotocoagulation on rubeosis iridis and neovascular glaucoma. Br J Ophthmol 61:278, 1977.

119. Laatikainen, L, Kohner, EM, Khoury, D, Blach, RK: Panretinal photocoagulation in central retinal vein occlusion: A randomised controlled clinical study. Br J Ophthmol 61:741, 1977.

120. Jacobson, DR, Murphy, RP, Rosenthal, AR: The treatment of angle neovascularization with panretinal photocoagulation. Ophthalmology 86:1270, 1979.

121. Murphy, RP, Egbert, PR: Regression of iris neovascularization following panretinal photocoagulation. Arch Ophthalmol 97:700, 1979.

122. Pavan, PR, Folk, JC, Weingeist, TA, et al: Diabetic rubeosis and panretinal photocoagulation. A prospective, controlled, masked trial using iris fluorescein angiography. Arch Ophthalmol 101:882, 1983.

123. Magargal, LE, Brown, GC, Augsburger, JJ, Parrish, RK II: Neovascular glaucoma following central retinal vein obstruction. Ophthalmology 88:1095, 1981.

124. Magargal, LE, Brown, GC, Augsburger, JJ, Donoso, LA: Efficacy of panretinal photocoagulation in preventing neovascular glaucoma following ischemic central retinal vein obstruction. Ophthalmology 89:780, 1982.

125. Laatikainen, L: A prospective follow-up study of panretinal photocoagulation in preventing neovascular glaucoma following ischaemic central retinal vein occlusion. Graefes Arch Clin Exp Ophthalmol 220:236, 1983.

126. Kaufman, SC, Ferris, FL, III, Swartz, M, et al: Intraocular pressure following panretinal photocoagulation for diabetic retinopathy. Diabetic retinopathy report no. 11. Arch Ophthalmol 105:807, 1987.

127. Weiter, JJ, Zuckerman, R: The influence of the photoreceptor-RPE complex on the inner retina. An explanation of the beneficial effects of photocoagulation. Ophthalmology 87:1133, 1980.

128. Murdoch, IE, Rosen, PH, Shilling, JS: Neovascular response in ischaemic central retinal vein occlusion after panretinal photocoagulation. Br J Ophthmol 75:459, 1991.

129. The Central Vein Occlusion Study Group: A randomized clinical trial of early panretinal photocoagulation for ischemic central vein occlusion. The Central Vein Occlusion Study Group N Report. Ophthalmology 102:1434, 1995.

130. Duker, JS, Brown, GC: The efficacy of panretinal photocoagulation for neovascularization of the iris after central retinal artery obstruction. Ophthalmology 96:92, 1989.

131. Teich, SA, Walsh, JB: A grading system for iris neovascularization. Prognostic implications for treatment. Ophthalmology 88:1102, 1981.

132. Flanagan, DW, Blach, RK: Place of panretinal photocoagulation and trabeculectomy in the management of neovascular glaucoma. Br J Ophthmol 67:526, 1983.

133. Goodart, R, Blankenship, G: Panretinal photocoagulation influence on vitrectomy results for complications of diabetic retinopathy. Ophthalmology 87:183, 1980.

134. Miller, JB, Smith, MR, Boyer, DS: Intraocular carbon dioxide laser photocautery. Indications and contraindications at vitrectomy. Ophthalmology 87:1112, 1980.

135. May, DR, Bergstrom, TJ, Parmet, AJ, Schwartz, JG: Treatment of neovascular glaucoma with transscleral panretinal cryotherapy. Ophthalmology 87:1106, 1980.

136. Vernon, SA, Cheng, H: Panretinal cryotherapy in neovascular disease. Br J Ophthmol 72:401, 1988.

137. Simmons, RJ, Dueker, DK, Kimbrough, RL, Aiello, LM: Goniophotocoagulation for neovascular glaucoma. Trans Am Acad Ophthalmol Otol 83:80, 1977.

138. Simmons, RJ, Deppermann, SR, Dueker, DK: The role of gonio-photocoagulation in neovascularization of the anterior chamber angle. Ophthalmology 87:79, 1980.

139. Drews, RC: Corticosteroid management of hemorrhagic glaucoma. Trans Am Acad Ophthalmol Otol 78:334, 1974.

140. Tano, Y, Chandler, D, Machemer, R: Treatment of intraocular proliferation with intravitreal injection of triamcinolone acetonide. Am J Ophthalmol 90:810, 1980.

141. Feibel, RM, Bigger, JF: Rubeosis iridis and neovascular glaucoma. Evaluation of cyclocryotherapy. Am J Ophthalmol 74:862, 1972.

142. Boniuk, M: Cryotherapy in neovascular glaucoma. Trans Am Acad Ophthalmol Otol 78:337, 1974.

143. Krupin, T, Mitchell, KB, Becker, B: Cyclocryotherapy in neovascular glaucoma. Am J Ophthalmol 86:24, 1978.

144. Faulborn, J, Birnbaum, F: Cyclocryotherapy of haemorrhagic glaucoma: clinical long time and histopathologic results. Klin Monatsbl Augenheilkd 170:651, 1977.

145. Faulborn, J, Hoster, K: Results of cyclocryotherapy in case of hemorrhagic glaucoma. Klin Monatsbl Augenheilkd 162:513, 1973.

146. Hampton, C, Shields, MB, Miller, KN, Blasini, M.: Evaluation of a protocol for transscleral Neodymium:YAG cyclophotocoagulation in one hundred patients. Ophthalmology 97:910, 1990.

147. Allen, RC, Bellows, AR, Hutchinson, BT, Murphy, SD: Filtration surgery in the treatment of neovascular glaucoma. Ophthalmology 89:1181, 1982.

148. Tsai, JC, Feuer, WJ, Parrish, II, RK, Grajewski, AL: 5-fluorouracil filtering surgery and neovascular glaucoma. Long-term follow-up of the original pilot study. Ophthalmology 102:887, 1995.

149. Herschler, J, Agness, D: A modified filtering operation for neovascular glaucoma. Arch Ophthalmol 97:2339, 1979.

150. Parrish, R, Herschler, J: Eyes with end-stage neovascular glaucoma. Natural history following successful modified filtering operation. Arch Ophthalmol 101:745, 1983.

151. L'Esperance, FA Jr, Mittl, RN, James, WA Jr: Carbon dioxide laser trabeculostomy for the treatment of neovascular glaucoma. Ophthalmology 90:821, 1983.

152. Molteno, ACB, Van Rooyen, MMB, Bartholomew, RS: Implants for draining neovascular glaucoma. Br J Ophthmol 61:120, 1977.

153. Egerer, I: Clinical experience in glaucoma surgery utilizing silicon catheters. Klin Monatsbl Aguenheilkd 174:434, 1979.

154. Ancker, E, Molteno, ACB: Molteno drainage implant for neovascular glaucoma. Trans Ophthalmol Soc UK 102:122, 1982.

155. Honrubia, RM, Gómez, ML, Hern–ndez, A, Grijalbo, MP: Long-term results of silicone tube in filtering surgery for eyes with neovascular glaucoma. Am J Ophthalmol 97:501, 1984.

156. Mermoud, A, Salmon, JF, Alexander, P, et al: Molteno tube implantation for neovascular glaucoma. Long-term results and factors influencing the outcome. Ophthalmology 100:897, 1993.

157. Sidoti, PA, Dunphy, TR, Baerveldt, G, et al: Experience with the Baerveldt glaucoma implant in treating neovascular glaucoma. Ophthalmology 102:1107, 1995.

158. Krupin, R, Kaufman, P, Mandell, A, et al: Filtering valve implant surgery for eyes with neovascuar glaucoma. Am J Ophthalmol 89:338, 1980.

159. McCuen, BW, II, Rinkoff, JS: Silicone oil for progressive anterior ocular neovascularization after failed diabetic vitrectomy. Arch Ophthalmol 107:677, 1989.

160. Packer, AJ, Tse, DT, Gu, X-Q, Hayreh, SS: Hematoporphyrin photoradiation therapy for iris neovascularization. A preliminary report. Arch Ophthalmol 102:1193, 1984.

161. Nanda, SK, Hatchell, DL, Tiedeman, JS, et al: A new method for vascular occlusion. Photochemical initiation of thrombosis. Arch Ophthalmol 105:1121, 1987.

162. Jampol, LM, Orlin, C, Cohen, SB, et al: Hyperbaric and transcorneal delivery of oxygen to the rabbit and monkey anterior segment. Arch Ophthalmol 106:825, 1988.

163. Miller, JW, Stinson, WG, Folkman, J: Regression of experimental iris neovascularization with systemic alpha-interferon. Ophthalmology 100:9, 1993.

164. Glacet-Bernard, A, Coscas, G, Chabanel, A, et al: A randomized, double-masked study on the treatment of retinal vein occlusion with troxerutin. Am J Ophthalmol 118:421, 1994.

165. Pederson, JE, MacLellan, HM: Experimental retinal detachment. I. Effect of subretinal fluid composition on reabsorption rate and intraocular pressure. Arch Ophthalmol 100:1150, 1982.

166. Cantrill, HL, Pederson, JE: Experimental retinal detachment. III. Vitreous fluorophotometry. Arch Ophthalmol 100:1810, 1982.

167. Tsuboi, S, Taki-Noie, J, Emi, K, Manabe, R: Fluid dynamics in eyes with rhegmatogenous retinal detachments. Am J Ophthalmol 99:673, 1985.

168. Campbell, DG: Iris retraction associated with rhegmatogenous retinal detachment syndrome and hypotony. A new explanation. Arch Ophthalmol 102:1457, 1984.

169. Phelps, CD, Burton, TC: Glaucoma and retinal detachment. Arch Ophthalmol 95:418, 1977.

170. Shammas, HF, Halasa, AH, Faris, BM: Intraocular pressure, cup-disc ratio, and steroid responsiveness in retinal detachment. Arch Ophthalmol 94:1108, 1976.

171. Pape, LG, Forbes, M: Retinal detachment and miotic therapy. Am J Ophthalmol 85:558, 1978.

172. Pemberton, JW: Schiøtz-applanation disparity following retinal detachment surgery. Arch Ophthalmol 81:534, 1969.

173. Burton, TC, Lambert, RW Jr: A predictive model for visual recovery following retinal detachment surgery. Ophthalmology 85:619, 1978.

174. Sebestyen, JG, Schepens, CL, Rosenthal, ML: Retinal detachment and glaucoma. I. Tonometric and gonioscopic study of 160 cases. Arch Ophthalmol 67:736, 1962.

175. Schwartz, A: Chronic open-angle glaucoma secondary to rhegmatogenous retinal detachment. Am J Ophthalmol 75:205, 1973.

176. Matsuo, N, Takabatake, M, Ueno, H, et al: Photoreceptor outer segments in the aqueous humor in rhegmatogenous retinal detachment. Am J Ophthalmol 101:673, 1986.

177. Netland, PA, Mukai, S, Covington, HI: Elevated intraocular pressure secondary to rhegmatogenous retinal detachment. Surv Ophthalmol 39:234, 1994.

178. Lambrou, FH, Vela, MA, Woods, W: Obstruction of the trabecular meshwork by retinal rod outer segments. Arch Ophthalmol 107:742, 1989.

179. Davidorf, FH: Retinal pigment epithelial glaucoma. Ophthalmol Digest 38:11, 1976.

180. Baba, H: Probability of the presence of glycosaminoglycans in aqueous humor. Graefes Arch Clin Exp Ophthalmol 220:117, 1983.

181. Yanoff, M: Glaucoma mechanisms in ocular malignant melanoma. Am J Ophthalmol 70:898, 1970.

182. Hyams, SW, Neumann, E: Transient angle-closure glaucoma after retinal vein occlusion. Report of two cases. Br J Ophthmol 56:353, 1972.

183. Grant, WM: Shallowing of the anterior chamber following occlusion of the central retinal vein. Am J Ophthalmol 75:384, 1973.

184. Bloome, MA: Transient angle-closure glaucoma in central retinal vein occlusion. Ann Ophthalmol 9:44, 1977.

185. Mendelsohn, AD, Jampol, LM, Shoch, D: Secondary angle-closure glaucoma after central retinal vein occlusion. Am J Ophthalmol 100:581, 1985.

186. Pesin, SR, Katz, LJ, Augsburger, JJ, et al: Acute angle-closure glaucoma from spontaneous massive hemorrhagic retinal or choroidal detachment. An updated diagnostic and therapeutic approach. Ophthalmology 97:76, 1990.

187. Steinemann, T, Goins, K, Smith, T, et al: Acute closed-angle glaucoma complicating hemorrhagic choroidal detachment associated with parenteral thrombolytic agents. Am J Ophthalmol 106:752, 1988.

188. Brockhurst, RJ: Nanophthalmos with uveal effusion. A new clinical entity. Arch Ophthalmol 93:1289, 1975.

187. Singh, OS, Simmons, RJ, Brockhurst, RJ, Trempe, CL: Nanophthalmos: a perspective on identification and therapy. Ophthalmology 89:1006, 1982.

190. Ryan, EA, Zwann, J, Chylack, LT Jr: Nanophthalmos with uveal effusion. Clinical and embryologic considerations. Ophthalmology 89:1013, 1982.

191. Ghose, S, Sachdev, MS, Kumar, H: Bilateral nanophthalmos, pigmentary retinal dystrophy, and angle closure glaucoma—a new syndrome? Br J Ophthmol 69:624, 1985.

192. MacKay, CJ, Shek, MS, Carr, RE, et al: Retinal degeneration with nanophthalmos, cystic macular degeneration, and angle closure glaucoma. A new recessive syndrome. Arch Ophthalmol 105:366, 1987.

193. Calhoun, FP Jr: The management of glaucoma in nanophthalmos. Trans Am Ophthalmol Soc 73:97, 1975.

194. Kimbrough, RL, Trempe, CS, Brockhurst, RJ, Simmons, RF: Angle-closure glaucoma in nonophthalmos. Am J Ophthalmol 88:572, 1979.

195. Trelstad, RL, Silbermann, NN, Brockhurst, RJ: Nonophthalmic sclera: ultrastructural, histochemical, and biochemical observations. Arch Ophthalmol 100:1935, 1982.

196. Yue, BYJT, Duvall, J, Goldberg, MF, et al: Nanophthalmic sclera. Morphologic and tissue culture studies. Ophthalmology 93: 534, 1986.

197. Stewart, DH, III, Streeten, BW, Brockhurst, RJ, et al: Abnormal scleral collagen in nanophthalmos. An ultrastructural study. Arch Ophthalmol 109:1017, 1991.

198. Yue, BYJT, Kurosawa, A, Duvall, J, et al: Nanophthalmic sclera. Fibronectin studies. Ophthalmology 95:56, 1988.

199. Shiono, T, Shoji, A, Mutoh, T, Tamai, M: Abnormal sclerocytes in nanophthalmos. Graefes Arch Clin Exp Ophthalmol 230:348, 1992.

200. Gass, JDM: Uveal effusion syndrome. A new hypothesis concerning pathogenesis and technique of surgical treatment. Retina 3:159, 1983.

201. Brockhurst, RJ: Vortex vein decompression for nanophthalmic uveal effusion. Arch Ophthalmol 98:1987, 1980.

202. Wax, MB, Kass, MA, Kolker, AE, Nordlund, JR: Anterior lamellar sclerectomy for nanophthalmos. J Glau 1:222, 1992.

203. Ward, RC, Gragoudas, ES, Pon, DM, Albert, DM: Abnormal scleral findings in uveal effusion syndrome. Am J Ophthalmol 106: 139, 1988.

204. Fourman, S: Angle-closure glaucoma complicating ciliochoroidal detachment. Ophthalmology 96:646, 1989.

205. Pollard, ZF: Secondary angle-closure glaucoma in cicatricial retrolental fibroplasia. Am J Ophthalmol 89:651, 1980.

206. Michael, AJ, Pesin, SR, Katz, LJ, Tasman, WS: Management of late-onset angle-closure glaucoma associated with retinopathy of prematurity. Ophthalmology 98:1093, 1991.

207. Smith, J, Shivitz, I: Angle-closure glaucoma in adults with cicatricial retinopathy of prematurity. Arch Ophthalmol 102:371, 1984.

208. Hartnett, ME, Gilbert, MM, Richardson, TM, et al: Anterior segment evaluation of infants with retinopathy of prematurity. Ophthalmology 97:122, 1990.

209. Kushner, BJ: Ciliary block glaucoma in retinopathy of prematurity. Arch Ophthalmol 100:1078, 1982.

210. Kushner, BJ, Sondheimer, S: Medical treatment of glaucoma associated with cicatricial retinopathy of prematurity. Am J Ophthalmol 94:313, 1982.

211. Hittner, HM, Rhodes, LM, McPherson, AR: Anterior segment abnormalities in cicatricial retinopathy of prematurity. Ophthalmology 86:803, 1979.

212. Pollard, ZF: Lensectomy for secondary angle-closure glaucoma in advanced cicatricial retrolental fibroplasia. Ophthalmology 91: 395, 1984.

213. Machemer, R: Closed vitrectomy for severe retrolental fibroplasia in the infant. Ophthalmology 90:436, 1983.

214. Trese, MT: Surgical results of stage V retrolental fibroplasia and timing of surgical repair. Ophthalmology 91:461, 1984.

215. Hartnett, ME, Gilbert, MM, Hirose, T, et al: Glaucoma as a cause of poor vision in severe retinopathy of prematurity. Graefes Arch Clin Exp Ophthalmol 231:433, 1993.

216. Hartnett, ME, Katsumi, O, Hirose, T, et al: Improved visual function in retinopathy of prematurity after lowering high intraocular pressure. Am J Ophthalmol 117:113, 1994.

217. Reese, AB: Persistent hyperplastic primary vitreous. Am J Ophthalmol 40:317, 1955.

218. Meisels, HI, Goldberg, MF: Vascular anastomoses between the iris and persistent hyperplastic primary vitreous. Am J Ophthalmol 88: 179, 1979.

219. Goldberg, MF, Mafee, M: Computed tomography for diagnosis of persistent hyperplastic primary vitreous (PHPV). Ophthalmology 90:442, 1983.

220. Alward, WLM, Krasnow, MA, Keech, RV, Pulido, JS: Persistent hyperplastic primary vitreous with glaucoma presenting in infancy. Arch Ophthalmol 109:1063, 1991.

221. Stark, WJ, Lindsey, PS, Fagadau, WR, Michels, RG: Persistent hyperplastic primary vitreous. Surgical treatment. Ophthalmology 90:452, 1983.

222. Smith, RE, Maumenee, AE: Persistent hyperplastic primary vitreous: results of surgery. Trans Am Acad Ophthalmol Otol 78:911, 1974.

223. Nankin, SJ, Scott, WE: Persistent hyperplastic primary vitreous. Roto-extraction and other surgical experience. Arch Ophthalmol 95: 240, 1977.

224. Laatikainen, L, Tarkkanen, A: Microsurgery of persistent hyperplastic primary vitreous. Ophthalmologica 185:193, 1982.

225. Federman, JL, Shields, JA, Altman, B, Koller, H: The surgical and nonsurgical management of persistent hyperplastic primary vitreous. Ophthalmology 89:20, 1982.

226. Volcker, HE, Lang, GK, Naumann, GOH: Surgery for posterior polar cataract in cases of persistent hyperplastic primary vitreous. Klin Monatsbl Augenheilkd 183:79, 1983.

227. Awan, KJ, Humayun, M: Changes in the contralateral eye in uncomplicated persistent hyperplastic primary vitreous in adults. Am J Ophthalmol 99:122, 1985.

228. Hoepner, J, Yanoff, M: Ocular anomalies in trisomy 13–15: An analysis of 13 eyes with two new findings. Am J Ophthalmol 74: 729, 1972.

229. Kogbe, OI, Follmann, P: Investigations into the aqueous humour dynamics in primary pigmentary degeneration of the retina. Ophthalmologica 171:165, 1975.

Chapter 17

GLAUCOMAS ASSOCIATED WITH ELEVATED EPISCLERAL VENOUS PRESSURE[a]

EPISCLERAL VENOUS PRESSURE

The episcleral venous pressure, as discussed in Chapter 2, is one factor which contributes to the intraocular pressure (IOP). The normal episcleral venous pressure is approximately 8–10 mm Hg (1–5), although values vary according to the measurement technique. The several instruments that have been devised for measuring episcleral venous pressure were described in Chapter 3 (1, 2, 4, 5).

It is commonly felt that the IOP rises mm Hg for mm Hg with an increase in the episcleral venous pressure, although it has been suggested that the magnitude of IOP rise may be greater than the rise in venous pressure (6). Studies of chronic open-angle glaucoma have revealed no abnormality of episcleral venous pressure (2, 5, 7). In fact, there appears to be a negative correlation between episcleral venous pressure and IOP, with one study suggesting that ocular hypertensives have significantly lower than normal episcleral venous pressures (5). There are, however, a variety of conditions in which elevated episcleral venous pressure can produce characteristic forms of associated glaucoma. These conditions are the subject of the present chapter.

GENERAL FEATURES OF ELEVATED EPISCLERAL VENOUS PRESSURE

The following findings are common to most cases of elevated episcleral venous pressure.

External Examination

The most consistent feature is variable degrees of dilatation and tortuosity of the episcleral and bulbar conjunctival vessels (Fig. 17.1). Additional findings may include chemosis, proptosis, and a bruit and pulsations over the orbit. However, the latter are inconsistent findings that depend upon the underlying cause of the elevated episcleral venous pressure, which are considered later in this chapter.

[a]Refer to Shields, MB: Color Atlas of Glaucoma. Baltimore, Williams & Wilkins, 1998, Plate II27.

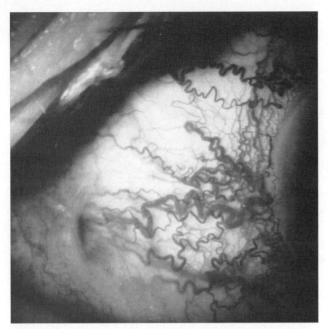

Figure 17.1. External view of patient with elevated episcleral venous pressure showing characteristic dilatation and tortuosity of the episcleral and bulbar conjunctival vessels.

Intraocular Pressure

As noted earlier, the rise in IOP is approximately equal to the rise in episcleral venous pressure. The resultant tension is typically in the mid-20s to mid-30s, and an increased ocular pulse is often present (8).

Gonioscopy

The anterior chamber angle is typically open, and the only abnormality may be blood reflux into Schlemm's canal. However, the latter feature has limited diagnostic value, since it is an inconsistent finding in cases of elevated episcleral venous pressure and may be seen in normal eyes.

Tonography

The facility of aqueous outflow is characteristically normal. In fact a study with monkeys revealed that elevated venous pressure was associated with increased outflow (9), which may, at least in part, result from a widening of Schlemm's canal. However, prolonged elevation of episcleral venous pressure often leads to a reduction in outflow facility, which may persist after normalization of the venous pressure (8).

CLINICAL FORMS OF ELEVATED EPISCLERAL VENOUS PRESSURE

The various causes of elevated episcleral venous pressure may be considered in three categories: (a) obstruction to venous flow, (b) arteriovenous fistulas, and (c) idiopathic episcleral venous pressure elevation (5). The mechanisms by which these conditions lead to glaucoma and their management are considered in separate sections at the end of this chapter.

Venous Obstruction

Thyrotropic Ophthalmopathy

This disorder is also referred to as endocrine exophthalmos or Graves' disease. The precise hormonal basis of the condition is uncertain, although the ocular pathology consists of orbital infiltration, primarily involving the extraocular muscles, with lymphocytes, mast cells, and plasma cells. This is the most common cause of unilateral, as well as bilateral, proptosis. In addition to glaucoma, other serious complications of thyrotropic ophthalmopathy include corneal exposure, due to proptosis and lid retraction, and optic nerve compression from the orbital mass.

The glaucoma may occur by several mechanisms. Elevated episcleral venous pressure may be present in severe cases of thyrotropic ophthalmopathy with marked proptosis and orbital congestion due to obstruction of venous flow through the orbit (Fig. 17.2). This, in turn, leads to a direct elevation of IOP. Another, less common, mechanism of glaucoma is the anterior chamber inflammation which may result from corneal exposure and ulceration.

Contracture of extraocular muscles, which occurs in the later phases of the infiltrative ophthalmopathy, may influence the IOP in different fields of gaze. Typically, fibrosis of the inferior rectus muscle causes resistance to upgaze, which is associated with a rise in the IOP when the patient looks up. In some cases, an artificial pressure elevation may be recorded with gaze in the usual straight-ahead position, and the patient should be allowed to change the direction of gaze to their "resting" position (10). Ideally, the IOP should be measured in several fields of gaze to avoid this potential testing artifact. It must also be kept in mind, as discussed in Chapter 4, that thyroid dysfunction may be associated with abnormal scleral rigidity, and the IOP in these individuals should be measured by applanation tonometry.

Superior Vena Cava Syndrome

Lesions of the upper thorax may obstruct venous return from the head, causing elevated episcleral venous pressure in association with exophthalmos, edema and cyanosis of the face and neck, and dilated veins of the head, neck, chest, and upper extremities (11).

Other conditions that may occasionally obstruct orbital venous drainage include *retrobulbar tumors* and *cavernous sinus thrombosis.*

Arteriovenous Fistulas

Carotid Cavernous Sinus Fistulas

Carotid cavernous sinus fistulas can be subdivided into two categories. The majority (about three-fourths) are secondary to trauma and are characterized by a direct vascular communication and high blood flow, while the remainder have a spontaneous etiology and typically have an indirect or dural communication with low flow (12).

TRAUMATIC. The typical trauma is severe head injury, which results in a large fistula between the internal carotid artery and the surrounding cavernous sinus venous plexus. This condition is characterized by pulsating exophthalmos, a bruit over the globe, conjunctival chemosis, engorgement of epibulbar veins, restriction of motility, and evidence of ocular ischemia (12–15). The shunting of the internal carotid cavernous sinus fistula causes high flow and high pressure (12, 16).

SPONTANEOUS. This form of carotid cavernous sinus fistula occurs most often in middle-aged to elderly women with no history of trauma. A small fistula in these cases is fed by a meningeal branch of the intracavernous internal carotid artery or external carotid artery, which empties directly into the cavernous sinus or an adjacent dural vein that connects with the cavernous sinus (16, 17). The mixing of arterial and venous blood leads to both a reduction in arterial pressure and an increase in orbital venous pressure, which increases the episcleral venous pressure. These patients have prominent episcleral and conjunctival veins, which is often the presenting complaint, but minimal proptosis and no pulsations or bruit. The small fistula results in low flow, low pressure shunting (16). The condition has been called "red-eyed shunt syndrome" (16), or "dural shunt syndrome" (17).

Orbital Varices

This condition is characterized by intermittent exophthalmos and elevated episcleral venous pressure, usually associated with stooping over or the Valsalva maneuver (6, 18). Since venous pressure is typically normal between episodes, associated glaucoma is not common. However, glaucomatous damage has been reported to occur, and it has been suggested that management with antiglaucoma medications may be effective and should be tried before considering surgical intervention (6).

Sturge-Weber Syndrome

One mechanism of IOP elevation in this condition is believed to be elevated episcleral venous pressure due to the episcleral hemangiomas with arteriovenous fistulas (19, 20). The Sturge-Weber syndrome is discussed in more detail in Chapter 18.

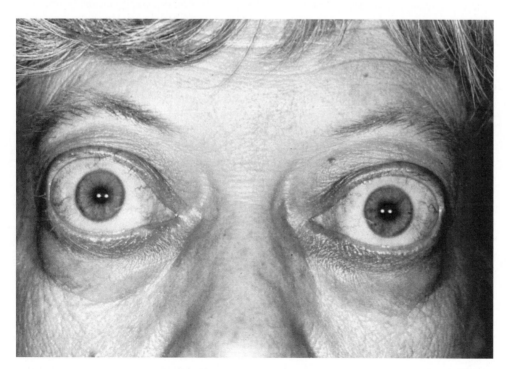

Figure 17.2. Patient with thyrotropic ophthalmopathy showing typical exophthalmos. Such patients may develop elevated episcleral venous pressure with associated glaucoma. (Courtesy of Jonathan Dutton, M.D.)

Idiopathic Episcleral Venous Pressure Elevation

Several cases have been reported of dilated episcleral veins and open-angle glaucoma without exophthalmos or any explanation for the venous congestion (21–27). The typical patient is elderly with no family history of the condition, although it may be seen in young adults and has been described in a mother and daughter (21). Most cases are unilateral, and those in which episcleral venous pressure has been measured have all had elevated venous pressures (21, 24, 27). The cause of the elevated episcleral venous pressure is unknown. In one series of five patients with unilateral elevation of episcleral venous pressure and open-angle glaucoma, venous outflow was normal by orbital venography, and the authors presumed the mechanism to be a localized venous obstruction in the region of the extraocular muscles (27). The associated glaucoma may be severe, with advanced glaucomatous damage.

MECHANISMS OF ASSOCIATED GLAUCOMA

There are several mechanisms by which elevated episcleral venous pressure may lead to glaucoma. Some are common to all forms of episcleral venous pressure elevation, while others are associated with specific conditions.

Direct Effect

As noted in the outset of this chapter, episcleral venous pressure is a component of the normal IOP, and a rise in episcleral venous pressure is associated with approximately the same amount of increase in IOP. These eyes typically have a wide open anterior chamber angle, often with blood in Schlemm's canal. This is the most common mechanism of glaucoma associated with episcleral venous pressure elevation. However, IOP elevation is not present in all patients with elevated venous pressure. For example, in patients with carotid cavernous sinus fistula, elevated IOP is more common in the atypical dural shunt syndrome, occurring in nearly all of these cases (16, 17).

Outflow Resistance

While facility of outflow is typically normal, if not improved (9), during elevated episcleral venous pressure, prolonged venous pressure elevation may lead to reduced outflow even after venous pressure is normalized (8). A trabeculectomy specimen from one idiopathic case revealed compression of the trabecular meshwork near Schlemm's canal, with extracellular deposits and hyalinization of the trabecular beams (26), although it is not clear as to whether this represented a primary or secondary alteration.

Acute Angle Closure

Angle-closure glaucoma has been associated with arteriovenous fistulae (28–30). The mechanism appears to be venous stasis within the vortex veins leading to either a serous choroidal detachment (28, 29, 31) or a suprachoroidal hemorrhage (30) and subsequent forward displacement of the lens-iris diaphragm. These have been reported in association with the dural shunt syndrome (28–30) and an orbital arteriovenous fistula (29).

Neovascular Glaucoma

The reduced arterial flow, especially associated with the dural shunt syndrome, may also lead to ocular ischemia with rubeosis iridis and neovascular glaucoma (14, 32, 33).

It has also been proposed, based on experimental models and mathematic analysis, that the visual field loss in glaucoma associated with elevated venous pressure is due to intraocular vein collapse and retardation of intraocular blood flow (34).

MANAGEMENT

Elevated Episcleral Venous Pressure

In many cases, the initial therapy should be directed toward eliminating the cause of the elevated episcleral venous pressure. This is particularly true in patients with thyrotropic ophthalmopathy, superior vena cava syndrome, retrobulbar tumors, or cavernous sinus thrombosis. However, in cases of carotid cavernous sinus fistula and orbital varices, the risk of surgical intervention may be such that other measures of glaucoma control should be considered first (6, 14, 15). Surgical intervention in the latter cases usually consists of intra-arterial balloon occlusion or embolization (12, 35). While reported success rates vary from 58% to 100% (12), complications do occur, including anterior segment ischemia, ischemia of the optic nerve, and cerebral ischemia (14, 15). More recently, a transvenous approach via the ipsilateral superior ophthalmic vein has been described as a safer way to pass a detachable balloon into the cavernous sinus (36). However, since many fistulae close spontaneously, especially with the dural shunt syndrome, conservative management is advisable in mild cases, with embolization for those with visual disability or progressive signs (35).

Associated Glaucoma

When treatment of the glaucoma is required, drugs which reduce aqueous production, such as β-blockers, α_2-agonists, and carbonic anhydrase inhibitors, should be used, since those which improve outflow are rarely effective. Cases with acute angle closure associated with the dural shunt syndrome and uveal effusion may also respond to these medications (29), while those with a suprachoroidal hemorrhage may require drainage of the blood (30). If surgical intervention becomes necessary, in most cases a filtering procedure should be employed. However, there is an increased risk of uveal effusion and expulsive hemorrhage when filtering eyes with elevated episcleral venous pressure, especially in the Sturge-Weber syndrome, and it has been recommended that prophylactic sclerostomies for drainage of any suprachoroidal fluid should be routinely performed at the time of surgery (37).

SUMMARY

The episcleral venous pressure normally contributes 8–10 mm Hg to the IOP. Elevated episcleral venous pressure may be associated with several forms of glaucoma. Conditions that may cause elevated episcleral venous pressure include (a) obstruction to venous flow, as with thyrotropic ophthalmopathy, superior vena cava syndrome, retrobulbar tumors, and cavernous sinus thrombosis, (b) arteriovenous fistulas, which include carotid cavernous sinus fistula, orbital varices, and the Sturge-Weber syndrome, and (c) idiopathic cases. Mechanisms of associated glaucoma include (a) the direct effect of elevated episcleral venous pressure on IOP, (b) chronic outflow obstruction, (c) acute angle closure, and (d) neovascular glaucoma. Management is usually directed first at the cause of the venous pressure elevation, with medical and surgical glaucoma therapy as required.

REFERENCES

1. Brubaker, RF: Determination of episcleral venous pressure in the eye. A comparison of three methods. Arch Ophthalmol 77:110, 1967.
2. Podos, SM, Minas, TF, Macri, FJ: A new instrument to measure episcleral venous pressure. Comparison of normal eyes and eyes with primary open-angle glaucoma. Arch Ophthalmol 80:209, 1968.
3. Krakau, CET, Widakowich, J, Wilke, K: Measurements of the episcleral venous pressure by means of an air jet. Acta Ophthalmol 51:185, 1973.
4. Phelps, CD, Armaly, MF: Measurement of episcleral venous pressure. Am J Ophthalmol 85:35, 1978.
5. Talusan, ED, Schwartz, B: Episcleral venous pressure. Differences between normal, ocular hypertensive, and primary open-angle glaucomas. Arch Ophthalmol 99:824, 1981.
6. Kollarits, CR, Gaasterland, D, Di Chiro, G, et al: Management of a patient with orbital varices, visual loss, and ipsilateral glaucoma. Ophthalmic Surg 8:54, 1977.
7. Linner, E: The outflow pressure in normal and glaucomatous eyes. Acta Ophthalmol 33:101, 1955.
8. Chandler, PA, Grant, WM: Glaucoma. 2nd ed. Philadelphia, Lea and Febiger, 1979, p. 267.
9. Barany, EH: The influence of extraocular venous pressure on outflow facility in Cercopithecus ethiops and Macaca fascicularis. Invest Ophthalmol Vis Sci 17:711, 1978.
10. Buschmann, W: Glaucoma and Graves' disease. Klin Monatsbl Augenheilkd 188:138, 1986.
11. Alfano, JE, Alfano, PA: Glaucoma and the superior vena caval obstruction syndrome. Am J Ophthalmol 42:685, 1956.
12. Keltner, JL, Satterfield, D, Dublin, AB, Lee, BCP: Dural and carotid cavernous sinus fistulas. Diagnosis, management, and complications. Ophthalmology 94:1585, 1987.
13. Henderson, JW, Schneider, RC: The ocular findings in carotid cavernous fistula in a series of 17 cases. Am J Ophthalmol 48:585, 1959.
14. Sanders, MD, Hoyt, WF: Hypoxic ocular sequelae of carotid-cavernous fistulae. Study of the causes of visual failure before and after neurosurgical treatment in a series of 25 cases. Br J Ophthalmol 53:82, 1969.
15. Palestine, AG, Younge, BR, Piepgras, DG: Visual prognosis in carotid-cavernous fistula. Arch Ophthalmol 99:1600, 1981.
16. Phelps, CD, Thompson, HS, Ossoinig, KC: The diagnosis and prognosis of atypical carotid-cavernous fistula (red-eyed shunt syndrome). Am J Ophthalmol 93:423, 1982.
17. Grove, AS Jr: The dural shunt syndrome. Pathophysiology and clinical course. Ophthalmology 90:31, 1983.
18. Wright, JE: Orbital vascular anomalies. Trans Am Acad Ophthalmol Otol 78:606, 1974.
19. Weiss, DI: Dual origin of glaucoma in encephalotrigeminal hemangiomatosis. Trans Ophthalmol Soc UK 93:477, 1971.
20. Phelps, CD: The pathogenesis of glaucoma in Sturge-Weber syndrome. Ophthalmology 85:276, 1978.
21. Minas, TF, Podos, SM: Familial glaucoma associated with elevated episcleral venous pressure. Arch Ophthalmol 80:202, 1968.
22. Radius, RL, Maumenee, AE: Dilated episcleral vessels and open-angle glaucoma. Am J Ophthalmol 86:31, 1978.
23. Benedikt, O, Roll, P: Dilatation and tortuosity of episcleral vessels in open-angle glaucoma. I: clinical picture. Klin Monatsbl Augenheilkd 176:292, 1980.
24. Talusan, ED, Fishbein, SL, Schwartz, B: Increased pressure of dilated episcleral veins with open-angle glaucoma without exophthalmos. Ophthalmology 90:257, 1983.
25. Ruprecht, KW, Naumann, GOH: Unilateral secondary open-angle glaucoma associated with idiopathically dilated episcleral vessels. Klin Monatsbl Augenheilkd 184:23, 1984.
26. Roll, P, Benedikt, O: Dilatation and Tortuosity of episcleral vessels in open-angle glaucoma. II: electron-microscopic findings in the trabecular lamellae. Klin Monatsbl Augenheilkd 176:297, 1980.
27. Jorgensen, JS, Guthoff, R: Pathogenesis of glaucoma in patients with idiopathically dilated episcleral vessels. Klin Mbl Augenheilk 190:428, 1987.
28. Harris, GJ, Rice, PR: Angle closure in carotid-cavernous fistula. Ophthalmology 86:1521, 1979.
29. Fourman, S: Acute closed-angle glaucoma after arteriovenous fistulas. Am J Ophthalmol 107:156, 1989.
30. Buus, DR, Tse, DT, Parrish, RK, II: Spontaneous carotid cavernous fistula presenting with acute angle closure glaucoma. Arch Ophthalmol 107:596, 1989.
31. Jorgensen, JS, Payer, H: Elevated episcleral venous pressure and uveal effusion. Klin Mbl Augenheilk. 195:14, 1989.
32. Spencer, WH, Thompson, HS, Hoyt, WF: Ischaemic ocular necrosis from carotid-cavernous fistula. Pathology of stagnant anoxic "inflammation" in orbital and ocular tissues. Br J Ophthalmol 57:145, 1973.
33. Weiss, DI, Shaffer, RN, Nehrenberg, TR: Neovascular glaucoma complicating carotid-cavernous fistula. Arch Ophthalmol 69:304, 1963.
34. Moses, RA, Grodzki, WJ Jr: Mechanism of glaucoma secondary to increased venous pressure. Arch Ophthalmol 103:1701, 1985.
35. Kupersmith, MJ, Berenstein, A, Choi, IS, et al: Management of nontraumatic vascular shunts involving the cavernous sinus. Ophthalmology 95:121, 1988.
36. Hanneken, AM, Miller, NR, Debrun, GM, Nauta, HJW: Treatment of carotid-cavernous sinus fistulas using a detachable balloon catheter through the superior ophthalmic vein. Arch Ophthalmol 107:87, 1989.
37. Bellows, RA, Chylack, LT, Epstein, DL, Hutchinson, BT: Choroidal effusion during glaucoma surgery in patients with prominent episcleral vessels. Arch Ophthalmol 97:493, 1979.

Chapter 18

GLAUCOMAS ASSOCIATED WITH INTRAOCULAR TUMORS

A variety of intraocular tumors can give rise to glaucoma. In one survey of 2597 patients with intraocular tumors, 5% of the tumor-containing eyes had tumor-induced elevated intraocular pressure (IOP) at the time of diagnosis of the tumor (1). In some cases, the mass lesions represent life-threatening malignancies, while other tumors are benign, creating critical problems with diagnosis and management. For patients with an intraocular malignancy, the emphasis shifts from the prevention of blindness to the preservation of life, while care must be taken in eyes with benign lesions to avoid loss of vision from unnecessary treatment. In this chapter, we consider the differential diagnosis and management of glaucomas associated with intraocular tumors.

PRIMARY UVEAL MELANOMAS[a]

Melanomas of the uveal tract, the most common primary intraocular malignancy, are frequently associated with glaucoma by several mechanisms and with a variety of clinical presentations. In one large histopathologic study of eyes with malignant melanomas involving one or more portions of the uveal tract, the overall prevalence of glaucoma was 20% (2). Anterior uveal melanomas lead to IOP elevation more frequently than posterior melanomas, with reports of 41% (2) and 45% (3) in two series, while choroidal melanomas were found to have associated glaucoma in 14% of one study (2). These figures are undoubtedly skewed, however, since one series represents histopathologic material (2), while the other represents patients primarily referred to a glaucoma service (3). A clinical series from an oncology service may provide more meaningful statistics, in which 3% of 2111 eyes with uveal melanomas had associated IOP elevation, including 7% with iris melanomas, 17% with ciliary body melanomas, and 2% with choroidal melanomas (1). Metastatic

[a]Refer to Shields, MB: Color Atlas of Glaucoma. Baltimore, Williams & Wilkins, 1998, Plates II28–31.

292

melanomas are rarely found in the eye, but can cause glaucoma and are discussed later in this chapter under "Systemic Malignancies."

Anterior Uveal Melanomas

Clinical Presentations and Mechanisms of Glaucoma

Melanomas of the anterior uveal tract most often arise from the ciliary body. These may be difficult to visualize directly, often presenting as a smooth-domed elevation of the overlying iris. Wide dilatation, however, may allow gonioscopic visualization of the lesion, which is typically seen as a chocolate-brown mass between the iris and lens. In other cases, a primary melanoma of the ciliary body may extend through the peripheral iris and become visible as a nodular mass on the iris stroma and in the anterior chamber angle (Fig. 18.1). Primary melanomas of the iris are usually easily seen by slitlamp biomicroscopy and gonioscopy, typically as slightly elevated, brown masses on the stroma (Fig. 18.2). Some melanomas of the iris, however, may be amelanotic, often with an associated secondary vasculature (Fig. 18.3).

Melanomas of the anterior uvea may lead to glaucoma by either open-angle or angle-closure mechanisms, with the former being more common. Aqueous humor outflow in the open anterior chamber angle can be obstructed by direct extension of the tumor, or by seeding of tumor cells or melanin granules (Fig. 18.4) (2–4). In some eyes, the melanoma may

arise from either iris, ciliary body, or the iridociliary junction and spread circumferentially, creating a *ring melanoma*. It may extend posteriorly, causing a retinal detachment and giving the impression of a choroidal tumor. Others may extend into the anterior chamber, causing elevated IOP due to infiltration of the angle with occasional iris nodularity and heterochromia (5).

In another condition, referred to as *melanomalytic glaucoma*, macrophages containing melanin from a necrotic melanoma obstruct the trabecular meshwork (2, 6). Ultrastructural studies reveal not only infiltration of the angle with melanin-laden macrophages, but also phagocytosis of melanin by trabecular endothelial cells, as well as tumor cells on the iris and in the meshwork (7, 8).

Yet another variation of anterior uveal melanoma and glaucoma occurs with a *tapioca melanoma*. This rare melanoma of the iris creates a nodular appearance resembling tapioca pudding (9), and typically consists of low grade spindle-type cells, although a case with epithelioid-type cells and metastases has been reported (10). Glaucoma is reported to occur in one-third of the cases with tapioca melanoma (9). Another reported mechanism of IOP elevation with an iris melanoma is neovascular glaucoma, which resolved after excision of the tumor (11).

Ciliary body melanomas may also cause an angle-closure form of glaucoma due to compression of the root of the iris into the anterior chamber angle (4) or forward displacement of the lens-iris diaphragm (Fig. 18.5). It should also be noted that some eyes with a melanoma confined to the ciliary body may have a slightly lower IOP than the fel-

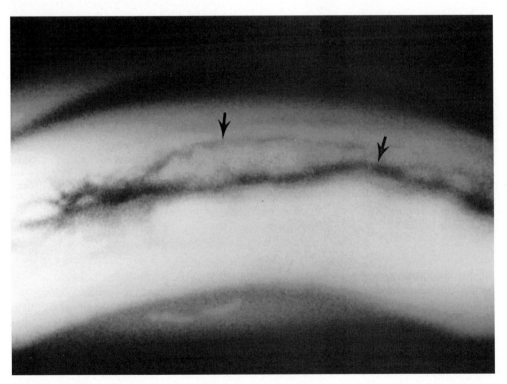

Figure 18.1. Gonioscopic view of malignant melanoma of the ciliary body presenting as multiple, pale tumors (*arrows*) on the peripheral iris and in the anterior chamber angle. (Reprinted with permission from The Secondary Glaucomas. Ritch R, Shields MB, eds. St. Louis, CV Mosby, 1982.)

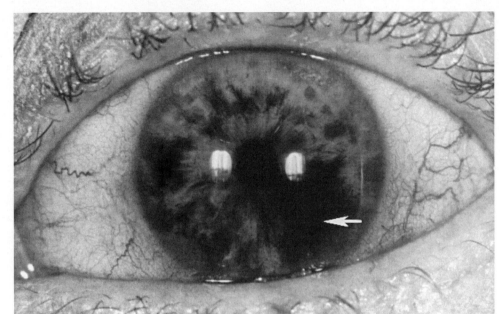

Figure 18.2. Slitlamp view of malignant melanoma of the iris *(arrow).* (Reprinted with permission from Shields, MB, Klintworth, GK: Anterior uveal melanomas and intraocular pressure. Ophthalmology 87:503, 1980.)

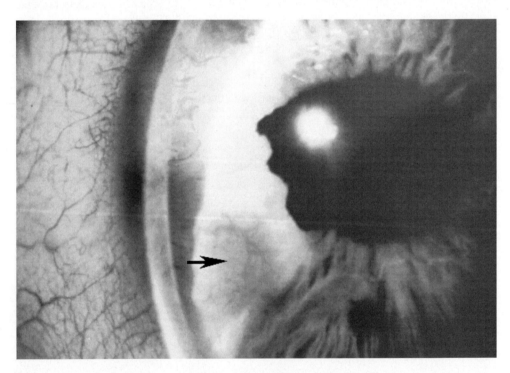

Figure 18.3. Slitlamp view of amelanotic malignant melanoma of the iris *(arrow).* (Courtesy of David G. Campbell, M.D.)

low eye (12). Any alteration in tension, therefore, can be an indication of an anterior uveal melanoma.

Differential Diagnosis

A number of conditions can be confused with glaucoma and an anterior uveal melanoma. Associated changes may mask an underlying melanoma, while other mass lesions may simulate an anterior uveal melanoma. For example, *iritis* may appear to be present in some cases of glaucoma and melanoma, which usually represents tumor cells in the anterior chamber (3), while other eyes may have pri-

mary iritis with inflammatory nodules that might be confused with a malignancy (13). In one large series, a primary *cyst of the iris* was the most common lesion to be confused with a melanoma of the iris (14). It is important to note, however, that anterior uveal melanomas can masquerade as cysts of the iris or ciliary body due to separation of the two epithelial layers by an eosinophilic exudate (Fig. 18.6) (3, 4). *Iris nevi* may be especially difficult to distinguish from iris melanomas not only clinically, but also histologically. A method for silver staining of nucleolar organizer regions has been shown to be helpful in making this distinction (15). Other benign tumors, as well as metastatic malignancies, must also be included in the differential diagnosis of uveal melanomas and will be discussed later in this chapter.

Choroidal Melanomas

Occasionally, a patient with a melanoma of the choroid may present with acute angle-closure glaucoma (2, 16). This is usually due to the forward displacement of the lens-iris diaphragm by a large posterior tumor, which is commonly associated with a total retinal detachment (2). The finding of a retinal detachment and glaucoma in the same eye, therefore, should alert the clinician to the possibility of an underlying malignant melanoma. Other reported mechanisms of IOP elevation in association with choroidal melanomas include neovascular glaucoma (2) and pigment dispersion in the vitreous with melanomalytic glaucoma (17). In addition to retinal detachment, other conditions that may mask the presence of a choroidal melanoma include intraocular inflammation and hemorrhage (18), while a dislocated lens nucleus may mimic a choroidal melanoma, especially when inflammatory glaucoma is also present (19).

Diagnostic Adjuncts

The difficulty in detecting a uveal melanoma and distinguishing it from other intraocular tumors occasionally necessitates the use of special diagnostic measures.

Ultrasonography

Ultrasonography may be useful in demonstrating the presence of a ciliary body melanoma (Fig. 18.7) or a choroidal melanoma when the latter is masked by a retinal detachment, vitreous hemorrhage, or other opacity in the ocular media. However, this technique does not, with absolute certainty, distinguish a neoplasm from other masses of the posterior ocular segment (20).

Radioactive Phosphorous Uptake

The ^{32}P test is said to be helpful in differentiating benign from malignant lesions of the choroid (21, 22). The study is not as useful, however, in diagnosing the smaller tumors of the iris (21) and ciliary body (22).

Fluorescein Angiography of the Iris

This test is reported to be useful in distinguishing melanomas from benign lesions of the iris, such as leiomyomas (23, 24) and benign melanocytic tumors (25). The angiographic characteristic of a melanoma of the iris is diffuse and eventually confluent fluorescence emanating from ill-defined vascular foci (25).

Cytopathologic Studies

An *aqueous or vitreous aspirate* may provide sufficient material for a histopathologic diagnosis of either a primary or

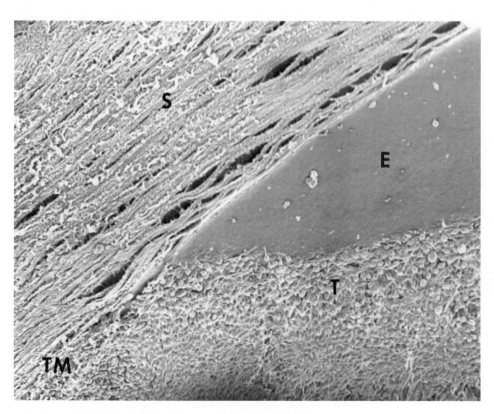

Figure 18.4. Scanning electron microscopic view of eye with malignant melanoma of the ciliary body showing tumor cells (T) in anterior chamber angle and on cornea, corneal endothelium *(E)*, corneal stroma *(S)*, and trabecular meshwork *(TM)*. (×120) (Reprinted with permission from Shields, MB, Klintworth, GK: Anterior uveal melanomas and intraocular pressure. Ophthalmology 87:503, 1980.)

metastatic malignancy (26, 27). This may be especially useful for suspected melanomas of the anterior uvea when cells can be seen in the aqueous by slitlamp biomicroscopy (Fig. 18.8). The technique involves aspiration of aqueous with a small-gauge needle through the limbus or peripheral cornea. For neoplastic cells, cytologic preservation is best with a Millipore filter (27).

A *fine needle aspiration biopsy* may also be used to obtain material for cytopathologic study from a suspected anterior uveal or choroidal melanoma (28). In one case, this allowed differentiation of a diffuse iris melanoma from a focal tumor (29).

Frozen Section Diagnoses

A frozen section may be helpful in identifying a tumor of the iris and in determining the surgical resection margins of the lesion (30). In sending the iridectomy specimen to the pathologist, care must be taken to identify the orientation of the tissue and to avoid curling of the edges (30).

Prognosis

When a uveal melanoma is associated with glaucoma, the prognosis appears to be worse for metastasis and death as opposed to a melanoma without glaucoma. In one study, three of four patients with a primary melanoma of the ciliary body and glaucoma died of metastatic disease within 2½ years after enucleation (3), while another investigation of uveal melanomas in children and adolescents identified glaucoma as a predominant factor relating to a fatal outcome (31). Histopathologic studies of eyes with a ciliary body melanoma and glaucoma often reveal tumor cells in the aqueous outflow system, which is a potential route of extraocular metastasis (3). Patients with choroidal melanomas and glaucoma also have a more guarded prognosis, because the tumor is usually large by the time the glaucoma has developed.

Melanomas of the iris, in general, have a better prognosis than that of other uveal melanomas (32, 33). The relatively

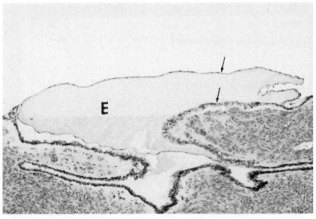

Figure 18.6. Light microscopic view of epithelial layers (*arrows*) of ciliary body separated by prominent eosinophilic exudate (*E*). Stroma of ciliary body contains malignant melanoma. (Hematoxylin & eosin, ×100) (Reprinted with permission from Shields, MB, Klintworth, GK: Anterior uveal melanomas and intraocular pressure. Ophthalmology 87:503, 1980.)

benign nature may be due to the earlier detection and small size at the time of detection allowed by the more obvious anterior location. However, metastases have been reported to occur (10, 32, 34–40). In one series of 1043 reported iris melanomas, 31 (3%) eventually metastasized (36). The cell type influences the rate of metastasis, with none among spindle A tumors in the above series, 2.6% with spindle B, 6.9% with epithelioid, and 10.5% with mixed-cell (36). The presence of glaucoma with an iris melanoma may also increase the risk of metastasis. Observed growth of iris lesions may be the best indicator of malignant potential. However, in one study of 175 patients with melanocytic tumors of the iris, followed for 1–12 years, there was only a 4.6% incidence of tumor growth, and the growth was not always indicative of the presence of malignant cells (37). This low incidence may be due, at least in part, to the slow growth of iris melanomas in some patients. In one case report, an iris melanoma was followed over 41 years before producing glaucoma and resulting in enucleation (40). Continued close observation, therefore, is essential in managing these cases.

Management

Considering the poor prognosis in cases of ciliary body or choroidal melanoma associated with glaucoma, the recommended management most often is enucleation. By the time glaucoma has developed, the melanoma is usually too large or diffuse for local treatment. However, there are exceptions, especially when the eye with the melanoma is the patient's only eye with useful vision. In such cases, local excision of an anterior uveal melanoma (41, 42) or radiotherapy of anterior or posterior tumors (43) is occasionally attempted. In one series of 52 patients undergoing iridocyclectomy for lesions of the iris or ciliary body, half of the excised lesions were benign and nearly one-third of the group eventually required enucleation

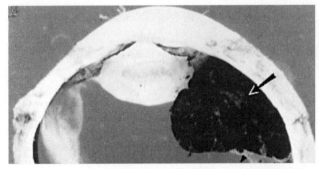

Figure 18.5. Gross appearance of sectioned eye showing malignant melanoma of the ciliary body (*arrow*) adjacent to the lens, creating closure of the anterior chamber angle. (Reprinted with permission from Shields, MB, Klintworth, GK: Anterior uveal melanomas and intraocular pressure. Ophthalmology 87:503, 1980.)

(42). Radiotherapy, especially with anterior tumors, may be complicated by hemorrhage and further pressure elevation, as well as failure to eradicate the melanoma (43).

Care must be taken to avoid artificial elevation of the IOP during both diagnostic and surgical maneuvers for fear that this may accelerate extraocular dissemination of tumor cells (44–47). Enucleation techniques have been developed to minimize intraoperative pressure elevation, which include manometric pressure regulating systems (45, 46), and the use of a wire snare to cut the optic nerve (47).

Cases of iris melanoma and glaucoma are usually managed more conservatively, since the tumors are typically small when first detected and can be observed for evidence of growth. However, as previously discussed, iris melanomas

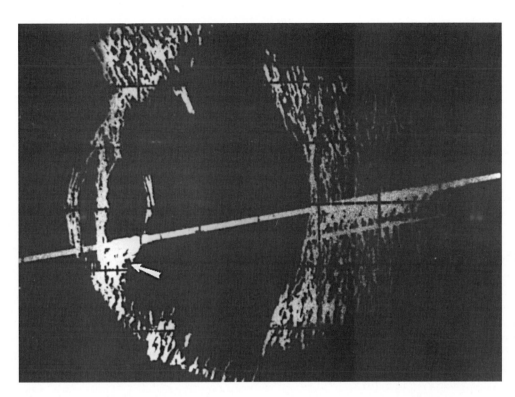

Figure 18.7. B-scan ultrasonographic view of ciliary body mass (*arrow*) in eye with malignant melanoma of ciliary body. (Reprinted with permission from The Secondary Glaucomas. Ritch R, Shields MB, eds. St. Louis, CV Mosby, 1982.)

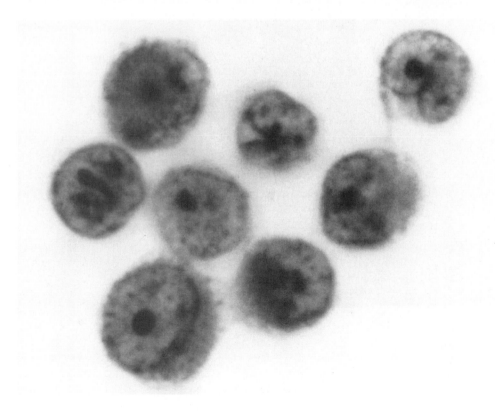

Figure 18.8. Light microscopic view of melanoma cells aspirated from aqueous of eye with anterior uveal melanoma. (Papanicolaou, ×400) (Reprinted with permission from The Secondary Glaucomas. Ritch R, Shields MB, eds. St. Louis, CV Mosby, 1982.)

may metastasize (10, 32, 34–40), and the degree to which associated glaucoma increases this risk is uncertain. In general, iris melanomas should be photographed and followed for evidence of growth. If slight growth is detected, continued close observation is still reasonable, whereas pronounced and progressive growth requires surgical intervention (38). This usually consists of complete excision by a sector iridectomy. Photocoagulation may be used to eradicate some iris melanomas (48). However, if the tumor has disseminated or diffusely extended in the anterior segment, as is often the case when associated glaucoma is present, enucleation is usually indicated.

The management of the associated glaucoma in eyes with a uveal melanoma is best limited to medical therapy. Filtering surgery should be avoided, since seeding of iris melanoma cells through a trabeculectomy site into the filtering bleb (49) with extraocular dissemination and fatal metastases (37) have been documented in such cases. When surgical intervention for the glaucoma is required, especially in eyes with iris melanomas, a cyclodestructive procedure is probably the procedure of choice.

SYSTEMIC MALIGNANCIES

Metastatic Carcinomas

Two large studies have been reported in which at least one eye from autopsy cases with known malignancies were examined for ocular metastases (50, 51). The most common

primary sites for metastasis to the eye were the lung and breast. The two studies agreed regarding the incidence of ocular metastases from the lung (6% (50) and 6.7% (51)), although the results differed for metastases from the breast (37% (50) and 9.7% (51)), as well as for the overall incidence of metastasis from all primary carcinomas (12% (50) and 4% (51)). In any event, metastatic carcinoma of the eye is not uncommon, and is said by some to be the most common form of intraocular malignancy (52).

The most common site of ocular metastasis is the posterior uvea (50, 51, 53), although glaucoma is more often associated with metastases to the anterior segment (54). In one study of 227 cases of carcinoma, metastatic to the eye and orbit, glaucoma was detected in 7.5% of the total group (53), and in 56% of the 26 with anterior ocular metastasis (54). In another series of 256 eyes with uveal metastases, associated IOP elevation was present in 5% of the total group, but in 64% and 67% of eyes with iris and ciliary body metastases, respectively (1). The clinical appearance of metastatic carcinomas of the anterior uvea is that of a gelatinous or translucent mass, which may be a single lesion or multiple nodules on the iris, often associated with rubeosis iridis, iridocyclitis, or hyphema (Fig. 18.9) (54–58).

Mechanisms of glaucoma in eyes with anterior uveal metastatic carcinoma include open-angle forms in which the trabecular meshwork may be covered by sheets of tumor cells or may be infiltrated with neoplastic tissue (1, 54). Other patients have angle-closure glaucoma due to compression of the iris by the tumor or due to peripheral anterior synechiae (1, 54). In some cases, ocular signs or

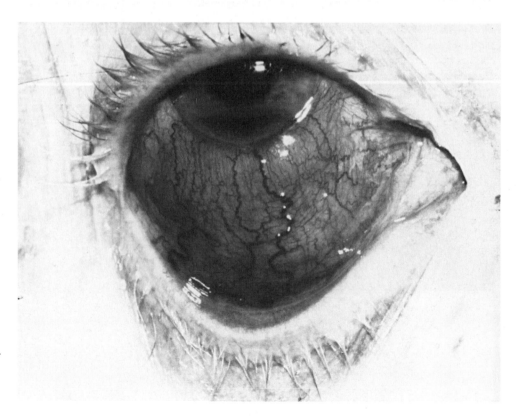

Figure 18.9. External view of patient with metastatic carcinoma showing inferior subconjunctival mass and layered hyphema and hypopyon, obscuring a mass of the ciliary body and iris. (Reprinted with permission from The Secondary Glaucomas. Ritch R, Shields MB, eds. St. Louis, CV Mosby, 1982.)

symptoms may be the first manifestation of metastatic malignancies. In one case report, a 54-year-old man, who was otherwise in good health, presented with angle-closure glaucoma and a hemorrhagic choroidal detachment. Suspected malignancy was confirmed by detection of squamous cell carcinoma of the lung and the patient died within 1 month of the ocular diagnosis with widespread metastases (59). An unusual case has also been described in which a nasal carcinoma caused bilateral glaucoma by infiltrating Schlemm's canal and intrascleral and episcleral collector channels (60).

In the management of metastatic carcinoma to the anterior uvea, paracentesis with aqueous aspiration for cytopathologic examination is often helpful in establishing the diagnosis (52, 57). When the cytology is nondiagnostic, a serologic tumor marker in the aqueous has been used to make the diagnosis (61). Treatment of the metastatic carcinoma usually includes radiation therapy and occasional chemotherapy (52, 56, 57). Enucleation is usually reserved for blind, painful eyes. If the associated glaucoma persists, it should be controlled medically whenever possible.

Metastatic Melanomas

Although ocular melanomas are nearly always primary malignancies, metastatic melanomas of the eye have been reported and may occasionally cause glaucoma (26). A unique form has been called *black hypopyon,* in which a disseminated cutaneous malignant melanoma metastasized to the eye where it became necrotic, possibly in response to immunotherapy or irradiation, resulting in a hypopyon of tumor cells and pigment-laden macrophages with associated glaucoma (62).

Leukemias

In an autopsy survey of 117 eyes of individuals who died of acute or chronic leukemia, the incidence of leukemic infiltrates in the ocular tissues was 28% (51). In a slitlamp study of 39 children with acute leukemia, the same percentage of cases were found to have flare or cells in the anterior chamber (63). In another series of childhood leukemias, the 5-year survival rate in patients with ocular manifestations was 21.4%, compared to 45.7% for those without ophthalmic involvement (64). Although this series began in 1972 when treatment was less effective than today (65), these findings still emphasize that any child with leukemia and apparent iritis should be regarded as having a relapse, and anterior chamber aspiration and iris biopsy are said to be essential procedures in establishing this diagnosis (65, 66). In a series of 135 patients who had fatal leukemia, ocular leukemic infiltration was found in one-third of the cases, most often in the choroid (67). A leukemic infiltration of the anterior ocular segment leads to glaucoma in some cases,

which may present in association with hyphema and hypopyon (68–70). These patients more often have acute lymphocytic leukemia. Both acute and chronic leukemias in adults may also have ocular involvement, with reported cases presenting variously as bilateral hypopyon (71, 72), or a massive subretinal hemorrhage with acute angle-closure glaucoma (73). As noted earlier, it may be necessary to study aqueous aspirates to confirm that the patient is in relapse (72). In most cases, after the diagnosis has been established by cytologic examination of the aqueous aspirate, treatment usually includes irradiation and chemotherapy. In one reported case, the glaucoma cleared after washing necrotic tumor cells from the anterior chamber (72).

Other Neoplasias

Lymphomas

An autopsy review of 60 eyes from patients with lymphomas revealed ocular involvement in four (6.7%) (51). The anterior ocular segment may be involved, presenting as iridocyclitis, with occasional IOP elevation (74). A case of open-angle glaucoma has also been reported in association with a subconjunctival malignant lymphoma (75).

Histiocytosis X

This uncommon multisystem disorder, characterized by accumulation of histiocytes in various tissues, includes three clinical subsets: eosinophilic granuloma (lesions confined to bone), Hand-Schuller-Christian disease (bone and soft tissue involvement), and Letterer-Siwe disease (predominantly soft tissue involvement in infants). Histiocytosis X has been reported to involve the anterior chamber with associated glaucoma (76). This is apparently extremely rare, however, since a study of 76 children with histiocytosis X revealed 18 with orbital, but none with intraocular, involvement (77).

Multiple Myeloma

Apparent nongranulomatous anterior uveitis with associated glaucoma in a patient with multiple myeloma was found by cytologic examination to represent an infiltrate of neoplastic plasma cells (78).

Myelodysplastic Syndrome

In this condition, hematopoietic precursors of all three cell lines (erythroid, myeloid, and megakaryocytic) are abundant, but morphologically abnormal, and 10–30% of cases are fatal due to acute blastic transformation of nonlymphotic leukemia. Cases have been reported in which patients presented with acute angle-closure glaucoma associated with uveal effusion and nonrhegmatogenous retinal detachment and hemorrhage (79, 80).

OCULAR TUMORS OF CHILDHOOD[b]

In addition to leukemia and other systemic neoplasia in which the eye may be involved secondarily, there are certain childhood tumors in which the ocular involvement is a primary part of the disorder. These include retinoblastoma, juvenile xanthogranuloma, and medulloepithelioma.

Retinoblastoma

Incidence of Glaucoma

Although glaucoma is not commonly recognized clinically in children with retinoblastoma, histopathologic studies suggest that glaucoma is a frequent complication of this disease. In one study of 149 eyes, there was histologic evidence of a glaucoma-inducing mechanism in 50% of the cases, although an elevated IOP had been clinically recorded in only 23% (81). In another series of 303 eyes with retinoblastoma, 17% had documented pressure elevation (1). Glaucoma was found in one study to be the presenting sign in 7% of eyes with retinoblastoma, with leukocoria (white pupillary reflex) and strabismus being the most common presentations, at 60% and 20%, respectively (82).

Mechanisms of Glaucoma

Neovascularization of the iris is a frequent histopathologic finding in eyes with retinoblastoma, and is the most common cause of the associated glaucoma (1, 81, 83, 84). Both the rubeosis iridis and neovascular glaucoma are frequently overlooked clinically and should be considered in all cases of retinoblastoma. Two additional causes of glaucoma are angle-closure due to massive exudative retinal detachment (1) and obstruction of the anterior chamber angle by inflammatory cells or necrotic tumor tissue (81). In a review of 1500 patients with retinoblastoma, anterior chamber involvement was seen in 30 cases and was found to indicate a poor prognosis (85). Specular microscopy has been shown to demonstrate clusters of retinoblastoma cells on the corneal endothelium as a bright, lacy network of reflections within a dark area (86).

Differential Diagnosis

Conditions which simulate retinoblastoma have been called "pseudogliomas" and include retinopathy of prematurity, persistent hyperplastic primary vitreous, retinal dysplasia, Coats' disease, toxocariasis, and infantile retinal detachment (87, 88). Each of these conditions also have a high incidence of rubeosis iridis so that this factor is not helpful in distinguishing retinoblastoma from the pseudogliomas (84, 87).

[b]Refer to Shields, MB: Color Atlas of Glaucoma. Baltimore, Williams & Wilkins, 1998, Plate II32.

Management

The presence of rubeosis iridis, with or without glaucoma, indicates a more grave prognosis in patients with retinoblastoma (84). This is also true when glaucoma is present without iris neovascularization, since it usually indicates a large tumor with angle closure or dissemination of tumor cells into the anterior chamber (85). In most of these cases, enucleation is indicated.

Juvenile Xanthogranuloma

This is a benign, self-limiting disease of infants and young children, with rare cases in young adults (89). It is characterized by discrete, yellow, papular cutaneous lesions primarily of the head and neck, as well as salmon-colored to lightly pigmented lesions of the iris (90, 91). The diagnosis is usually established by a biopsy of a skin lesion or an aqueous tap and iris biopsy, the histology of which reveals foamy histiocytes and Touton giant cells. The iris lesions are typically unilateral and may cause spontaneous hyphema. Glaucoma may occur from invasion of the anterior chamber angle with histiocytes or from the hyphema or a secondary uveitis. Treatment for eyes with juvenile xanthogranuloma and associated glaucoma includes topical and subconjunctival corticosteroids and occasional external beam irradiation (92–97). Invasive surgery should be avoided if possible. Attempted trabeculectomies in one child resulted in only light perception (97).

Medulloepithelioma

A medulloepithelioma, or diktyoma, is a primary tumor of childhood, which arises most often from nonpigmented ciliary epithelium. The clinical appearance is that of a whitish-gray mass or cyst of the iris or ciliary body. In a study of 56 cases, glaucoma was observed clinically in 26 eyes (98). Histopathologic evidence of glaucoma was seen in 18 cases, 11 of which had rubeosis iridis. Peripheral anterior synechiae and shallow anterior chambers were also commonly observed. In one report, glaucoma was associated with two white flocculi floating in the anterior chamber, delicate iris neovascularization, and a globular ciliary body mass (99). Some medulloepitheliomas are malignant, although the mortality rate is low. While enucleation is the most common treatment, success has been reported with iridocyclectomy, and local excision has been recommended when the tumor is small and well-circumscribed (98).

Rhabdomyosarcoma

Rhabdomyosarcoma is the most common malignant orbital tumor of childhood. It is rarely intraocular, but has been reported to arise from the iris or ciliary body (100).

BENIGN TUMORS OF THE ANTERIOR UVEA

In the differential diagnosis of anterior uveal tumors, several benign lesions must be considered. These include nevi, cysts, melanocytoses, melanocytomas, adenomas, and leiomyomas. Glaucoma may be associated with several of these conditions, further compounding the diagnostic problem.

Nevi of the Iris

One or more nevi on the stromal surface of the iris is not an uncommon clinical finding. They are usually recognized as small, discrete, flat or slightly elevated lesions of variable pigmentation. Some, however, may be confused with melanomas, which has led to unnecessary surgical intervention. In a retrospective clinicopathologic study of 189 lesions of the anterior uvea that were originally diagnosed as melanomas, 80% were reclassified as nevi of several cell types (101). These authors found no clinical features to distinguish benign from malignant tumors, including diffuse spread or the presence of glaucoma. In another study of melanocytic iris tumors, however, five clinical variables were associated with a higher risk of malignancy: (a) diameter greater than 3 mm; (b) pigment dispersion; (c) prominent tumor vascularity; (d) elevated IOP; and (e) tumor-related ocular symptoms (102). As previously noted in this chapter, fluorescein angiography of the iris, aqueous aspiration for cytologic examination, or a biopsy may aid in the important differentiation between melanomas and benign lesions of the iris. Diffuse, pigmented and nonpigmented nevi of the iris can cause glaucoma by direct extension across the trabecular meshwork (101, 103). This is rare in children, but the case of a 16-year-old girl has been reported in which an aggressive iris nevus caused glaucoma by invading the trabecular meshwork (104).

A specific form of iris nevus with associated glaucoma is the *iris nevus syndrome*. In these cases, diffuse nevi of the iris are associated with progressive synechial closure of the angle and subsequent IOP elevation (105). A subset of the iridocorneal endothelial syndrome, the *Cogan-Reese syndrome*, has a similar clinical appearance, but the pedunculated nodules on the surface of the iris are composed of tissue resembling iris stroma (106). The benign lesions of the iris in both of these conditions have been mistaken for malignant melanomas, which has led to enucleation in some patients. These conditions are discussed further in Chapter 13.

Cysts

Cysts of the iris have been classified as primary and secondary, with the former arising from the epithelial layers of the iris and ciliary body or, less often, from the iris stroma (107). The majority of the primary cysts are stationary lesions, rarely progressing or causing visual complications. However, families have been described in which multiple cysts of the iris and ciliary body, presumably of autosomal dominant inheritance, caused angle-closure glaucoma (108). Other reported mechanisms of IOP elevation associated with iris cysts include pigment dispersion (109) and a mucus-producing epithelial cyst of the iris stroma of unknown origin (110). Iris cysts have been successfully treated by laser cystotomy (108, 111), although others may require surgical excision if uncontrolled IOP or other symptoms persist. Secondary cysts of the iris may result from surgery, trauma or neoplasia, and are more likely than primary cysts to lead to inflammation and glaucoma (107, 112). Ultrasound has been shown to be a useful diagnostic adjunct for both primary and secondary iris cysts (112, 113).

Melanocytomas

These tumors are classified as benign nevi and are seen clinically as darkly pigmented lesions, usually on the optic nerve head and less often in the choroid, ciliary body, or iris. Those in the latter location have been reported to cause glaucoma, either by direct spread into the anterior chamber angle (114) or dispersion of pigment into the angle from a necrotic melanocytoma (115).

Melanoses

Melanosis iridis is characterized by verrucous-like elevations on the surface of a darkly pigmented, velvety iris. It is usually unilateral and sometimes sectorial, although bilateral involvement has been reported (116). *Melanosis oculi* has additional hyperpigmentation of the episclera, choroid or both and has been reported in association with open-angle glaucoma, in which the mechanism appears to be heavy pigmentation of the trabecular meshwork (117). A similar condition has been observed in oculodermal melanocytosis (nevus of Ota), which is considered further in the next section of this chapter.

Adenomas

Benign adenomas may arise from the epithelium of the anterior uvea, especially the ciliary body (Fuchs' adenoma) (118). They occur predominantly in adults, although adenomas have been observed in a child with associated hyperplastic primary vitreous (119). While common among the elderly, they are rarely noted clinically (120). Some, however, can involve the iris, primarily or secondarily (121), and have been reported to cause glaucoma from pigment dispersion (122). Adenomas must be distinguished from anterior uveal cysts and melanomas (121). Adenocarcinomas may also arise from the ciliary body epithelium and have been reported to cause glaucoma (123).

Leiomyomas

These rare tumors may appear as a slow-growing grayish white, vascularized nodule on the surface of the iris. Glaucoma is not a typical complication.

PHAKOMATOSES[c]

In 1932, Van der Hoeve (124) coined the term "phakomatosis," meaning "motherspot" or "birthmark," to denote a group of disorders that are characterized by *hamartomas,* which are congenital tumors arising from tissue that is normally found in the involved area. The hamartomas primarily involve the eye, skin, and nervous system, although other systems may be involved to a lesser degree, including pulmonary, cardiovascular, gastrointestinal, renal, and skeletal. In some cases, the anomalies are present at birth, while others become manifest later in life. The four conditions that traditionally comprise the phakomatoses are (a) von Hippel-Lindau syndrome, (b) von Recklinghausen's neurofibromatosis, (c) tuberous sclerosis or Bourneville's disease, and (d) Sturge-Weber syndrome. Several other disorders subsequently have been included by various authors. The following discussion is limited to those phakomatoses which frequently, or occasionally, may have associated glaucoma.

Sturge-Weber Syndrome (Encephalotrigeminal Angiomatosis)

General Features

The hamartoma in this condition arises from vascular tissue and produces a characteristic port-wine hemangioma of the skin along the trigeminal distribution (Fig. 18.10) and an ipsilateral leptomeningeal angioma. The angiomata are present at birth and are usually unilateral, although bilateral cases also occur. In one review of 51 patients, the condition was recognized before 24 months of age in more than half the cases (125). The nervous system involvement frequently causes seizure disorders, hemispheric motor or sensory defects, and intellectual deficiency. A characteristic radiographic finding is cortical calcifications that develop after several years and appear as double densities or "railroad tracks." There is no race or sex predilection, and no hereditary pattern has been established.

[c]Refer to Shields, MB: Color Atlas of Glaucoma. Baltimore, Williams & Wilkins, 1998, Plates II33–35.

Ocular Features

In approximately half of the cases in which the port-wine stain involves both the ophthalmic and maxillary divisions of the trigeminal nerve, glaucoma will be present. Slitlamp examination typically reveals a dense episcleral vascular plexus and occasional ampulliform dilatations of conjunctival vessels. These findings are always on the side of the cutaneous lesion. Some patients also have a choroidal hemangioma. In the study of 51 patients noted above, 69% had conjunctival or episcleral hemangiomas, and 55% had choroidal hemangiomas (125). Glaucoma was present in 71% of the patients (125).

Theories of Glaucoma Mechanism

The cause of glaucoma in the Sturge-Weber syndrome has been a controversial issue. Weiss (126) described two mechanisms, the more common of which occurs in infants, with a developmental anomaly of the anterior chamber angle similar to that of congenital glaucoma. One histopathologic report described a partial developmental anomaly of the anterior chamber angle (127), while another study revealed

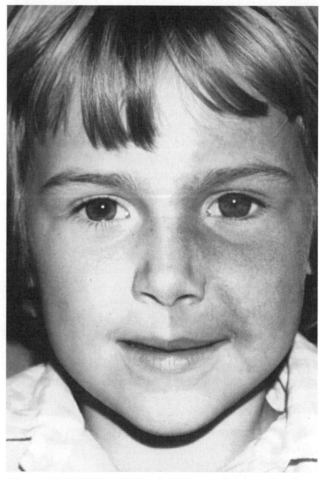

Figure 18.10. Child with Sturge-Weber syndrome and unilateral glaucoma showing typical port-wine hemangioma of the skin along the distribution of the left trigeminal nerve.

neovascularization in the trabecular meshwork (128). Cibis and associates (129) found aging changes, similar to those seen in chronic open-angle glaucoma, in the trabecular meshwork of three eyes with Sturge-Weber syndrome.

The other mechanism of glaucoma appears later in life and is associated with an open anterior chamber angle and small arteriovenous fistulas in the episcleral vessels. Phelps (130) observed episcleral hemangiomas in all cases and elevated episcleral venous pressure whenever this parameter could be studied, but saw no abnormalities of the anterior chamber angle. He felt that elevated episcleral venous pressure was the most common glaucoma mechanism in all ages of patients with the Sturge-Weber syndrome.

Management

Medical therapy may suffice to control the glaucoma that occurs in later life, while the infantile form usually requires surgical intervention (126). Success has been reported with a trabeculectomy in children and adults (131, 132). However, filtering surgery in these patients is commonly associated with intraoperative choroidal effusion (132–134), and occasionally with expulsive hemorrhage (127, 133–135). In one study of 30 patients, goniotomy was not associated with these complications and was the author's first choice in most cases (132). Since it may not be certain whether the glaucoma is due to an anterior chamber angle anomaly or elevated episcleral venous pressure, a combined trabeculotomy-trabeculectomy may improve the chances of success, by treating both possible sources of elevated IOP (133, 136), although it does not reduce the potential for serious complications. Another alternative to reduce the risk of massive choroidal effusion and expulsive hemorrhage is a cyclodestructive procedure.

von Recklinghausen's Neurofibromatosis

General Features

The principal systemic lesions in this condition involve the skin and include café au lait spots, which are flat, hyperpigmented lesions with well-circumscribed borders, and neurofibromas, that appear as soft, flesh-colored, pedunculated masses. The latter lesions arise from Schwann cells. Central nervous system involvement is uncommon, although neurofibromas may develop from cranial nerves, especially the acoustic nerve. Two subsets of neurofibromatosis have been distinguished: *peripheral* (von Recklinghausen's), characterized by the skin lesions, and *central,* characterized by bilateral acoustic Schwannomas (137). Both are inherited by an autosomal dominant mode with variable expressivity. Genetic analysis of a kindred with von Recklinghausen's neurofibromatosis indicated that the responsible gene is located near the centromere on chromosome 17 (138).

Ocular Features

In the peripheral form, the eyelids, conjunctiva, iris, ciliary body, and choroid may be involved with the neurofibromas. The hamartomatous lesions of the iris are called *Lisch nodules* (139). They are usually bilateral and characterized by well-defined, clear to yellow, or brown, dome-shaped, gelatinous elevations on the iris stroma (Fig 18.11). An ultrastructural study indicates that they are of melanocytic origin (140). Lisch nodules are a nearly constant feature of von Recklinghausen's neurofibromatosis, occurring in 92% of one series of 77 patients (141). In another study of 64 patient, the nodules were seen in 95% and in all patients aged 16 years or older (142). In addition, chorioretinal hamartomas and gliomas of the optic nerve are occasionally present. A fluorescein angiographic study of the choroidal lesions revealed avascular patches of hypofluorescence similar to multiple small choroidal nevi (142). The central form of neurofibromatosis does not typically have ocular findings, other than presenile posterior subcapsular or nuclear cataracts (137).

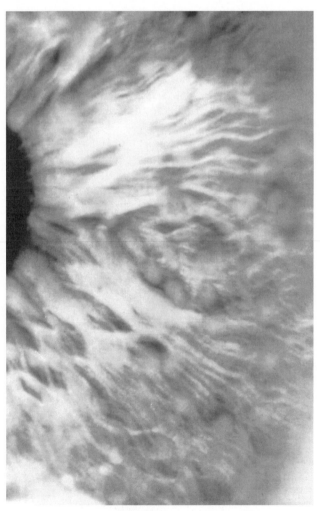

Figure 18.11. Slitlamp view of Lisch nodules on the iris of a patient with von Recklinghausen's neurofibromatosis. (Courtesy of George Rosenwasser, M.D.)

Intraocular pressure elevation is more likely to occur in neurofibromatosis when the lids are involved with neurofibromas. The several possible mechanisms of glaucoma include (a) infiltration of the angle with neurofibromatous tissue, (b) closure of the anterior chamber angle due to nodular thickening of the ciliary body and choroid, (c) fibrovascular membrane resembling neovascular glaucoma, and (d) failure of normal anterior chamber angle development (143, 144).

Management

In treating the glaucoma, medical measures should be attempted first, since surgical approaches are often not satisfactory. An infant with unilateral glaucoma underwent five unsuccessful operations before ocular neurofibromatosis was discovered 2 years later (145).

von Hippel-Lindau Disease

This phakomatosis is characterized by angiomatosis of the retina and, in a small percentage of cases, the cerebellum. Most cases are not familial. Glaucoma may occur as a late sequelae due to rubeosis iridis or iridocyclitis.

Nevus of Ota (Oculodermal Melanocytosis)

This condition is not included in all reported classifications of the phakomatoses, but does fit the broader definition of the disease group.

General Features

The hamartoma in this condition represents an abnormally large accumulation of melanocytes in ocular tissues, especially the episclera (Fig. 18.12), as well as the skin in the distribution of the trigeminal nerve, and occasionally the nasal or buccal mucosa. In a study of 194 patients, 67 had only dermal involvement, 12 had only ocular involvement, and 115 had both (146). It is nearly always unilateral with a preponderance of females and a tendency toward races with darker pigmentation (147). Degeneration to malignant melanomas may occur in Caucasian patients, but rarely in non-Caucasians (148–151).

Glaucoma

Evidence of chronic glaucoma has been observed in patients with the nevus of Ota (152–156). Elevated IOP, with or without glaucomatous damage, was seen in 10% of one series (146). The involved eye typically has unusually heavy pigmentation of the trabecular meshwork, and histopathologic studies have revealed melanocytes in the meshwork (154, 155).

Management

Medical management, as with other forms of open-angle glaucoma, should be tried first. When this fails, laser trabeculoplasty may be effective (117), although filtering surgery will most likely be required.

SUMMARY

Primary malignant melanomas of the uvea may cause open-angle forms of glaucoma by either direct extension or seed-

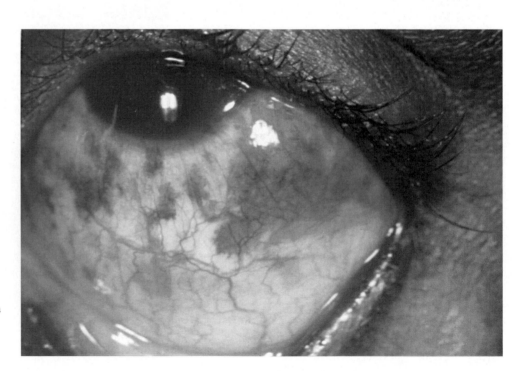

Figure 18.12. Abnormal pigmentation of the episclera in a patient with oculodermal melanocytosis (Nevus of Ota).

ing of tumor cells, pigment granules, or macrophages into the anterior chamber angle. Less often, these tumors may cause angle-closure glaucoma by a mass effect behind the iris or lens. Ultrasonography and cytology of aqueous aspirates are useful diagnostic adjuncts, and most confirmed cases are managed by enucleation. Systemic malignancies, including metastatic carcinomas and melanomas, leukemias, and lymphomas, may occasionally cause glaucoma, usually by invasion of the anterior chamber angle. Ocular tumors of childhood that may cause glaucoma include retinoblastoma, juvenile xanthogranuloma, and medulloepithelioma. Other benign tumors of the anterior uvea that may be associated with glaucoma are nevi, cysts, melanocytomas, melanosis, adenomas, and leiomyomas. Some of the phakomatoses, most notably the Sturge-Weber syndrome, von Recklinghausen's neurofibromatosis, and the nevus of Ota, may also have associated glaucoma.

REFERENCES

1. Shields, CL, Shields, JA, Shields, MB, Augsburger, JJ: Prevalence and mechanisms of secondary intraocular pressure elevation in eyes with intraocular tumors. Ophthalmology 94:839, 1987.
2. Yanoff, M: Glaucoma mechanisms in ocular malignant melanomas. Am J Ophthalmol 70:898, 1970.
3. Shields, MB, Klintworth, GK: Anterior uveal melanomas and intraocular pressure. Ophthalmology 87:503, 1980.
4. Hopkins, RE, Carriker, FR: Malignant melanoma of the ciliary body. Am J Ophthalmol 45:835, 1958.
5. Omulecki, W, Pruszczynski, M, Borowski, J: Ring melanoma of the iris and ciliary body. Br J Ophthalmol 69:514, 1985.
6. Yanoff, M, Scheie, HG: Melanomalytic glaucoma. Report of a case. Arch Ophthalmol 84:471, 1970.
7. Van Buskirk, EM, Leure-duPree, AE: Pathophysiology and electron microscopy of melanomalytic glaucoma. Am J Ophthalmol 85:160, 1978.
8. McMenamin, PG, Lee, WR: Ultrastructural pathology of melanomalytic glaucoma. Br J Ophthalmol 70:895, 1986.
9. Reese, AB, Mund, ML, Iwamoto, T: Tapioca melanoma of the iris. Part 1. Clinical and light microscopy studies. Am J Ophthalmol 74:840, 1972.
10. Zakka, KA, Foos, RY, Sulit, H: Metastatic tapioca iris melanoma. Br J Ophthalmol 63:744, 1979.
11. Shields, MB, Proia, AD: Neovascular glaucoma associated with an iris melanoma. A clinicopathologic report. Arch Ophthalmol 105:672, 1987.
12. Foos, RY, Hull, SN, Straatsma, BR: Early diagnosis of ciliary body melanomas. Arch Ophthalmol 81:336, 1969.
13. Gupta, K, Hoepner, JA, Streeten, BW: Pseudomelanoma of the iris in herpes simplex keratoiritis. Ophthalmology 93:1524, 1986.
14. Shields, JA, Sanborn, GE, Augsburger, JJ: The differential diagnosis of malignant melanoma of the iris. A clinical study of 200 patients. Ophthalmology 90:716, 1983.
15. Marcus, DM, Mawn, LA, Egan, KM, Albert, DM: Nucleolar organizer regions in iris nevi and melanomas. Am J Ophthalmol 114:202, 1992.
16. Singer, PR, Krupin, T, Smith, ME, Becker, B: Recurrent orbital and metastatic melanoma in a patient undergoing previous glaucoma surgery. Am J Ophthalmol 87:766, 1979.
17. El Baba, F, Hagler, WS, De La Cruz, A, Green, WR: Choroidal melanoma with pigment dispersion in vitreous and melanomalytic glaucoma. Ophthalmology 95:370, 1988.
18. Fraser, DJ, Font, RL: Ocular inflammation and hemorrhage as initial manifestations of uveal malignant melanoma. Incidence and prognosis. Arch Ophthalmol 97:1311, 1979.
19. Alward, WLM, Frazier Byrne, S, Hughes, JR, Hodapp, EA: Dislocated lens nuclei simulating choroidal melanomas. Arch Ophthalmol 107:1463, 1989.
20. Gitter, KA, Meyer, D, Sarin, LK: Ultrasound to evaluate eyes with opaque media. Am J Ophthalmol 64:100, 1967.
21. Shields, JA: Accuracy and limitations of the ^{32}P test in the diagnosis of ocular tumors: an analysis of 500 cases. Ophthalmology 85:950, 1978.
22. Goldberg, B, Kara, GB, Previte, LR: The use of radioactive phosphorus (^{32}P) in the diagnosis of ocular tumors. Am J Ophthalmol 90:817, 1980.
23. Christiansen, JM, Wetzig, PC, Thatcher, DB, Green, WR: Diagnosis and management of anterior uveal tumors. Ophthalmic Surg 10:81, 1979.
24. Brovkina, AF, Chichua, AG: Value of fluorescein iridography in diagnosis of tumours of the iridociliary zone. Br J Ophthalmol 63:157, 1979.
25. Jakobiec, FA, Depot, MJ, Henkind, P, Spencer, WH: Fluorescein angiographic patterns of iris melanocytic tumors. Arch Ophthalmol 100:1288, 1982.
26. Char, DH, Schwartz, A, Miller, TR, Abele, JS: Ocular metastases from systemic melanoma. Am J Ophthalmol 90:702, 1980.
27. Green, WR: Diagnostic cytopathology of ocular fluid specimens. Ophthalmology 91:726, 1984.
28. Midena, E, Segato, T, Piermarocchi, S, Boccato, P: Fine needle aspiration biopsy in ophthalmology. Surv Ophthalmol 29:410, 1985.
29. Char, DH, Crawford, JB, Gonzales, J, Miller, T: Iris melanoma with increased intraocular pressure. Differentiation of focal solitary tumors from diffuse or multiple tumors. Arch Ophthalmol 107:548, 1989.
30. Karcioglu, ZA, Caldwell, DR: Frozen section diagnosis in ophthalmic surgery. Surv Ophthalmol 28:323, 1984.
31. Barr, CC, McLean, IW, Zimmerman, LE: Uveal melanoma in children and adolescents. Arch Ophthalmol 99:2133, 1981.
32. Rones, B, Zimmerman, LE: The prognosis of primary tumors of the iris treated by iridectomy. Arch Ophthalmol 60:193, 1958.
33. Dunphy, EB, Dryja, TP, Albert, DM, Smith, TR: Melanocytic tumor of the anterior uvea. Am J Ophthalmol 86:680, 1978.
34. Sunba, MSN, Rahi, AHS, Morgan, G: Tumors of the anterior uvea. I. Metastasizing malignant melanoma of the iris. Arch Ophthalmol 98:82, 1980.
35. Kersten, RC, Tse, DT, Anderson, R: Iris melanoma. Nevus or malignancy? Surv Ophthalmol 29:423, 1985.
36. Geisse, LJ, Robertson, DM: Iris melanomas. Am J Ophthalmol 99:638, 1985.
37. Territo, C, Shields, CL, Shields, JA, et al: Natural course of melanocytic tumors of the iris. Ophthalmology 95:1251, 1988.
38. McGalliard, JN, Johnston, PB: A study of iris melanoma in Northern Ireland. Br J Ophthalmol 73:591, 1989.
39. Shields, JA, Shields, CL: Hepatic metastases of diffuse iris melanoma 17 years after enucleation. Am J Ophthalmol 106:749, 1989.
40. Charteris, DG: Progression of an iris melanoma over 41 years. Br J Ophthalmol 74:566, 1990.
41. Sugar, HS: Removal of some intraocular tumors: report of twelve cases. Ann Ophthalmol 13:633, 1981.
42. Memmen, JE, McLean, IW: The long-term outcome of patients undergoing iridocyclectomy. Ophthalmology 97:429, 1990.
43. Foulds, WS, Lee, WR: The significance of glaucoma in the management of melanomas of the anterior segment. Trans Ophthalmol Soc UK 103:59, 1983.
44. Zimmerman, LE, McLean, IW, Foster, WD: Statistical analysis of follow-up data concerning uveal melanomas, and the influence of enucleation. Ophthalmology 87:557, 1980.
45. Kramer, KK, LaPiana, FG, Whitmore, PV: Enucleation with stabilization of intraocular pressure in the treatment of uveal melanomas. Ophthalmic Surg 11:39, 1980.

46. Blair, CJ, Guerry, RK, Stratford, TP: Normal intraocular pressure during enucleation for choroidal melanoma. Arch Ophthalmol 101:1900, 1983.

47. Migdal, C: Effect of the method of enucleation on the prognosis of choroidal melanoma. Br J Ophthalmol 67:385, 1983.

48. Cleasby, GW, Van Westenbrugge, JA: Treatment of iris melanoma by photocoagulation: a case report. Ophthalmic Surg 18:42, 1987.

49. Grossniklaus, HE, Brown, RH, Stulting, RD, Blasberg, RD: Iris melanoma seeding through a trabeculectomy site. Arch Ophthalmol 108:1287, 1990.

50. Bloch, RS, Gartner, S: The incidence of ocular metastatic carcinoma. Arch Ophthalmol 85:673, 1971.

51. Nelson, CC, Hertzberg, BS, Klintworth, GK: A histopathologic study of 716 unselected eyes in patients with cancer at the time of death. Am J Ophthalmol 95:788, 1983.

52. Scholz, R, Green, WR, Baranano, EC, et al: Metastatic carcinoma to the iris. Diagnosis by aqueous paracentesis and response to irradiation and chemotherapy. Ophthalmology 90:1524, 1983.

53. Ferry, AP, Font, RL: Carcinoma metastatic to the eye and orbit. I. A clinicopathologic study of 227 cases. Arch Ophthalmol 92:276, 1974.

54. Ferry, AP, Font, RL: Carcinoma metastatic to the eye and orbit. II. A clinicopathological study of 26 patients with carcinoma metastatic to the anterior segment of the eye. Arch Ophthalmol 93:472, 1975.

55. Freeman, TR, Friedman, AH: Metastatic carcinoma of the iris. Am J Ophthalmol 80:947, 1975.

56. Frank, KW, Sugar, HS, Sherman, AI, et al: Anterior segment metastases from an ovarian choriocarcinoma. Am J Ophthalmol 87:778, 1979.

57. Woog, JJ, Chess, J, Albert, DM, et al: Metastatic carcinoma of the iris simulating iridocyclitis. Br J Ophthalmol 68:167, 1984.

58. Kurosawa, A, Sawaguchi, S: Iris metastasis from squamous cell carcinoma of the uterine cervix. Arch Ophthalmol 105:618, 1987.

59. Khawly, JA, Shields, MB: Metastatic carcinoma manifesting as angle-closure glaucoma. Am J Ophthalmol 118:116, 1994.

60. Johnson, BL: Bilateral glaucoma caused by nasal carcinoma obstructing Schlemm's canal. Am J Ophthalmol 96:550, 1983.

61. Rotkis, WM, Kulander, BG, Chandler, JW, Kaiser, FS: Diagnosis of anterior chamber metastasis by serologic marker found during anterior chamber paracentesis. Am J Ophthalmol 102:179, 1986.

62. Wormald, RPL, Harper, JI: Bilateral black hypopyon in a patient with self-healing cutaneous malignant melanoma. Br J Ophthalmol 67:231, 1983.

63. Abramson, A: Anterior chamber activity in children with acute leukemia. Ann Ophthalmol 12:553, 1980.

64. Ohkoshi, K, Tsiaras, WG: Prognostic importance of ophthalmic manifestations in childhood leukaemia. Br J Ophthalmol 76:651, 1992.

65. Rennie, I: Ophthalmic manifestations of childhood leukaemia. Br J Ophthalmol 76:641, 1992.

66. Novakovic, P, Kellie, SJ, Taylor, D: Childhood leukaemia: relapse in the anterior segment of the eye. Br J Ophthalmol 73:354, 1989.

67. Leonardy, NJ, Rupani, M, Dent, G, Klintworth, GK: Analysis of 135 autopsy eyes for ocular involvement in leukemia. Am J Ophthalmol 109:436, 1990.

68. Zakka, KA, Yee, RD, Shorr, N, et al: Leukemic iris infiltration. Am J Ophthalmol 89:204, 1980.

69. Kincaid, MC, Green, WR: Ocular and orbital involvement in leukemia. Surv Ophthalmol 27:211, 1983.

70. Rosenthal, AR: Ocular manifestations of leukemia. A review. Ophthalmology 90:899, 1983.

71. Santoni, G, Fiore, C, Lupidi, G, Bibbiani, U: Recurring bilateral hypopyon in chronic myeloid leukemia in blastic transformation. A case report. Graefes Arch Clin Exp Ophthalmol 223:211, 1985.

72. Ayliffe, W, Foster, CS, Marcoux, P, et al: Relapsing acute myeloid leukemia manifesting as hypopyon uveitis. Am J Ophthalmol 119:361, 1995.

73. Kozlowski, IMD, Hirose, T, Jalkh, AE: Massive subretinal hemorrhage with acute angle-closure glaucoma in chronic myelocytic leukemia. Am J Ophthalmol 103:837, 1987.

74. Saga, T, Ohno, S, Matsuda, H, et al: Ocular involvement by a peripheral T-cell lymphoma. Arch Ophthalmol 102:399, 1984.

75. Sato, M, Futa, R: A case of secondary open-angle glaucoma associated with subconjunctival malignant melanoma. Jpn J Clin Ophthalmol 40:57, 1986.

76. Epstein, DL, Grant, WM: Secondary open-angle glaucoma in histiocytosis X. Am J Ophthalmol 84:332, 1977.

77. Moore, AT, Pritchard, J, Taylor, DSI: Histiocytosis X: an ophthalmological review. Br J Ophthalmol 69:7, 1985.

78. Shakin, EP, Augsburger, JJ, Eagle, RC Jr, et al: Multiple myeloma involving the iris. Arch Ophthalmol 106:524, 1988.

79. Smith, DL, Skuta, GL, Trobe, JD, Weinberg, AB: Angle-closure glaucoma as initial presentation of myelodysplastic syndrome. Can J Ophthalmol 25:306, 1990.

80. Wohlrab, T-M, Pleyer, U, Rohrbach, JM, et al: Sudden increase in intraocular pressure as an initial manifestation of myelodysplastic syndrome. Am J Ophthalmol 119:370, 1995.

81. Yoshizumi, MO, Thomas, JV, Smith, TR: Glaucoma-inducing mechanisms in eyes with retinoblastoma. Arch Ophthalmol 96:105, 1978.

82. Ellsworth, RM: The practical management of retinoblastoma. Trans Am Ophthalmol Soc 67:462, 1969.

83. Walton, DS, Grant, WM: Retinoblastoma and iris neovascularization. Am J Ophthalmol 65:598, 1968.

84. Spaulding, AG: Rubeosis iridis in retinoblastoma and pseudoglioma. Trans Am Ophthalmol Soc 76:584, 1978.

85. Haik, BG, Dunleavy, SA, Cooke, C, et al: Retinoblastoma with anterior chamber extension. Ophthalmology 94:367, 1987.

86. Roberts, CW, Iwamoto, M, Haik, BC: Ultrastructural correlation of specular microscopy in retinoblastoma. Am J Ophthalmol 102:182, 1986.

87. Moazed, K, Albert, D, Smith, TR: Rubeosis iridis in "pseudogliomas." Surv Ophthalmol 25:85, 1980.

88. Shields, JA: Ocular toxocariasis. A review. Surv Ophthalmol 28:361, 1984.

89. Bruner, WE, Stark, WJ, Green, WR: Presumed juvenile xanthogranuloma of the iris and ciliary body in an adult. Arch Ophthalmol 100:457, 1982.

90. Zimmerman, L: Ocular lesions of juvenile xanthogranuloma (nevoxanthoendothelioma). Trans Am Acad Ophthalmol Otol 69:412, 1965.

91. Schwartz, LW, Rodrigues, MM, Hallett, JW: Juvenile xanthogranuloma diagnosed by paracentesis. Am J Ophthalmol 77:243, 1974.

92. Gass, JDM: Management of juvenile xanthogranuloma of the iris. Arch Ophthalmol 71:344, 1964.

93. Hadden, OB: Bilateral juvenile xanthogranuloma of the iris. Br J Ophthalmol 59:699, 1975.

94. Witmer, R, Landolt, E: Juvenile xanthogranuloma of the iris. Klin Monatsbl Augenheilkd 176:658, 1980.

95. Thieme, R, Lukassek, B, Keinert, K: Problems in juvenile xanthogranuloma of the anterior uvea. Klin Monatsbl Augenheilkd 176:893, 1980.

96. Cadera, W, Silver, MM, Burt, L: Juvenile xanthogranuloma. Can J Ophthalmol 18:169, 1983.

97. Casteels, I, Olver, J, Malone, M, Taylor, D: Early treatment of juvenile xanthogranuloma of the iris with subconjunctival steroids. Br J Ophthalmol 77:57, 1993.

98. Broughton, WL, Zimmerman, LE: A clinicopathologic study of 56 cases of intraocular medulloepitheliomas. Am J Ophthalmol 85:407, 1978.

99. Jakobiec, FA, Howard, GM, Ellsworth, RM, Rosen, M: Electron microscopic diagnosis of medulloepithelioma. Am J Ophthalmol 79:321, 1975.

100 Wilson, ME, McClatchey, SK, Zimmerman, LE: Rhabdomyosarcoma of the ciliary body. Ophthalmology 97:1484, 1990.

101. Jakobiec, FA, Silbert, G: Are most iris "melanomas" really nevi? A clinicopathologic study of 189 lesions. Arch Ophthalmol 99:2117, 1981.

102. Harbour, JW, Augsburger, JJ, Eagle, RC Jr: Initial management and follow-up of melanocytic iris tumors. Ophthalmology 102:1987, 1995.

103. Nik, NA, Hidayat, A, Zimmerman, LE, Fine, BS: Diffuse iris nevus manifested by unilateral open angle glaucoma. Arch Ophthalmol 99:125, 1981.

104. Carlson, DW, Alward, WLM, Folberg, R: Aggressive nevus of the iris with secondary glaucoma in a child. Am J Ophthalmol 119:367, 1995.

105. Scheie, HG, Yanoff, M: Iris nevus (Cogan-Reese) syndrome. A cause of unilateral glaucoma. Arch Ophthalmol 93:963, 1975.

106. Cogan, DG, Reese, AB: A syndrome of iris nodules, ectopic Descemet's membrane, and unilateral glaucoma. Doc Ophthalmol 26:424, 1969.

107. Shields, JA, Kline, WM, Augsburger, JJ: Primary iris cysts: a review of the literature and report of 62 cases. Br J Ophthalmol 68:152, 1984.

108. Vela, A, Rieser, JC, Campbell, DG: The heredity and treatment of angle-closure glaucoma secondary to iris and ciliary body cysts. Ophthalmology 91:332, 1983.

109. Alward, WLM, Ossoinig, KC: Pigment dispersion secondary to cysts of the iris pigment epithelium. Arch Ophthalmol 113:1574, 1995.

110. Albert, DL, Brownstein, S, Kattleman, BS: Mucogenic glaucoma caused by an epithelial cyst of the iris stroma. Am J Ophthalmol 114:222, 1992.

111. Bron, AJ, Wilson, CB, Hill, AR: Laser treatment of primary ring-shaped epithelial iris cyst. Br J Ophthalmol 68:859, 1984.

112. Finger, PT, McCormick, SA, Lombardo, J, et al: Epithelial inclusion cyst of the iris. Arch Ophthalmol 113:777, 1995.

113. Sidoti, PA, Valencia, M, Chen, N, et al: Echographic evaluation of primary cysts of the iris pigment epithelium. Am J Ophthalmol 120:161, 1995.

114. Nakazawa, M, Tamai, M: Iris melanocytoma with secondary glaucoma. Am J Ophthalmol 97:797, 1984.

115. Shields, JA, Annesley, WH Jr, Spaeth, GL: Necrotic melanocytoma of iris with secondary glaucoma. Am J Ophthalmol 84:826, 1977.

116. Traboulsi, EI, Maumenee, IH: Bilateral melanosis of the iris. Am J Ophthalmol 103:115, 1987.

117. Goncalves, V, Sandler, T, O'Donnell, FE Jr: Open angle glaucoma in melanosis oculi: response to laser trabeculoplasty. Ann Ophthalmol 17:33, 1985.

118. Lieb, WE, Shields, JA, Eagle, RC Jr, et al: Cystic adenoma of the pigmented ciliary epithelium. Clinical, pathologic, and immunohistopathologic findings. Ophthalmology 97:1489, 1990.

119. Doro, S, Werblin, TP, Haas, B, et al: Fetal adenoma of the pigmented ciliary epithelium associated with persistent hyperplastic primary vitreous. Ophthalmology 93:1343, 1986.

120. Zaidman, GW, Johnson, BL, Salamon, SM, Mondino, BJ: Fuchs' adenoma affecting the peripheral iris. Arch Ophthalmol 101:771, 1983.

121. Shields, CL, Shields, JA, Cook, GR, et al: Differentiation of adenoma of the iris pigment epithelium from iris cyst and melanoma. Am J Ophthalmol 100:678, 1985.

122. Shields, JA, Augsburger, JJ, Sanborn, GE, Klein, RM: Adenoma of the iris-pigment epithelium. Ophthalmology 90:735, 1983.

123. Papale, JJ, Akiwama, K, Hirose, T, et al: Adenocarcinoma of the ciliary body pigment epithelium in a child. Arch Ophthalmol 102:100, 1984.

124. Van der Hoeve, J: Eye symptoms in phakomatoses. Trans Ophthalmol Soc UK 52:380, 1932.

125. Sullivan, TJ, Clarke, MP, Morin, JD: The ocular manifestations of the Sturge-Weber syndrome. J Pediatr Ophthalmol Strabismus 29:349, 1992.

126. Weiss, DI: Dual origin of glaucoma in encephalotrigeminal haemangiomatosis. Trans Ophthalmol Soc UK 93:477, 1973.

127. Christensen, GR, Records, RE: Glaucoma and expulsive hemorrhage mechanisms in the Sturge-Weber syndrome. Ophthalmology 86:1360, 1979.

128. Mwinula, JH, Sagawa, T, Tawara, A, Inomata, H: Anterior chamber angle vascularization in Sturge-Weber syndrome. Report of a case. Graefes Arch Clin Exp Ophthalmol 232:387, 1994.

129. Cibis, GW, Tripathi, RC, Tripathi, BJ: Glaucoma in Sturge-Weber syndrome. Opthalmology 91:1061, 1984.

130. Phelps, CD: The pathogenesis of glaucoma in Sturge-Weber syndrome. Ophthalmology 85:276, 1978.

131. Ali, MA, Fahmy, IA, Spaeth, GL: Trabeculectomy for glaucoma associated with Sturge-Weber syndrome. Ophthalmic Surg 21:352, 1990.

132. Iwach, AG, Hoskins, HD Jr, Hetherington, J Jr, Shaffer, RN: Analysis of surgical and medical management of glaucoma in Sturge-Weber syndrome. Ophthalmology 97:904, 1990.

133. Board, RJ, Shields, MB: Combined trabeculotomy-trabeculectomy for the mangagement of glaucoma associated with Sturge-Weber syndrome. Ophthalmic Surg 12:813, 1981.

134. Bellows, AR, Chylack, LT Jr, Epstein, DL, Hutchinson, BT: Choroidal effusion during glaucoma surgery in patients with prominent episcleral vessels. Arch Ophthalmol 97:493, 1979.

135. Theodossiadis, G, Damanakis, A, Koutsandrea, C: Expulsive choroidal effusion during glaucoma surgery in a child with Sturge-Weber syndrome. Klin Monatsbl Augenheilkd 186:300, 1985.

136. Agarwal, HC, Sandramouli, S, Sihota, R, Sood, NN: Sturge-Weber syndrome: management of glaucoma with combined trabeculotomy-trabeculectomy. Ophthalmic Surg 24:399, 1993.

137. Pearson-Webb, MA, Kaiser-Kupfer, MI, Eldridge, R: Eye findings in bilateral acoustic (central) neurofibromatosis: Association with presenile lens opacities and cataracts but absence of Lisch nodules. N Engl J Med 315:1553, 1986.

138. Barker, D, Wright, E, Nguyen, K, et al: Gene for von Recklinghausen neurofibromatosis is in the pericentromeric region of chromosome 17. Science 236:1100, 1987.

139. Lubs, M-L E, Bauer, MSA, Formas, ME, Djokic, B: Lisch nodules in neurofibromatosis type I. New Eng J Med 324:1264, 1991.

140. Perry, HD, Font, RL: Iris nodules in von Recklinghausen's neurofibromatosis. Electron microscopic confirmation of their melanocytic origin. Arch Ophthalmol 100:1635, 1982.

141. Lewis, RA, Riccardi, VM: von Recklinghausen neurofibromatosis. Incidence of iris hamartomata. Ophthalmology 88:348, 1981.

142. Huson, S, Jones, D, Beck, L: Ophthalmic manifestations of neurofibromatosis. Br J Ophthalmol 71:235, 1987.

143. Grant, WM, Walton, DS: Distinctive gonioscopic findings in glaucoma due to neurofibromatosis. Arch Ophthalmol 79:127, 1968.

144. Wolter, JR, Butler, RG: Pigment spots of the iris and ectropion uveae. With glaucoma in neurofibromatosis. Am J Ophthalmol 56:964, 1963.

145. Brownstein, S, Little, JM: Ocular neurofibromatosis. Ophthalmology 90:1595, 1983.

146. Teekhasaenee, C, Ritch, R, Rutnin, U, Leelawongs, N: Ocular findings in oculodermal melanocytosis. Arch Ophthalmol 108:1114, 1990.

147. Mishima, Y, Mevorah, B: Nevus Ota and nevus Ito in American Negroes. J Invest Dermatol 36:133, 1961.

148. Albert, DM, Scheie, HG: Nevus of Ota with malignant melanoma of the choroid. Report of a case. Arch Ophthalmol 69:774, 1963.

149. Font, RL, Reynolds, AM, Zimmerman, LE: Diffuse malignant melanoma of the iris in the nevus of Ota. Arch Ophthalmol 77:513, 1967.

150. Sabates, FN, Yamashita, T: Congenital melanosis oculi. Complicated by two independent malignant melanomas of the choroid. Arch Ophthalmol 77:801, 1967.

151. Velazquez, N, Jones, IS: Ocular and oculodermal melanocytosis associated with uveal melanoma. Ophthalmology 90:1472, 1983.

152. Fishman, GRA, Anderson, R: Nevus of Ota. Report of two cases, one with open-angle glaucoma. Am J Ophthalmol 54:453, 1962.

153. Foulks, GN, Shields, MB: Glaucoma in oculodermal melanocytosis. Ann Ophthalmol 9:1299, 1977.

154. Sugar, HS: Glaucoma with trabecular melanocytosis. Ann Ophthalmol 14:374, 1982.

155. Futa, R, Shimizu, T, Okura, F, Yasutake, T: A case of open-angle glaucoma associated with nevus Ota—electron microscopic study of the anterior chamber angle and iris. Folia Ophthalmol Jpn 35:501, 1984.

156. Khawly, JA, Imami, N, Shields, MB: Glaucoma associated with the nevus of Ota. Arch Ophthalmol 113:1208, 1995.

Chapter 19

GLAUCOMAS ASSOCIATED WITH OCULAR INFLAMMATION

Any portion of the eye can be affected by inflammatory processes, including the uveal tract (uveitis), cornea (keratitis), sclera (scleritis), and episclera (episcleritis). Uveitis is by far the most common of these disease categories and can have either an acute or chronic course. Most of the acute cases involve the anterior uvea (iritis or iridocyclitis), while the chronic forms, which have been defined as persisting for three months or longer, have been subclassified into four groups: (a) anterior uveitis (iritis or iridocyclitis); (b) intermediate uveitis (pars planitis); (c) posterior uveitis (choroiditis or chorioretinitis); and (d) anterior and posterior uveitis (panuveitis) (1). The relative frequencies of these four types of chronic uveitis, based on a survey of 400 consecutive patients from a uveitis service in Israel, was 45.8%, 15.3%, 14.5%, and 24.5%, respectively (1), which is similar to reported studies from the United States and England (2–4).

The form of ocular inflammation which most frequently produces intraocular pressure (IOP) elevation is iridocyclitis. In addition, when glaucoma is associated with other types of ocular inflammation, there is usually secondary involvement of the anterior uveal tract. We therefore consider first the clinical forms of iridocyclitis and the mechanisms and management of the associated glaucomas, and then review the other forms of ocular inflammation that may be associated with glaucoma.

IRIDOCYCLITIS[a]

Terminology

The general forms of iridocyclitis are classified primarily according to the clinical presentation and duration of active disease. A specific case of iridocyclitis, however, may manifest one or all of these clinical forms at different times during the course of the disease.

Acute Iridocyclitis

The characteristic history for this type of iridocyclitis is the sudden onset of mild to moderate ocular pain, photophobia, and blurred vision. Physical examination typically reveals ciliary flush and a slight constriction of the pupil (Fig. 19.1). Slitlamp biomicroscopy shows variable degrees of aqueous flare and cells, and fine inflammatory precipitates may be seen on the corneal endothelium (keratic precipitates). The IOP is often lower than in the fellow eye, although some patients will present with a marked elevation of the pressure, which may be associated with severe pain and corneal edema.

Subacute Iridocyclitis

Some cases of ocular inflammation produce minimal or no symptoms. The diagnosis may be made during a routine eye examination or as part of a workup for a related sys-

[a]Refer to Shields, MB: Color Atlas of Glaucoma. Baltimore, Williams & Wilkins, 1998, Plates II36–37.

temic disease. This form of iridocyclitis can have serious consequences because complications such as associated glaucoma may go undetected until advanced damage has occurred.

Chronic Iridocyclitis

The clinical presentation in this form of iridocyclitis ranges from acute to subacute, but is characterized by a protracted course of months to years, often with remissions and exacerbations. Complicating sequelae include the formation of posterior and peripheral anterior synechiae, cataracts, and band keratopathy (Fig. 19.2). It is this form of iridocyclitis that is particularly prone to cause glaucoma. In a study of 100 patients with uveitis, all of whom had anterior uveal involvement, glaucoma was present in 23 cases, of which 20 represented chronic uveitis and three acute uveitis (5).

Clinical Forms of Iridocyclitis and Glaucoma

Acute Anterior Uveitis

This is the most common form of ocular inflammation, with a lifetime cumulative incidence of approximately 0.2% in the general population (6). It probably represents a group of conditions characterized by acute iridocyclitis, although the pathogenesis of most cases is unknown except for the close association in many patients with the genetic marker HLA-B27. Acute anterior uveitis is often classified as *HLA-B27-positive* and *HLA-B27-negative* populations. HLA-B27-positive acute anterior uveitis appears to represent a distinct clinical entity,

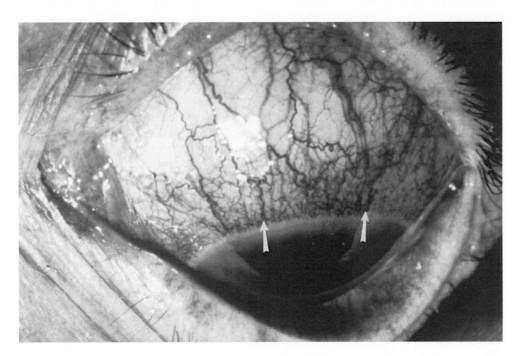

Figure 19.1. Slitlamp view of eye with acute iritis showing typical ciliary flush *(arrows)*. (Courtesy of Gary N. Foulks, M.D.)

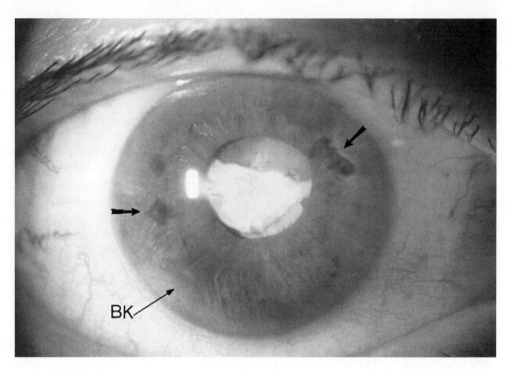

Figure 19.2. Slitlamp view of eye with chronic iritis showing anterior synechiae *(arrows)*, dense cataract, and band keratopathy *(BK)*.

accounting for approximately half of all cases in white patients (7). As compared to patients with HLA-B27-negative acute anterior uveitis, the HLA-B27-positive form occurs more in white individuals, has a younger age of onset (with a median age in the early 30s), a slight preponderance of men, and is typically unilateral or unilateral alternating, although bilateral cases do occur (8–10). Ocular findings may be severe, such as fibrin in the anterior chamber, although mutton fat keratic precipitates are not a typical finding (8). Ocular complications, including cataracts, posterior synechiae, elevated IOP, and cystoid macular edema, are also more common than in HLA-B27-negative cases (8–10), although the long-term visual outcome is not significantly different (8, 9). Anterior segment fluorophotometry suggests that HLA-B27-positive patients have more severe inflammation on the basis of blood-aqueous barrier disruption (11).

Rheumatologic complications, including ankylosing spondylitis, are seen in one-half to two-thirds of the HLA-B27-positive patients, while it is uncommon in the HLA-B27-negative population (8–10). The former patients also have a higher than normal prevalence of first-degree relatives with HLA-B27-positive acute anterior uveitis and ankylosing spondylitis (10, 12).

Patients with acute anterior uveitis usually respond to non-specific anti-inflammatory therapy, as discussed later in this chapter, although it is important to rule out related ocular or systemic disease, which may require more specific therapy.

Sarcoidosis

This is a multisystem inflammatory disorder of uncertain etiology, which has a predilection for young adults and black individuals. The typical histopathologic finding is noncaseating

granulomas, and systemic involvement commonly includes pulmonary hilar lymphadenopathy, peripheral lymphadenopathy, and cutaneous lesions. In a review of 532 cases of sarcoidosis, 202 (38%) had ocular involvement (13), while in another survey of 159 patients with systemic sarcoidosis, more than half presented with ocular lesions as the initial manifestation (14). Ocular findings include chorioretinitis, retinal periphlebitis, and occasional involvement of the optic nerve, orbit, or lacrimal glands, although by far the most common ocular abnormality is anterior uveitis (13, 14).

IRIDOCYCLITIS. Acute iridocyclitis with the previously described features of ciliary flush, aqueous flare and cells, and occasional fine or large (mutton-fat) keratic precipitates, was noted in approximately 15% of 202 patients with ocular sarcoid (13). In the acute phase, the inflammation was usually unilateral. A more frequent finding, indeed the most common ocular manifestation of sarcoidosis, is a *chronic granulomatous uveitis,* which was reported in more than half of the 202 cases (13). This is more often bilateral, has a protracted course, and is typified by mutton-fat keratic precipitates, synechiae, and iris nodules (Fig. 19.3). The nodules, which were seen in 23 (11.4%) of the 202 cases of ocular sarcoid (13), may involve the pupillary border (Koeppe nodules) and stroma of the iris (Busacca nodules), as well as the anterior chamber angle and the ciliary body (14, 15). In one series of 102 eyes of 52 patients with ocular sarcoidosis, 35% of eyes had iris nodules, 49% had nodules in the angle, and 42% had ciliary nodules (15). Gonioscopy may also reveal inflammatory precipitates on the trabecular meshwork (16) and whitish spots on the ciliary body band, which hyperfluoresce during fluorescein gonioangiography and may represent granulomas of the ciliary body (17).

Chronic ocular sarcoidosis is associated with a worse visual prognosis than the acute form. In a series of 21 patients with sarcoid uveitis, eight had a monophasic course and a favorable visual outcome, while 13 had a relapsing course with severe visual loss in five eyes (18). The course of the ocular disease does not always parallel that of the systemic manifestations. In one series of 33 patients with ocular and systemic sarcoidosis, all had chronic systemic manifestations, defined as a minimum duration of 5 years, while the anterior uveitis was chronic in only 18 patients (19). In another series of patients with chronic ocular sarcoidosis, approximately half had no systemic manifestations (18). Sarcoidosis may also masquerade as many other conditions. In one report, five patients with clinical signs compatible with Fuchs' heterochromic uveitis (discussed later in this chapter) were found to have sarcoidosis on the basis of elevated serum angiotensin converting enzyme levels or a positive Kveim test (20).

GLAUCOMA. This complication of the iridocyclitis occurred in 22 (10.9%) of the 202 patients with ocular sarcoid (13). Chronic uveitis and associated glaucoma are poor prognostic signs, with 8 of 11 such patients suffering severe visual loss in one study (19). The most common mechanism of glaucoma associated with the iridocyclitis of sarcoidosis is obstruction of the trabecular meshwork by inflammatory debris or nodules (21). A more chronic form of glaucoma may also occur in association with iris bombé or goniosynechiae (21), and a subacute form has been described with the pre-

cipitates on the trabecular meshwork (16). Neovascularization of the iris and angle has also been reported as a mechanism of glaucoma in association with sarcoidosis (22).

Juvenile Rheumatoid Arthritis

Juvenile rheumatoid arthritis (JRA) is a spectrum of arthritic disorders in children. One form is characterized by monarticular, or pauciarticular (involvement of four joints or less) onset, a predilection for girls, and minimal additional systemic manifestations. Other types of JRA have polyarticular onset or additional acute systemic involvement.

IRIDOCYCLITIS. The prevalence of iridocyclitis in patients with the monarticular or pauciarticular form of JRA has been variously reported at 16% (23), 19% (24), and 29% (25), while the other types of JRA are rarely associated with this ocular finding (24–28). In addition, JRA is by far the most common systemic finding in children who have anterior uveitis associated with a specific systemic disease, accounting for 81% of one large series (29). The ocular inflammation may have an acute onset, with the typical features of acute iridocyclitis. However, many cases are asymptomatic, emphasizing the need for periodic ocular examinations of children with JRA (24, 25). The onset of the arthritis typically precedes that of the uveitis, although iridocyclitis may persist in adult life whereas the arthritis usually disappears (26). Children with iridocyclitis rarely have a positive serology for

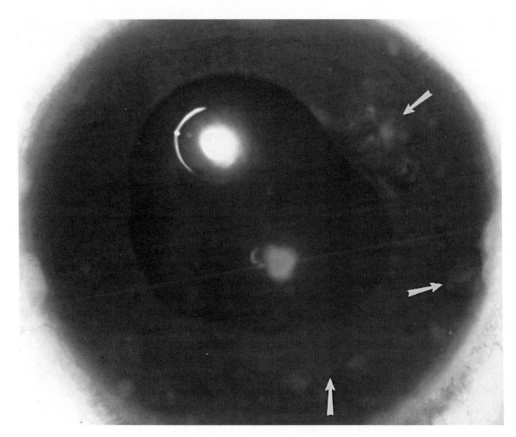

Figure 19.3. Slitlamp view of eye with sarcoid uveitis showing typical iris nodules (*arrows*). (Courtesy of John W. Reed, M.D.)

rheumatoid factor, but they frequently have antinuclear antibody (26, 28) and HLA-B27 antigen (28), and some eventually are found to have typical ankylosing spondylitis (28).

Complications that may cause significant visual loss in children with iridocyclitis and JRA include cataracts, band keratopathy, and glaucoma. These are more common when the uveitis is the initial manifestation. In one series, 67% of such patients had a poor visual outcome, compared to only 6% of those in whom the arthritis preceded the uveitis (30). The prevalence and severity of the complications and visual loss also correlate with the degree and duration of the ocular inflammation. In one report of 60 patients, an aggressive stepladder, steroid-sparing, therapeutic algorithm (topical and regional corticosteroids, systemic nonsteroidal anti-inflammatory drugs, systemic steroids, and systemic immunosuppressive chemotherapy) was felt to control the iridocyclitis, while reducing the prevalence of cataract formation and retinal pathology (31). Those cases requiring cataract surgery responded well to phacoemulsification and anterior vitrectomy after at least 3 months of complete freedom from inflammation (31).

GLAUCOMA. The reported prevalence of glaucoma in children with JRA and iridocyclitis ranges from 14% to 27% (26–28, 30). Glaucoma is a particularly serious complication, with half of the eyes in one study having a vision of 20/200 or less (28). The glaucoma mechanism is usually a pupillary block, although it may also be related to alterations in the trabecular meshwork early in the course of the disease. Histopathologic studies of two advanced cases revealed peripheral anterior synechiae and occlusion of the pupil in one (32), and a dense inflammatory infiltrate composed primarily of plasma cells in the iris and ciliary body with angle closure in the other patient (33). Treatment is typically difficult, with many eyes responding only partially to corticosteroids. The addition of nonsteroidal anti-inflammatory agents may be helpful in these cases (27, 28). Antiglaucoma drugs may be required to control IOP elevation, and glaucoma surgery is occasionally needed, although reported results in these cases are poor (26).

Ankylosing Spondylitis (Marie-Strumpell Disease)

This form of arthritis typically involves the cervical or lumbosacral spine and is associated with an intermittent acute iridocyclitis in 3.5–12.5% of reported cases (34). A high percentage of these patients have the HLA-B27 antigen (35). Recurrent uveitis may precede the arthritic symptoms, and there is evidence, based on HLA typing and sensitive bone scans, that the ocular inflammation may occur in the absence of overt symptoms or radiologic evidence of the spondylitis (34). As previously noted, there is an apparent overlap between this condition and HLA-B27-positive acute anterior uveitis (8–12) and the iridocyclitis with JRA (28). Glaucoma may result from trabecular damage or synechiae formation.

Pars Planitis

This protracted ocular inflammatory disorder, which has also been referred to as intermediate uveitis (1) or chronic cyclitis (36), primarily involves the ciliary body. Typical findings include a "snowbank" appearance of the vitreous base overlying the pars plana inferiorly, retinal phlebitis, and a cystoid maculopathy (37). In a series of 100 cases with a 4–20 year followup, the incidence of glaucoma was 8% (36), while another group of 58 eyes had glaucoma in 7% (37). A clinicopathologic study of seven cases of pars planitis revealed glaucoma in five, and possible mechanisms of pressure elevation included peripheral anterior synechiae, iris bombé, and rubeosis iridis (38). Topical corticosteroid and antiglaucoma therapy may be effective in some cases. Decreased visual acuity, which is usually due to cystoid maculopathy may require the chronic use of oral and/or periocular steroids, cryotherapy in the area of the "snowbank," and systemic antimetabolites as the final step (37).

Glaucomatocyclitic Crisis (Posner-Schlossman Syndrome)

In 1948, Posner and Schlossman (39) described a uniocular disease in young to middle-aged adults, which was characterized by recurrent attacks of mild anterior uveitis with marked elevations of IOP. Many patients have associated systemic disorders, including various allergic conditions and gastrointestinal diseases, most notably peptic ulcers (40). In one series of 22 patients, HLA-Bw54 was present in 41%, suggesting that immunogenetic factors play an important role in the pathogenesis of glaucomatocyclitic crisis (41). The possible role of herpes simplex virus was also suggested by a study which revealed DNA evidence of the virus in all aqueous specimens of three patients during acute attacks, but in none of 10 normal controls (42).

IRIDOCYCLITIS. The typical symptoms are slight ocular discomfort, blurred vision, and halos, which last from several hours up to a few weeks, or, rarely, more, and tend to recur on a monthly or yearly basis (39). Physical findings are minimal, with occasional mild ciliary flush, slight pupillary constriction, and corneal epithelial edema. Hypochromia of the iris is not a consistent finding, but has been reported in up to 40% of various series (43). Early segmental iris ischemia with late congestion and leakage on fluorescein angiography has also been described (44). Slitlamp biomicroscopy reveals occasional faint flare and a few fine, nonpigmented keratic precipitates, while gonioscopy shows a normal, open angle with occasional debris and the characteristic absence of synechiae (39, 43).

GLAUCOMA. The IOP is typically elevated in the range of 40–60 mm Hg and coincides with the duration of the uveitis. Intraocular pressure and facility of aqueous outflow usually return to normal between attacks, although severe cases with optic nerve head and visual field damage have been reported (45, 46). The glaucoma may be related to inflammatory changes in the trabecular meshwork. Histologic evaluation of a trabeculectomy specimen obtained during an acute attack revealed numerous mononuclear cells in the meshwork (47). Other theories of mechanism include increased aqueous production, possibly due to elevated levels of aqueous prostaglandins (48), and an association with chronic open-angle glaucoma (44, 45). Most cases can be controlled during attacks with corticosteroids and antiglaucoma agents which reduce aqueous production (43, 49). Apraclonidine has been reported to be especially effective during acute attacks (50). Rare, severe cases, however, may require filtering surgery (46, 47).

Fuchs' Heterochromic Cyclitis

In 1906, Fuchs (51) described a condition characterized by mild anterior uveitis, heterochromia, cataracts, and occasional glaucoma. The similarities and differences between this disease and glaucomatocyclitic crisis should be noted to avoid confusing the two. Fuchs' heterochromic cyclitis (also referred to as uveitis or iridocyclitis) is usually unilateral, although bilateral involvement has been reported in up to 13% of the cases (52). The typical age of onset is in the third or fourth decade (53) and there is an equal incidence among men and women (52). It is said to be the most commonly misdiagnosed form of uveitis (54), especially in black patients in whom the heterochromia may be less obvious (55).

Several theories of etiology have been considered, with the most likely being a true inflammation of immunologic origin, possibly related to depression of suppressor T-cell activity (54). Cellular immunity to corneal antigens has been found in the majority of patients (56), with autoantibodies against corneal epithelium in almost 90% of cases (57). Immune deposits have been found in the vessel walls of iris biopsy specimens (58). The search for HLA-linked genetic factors is inconclusive, although preliminary evidence suggests a decrease in the frequency of HLA-CW3 (59). Fuchs' heterochromic cyclitis has been reported in a father and son with associated retinitis pigmentosa (60), although the reported discordance in monozygotic twins suggests little or no genetic predisposition (61). A few patients have associated congenital Horner's syndrome, suggesting the possibility of a neurogenic mechanism in these cases (62). A clinical association between Fuchs' heterochromic cyclitis and toxoplasmosis raised the possibility of a causal relationship (63, 64), although a study of 88 patients with the former condition revealed no association with toxoplasmosis by indirect immunofluorescence antibody tests, enzyme-linked immunosorbent assay, or cellular immunity tests to toxoplasma antigen (65). As previously noted, clinical similarities with sarcoidosis have also been reported (20).

IRIDOCYCLITIS. The uveitis in this disease is mild and tends to run a single, very protracted course, although it may be inter-mittent initially. The patient is usually unaware of any difficulty until visual disturbance, primarily from cataract formation, becomes apparent. While hypochromia of the iris is more common than in glaucomatocyclitic crisis, it is not a constant feature, and tends to develop gradually during the course of the disease (52, 53). In one series, it was seen in 92% of 54 white patients and 76% of 13 black individuals (55).

Gross signs of ocular inflammation are typically absent, although slitlamp biomicroscopy may reveal minimal aqueous flare and cells. Characteristic fine stellate keratic precipitates are usually seen on the lower half of the cornea, but may involve the upper half also (66). The iris frequently has extensive stromal atrophy, and transillumination of the iris is reported to demonstrate a characteristic light, even translucence (67). One study revealed translucency not only of the iris but also of the surrounding ocular wall (68). Electron microscopic studies of the iris have revealed a scant number of deep stromal melanocytes with immature melanin granules, abundant plasma cells, an increase in mast cells and a membranous degeneration of nerve fibers (69, 70).

Patients may also have neovascularization of both the anterior chamber angle and iris, as well as nodules on the iris (59). The nodules typically occur along the pupillary border, similar to the Koeppe nodules of sarcoidosis, although may appear across the whole surface of the iris (71). In one series, the nodules were seen in 20% of white and 30% of black patients (55). The finding of unilateral iris nodules may be especially helpful in making the diagnosis of Fuchs' cyclitis in black individuals, in whom the heterochromia may be less apparent (71). Anterior segment fluorescein angiography has shown delayed filling, sector ischemia, leakage, and neovascularization (72, 73), and fluorophotometry has revealed an abnormal permeability of the blood-aqueous barrier (74). A high percentage of patients may also have chorioretinal scars which, as previously noted, are often consistent with toxoplasmosis (63, 64, 75, 76).

CATARACT. As previously noted, cataract formation is also a typical feature of Fuchs' heterochromic cyclitis. In approaching cataract surgery in these patients, intensive perioperative steroid therapy is advised and synechia lysis may be required during the procedure (77). Postoperative complications of marked anterior uveitis, hyphema, IOP elevation, and cystoid macular edema are more common than in routine cataract surgery (77). However, most reports describe good visual outcomes with extracapsular cataract extraction and posterior chamber intraocular lens implantation (77–79).

GLAUCOMA. Intraocular pressure elevation is not as common as with glaucomatocyclitic crisis, but may occur as a late, serious complication. The reported incidence varies from 13% to 59% (66, 80–82), with the higher figures seen in series with long-term followup. The glaucoma typically persists after the uveitis has subsided. The anterior chamber angle is open and characteristically free of synechiae, although fine vessels, which may hemorrhage, are often seen extending onto the trabecular meshwork (80). Histopathologic examination of the anterior chamber angle structures in one case revealed rubeosis, trabeculitis, and an inflammatory membrane over the angle (83), while another study showed extensive atrophy of Schlemm's canal and the trabecular endothelium (84). The glaucoma typically does not respond to steroid therapy, but requires standard medical or surgical management (53, 66, 82). In one series of 30 patients, maximum medical therapy was unsuccessful in 73%, but surgical interventions (mostly trabeculectomy, half with 5-fluorouracil) was successful in 72% of the cases (82).

Behçet's Disease

This multiple system disease is due to an occlusive vasculitis, and is characterized by uveitis, aphthous lesions of the mouth, and ulcerations of the genitalia (85, 86). Additional systemic findings include erythema nodosum, arthropathy, thrombophlebitis, and a necrotizing vasculitis of the central nervous system, which may be fatal. The most common ocular disorder is iridocyclitis. Behçet's disease is relatively common in the Mediterranean basin and was found to be the most common associated condition with chronic uveitis in a uveitis service in Israel (1), although it is much less common in the United States and England (2–4). The iridocyclitis may be associated with a sterile hypopyon. In a study of 49 patients, followed over a 10-year period, 17 developed a hypopyon, which typically appears late in the course of the disease but was the initial finding in three patients (87). Posterior uveitis and necrotizing retinal vasculitis are also commonly found in this disorder (86, 88). In the 10-year study, all patients developed both anterior and posterior involvement within 2 years (87). The uveitis tends to occur late in the course of the disease and is eventually bilateral. The anterior uveitis may lead to glaucoma. All patients initially respond to steroid treatment, although the uveitis, in most cases, eventually requires cytotoxic-immunosuppressive agents such as chlorambucil (87). Even with this therapy, the prognosis is poor, with loss of useful visual acuity in 74% of eyes in the 10-year study (87).

Reiter's Syndrome

This multisystem disease is characterized by conjunctivitis, urethritis, arthritis, and mucocutaneous lesions. It typically afflicts young men, with a high frequency of the HLA-B27 genotype (89). In a review of 113 patients, there were 98% with rheumatologic manifestations, 74% with genitourinary, 58% with ocular, and 42% with mucocutaneous findings (89). Conjunctivitis was seen in all patients with ocular manifestations and is characterized by a papillary reaction with a mucopurulent discharge. A nongranulomatous iridocyclitis without hypopyon was the second most common ocular manifestation, occurring in 12% of the total group, although glaucoma was only seen in one of the 113 patients.

Grant's Syndrome (Glaucoma Associated with Precipitates on the Trabecular Meshwork)

Chandler and Grant (90) described an uncommon form of open-angle glaucoma in which the only evidence of ocular inflammation is precipitates on the trabecular meshwork. Since the condition is usually bilateral, it may be mistaken for chronic open-angle glaucoma. However, careful gonioscopy reveals gray or slightly yellow precipitates on the meshwork and irregular peripheral anterior synechiae, which often attach to the trabecular precipitates (16). The cause is unknown, although some patients eventually develop sarcoidosis, rheumatoid arthritis, ankylosing spondylitis, episcleritis, glaucomatocyclitic crisis, or chronic uveitis (16). The glaucoma, which is presumed to be due to inflammatory changes in the trabecular meshwork, usually clears promptly with topical corticosteroid therapy, although antiglaucoma drugs which reduce aqueous production may be temporarily required for pressure control. The condition often recurs, and the patients must be followed closely. Untreated cases may progress to synechial closure of the angle.

Epidemic Dropsy

This acute toxic disease, which results from the unintentional ingestion of sanguinarine in *Argemone mexicana* oil as an adulterant of cooking oils, is characterized by the explosive onset of leg edema, with tenderness, erythema, and rash over the edematous parts, gastrointestinal symptoms, low-grade fever, and congestive heart failure which may be fatal (91, 92). Ocular features include glaucoma and retinal vascular dilatation, tortuosity, and hemorrhage (91). The glaucoma is bilateral with open angles, normal outflow facility, and normal trabecular meshwork by histopathologic and histochemical testing (92). Although there are no signs of anterior segment inflammation, aqueous assays reveal elevated prostaglandin E_2 levels, histamine activity, and total protein levels, suggesting hypersecretion as the mechanism of the elevated IOP (92).

Infectious Diseases

The following infectious processes may cause an iridocyclitis with the occasional association of glaucoma.

CONGENITAL RUBELLA. This disorder predominantly affects the heart, auditory apparatus, and eyes (93), although virtually any organ may be involved. Ocular defects occur in 30–60% of the cases and include cataracts, microphthalmia, retinopathy, and glaucoma (94). Corneal edema may occur due to coexistent glaucoma or in the absence of elevated IOP (95). The associated glaucoma is reported to occur in 2–15% of children with congenital rubella (96). Contrary to earlier reports, the cataracts and glaucoma occur together at a frequency that would be anticipated with each occurring independently (96). The glaucoma may be associated with hypoplasia of the iris stroma and hypoperfusion by iris angiography (97). The glaucoma is particularly severe, with blindness occurring in 8 of 15 children in one followup study (98). Mechanisms of the glaucoma include iridocyclitis, angle anomalies, and angle-closure glaucoma due to microphthalmia, an intumescent lens, or pupillary block after cataract extraction. Although the ocular abnormalities are most often observed in the neonatal period, the glaucoma may also occur later in childhood, or in young adults, usually in association with microphthalmia and cataracts (99).

SYPHILIS. Congenital syphilis may cause iridocyclitis with glaucoma in either the early or late stages of the disease. Glaucoma associated with the interstitial keratitis of congenital syphilis is discussed later in this chapter. Acquired syphilis in adults may also cause iridocyclitis and IOP elevation (100). Mass lesions of the iris and ciliary body have also been associated with this condition (101).

HANSEN'S DISEASE. Uveitis is common in *lepromatous leprosy* and typically involves the iris and ciliary body (102–104), with four forms having been described: (a) chronic iridocyclitis, (b) acute plastic iridocyclitis, (c) iris pearls or miliary lepromata, which is pathognomonic of the disease, and (d) nodular lepromata, characterized by larger, less discrete masses on the iris (102). Complications of keratitis and iridocyclitis are the main causes of blindness in this disease (104). The chronic iridocyclitis may be associated with iris atrophy and small nonreacting pupils, which aggravate the visual impairment (105, 106). In a study of 100 cases, 19 had acute or chronic iridocyclitis and 12 had evidence of glaucoma, which was usually associated with chronic anterior uveitis (107). In another study of 193 patients, glaucoma was found in 10%, half of whom had associated uveitis, despite the fact that all had been previously treated with dapsone and/or clofazimine (108).

Patients with Hansen's disease more typically have lower than normal IOP and a significant postural change in IOP from the upright to the supine position. In some cases, this may be associated with chronic plastic iridocyclitis (106, 109, 110). However, these same IOP anomalies may be seen in patients without clinical evidence of anterior uveal inflammation and even in household contacts of patients with Hansen's disease (111). These findings are felt to suggest early subclinical ciliary body autonomic neuropathy and may be useful in the early diagnosis of the disease. In cases with active anterior uveitis, however, the mechanism for the hypotension may be reduced aqueous production or increased uveoscleral outflow secondary to the inflammation (106, 110).

Active iridocyclitis is reported to respond to treatment with dapsone, corticosteroids, and rifampin (102). There is evidence that effective antimicrobial and antiinflammatory therapy may significantly minimize the ocular complications (112).

DISSEMINATED MENINGOCOCCEMIA. These patients may have associated iridocyclitis (113) or endophthalmitis (114)

with acute glaucoma, which is presumably due to obstruction of the anterior chamber by a blanket of cells.

HEMORRHAGIC FEVER WITH RENAL SYNDROME (NEPHROPATHIA EPIDEMICA). This disease is caused by the Puumala virus and is characterized by fever, chills, malaise, nausea, vomiting, and headache, which progresses to back and abdominal pain, uremia, hematuria, oliguria, and proteinuria. Three patients have been described with associated transient angle-closure glaucoma, which was felt to be due to swelling of the ciliary body (115). However, in a prospective study of 37 patients during the acute phase of the disease, the anterior chamber was shallower than after clinical recovery, but the IOP was below baseline and there were no cases of acute angle-closure attacks (116).

ACQUIRED IMMUNE DEFICIENCY SYNDROME (AIDS). This viral disorder has severe defects of immunoregulation, leading to life-threatening opportunistic infections, Kaposi's sarcoma, or both. Bilateral acute angle-closure glaucoma has been reported in these patients, which appears to be due to choroidal effusion with anterior rotation of the ciliary body (117–120). B-scan echography is helpful in establishing the diagnosis by demonstrating diffuse choroidal thickening with ciliochoroidal effusion (119, 120). These cases do not respond to miotics or iridotomy, although peripheral iridoplasty was successful in one case (118). Treatment with aqueous suppressants, cycloplegics, and topical steroids has been reported to achieve complete resolution of the angle closure (119).

LISTERIA MONOCYTOGENES. Listeria monocytogenes endophthalmitis may present with a "dark hypopyon" and markedly elevated IOP. The dark appearance is due to associated pigment dispersion, and the diagnosis can be established by culture and histopathologic examination of ocular fluid (121).

Theories of Mechanisms for Associated Glaucoma

The possible mechanisms by which iridocyclitis may lead to an elevated IOP already have been mentioned with regard to certain specific forms of iridocyclitis and are now summarized. In general, iridocyclitis affects both aqueous production and resistance to aqueous outflow, with the subsequent change in IOP representing a balance between these two factors.

Aqueous Production

Inflammation of the ciliary body usually leads to reduced aqueous production. If this outweighs a concomitant increased resistance to outflow, the IOP will be reduced, which is often the case with acute iridocyclitis. Experimental iridocyclitis in monkeys suggests that the hypotony may be due to both a reduction in aqueous humor flow and an increase in uveoscleral outflow (122). However, prostaglandins, which have been demonstrated in the aqueous of eyes with uveitis, are known to cause elevated IOP without a reduction in outflow facility (123–126), suggesting that increased aqueous production may possibly occur in some cases of uveitis.

Aqueous Outflow

When the aqueous outflow system is involved in an ocular inflammatory disease, increased resistance to outflow may result from a variety of acute and chronic mechanisms.

ACUTE MECHANISMS OF OBSTRUCTION. During the active phase of iridocyclitis several mechanisms of obstruction to aqueous outflow may lead to a relatively sudden, but usually reversible, rise in IOP. In the majority of cases, the anterior chamber angle is open, which is an important observation in ruling out pupillary-block glaucoma. Obstruction of the trabecular meshwork may occur in several ways.

A disruption in the blood-aqueous barrier allows inflammatory cells and fibrin to enter the aqueous and accumulate in the trabecular meshwork. Normal serum components have been shown to reduce outflow when perfused in enucleated human eyes (127). Prostaglandins were demonstrated to increase aqueous protein content (125, 126, 128, 129), and it has been suggested that an accumulation of cyclic adenosine monophosphate (cAMP), due to prostaglandins or certain nonprostaglandin agents, causes the barrier damage (130).

In other cases, swelling or dysfunction of the trabecular lamellae or endothelium may lead to aqueous outflow obstruction. Precipitates on the trabecular meshwork, as previously discussed, may also occur in eyes with ocular inflammation and elevated IOP (16, 90). It must also be kept in mind that the use of corticosteroids in treating the inflammation may create yet another mechanism of IOP elevation (steroid-induced glaucoma), which is discussed in the next chapter.

Much less commonly, ocular inflammation may lead to acute closure of the anterior chamber angle by uveal effusion with forward rotation of the ciliary body. In addition, if a significant posterior uveitis is present, angle-closure may result from displacement of the lens-iris diaphragm due to massive exudative retinal detachment.

CHRONIC MECHANISMS OF OBSTRUCTION. Several sequelae of inflammation may lead to a chronic elevation of IOP. Obstruction of aqueous outflow may result from scarring and obliteration of outflow channels, or from the overgrowth of an endothelial-cuticular or fibrovascular membrane in the open angle. The membranes may eventually contract, leading to synechial closure of the angle. In addition to the influence of membrane contraction, peripheral anterior synechiae may result from the protein and inflammatory cells in the angle, which pull the iris toward the cornea. Posterior synechiae

may also be a sequelae of anterior uveitis and can cause iris bombé with closure of the anterior chamber angle.

Management

In treating an eye with iridocyclitis and glaucoma, control of the inflammatory component alone frequently leads to normalization of the IOP, and this is usually the first approach in the treatment plan. However, if the magnitude of the pressure elevation poses an immediate threat to vision, or if the IOP does not respond adequately to anti-inflammatory therapy, medical, and even surgical, management of the glaucoma may be indicated. The following basic principles of management apply to most cases of iridocyclitis, as well as other forms of ocular inflammation, with exceptions as noted in the discussions of the specific diseases.

Management of the Inflammation

CORTICOSTEROIDS. This group of drugs constitutes the first-line of defense in most cases of ocular inflammation. Topical administration is preferred for anterior segment disease and commonly used steroids include prednisolone 1.0% and dexamethasone 0.1%. In a rabbit model of anterior uveitis, frequent topical administration of prednisolone acetate 1.0% caused a significant decrease in protein levels and leukocytes in the anterior chamber (131). Administration of the steroid every hour may be required initially, with gradual reduction in frequency as the inflammation subsides. In a rabbit model of keratitis, instillation every 15 minutes was even more effective than the hourly regimen, although five doses at 1-minute intervals each hour was equivalent to the effect achieved by administration every 15 minutes (132). When the response to topical administration is insufficient, periocular injections (e.g., dexamethasone phosphate, prednisolone succinate, triamcinolone acetate, or methylprednisolone acetate) or a systemic corticosteroid (e.g., prednisone) may be required. With any form of administration, the many side effects of corticosteroids must be considered, including steroid-induced glaucoma.

NONSTEROIDAL ANTI-INFLAMMATORY AGENTS. When the use of corticosteroids are contraindicated or inadequate, other anti-inflammatory drugs may be helpful. *Prostaglandin synthetase inhibitors* such as aspirin (133), imidazole (134), indoxyl (135), indomethacin (135), and dipyridamole (136) have been effective in some cases of uveitis. With severe cases, *immunosuppressive agents* such as methotrexate (137), azathioprine (138), or chlorambucil (138) may be indicated. In a study of 25 patients with severe chronic uveitis who were poorly responsive or unresponsive to corticosteroid therapy, all responded to long-term daily administration of prednisone 10–15 mg combined with azathioprine 2.0–2.5 mg or chlorambucil 6–8 mg (138). These patients must be monitored closely for hematologic reactions.

New anti-inflammatory drugs are also being evaluated, which may prove to be beneficial in the treatment of uveitis. For example, the newer cyclooxygenase inhibitors such as flurbiprofen, ketorolac, suprofen, and diclofenac may provide useful anti-inflammatory effects without the risk of steroid-induced IOP elevation. Another new class of anti-inflammatory agents are the 21-aminosteroids, which have been developed as free radical scavengers and have shown promise in rabbit models (139).

In conjunction with anti-inflammatory agents, a mydriatic-cycloplegic drug such as atropine 1%, homatropine 1–5%, or cyclopentolate 0.5–1% is usually indicated to avoid posterior synechiae and to relieve the discomfort of ciliary muscle spasm.

Management of the Glaucoma

MEDICAL. Since miotics are generally contraindicated in the inflamed eye, a topical β-blocker, α_2-agonist, carbonic anhydrase inhibitor, or epinephrine compound is usually the first-line antiglaucoma drug in the treatment of glaucoma associated with ocular inflammation. An oral carbonic anhydrase inhibitor may also be needed, and a hyperosmotic agent is occasionally required as a short-term emergency measure.

SURGICAL. Intraocular surgery should be avoided whenever possible in eyes with active inflammation. However, when medical therapy is inadequate, surgery may be required. In these cases, it is best to do the least amount of surgery possible. A laser iridotomy is safer than an incisional iridectomy when an angle closure mechanism if present, although fibrin may tend to close a small iridotomy in an inflamed eye. Laser trabeculoplasty is not only ineffective in eyes with uveitis and open-angle glaucoma, but may cause an additional, significant rise in IOP and is generally contraindicated in these cases. Filtering surgery with heavy steroid therapy is usually indicated in open-angle cases that are uncontrolled on maximum tolerable medical therapy. Adjuvant use of subconjunctival 5-fluorouracil (5-FU) has been shown to significantly improve the success rate in these cases (140, 141), and adjunctive mitomycin-c is probably even more effective than 5-FU in these cases (142). Aqueous drainage devices, such as the Molteno implant, have also been reported to be useful, especially when significant postoperative inflammation is likely (143).

A technique called *trabeculodialysis,* in which a goniotomy knife is used to incise above the trabecular meshwork and then peel the meshwork downward, has also been described (144). This was successful in a preliminary series of eyes with anterior uveitis and glaucoma (144), although a subsequent study of 30 eyes in 23 children and young adults achieved success in only 60%, with most of these requiring concomitant antiglaucoma medication (145). Cyclodestructive surgery, such as transscleral Nd:YAG cyclophotocoagulation, may be another reasonable surgical option, especially in aphakic and pseudophakic eyes.

OTHER FORMS OF OCULAR INFLAMMATION

Choroiditis and Retinitis

In the following conditions, an inflammation that is predominantly posterior may cause glaucoma either by an associated anterior inflammatory component or by angle closure from a posterior mass effect.

Vogt-Koyanagi-Harada Syndrome

The systemic findings in this disorder include alopecia, poliosis, vitiligo, and central nervous system and auditory signs. Ocular manifestations consist of bilateral, diffuse granulomatous uveitis with exudative retinal detachment. In two reviews of 51 and 42 patients, glaucoma was found in 20% (146) and 38% (147), respectively. In the first of these groups, a mild anterior uveitis was seen in all patients, posterior synechiae occurred in 36%, keratic precipitates in 30%, and nodules on the iris in 8.4% (146). Mechanisms of glaucoma may be open-angle in association with anterior uveitis, or angle-closure, which is apparently due to swelling of the ciliary body secondary to severe choroiditis (147–150). In the series of 42 patients, those with glaucoma had open-angles in 56.3% and angle-closure in 43.7% (147). These conditions may respond to corticosteroid therapy (148) and antiglaucoma medication, although a high percentage require surgical intervention (147).

Sympathetic Ophthalmia

This form of ocular inflammation typically occurs weeks or months after traumatic or surgical penetration of the fellow eye. The severity of the inflammation is related to the degree of ocular pigmentation, and the choroid is predominantly affected with frequent involvement of the overlying retina (151, 152). The condition bears striking clinical and histopathologic similarities to the Vogt-Koyanagi-Harada syndrome and the two disorders may share a common immunopathologic inflammatory mechanism (152). In a study of 17 cases with an average followup of 10.6 years, seven (43%) had glaucoma (151). The mechanism of the glaucoma is unknown, although in a histopathologic study of 105 cases, a high percentage had plasma cell infiltration of the iris and ciliary body (151) suggesting an immune reaction near the area of aqueous outflow. Whatever the cause, the glaucoma is typically difficult to treat, requiring frequent adjustments of corticosteroids and occasional surgical intervention (153).

Cytomegalic Inclusion Retinitis

This disorder was described in two adult renal transplant patients, both of whom developed open-angle glaucoma presumably due to an associated anterior uveitis (154).

Toxocariasis

The common ocular form of this disease, characterized by retinitis and vitreitis, may also have anterior uveitis with posterior synechiae, iris bombé, and associated glaucoma (155).

Keratitis

Interstitial Keratitis

As a feature of *congenital syphilis,* interstitial keratitis typically appears late in the course of the disease, between 5 and 16 years of age, although it may appear as early as birth or as late as 30 years of age (156). The presenting symptoms of interstitial keratitis include marked ciliary flush, lacrimation, photophobia, and pain. The mechanisms of glaucoma associated with interstitial keratitis, in addition to the previously discussed concomitant iridocyclitis, include open-angle and angle-closure forms that usually appear later in life (157, 158).

With the open-angle glaucomas, the eye may have irregular pigmentation of the anterior chamber angle, with occasional columnar peripheral anterior synechiae, and one histopathologic study revealed endothelium and a glassy membrane over the angle (157). This condition responds poorly to medical therapy, but may be controlled by filtering surgery. Another mechanism of open-angle glaucoma in the adult is the recurrence of iridocyclitis in an eye that had interstitial keratitis in younger life (157). The residual ghost vessels in the cornea may help in making this diagnosis.

Eyes with interstitial keratitis in infancy often have small anterior segments and narrow angles, which can lead to angle-closure glaucoma later in life. This is usually subacute and responds well to peripheral iridotomy (157, 159). In some cases, multiple cysts of the iris may lead to angle-closure.

Interstitial keratitis may also be associated with vertigo, tinnitus, and deafness, which is referred to as *Cogan's syndrome.* An atypical form may have noncorneal ocular inflammation (160), which may involve the anterior uvea with associated glaucoma.

Herpes Simplex Keratouveitis

This viral infection may cause recurrent conjunctivitis, keratitis, and uveitis. In one study of patients with herpes simplex keratouveitis, 28% had IOP elevation, and 10% had glaucomatous damage (161). The keratitis in cases with associated IOP elevation is typically disciform or stromal, rather than a superficial ulcer (161). The pressure usually remains elevated for several weeks, and a rabbit model suggests a biphasic IOP response in which the uveitis during the first few days represents active infection, but subsequently is due to immune mechanisms (162). An analysis of aqueous from 33 herpes patients revealed herpes simplex virus in eight cases, all of which had associated glaucoma (163). Histopathology of rabbit eyes with experimental herpetic keratouveitis showed mononuclear cells in the trabecular meshwork and peripheral anterior synechiae (164).

Management of this condition requires attention to the infection, inflammation, and glaucoma, and one suggested regimen includes topical trifluorothymidine, corticosteroids, and cycloplegics along with antiglaucoma agents that reduce aqueous production (163). One study indicated that the severity of the uveitis and IOP rise in experimental secondary herpes simplex uveitis was lessened with dexamethasone 0.1% twice daily, but not with aspirin or cyclophosphamide (165).

Herpes Zoster Keratouveitis

In addition to causing the characteristic cutaneous vesicular eruptions along the trigeminal distribution, this viral disease may produce a keratitis and uveitis. The anterior uveitis not uncommonly leads to glaucoma. In one series of 86 patients with herpes zoster ophthalmicus, 37 had uveitis and 10 of these had associated glaucoma (166). In another study, 5 of 14 patients with keratouveitis had transient high IOP (167). Topical acyclovir has been shown to be superior to topical steroids in the treatment of herpes zoster keratouveitis (168).

Adenovirus Type 10

This viral agent has been reported to cause keratoconjunctivitis with a transient increased IOP (169).

Scleritis

This is an extremely painful, potentially disastrous form of ocular inflammation, which may primarily involve either the anterior or posterior segment of the eye (170). The anterior forms may present as *diffuse* or *nodular anterior scleritis,* characterized by episcleral congestion and scleral edema. These are painful and often recurrent, but relatively benign. *Necrotizing scleritis* is a more severe condition, with extensive granulomatous infiltration of the conjunctiva, episclera, and sclera and degradation of scleral collagen (171, 172). It is typically painful and progressive, although a variation, *scleromalacia perforans,* which is seen primarily in patients with rheumatoid arthritis, has no pain or redness. Anterior segment fluorescein angiography helps to distinguish the more benign forms, which have vasodilatation and rapid flow, from the necrotizing cases, which have gross vascular abnormalities and delayed flow (173). Posterior scleritis, which is more difficult to diagnose, may present with pars planitis, exudative retinal detachment, optic nerve head edema, or proptosis.

In two large studies, the prevalence of glaucoma was 11.6% (170) and 13% (174), while in another series, elevated IOP was present in 18.7% with rheumatoid scleritis and 12% with nonrheumatoid scleritis (175). A histopathologic study of 92 enucleated eyes revealed evidence of increased IOP in

49% (176). In the vast majority of cases, the glaucoma is associated with anterior scleritis, and mechanisms of pressure elevation in these patients include trabecular meshwork damage by iridocyclitis, overlying corneoscleral inflammation, and peripheral anterior synechiae (176). Other reported mechanisms include steroid-induced glaucoma, iris neovascularization (176), and elevated episcleral venous pressure in an eye with anterior diffuse scleritis in relapsing polychondritis (177). Bilateral glaucoma with marked IOP elevations, presumably of an open-angle mechanism, has also been described in a 14-year-old boy with scleritis, a fibrinous anterior uveitis and rheumatic fever (178). Glaucoma associated with posterior scleritis is much less common, but angle-closure mechanisms may result from a forward shift of the lens-iris diaphragm or an anterior rotation of the ciliary body in association with choroidal effusion (179, 180).

Treatment of the scleritis generally consists of topical and systemic corticosteroids, and nonsteroidal anti-inflammatory agents. A combination of oral prednisone and indomethacin proved to be more effective than either drug used alone and allowed lower doses of each (10–60 mg and 50–150 mg daily, respectively) (181). Antiglaucoma agents are used as needed and surgical intervention for the glaucoma should be resorted to only when absolutely necessary.

Episcleritis

In contrast to scleritis, episcleritis produces only mild discomfort and does not typically lead to serious sequelae. The characteristic appearance is congestion of the episcleral vessels, which may be diffuse with chemosis and occasional lid edema (simple episcleritis), or localized with nodules in the episcleral tissue (nodular episcleritis) (170). Associated glaucoma is uncommon in this condition (170, 175), but has been reported (174, 182). In one series of 127 eyes of 94 patients, glaucoma was present in 4% (174). Presumed mechanisms of open-angle glaucoma include inflammation of the angle structures (182) and steroid-induced glaucoma (170). Angle-closure glaucoma has also been observed in association with episcleritis (175, 183), which was due to ciliochoroidal effusion in one patient with immunoglobulin A nephropathy (183). In most cases, both the episcleritis and the secondary glaucoma respond to topical corticosteroids, although iridotomy may be required for an angle-closure mechanism (183).

SUMMARY

The type of ocular inflammation most often associated with IOP elevation is iridocyclitis, either in a primary form or secondary to inflammation elsewhere in the eye. The anterior uveitis may be acute, subacute, or chronic, and may occur as an isolated finding of uncertain etiology (e.g., acute anterior uveitis, pars planitis, glaucomatocyclitic crises, and Fuchs' heterochromic cyclitis), or in association with a systemic inflammatory disorder (e.g., sarcoidosis, some forms of rheumatoid arthritis, Behçet's disease, and many infectious conditions). The mechanisms by which iridocyclitis leads to obstruction of aqueous outflow include acute, usually reversible forms (e.g., accumulation of inflammatory elements in the intertrabecular spaces, edema of the trabecular lamellae, or angle closure due to ciliary body swelling) and chronic forms (e.g., scar formation or membrane overgrowth in the anterior chamber angle). There is also a suggestion that uveitis may cause increased aqueous production in some cases. Treatment of combined iridocyclitis and glaucoma involves steroidal and nonsteroidal anti-inflammatory agents and antiglaucoma drugs, with surgical intervention reserved for medical failures. Other forms of ocular inflammation that may be associated with glaucoma include choroiditis and retinitis, keratitis, scleritis, and episcleritis.

REFERENCES

1. Weiner, A, BenEzra, D: Clinical patterns and associated conditions in chronic uveitis. Am J Ophthalmol 112:151, 1991.
2. Darrel, RW, Wagener, HP, Kurland, LT: Epidemiology of uveitis. Incidence and prevalence in a small urban community. Arch Ophthalmol 68:502, 1962.
3. Perkins, ES, Folk, J: Uveitis in London and Iowa. Ophthalmologica 189:36, 1984.
4. Henderly, DE, Genstler, AJ, Smith, RE, Rao, NA: Changing patterns of uveitis. Am J Ophthalmol 103:131, 1987.
5. Panek, WC, Holland, GN, Lee, DA, Christensen, RE: Glaucoma in patients with uveitis. Br J Ophthalmol 74:223, 1990.
6. Linssen, A, Rothova, A, Valkenburg, HA, et al: The lifetime cumulative incidence of acute anterior uveitis in a normal population and its relation to ankylosing spondylitis and histocompatibility antigen HLA-B27. Invest Ophthalmol Vis Sci 32:2568, 1991.
7. Brewerton, DA, Caffrey, M, Nicholls, A, et al: Acute anterior uveitis and HLA 27. Lancet 2:994, 1973.
8. Rothova, A, van Veenedaal, WG, Linssen, A, et al: Clinical features of acute uveitis. Am J Ophthalmol 103:237, 1987.
9. Linssen, A, Meenken, C: Outcomes of HLA-B27-positive and HLA-B27-negative acute anterior uveitis. Am J Ophthalmol 120:351, 1995.
10. Tay-Kearney, M-L, Schwam, BL, Lowder, C, et al: Clinical features and associated systemic diseases of HLA-B27 uveitis. Am J Ophthalmol 121:47, 1996.
11. Fearnley, IR, Spalton, DJ, Smith, SE: Anterior segment fluorophotometry in acute anterior uveitis. Arch Ophthalmol 105:1550, 1987.
12. Derhaag, PJFM, Linssen, A, Broekema, N, et al: A familial study of the inheritance of HLA-B27-positive acute anterior uveitis. Am J Ophthalmol 105:603, 1988.
13. Obenauf, CD, Shaw, HE, Sydnor, CF, Klintworth, GK: Sarcoidosis and its ophthalmic manifestations. Am J Ophthalmol 86:648, 1978.
14. Ohara, K, Okubo, A, Sasaki, H, Kamara, K: Intraocular manifestations of systemic sarcoidosis. Jpn J Ophthalmol 36:452, 1992.
15. Mizuno, K, Takahashi, J: Sarcoid cyclitis. Ophthalmology 93:511, 1986.
16. Roth, M, Simmons, RJ: Glaucoma associated with precipitates on the trabecular meshwork. Ophthalmology 86:1613, 1979.
17. Kimura, R: Hyperfluorescent dots in the ciliary body band in patients with granulomatous uveitis. Br J Ophthalmol 66:322, 1982.
18. Karma, A, Huhti, E, Poukkula, A: Course and outcome of ocular sarcoidosis. Am J Ophthalmol 106:467, 1988.
19. Jabs, DA, Johns, CJ: Ocular involvement in chronic sarcoidosis. Am J Ophthalmol 102:297, 1986.

20. Goble, RR, Murray, PI: Fuchs' heterochromic uveitis and sarcoidosis. Br J Ophthalmol 79:1021, 1995.

21. Iwata, K, Nanba, K, Sobue, K, Abe, H: Ocular sarcoidosis: evaluation of intraocular findings. Ann NY Acad Sci 278:445, 1976.

22. Mayer, J, Brouillette, G, Corriveau, LA: Sarcoidose et rubeosis iridis. Can J Ophthalmol 18:197, 1983.

23. Korner-Stiefbold, U, Sauvain MJ, Gerber, N, et al: Ophthalmological complications in patients with juvenile chronic arthritis (JCA). Klin Monatsbl Augenheilkd 202:269, 1993.

24. Calabro, JJ, Parrino, GR, Atchoo, PD, et al: Chronic iridocyclitis in juvenile rheumatoid arthritis. Arthritis Rheum 13:406, 1970.

25. Schaller, J, Kupfer, C, Wedgwood, RJ: Iridocyclitis in juvenile rheumatoid arthritis. Pediatrics 44:92, 1969.

26. Key, SN III, Kimura, SJ: Iridocyclitis associated with juvenile rheumatoid arthritis. Am J Ophthalmol 80:425, 1975.

27. Chylack, LT Jr, Bienfang, DC, Bellows, R, Stillman, JS: Ocular manifestations of juvenile rheumatoid arthritis. Am J Ophthalmol 79:1026, 1975.

28. Kanski, JJ: Anterior uveitis in juvenile rheumatoid arthritis. Arch Ophthalmol 95:1794, 1977.

29. Kanski, JJ, Shun-Shin, GA: Systemic uveitis syndromes in childhood: an analysis of 340 cases. Ophthalmology 91:1247, 1984.

30. Wolf, MD, Lichter, PR, Ragsdale, CG: Prognostic factors in the uveitis of juvenile rheumatoid arthritis. Ophthalmology 94:1242, 1987.

31. Foster, CS, Barrett, F: Cataract development and cataract surgery in patients with juvenile rheumatoid arthritis-associated iridocyclitis. Ophthalmology 100:809, 1993.

32. Sabates, R, Smith, T, Apple, D: Ocular histopathology in juvenile rheumatoid arthritis. Ann Ophthalmol 11:733, 1979.

33. Merriam, JC, Chylack, LT, Albert, DM: Early-onset pauciarticular juvenile rheumatoid arthritis. A histopathologic study. Arch Ophthalmol 101:1085, 1983.

34. Russell, AS, Lentle, BC, Percy, JS, Jackson, FI: Scintigraphy of sacroiliac joints in acute anterior uveitis. A study of thirty patients. Ann Intern Med 85:606, 1976.

35. Brewerton, DA, Hart, FD, Nicholls, A, et al: Ankylosing spondylitis and HL-A 27. Lancet 1:904, 1973.

36. Smith, RE, Godfrey, WA, Kimura, SJ: Complications of chronic cyclitis. Am J Ophthalmol 82:277, 1976.

37. Henderly, DE, Genstler, AJ, Rao, NA, and Smith, RE: Pars planitis. Trans Ophthalmol Soc UK 105:227, 1986.

38. Pederson, JE, Kenyon, KE, Green, WR, Maumenee, AE: Pathology of pars planitis. Am J Ophthalmol 86:762, 1978.

39. Posner, A, Schlossman, A: Syndrome of unilateral recurrent attacks of glaucoma with cyclitic symptoms. Arch Ophthalmol 39:517, 1948.

40. Knox, DL: Glaucomatocyclitic crises and systemic disease: peptic ulcer, other gastrointestinal disorders, allergy and stress. Trans Am Ophthalmol Soc 86:473, 1988.

41. Hirose, S, Ohno, S, Matsuda, H: HLA-Bw54 and glaucomatocyclitic crisis. Arch Ophthalmol 103:1837, 1985.

42. Yamamoto, S, Pavan-Langston, D, Tada, R, et al: Possible role of herpes simplex virus in the origin of Posner-Schlossman syndrome. Am J Ophthalmol 119:796, 1995.

43. Hollwich, F: Clinical aspects and therapy of the Posner-Schlossmann-syndrome. Klin Monatsbl Augenheilkd 172:736, 1978.

44. Raitta, C, Vannas, A: Glaucomatocyclitic crisis. Arch Ophthalmol 95:608, 1977.

45. Kass, MA, Becker, B, Kolker, AE: Glaucomatocyclitic crisis and primary open-angle glaucoma. Am J Ophthalmol 75:668, 1973.

46. Hung, PT, Chang, JM: Treatment of glaucomatocyclitic crises. Am J Ophthalmol 77:169, 1974.

47. Harstad, HK, Ringvold, A: Glaucomatocyclitic crises (Posner-Schlossman syndrome). A case report. Acta Ophthalmol 64:146, 1986.

48. Nagataki, S, Mishima, S: Aqueous humor dynamics in glaucomatocyclitic crisis. Invest Ophthalmol 15:365, 1976.

49. de Roeth, A Jr: Glaucomatocyclitic crisis. Am J Ophthalmol 69:370, 1970.

50. Hong, C, Yung Song, KY: Effect of apraclonidine hydrochloride on the attack of Posner-Schlossman syndrome. Korean J Ophthalmol 7:28, 1993.

51. Fuchs, E: Uber Komplikationen der Heterochromie. Ztschr Augenh 15:191, 1906.

52. Franceschetti, A: Heterochromic cyclitis (Fuchs' syndrome). Am J Ophthalmol 39:50, 1955.

53. Kimura, SJ, Hogan, MJ, Thygeson, P: Fuchs' syndrome of heterochromic cyclitis. Arch Ophthalmol 54:179, 1955.

54. O'Connor, GR: Heterochromic iridocyclitis. Trans Ophthalmol Soc UK 104:219, 1985.

55. Tabbut, BR, Tessler, HH, Williams, D: Fuchs' heterochromic iridocyclitis in blacks. Arch Ophthalmol 106:1688, 1988.

56. van der Gaag, R, Broersma, L, Rothova, A, et al: Immunity to a corneal antigen in Fuchs' heterochromic cyclitis patients. Invest Ophthalmol Vis Sci 30:443, 1989.

57. La Hey, E, Baarsma, GS, Rothova, A, et al: High incidence of corneal epithelium antibodies in Fuchs' heterochromic cylitis. Br J Ophthalmol 72:921, 1988.

58. La Hey, E, Mooy, CM, Baarsma, GS, et al: Immune deposits in iris biopsy specimens from patients with Fuchs' heterochromic iridocyclitis. Am J Ophthalmol 113:75, 1992.

59. De Bruyere, M, Dernouchamps, J-P, Sokal, G: HLA antigens in Fuchs' heterochromic iridocyclitis. Am J Ophthalmol 102:392, 1986.

60. van den Born, LI, van Schooneveld, MJ, de Jong, PTVM, Bleeker-Wagemakers, EM: Fuchs' heterochromic uveitis associated with retinitis pigmentosa in a father and son. Br J Ophthalmol 78:504, 1994.

61. Jones, NP, Read, AP: Is there a genetic basis for Fuchs' heterochromic uveitis? Discordance in monozygotic twins. Br J Ophthalmol 76:22, 1992.

62. Regenbogen, LS, Naveh-Floman, N: Glaucoma in Fuchs' heterochromic cyclitis associated with congenital Horner's syndrome. Br J Ophthalmol 71:844, 1987.

63. Schwab, IR: The epidemiologic association of Fuchs' heterochromic iridocyclitis and ocular toxoplasmosis. Am J Ophthalmol 111:356, 1991.

64. La Heiji, E, Rothova, A: Fuchs' heterochromic cyclitis in congenital ocular toxoplasmosis. Br J Ophthalmol 75:372, 1991.

65. La Hey, E, Rothova, A, Baarsma, GS, et al: Fuchs' heterochromic iridocyclitis is not associated with ocular toxoplasmosis. Arch Ophthalmol 110:806, 1992.

66. Liesegang, TJ: Clinical features and prognosis in Fuchs' uveitis syndrome. Arch Ophthalmol 100:1622, 1982.

67. Saari, M, Vuorre, I, Nieminen, H: Infra-red transillumination stereophotography of the iris in Fuchs's heterochromic cyclitis. Br J Ophthalmol 62:110, 1978.

68. La Hey, E, Ijspeert, JK, van den Berg, TJTP, Kijlstra, A: Quantitative analysis of iris translucency in Fuchs' heterochromic cyclitis. Invest Ophthalmol Vis Sci 34:2931, 1993.

69. Melamed, S, Lahav, M, Sandbank, U, et al: Fuch's heterochromic iridocyclitis: an electron microscopic study of the iris. Invest Ophthalmol Vis Sci 17:1193, 1978.

70. McCartney, ACE, Bull, TB, Spalton, DJ: Fuchs' heterochromic cyclitis: an electron microscopy study. Trans Ophthalmol Soc UK 105:324, 1986.

71. Rothova, A, La Hey, E, Baarsma, GS, Breebaart, AC: Iris nodules in Fuchs' heterochromic uveitis. Am J Ophthalmol 18:338, 1994.

72. Saari, M, Vuorre, I, Nieminen, H: Fuchs' heterochromic cyclitis: a simultaneous bilateral fluorescein angiographic study of the iris. Br J Ophthalmol 62:715, 1978.

73. Berger, BB, Tessler, HH, Kottow, MH: Anterior segment ischemia in Fuchs' heterochromic cyclitis. Arch Ophthalmol 98:499, 1980.

74. Johnson, D, Liesegang, TJ, Brubaker, RF: Aqueous humor dynamics in Fuchs' uveitis syndrome. Am J Ophthalmol 95:783, 1983.

75. Arffa, RC, Schlaegel, TF: Chorioretinal scars in Fuchs' heterochromic iridocyclitis. Arch Ophthalmol 102:1153, 1984.

76. De Abreu, MT, Belfort, R Jr, Hirata, PS: Fuchs' heterochromic cyclitis and ocular toxoplasmosis. Am J Ophthalmol 93:739, 1982.

77. Daus, W, Schmidbauer, J, Buschendorff, P, et al: Results of extracapsular cataract extraction with intraocular lens implantation in eyes with uveitis and Fuchs' heterochromic iridocyclitis. Ger J Ophthalmol 1:399, 1992.

78. Baarsma, GS, de Vries, J, Hammudoglu, CD: Extracapsular cataract extraction with posterior chamber lens implantation in Fuchs's heterochromic cyclitis. Br J Ophthalmol 75:306, 1991.

79. O'Neill, D, Murray, PI, Patel, BC, Hamilton, AMP: Extracapsular cataract surgery with and without intraocular lens implantation in Fuchs' heterochromic cyclitis. Ophthalmology 102:1362, 1995.

80. Huber, A: Das Glaukom bei komplizierter heterochromic Fuchs. Ophthalmologica 142:66, 1961.

81. Daus, W, Kraus-Mackiw, E: Fuchs' heterochromic cyclitis. Case reports of patients treated at Heidelberg University Eye Hospital since 1978. Klin Monatsbl Augenheilkd 185:410, 1984.

82. La Hey, E, de Vries, J, Langerhorst, CT, et al: Treatment and prognosis of secondary glaucoma in Fuchs' heterochromic iridocyclitis. Am J Ophthalmol 116:327, 1993.

83. Perry, HD, Yanoff, M, Scheie, HG: Rubeosis in Fuchs heterochromic iridocyclitis. Arch Ophthalmol 93:337, 1975.

84. Benedikt, O, Roll, P, Zirm, M: The glaucoma in heterochromic cyclitis Fuchs. Gonioscopic studies and electron microscopic investigations of the trabecular meshwork. Klin Monatsbl Augenheilkd 173:523, 1978.

85. Colvard, DM, Robertson, DM, O'Duffy, JD: The ocular manifestations of Behçet's disease. Arch Ophthalmol 95:1813, 1977.

86. Michelson, JB, Chisari, FV: Behçet's disease. Surv Ophthalmol 26:190, 1982.

87. Benezra, D, Cohen, E: Treatment and visual prognosis in Behçet's disease. Br J Ophthalmol 70:589, 1986.

88. James, DG, Spiteri, MA: Behçet's disease. Ophthalmology 89:1279, 1982.

89. Lee, DA, Barker, SM, Su, WPD, et al: The clinical diagnosis of Reiter's syndrome. Ophthalmic and nonophthalmic aspects. Ophthalmology 93:350, 1986.

90. Chandler, PA, Grant, WM: Lectures on Glaucoma. Philadelphia, Lea and Febiger, 1954, p. 257.

91. Rathore, MK: Ophthalmological study of epidemic dropsy. Br J Ophthalmol 66:573, 1982.

92. Sachdev, MS, Sood, NN, Verma, LK, et al: Pathogenesis of epidemic dropsy glaucoma. Arch Ophthalmol 106:1221, 1988.

93. Cooper, LZ, Ziring, PR, Ockerse, AB, et al: Rubella. Clinical manifestations and management. Am J Dis Child 118:18, 1969.

94. Rudolph, AJ, Desmond, MM: Clinical manifestations of the congenital rubella syndrome. Int Ophthalmol Clin 12:3, 1972.

95. deLuise, VP, Cobo, LM, Chandler, D: Persistent corneal edema in the congenital rubella syndrome. Ophthalmology 90:835, 1983.

96. Boniuk, M: Glaucoma in the congenital rubella syndrome. Int Ophthalmol Clin 12:121, 1972.

97. Brooks, AMV, Gillies, WE: Glaucoma associated with congenital hypoplasia of the iris stroma in rubella. Glaucoma 11:36, 1989.

98. Wolff, SMacK: The ocular manifestations of congenital rubella. Trans Am Ophthalmol Soc 70:577, 1972.

99. Boger, WP III: Late ocular complications in congenital rubella syndrome. Ophthalmology 87:1244, 1980.

100. Schwartz, LK, O'Connor, GR: Secondary syphilis with iris papules. Am J Ophthalmol 90:380, 1980.

101. Scully, RE, Mark, EJ, McNeely, BU: Mass in the iris and a skin rash in a young man. N Engl J Med 310:972, 1984.

102. Michelson, JB, Roth, AM, Waring, GO III: Lepromatous iridocyclitis diagnosed by anterior chamber paracentesis. Am J Ophthalmol 88:674, 1979.

103. Malla, OK, Brandt, F, Anten, JGF: Ocular findings in leprosy patients in an institution in Nepal (Khokana). Br J Ophthalmol 65:226, 1981.

104. Joffrion, VC, Brand, ME: Leprosy of the eye—a general outline. Lepr Rev 55:105, 1984.

105. Ffytche, TJ: Role of iris changes as a cause of blindness in lepromatous leprosy. Br J Ophthalmol 65:231, 1981.

106. Lewallen, S, Courtright, P, Lee, H-S: Ocular autonomic dysfunction and intraocular pressure in leprosy. Br J Ophthalmol 73:946, 1989.

107. Shields, JA, Waring, GO III, Monte, LG: Ocular findings in leprosy. Am J Ophthalmol 77:880, 1974.

108. Walton, RC, Ball, SF, Joffrion, VC: Glaucoma in Hansen's disease. Br J Ophthalmol 75,270, 1991.

109. Brandt, F, Malla, OK, Anten, JGF: Influence of untreated chronic plastic iridocyclitis on intraocular pressure in leprous patients. Br J Ophthalmol 65:240, 1981.

110. Hussein, N, Courtright, P, Ostler, HB, et al: Low intraocular pressure and postural changes in intraocular pressure in patients with Hansen's Disease. Am J Ophthalmol 108:80, 1989.

111. Hussein, N, Chiang, T, Ehsan, Q, Hussain, R: Intraocular pressure decrease in household contacts of patients with Hansen's disease and endemic control subjects. Am J Ophthalmol 114:479, 1992.

112. Spaide, R, Nattis, R, Lipka, A, D'Amico, R: Ocular findings in leprosy in the United States. Am J Ophthalmol 100:411, 1985.

113. deLuise, VP, Stern, JT, Paden, P: Uveitic glaucoma caused by disseminated meningococcemia. Am J Ophthalmol 95:707, 1983.

114. Jensen, AD, Naidoff, MA: Bilateral meningococcal endophthalmitis. Arch Ophthalmol 90:396, 1973.

115. Saari, KM: Acute glaucoma in hemorrhagic fever with renal syndrome (nephropathia epidemica). Am J Ophthalmol 81:455, 1976.

116. Kontkanen, MI, Puustjarvi, TJ, Lähdevirta, JK: Intraocular pressure changes in nephropathia epidemica. Ophthalmology 102:1813, 1995.

117. Ullman, S, Wilson, RP, Schwartz, L: Bilateral angle-closure glaucoma in association with the acquired immune deficiency syndrome. Am J Ophthalmol 101:419, 1986.

118. Koster, HR, Liebmann, JM, Ritch, R, Hudock, S: Acute angle-closure glaucoma in a patient with acquired immunodeficiency syndrome successfully treated with argon laser peripheral iridoplasty. Ophthalmol Surg 21:501, 1990.

119. Nash, RW, Lindquist, TD: Bilateral angle-closure glaucoma associated with uveal effusion: presenting sign of HIV infection. Surv Ophthalmol 36:255, 1992.

120. Joshi, N, Constable, PH, Margolis, TP, et al: Bilateral angle closure glaucoma and accelerated cataract formation in a patient with AIDS. Br J Ophthalmol 78:656, 1994.

121. Eliott, D, O'Brien, TP, Green, WR, et al: Elevated introcular pressure, pigment dispersion and dark hypopyon in endogenous endophthalmitis from *Listeria* monocytogenes. Surv Ophthalmol 37:117, 1992.

122. Toris, CB, Pederson, JE: Aqueous humor dynamics in experimental iridocyclitis. Invest Ophthalmol Vis Sci 28:477, 1987.

123. Chiang, TS, Thomas, RP: Ocular hypertension following intravenous infusion of prostaglandin E$_1$. Arch Ophthalmol 88:418, 1972.

124. Chiang, TS, Thomas, RP: Consensual ocular hypertensive response to prostaglandin E$_2$. Invest Ophthalmol 11:845, 1972.

125. Kass, MA, Podos, SM, Moses, RA, Becker, B: Prostaglandin E$_1$ and aqueous humor dynamics. Invest Ophthalmol 11:1022, 1972.

126. Podos, SM, Becker, B, Kass, MA: Prostaglandin synthesis, inhibition, and intraocular pressure. Invest Ophthalmol 12:426, 1973.

127. Epstein, DL, Hashimoto, JM, Grant, WM: Serum obstruction of aqueous outflow in enucleated eyes. Am J Ophthalmol 86:101, 1978.

128. Neufeld, AH, Sears, ML: The site of action of prostaglandin E$_2$ on the disruption of the blood-aqueous barrier in the rabbit eye. Exp Eye Res 7:445, 1973.

129. Kulkarni, PS, Srinivasan, BD: The effect of intravitreal and topical prostaglandins on intraocular inflammation. Invest Ophthalmol Vis Sci 23:383, 1982.

130. Bengtsson, E: The effect of theophylline on the breakdown of the blood-aqueous barrier in the rabbit eye. Invest Ophthalmol Vis Sci 16:636, 1977.

131. Bolliger, GA, Kupferman, A, Leibowitz, HM: Quantitation of anterior chamber inflammation and its response to therapy. Arch Ophthalmol 98:1110, 1980.

132. Leibowitz, HM, Kupferman, A: Optimal frequency of topical prednisolone administration. Arch Ophthalmol 97:2154, 1979.

133. Marsetio, M, Siverio, CE, Oh, JO: Effects of aspirin and dexamethasone on intraocular pressure in primary uveitis produced by herpes simplex virus. Am J Ophthalmol 81:636, 1976.

134. Kass, MA, Palmberg, P, Becker, B: The ocular anti-inflammatory action of imidazole. Invest Ophthalmol Vis Sci 16:66, 1977.

135. Spinelli, HM, Krohn, DL: Inhibition of prostaglandin-induced iritis. Topical indoxole vs. indomethacin therapy. Arch Ophthalmol 98:1106, 1980.

136. Podos, SM: Effect of dipyridamole on prostaglandin-induced ocular hypertension in rabbits. Invest Ophthalmol Vis Sci 18:646, 1979.

137. Wong, VG, Hersh, EM: Methotrexate in the therapy of cyclitis. Trans Am Acad Ophthalmol Otol 69:279, 1965.

138. Andrasch, RH, Pirofsky, B, Burns, RP: Immunosuppressive therapy for severe chronic uveitis. Arch Ophthalmol 96:247, 1978.

139. Fiscella, R, Gagliano, DA, Peachey, NS, et al: Intravitreal U75412E: a new free radical scavenger. Ophthalmol Surg 22:740, 1991.

140. Jampel, HD, Jabs, DA, Quigley, HA: Trabeculectomy with 5-fluorouracil for adult inflammatory glaucoma. Am J Ophthalmol 109:68, 1990.

141. Patitsas, CJ, Rockwood, EJ, Meisler, DM, Lowder, CY: Glaucoma filtering surgery with postoperative 5-fluorouracil in patients with intraocular inflammatory disease. Ophthalmology 99:594, 1992.

142. Prata, JA, Neves, RA, Minckler, DS et al: Trabeculectomy with mitomycin C in glaucoma associated with uveitis. Ophthalmol Surg 25:616, 1994.

143. Hill, RA, Nguyen, QH, Baerveldt, G, et al: Trabeculectomy and Molteno implantation for glaucomas associated with uveitis. Ophthalmology 100:903, 1993.

144. Hoskins, HD Jr, Hetherington, J Jr, Shaffer, RN: Surgical managment of the inflammatory glaucomas. Perspect Ophthalmol 1:173, 1977.

145. Kanski, JJ, McAllister, JA: Trabeculodialysis for inflammatory glaucoma in children and young adults. Ophthalmology 92:927, 1985.

146. Ohno, S, Char, DH, Kimura, SJ, O'Connor, GR: Vogt-Koyanagi-Harada syndrome. Am J Ophthalmol 83:735, 1977.

147. Forster, DJ, Rao, NA, Hill, RA, et al: Incidence and management of glaucoma in Vogt-Koyanagi-Harada syndrome. Ophthalmology 100:613, 1993.

148. Shirato, S, Hayashi, K, Masuda, K: Acute angle closure glaucoma as an initial sign of Harada's disease: report of two cases. Jpn J Ophthalmol 24:260, 1980.

149. Kimura, R, Sakai, M, Okabe, H: Transient shallow anterior chamber as initial symptom in Harada's syndrome. Arch Ophthalmol 99:1604, 1981.

150. Kimura, R, Kasai, M, Shoji, K, Kanno, C: Swollen ciliary processes as an initial symptom in Vogt-Koyanagi-Harada syndrome. Am J Ophthalmol 95:402, 1983.

151. Lubin, JR, Albert, DM, Weinstein, M: Sixty-five years of sympathetic ophthalmia. A clinicopathologic review of 105 cases (1913–1978). Ophthalmology 87:109, 1980.

152. Marak, GE Jr: Recent advances in sympathetic ophthalmia. Surv Ophthalmol 24:141, 1979.

153. Makley, TA Jr, Azar, A: Sympathetic ophthalmia. A long-term follow-up. Arch Ophthalmol 96:257, 1978.

154. Merritt, JC, Callender, CO: Adult cytomegalic inclusion retinitis. Ann Ophthalmol 10:1059, 1978.

155. Shields, JA: Ocular toxocariasis. A review. Surv Ophthalmol 28:361, 1984.

156. Tavs, LE: Syphilis. Maj Prob Clin Ped 19:222, 1978.

157. Grant, WM: Late glaucoma after interstitial keratitis. Am J Ophthalmol 79:87, 1975.

158. Tsukahara, S: Secondary glaucoma due to inactive congenital syphilitic interstitial keratitis. Ophthalmologica 174:188, 1977.

159. Sugar, HS: Late glaucoma associated with inactive syphilitic interstitial keratitis. Am J Ophthalmol 53:602, 1962.

160. Cobo, LM, Haynes, BF: Early corneal findings in Cogan's syndrome. Ophthalmology 91:903, 1984.

161. Falcon, MG, Williams, HP: Herpes simplex kerato-uveitis and glaucoma. Trans Ophthalmol Soc UK 98:101, 1978.

162. Oh, JO: Effect of cyclophosphamide on primary herpes simplex uveitis in rabbits. Invest Ophthalmol Vis Sci 17:769, 1978.

163. Sundmacher, R, Neumann-Haefelin, D: Herpes simplex virus isolations from the aqueous of patients suffering from focal iritis, endotheliitis, and prolonged disciform keratitis with glaucoma. Klin Monatsbl Augenheilkd 175:488, 1979.

164. Townsend, WM, Kaufman, HE: Pathogenesis of glaucoma and endothelial changes in herpetic kerato-uveitis in rabbits. Am J Ophthalmol 71:904, 1971.

165. Dennis, RF, Oh, JO: Aspirin, cyclophosphamide, and dexamethasone effects on experimental secondary herpes simplex uveitis. Arch Ophthalmol 97:2170, 1979.

166. Womack, LW, Liesegang, TJ: Complications of herpes zoster ophthalmicus. Arch Ophthalmol 101:42, 1983.

167. Reijo, A, Antti, V, Jukka, M: Endothelial cell loss in herpes zoster keratouveitis. Br J Ophthalmol 67:751, 1983.

168. McGill, J, Chapman, C: A comparison of topical acyclovir with steroids in the treatment of herpes zoster keratouveitis. Br J Ophthalmol 67:746, 1983.

169. Hara, J, Ishibashi, T, Fujimoto, F, et al: Adenovirus type 10 keratoconjunctivitis with increased intraocular pressure. Am J Ophthalmol 90:481, 1980.

170. Watson, PG, Hayreh, SS: Scleritis and episcleritis. Br J Ophthalmol 60:163, 1976.

171. Young, RD, Watson, PG: Microscopical studies of necrotising scleritis. I. Cellular aspects. Br J Ophthalmol 68:770, 1984.

172. Young, RD, Watson, PG: Microscopical studies of necrotising scleritis. II. Collagen degradation in the scleral stroma. Br J Ophthalmol 68:781, 1984.

173. Watson, PG, Bovey, E: Anterior segment fluorescein angiography in the diagnosis of scleral inflammation. Ophthalmology 92:1, 1985.

174. de La Maza, MS, Jabbur, NS, Foster, CS: Severity of scleritis and episcleritis. Ophthal 101:389, 1994.

175. McGavin, DDM, Williamson, J, Forrester, JV, et al: Episcleritis and scleritis. A study of their clinical manifestations and association with rheumatoid arthritis. Br J Ophthalmol 60:192, 1976.

176. Wilhelmus, KR, Grierson, I, Watson, PG: Histopathologic and clinical associations of scleritis and glaucoma. Am J Ophthalmol 91:697, 1981.

177. Chen, CJ, Harisdangkul, V, Parker, L: Transient glaucoma associated with anterior diffuse scleritis in relapsing polychondritis. Glaucoma 4:109, 1982.

178. Ortiz, JM, Kamerling, JM, Fischer, D, Baxter, J: Scleritis, uveitis, and glaucoma in a patient with rheumatic fever. Am J Ophthalmol 120:538, 1995.

179. Quinlan, MP, Hitchings, RA: Angle-closure glaucoma secondary to posterior scleritis. Br J Ophthalmol 62:330, 1978.

180. Mangouritsas, G, Ulbig, M: Secondary angle closure glaucoma in posterior scleritis. Klin Monatsbl Augenheilkd 199:40, 1991.

181. Mondino, BJ, Phinney, RB: Treatment of scleritis with combined oral prednisone and indomethacin therapy. Am J Ophthalmol 106:473, 1988.

182. Harbin, TS Jr, Pollack, IP: Glaucoma in episcleritis. Arch Ophthalmol 93:948, 1975.

183. Pavlin, CJ, Easterbrook, M, Harasiewicz, K, Foster, FS: An ultrasound biomicroscopic analysis of angle-closure glaucoma secondary to ciliochoroidal effusion in IgA nephropathy. Am J Ophthalmol 116:341, 1993.

Chapter 20

STEROID-INDUCED GLAUCOMA

As discussed in Chapter 9, a certain percent of the general population will respond to repeated instillation of topical corticosteroids with a variable increase in the intraocular pressure (IOP). This occurs more commonly in individuals who have chronic open-angle glaucoma or a family history of the disease. There are many unknown facets regarding the pressure response to steroids, such as the precise distribution of steroid responders in the general population, the reproducibility of these responses, and hereditary influences. Nevertheless, the critical fact is that certain people do manifest this response to chronic steroid therapy, and the IOP elevation can lead to glaucomatous optic atrophy and loss of vision. Such a condition is referred to as steroid-induced glaucoma.

HISTORIC BACKGROUND

In 1950, McLean (1) reported an IOP rise in response to the systemic administration of ACTH for the treatment of uveitis. Francois (2), in 1954, noted that a similar elevation in tension could occur after local therapy with cortisone. Numerous reports followed these early observations, which confirmed that IOP rise may occur with topical, systemic, or periocular administration of corticosteroids, although more often after local therapy.

CLINICAL FEATURES

The typical clinical presentation is associated with topical steroid therapy. Intraocular pressure elevation usually develops within a few weeks with potent corticosteroids, or in months with the weaker steroids (3). The clinical picture resembles that of chronic open-angle glaucoma with an open, normal appearing anterior chamber angle and absence of symptoms. Much less often, the condition may have an acute presentation, in which pressure rises have been observed within hours after steroid administration in eyes with open angles (3, 4). This has been seen with intensive systemic steroid therapy or with the topical use of potent corticosteroids.

Although children are reported to have a lower incidence of positive steroid responders than adults (5), IOP elevation has been precipitated by treating external diseases in infants with corticosteroids (6), or by the use of corticosteroid eyedrops after strabismus surgery in children under 10 years of age (7). However, long-term, low-dose oral prednisone therapy in children was not associated with higher than normal IOPs in one study (8). It has been reported that IOP elevation may occur in the first few weeks after a trabeculectomy despite a good filtering bleb, possibly due to the influence of topical steroid therapy (9). Steroid-induced glaucoma may also mimic low-tension glaucoma, when the steroid-induced pressure elevation has damaged the optic nerve head and visual field, but the IOP has subsequently returned to normal with cessation of the steroid (10).

THEORIES OF MECHANISM

It is generally agreed that the IOP elevation due to steroid administration results from reduction in facility of aqueous outflow (11–13). In the rabbit eye, intravenously administered glucocorticoids are specifically bound in the nuclei of cells in the outflow pathway (14). When cultured human trabecular cells were incubated with dexamethasone, a high binding affinity for the glucocorticoid was demonstrated, with two-thirds of the binding occurring in the nuclear fraction (15). The binding affinity of rabbit iris-ciliary body for dexamethasone was found to be virtually identical to that of rabbit liver, although the concentration of glucocorticoid receptors was nearly two-fold higher in the ocular tissue (16). It has also been shown that topical administration of steroids in rabbits is associated with a translocation of glucocorticoid receptors from the cytoplasm to the nucleus in iris-ciliary body and adjacent corneoscleral tissue (17). This may be a necessary event in steroid-induced elevation of IOP since the degree to which a glucocorticoid is able to produce translocation correlates with the in vivo pressure-inducing tendency of that drug (17). Other studies have shown that dihydrocortisols, which are intermediate glucocorticoid metabolites, accumulate abnormally in trabecular cells from patients with chronic open-angle glaucoma and potentiate the effect of topical dexamethasone on IOP elevation in rabbits (18).

The above studies suggest that trabecular and anterior uveal tissue have a high concentration of glucocorticoid receptors and probably represent the target tissue in the steroid-induced mediation of reduced aqueous outflow facility. The precise mechanism responsible for the obstruction to outflow is unknown, but the following observations and theories have been reported.

Influence on Extracellular Matrix

Hyaluronidase-sensitive glycosaminoglycans (mucopolysaccharides) are normally present in the aqueous outflow system. Francois (19–21) postulated that glycosaminoglycans in the polymerized form become hydrated, producing a "biological edema" which may increase resistance to aqueous outflow. Hyaluronidase within lysosomes depolymerizes hyaluronate, and corticosteroids stabilize the lysosomal membrane, which leads to an accumulation of polymerized glycosaminoglycans in the trabecular meshwork. Francois also suggested that the lysosomes reside primarily in fibroblasts in the meshwork, which he called goniocytes. He felt that clones of goniocytes may have variable sensitivity to corticosteroids, accounting for the differences in individual pressure responses. Lysosomal hyaluronidase activity has been demonstrated in the corneoscleral junction of rabbit and human eyes, although the role of the enzyme in aqueous outflow regulation is unclear (22). Examinations of trabecular specimens from eyes with steroid-induced glaucoma have also been inconclusive, although there is some evidence, both in human eyes (23), as well as in experimental rabbit studies (24), that an excess accumulation of glycosaminoglycans in the aqueous outflow system may be an important factor in steroid-induced glaucoma.

Topical dexamethasone-induced IOP elevation in rabbits was associated with an increase in chondroitin sulfate within the aqueous outflow pathway, but a decrease in hyaluronic acid (25). Dexamethasone-induced ocular hypertension has also been produced in perfusion-cultured human eyes, in which the morphologic changes in the trabecular meshwork were similar to those reported in steroid-induced glaucoma and chronic open-angle glaucoma (26), and a time-dependent increase was observed in the undigestible glycosaminoglycans incorporation profile in the meshwork (27). Dexamethasone has also been shown to decrease the synthesis of collagen in normal human trabecular meshwork explants (28). In both organ explants and cell cultures containing trabecular meshwork, dexamethasone decreased the extracellular activity of tissue plasminogen activator (29). In cultured human trabecular meshwork cells, glucocorticoids increased the expression of the extracellular matrix protein fibronectin, increased depositions of which are also seen in the outflow pathways of patients with chronic open-angle glaucoma (30). It also caused the formation of cross-linked actin network in the trabecular meshwork cytoskeleton (31).

Influence on Phagocytosis

Endothelial cells lining the trabecular meshwork have phagocytic properties, which may help to clean the aqueous of debris before it reaches the inner wall of Schlemm's canal. Corticosteroids are known to suppress phagocytic activity, and the possibility has been raised that suppressed phagocytosis of the trabecular endothelium may allow debris in the aqueous to accumulate in the meshwork and act as a barrier to outflow (32). This theory is consistent with ultrastructural studies showing marked depositions of amorphous and fibrous or linear material in the juxtacanalicular meshwork of eyes with steroid-induced glaucoma (33, 34).

Additional Observations

The influence of corticosteroid therapy on aqueous production is uncertain, with one fluorophotometric study showing an increased rate of aqueous flow associated with the oral administration of hydrocortisone (35), while another study found no alteration in flow after 1 week of topical dexamethasone therapy (36). It has been observed in rabbits that long-term topical steroid administration is associated with a shift toward an alkaline aqueous and reduced ascorbic acid content (37, 38). Additional ocular responses that may occur in some individuals on chronic topical corticosteroid therapy include a slight mydriasis and ptosis, and an increase in corneal thickness, although none of these changes appear to correlate with the IOP response (12, 39).

PREVENTION

To avoid loss of vision from steroid-induced glaucoma, physicians must know how to prevent or minimize the chances of its occurrence. This requires close attention to the patient's history and to the selection and use of steroids.

Patient Selection

As previously noted, individuals with chronic open-angle glaucoma or a family history of the disease are more likely to respond to chronic steroid therapy with a significant rise in IOP. In addition, it has been noted that high myopes (40), diabetics (41), and patients with connective tissue diseases (especially rheumatoid arthritis) (42) have a similar predisposition. These patients, therefore, are at a somewhat higher risk of developing steroid-induced glaucoma. However, since it is not possible to predict which additional individuals without these predisposing factors will also have a pressure rise, all patients must be treated cautiously. This involves avoiding steroids when a safer drug will suffice, using the least amount of steroid necessary, establishing a baseline IOP before initiating therapy, and monitoring the tension closely for the duration of the corticosteroid therapy.

Drug Selection

When corticosteroid therapy is required for any disorder, the optimum drug is the one which will achieve the desired therapeutic response by the safest route of administration, in the lowest concentration, and with the fewest potential adverse reactions. With regard to the IOP response, these facts should be considered.

Routes of Administration

TOPICAL. Topical corticosteroid therapy is more often associated with an IOP rise than is the case with systemic administration. This may occur not only with drops or ointment applied directly to the eye, but also with steroid preparations used in treating the skin of the eyelids (43–45).

PERIOCULAR. Periocular injection is the most dangerous route of corticosteroid administration from the standpoint of steroid-induced glaucoma. Intraocular pressure elevation may occur in response to subconjunctival, sub-Tenons, or retrobulbar injections of steroids (46–50). The patient's response to earlier topical steroid therapy does not always predict how that individual will respond to periocular corticosteroids (49). Repository steroids are particularly dangerous because of their prolonged duration of action, and it may occasionally be necessary to surgically excise the remaining drug before the pressure can be brought under control (48–50). Histopathologic study of excised specimens has revealed granular or foamy, eosinophilic material in the subepithelial connective tissue (50). If repository steroids must be used, they should be injected in an inferior quadrant to avoid compromising the superior sites for possible future filtering surgery.

SYSTEMIC. Systemic administration of corticosteroids is least likely to induce glaucoma, although cases have been described (51–55). In one study of 62 patients receiving systemic steroids following renal transplantation, six developed IOP elevation, and five of these had HLA-B12 (55). It is reported that this response does not correlate with the dosage or duration of treatment, but is associated with the degree of pressure response to topical steroids (53, 54). Intraocular pressure elevation has been noted in association with inhalation and nasal corticosteroids (56), and it has been reported that amounts of corticosteroids, sufficient to influence the IOP, can be absorbed from skin application in areas remote from the eyes (23).

Relative Pressure-Inducing Effects of Topical Steroids

Although topical corticosteroids are more likely to cause an elevation of the IOP than are systemic steroids, the topical route of administration is still generally preferred to avoid the additional dangers associated with systemic corticosteroid therapy. While no topical steroid is totally free of a pressure-inducing effect, the following observations have been reported regarding the relative tendencies of these drugs to induce an elevation of the IOP.

CORTICOSTEROIDS. In general, the pressure-inducing effect of a topical steroid is proportional to its anti-inflammatory potency. *Betamethasone, dexamethasone,* and *prednisolone* are commonly used, potent corticosteroids with a significant tendency to produce steroid-induced glaucoma. However, as might be anticipated, the pressure-inducing potency is related to the dosage of the drug. In a study of high topical steroid responders, betamethasone 0.01% caused significantly less pressure elevation than the 0.1% concentration (57). In addition, the formulation may cause some dissociation of anti-inflammatory and pressure-inducing effects. In a rabbit study, dexamethasone acetate 0.1% had a better anti-inflammatory effect than dexamethasone alcohol 0.1% or dexamethasone sodium phosphate 0.1%, while the acetate and sodium phosphate preparations had the same effect on IOP elevation in humans (58).

Flurandrenolide, a less commonly used corticosteroid, has also been reported to cause steroid-induced glaucoma (59). A newer corticosteroid with high topical activity, *clobetasone butyrate* 0.1%, was compared with prednisolone phosphate 0.5% and betamethasone phosphate 0.1% (60–63). While the results varied somewhat among studies, clobetasone butyrate was comparable or slightly weaker in anti-inflammatory action, but also had less of a tendency to produce IOP elevation.

NONADRENAL STEROIDS. A group of drugs closely related to progesterone has been shown to have useful anti-inflammatory properties with significantly less pressure-inducing effects than most corticosteroids. *Medrysone* is primarily of value in the treatment of extraocular disorders, since it has limited corneal penetration, although one study found it to be effective in treating iritis (64). Most reports describe little or no associated IOP elevation (64–66), although a slight pressure response in some patients has been observed (57, 67). The steroid antagonist, mifepristone, has been shown to reduce the hypertensive effect of medrysone in rabbits (68). *Fluorometholone* 0.1% is more efficacious than medrysone in treating inflammation of the anterior ocular segment. Although the pressure-inducing effect of fluorometholone is substantially less than that of the potent corticosteroids (63, 67, 71), significant pressure rises have been observed with the use of this drug (71, 72). Fluorometholone 0.25% is also less likely to increase IOP in corticosteroid responders than dexamethasone 0.1% (73), although the increased concentration does not appear to significantly enhance its anti-inflammatory effect (63). Formulation of fluorometholone as an acetate derivative, however, does appear to increase its effectiveness, rendering it as effective as 1.0% prednisolone acetate in one study (63). Despite the greater margin of safety with regard to IOP elevation, the same precautions must be taken with the nonadrenal steroids as with the corticosteroids.

NONSTEROIDAL ANTI-INFLAMMATORY DRUGS. Topical nonsteroidal anti-inflammatory drugs (NSAIDs), which act primarily as cyclooxygenase inhibitors, may be effective in treating anterior ocular segment inflammation, apparently by reducing the breakdown of the blood-aqueous barrier. Preliminary experience with topical *oxyphenbutazone* (74), *flurbiprofen* (75), and *diclofenac* (76) indicates that these NSAID agents do not cause an elevation of IOP. Other commercially available drugs in this class include *suprofen* and *ketorolac*. It has also been shown that flurbiprofen does not block corticosteroid-induced pressure elevation (75).

MANAGEMENT

Discontinuation of the Steroid

Discontinuation of the steroid is the first line of defense and is often all that is required. The chronic form is said to normalize in 1–4 weeks, while the acute form typically resolves within days of stopping the steroid (4). In rare cases, the glaucoma may persist despite stopping all steroids. The latter situation occurred in 6 of 210 patients (2.8%) in one series, and all of these patients had a family history of glaucoma (3). The duration of steroid therapy also appears to influence the reversibility of the IOP elevation. In a study of 22 patients with steroid-induced glaucoma, the pressures normalized in all cases in which the drug was used for less than 2 months, while the tension remained chronically elevated in all patients who used the steroid for more than 4 years (77). If continued corticosteroid therapy is essential,

it may be possible to control the IOP with the additional use of antiglaucoma medications or by changing to a steroid with less pressure-inducing potential.

Glaucoma Therapy

The medical management of these cases is essentially the same as for chronic open-angle glaucoma. Surgical intervention is indicated when the glaucoma is uncontrolled on maximum tolerable medication. As previously noted, it may occasionally be necessary to excise a depot of periocular steroid if this appears to be responsible for the persistent pressure elevation (48–50). In other cases of medically uncontrollable glaucoma, laser trabeculoplasty is usually indicated, followed by filtering surgery if necessary.

SUMMARY

The prolonged use of steroids, especially the topical administration of corticosteroids, will cause an IOP elevation in some patients, with clinical findings that typically resemble chronic open-angle glaucoma. The mechanism of the glaucoma is uncertain, although an unusual sensitivity to steroids in the aqueous outflow pathways may lead to increased resistance to outflow, possibly through an influence on the extracellular matrix or endothelial cells of the trabecular meshwork. The problem is best managed by attempting to prevent it through the judicious use of anti-inflammatory agents. When steroid-induced glaucoma does occur, the steroid should be stopped, if possible, and persisting pressure elevation should be managed with medication or surgery as required.

REFERENCES

1. McLean, JM: Use of ACTH and cortisone. Discussion of paper of Woods, AC. Trans Am Ophthalmol Soc 48:293, 1950.
2. Francois, J: Cortisone et tension oculaire. Ann D'Oculist 187: 805, 1954.
3. Francois, J: Corticosteroid glaucoma. Ann Ophthalmol 9:1075, 1977.
4. Weinreb, RN, Polansky, JR, Kramer, SG, Baxter, JD: Acute effects of dexamethasone on intraocular pressure in glaucoma. Invest Ophthalmol Vis Sci 26:170, 1985.
5. Biedner, B-A, David, R, Grudsky, A, Sachs, U: Intraocular pressure response to corticosteroids in children. Br J Ophthalmol 64:430, 1980.
6. Gnad, HD, Martenet, AC: Kongenitales Glaukom and Cortison. Klin Monatsbl Augenheilkd 162:86, 1973.
7. Ohji, M, Kinoshita, S, Ohmi, E, Kuwayama, Y: Marked intraocular pressure to instillation of corticosteroids in children. Am J Ophthalmol 112:450, 1991.
8. Kaye, LD, Kalenak, JW, Price, RL, Cunningham, R: Ocular implications of long-term prednisone therapy in children. J Pediatr Ophthalmol Strabismus 30:142, 1993.
9. Wilensky, JT, Snyder, D, Gieser, D: Steroid-induced ocular hypertension in patients with filtering blebs. Ophthalmology 87:240, 1980.
10. Sugar, HS: Low tension glaucoma: a practical approach. Ann Ophthalmol 11:1155, 1979.

11. Armaly, MF: Effect of corticosteroids on intraocular pressure and fluid dynamics. II. The effect of dexamethasone in the glaucomatous eye. Arch Ophthalmol 70:492, 1963.

12. Miller, D, Peczon, JD, Whitworth, CG: Corticosteroids and functions in the anterior segment of the eye. Am J Ophthalmol 59:31, 1965.

13. Kupfer, C, Ross, K: Studies of aqueous humor dynamics in man. I. Measurements in young normal subjects. Invest Ophthalmol 10:518, 1971.

14. Tchernitchin, A, Wenk, EJ, Hernandez, et al: Glucocorticoid localization by radioautography in the rabbit eye following systemic administration of ³H-dexamethasone. Invest Ophthalmol Vis Sci 19:1231, 1980.

15. Weinreb, RN, Bloom, E, Baxter, JD, et al: Detection of glucocorticoid receptors in cultured human trabecular cells. Invest Ophthalmol Vis Sci 21:403, 1981.

16. McCarty, GR, Schwartz, B: Increased concentration of glucocorticoid receptors in rabbit iris-ciliary body compared to rabbit liver. Invest Ophthalmol Vis Sci 23:525, 1982.

17. Southren, AL, Dominguez, MO, Gordon, GG, et al: Nuclear translocation of the cytoplasmic glucocorticoid receptor in the iris-ciliary body and adjacent corneoscleral tissue of the rabbit following topical administration of various glucocorticoids. Invest Ophthalmol Vis Sci 24:147, 1983.

18. Southren, AL, Gordon, GG, l'Hommedieu, D, et al: 5B-dihydrocortisol: possible mediator of the ocular hypertension in glaucoma. Invest Ophthalmol Vis Sci 26:393, 1985.

19. Francois, J, Victoria-Troncoso, V: Mucopolysaccharides and pathogenesis of cortisone glaucoma. Klin Monatsbl Augenheilkd 165:5, 1974.

20. Francois, J: The importance of the mucopolysaccharides in intraocular pressure regulation. Invest Ophthalmol 14:173, 1975.

21. Francois, J: Tissue culture of ocular fibroblasts. Ann Ophthalmol 11:1551, 1975.

22. Hayasaka, S: Lysosomal enzymes in ocular tissues and diseases. Surv Ophthalmol 27:245, 1983.

23. Spaeth, GL, Rodrigues, MM, Weinreb, S: Steroid-induced glaucoma: A. Persistent elevation of intraocular pressure. B. Histopathological aspects. Trans Am Ophthalmol Soc 75:353, 1977.

24. Ticho, U, Lahav, M, Berkowitz, S, Yoffe, P: Ocular changes in rabbits with corticosteroid-induced ocular hypertension. Br J Ophthalmol 63:646, 1979.

25. Knepper, PA, Collins, JA, Frederick, R: Effect of dexamethasone, progesterone, and testosterone on IOP and GAGs in the rabbit eye. Invest Ophthalmol Vis Sci 26:1093, 1985.

26. Clark, AF, Wilson, K, de Kater, AW, et al: Dexamethasone-induced ocular hypertension in perfusion-cultured human eyes. Invest Ophthalmol Vis Sci 36:478, 1995.

27. Johnson, DH, Bradley, JMB, Acott, TS: The effect of dexamethasone on glycosaminoglycans of human tabecular meshwork in perfusion organ culture. Invest Ophthalmol Vis Sci 31:2568, 1990.

28. Hernandez, MR, Weinstein, BI, Dunn, MW, et al: The effect of dexamethasone on the synthesis of collagen in normal human trabecular meshwork explants. Invest Ophthalmol Vis Sci 26:1784, 1985.

29. Seftor, REB, Stamer, WD, Seftor, EA, Snyder, RW: Dexamethasone decreases tissue plasminogen activator activity in trabecular meshwork organ and cell cultures. J Glau 3:323, 1994.

30. Steely, HT, Browder, SL, Julian, MB, et al: The effects of dexamethasone on fibronectin expression in cultured human trabecular meshwork cells. Invest Ophthalmol Vis Sci 33:2242, 1992.

31. Clark, AF, Wilson, K, McCartney, MD, et al: Glucocorticoid-induced formation of cross-linked actin networks in cultured human trabecular meshwork cells. Invest Ophthalmol Vis Sci 35:281, 1994.

32. Bill, A: The drainage of aqueous humor. Invest Ophthalmol 14:1, 1975.

33. Rohen, JW, Linner, E, Witmer, R: Electron microscopic studies on the trabecular meshwork in two cases of corticosteroid-glaucoma. Exp Eye Res 17:19, 1973.

34. Roll, P, Benedikt, O: Electronmicroscopic investigation of the trabecular meshwork in cortisone glaucoma. Klin Monatsbl Augenheilkd 174:421, 1979.

35. Kimura, R, Honda, M: Effect of orally administered hydrocortisone on the rate of aqueous flow in man. Acta Ophthalmol 60:584, 1982.

36. Rice, SW, Bourne, WM, Brubaker, RF: Absence of an effect of topical dexamethasone on endothelial permeability and flow of aqueous humor. Invest Ophthalmol Vis Sci 24:1307, 1983.

37. Schirru, A, Pecori-Giraldi, J, Pellegrino, N: Topical corticosteroids and vitreous dynamics in the rabbit. Acta Ophthalmol 51:811, 1973.

38. Virno, M, Schirru, A, Pecori-Giraldi, J, Pellegrino, N: Aqueous humor alkalosis and marked reduction in ocular ascorbic acid content following long-term topical cortisone (9ₐ-fluoro-16ₐ-methylprednisolone). Ann Ophthalmol 6:983, 1974.

39. Spaeth, GL: The effect of autonomic agents on the pupil and the intraocular pressure of eyes treated with dexamethasone. Br J Ophthalmol 64:426, 1980.

40. Podos, SM, Becker, B, Morton, WR: High myopia and primary open-angle glaucoma. Am J Ophthalmol 62:1039, 1966.

41. Becker, B: Diabetes mellitus and primary open-angle glaucoma. Am J Ophthalmol 71:1, 1971.

42. Gaston, H, Absolon, MJ, Thurtle, OA, Sattar, MA: Steroid responsiveness in connective tissue diseases. Br J Ophthalmol 67:487, 1983.

43. Cubey, RB: Glaucoma following the application of corticosteroid to the skin of the eyelids. Br J Dermatol 95:207, 1976.

44. Zugerman, C, Sauders, D, Levit, F: Glaucoma from topically applied steroids. Arch Dermatol 112:1326, 1976.

45. Vie, R: Glaucoma and amaurosis associated with long-term application of topical corticosteroids to the eyelids. Acta Derm Venereol 60:541, 1980.

46. Kalina, RE: Increased intraocular pressure following subconjunctival corticosteroid administration. Arch Ophthalmol 81:788, 1969.

47. Nozik, RA: Periocular injection of steroids. Trans Am Acad Ophthalmol Otol 76:695, 1972.

48. Herschler, J: Intractable intraocular hypertension induced by repository triamcinolone acetonide. Am J Ophthalmol 74:501, 1972.

49. Herschler, J: Increased intraocular pressure induced by repository corticosteroids. Am J Ophthalmol 82:90, 1976.

50. Ferry, AP, Harris, WP, Nelson, MH: Histopathologic features of subconjunctivally injected corticosteroids. Am J Ophthalmol 103:716, 1987.

51. Stern, JJ: Acute glaucoma during cortisone therapy. Am J Ophthalmol 36:389, 1953.

52. Covell, LL: Glaucoma induced by systemic steroid therapy. Am J Ophthalmol 45:108, 1958.

53. Godel, V, Feiler-Ofry, V, Stein, R: Systemic steroids and ocular fluid dynamics. I. Analysis of the sample as a whole. Influence of dosage and duration of therapy. Acta Ophthalmol 50:655, 1972.

54. Godel, V, Feiler-Ofry, V, Stein, R: Systemic steroids and ocular fluid dynamics. II. Systemic versus topical steroids. Acta Ophthalmol 50:664, 1972.

55. Adhikary, HP, Sells, RA, Basu, PK: Ocular complications of systemic steroid after renal transplantation and their association with HLA. Br J Ophthalmol 66:290, 1982.

56. Opatowsky, I, Feldman, RM, Gross, R, Feldman, ST: Intraocular pressure elevation associated with inhalation and nasal corticosteroids. Ophthalmology 102:177, 1995.

57. Kitazawa, Y: Increased intraocular pressure induced by corticosteroids. Am J Ophthalmol 82:492, 1976.

58. Leibowitz, HM, Kupperman, A, Stewart, RH, Kimbrough, RL: Evaluation of dexamethasone acetate as a topical ophthalmic formulation. Am J Ophthalmol 86:418, 1978.

59. Brubaker, RF, Halpin, JA: Open-angle glaucoma associated with topical administration of flurandrenolide to the eye. Mayo Clin Proc 50:322, 1975.

60. Ramsell, TG, Bartholomew, RS, Walker, SR: Clinical evaluation of clobetasone butyrate: a comparative study of its effects in postoperative inflammation and on intraocular pressure. Br J Ophthalmol 64:43, 1980.

61. Dunne, JA, Travers, JP: Double-blind clinical trial of topical steroids in anterior uveitis. Br J Ophthalmol 63:762, 1979.

62. Eilon, LA, Walker, SR: Clinical evaluation of clobetasone butyrate eye drops in the treatment of anterior uveitis and its effect on intraocular pressure. Br J Ophthalmol 65:644, 1981.

63. Leibowitz, HM, Ryan, WJ Jr, Kupferman, A: Comparative anti-inflammatory efficacy of topical corticosteroids with low glaucoma-inducing potential. Arch Ophthalmol 110:118, 1992.

64. Bedrossian, RH, Eriksen, SP: The treatment of ocular inflammation with medrysone. Arch Ophthalmol 99:184, 1969.

65. Spaeth, GL: Hydroxymethylprogesterone. An anti-inflammatory steroid without apparent effect on intraocular pressure. Arch Ophthalmol 75:783, 1966.

66. Dorsch, W, Thygeson, P: The clinical efficacy of medrysone, a new ophthalmic steroid. Am J Ophthalmol 65:74, 1968.

67. Mindel, JS, Tavitian, HO, Smith, H Jr, Walker, EC: Comparative ocular pressure elevation by medrysone, fluorometholone, and dexamethasone phosphate. Arch Ophthalmol 98:1577, 1980.

68. Green, K, Cheeks, L, Slagle, T, Phillips, CI: Interaction between progesterone and mifepristone on intraocular pressure in rabbits. Curr Eye Res 8:317, 1989.

69. Fairbairn, WD, Thorson, JC: Fluorometholone. Anti-inflammatory and intraocular pressure effects. Arch Ophthalmol 86:138, 1971.

70. Akingbehin, AO: Comparative study of the intraocular pressure effects of fluorometholone 0.1% versus dexamethasone 0.1%. Br J Ophthalmol 67:661, 1983.

71. Morrison, E, Archer, DB: Effect of fluorometholone (FML) on the intraocular pressure of corticosteroid responders. Br J Ophthalmol 68:581, 1984.

72. Stewart, RH, Kimbrough, RL: Intraocular pressure response to topically administered fluorometholone. Arch Ophthalmol 97:2139, 1979.

73. Kass, M, Cheetham, J, Duzman, E, Burke, PJ: The ocular hypertensive effect of 0.25% fluorometholone in corticosteroid responders. Am J Ophthalmol 102:159, 1986.

74. Wilhemi, E: Experimental and clinical investigation of a non-hormonal anti-inflammatory eye ointment. Ophthalmic Res 5:253, 1973.

75. Gieser, DK, Hodapp, E, Goldberg, I, et al: Flurbiprofen and intraocular pressure. Ann Ophthalmol 13:831, 1981.

76. Strelow, SA, Sherwood, MB, Broncato, LJB, et al: The effect of diclofenac sodium ophthalmic solution on intraocular pressure following cataract extraction. Ophthalmic Surg 23:170, 1992.

77. Espildora, J, Vicuna, P, Diaz, E: Cortisone-induced glaucoma: a report on 44 affected eyes. J Fr Ophthalmol 4:503, 1981.

Chapter 21

GLAUCOMAS ASSOCIATED WITH INTRAOCULAR HEMORRHAGE[a]

Intraocular hemorrhage is most commonly caused by trauma or surgery. In addition, hyphemas may occur spontaneously in association with several ocular disorders, most of which were discussed in previous chapters. Whatever the initial cause of the intraocular hemorrhage may be, it frequently leads to intraocular pressure (IOP) elevation when the aqueous outflow channels become obstructed by blood in various forms. In this chapter, we consider the mechanisms and management of the blood-induced glaucomas, as well as some specific causes of intraocular hemorrhage that are not covered in other chapters.

GLAUCOMAS ASSOCIATED WITH HYPHEMA

Blunt Trauma

A common source of hyphema, or blood in the anterior chamber, is blunt trauma. This usually results from a tear in

the ciliary body, causing bleeding from the small branches of the major arterial circle.

General Features

Young age and male gender appear to be risk factors for blunt ocular trauma. In one large series, 77% of the patients with traumatic hyphemas were under 30 years of age (1). In another large study, the annual incidence of traumatic hyphema was significantly higher in men, and sports-related injuries were identified as a cause for a recent increase in the incidence rate (2).

The initial clinical finding may be a microscopic hyphema, which is characterized by red blood cells circulating in the aqueous. In other cases, the quantity of blood may be sufficient to create a layered hyphema. These range in size from a small layer of blood in the inferior quadrant of the anterior chamber, which is the more common situation, to a

[a]Refer to Shields, MB: Color Atlas of Glaucoma. Baltimore, Williams & Wilkins, 1998, Plate II38.

total hyphema in which the entire anterior chamber is filled with blood. In most cases, the blood clears within a few days, primarily through the trabecular meshwork, and the prognosis is good unless the associated trauma has caused other ocular injuries. However, complications may occur during the postinjury course which can have devastating results.

Complications

RECURRENT HEMORRHAGE. The reported frequency with which eyes rebleed after traumatic hyphema ranges from 4% to 35%, with a rate of less than 10% in most reported series (2–28). Rebleeding usually occurs during the first week after the initial injury, which is probably related to the normal lysis and retraction of the clot. There is considerable variation among studies regarding risk factors for recurrent bleeding. Some investigators found no identifiable factors (22, 23), while others observed a higher frequency to be associated with the size of the initial hyphema, the degree of reduced visual acuity, and the delay in medical attention (24). Aspirin has also been shown to have a detrimental effect on the frequency of rebleeding (9, 14, 29). Elevated IOP has been identified as a risk factor for recurrent hemorrhage (24), but there is a suggestion that hypotony may also increase the chances of rebleeding (3, 5). One study found black race to be another risk factor for recurrent hemorrhage (21).

While studies may differ regarding the frequency of rebleeding and the risk factors by which this complication can be predicted, nearly all reported series agree that recurrent hemorrhage, as compared to the initial hyphema, is associated with significantly more complications and a more frequent need for surgical intervention.

ASSOCIATED GLAUCOMA. Although IOP elevation may occur following the initial bleed, it is more common after a recurrent hemorrhage, and constitutes the most serious complication of a traumatic hyphema. The incidence of glaucoma associated with a traumatic hyphema is partially related to the size of the hemorrhage. In one study of 235 cases, glaucoma occurred in 13.5% of the eyes in which the hyphema filled less than one-half of the anterior chamber, 27% of those with a bleed involving greater than half the chamber, and in 52% of the cases with a total hyphema (17). It is important to distinguish between a total hyphema with bright red blood, and an "eight-ball" or "black-ball" hyphema, which is characterized by dark reddish-black blood (Fig. 21.1), since the latter carries a more grave prognosis relative to associated glaucoma (4). In one series of 113 cases, elevated IOP occurred in one-third of those with a rebleed, but in all cases with eight-ball hyphemas (4).

The mechanism of pressure elevation is related to obstruction of the trabecular meshwork in most cases of traumatic hyphema. Although fresh red blood cells are known to pass through the conventional aqueous outflow system with relative ease, it appears to be the overwhelming numbers of cells, combined with plasma, fibrin, and debris, that may lead to a transient obstruction of aqueous outflow (30). In cases of eight-ball hyphema, it is presumably the formation of a clot, occasionally with degenerated red blood cells from an associated vitreous hemorrhage, which further impedes outflow.

Sickle cell hemoglobinopathies, including sickle cell trait, increase the incidence of glaucoma in association with hyphema (31–33). Erythrocytes in these disorders have a greater tendency to sickle in the aqueous humor (31, 32, 34),

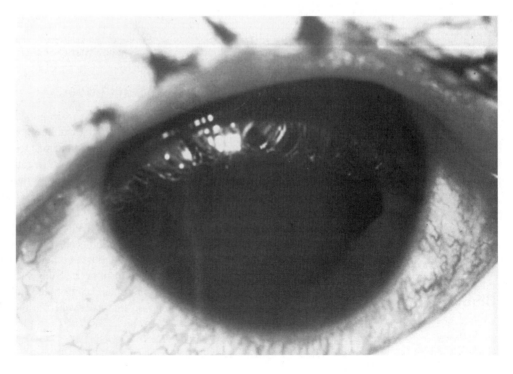

Figure 21.1. Slitlamp view of eye with total, "eight-ball" hyphema and associated glaucoma.

and the elongated, rigid cells pass more slowly through the trabecular meshwork (35), leading to IOP elevation even with small amounts of intracameral blood (31, 32). In addition, even moderate elevations of pressure may have a more deleterious effect on the optic nerve head in patients with sickle cell anemia, possibly due to reduced vascular perfusion (31, 32). Another mechanism of glaucoma associated with sickle cell hemoglobinopathies is obstruction to aqueous outflow due to sickled erythrocytes in Schlemm's canal, which has been observed following blunt trauma and in one case with no antecedent trauma (33).

Another condition that may be associated with delayed clearing of blood from the anterior chamber is diabetes. Erythrocytes from diabetic patients have decreased deformability and increased adherence, resulting in delayed clearance time from the rabbit anterior chamber, as compared to red blood cells from healthy human subjects (36).

CORNEAL BLOODSTAINING. Corneal bloodstaining is typically the result of a prolonged, total hyphema that is usually, but not always (37), associated with elevated IOP. This complication occurred in 6 of 289 patients (2%) with traumatic hyphema, all of whom had a recurrent, total hyphema (35). The earliest pathologic event may be corneal endothelial decompensation associated with the passage of hemoglobin and hemoglobin products into the stroma (38). The cornea may initially have a red discoloration, which was found in rabbit studies to be associated with extracellular hemoglobin particles and oxyhemoglobin (38). The hemoglobin is apparently phagocytized by keratocytes and degraded to hemosiderin (38, 39). The cornea takes on a brownish discoloration at this stage, which is associated with methemoglobin in the stroma (38). Clearing of the corneal bloodstaining begins in the peripheral and posterior stroma, apparently due to diffusion of hemoglobin breakdown products out of the cornea and may take up to 3 years for total clearing (39, 40).

Management

CONSERVATIVE MANAGEMENT OF HYPHEMA. There is general agreement that the uncomplicated hyphema should be managed nonsurgically with an aim toward accelerating resorption of the hyphema and minimizing rebleeding. Opinions vary, however, as to the best means of accomplishing these goals. A traditional approach was to admit the patient for approximately 5 days of bed rest with elevation of the head of the bed and monocular or binocular patching (4, 10). However, one study showed no significant difference between patients treated with strict bed rest and patching as compared to a group that was allowed limited activity without patching (41). A comparison of monocular and binocular patching also revealed no difference in outcome (42). It is reasonable, therefore, to allow limited ambulation, with a shield simply to protect the injured eye. Hospitalization is not always necessary, unless the hyphema is large, there is associated ocular trauma, sickle cell disease or trait is pres-

ent, or the patient cannot be relied upon to maintain limited activity or to return for recommended followup visits.

ACCELERATION OF HYPHEMA CLEARANCE. Various drugs have been used by some physicians to accelerate resorption of the hyphema, but none of these have proven value in this regard. Rabbit studies have not supported the efficacy of atropine (43), pilocarpine (44), or acetazolamide (45) for this purpose, although there is a suggestion that hyperosmotics may accelerate resorption of a clotted hyphema (46). Intracameral tissue plasminogen activator, a clot-specific fibrinolytic agent, has been shown to accelerate the clearance of experimental hyphema in rabbits (46, 47), although it may also increase the risk of rebleeding (47, 48). At the present time, therefore, there is no drug with proven efficacy for safely accelerating hyphema resorption.

PREVENTION OF REBLEEDING. Numerous drugs have also been evaluated regarding their ability to prevent a rebleed, with reported results that have been conflicting. Some investigators found that oral prednisone significantly lowered the rebleed rate (8), while others found neither steroids (15) nor estrogen (4) to be of value in this regard. *Antifibrinolytic agents* (including *tranexamic acid* (12, 13, 28, 49–51) and *aminocaproic acid* (11, 21, 26, 27, 52–56)) have been used in an effort to minimize rebleeding by delaying the natural lysis of the clot. Most reports indicate that the use of either drug is associated with a significant reduction in rebleeds (11, 13, 26, 28, 49–53). Tranexamic acid has been evaluated in several series of traumatic hyphemas in children (28, 50, 51). In a study of hospitalized children, the rebleeding rate was 3% with tranexamic acid, 25 mg/kg every 8 hours for 5 days, compared to 8% without antifibrinolytic therapy (28). One group of children with small hyphemas treated with systemic tranexamic acid therapy and limited activity at home had no recurrent hemorrhage (51).

Some studies have found no significant difference between either tranexamic acid (12) or aminocaproic acid (54) and placebo therapy. Aminocaproic acid is typically given as 100 mg/kg every 4 hours up to a maximum of 30 g/day for 5 days, which is associated with frequent side effects including light-headedness, nausea and vomiting, and systemic hypotension. A half dose of 50 mg/kg reduced the incidence of dizziness and hypotension, without adversely affecting the reduced rate of recurrent hemorrhage, but did not lower the incidence of nausea and vomiting (55). In a randomized comparison of aminocaproic acid 50 mg/kg every 4 hours for 5 days versus oral prednisone 40 mg daily, the rebleed rate was 7.1% in each group (27). Another reported complication is elevated IOP associated with the accelerated clot dissolution (56). Preliminary evidence in rabbit studies suggests that topical aminocaproic acid may be an effective alternative to systemic treatment, which may at least reduce the systemic side effects (57–59).

The influence of hydrostatic pressure on the damaged vessels has also been studied, and one report described fewer rebleeds with medical reduction of systemic blood pressure and elevation of the head of the bed (60). As previously noted, the use of aspirin may increase the chances of recurrent hemorrhage (9, 14), and any drug that may increase the risk of bleeding should be avoided, whenever possible, for the first week after the trauma or until the hyphema has completely cleared.

MANAGEMENT OF ASSOCIATED INTRAOCULAR PRESSURE ELEVATION. *Medical treatment* of elevated IOP is occasionally needed to protect the optic nerve head and enhance the resorption of the hyphema. Pressure reduction is best accomplished with topical β-blocker therapy. Caution should be given to the use of carbonic anhydrase inhibitors in patients with sickle cell hemoglobinopathies, since they increase the concentration of ascorbic acid in the aqueous humor, leading to more sickling in the anterior chamber (61). Epinephrine may increase intravascular and intracameral sickling by its vasoconstrictive and subsequent deoxygenating effect, although the drug had no effect on the duration of the hyphema or percentage of sickled cells in the anterior chamber when human sickle cell thalassemia blood was injected into the anterior chamber of rabbits (62). In the management of patients with sickle cell trait, control of the IOP during the first 24 hours was found to be associated with a good prognosis, while lack of control during that time period was associated with continued difficulty in managing the pressure (63). Hyperbaric oxygen therapy has been shown to significantly reduce the percentage of sickled cells injected intracamerally in rabbits by raising the aqueous pO_2, which may be of value in patients with sickle cell hyphema (64).

Surgical intervention becomes necessary when a sustained IOP elevation cannot be controlled medically and threatens to damage the optic nerve or is associated with corneal bloodstaining. The critical pressure level depends on the status of the optic nerve head (if this is known), with healthy discs usually tolerating pressures of 40–50 mm Hg for 5 or 6 days, while a nerve head with preexisting glaucomatous optic atrophy may undergo further damage at pressures under 30 mm Hg within 24–48 hours. A total hyphema for more than 4 days is an additional indication for surgical intervention. As noted earlier, special attention must be given to patients with sickle cell anemia or trait since their nerve heads are especially vulnerable to damage at minimal to moderate elevations in IOP. A pressure in the mid-20s for more than 1 day may be an indication to surgically intervene in these patients (63).

The surgical approach most often used is evacuation of the hyphema, which usually includes clotted blood, from the anterior chamber. It is also possible to remove the liquified portion of the hyphema by gentle anterior chamber washout through a paracentesis wound and allow the clot to resorb (65). This technique is of particular value when a sudden increase in pressure requires emergency measures to avoid irreversible loss of vision, as may occur with sickle cell dis-

ease (66). A corneal transfixing needle has been developed for simultaneous irrigation of the anterior chamber and evacuation of a fluid hyphema (67).

Many surgeons prefer to also remove the clot, and fibrinolytic agents such as urokinase (68, 69) and fibrinolysin (70–74) have been used to facilitate clot lysis and irrigation. Other reported surgical techniques to remove the clot include cryoextraction (75), ultrasonic emulsification and extraction (76), and removal with vitrectomy instruments (77–79). Viscoelastic agents, such as sodium hyaluronate, have also been used to mechanically dissect a clot from the iris and express it through a corneoscleral incision (80, 81). The fourth day after injury is said to be the optimum time for removal of the clot, because it has usually retracted from the adjacent structures (82, 83).

Other surgeons have advocated a trabeculectomy and iridectomy combined with gentle irrigation of the anterior chamber (84, 85). The iris may prolapse into the incision during any surgical attempt to evacuate the hyphema, due to a pupillary block, necessitating an iridectomy (86), and it has been reported that complete resorption of the hyphema may follow iridectomy alone (87). When recurrent bleeding occurs during clot extraction, raising the IOP to 50 mm Hg for 5 minutes has been used to stop the bleeding (79).

Penetrating Injuries

Intraocular hemorrhage is also frequently associated with penetrating injuries, although associated glaucoma is less common than with blunt trauma during the early postinjury period due to the open wound. However, IOP elevation may follow closure of the wound, especially if meticulous care is not given to reconstruction of the anterior chamber and treatment of the associated inflammation in the early postoperative period (88).

Hyphemas Associated with Intraocular Surgery

Bleeding within the eye can be a serious complication of any intraocular procedure and may occur during the operation or in the early or even late postoperative period.

During Surgery

As an intraoperative complication, bleeding is usually associated with damage to the ciliary body, as can occur when performing a cyclodialysis, filtering procedure, or iridectomy. This bleeding can usually be controlled by placing a large air bubble in the anterior chamber for a few minutes, which raises the IOP and acts as a tamponade. Direct, gentle pressure with the tip of a sponge or Gel-Foam or the application of epinephrine 1:1000 to the ciliary body for

1–2 minutes can also be helpful in stopping ciliary body bleeding. Cautery is generally avoided in these cases, although use of an intraocular, bipolar unit may be effective.

Postoperatively

Bleeding in the *early* postoperative period is usually not associated with serious sequelae and should be managed conservatively with limited activity and elevation of the head. Small hyphemas after intraocular surgery normally clear rapidly, although the time may be considerably longer in eyes with preexisting glaucoma, due to delayed passage of red blood cells through the trabecular meshwork. When a postoperative hyphema is associated with elevated IOP, conservative medical management should be instituted as required, using drugs that lower aqueous production or hyperosmotics if necessary. Surgical intervention is reserved for critical cases, although the indications may be somewhat more liberal than with a traumatic hyphema if there is danger of rupturing a corneoscleral wound or causing further atrophy to an optic nerve that has previously been damaged by glaucoma.

Hemorrhage during the *late* postoperative period may result from reopening of a uveal wound or from disruption of new vessels growing across a corneoscleral incision (89). In a study of 58 eyes, 5–10 years after cataract extraction, 12% had vessels in the inner aspects of the incision site and nearly half of these had evidence of mild intraocular hemorrhage (90). Direct argon laser therapy may be used to treat such vessels when they can be visualized gonioscopically (89), and transscleral Nd:YAG photocoagulation may be effective when the former fails (91). Penetrating cyclodiathermy (92) and cryotherapy (90) are also reported to be useful in managing the intraocular hemorrhage.

Spontaneous Hyphemas

Hyphemas may also develop spontaneously in a variety of conditions, most of which were considered in previous chapters. In some cases, the hyphema may cause or contribute to an elevation of the IOP.

Intraocular Tumors

As noted in Chapter 18, a spontaneous hyphema may occur in a child with juvenile xanthogranuloma, and intraocular hemorrhage may also be a manifestation of an ocular malignant melanoma.

Neovascularization

New blood vessels in the anterior ocular segment, which may lead to a spontaneous hyphema, are seen in neovascular glaucoma (Chapter 16) and in Fuchs' heterochromic cyclitis (Chapter 19).

Vascular Tufts at the Pupillary Margin

This condition is also referred to as neovascular tufts, or iris microhemangiomas, and represents yet another source of spontaneous hyphema. Slitlamp biomicroscopy may reveal multiple vascular tufts along the pupillary margin, and fluorescein angiography of the iris is reported to demonstrate small areas of staining and leakage from the lesions (93). One histopathologic study revealed thin-walled new vessels at the pupillary margin of the iris with a mild inflammatory cell infiltration (94), while another report described the vascular abnormality as a hamartoma of the capillary hemangioma type (95). The condition is typically seen in elderly individuals, but may be found in young adults. Most of these patients have no systemic disease (93), although associations with diabetes mellitus (93, 96) and myotonic dystrophy (96, 97) have been reported. Spontaneous hyphemas occur in a small number of these cases, occasionally causing transient IOP elevation (98, 99). Laser photocoagulation has been reported to successfully eradicate bleeding vascular tufts (94, 100). However, since it is rare to have recurrent hyphemas or permanent damage related to the transiently elevated IOP, it is best to withhold treatment until one or more recurrences of bleeding are documented.

GLAUCOMAS ASSOCIATED WITH DEGENERATED OCULAR BLOOD

Ghost Cell Glaucoma

In 1976, Campbell and coworkers (101) described a form of glaucoma in which degenerated red blood cells (ghost cells) develop in the vitreous cavity and subsequently enter the anterior chamber where they temporarily obstruct aqueous outflow.

Theories of Mechanism (101)

Having entered the vitreous cavity by one of several mechanisms (trauma, surgery, or retinal disease), fresh erythrocytes are transformed from their typical biconcave, pliable nature to tan- or khaki-colored, spherical, less pliable structures, referred to as ghost cells. Histologically, these cells have thin walls and appear hollow except for clumps of denaturized hemoglobin, called Heinz bodies (Fig. 21.2). Unlike fresh red blood cells, ghost cells do not pass readily through a 5-μm Millipore filter or human trabecular meshwork. The ghost cells develop within a matter of weeks and may then remain in the vitreous cavity for many months until a disruption of the anterior hyaloid allows them to enter the anterior chamber. Once in the anterior chamber, the abnormal cells accumulate in the trabecular meshwork where they may cause a temporary, but occasionally marked, elevation of IOP.

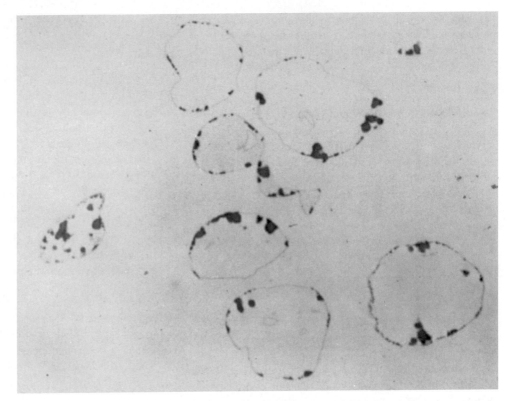

Figure 21.2. Transmission electron microscopic appearance of red blood cell ghosts from eye of patient with ghost cell glaucoma. Dark areas at cell periphery are Heinz bodies (×23,000). (Courtesy of David G. Campbell, M.D.)

Specific Causes

Several situations have been described which may lead to ghost cell glaucoma.

CATARACT EXTRACTION. Cataract extraction may be associated with glaucoma due to ghost cells in one of three ways (102): (a) A large hyphema with vitreous hemorrhage occurs in the early postoperative period. As the hyphema clears, ghost cells, which developed in the vitreous, come forward and obstruct aqueous outflow. (b) A vitreous hemorrhage is present before cataract surgery, and disruption of the anterior hyaloid as a result of the operation allows the ghost cells to enter the anterior chamber. (c) A vitreous hemorrhage develops at some point after cataract extraction due to retinal disease, and the ghost cells develop and come forward through previously made defects in the anterior hyaloid. Ghost cell glaucoma has also been associated with intraocular lens implantation, especially when anterior chamber or iris-fixation lenses were used (103).

VITRECTOMY. Vitrectomy may lead to ghost cell glaucoma in eyes with preexisting vitreous hemorrhage if the anterior hyaloid is disrupted and the vitreous and cells are not completely removed (104).

VITREOUS HEMORRHAGE WITHOUT SURGERY. Vitreous hemorrhage without surgery may also lead to ghost cell glaucoma. The vitreous hemorrhage may be due to trauma, or may be associated with a retinal disorder such as diabetic retinopathy (105, 106). The traumatic cases may have associated hyphema, which may have cleared before the ghost cell glaucoma develops or which may persist and mask the actual mechanism of the glaucoma. The route of ghost cells to the anterior chamber in these phakic eyes is presumed to be a defect in the anterior hyaloid face (105, 106).

Clinical Features (101)

Depending on the number of ghost cells in the anterior chamber, the IOP ranges from normal to marked elevation with pain and corneal edema. Slitlamp biomicroscopy reveals characteristic khaki-colored cells in the aqueous and on the corneal endothelium. If present in large quantities, the ghost cells may layer out inferiorly creating a pseudohypopyon, which is occasionally associated with a layer of fresher red blood cells (candy-stripe sign) (Fig. 21.3). The anterior chamber angle on gonioscopy is typically open and may appear normal, or may be covered by scant to heavy amounts of khaki-colored cells.

Differential Diagnosis

Glaucoma due to ghost cells may be confused with the less common hemolytic and hemosiderotic glaucomas, which are discussed next. In addition, neovascular glaucoma and glaucoma due to inflammation must be ruled out. Although the diagnosis is usually easily made on the basis of history and clinical features, it may be confirmed by examination of an aqueous aspirate, which reveals the typical ghost cells. This examination may be performed with phase contrast microscopy (101) or by routine light microscopy of a paraffin-embedded specimen stained with hematoxylin and eosin (107).

Management

Glaucoma due to ghost cells is not a permanent condition, but may last for months before the abnormal cells eventually clear from the anterior chamber angle. In the interim, it is often possible to control the IOP with standard antiglaucoma medication. Other cases, however, require surgical intervention, which usually involves removal of the ghost cells from the anterior chamber by irrigation (101) or removal of all ocular ghost cells by vitrectomy (108).

Hemolytic Glaucoma

Fenton and Zimmerman (109) described a form of glaucoma associated with intraocular hemorrhage in which macrophages ingest contents of the red blood cells and then accumulate in the trabecular meshwork where they temporarily obstruct aqueous outflow. Clinically, numerous red-tinted cells are seen floating in the aqueous, and the anterior chamber angle is typically open, with reddish brown pigment covering the trabecular meshwork (110). Cytologic examination of the aqueous reveals *macrophages* containing golden-brown pigment (110), and an ultrastructural study of seven eyes revealed red blood cells and macrophages with phagocytized blood and pigment in the trabecular spaces (111). The endothelial cells of the trabecular meshwork were degenerated and also had phagocytized blood (111). The condition is self-limiting and should be managed medically if possible. When surgical intervention is required, anterior chamber lavage has been recommended (110).

Hemosiderotic Glaucoma

This is a rare condition in which hemoglobin from lysed red blood cells in the anterior chamber is phagocytized by endothelial cells of the trabecular meshwork. Iron in the hemoglobin subsequently causes siderosis, which is believed to produce tissue alterations in the trabecular meshwork, eventually resulting in obstruction to aqueous outflow (112). However, an association between iron-staining of the trabecular meshwork and impairment of aqueous outflow has yet to be clearly established.

SUMMARY

Red blood cells in the anterior chamber, in either a fresh or degenerated form, may lead to elevated IOP by obstructing aqueous outflow through the trabecular meshwork. The most common cause of a fresh hyphema is blunt trauma. Glaucoma may result from the initial hemorrhage, but more often from a rebleed, and initial therapy is directed toward accelerating resorption of the hyphema and minimizing rebleeding. When glaucoma occurs, medical management may control the IOP until the hyphema clears, although some cases require surgical intervention, which includes removal of the blood. Other causes of fresh hyphema include spontaneous bleeding from tumors, neovascularization, or vascular tufts at the pupillary margin. The most common form of glaucoma associated with degenerated ocular blood

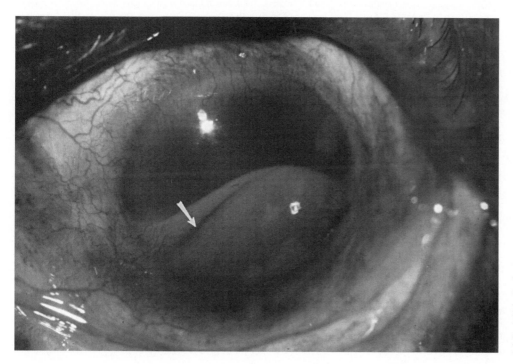

Figure 21.3. Slitlamp view of eye with ghost cell glaucoma showing typical layered hyphema of dark (*arrow*) and light colored cells (candy-stripe sign). (Courtesy of David G. Campbell, M.D.)

is ghost cell glaucoma, in which erythrocytes in the vitreous degenerate to a rigid, spherical state and then enter the anterior chamber to obstruct aqueous outflow. This may follow cataract extraction, vitrectomy, or trauma. Other situations in which degenerated blood may lead to glaucoma include hemolytic glaucoma and hemosiderotic glaucoma.

REFERENCES

1. Pilger, IS: Medical treatment of traumatic hyphema. Surv Ophthalmol 20:28, 1975.
2. Kennedy, RH, Brubaker, RF: Traumatic hyphema in a defined population. Am J Ophthalmol 106:123, 1988.
3. Howard, GM, Hutchinson, BT, Frederick, AR Jr: Hyphema resulting from blunt trauma. Gonioscopic, tonographic, and ophthalmoscopic observations following resolution of the hemorrhage. Trans Am Acad Ophthalmol Otol 69:294, 1965.
4. Spaeth, GL, Levy, PM: Traumatic hyphema: its clinical characteristics and failure of estrogens to alter its course. A double-blind study. Am J Ophthalmol 62:1098, 1966.
5. Milstein, BA: Traumatic hyphema: a study of 83 consecutive cases. South Med J 64:1081, 1971.
6. Giles, CL, Bromley, WG: Traumatic hyphema. A retrospective analysis from the University of Michigan Teaching Hospitals. J Pediatr Ophthalmol 9:90, 1972.
7. Edwards, WC, Layden, WE: Traumatic hyphema. A report of 184 consecutive cases. Am J Ophthalmol 75:110, 1973.
8. Yasuna, E: Management of traumatic hyphema. Arch Ophthalmol 91:190, 1974.
9. Crawford, JS, Lewandowski, RL, Chan, W: The effect of aspirin on rebleeding in traumatic hyphema. Am J Ophthalmol 80:543, 1975.
10. Fritch, CD: Traumatic hyphema. Ann Ophthalmol 8:1223, 1976.
11. Crouch, ER Jr, Frenkel, M: Aminocaproic acid in the treatment of traumatic hyphema. Am J Ophthalmol 81:355, 1976.
12. Mortensen, KK, Sjølie, AK: Secondary hemorrhage following traumatic hyphaema. A comparative study of conservative and tranexamic acid treatment. Acta Ophthalmol 56:763, 1978.
13. Bramsen, T: Fibrinolysis and traumatic hyphaema. Acta Ophthalmol 57:447, 1979.
14. Gorn, RA: The detrimental effect of aspirin on hyphema rebleed. Ann Ophthalmol 11:351, 1979.
15. Spoor, TC, Hammer, M, Belloso, H: Traumatic hyphema. Failure of steroids to alter its course: a double-blind prospective study. Arch Ophthalmol 98:116, 1980.
16. Rakusin, W: Traumatic hyphema. Am J Ophthalmol 74:284, 1972.
17. Coles, WH: Traumatic hyphema: an analysis of 235 cases. South Med J 61:813, 1968.
18. Cassel, GH, Jeffers, JB, Jaeger, EA: Wills Eye Hospital traumatic hyphema study. Ophthalmic Surg 16:441, 1985.
19. Thomas, MA, Parrish, RK II, Feuer, WJ: Rebleeding after traumatic hyphema. Arch Ophthalmol 104:206, 1986.
20. Agapitos, PJ, Noel, L-P, Clarke, WN: Traumatic hyphema in children. Ophthalmology 94:1238, 1987.
21. Spoor, TC, Kwitko, GM, O'Grady, JM, Ramocki, JM: Traumatic hyphema in an urban population. Am J Ophthalmol 109:23, 1990.
22. Kearns, P: Traumatic hyphaema: a retrospective study of 314 cases. Br J Ophthalmol 75:137, 1991.
23. Ng, CS, Strong, NP, Sparrow, JM, Rosenthal, AR: Factors related to the incidence of secondary haemorrhage in 462 patients with traumatic hyphema. Eye 6:308, 1992.
24. Fong, LP: Secondary hemorrhage in traumatic hyphema. Ophthalmology 101:1583, 1994.
25. Volpe, NJ, Larrison, WI, Hersh, PS, Kim, T, Shingleton, BJ: Secondary hemorrhage in traumatic hyphema. Am J Ophthalmol 112:507, 1991.
26. Wilson, TW, Jeffers, JB, Nelson, LB: Aminocaproic acid prophylaxis in traumatic hyphema. Ophthalmic Surg 21:807, 1990.
27. Farber, MD, Fiscella, R, Goldberg, MF: Aminocaproic acid versus prednisone for the treatment of traumatic hyphema. A randomized clinical trial. Ophthalmology 98:279, 1991.
28. Deans, R, Noël, L-P, Clarke, WN: Oral administration of tranexamic acid in the management of traumatic hyphema in children. Can J Ophthalmol 27:181, 1992.
29. Ganley, JP, Geiger, JM, Clement, JR, Rigby, et al: Aspirin and recurrent hyphema after blunt ocular trauma. Am J Ophthalmol 96:797, 1983.
30. Sternberg, P Jr, Tripathi, RC, Tripathi, BJ, Chilcote, RR: Changes in outflow facility in experimental hyphema. Invest Ophthalmol Vis Sci 19:1388, 1980.
31. Goldberg, MF: The diagnosis and treatment of secondary glaucoma after hyphema in sickle cell patients. Am J Ophthalmol 87:43, 1979.
32. Goldberg, MF: Sickled erythrocytes, hyphema, and secondary glaucoma: 1. The diagnosis and treatment of sickled erythrocytes in human hyphemas. Ophthalmic Surg 10:17, 1979.
33. Friedman, AH, Halpern, BL, Friedberg, DN, et al: Transient open-angle glaucoma associated with sickle cell trait: report of 4 cases. Br J Ophthalmol 63:832, 1979.
34. Goldberg, MF: Sickled erythrocytes, hyphema, and secondary glaucoma: IV. The rate and percentage of sickling of erythrocytes in rabbit aqueous humor, in vitro and in vivo. Ophthalmic Surg 10:62, 1979.
35. Goldberg, MF, Tso, MOM: Sickled erythrocytes, hyphema, and secondary glaucoma: VII. The passage of sickled erythrocytes out of the anterior chamber of the human and monkey eye: light and electron microscopic studies. Ophthalmic Surg 10:89, 1979.
36. Williams, GA, Hatchell, DL, Collier, BD, Knobel, J: Clearance from the anterior chamber of RBCs from human diabetics. Arch Ophthalmol 102:930, 1984.
37. Beyer, TL, Hirst, LW: Corneal blood staining at low pressures. Arch Ophthalmol 103:654, 1985.
38. Gottsch, JD, Messmer, EP, McNair, DS, Font, RL: Corneal blood staining. An animal model. Ophthalmology 93:797, 1986.
39. McDonnell, PJ, Green, WR, Stevens, RE, et al: Blood staining of the cornea. Light microscopic and ultrastructural features. Ophthalmology 92:1668, 1985.
40. Brodrick, JD: Corneal blood staining after hyphaema. Br J Ophthalmol 56:589, 1972.
41. Read, J, Goldberg, MF: Comparison of medical treatment for traumatic hyphema. Trans Am Acad Ophthalmol Otol 78:799, 1974.
42. Edwards, WC, Layden, WE: Monocular versus binocular patching in traumatic hyphema. Am J Ophthalmol 76:359, 1973.
43. Rose, SW, Coupal, JJ, Simmons, G, Kielar, RA: Experimental hyphema clearance in rabbits. Drug trials with 1% atropine and 2% and 4% pilocarpine. Arch Ophthalmol 95:1442, 1977.
44. Masket, S, Best, M: Therapy in experimental hyphema. II. Acetazolamide. Arch Ophthalmol 87:222, 1972.
45. Masket, S, Best, M, Fisher, LV, et al: Therapy in experimental hyphema. Arch Ophthalmol 85:329, 1971.
46. Lambrou, FH, Snyder, RW, Williams, GA: Use of tissue plasminogen activator in experimental hyphema. Arch Ophthalmol 105:995, 1987.
47. Howard, GR, Vukich, J, Fiscella, RG, et al: Intraocular tissue plasminogen activator in a rabbit model of traumatic hyphema. Arch Ophthalmol 109:272, 1991.
48. Williams, DF, Han, DP, Abrams, GW: Rebleeding in experimental traumatic hyphema treated with intraocular tissue plasminogen activator. Arch Ophthalmol 108:264, 1990.
49. Bramsen, T: Traumatic hyphaema treated with the antifibrinolytic drug tranexamic acid. Acta Ophthalmol 54:250, 1976.
50. Uusitalo, RJ, Ranta-Kemppainen, L, Tarkkanen, A: Management of traumatic hyphema in children. An analysis of 340 cases. Arch Ophthalmol 106:1207, 1988.

51. Clarke, WN, Noel, L-P: Outpatient treatment of microscopic and rim hyphemas in children with tranexamic acid. Can J Ophthalmol 28:325, 1993.

52. McGetrick, JJ, Jampol, LM, Goldberg, MF, et al: Aminocaproic acid decreases secondary hemorrhage after traumatic hyphema. Arch Ophthalmol 101:1031, 1983.

53. Kutner, B, Fourman, S, Brein, K, et al: Aminocaproic acid reduces the risk of secondary hemorrhage in patients with traumatic hyphema. Arch Ophthalmol 105:206, 1987.

54. Kraft, SP, Christianson, MD, Crawford, JS, et al: Traumatic hyphema in children. Treatment with epsilon-aminocaproic acid. Ophthalmology 94:1232, 1987.

55. Palmer, DJ, Goldberg, MF, Frenkel, M, et al: A comparison of two dose regimens of epsilon aminocaproic acid in the prevention and management of secondary traumatic hyphemas. Ophthalmology 93:102, 1986.

56. Dieste, MC, Hersh, PS, Kylstra, JA, et al: Intraocular pressure increase associated with epsilon-aminocaproic acid therapy for traumatic hyphema. Am J Ophthalmol 106:383, 1988.

57. Allingham, RR, Williams, PB, Crouch, ER Jr, et al: Topically applied aminocaproic acid concentrates in the aqueous humor of the rabbit in therapeutic levels. Arch Ophthalmol 105:1421, 1987.

58. Allingham, RR, Crouch, ER Jr, Williams, PB, et al: Topical aminocaproic acid significantly reduces the incidence of secondary hemorrhage in traumatic hyphema in the rabbit model. Arch Ophthalmol 106:1436, 1988.

59. Ehlers, WH, Crouch, ER, Williams, PB, Riggs, PK: Factors affecting therapeutic concentration of topical aminocaproic acid in traumatic hyphema. Invest Ophthalmol Vis Sci 31:2389, 1990.

60. Macdougald, TJ: The treatment of traumatic hyphaema. Trans Ophthalmol Soc UK 92:815, 1972.

61. Goldberg, MF: Sickled erythrocytes, hyphema, and secondary glaucoma: V. The effect of vitamin C on erythrocyte sickling in aqueous humor. Ophthalmic Surg 10:70, 1979.

62. Vernot, JA, Barron, BA, Goldberg, MF: Effects of topical epinephrine on experimental sickle cell hyphema. Arch Ophthalmol 103:280, 1985.

63. Deutsch, TA, Weinreb, RN, Goldberg, MF: Indications for surgical management of hyphema in patients with sickle cell trait. Arch Ophthalmol 102:566, 1984.

64. Wallyn, CR, Jampol, LM, Goldberg, MF, Zanetti, CL: The use of hyperbaric oxygen therapy in the treatment of sickle cell hyphema. Invest Ophthalmol Vis Sci 26:1155, 1985.

65. Belcher, CD III, Brown, SVL, Simmons, RJ: Anterior chamber washout for traumatic hyphema. Ophthalmic Surg 16:475, 1985.

66. Wax, MB, Ridley, ME, Magargal, LE: Reversal of retinal and optic disc ischemia in a patient with sickle cell trait and glaucoma secondary to traumatic hyphema. Ophthalmology 89:845, 1982.

67. Tripathi, RC: A corneal transfixing irrigation/perfusion device: a new method for evacuation of hyphema. Ophthalmic Surg 11:569, 1980.

68. Rakusin, W: The role of urokinase in the management of traumatic hyphaema. Ophthalmologica 167:373, 1973.

69. Leet, DM: Treatment of total hyphemas with urokinase. Am J Ophthalmol 84:79, 1977.

70. Oosterhuis, JA: Fibrinolysin irrigation in traumatic secondary hyphema. Ophthalmologica 155:357, 1968.

71. Podos, S, Liebman, S, Pollen, A: Treatment of experimental total hyphemas with intraocular fibrinolytic agents. Part II. Arch Ophthalmol 71:537, 1964.

72. Scheie, HG, Ashley, BJ Jr, Burns, DT: Treatment of total hyphema with fibrinolysin. Arch Ophthalmol 69:147, 1963.

73. Polychronakos, D, Razoglou, C: Treatment of total hyphema with fibrinolysin. Ophthalmologica 154:31, 1967.

74. Horven, I: Fibrinolysis and hyphema. The effect of "thrombolysin" and "kabikinas" on clotted blood in cameral anterior of the eye in rabbits. Acta Ophthalmol 46:320, 1962.

75. Hill, K: Cryoextraction of total hyphema. Arch Ophthalmol 80:368, 1968.

76. Kelman, CD, Brooks, DL: Ultrasonic emulsification and aspiration of traumatic hyphema. A preliminary report. Am J Ophthalmol 71:1289, 1971.

77. McCuen, BW, Fung, WE: The role of vitrectomy instrumentation in the treatment of severe traumatic hyphema. Am J Ophthalmol 88:930, 1979.

78. Diddie, KR, Ernest, JT: Rotoextractor evacuation of total hyphema. Ophthalmic Surg 7:49, 1976.

79. Stern, WH, Mondal, KM: Vitrectomy instrumentation for surgical evacuation of total anterior chamber hyphema and control of recurrent anterior chamber hemorrhage. Ophthalmic Surg 10:34, 1979.

80. Sholiton, DB, Solomon, OD: Surgical management of black ball hyphema with sodium hyaluronate. Ophthalmic Surg 12:820, 1981.

81. Bartholomew, RS: Viscoelastic evacuation of traumatic hyphaema. Br J Ophthalmol 71:27, 1987.

82. Sears, ML: Surgical management of black ball hyphema. Trans Am Acad Ophthalmol Otol 74:820, 1970.

83. Wolter, JR, Henderson, JW, Talley, TW: Histopathology of a black ball blood clot removed four days after total traumatic hyphema. J Pediatr Ophthalmol 8:15, 1971.

84. Weiss, JS, Parrish, RK, Anderson, DR: Surgical therapy of traumatic hyphema. Ophthalmic Surg 14:343, 1983.

85. Graul, TA, Ruttum, MS, Lloyd, MA, et al: Trabeculectomy for traumatic hyphema with increased intraocular pressure. Am J Ophthalmol 117:155, 1994.

86. Heinze, J: The surgical management of total hyphaema. Aust J Ophthalmol 3:20, 1975.

87. Parrish, R, Bernardino, V Jr: Iridectomy in the surgical management of eight-ball hyphema. Arch Ophthalmol 100:435, 1982.

88. Richardson, K: Acute glaucoma after trauma. In: Ocular Trauma. Freeman, H MacK, ed. New York, Appleton-Century-Croft, 1979, p. 161.

89. Bene, C, Hutchins, R, Kranias, G: Cataract wound neovascularization. An often overlooked cause of vitreous hemorrhage. Ophthalmology 96:50, 1989.

90. Watzke, RC: Intraocular hemorrhage from vascularization of the cataract incision. Ophthalmology 87:19, 1980.

91. Kramer, TR, Brown, RH, Lynch, MG, Martinez, L: Transcleral Nd:YAG photocoagulation for cataract incision vascularization associated with recurrent hyphema. Am J Ophthalmol 107:681, 1989.

92. Lieppman, M, Goldberg, MF: The treatment of postoperative hyphema by cyclodiathermy. Surv Ophthalmol 26:253, 1982.

93. Cobb, B: Vascular tufts at the pupillary margin: a preliminary report on 44 patients. Trans Ophthalmol Soc UK 88:211, 1968.

94. Coleman, SL, Green, WR, Partz, A: Vacular tufts of pupillary margin of iris. Am J Ophthalmol 83:881, 1977.

95. Meades, KV, Francis, IC, Kappagoda, MB, Filipic, M: Light microscopic and electron microscopic histopathology of an iris microhaemangioma. Br J Ophthalmol 70:290, 1986.

96. Mason, GI: Iris neovascular tufts. Relationship to rubeosis, insulin, and hypotony. Arch Ophthalmol 97:2346, 1979.

97. Cobb, B, Shilling, JS, Chisholm, IH: Vascular tufts at the pupillary margin in myotonic dystrophy. Am J Ophthalmol 69:573, 1970.

98. Perry, HD, Mallen, FJ, Sussman, W: Microhaemangiomas of the iris with spontaneous hyphaema and acute glaucoma. Br J Ophthalmol 61:114, 1977.

99. Mason, GI, Ferry, AP: Bilateral spontaneous hyphema arising from iridic microhemangiomas. Ann Ophthalmol 11:87, 1979.

100. Hagen, AP-V, Williams, GA: Argon laser treatment of a bleeding iris vascular tuft. Am J Ophthalmol 101:379, 1986.

101. Campbell, DG, Simmons, RJ, Grant, WM: Ghost cells as a cause of glaucoma. Am J Ophthalmol 81:441, 1976.

102. Campbell, DG, Essigmann, EM: Hemolytic ghost cell glaucoma. Further studies. Arch Ophthalmol 97:2141, 1979.

103. Summers, CG, Lindstrom, RL: Ghost cell glaucoma following lens implantation. Am Intra-Ocular Implant Soc J 9:429, 1983.

104. Campbell, DG, Simmons, RJ, Tolentino, FI, McMeel, JW: Glaucoma occurring after closed vitrectomy. Am J Ophthalmol 83:63, 1977.

105. Brooks, AMV, Gillies, WE: Haemolytic glaucoma occurring in phakic eyes. Br J Ophthalmol 70:603, 1986.

106. Mansour, AM, Chess, J, Starita, R: Nontraumatic ghost cell glaucoma—a case report. Ophthalmic Surg 17:34, 1986.

107. Cameron, JD, Havener, VR: Histologic confirmation of ghost cell glaucoma by routine light microscopy. Am J Ophthalmol 96:251, 1983.

108. Singh, H, Grand, MG: Treatment of blood-induced glaucoma by trans pars plana vitrectomy. Retina 1:255, 1981.

109. Fenton, RH, Zimmerman, LE: Hemolytic glaucoma. An unusual cause of acute open-angle secondary glaucoma. Arch Ophthalmol 70:236, 1963.

110. Phelps, CD, Watzke, RC: Hemolytic glaucoma. Am J Ophthalmol 80:690, 1975.

111. Grierson, I, Lee, WR: Further observations on the process of haemophagocytosis in the human outflow system. Graefes Arch Clin Exp Ophthalmol 208:49, 1978.

112. Vannas, S: Hemosiderosis in eyes with secondary glaucoma after delayed intraocular hemorrhages. Acta Ophthalmol 38:254, 1960.

GLAUCOMAS ASSOCIATED WITH OCULAR TRAUMA[a]

CONTUSION INJURIES

General Features

Blunt injuries involving the eye are not uncommon. A survey of data derived from hospital discharge abstracts in the United States between 1984 and 1987 revealed a rate of 13.2 per 100,000 for any ocular trauma as a principal diagnosis, of which approximately 40% were coded as contusion of the eyeball, or adnexa, or orbital blowout fracture (1). Young men appear to be most prone to such trauma. In a series of 205 patients with ocular contusion injuries, 85% were males and 75% were less than 30 years of age (2). Sporting and domestic accidents accounted for nearly two-thirds of these injuries, with the remaining known causes being divided between industrial accidents and malicious acts. Among 32 patients who were hospitalized for sport-related ocular contusion, ball games were the most common cause (3). Boxing is an especially high-risk sport for ocular trauma, which was seen in 66% of one series of 74 boxers (4). Another potential source of severe ocular trauma, which is being seen more in recent years, is air bag inflation during a motor vehicle accident (5).

[a]Refer to Shields, MB: Color Atlas of Glaucoma. Baltimore, Williams & Wilkins, 1998, Plate II39.

Clinical Findings

The anterior segment is the portion of the eye most frequently damaged by blunt trauma, and *hyphema* is the most common mode of clinical presentation, occurring in 81% of the eyes in one series (2). The management of traumatic hyphema was discussed in Chapter 21. As the blood clears, ruptures in various structures of the anterior segment may be found (Fig. 22.1). The most common of these is *angle recession,* which is seen by gonioscopy as an irregular widening of the ciliary body band (Fig. 22.2). Histologically, this represents a tear between the longitudinal and circular muscles of the ciliary body. The reported prevalence of angle recession in eyes with traumatic hyphemas ranges from 60% to 94% (6–10). Angle abnormalities were noted in over half of the 32 patients with sport-related ocular contusion (3), and in 19% of the 74 boxers (4). When gonioscopy was included in a population-based glaucoma survey, some degree of angle recession was found in 14.8% of the people studied, 5.5% of whom had glaucoma (11). Other associated injuries include *iridodialysis,* a tear in the root of the iris (Fig. 22.3), and *cyclodialysis,* which is a separation of the ciliary body from the scleral spur. Another finding that has been reported in association with recurrent trauma, angle-recession, and glaucoma is *iridoschisis,* or separation of layers of iris stroma, which appears to differ from that seen in the elderly by being more patchy and involving both superior and inferior quadrants (12). Patients with blunt ocular trauma may

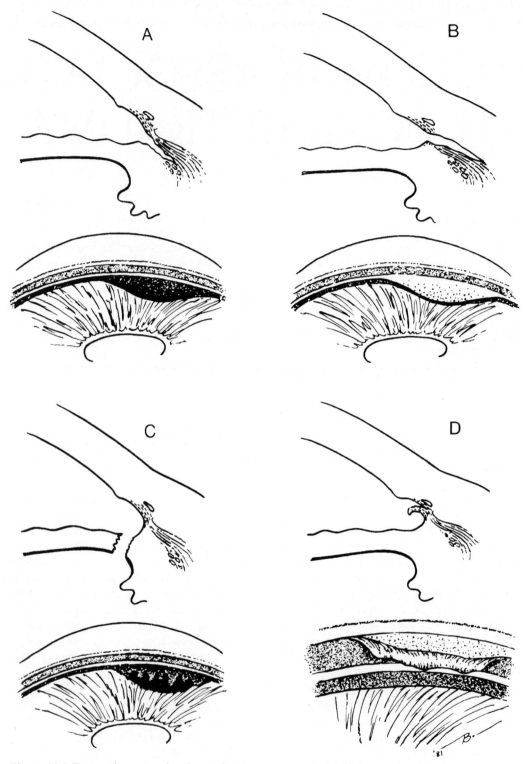

Figure 22.1. Forms of anterior chamber angle injury associated with blunt trauma, showing cross-sectional and corresponding gonioscopic appearance. **A.** Angle recession (tear between longitudinal and circular muscles of ciliary body). **B.** Cyclodialysis (separation of ciliary body from scleral spur, with widening of suprachoroidal space). **C.** Iridodialysis (tear in root of iris). **D.** Trabecular damage (tear in anterior portion of meshwork, creating a flap that is hinged at the scleral spur).

also present with iritis, cataracts, dislocation of the lens, or chorioretinal trauma.

Mechanisms of Glaucoma

Early Postinjury Period

A patient with a recent blunt ocular injury may present with a slightly reduced intraocular pressure (IOP). This may result from a reduction in aqueous production due to the associated iritis or possibly a temporary increase in outflow facility as a consequence of the disruption of structures in the anterior chamber angle.

Other patients may have an elevated IOP during the early postcontusion period. In some cases, this may be a transient elevation, which lasts for up to several weeks and

occurs in the absence of any other obvious damage to the eye. However, there is usually an associated traumatic iritis, hyphema, or dislocation of the lens, the mechanisms of which were discussed previously (Chapters 19, 21, and 15, respectively). Other reported mechanisms of elevated IOP associated with blunt trauma to the eye include shallowing of the anterior chamber due to uveal effusion (13, 14), and vitreous filling a deep anterior chamber (15).

Late Postinjury Period

Although the elevated IOP following blunt ocular trauma is transient in most cases, it is important to follow these patients indefinitely, since a reported 4–9% of those with angle recessions greater than 180° will eventually, often many years later, develop a chronic glaucoma (7, 9, 16, 17). This condition has been called *angle recession glau-*

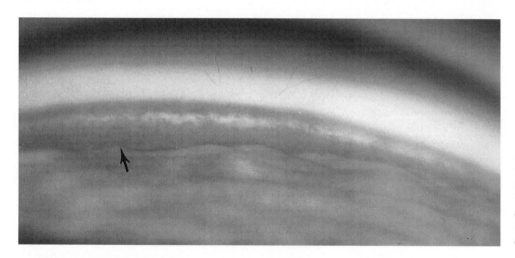

Figure 22.2. Gonioscopic view of eye with angle recession, characterized by the irregular widening of the ciliary body band *(arrow)*. (Courtesy of L. Frank Cashwell, M.D.)

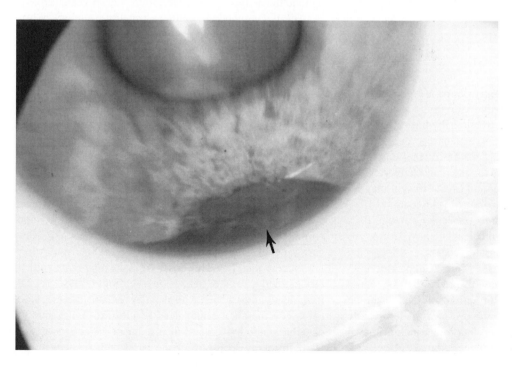

Figure 22.3. Slitlamp view of eye with iridodialysis *(arrow)*.

coma, although the term is somewhat of a misnomer, since the angle recession is not the actual cause of the obstruction to aqueous outflow. The clinicopathologic correlation between blunt injury to the eye and the delayed development of glaucoma was noted by Wolff and Zimmerman (18), who suggested that the angle recession provided evidence of past injury, but was not the actual cause of the glaucoma. They suggested that initial trauma to the trabecular meshwork stimulated proliferative and/or degenerative changes in the trabecular tissue, which led to obstruction of aqueous outflow. Herschler (19) supported this concept by observations of clinical cases and animal studies, which revealed tears in the trabecular meshwork just posterior to Schwalbe's line during the early posttrauma period. This produced a flap of trabecular tissue, which was hinged at the scleral spur (Fig. 22.1). With time, scarring ensued, causing the initial trabecular injury to be less apparent, but also leading to chronic obstruction in portions of the aqueous outflow system.

Another mechanism of delayed IOP elevation, in addition to alterations within the trabecular meshwork, is the extension of an endothelial layer with a Descemet's-like membrane from the cornea over the anterior chamber angle (18, 20, 21). Additional factors may influence which eyes with a history of blunt trauma will develop chronic glaucoma. For example, the majority of eyes which eventually develop glaucoma after blunt injury appear to have an underlying predisposition to reduced aqueous outflow, as evidenced by frequent alterations of IOP in the fellow eye (10, 19, 22). Among 13 patients who developed angle recession glaucoma an average of 34 years following trauma, seven had definite or suspicious glaucomatous visual field loss in the fellow eye (22). It has also been noted that elderly patients are more susceptible to late postcontusion pressure elevation (17).

Management of Glaucoma

Elevated IOP in the early postinjury period is best controlled medically, if possible, primarily with drugs that reduce aqueous production such as carbonic anhydrase inhibitors, β-blockers, and α₂-agonists. Concomitant disorders such as inflammation, hyphema, and dislocation of the lens, must also be managed as discussed in the previous chapters. Eyes with a shallow anterior chamber and uveal effusion may respond to corticosteroids and mydriatic-cycloplegics (13).

Chronic IOP elevation due to trabecular damage does not respond well to standard medical therapy. In one reported case with associated angle recession, pilocarpine caused a paradoxic pressure rise, while cycloplegics lowered the tension (23). The authors theorized that the reduction in conventional outflow, combined with the tear in the ciliary body, may have shifted the eye to a predominantly uveoscleral mechanism of aqueous outflow, which is known to be impaired by miotics. They suggested that cycloplegics

may have therapeutic value in these cases. In addition, drugs which reduce aqueous production may be more efficacious in eyes with scarring of the trabecular meshwork.

Laser trabeculoplasty does not have a high success rate in this form of glaucoma, although it should usually be tried when medical therapy is ineffective, before going to filtering surgery. An alternative laser procedure, Nd:YAG trabeculopuncture, in which an energy of 1.0–2.5 mJ is applied to the meshwork in a manner similar to argon laser trabeculoplasty, has been reported to offer significant advantages over trabeculoplasty in the treatment of angle recession glaucoma (24).

When both medical and laser therapy have failed, an incisional outflow operation is usually indicated. In a study comparing three procedures (trabeculectomy without antimetabolite, trabeculectomy with adjunctive 5-fluorouracil or mitomycin C, or a Molteno single-plate implantation), trabeculectomy with antimetabolite therapy was the most effective, although late bleb infection is a significant risk (25). An alternative to outflow surgery, especially in eyes with limited visual potential, is transscleral cyclophotocoagulation or one of the other cyclodestructive procedures.

PENETRATING INJURIES

General Features

Penetrating injuries of the eye may result from blunt force, sharp lacerations, or missiles. In a study of 453 patients, the relative frequency of these three sources of trauma was 22%, 37%, and 41%, respectively (26). As with the nonpenetrating injuries, young men are most vulnerable to these types of accidents. Of the patients in the study, 86% were males and the mean age of the entire group was 26 years (26).

The IOP immediately after a penetrating injury is usually reduced due to the open wound, or the associated iridocyclitis. Following closure of the corneal or scleral wound, however, glaucoma may develop as a result of intraocular tissue changes induced by the penetrating injury.

Mechanisms of Glaucoma

Tissue Disruption

During the early postinjury period, the IOP may be elevated due to inflammation, hyphema, or angle closure from a swollen, disrupted lens. As these conditions subside, more chronic mechanisms of glaucoma may follow. In some cases, a cyclitic membrane may develop as the result of inflammatory material. This arises from the nonpigmented ciliary epithelium and organizes on a scaffold of lens, iris, anterior hyaloid, or whatever tissue may remain after the injury (27). The membrane may lead to closure of the anterior chamber angle by forward displacement of the lens-iris diaphragm or by seclusion of the pupil with subsequent iris bombé. Failure to reform a flat anterior chamber or adequately treat the inflammation may lead to chronic pressure elevation due to peripheral anterior synechiae. Additional, rare causes of delayed elevation of IOP include sympathetic ophthalmia and epithelial ingrowth, which are discussed in Chapters 19 and 23, respectively.

Retained Intraocular Foreign Bodies

Retained intraocular foreign bodies may be associated with the same tissue disruption and associated glaucoma as noted earlier. In addition, prolonged intraocular retention of certain metallic foreign bodies may lead to delayed tissue alterations. *Siderosis* results from the intraocular retention of ferrous metal (iron), but may also be due to intraocular hemorrhage (the ionized form of iron is indistinguishable from hemosiderin). This material can cause structural alterations in tissues throughout the eye. Glaucoma may be a complication of advanced cases, although there is no proof that trabecular outflow is impaired by iron-staining of the trabecular structures. Copper is also oxidized within the eye and can lead to *chalcosis,* with tissue damage that is nearly as severe as that encountered with ferrous foreign bodies. Glaucoma appears to be less common in these patients, although retinal changes may lead to visual field defects that might be confused with those of glaucoma (28).

Management of Glaucoma

The best way to avoid loss of vision from glaucoma following penetrating ocular injuries is to minimize the development of chronic aqueous outflow obstruction by proper treatment of the initial injury. This may include removal of portions of incarcerated uveal tissue, aspiration of the lens if disrupted or swollen, anterior vitrectomy, removal of foreign bodies, meticulous closure of the wound, and reformation of the anterior chamber. In some cases, it is necessary to close the wound initially and perform the intraocular surgery with vitreous instruments at a later date. In a series of 112 such patients, the final visual result was best when the vitrectomy was done within 72 hours of the injury (27). Corticosteroid therapy to avoid cyclitic membranes and scarring in the anterior chamber angle are also important during the early postinjury period and antibiotic therapy is required as prophylaxis against endophthalmitis.

Antiglaucoma medication may be required for control of transient pressure elevations during the early postinjury period, as well as subsequent chronic glaucoma, and drugs which reduce aqueous production are preferable in both situations. When medical therapy is insufficient, especially in the chronic cases, surgical intervention is indicated. Laser trabeculoplasty is usually not possible due to peripheral anterior synechia, in which case filtering surgery should be recommended. In siderosis bulbi, removal of the intraocular foreign body by vitrectomy techniques may be beneficial in some cases (29).

CHEMICAL AND THERMAL BURNS

Alkali Burns

Alkali burns of the eye may produce a rapid initial rise in the IOP. This is often followed by a return to normal or subnormal pressure and then a slower, sustained elevation of the ocular tension (30). Possible mechanisms of the early pressure rise include shrinkage of the cornea and sclera (30) and an increase in uveal blood flow (31). The altered blood flow dynamics may be mediated by prostaglandins (31), which may also be associated with the later IOP elevation (30). A hypopyon may also develop and contribute to the pressure rise.

In managing the glaucoma associated with an alkali burn of the cornea, topical corticosteroids may be helpful if a significant inflammatory component is present. It has been shown in rabbits that topical steroids can be used for the first week without increasing the risk of corneal melting, but not thereafter (32). In addition, the presence of prostaglandins during the delayed pressure rise suggests that the early use of drugs such as indomethacin and imidazole, which inhibit prostaglandin synthesis, may be beneficial. Antiglaucoma agents, especially those that reduce aqueous production, are also frequently required in these cases. As with other forms of anterior uveitis, miotics should usually be avoided.

Acid Burns

Acid burns of the cornea have been shown to cause an IOP response in rabbits similar to that seen with alkali burns (33). A rapid tension increase, lasting up to 3 hours, is felt to result from shrinkage of the outer ocular coats, while a subsequent sustained rise is considered to be mediated by prostaglandin release (33). Treatment of the associated glaucoma in these cases is similar to that for alkali burns.

Thermal Burns

Thermal burns of the face often involve the eyelids, although the globes tend to be spared except for occasional corneal injury. However, in severely burned patients, in which the administration of large quantities of intravenous fluids to maintain blood pressure is the key therapeutic measure, orbital congestion and massive periorbital swelling may lead to marked IOP elevations (34). In three reported cases, lateral canthotomies resulted in a significant relief of the potentially damaging high pressures (34).

RADIATION DAMAGE

Radiation therapy to structures near the eyes may lead to elevation of IOP (35). The mechanism of pressure rise is not understood in all cases, although some are due to neovascular glaucoma or intraocular hemorrhage secondary to retinal radiation damage. Medical therapy should be used when possible, although surgical intervention, such as filtering surgery or a cyclodestructive procedure, is often required, and the prognosis is generally poor.

SUMMARY

The most common form of ocular trauma that may lead to IOP elevation is blunt, or contusion injuries. These may cause an early pressure rise due to iritis, hyphema, or lens dislocation, or delayed development of glaucoma from scarring of the damaged trabecular meshwork. Penetrating injuries may also cause an elevation of tension due to tissue disruption in the anterior chamber angle, or in association with the retention of intraocular foreign bodies such as iron and copper. In addition, either alkali or acid burns may cause a pressure rise, the mechanisms of which may include collagen shrinkage and prostaglandin release. Thermal burns and radiation damage are other, rare causes of elevated intraocular pressure.

REFERENCES

1. Kopfer, J, Tielsch, JM, Vitale, S, et al: Ocular trauma in the United States. Eye injuries resulting in hospitalization, 1984 through 1987. Arch Ophthalmol 110:838, 1992.
2. Canavan, YM, Archer, DB: Anterior segment consequences of blunt ocular injury. Br J Ophthalmol 66:549, 1982.
3. Gracner, B, Kurelac, Z: Gonioscopic changes in ocular contusions sustained in sports. Klin Monatsbl Augenheilkd 186:128, 1985.
4. Giovinazzo, VJ, Yannuzzi, LA, Sorenson, JA, et al: The ocular complications of boxing. Ophthalmology 94:587, 1987.
5. Lesher, MP, Durrie, DS, Stiles, MC: Corneal edema, hyphema, and angle recession after air bag inflation. Arch Ophthalmol 111:1320, 1993.
6. Howard, GM, Hutchinson, BT, Frederick, AR: Hyphema resulting from blunt trauma. Gonioscopic, tonographic, and ophthalmoscopic observations following resolution of the hemorrhage. Trans Am Acad Ophthalmol Otol 69:294, 1965.
7. Blanton, FM: Anterior chamber angle recession and seconday glaucoma. A study of the after effects of traumatic hyphemas. Arch Ophthalmol 72:39, 1964.
8. Tonjum, AM: Gonioscopy in traumatic hyphema. Acta Ophthalmol 44:650, 1966.
9. Mooney, D: Angle recession and secondary glaucoma. Br J Ophthalmol 57:608, 1973.
10. Spaeth, GL: Traumatic hyphema, angle recession, dexamethasone hypertension, and glaucoma. Arch Ophthalmol 78:714, 1967.
11. Salmon, JF, Mermoud, A, Ivey, A, et al: The detection of post-traumatic angle recession by gonioscopy in a population-based glaucoma survey. Ophthalmology 101:1844, 1994.
12. Salmon, JF: The association of iridoschisis and angle-recession glaucoma. Am J Ophthalmol 114:766, 1992.
13. Dotan, S, Oliver, M: Shallow anterior chamber and uveal effusion after nonperforating trauma to the eye. Am J Ophthalmol 94:782, 1982.
14. Kutner, BN: Acute angle closure glaucoma in nonperforating blunt trauma. Arch Ophthalmol 106:19, 1988.
15. Samples, JR, Van Buskirk, EM: Open-angle glaucoma associated with vitreous humor filling the anterior chamber. Am J Ophthalmol 102:759, 1986.
16. Kaufman, JH, Tolpin, DW: Glaucoma after traumatic angle recession. A ten-year prospective study. Am J Ophthalmol 79:648, 1974.
17. Thiel, H-J, Aden, G, Pulhorn, G: Changes in the chamber angle following ocular contusions. Klin Monatsbl Augenheilkd 177:165, 1980.
18. Wolff, SM, Zimmerman, LE: Chronic secondary glaucoma. Associated with retrodisplacement of iris root and deepening of the anterior chamber angle secondary to contusion. Am J Ophthalmol 54:547, 1962.
19. Herschler, J: Trabecular damage due to blunt anterior segment injury and its relationship to traumatic glaucoma. Trans Am Acad Ophthalmol Otol 83:239, 1977.
20. Lauring, L: Anterior chamber glass membranes. Am J Ophthalmol 68:308, 1969.
21. Iwamoto, T, Witmer, R, Landolt, E: Light and electron microscopy in absolute glaucoma with pigment dispersion phenomena and contusion angle deformity. Am J Ophthalmol 72:420, 1971.
22. Tesluk, GC, Spaeth, GL: The occurrence of primary open-angle glaucoma in the fellow eye of patients with unilateral angle-cleavage glaucoma. Ophthalmology 92:904, 1985.
23. Bleiman, BS, Schwartz, AL: Paradoxical intraocular pressure response to pilocarpine. A proposed mechanism and treatment. Arch Ophthalmol 97:1305, 1979.
24. Fukuchi, T, Iwata, K, Sawaguchi, S, et al: Nd:YAG laser trabeculopuncture (YLT) for glaucoma with traumatic angle recession. Graefes Arch Clin Exp Ophthalmol 231:571, 1993.
25. Mermoud, A, Salmon, JF, Barron, A, et al: Surgical management of post-traumatic angle recession glaucoma. Ophthalmology 100:634, 1993.
26. deJuan, E Jr, Sternberg, P Jr, Michels, RG: Penetrating ocular injuries. Types of injuries and visual results. Ophthalmology 90:1318, 1983.
27. Coleman, DJ: Early vitrectomy in the management of the severely traumatized eye. Am J Ophthalmol 93:543, 1982.
28. Rosenthal, AR, Marmor, MF, Leuenberger, P, Hopkins, JL: Chalcosis: a study of natural history. Ophthalmology 86:1956, 1979.
29. Sneed, SR, Weingeist, TA: Management of siderosis bulbi due to a retained iron-containing intraocular foreign body. Ophthalmology 97:375, 1990.
30. Paterson, CA, Pfister, RR: Intraocular pressure changes after alkali burns. Arch Ophthalmol 91:211, 1974.
31. Green, K, Paterson, CA, Siddiqui, A: Ocular blood flow after experimental alkali burns and prostaglandin administration. Arch Ophthalmol 103:569, 1985.
32. Donshik, PC, Berman, MB, Dohlman, CH, et al: Effect of topical corticosteroids on ulceration in alkali-burned corneas. Arch Ophthalmol 96:2117, 1978.
33. Paterson, CA, Eakins, KE, Paterson, E, et al: The ocular hypertensive response following experimental acid burns in the rabbit eye. Invest Ophthalmol Vis Sci 18:67, 1979.
34. Evans, LS: Increased intraocular pressure in severely burned patients. Am J Ophthalmol 111:56, 1991.
35. Barron, A, McDonald, JE, Hughes, WF: Long-term complications of beta radiation therapy in ophthalmology. Trans Am Ophthalmol Soc 68:112, 1970.

GLAUCOMAS FOLLOWING OCULAR SURGERY

Another large group of glaucomas are those which occur as complications of various ocular surgical procedures including glaucoma surgery, cataract extraction and related procedures, corneal transplantation, and vitreoretinal surgery.

MALIGNANT (CILIARY BLOCK) GLAUCOMA[a]

Terminology

In 1869, von Graefe (1) described a rare complication of certain ocular procedures, which was characterized by shal-

lowing or flattening of the anterior chamber and an elevation of the intraocular pressure (IOP). He called the condition *malignant glaucoma* because of the poor response to conventional therapy. Today, the concept of malignant glaucoma has been expanded to include a variety of clinical situations, which have these common denominators: (a) shallowing or flattening of both the central and peripheral anterior chamber; (b) elevation of the IOP; and (c) unresponsiveness to or aggravation by miotics, but frequent relief with cycloplegic-mydriatic therapy (2, 3).

---

[a]Refer to Shields, MB: Color Atlas of Glaucoma. Baltimore, Williams & Wilkins, 1998, Plate II40.

Studies regarding the mechanism of malignant glaucoma, which are considered later in this chapter, have led some authors to recommend new terms for this group of diseases. Based on the theory that obstruction of normal aqueous flow is due to apposition of the ciliary processes against the equator of the lens or the anterior hyaloid, the name, *ciliary block glaucoma,* was proposed (4, 5). The term, *aqueous misdirection,* is also commonly used to denote the concept of posterior diversion of the aqueous due to the ciliary block. To describe the concept that a forward shift of the lens pushes peripheral iris into the anterior chamber angle, the term *direct lens block angle closure* has been suggested (6). At present, there is no universal agreement regarding the terminology for this group of conditions, and the traditional term, malignant glaucoma, is retained for purposes of discussion in this text.

Clinical Forms

It has yet to be established whether all clinical conditions that are called malignant glaucoma should actually be included within a single disease category. Nevertheless, the following disorders have been described under that name.

Classic Malignant Glaucoma

This is the prototype and most common form of the disease group. It typically follows incisional surgical intervention for angle-closure glaucoma, and is reported to complicate 0.6–4% of these cases (2, 3, 7). Neither the type of surgery nor the level of IOP immediately prior to surgical intervention appear to be related to the postoperative development of malignant glaucoma (3). However, partial or total closure of the anterior chamber angle at the time of surgery is associated with an increased incidence of this complication (3). Furthermore, an acute angle-closure attack may be a predisposing factor, since malignant glaucoma, when it occurs, nearly always does so in an eye that has had an attack, even though the angle may be open preoperatively (7). Conversely, the condition rarely if ever follows a prophylactic iridectomy, when the angle is open at the time of surgery (7).

While the classic presentation is a unilateral disorder in the early postoperative period following incisional surgery, there are several exceptions. Cases have been reported following laser iridotomy (8, 9), and bilateral cases have been reported with both incisional and laser procedures (8–10). In addition, some cases following either incisional or laser surgery may be seen months to years later, often, but not always, corresponding to the cessation of cycloplegic therapy or the institution of miotic drops (2, 3, 10).

Malignant Glaucoma in Aphakia

Although classic malignant glaucoma typically occurs in phakic eyes, it may persist after lens removal for treatment of the disease, or develop after cataract extraction in eyes without preexisting glaucoma (3). It is important to distinguish malignant glaucoma in aphakia, as well as in its other forms, from pupillary block glaucoma and delayed suprachoroidal hemorrhage, which is considered later in this chapter.

Malignant Glaucoma in Pseudophakia

Malignant glaucoma may occur in association with an anterior chamber intraocular lens implant, presumably by the same mechanism as with malignant glaucoma in aphakia (11). More recently, it has also been observed in eyes with posterior chamber implants, with or without an associated glaucoma filtering procedure (12–16). A large posterior chamber intraocular lens optic (7 mm) in an eye with a short axial length was felt to be responsible for malignant glaucoma in one case, and caution is advised in these patients (16). Malignant glaucoma has also been reported in an 8-year-old child following extracapsular cataract extraction and posterior chamber lens implantation (17).

Miotic-Induced Malignant Glaucoma

As noted earlier, the onset of classic malignant glaucoma may correspond to the institution of miotic therapy, suggesting a causal relationship (18). In addition, similar clinical pictures have been described in unoperated eyes that were receiving miotic therapy (19), and in an eye treated with miotics after a filtering procedure for open-angle glaucoma (20).

Malignant Glaucoma Associated with Inflammation

Inflammation and trauma have also been reported as precipitating factors of malignant glaucoma (6). A form of malignant glaucoma has been reported in association with endophthalmitis secondary to fungal keratomycosis (21) and the atypical bacterium, nocardia asteroides (22).

Malignant Glaucoma Associated with Other Ocular Disorders

Retinal detachment surgery was said to cause the "malignant glaucoma syndrome" in a patient who developed choroidal detachments after a buckling procedure (23). The condition has also been reported in children with retinopathy of prematurity (24) and in a patient with corneal hydrops in keratoconus (25).

Spontaneous Malignant Glaucoma

It has also been reported that malignant glaucoma may develop in an eye without previous surgery, miotic therapy, or other apparent cause (26).

Theories of Mechanism

There is a lack of general agreement regarding the sequence of events responsible for the development of malignant glaucoma, although the following are the more popular theories.

Posterior Pooling of Aqueous

Shaffer (27) hypothesized that an accumulation of aqueous behind a posterior vitreous detachment causes the forward displacement of the iris-lens or iris-vitreous diaphragm. The concept was subsequently expanded to include the pooling of aqueous within vitreous pockets. This theory has been supported by an ultrasonographic study of eyes with malignant glaucoma in aphakia, demonstrating echo-free zones in the vitreous from which aqueous was reportedly aspirated (28). The mechanism(s) leading to the posterior diversion of aqueous is uncertain, although there is strong evidence to support the following possibilities.

CILIOLENTICULAR (OR CILIOVITREAL) BLOCK. It has been observed in cases of malignant glaucoma that the tips of the ciliary processes rotate forward and press against the lens equator in the phakic eye, or against the anterior hyaloid in aphakia, which might create the obstruction to forward flow of aqueous (Figs. 23.1 and 23.2) (4, 29). Ultrasound biomicroscopic studies have confirmed the anterior rotation of the ciliary processes (30, 31), with one study also showing a shallow supraciliary fluid level (31). As previously noted, it was this concept that led to the proposed term, "ciliary block glaucoma," as a substitute for malignant glaucoma (4).

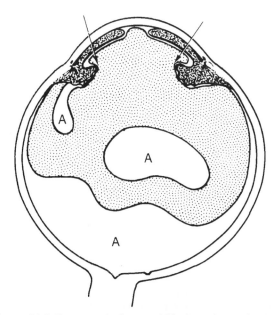

Figure 23.2. Concept of ciliovitreal block as the mechanism of malignant glaucoma in aphakia. Apposition of ciliary processes against the anterior hyaloid (*arrows*) leads to posterior diversion of aqueous (*A*), which causes a forward shift of the vitreous and iris.

ANTERIOR HYALOID OBSTRUCTION. It has also been suggested that the anterior hyaloid may contribute to ciliolenticular block and that breaks in the hyaloid near the vitreous base possibly allow the posterior diversion of aqueous (Fig. 21.3) (5). The hyaloid breaks, however, have a one-way valve effect, since fluid coming anteriorly closes the vitreous face against the ciliary body, preventing forward flow (5). Some investigators have observed the ciliolenticular contact, but note that the spaces between the ciliary processes are open, with vitreous visible behind them, suggesting that the obstruction to anterior aqueous flow is the anterior vitreous face, which is compressed forward against the ciliary processes in both phakic and aphakic forms of malignant glaucoma (3).

Perfusion studies with both animal (32) and human (33, 34) eyes have shown that resistance to flow of a fluid through vitreous increases significantly with an elevation of pressure in the eye. It has been postulated that the increased resistance might be due to compression of the vitreous, as well as its displacement against the ciliary body, lens, and iris, thereby reducing the available area of anterior hyaloid through which fluid could flow (33, 34). These clinical and laboratory observations support the concept that an intact anterior hyaloid may be important in preventing the forward movement of aqueous that has been trapped in or behind the vitreous.

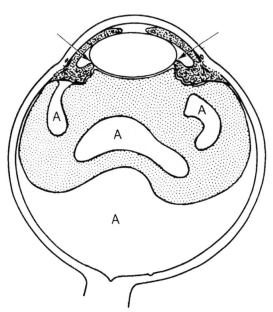

Figure 23.1. Concept of ciliolenticular block as the mechanism of malignant glaucoma. Apposition of ciliary processes to the lens equator (*arrows*) causes a posterior diversion of aqueous (*A*) which pools in and behind the vitreous with a forward shift of the lens-iris diaphragm.

Slackness of Lens Zonules

Chandler and Grant (35) have postulated that the forward movement of the lens-iris diaphragm in malignant glaucoma might be due to abnormal slackness or weakness of the zonules of the lens, as well as pressure from the vitre-

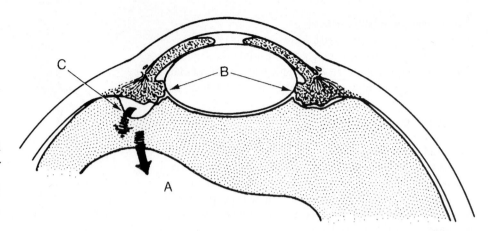

Figure 23.3. The anterior hyaloid may contribute to the ciliolenticular block *(B)*, and breaks in the hyaloid near the vitreous base *(C)* may allow the aqueous *(A)* to be diverted posteriorly *(arrows)*.

ous. Others have also advocated this theory and suggested that the laxity of the zonules might be the result of severe, prolonged angle closure (7), or ciliary muscle spasm induced by surgery, miotics, inflammation, trauma, or unknown factors (6). The concept that the lens subsequently pushes the peripheral iris into the anterior chamber angle, as noted earlier, led to the proposed term "direct lens block angle closure" (6).

It seems very likely that malignant glaucoma is a multifactorial disorder, in which elements of all the aforementioned mechanisms may be involved to variable degrees.

Differential Diagnosis

The diagnosis of malignant glaucoma requires the exclusion of the following conditions (3, 5).

Pupillary Block Glaucoma

Pupillary block is the most difficult entity to distinguish from malignant glaucoma, but must be ruled out before the latter diagnosis can be made. During slitlamp biomicroscopy, attention should be directed to two questions. First, is there moderate depth to the central anterior chamber with bowing of the peripheral iris into the chamber angle as with pupillary block, or is the entire iris-lens or iris-vitreous diaphragm shifted forward with marked shallowing or loss of the central anterior chamber as with malignant glaucoma (Fig. 23.4)? Second, and probably of more diagnostic value, is a patent iridectomy present? If the iridectomy is clearly patent, a pupillary block is unlikely. However, if patency cannot be confirmed, the diagnosis of pupillary block cannot be ruled out, and one should proceed with a laser iridotomy.

Choroidal Detachments

Choroidal separation with serous fluid is common after glaucoma filtering procedures and might be confused with malignant glaucoma due to the shallow or flat anterior

chamber. These eyes are typically hypotonus. However, when the anterior chamber is flat, IOP measurements by either Goldmann applanation tonometry, pneumotonometry, or a Tono-pan are grossly inaccurate, tending to overestimate at low pressures and underestimate at high pressures, and therefore cannot be relied upon to distinguish between excessive filtration and malignant glaucoma (36). A more helpful diagnostic finding is the light-brown choroidal detachments, which are easily seen if there is adequate visibility of the posterior ocular segment or otherwise can be diagnosed by ultrasonography.

Most serous choroidal detachments will resolve spontaneously. However, those that are persistent or massive with central touch can be approached surgically by making scleral incisions in the inferior quadrants. If a characteristic straw-colored fluid is obtained from the suprachoroidal space, the diagnosis of serous choroidal detachment is confirmed, and the procedure is completed by draining as much suprachoroidal fluid as possible and reforming the anterior chamber with air and/or saline.

Suprachoroidal Hemorrhage

This may occur hours or days after ocular surgery and create shallowing or loss of the anterior chamber, which is typically associated with pain and elevated IOP. The eye is usually more inflamed than with serous choroidal detachment and the choroidal elevation is frequently dark reddish-brown. The surgical approach is the same as for serous choroidal detachments, with drainage of the blood from the suprachoroidal space via the sclerotomies and reformation of the anterior chamber.

Management

Medical

Chandler and Grant (35) reported in 1962 that mydriatic-cycloplegic treatment was effective for malignant glaucoma, and the following year, Weiss and coworkers (37) recommended the use of hyperosmotics to combat this condition. The value of a cycloplegic may be both to pull the lens back by tightening the zonules (35) and to break a ciliary block (5), while the presumed benefit of a hyperosmotic is to reduce the pressure exerted by the vitreous (37). These two measures, along with a carbonic anhydrase inhibitor, and/or topical β-blocker or α₂-agonist, to reduce the amount of aqueous that may be pooling posteriorly, constitute the standard medical approach to malignant glaucoma. A standard medical regimen includes the use of topical atropine four times daily, oral glycerol or intravenous mannitol, a topical β-blocker and/or α₂-agonist, and oral acetazolamide, or methazolamide, or topical dorzolamide. The patient should be maintained on atropine indefinitely after the attack is broken to prevent recurrences.

Surgical

The above medical regimen is curative in approximately half of the cases within 5 days (2, 3). If the condition persists beyond this time, surgical intervention is usually indicated. There is no clear-cut evidence as to which of several surgical approaches for malignant glaucoma is superior. In general, it is best to try one of the more conservative laser approaches first if circumstances permit. If this is not effective or feasible, the next step is either a posterior sclerotomy

with air injection or an anterior vitrectomy, followed by lens removal if necessary.

LASER TECHNIQUES. Argon laser photocoagulation of the ciliary processes that can be visualized through an iridectomy, followed by medical therapy, has been reported to relieve malignant glaucoma, presumably by breaking the ciliolenticular block (38). Other investigators have also found this approach to be effective, even without the concomitant use of cycloplegics (39), although the latter drug should remain a standard part of the therapy for malignant glaucoma. The Nd:YAG laser has also been effective in treating aphakic and pseudophakic malignant (ciliovitreal block) glaucoma by disrupting the anterior hyaloid face (40, 41) or the posterior lens capsule and hyaloid face (15, 42, 43).

POSTERIOR SCLEROTOMY AND AIR INJECTION. A pars plana incision with aspiration of fluid from the vitreous and reformation of the anterior chamber with an air bubble (Fig. 23.5) is felt by some to be the incisional surgical procedure of choice for classic malignant glaucoma (2, 3, 5). It has been suggested that the sclerotomy should be placed 3 mm posterior to the limbus to break the anterior hyaloid, thereby reducing its contribution to the blockade (5). Postoperatively, the patients are generally maintained on atropine to avoid recurrence.

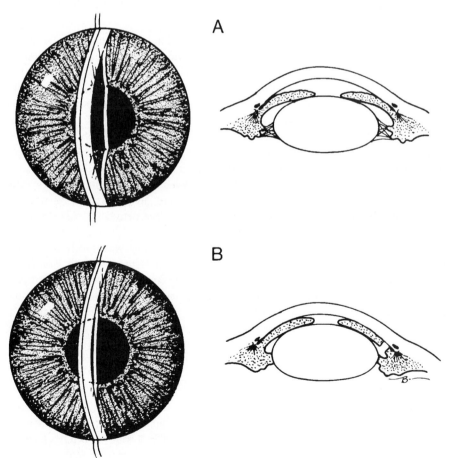

A

B

Figure 23.4. Distinctions between pupillary block glaucoma and malignant glaucoma. **A.** In pupillary block glaucoma, there is moderate depth to the central anterior chamber with forward bowing of the peripheral iris and absence of a patent iridectomy. **B.** In malignant glaucoma, the entire lens-iris diaphragm is shifted forward with marked shallowing, or loss of the central anterior chamber, and a patent peripheral iridectomy may be present.

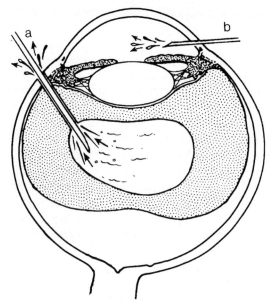

Figure 23.5. Posterior sclerotomy and air injection in the management of malignant glaucoma. Fluid is drained or aspirated from the vitreous via a pars plana incision *(a)*, and the anterior chamber is deepened with air *(b)*.

ANTERIOR PARS PLANA VITRECTOMY. Other surgeons prefer a careful removal of the anterior vitreous with vitrectomy instruments (44–48). The reported results with both the posterior sclerotomy and the anterior vitrectomy techniques are favorable, while both also have a potential for serious complications. The choice in most cases will depend upon the surgeon's experience and preference.

LENS EXTRACTION. This is favored by some surgeons as the incisional surgical procedure of choice, while others utilize the approach if the posterior sclerotomy and air injection or anterior vitrectomy fails (49). To be effective, lens extraction should be combined with an incision of the anterior hyaloid and possibly with deep incisions into fluid pockets in the vitreous (2, 3).

OTHER SURGICAL APPROACHES. Cyclocryotherapy has also been advocated, with the presumed mechanism being alteration in the ciliary body or vitreous (50). Perilenticular incision of the vitreous was described by Chandler (51), but the procedure was generally abandoned due to the significant risks involved.

Management of the Fellow Eye

When malignant glaucoma has occurred in one eye, there is a significant chance that it will develop in the fellow eye if surgery is performed following an acute angle closure attack. For this reason, it is best to do a prophylactic laser iridotomy early. However, if angle-closure glaucoma is present, every effort should be made to break the attack before surgery and, if the attack cannot be broken, mydriatic-

cycloplegic therapy should be used vigorously postiridotomy and continued indefinitely.

GLAUCOMAS IN APHAKIA OR PSEUDOPHAKIA

Terminology

The term "aphakic or pseudophakic glaucoma" is occasionally seen in the literature. It is mentioned in this text only to discourage its use since it implies that a single form of glaucoma is associated with aphakia or pseudophakia. As will be seen in the following discussion, there are many mechanisms by which cataract extraction, with or without intraocular lens implantation, can lead to glaucoma, and it is best to refer to these glaucomas in aphakia or pseudophakia by terms which describe the particular events leading to the IOP elevation.

Incidence

The IOP may be elevated transiently in the early postoperative period or may become chronically elevated at any time after cataract surgery.

Aphakia

In the days before intraocular lens implantation, a rise in IOP during the first several days after cataract extraction was not uncommon, although the frequency of this complication undoubtedly varied according to the surgical technique. Early studies in which the corneoscleral incision was approximated with various numbers of silk or gut sutures revealed no significant difference between pre- and postoperative pressures (52) and only occasional, minor fluctuations in tonographic facilities of outflow (53). However, in later series, in which multiple, fine sutures were used for tight wound closure, a significant IOP rise occurred in the early postoperative period in a high percentage of the eyes (54, 55).

Chronic glaucoma in aphakia was much less common than the early, transient pressure rise. In one series of 203 uncomplicated cataract extractions, persistent glaucoma occurred in 3% of the eyes (56). However, these chronic cases posed a much greater threat to vision, as well as a much more difficult therapeutic challenge, than the eyes with transient pressure elevation.

Pseudophakia

The advent of extracapsular cataract extraction and posterior chamber intraocular lens implantation was, in general, associated with a reduced incidence of long-term IOP elevation (57, 58). In one series of 373 eyes undergoing cataract surgery, those receiving intracapsular extraction and anterior chamber (133) or iris fixation (31) lenses had a late mean IOP rise of 0.8 mm Hg, while those undergoing extracapsular surgery with posterior chamber implants (209) had a mean IOP fall of 0.6 mm Hg (59). However, the latter procedure is not without pressure complications in both the early and late postoperative periods. In eyes without preexisting glaucoma, more than half of one series had an IOP of 25 mm Hg or more 2–3 hours postoperatively (60), while a pressure above 23 mm Hg on the first postoperative day was seen in 29% of eyes in another study (61). Chronic glaucoma was seen in 4% of eyes following standard extracapsular extraction in one series (61), and in 2.1% of another large series (62). Postoperative glaucoma also occurred in 11.3% of eyes receiving secondary anterior chamber implants (63).

Extracapsular cataract extraction and posterior chamber intraocular lens implantation, as compared to intracapsular surgery, has also reduced, but not eliminated, IOP complications in eyes with preexisting glaucoma (64). In one comparative study, the former procedure was associated with a slightly more favorable pressure course, although an IOP above 21 mm Hg on the first postoperative day was seen with approximately half the eyes undergoing either operation (65). However, late results indicate that most patients require the same or less medication as preoperatively to control their IOP (64, 66, 67). While long-term results of large series are not yet available, it is likely that phacoemulsification and posterior chamber lens implantation in eyes with or without preexisting glaucoma has the same, if not better, IOP course as with extracapsular surgery. With any cataract procedures, however, both early and late postoperative IOP elevation can occur by a wide variety of mechanisms, which include the following.

Mechanism of Intraocular Pressure Elevation

Distortion of the Anterior Chamber Angle

Kirsch and coworkers (68, 69) described the gonioscopic appearance of an internal white ridge resembling an inverted snow bank along the inner margins of the corneoscleral incision following routine cataract extraction. For about the first 2 weeks, the ridge typically obscures visualization of the trabecular meshwork and then gradually recedes over the next few months. There is some controversy regarding the pathogenesis of the internal ridge. Campbell and Grant (70) provided evidence that distortion of the anterior chamber angle is induced by tight corneoscleral sutures (Fig. 23.6), while Kirsch and coworkers (69) suggested that edema of the deep corneal stroma is the mechanism. Whatever the initiating factor(s) may be, the ridge is known to be associated with the formation of peripheral anterior synechiae, vitreous adhesions, and hyphema (68). In addition, it is quite likely that the white ridge contributes, at least in some cases, to the early, transient pressure elevation after cataract surgery. In one study of 95 cataract extractions, early IOP rise occurred in 23% of the cases with limbal incisions, but in none with corneal incisions, suggesting that distortion produced by the corneoscleral wound temporarily influences the adjacent trabecular meshwork and aqueous outflow (71).

Influence of Viscoelastic Substances

To protect the corneal endothelium and maintain anterior chamber depth during certain stages of cataract extraction and intraocular lens implantation, it has become common practice

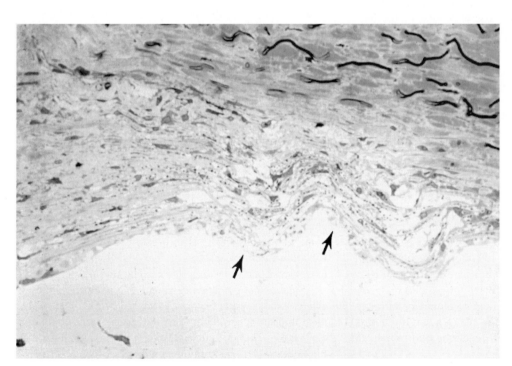

Figure 23.6. Light microscopic view of autopsy eye showing distortion of trabecular meshwork *(arrows)* due to placement of corneoscleral sutures as performed in routine cataract surgery. (Courtesy of David G. Campbell, M.D.)

to fill the anterior chamber with a viscous aqueous substitute. The viscoelastic substance that has received the most extensive evaluation for this purpose is *sodium hyaluronate* (Healon). While some surgeons have noted no significant postoperative pressure rises associated with the use of sodium hyaluronate (72, 73), others have documented high pressures in the first few days after surgery (74–77). Sodium hyaluronate injected into the anterior chamber of rabbit and monkey eyes caused marked pressure rises (78), and perfusion in enucleated human eyes decreased the outflow facility by 65% (79). This was not reversed by vigorous anterior chamber irrigation, but facility was restored to baseline by irrigation with hyaluronidase (79). Clinically, aspiration of sodium hyaluronate at the end of cataract surgery did not significantly reduce the incidence or degree of postoperative IOP rise in one study (80). The most likely mechanism of the IOP elevation is temporary obstruction of the trabecular meshwork by the viscoelastic, although sodium hyaluronate has also been shown to exacerbate postoperative inflammation (81).

Alternative viscoelastic substances have also been evaluated. *Chondroitin sulfate* was shown to cause minimal pressure elevation when used during lens implantation in a variety of animal eyes (82) or when injected as a 10% concentration into the anterior chamber of rabbit and monkey eyes (78). A formulation of *chondroitin sulfate and sodium hyaluronate* (Viscoat) has been compared to sodium hyaluronate and was found to be less advantageous during cataract surgery in one study and yet to still cause IOP rises in the immediate postoperative period in many patients (83), although another study found the duration of IOP elevation to be shorter with the former agent (84). A modified sodium hyaluronate viscoelastic (Healon GV), which has a higher molecular weight, viscosity, and sodium hyaluronate concentration than Healon, was found to be associated with a comparable postoperative IOP course to that of the latter agent (85). *Methylcellulose* 1–2% has not been found to cause a significant postoperative pressure rise in either animal (79) or human (86) eyes, and appears to provide good protection of the corneal endothelium (86). In comparative trials, hydroxypropyl methylcellulose 2% was found to have the same effect on corneal thickness as balanced salt solution with no rise in IOP (87), and the same early, mild IOP elevation as with sodium hyaluronate 1% (88).

In the early 1990s, a significant problem was encountered with a synthetic viscoelastic containing *polyacrylamide* 4% (Orcolon). Although preliminary comparisons with Healon revealed either no difference in postoperative IOP (89) or a slight, but significant increase in IOP on the first postoperative day (90), subsequent experience disclosed a small percentage of patients with severe, refractory glaucoma that often required filtering surgery and, in many cases, led to significant visual loss (91, 92). Laboratory studies in bovine, monkey, and human eyes showed an accumulation of microgels in the trabecular meshwork as the apparent mechanism of the glaucoma induced by the viscoelastic (93), which was subsequently withdrawn from the market.

Inflammation and Hemorrhage

Transient postoperative inflammation occurs to some degree after every cataract extraction. When excessive, obstruction of the trabecular meshwork by inflammatory cells and fibrin may lead to IOP elevations. The inflammatory response and associated glaucoma may be particularly prominent when lens fragments are retained in the vitreous following extracapsular cataract extraction (94).

Intraocular lens implants increase the risk of serious postoperative uveitis, especially with anterior chamber and iris-supported lenses (95). This may be associated with hyphema and glaucoma, which has been referred to as the "UGH" (uveitis, glaucoma, and hemorrhage) syndrome (96, 97). Uveitis was particularly common with the iris-supported lenses, apparently due to the movement of the lens against the iris and the subsequent cellular reaction (98, 99). The mechanism of inflammation and hemorrhage with anterior chamber lenses is felt to be related to contact of the rough posterior surface of the lens with the iris. The degree to which this occurs is apparently related to the design and quality of the specific lens (96, 97, 100). Posterior chamber lenses are least likely to induce uveitis. Fluorophotometric studies have shown that pseudophakic eyes with a posterior chamber lens and an intact posterior lens capsule have minimal alteration in the blood-aqueous barrier (101–103). Nevertheless, the UGH syndrome after posterior chamber lens implantation has been described (104).

In addition to the hyphema associated with uveitis, bleeding in the aqueous or vitreous compartments may be seen immediately after cataract surgery or as a late or recurring complication. One source of the late hemorrhage is new vessels in the corneoscleral wound (105). Intraocular lens implantation may also be complicated by late or recurrent hemorrhage, which has been reported with anterior chamber (106), iris fixation (107), and posterior chamber implants (108, 109). The latter usually have sulcus fixation, and the mechanism in all cases is presumably an erosion into the adjacent tissue (110). Postoperative bleeding from any source may lead to IOP elevation by the mechanisms discussed in Chapter 21, including ghost cell glaucoma from a vitreous hemorrhage (111).

Pigment Dispersion

Variable amounts of pigment granules, primarily from the iris pigment epithelium, are dispersed into the anterior chamber with all cataract operations. If the degree of pigment dispersion is excessive, it can lead to a transient IOP elevation in either aphakic or pseudophakic eyes, with the latter occasionally leading to a chronic form of glaucoma.

Pseudophakic pigmentary glaucoma is most often associated with posterior chamber lenses (112–115). The mechanism appears to be rubbing of the iris pigment epithelium against the periphery and haptics of the intraocular lens, leading to the dispersion of pigment granules which obstruct the trabecular meshwork, similar to the situation with phakic pigmentary glaucoma. Pigment granules on the central corneal endothelium (Krukenberg spindle) is an occasional, but not consistent, finding. The granules may also be seen circulating in the aqueous of the anterior chamber, especially after pupillary dilatation. The most diagnostic finding, however, is iris transillumination defects at the sites of contact with the implant. The iris may also have pigment granules on the stroma, and blue irides may have a grayish discoloration (113). Gonioscopy will reveal heavy pigmentation of the trabecular meshwork.

Vitreous Filling the Anterior Chamber

Grant (116) described a mechanism of acute open-angle glaucoma in which vitreous humor fills the anterior chamber after cataract surgery. He reported that this can be cured in some cases by mydriasis to minimize pupillary block, while other eyes require miosis to draw the vitreous from the angle. Simmons (117) noted that many cases will resolve spontaneously in several months. When surgical intervention is required, an iridotomy may be curative, while other eyes will require an anterior vitrectomy (118).

Pupillary Block

IN APHAKIA. This is a relatively rare complication of cataract extraction, but tends to occur more commonly with round

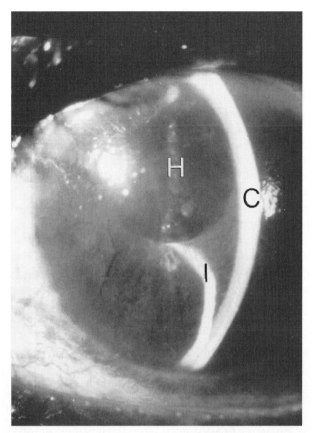

Figure 23.8. Slitlamp view of eye with pupillary block in aphakia showing hyaloid face *(H)* well back from cornea *(C)* centrally, but peripheral anterior bowing of iris *(I)* with closure of anterior chamber angle.

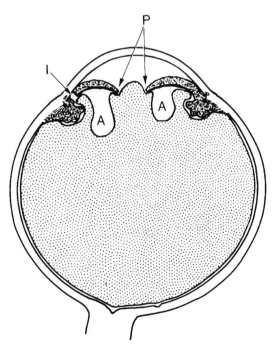

Figure 23.7. Pupillary block in aphakia. An adherence between the iris and anterior vitreous face blocks the flow of aqueous into the anterior chamber at both the pupil *(P)* and iridectomy site *(I)*. The posterior accumulation of aqueous *(A)* causes forward bowing of the peripheral iris with closure of the anterior chamber angle.

pupil extractions (119, 120). It is particularly likely to occur weeks after a transient flat anterior chamber secondary to a wound leak. The condition may also be more common following surgery for congenital cataracts, and a combination of sector and peripheral iridectomies with multiple sphincterotomies was reported to minimize this complication (121). With modern techniques of congenital cataract surgery, such measures are probably not necessary, although a peripheral iridectomy is still advisable.

The pathogenesis of pupillary block in aphakia is felt to be an adherence between the iris and anterior vitreous face, which prevents aqueous flow into the anterior chamber either through the pupil or iridectomy. The aqueous accumulates in pools behind the iris, causing a forward shift of the iris and closure of anterior chamber angle (Fig. 23.7). The mechanism may be dependent on an intact anterior hyaloid, since fluorescein studies have shown that aqueous will flow through spontaneous openings in the vitreous face (122). It may be possible to distinguish this condition from the much less common malignant glaucoma in aphakia by the deeper central anterior chamber and forward bowing of the peripheral iris in the former situation (Fig. 23.8) (123).

IN PSEUDOPHAKIA. Pupillary block glaucoma in pseudophakia was once seen most often with anterior chamber

(124–126) and iris-supported (127, 128) lenses, although there have now been numerous reports of this complication following posterior chamber lens implantation (124, 129–133). It usually appears in the early period after surgery, but may occur months or years later. Many cases are asymptomatic and are discovered during a routine postoperative examination. Some may even have a normal IOP although peripheral anterior synechiae and chronic pressure elevation usually follow if the peripheral anterior chamber depth is not promptly restored. With anterior chamber lenses, the iris bulges forward on either side of the lens (Fig. 23.9), while the mechanism with posterior chamber lenses appears to be excessive inflammation with posterior synechiae to the intraocular lens or the anterior capsule (133).

With modern cataract techniques and posterior chamber intraocular lens implants, the incidence of pupillary block glaucoma in pseudophakia is sufficiently low that a peripheral iridectomy is no longer a routine part of cataract surgery for most surgeons (134, 135). However, when excessive

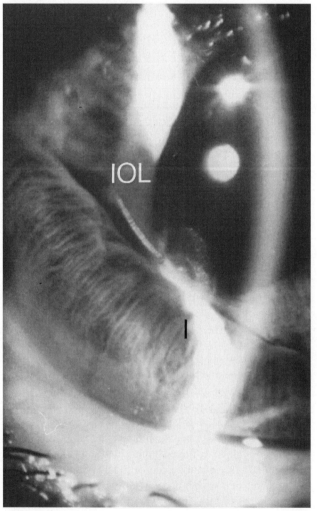

Figure 23.9. Slitlamp view of pupillary block in pseudophakia showing forward bulging of iris (*I*) peripheral to margin of anterior chamber intraocular lens (*IOL*).

postoperative inflammation is anticipated, and especially when combining the cataract surgery with a filtering procedure, an iridectomy, is still advisable.

Peripheral Anterior Synechiae and/or Trabecular Damage

In most cases of chronic glaucoma in aphakia or pseudophakia, peripheral anterior synechiae are present, presumably due to a flat anterior chamber and/or excessive inflammation in the early postoperative period. Flat anterior chambers after cataract surgery may be due to a *wound leak* with subsequent hypotony and choroidal detachments. This leads to a vicious cycle, since the choroidal detachments cause decreased aqueous production with further hypotony and also contribute to the forward shift of the iris and vitreous. To avoid the complication of peripheral anterior synechiae and chronic glaucoma, a flat anterior chamber should be corrected promptly. In one series of 203 uncomplicated cataract extractions, 47% had some degree of peripheral anterior synechiae, and all of those with associated glaucoma had goniosynechiae in more than one-fourth of the angle (56). In some cases, peripheral anterior synechiae may develop over the haptics of an anterior chamber lens months after the surgery and continue to progress over time (136).

In other cases of glaucoma in aphakia or pseudophakia, the angle may be open in all quadrants and appear normal, except for variable degrees of increased pigmentation. The mechanism of aqueous outflow obstruction in cases of chronic open-angle glaucoma in aphakia or pseudophakia is uncertain, but most likely relates to alterations within the trabecular meshwork as a result of the surgery and possibly to a preexisting reduction in outflow facility.

Glaucoma after Congenital Cataract Surgery

Children tend to have a higher incidence of glaucoma after cataract extraction than adults. In various series, the reported prevalences range from 6.1% to 24% (137–139). Most of these have an open-angle mechanism (139, 140). As previously noted, however, a pupillary-block mechanism is not uncommon in aphakic children (121), and pseudophakic pupillary-block glaucoma in children has also been reported (141). It may be, therefore, that this is another situation in which an iridectomy is still indicated as a part of the cataract surgery. It has also been suggested that the use of a vitrectomy instrument to aspirate the cataract, with wide excision of the posterior capsule, may reduce the incidence of postoperative glaucoma in children (137). However, even with automated lensectomy and vitrectomy in children, some studies reveal glaucoma rates of 12.5% to 24% (138, 139).

Influence of α-Chymotrypsin

This mechanism is rarely seen today, but was common during the era of intracapsular surgery. Barraquer (142), in

1958, demonstrated the value of the enzymatic zonulolysis with α-chymotrypsin in facilitating intracapsular cataract extraction, and the enzyme was commonly used for that purpose. In 1964, Kirsch (143) reported a transient pressure rise in 75% of the eyes in which 2–4 cc of a 1:5,000 dilution of the enzyme was used, compared to a 24% incidence of high pressures in a group without enzyme. The complication was somewhat more common in patients with preexisting open-angle glaucoma (144). Tonographic studies showed a decrease in aqueous outflow facility (145, 146), although no abnormal parameters were noted 2–4 months postoperatively (147). The enzyme-induced pressure response could be produced experimentally in monkeys (148–150), and histologic studies of those eyes suggested that the pressure rise was due to an accumulation of lens zonule fragments, characterized by uniform segments of approximately 1000 Å (151) in the trabecular meshwork (150, 152).

Based on the above clinical and laboratory observations, the term *enzyme glaucoma* was often applied to those cases of early, transient IOP elevation with deep anterior chambers in which the enzyme was used to facilitate intracapsular lens extraction. Several studies, however, revealed no difference in the postoperative pressure course in groups with and without enzyme (55, 71, 153), even in eyes with preexisting glaucoma (154), which may have been related to the volume or concentration of α-chymotrypsin. Eyes receiving 0.25–0.5 cc of 1:5000–1:10,000 dilution had pressure responses similar to cases without enzyme (153). Kirsch (155) also observed the apparent dose relationship, but still found a 55% incidence of high pressures in the early postoperative period following the use of 0.25 cc of 1:5000 α-chymotrypsin.

Neodymium:YAG Laser Posterior Capsulotomy

Another cause of IOP elevation after extracapsular cataract extraction or phacoemulsification is the use of Nd:YAG laser to perform a discission in the posterior lens capsule when that structure becomes significantly opacified following the initial surgery. Numerous studies have confirmed that the procedure may be associated with significant pressure elevation (156–168). The pressure rise may be detected within the first few hours and usually returns to baseline within 1 week, although some may last for several weeks, and several large series have revealed persistent or late-onset pressure elevations in 0.8–6% of the cases (158, 167, 168). Cases have been reported in which the laser-induced pressure elevation caused progressive glaucomatous visual field loss (159) or transient loss of light perception requiring emergency paracentesis (160). It should also be kept in mind that other causes of visual loss following Nd:YAG capsulotomy include cystoid macular edema and retinal detachment (167). Risk factors for significant IOP elevations after Nd:YAG capsulotomy differ among studies, but those which have been reported include preexisting glaucoma or a preoperative pressure above 20 mm Hg, larger capsulotomies, a sulcus, rather than cap-

sular, fixed posterior chamber lens (166), the absence of a posterior chamber lens, myopia, vitreoretinal disease, vitreous prolapse into the anterior chamber (169), and the total laser energy used (170).

The mechanism of IOP elevation following Nd:YAG capsulotomy is not fully understood, although tonographic studies have shown that it is related to reduced aqueous outflow (161, 170). Most cases have an open-angle mechanism, and the obstruction of the trabecular meshwork may be with fibrin and inflammatory cells due to a breakdown in the blood-aqueous barrier or debris from the capsule or cortical remnants (171, 172). A study in a rabbit model suggests that the release of calcitonin gene-related peptide (a neuropeptide responsible for neurogenic irritative responses in rabbits) is partly responsible for the disruption of the blood-aqueous barrier and IOP elevation (173). Other reported mechanisms of IOP elevation include pupillary block due to forward movement of the vitreous (164), and herniated vitreous occluding a preexisting glaucoma surgical fistula (165). Pretreatment with indomethacin was not found to reduce the postoperative pressure rise (174). However, pretreatment with timolol (174, 175) or acetazolamide (176), and especially pre- and/or posttreatment with 1.0% or 0.5% apraclonidine (177–180), have been shown to minimize the early postoperative rise in IOP.

Anterior capsulotomies have also been evaluated in animal eyes, which produced pressure rises in all cases, presumably due to outflow obstruction by liquified cortical material (181). In human cases, IOP elevations occurred at varying intervals after laser surgery, but were usually transient (182).

Management

Preoperative Considerations

In preparing for a cataract operation, there are certain considerations that may help to minimize the risk of postoperative complications related to glaucoma, particularly in eyes with preexisting glaucoma. For example, in administering retrobulbar anesthesia, it may be best to not include *epinephrine* in the anesthetic mixture for fear of the influence this could have on perfusion of the optic nerve head.

PRESSURE REDUCERS. Many surgeons elect to reduce the vitreous volume and IOP by applying external pressure to the globe before surgery to maintain a deep anterior chamber and to minimize the potential complications of vitreous loss and expulsive hemorrhage. The external force may be accomplished by digital pressure, a rubber ball with an elastic band around the head, or a pneumatic rubber balloon (Honan intraocular pressure reducer). Each technique has the potential risk of optic atrophy or arterial occlusion from the excessive or prolonged application of pressure, and the Honan device may be the safest in this regard by allowing monitoring of the pressure in the balloon. Although the IOP does not correlate directly or linearly with the pressure in the Honan balloon, studies suggest that it is safe in normotensive eyes, especially when the instrument is set at 30 mm Hg for 5 minutes (183). However, the induced IOP rise is a function of the initial ocular tension, and marked pressure elevations may occur in eyes with initial levels above 30 mm Hg, indicating the need for extreme caution in these cases (183).

SELECTION OF INTRAOCULAR LENS. As noted earlier, posterior chamber intraocular lens implantation in association with extracapsular cataract extraction (and phacoemulsification), while not devoid of potential glaucoma-related complications, is generally associated with a slight reduction in postoperative IOP and is well-tolerated even in eyes with advanced preexisting glaucoma. Anterior chamber lenses, however, are more problematic, and preoperative glaucoma or anterior chamber angle abnormalities are relative contraindications to their use. In one study of 18 normotensive eyes with angle-supported lenses, synechiae developed around the haptics in 12 cases (184), which can lead to aqueous outflow obstruction, especially in eyes with preexisting glaucoma. In another study, anterior chamber lens implantation in eyes with preoperative peripheral anterior synechiae was associated with corneal endothelial cell loss, fibrous endothelial metaplasia, and angle cicatrization (185).

Intraoperative Considerations

Attention to gentle handling of tissues, hemostasis, and minimal intraocular manipulation may reduce the risk of postoperative IOP rise associated with hemorrhage or excessive inflammation or pigment dispersion. One study found that the technique of wound closure (specifically a sutureless sclerocorneal tunnel incision) and the surgeon's experience were more important than prophylactic medications in preventing IOP elevation after phacoemulsification (186). In addition, judicious use of intraocular agents such as viscoelastic substances, especially in eyes with preexisting glaucoma, may help to minimize the risk of postoperative glaucoma complications.

Another class of agents often injected into the eye during cataract surgery are the miotics, *acetylcholine* and *carbachol,* which are used to constrict the pupil, especially after posterior chamber intraocular lens implantation. Acetylcholine, as compared to balanced salt solution, was associated with lower IOPs at 3 and 6 hours postoperatively, although the difference was not statistically significantly different at 24 hours (187). The combination of preoperative acetazolamide and intraoperative acetylcholine was more effective than either drug alone in controlling postoperative IOP elevation (188). Carbachol, on the other hand, was associated with lower postoperative pressures, as compared to either acetylcholine or balanced salt solution, at 24 hours, 2 days, and 3 days postoperatively (189–194). The intracameral use

of carbachol, therefore, may be helpful in avoiding early IOP rises, especially in eyes with preexisting glaucoma.

Early Postoperative Period

The IOP has been noted to rise within 6–7 hours after routine cataract extraction, and generally returns to normal within 1 week. A modest pressure rise, e.g., less than 30 mm Hg, in a nonglaucomatous eye with a deep anterior chamber is usually of no consequence and requires no antiglaucoma therapy. However, high pressures may cause pain and occasional disruption of the corneoscleral wound. Furthermore, eyes with preexisting glaucoma and advanced glaucomatous optic atrophy may have further nerve damage with even short episodes of pressure elevation. In addition, anterior ischemic optic neuropathy has been reported to occur during these periods of elevated pressure in eyes with vulnerable optic nerve head circulation (195). Therefore, if there is pain or a threat to the optic nerve head, cornea, or cataract incision, temporary medical measures should be employed.

A number of drugs have been evaluated for efficacy in controlling the early IOP rise in eyes with *open anterior chamber angles.* While the results are somewhat conflicting, both acetazolamide (196–198) and timolol (198–204) are generally felt to be useful in these cases. One study found timolol to be more effective than acetazolamide (204), while another study compared levobunolol, timolol, and betaxolol, and found the former to be the most effective of the three β-blockers in controlling the early postcataract IOP rise (205). Apraclonidine 1% has also been shown to be useful in controlling postoperative IOP elevation (206), but is more effective when given 1 hour (207) preoperatively than immediately after the surgery. Apraclonidine also appears to reduce aqueous flare after cataract surgery (206).

Pilocarpine drops were not felt to be of value in one study (197), although pilocarpine gel was found to be effective in another study, without significantly increasing postoperative inflammation (208). However, pilocarpine gel was not as effective as intracameral carbachol in one study (193). Epinephrine is generally avoided due to the danger of macular edema (209). Steroids were reported to be ineffective in one study (197), but may be helpful in controlling the pressure when inflammation is excessive. Indomethacin and aspirin have also been shown to reduce the postoperative pressure rise, presumably by inhibiting prostaglandin synthesis (210). When uveitis and glaucoma are associated with retained lens fragments in the vitreous, pars plana vitrectomy is reported to yield good results (94).

Uveitis, glaucoma, and *hyphema* may be managed with either mydriatics or miotics to minimize iris movement against the lens in mild cases. In more severe cases, steroids should be employed for the iritis and a carbonic anhydrase inhibitor or topical β-blocker or α_2-agonist for the glaucoma. Argon laser photocoagulation may be effective in controlling the hemorrhage if the bleeding sites are visible (108). Recurrent hyphema and glaucoma is usually an indication to remove the lens, although this is often difficult and can lead to significant intraoperative complications. When glaucoma and hyphema are associated with vitreous hemorrhage, pars plana vitrectomy has been recommended (211). *Pigment dispersion in pseudophakia* can usually be controlled medically and gradually becomes easier to manage in most cases. Removal of the lens is rarely required.

Pupillary block in aphakia may initially be treated with mydriasis to break the block, although an iridotomy is usually required (119, 120). To be effective, the iridotomy must be placed over a pocket of aqueous behind the iris, rather than an area in which the vitreous is in broad apposition to the posterior surface of the iris. The laser is particularly useful in these cases, since more than one iridotomy can be made until an aqueous pocket is found as evidenced by a deepening of the peripheral anterior chamber. Suggested alternative surgical approaches include separating the iris from the vitreous adhesions with laser iridoplasty (212) or an iris repositor (213) and pars plana vitrectomy (214).

Pupillary block in pseudophakia may be broken with mydriatic therapy by enlarging the pupil beyond the edges of an anterior chamber lens or by lysing posterior synechiae from a posterior chamber lens. Carbonic anhydrase inhibitors, hyperosmotics, a β-blocker or an α_2-agonist may also be required as emergency measures. The definitive treatment is an iridotomy, which is best achieved with a laser when possible. The laser may also be used to break the block by dilating the pupil (215). Closed vitrectomy has also been used to relieve pseudophakic pupillary block (216).

Late Postoperative Period

The majority of patients with chronic glaucoma in aphakia or pseudophakia can and should be managed medically. Miotic therapy is frequently effective, as is the use of drugs which reduce aqueous production, such as carbonic anhydrase inhibitors, β-blockers and α_2-agonists. Epinephrine is usually avoided due to the danger of macular edema (209). Surgical intervention is reserved for cases that are uncontrolled on maximum tolerable medical therapy. Laser trabeculoplasty may be effective in cases which do not have extensive peripheral anterior synechiae and is the initial surgical procedure of choice (217). When strict IOP and visual acuity criteria were used to define success in one study, no surgical procedure was highly effective for chronic glaucoma in aphakia or pseudophakia (218). In one series of trabeculectomies in 82 aphakic eyes, less than half were successful (219). Other surgeons, however, have had somewhat better results and feel that trabeculectomy is the procedure of choice if trabeculoplasty fails or is not possible (217). The postoperative use of 5-fluorouracil has been shown to increase the success rate of filtering surgery in aphakic eyes (220), and intraoperative mitomycin C may be even more effective in these cases. When conjunctival scarring does not allow performance of a trabeculectomy in a superior quadrant, a drainage implant device is usually the best next step. Transscleral Nd:YAG

cyclophotocoagulation has also been shown to be effective in chronic glaucoma in aphakia and pseudophakia (221), although should usually be reserved for patients with poor visual potential or in whom incisional surgery is not possible or felt to have a poor chance of success.

As previously noted, when Nd:YAG capsulotomy is required in the late postoperative period, apraclonidine 1.0% or 0.5% given one before and/or immediately after the procedure is effective in minimizing the postlaser pressure rise (177–180). Other drugs that have also been reported to be effective include timolol (174, 175), acetazolamide (176) and pilocarpine (222).

GLAUCOMAS ASSOCIATED WITH EPITHELIAL INGROWTH AND OTHER CELLULAR PROLIFERATIONS

There is a group of rare, but potentially devastating, conditions that may complicate cataract surgery, incisional glaucoma procedures, and any other incisional operation, as well as some forms of trauma. These conditions have as their common denominator a proliferation of cells into the anterior chamber.

Epithelial Ingrowth

Clinical Features

In this condition, also referred to as *epithelial downgrowth,* an epithelial membrane grows into the eye through a penetrating wound. It extends over the posterior surface of the cornea, causing corneal edema, and also grows down across the anterior chamber angle and onto the iris, which may lead to a refractory form of glaucoma. It is reported to occur in 0.09–0.12% of eyes after cataract surgery (223–226). The incidence appears to be declining with newer cataract techniques (225), although a case has been reported with a sutureless scleral tunnel incision (226). It may also occur after penetrating trauma (227, 228), penetrating keratoplasty (229), and glaucoma surgery (230).

Early in the disease process, a wound leak may be demonstrated by the Seidel test. By slitlamp biomicroscopy, the epithelial ingrowth on the cornea is seen as a thin gray translucent or transparent membrane with a scalloped, thickened leading edge. Specular microscopy is reported to reveal a characteristic pattern of cell borders, which may have some diagnostic value (226, 230). Fluorophotometry has also been reported to have diagnostic value by showing a delayed disappearance of the topically applied fluorescein in the area overlying the membrane (226). The membrane on the iris is more difficult to see, but it typically causes a flattening of the stroma and can be delineated by the characteristic white burns that result from diagnostic application of argon laser photocoagulation (231). In one case with a penetrating foreign body, the membrane had a gelatinous appearance, which by histology revealed goblet cells and mucinous material (228). Gonioscopy often reveals peripheral anterior synechiae. Cytologic evaluation of an aqueous aspirate has been described as a diagnostic aid (232, 233), although the clinical features are usually sufficient to establish the diagnosis.

Mechanisms of Ingrowth and Glaucoma

A wound leak is generally felt to be the initial factor leading to epithelial ingrowth and is frequently seen at the time of diagnosis (231, 234, 235). Reports differ as to whether the condition is more likely to occur with a fornix-based conjunctival flap during cataract surgery as opposed to a limbus-based flap (223, 224). Ultrastructural studies show well-developed epithelium, resembling that of the bulbar conjunctiva, growing over posterior cornea, anterior chamber angle, and the iris (236–239). Mechanisms that have been proposed for the glaucoma associated with epithelial ingrowth include the growth of epithelium over the trabecular meshwork, areas of necrosis in the trabecular meshwork, peripheral anterior synechiae, pupillary block, and desquamated epithelium or mucinous material in the aqueous outflow system (223, 228, 236, 239, 240).

Management

When epithelial ingrowth is present, radical surgical intervention is usually required. Maumenee (231) described a technique of excising the fistula and involved iris and destroying the epithelium on the posterior cornea with cryotherapy. Subsequent modifications have included en bloc excision of the involved chamber angle tissues (241–244), excision of all involved tissue followed by keratoplasty (242, 243), and the use of vitrectomy instruments to remove involved iris and vitreous (235). In a case treated with filtering surgery and adjunctive subconjunctival 5-fluorouracil, the epithelial membrane grew rapidly to involve the entire posterior cornea when the injections were stopped (245). The implantation of a Molteno drainage device has also been shown to be effective palliative treatment for the associated glaucoma in these cases (246), and a double-plate Molteno shunt combined with penetrating keratoplasty provided IOP control and restoration of vision in two cases (247).

Fibrous Proliferation

Two forms of this condition have been described: fibrous ingrowth and retrocorneal membranes. *Fibrous ingrowth* is the result of inadequate wound closure after intraocular surgery or penetrating trauma. It has been reported to occur in approximately one-third of eyes enucleated after cataract extraction (248, 249). The hallmark of this form of fibrous proliferation is a break in the corneal endothelium and Descemet's membrane, which allows fibroblasts to enter the anterior chamber from subepithelial connective tissue (250), or from corneal or limbal stroma (251, 252). The fibrous tissue, which is often vascularized, may grow over the corneal endothelium, the anterior chamber angle, and iris, and into the vitreous cavity. Peripheral anterior synechiae are frequently seen in these cases (252). Clinically, the condition may be difficult to distinguish from epithelial ingrowth, although it is usually less progressive and less destructive. When glaucoma is present, it may either be the result of damage from the surgery or trauma or from the direct effect of the fibrous tissue in the anterior chamber angle. Treatment is generally confined to controlling the IOP, preferably with medications, although surgery, such as a cyclodestructive procedure, may be necessary.

Retrocorneal membranes may result from a variety of inflammatory or traumatic insults to the cornea. Descemet's membrane is typically intact and the fibrous tissue is believed to represent metaplastic endothelial cells (253). Glaucoma is not commonly associated, but may result from the initial insult.

Melanocyte Proliferation

A proliferation of melanocytes from the iris across the trabecular meshwork and posterior surface of the cornea has also been described as a mechanism of glaucoma following cataract extraction (254).

GLAUCOMAS ASSOCIATED WITH PENETRATING KERATOPLASTY

Incidence

Penetrating keratoplasty, utilizing modern techniques of tight wound closure, is complicated by a significant incidence of IOP elevation in both the early and late postoperative periods, although reported incidences vary considerably (255–257). One study revealed a 31% incidence of early increases in IOP and a 29% incidence of late (more than 3 months) increases (255), while another large survey had a 9% incidence of immediate postoperative glaucoma and an 18% incidence of chronic postkeratoplasty glaucoma (257). Late, chronic glaucoma is more likely to occur in those eyes that had an early postoperative pressure rise (256). Factors associated with glaucoma after penetrating keratoplasty include aphakia and preexisting glaucoma (255–258). In one series, the average maximum pressure in the first week was 24 mm Hg in phakic eyes, 40 mm Hg in aphakic eyes, and 50 mm Hg in those with combined cataract extraction and keratoplasty (259). When keratoplasty was combined with cataract extraction, the incidence of glaucoma was higher when an intracapsular extraction was used as compared to extracapsular surgery (260). The incidence of postkeratoplasty glaucoma is also higher following repeated penetrating keratoplasty (261). Glaucoma after corneal grafting is dangerous not only from the standpoint of glaucomatous optic atrophy, but also from the high incidence of associated graft failures (262).

Clinical Findings and Glaucoma Mechanisms

Early Postoperative Period

In some cases, the postoperative glaucoma after penetrating keratoplasty has the same pressure elevating mechanisms that are associated with other intraocular procedures, including uveitis, hemorrhage, pupillary block, and steroid-induced glaucoma (263). However, additional mechanisms of glaucoma occur early in the postoperative period, which are unique to eyes having undergone penetrating keratoplasty, especially when aphakia is also present. Two such mechanisms have been postulated.

COLLAPSE OF THE TRABECULAR MESHWORK. Collapse of the trabecular meshwork may result from the loss of anterior support due to the incision in Descemet's membrane, which may be compounded in the aphakic eye by a reduction in posterior support from the loss of zonular tension (264, 265). This hypothesis is felt to be supported by the observation that through-and-through suturing in one study was associated with better facility of outflow in autopsy eyes (264) and lower early postoperative IOP, as compared to eyes with conventional suturing (265). Other surgeons, however, reported less postoperative pressure rise with superficial sutures, which they believed prevented angle distortion (266).

COMPRESSION OF THE ANTERIOR CHAMBER ANGLE. Compression of the anterior chamber angle may be caused by the conventional techniques of penetrating keratoplasty, causing an early postoperative IOP rise as well as subsequent chronic glaucoma due to peripheral anterior synechiae (266, 267). Modified techniques that may help to avoid this complication are discussed under Management.

Late Postoperative Period

Gradual flattening of the anterior chamber several months after aphakic keratoplasty has been described (268). This phenomenon appears to be related to an intact anterior vitreous face, and prophylactic vitrectomy has been suggested to avoid this complication. Intraocular pressure elevation may also occur in association with graft rejection, which may require long-term steroid and antiglaucoma therapy (269). The pigment dispersion syndrome may also be seen with pseudophakic corneal transplant, which has the unique feature of an inferior linear pigmented endothelial line and which must not be confused with an allograft reaction (270). Another late-developing glaucoma occurs after keratoplasty for congenitally opaque corneas (271). It is not associated with peripheral anterior synechiae, and the mechanism is unknown. Other forms of late-onset glaucoma may be due to peripheral anterior synechiae, steroid-induced glaucoma (263), and epithelial ingrowth (229, 272).

Management

Preventative Measures

Based on a mathematical model, it has been postulated that these factors may minimize angle compression and also improve trabecular support: (a) a donor graft that is larger than the recipient trephine; (b) looser or shorter suture bites to minimize tissue compression; (c) smaller trephine size; (d) a thinner peripheral host cornea; and (e) a larger host corneal diameter (267, 273). Reports are conflicting as to whether an oversized corneal donor graft improves outflow and reduces postkeratoplasty glaucoma. A perfusion study with autopsy eyes did not reveal an improvement in outflow (274), and the use of 0.5-mm oversized grafts in one clinical series did not afford any protection against postoperative glaucoma (275). However, other clinical studies indicate that oversized grafts are associated with deeper anterior chamber depths (276), a lower incidence of progressive angle closure (277), and significantly lower postoperative pressures as compared to eyes with same sized grafts (278, 279). Oversized grafts, however, are contraindicated in treating keratoconus since they cause a significant increase in myopia (280). Another technique to prevent postkeratoplasty angle-closure glaucoma is the placement of sutures near the pupillary portion of a flaccid iris to create a taut iris (281). It has also been emphasized that glaucoma following keratoplasty can be minimized by using meticulous wound closure, and extensive postoperative steroids (282) (with caution for steroid-responsive patients).

Treatment of Glaucoma

MEDICAL THERAPY. Medical therapy should be tried first, unless a specific, treatable condition, such as pupillary block, is apparent. However attempts to alter the early postoperative pressure rise are frequently unsuccessful. Carbonic anhydrase inhibitors were not found to be significantly efficacious in this situation (283, 284), although they may be useful in treating the chronic glaucoma. Reported results with timolol have been conflicting (266, 284), although it does appear to have some value, especially in controlling chronic glaucoma after keratoplasty (263). Apraclonidine may be effective in some patients in the early, and possibly in the late, course. Hyperosmotic agents may be useful for the temporary control of extreme pressure elevation in the early post-operative period (283). Miotics and epinephrine may also occasionally be of value.

SURGICAL THERAPY. Surgical therapy is indicated when either the optic nerve head or the graft is threatened by a persistent elevation of IOP. No glaucoma operation has been found to be entirely suitable for controlling IOP and preserving graft clarity. Cyclodialysis was successful in only 22 of 100 such cases in one study (285), and another investigation found a 30% incidence of graft failure after any intraocular procedure (286). When penetrating keratoplasty was performed after trabeculectomy in one series, the 5-year probability of maintaining IOP control and a clear graft was only 0.27, which increased to 0.5 in another series of combined trabeculectomy and penetrating keratoplasty (287). Implantation of a Molteno drainage tube achieved IOP control of 21 mm Hg or less with one or more procedures in a series of 17 eyes, although seven had allograft rejections (288), while another series of drainage tubes implants had a final IOP below 18 mm Hg in 96%, but graft failure occurred in 42% (289). Cyclocryotherapy was once the most commonly used surgical procedure for glaucoma following penetrating keratoplasty (290), although the high incidence of serious complications limits its usefulness. Transscleral cyclophotocoagulation has largely replaced cyclocryotherapy as the cyclodestructive procedure of choice. However, in one series of 39 patients, 77% had a final IOP between 7 and 21 mm Hg, but 44% of those with clear grafts before cyclophotocoagulation had graft decompensation (291).

GLAUCOMAS ASSOCIATED WITH VITREOUS AND RETINAL PROCEDURES

Glaucomas Following Pars Plana Vitrectomy

Incidence

Intraocular pressure elevation is the most common major complication following pars plana vitreous surgery (292–297). The reported incidence of postoperative glaucoma ranges from 20% to 26% (294–296). In a prospective study of 222 cases, an IOP rise of 5–22 mm Hg during the first 48 hours occurred in 61.3% of eyes, with a 30 mm Hg rise in 35.6% (297).

Clinical Findings and Glaucoma Mechanisms

Many of the factors that lead to IOP elevation after pars plana vitrectomy and the management of these conditions were considered in other chapters. It may be helpful to review these various mechanisms according to the time frame in which they occur after vitreous surgery:

FIRST DAY. *Air,* or long-acting gases such as *sulfur hexafluoride* and *perfluorocarbons* (perfluoropropane and perfluoroethane), are occasionally injected into the vitreous cavity to tamponade the retina. The expansion of these gases during the early postoperative period not uncommonly leads to significant IOP elevation (294–301). Perfluorocarbons are capable of greater expansion and longevity than sulfur hexafluoride (302). In one study of 10 patients receiving 0.3 ml perfluoropropane, all eyes had an immediate IOP rise, which was sufficient in four eyes to collapse the central retinal artery (301). However, the pressure fell to baseline in 30–60 minutes and did not rise again for the subsequent 5 days.

Monitoring of IOP in the early postoperative period is important when using any long-acting gas and attention must be given to the tonometer used. Studies with living rabbit and enucleated human eyes indicate that the Schiøtz tonometer gives falsely low readings (303, 304), which is apparently due to low scleral rigidity (305). Pneumatic tonometry also underestimates IOP in gas-filled human autopsy eyes, while Perkins applanation tonometry gave the most accurate readings when using a mercury manometer as a reference standard (304). In a clinical study of 84 gas-filled eyes, the Tono-Pen gave pressure readings that were comparable to those obtained by Goldmann applanation tonometry, while pneumatic tonometry again underestimated the IOP (306).

Occasionally, it is necessary to remove a portion of the gas to relieve extremely high IOPs (294). Patients with a gas-filled eye should be cautioned regarding air travel, although expansion of a 0.6-ml bubble during ascent is usually compensated for by accelerated aqueous outflow without a significant IOP rise (307, 308). If the patient does notice pain or dimness of vision, the pilot should be asked to adjust the altitude to the next flight level (308). On descent, the eye may become hypotonus, and drugs which reduce aqueous production should be avoided, since they may prolong the hypotony, leading to uveal effusion (308).

Another class of agents, heavier-than-water perfluorocarbon liquids, can be used to hydrokinetically manipulate the retina, remove dislocated intraocular lenses and lens fragments, and as short-term tamponade. One of these, *perfluoroperhydrophenanthrene* (Vitreon), was associated with chronically elevated IOP in 11% of cases (309). The mechanism of the associated glaucoma appears to be angle closure (310).

Severe choroidal and ciliary body *hemorrhage,* the equivalent of an expulsive hemorrhage in open-eye surgery, can also cause angle closure glaucoma in the immediate postoperative period (295).

FIRST WEEK. Intraocular pressure elevation during this period is most likely due to one of the following, all of which are discussed in other chapters: (a) hyphema, ghost cells, or hemolytic glaucoma (Chapter 21); (b) retained lens material with phacolytic glaucoma (Chapter 15); (c) uveitis (Chapter 19); and (d) preexisting glaucoma. Yet another cause of IOP elevation in the early postvitrectomy period is *fibrin pupillary block* (311, 312). This has been successfully treated by making holes in the fibrin pupillary membrane with argon laser (311) and by the intracameral injection of recombinant tissue plasminogen activator to dissolve the fibrin clot (312).

TWO TO FOUR WEEKS POSTOPERATIVELY. Two to four weeks postoperatively, the cause of newly developed glaucoma is most often *neovascular glaucoma,* which is discussed in Chapter 16.

Silicone oil is occasionally used as a retinal tamponade in unusually difficult vitreoretinal procedures. The reported frequencies with which this technique is associated with postoperative IOP elevation varies widely among studies from 5% to 50% (313–320), while one series showed no influence of silicone or ocular tension (321). This discrepancy may relate to the numerous variables induced by the intraocular silicone, as well as the underlying disease of the eye, which may reduce both aqueous outflow and inflow, with the resulting IOP representing a balance of the two. Most studies, however, suggest that a high percentage of patients do have a transient postoperative pressure rise, with a small number retaining chronic glaucoma.

Mechanisms of IOP elevation that are directly attributable to the silicone include pupillary block (322–325) and silicone oil in the anterior chamber (323, 325, 326–328). Histologic studies have shown obstruction of the trabecular meshwork by minute silicone bubbles, pigmented cells, and silicone-laden macrophages (329, 330). However, these findings are not always associated with glaucoma. In one study of eyes with emulsified silicone oil in the anterior chamber, new glaucoma developed in 10% (327). The absence of glaucoma in other cases may be due to the pressure lowering effect of ciliary body detachment by cyclitic membranes (315) or total retinal detachments (331). Fibrous tissue has been shown to form around silicone vesicles, the retraction of which may lead to these detachments (331).

An iridectomy may relieve not only the pupillary block mechanism, but also some cases of open angle glaucoma, by allowing the silicone to fall back into the vitreous cavity (322–325). Since the silicone oil rises to the top of the eye, the iridectomy should be placed inferiorly, and this should be a standard part of all vitreoretinal procedures that include use of silicone oil. It has been suggested, however, that the iridectomy should be placed peripherally and be no larger than 2 mm, since a larger, more centrally located inferior iridectomy may allow silicone oil to enter the anterior chamber, creating a form of reverse pupillary block with a deep anterior chamber (328). When the iridectomy does not relieve the chronic IOP elevation, antiglaucoma medications may be adequate, while other patients may require surgical intervention, including removal of the silicone oil, a drainage implant device, or cyclodestructive procedure (319).

Glaucomas Following Scleral Buckling Procedures

Scleral buckling procedures are reported to cause a transient shallowing of the anterior chamber with elevation of the IOP in 4–7% of the cases (332). However, this is frequently asymptomatic and may go undetected unless slitlamp biomicroscopy and tonometry are performed in the early postoperative period. Experimental studies with monkeys suggest that occlusion of the vortex veins by an encircling band or sectoral scleral indentation causes congestion and forward rotation of the ciliary body with subsequent shallowing of the anterior segment (333). The same study showed that occlusion of the vortex veins also caused the ciliary processes to produce a protein-rich aqueous, which might further reduce outflow (333). These changes in the early postoperative period rarely lead to serious sequelae. In fact, many eyes have reduced IOP months after retinal detachment surgery, which is due to a decrease in aqueous production (334). However, peripheral anterior synechiae may develop with subsequent chronic glaucoma. The physician must be alert for this since reduced scleral rigidity in these patients may give falsely low IOP readings, especially with indentation tonometry (335).

Treatment of angle closure following scleral buckling includes atropine to relieve ciliary muscle spasm and corticosteroids to reduce the inflammation and prevent synechia formation. Carbonic anhydrase inhibitors, β-blockers, α_2-agonists, and epinephrine compounds may also be used when necessary for temporary pressure control. When surgical intervention is required, drainage of suprachoroidal fluid is usually the procedure of choice. A peripheral iridectomy is rarely of value in these cases.

Scleral buckling surgery has also been shown to cause marked intraoperative IOP elevations. One study, using a pars plana infusion cannula attached to an electronic pressure transducer, documented pressures up to 210 mm Hg during scleral depression and cryopexy, although the long-term consequences of these pressure elevations are not known (336). Scleral buckling also may decrease ocular blood flow due to decreased ophthalmic perfusion pressure (337).

Glaucomas Following Retinal Photocoagulation

An elevated IOP may follow extensive xenon or laser photocoagulation of the retina (338–340). In many cases, the anterior chamber angle remains open, and the mechanism of pressure elevation in these eyes is unknown. Other patients will have a closed angle either initially or later in the course of the pressure elevation. The mechanism of angle closure is felt to be either swelling of the ciliary body (338) or an outpouring of fluid from the choroid to the vitreous with subsequent forward displacement of the lens-iris diaphragm (338). The condition is temporary, with normal or slightly reduced pressures having been recorded after 1 month (341), although an analysis of data from the Diabetic Retinopathy Study did not support the belief that panretinal photocoagulation may reduce IOP (342). Pretreatment with apraclonidine reduced the incidence of IOP elevations greater than 6 mm Hg during the first 3 hours after laser surgery, as compared to placebo drops (25% vs. 32%, respectively), although the difference was not statistically significant (343). The pressure rise should be managed medically in the same manner described for the early pressure rise and shallow anterior chamber after scleral buckling.

SUMMARY

Malignant, or ciliary block, glaucoma occurs most often as a complication of incisional surgery for angle-closure glaucoma. The mechanism appears to be a posterior diversion of aqueous, leading to a collapse of the anterior chamber from forward vitreous displacement. Atropine is the mainstay of the medical therapy, although about half of the patients require surgical intervention. Another group of procedures that may be complicated by IOP elevation is cataract surgery. Causes of increased pressure during the early postoperative period include inflammation, hemorrhage, pigment dispersion, anterior chamber angle distortion, angle closure, vitreous in the anterior chamber, and the use of sodium hyaluronate. Chronic glaucoma following cataract surgery may result from peripheral anterior synechiae or trabecular meshwork damage. The implantation of an intraocular lens may induce some additional mechanisms of glaucoma, associated with pupillary block, inflammation, hemorrhage, or pigment dispersion. Discission of the posterior lens capsule with a Nd:YAG laser is yet another cause of IOP elevation in association with cataract surgery. Epithelial ingrowth and other cellular proliferations in the anterior chamber may be the mechanism of glaucoma after anterior segment incisional procedures, as well as some forms of trauma. Penetrating keratoplasty may be complicated by associated glaucoma, with the common glaucoma mechanism being angle closure. Vitreoretinal procedures, including vitrectomy, the intravitreal injection of gas or silicone oil, scleral buckling, and retinal photocoagulation, may also be associated with postoperative IOP elevation.

REFERENCES

1. von Graefe, A: Beitrage zur pathologie und therapie des glaucoms. Arch Fur Ophthalmol 15:108, 1869.
2. Chandler, PA, Simmons, RJ, Grant, WM: Malignant glaucoma. Medical and surgical treatment. Am J Ophthalmol 66:495, 1968.
3. Simmons, RJ: Malignant glaucoma. Br J Ophthalmol 56:263, 1972.
4. Weiss, DI, Shaffer, RN: Ciliary block (malignant) glaucoma. Trans Am Acad Ophthalmol Otol 76:450, 1972.
5. Shaffer, RN, Hoskins, HD Jr: Ciliary block (malignant) glaucoma. Ophthalmology 85:215, 1978.
6. Levene, R: A new concept of malignant glaucoma. Arch Ophthalmol 87:497, 1972.
7. Lowe, RF: Malignant glaucoma related to primary angle closure glaucoma. Aust J Ophthalmol 7:11, 1979.
8. Cashwell, LF, Martin, TJ: Malignant glaucoma after laser iridotomy. Ophthalmology 99:651, 1992.
9. Aminlari, A, Sassani, JW: Simultaneous bilateral malignant glaucoma following laser iridotomy. Graefes Arch Clin Exp Ophthalmol 231:12, 1993.
10. Saunders, PPR, Douglas, GR, Feldman, F, Stein, RM: Bilateral malignant glaucoma. Can J Ophthalmol 27:19, 1992.
11. Hanish, SJ, Lamberg, RL, Gordon, JM: Malignant glaucoma following cataract extraction and intraocular lens implant. Ophthalmic Surg 13:713, 1982.
12. Tomey, KF, Senft, SH, Antonios, SR, et al: Aqueous misdirection and flat chamber after posterior chamber implants with and without trabeculectomy. Arch Ophthalmol 105:770, 1987.
13. Duy, TP, Wollensak, J: Ciliary block (malignant) glaucoma following posterior chamber lens implantation. Ophthalmic Surg 18:741, 1987.
14. Dickens, CJ, Shaffer, RN: The medical treatment of ciliary block glaucoma after extracapsular cataract extraction. Am J Ophthalmol 103:237, 1987.
15. Risco, JM, Tomey, KF, Perkins, TW: Laser capsulotomy through intraocular lens positioning holes in anterior aqueous misdirection. Arch Ophthalmol 107:1569, 1989.
16. Reed, JE, Thomas, JV, Lytle, RA, Simmons, RJ: Malignant glaucoma induced by an intraocular lens. Ophthalmic Surg 21:177, 1990.
17. Vajpayee, RB, Talwar, D: Pseudophakic malignant glaucoma in a child. Ophthalmic Surg 22:266, 1991.
18. Pecora, JL: Malignant glaucoma worsened by miotics in a postoperative angle-closure glaucoma patient. Ann Ophthalmol 11:1412, 1979.
19. Rieser, JC, Schwartz, B: Miotic-induced malignant glaucoma. Arch Ophthalmol 87:706, 1972.
20. Merritt, JC: Malignant glaucoma induced by miotics postoperatively in open-angle glaucoma. Arch Ophthalmol 95:1988, 1977.
21. Jones, BR: Principles in the management of oculomycosis. Trans Am Acad Ophthalmol Otol 79:15, 1975.
22. Lass, JH, Thoft, RA, Bellows, AR, Slansky, HH: Exogenous nocardia asteroids endophthalmitis associated with malignant glaucoma. Ann Ophthalmol 13:317, 1981.
23. Weiss, IS, Deiter, PD: Malignant glaucoma syndrome following retinal detachment surgery. Ann Ophthalmol 6:1099, 1974.
24. Kushner, BJ: Ciliary block glaucoma in retinopathy of prematurity. Arch Ophthalmol 100:1078, 1982.
25. Jacoby, B, Reed, JW, Cashwell, LF: Malignant glaucoma in a patient with Down's syndrome and corneal hydrops. Am J Ophthalmol 110:434, 1990.
26. Schwartz, AL, Anderson, DR: "Malignant glaucoma" in an eye with no antecedent operation or miotics. Arch Ophthalmol 93:379, 1975.
27. Shaffer, RN: The role of vitreous detachment in aphakic and malignant glaucoma. Trans Am Acad Ophthalmol Otol 58:217, 1954.
28. Buschmann, W, Linnert, D: Echography of the vitreous body in case of aphakia and malignant aphakic glaucoma. Klin Monatsbl Augenheilkd 168:453, 1976.
29. Lippas, J: Mechanics and treatment of malignant glaucoma and the problem of a flat anterior chamber. Am J Ophthalmol 57:620, 1964.
30. Tello, C, Chi, T, Shepps, G, et al: Ultrasound biomicroscopy in pseudophakic malignant glaucoma. Ophthalmology 100:1330, 1993.
31. Trope, GE, Pavlin, CJ, Bau, A, et al: Malignant glaucoma. Clinical and ultrasound biomicroscopic features. Ophthalmology 101:1030, 1994.
32. Fatt, I: Hydraulic flow conductivity of the vitreous gel. Invest Ophthalmol Vis Sci 16:555, 1977.
33. Epstein, DL, Hashimoto, JM, Anderson, PJ, Grant, WM: Experimental perfusions through the anterior and vitreous chambers with possible relationships to malignant glaucoma. Am J Ophthalmol 88:1078, 1979.
34. Quigley, HA: Malignant glaucoma and fluid flow rate. Am J Ophthalmol 89:879, 1980.

35. Chandler, PA, Grant, WM: Mydriatic-cycloplegic treatment in malignant glaucoma. Arch Ophthalmol 68:353, 1962.

36. Wright, MM, Grajewski, AL: Measurement of intraocular pressure with a flat anterior chamber. Ophthalmology 98:1854, 1991.

37. Weiss, DI, Shaffer, RN, Harrington, DO: Treatment of malignant glaucoma with intravenous mannitol infusion. Medical reformation of the anterior chamber by means of an osmotic agent: a preliminary report. Arch Ophthalmol 69:154, 1963.

38. Herschler, J: Laser shrinkage of the ciliary processes. A treatment for malignant (ciliary block) glaucoma. Ophthalmology 87:1155, 1980.

39. Weber, PA, Henry, MA, Kapetansky, FM, Lohman, LF: Argon laser treatment of the ciliary processes in aphakic glaucoma with flat anterior chamber. Am J Ophthalmol 97:82, 1984.

40. Epstein, DL, Steinert, RF, Puliafito, CA: Neodymium-YAG laser therapy to the anterior hyaloid in aphakic malignant (ciliovitreal block) glaucoma. Am J Ophthalmol 98:137, 1984.

41. Melamed, S, Ashkenazi, I, Blumenthal, M: Nd-YAG laser hyaloidotomy for malignant glaucoma following one-piece 7-mm intraocular lens implantation. Br J Ophthalmol 75:501, 1991.

42. Halkias, A, Magauran, DM, Joyce, M: Ciliary block (malignant) glaucoma after cataract extraction with lens implant treated with YAG laser capsulotomy and anterior hyaloidotomy. Br J Ophthalmol 76:569, 1992.

43. Little, BC: Treatment of aphakic malignant glaucoma using Nd:YAG laser posterior capsulotomy. Br J Ophthalmol 78:499, 1994.

44. Sugar, HS: Bilateral aphakic malignant glaucoma. Arch Ophthalmol 87:347, 1972.

45. Koerner, FH: Anterior pars plana vitrectomy in ciliary and iris block glaucoma. Graefes Arch Clin Exp Klin Exp Ophthal 214:119, 1980.

46. Boke, W, Teichmann, K-D, Junge, W: Experiences with ciliary block ("malignant") glaucoma. Klin Monatsbl Augenheilkd 177:407, 1980.

47. Momeda, S, Hayashi, H, Oshima, K: Anterior pars plana vitrectomy for phakic malignant glaucoma. Jpn J Ophthalmol 27:73, 1983.

48. Byrnes, GA, Leen, MM, Wong, TP, Benson, WE: Vitrectomy for ciliary block (malignant) glaucoma. Ophthalmology 102:1308, 1995.

49. Bastian, A, Kohler, U: Therapy and functional results in malignant glaucoma. Klin Monatsbl Augenheilkd 161:316, 1972.

50. Benedikt, O: A new operative method for the treatment of malignant glaucoma. Klin Monatsbl Augenheilkd 170:665, 1977.

51. Chandler, PA: A new operation for malignant glaucoma: a preliminary report. Trans Am Ophthalmol Soc 62:408, 1964.

52. Galin, MA, Baras, I, Perry, R: Intraocular pressure following cataract extraction. Arch Ophthalmol 66:80, 1961.

53. Lee, P-F, Trotter, RR: Tonographic and gonioscopic studies before and after cataract extraction. Arch Ophthalmol 58:407, 1957.

54. Tuberville, A, Tomoda, T, Nissenkorn, I, Wood, TO: Postsurgical intraocular pressure elevation. Am Intra-Ocular Implant Soc J 9:309, 1983.

55. Rich, WJ, Radtke, ND, Cohan, BE: Early ocular hypertension after cataract extraction. Br J Ophthalmol 58:725, 1974.

56. Racz, P, Szilvassy, I, Pinter, E: Findings in the anterior chamber angle after cataract extraction without complication. Klin Monatsbl Augenheilkd 164:218, 1974.

57. Hansen, TE, Naeser, K, Nilsen, NE: Intraocular pressure 2½ years after extracapsular cataract extraction and sulcus implantation of posterior chamber intraocular lens. Acta Ophthalmol 69:225, 1991.

58. Hansen, MH, Gyldenkerne, GJ, Otland, NW, et al: Intraocular pressure seven years after extracapsular cataract extraction and sulcus implantation of a posterior chamber intraocular lens. J Cataract Refract Surg 21:676, 1995.

59. Radius, RL, Schultz, K, Sobocinski, K, et al: Pseudophakia and intraocular pressure. Am J Ophthalmol 97:738, 1984.

60. Gross, JG, Meyer, DR, Robin, AL, et al: Increased intraocular pressure in the immediate postoperative period after extracapsular cataract extraction. Am J Ophthalmol 105:466, 1988.

61. Kooner, KS, Dulaney, DD, Zimmerman, TJ: Intraocular pressure following extracapsular cataract extraction and posterior chamber intraocular lens implantation. Ophthalmic Surg 19:471, 1988.

62. David, R, Tessler, Z, Yagev, R, et al: Persistently raised intraocular pressure following extracapsular cataract extraction. Br J Ophthalmol 74:272, 1990.

63. Kooner, KS, Dulaney, DD, Zimmerman, TJ: Intraocular pressure following secondary anterior chamber lens implantation. Ophthalmic Surg 19:274, 1988.

64. Onali, T, Raitta, C: Extracapsular cataract extraction and posterior chamber lens implantation in controlled open-angle glaucoma. Ophthalmic Surg 22:381, 1991.

65. Vu, MT, Shields, MB: The early postoperative pressure course in glaucoma patients following cataract surgery. Ophthalmic Surg 19:467, 1988.

66. Handa, J, Henry, JC, Krupin, T, Keates, E: Extracapsular cataract extraction with posterior chamber lens implantation in patients with glaucoma. Arch Ophthalmol 105:765, 1987.

67. Kooner, KS, Dulaney, DD, Zimmerman, TJ: Intraocular pressure following ECCE and IOL implantation in patients with glaucoma. Ophthalmic Surg 19:570, 1988.

68. Kirsch, RE, Levine, O, Singer, JA: Ridge at internal edge of cataract incision. Arch Ophthalmol 94:2098, 1976.

69. Kirsch, RE, Levine, O, Singer, JA: Further studies on the ridge at the internal edge of the cataract incision. Trans Am Acad Ophthalmol Otol 83:224, 1977.

70. Campbell, DG, Grant, WM: Trabecular deformation and reduction of outflow facility due to cataract and penetrating keratoplasty sutures. Invest Ophthalmol Vis Sci (Suppl):126, 1977.

71. Rothkoff, L, Biedner, B, Blumenthal, M: The effect of corneal section on early increased intraocular pressure after cataract extraction. Am J Ophthalmol 85:337, 1978.

72. Holmberg, ÅS, Philipson, BT: Sodium hyaluronate in cataract surgery. I. Report on the use of Healon in two different types of intracapsular cataract surgery. Ophthalmology 91:45, 1984.

73. Holmberg ÅS, Philipson, BT: Sodium hyaluronate in cataract surgery. II. Report on the use of Healon in extracapsular cataract surgery using phacoemulsification. Ophthalmology 91:53, 1984.

74. Binkhorst, CD: Inflammation and intraocular pressure after the use of Healon in intraocular lens surgery. Am Intra-Ocular Implant Soc J 6:340, 1980.

75. Pape, LG: Intracapsular and extracapsular technique of lens implantation with Healon. Am Intra-Ocular Implant Soc J 6:342, 1980.

76. Ruusuvaara, P, Pajari, S, Setala, K: Effect of sodium hyaluronate on immediate postoperative intraocular pressure after extracapsular cataract extraction and IOL implantation. Acta Ophthalmol 68:721, 1990.

77. Anmarkrud, N, Bergaust, B, Bulie, T: The effect of Healon and timolol on early postoperative intraocular pressure after extracapsular cataract extraction with implantation of a posterior chamber lens. Acta Ophthalmol 70:96, 1992.

78. Mac Rae, SM, Edelhauser, HF, Hyndiuk, RA, et al: The effects of sodium hyaluronate, chondroitin sulfate, and methylcellulose on the corneal endothelium and intraocular pressure. Am J Ophthalmol 95:332, 1983.

79. Berson, FG, Patterson, MM, Epstein, DL: Obstruction of aqueous outflow by sodium hyaluronate in enucleated human eyes. Am J Ophthalmol 95:668, 1983.

80. Stamper, RL, DiLoreto, D, Schacknow, P: Effect of intraocular aspiration of sodium hyaluronate on postoperative intraocular pressure. Ophthalmic Surg 21:486, 1990.

81. Tsurimaki, Y, Shimizu, H: Effects of residual sodium hyaluronate on postsurgical blood-aqueous barrier. Jpn J Ophthalmol 35:446, 1991.

82. Harrison, SE, Soll, DB, Shayegan, M, Clinch, T: Chondroitin sulfate: a new and effective protective agent for intraocular lens insertion. Ophthalmology 89:1254, 1982.

83. Alpar, JJ, Alpar, AJ, Baca, J, Chapman, D: Comparison of Healon and Viscoat in cataract extraction and intraocular lens implantation. Ophthalmic Surg 19:636, 1988

84. Burke, S, Sugar, J, Farber, MD: Comparison of the effects of two viscoelastic agents, Healon and Viscoat, on postoperative intraocular pressure after penetrating keratoplasty. Ophthalmic Surg 21:821, 1990.

85. Caporossi, A, Baiocchi, S, Sforzi, C, Frezzotti, R: Healon GV versus Healon in demanding cataract surgery. J Cataract Refract Surg 21:710, 1995.

86. Aron-Rosa, D, Cohn, HC, Aron, J-J, Bouquety, C: Methylcellulose instead of Healon in extracapsular surgery with intraocular lens implantation. Ophthalmology 90:1235, 1983.

87. Bigar, F, Gloor, B, Schimmelpfennig, B, Thumm, D: Tolerance and safety of intraocular use of 2% hydroxypropylymethylcellulose. Klin Monatsbl Augenheil 193:21, 1988.

88. Storr-Paulsen, A: Analysis of the short-term effect of two viscoelastic agents on the intraocular pressure after extracapsular cataract extraction. Sodium hyaluronate 1% vs hydroxypropyl methylcellulose 2%. Acta Ophthalmol 71:173, 1993.

89. Mortimer, C, Sutton, H, Henderson, C: Efficacy of polyacrylamide vs sodium hyaluronate in cataract surgery. Can J Ophthalmol 26:144, 1991.

90. Laflamme, MY, Swieca, R: A prospective comparison of 4% polyacrylamide (Orcolon) and 1% sodium hyaluoronate (Healon) in cataract and intraocular lens implant surgery. Can J Ophthalmol 25:229, 1990.

91. Siegel, MJ, Spiro, HJ, Miller, JA, Siegel, LI: Secondary glaucoma and uveitis associated with Orcolon. Arch Ophthalmol 109:1496, 1991.

92. Herrington, RG, Ball, SF, Updegraff, SA: Delayed sustained increase in intraocular pressure secondary to the use of polyacrylamide gel (Orcolon) in the anterior chamber. Ophthalmic Surg 24:658, 1993.

93. Kaufman, PL, Lütjen-Drecoll, E, Hubbard, WC, Erickson, KA: Obstruction of aqueous humor outflow by cross-linked polyacrylamide microgels in bovine, monkey, and human eyes. Ophthalmology 101:1672, 1994.

94. Hutton, WL, Snyder, WB, Vaiser, A: Management of surgically dislocated intravitreal lens fragments by pars plana vitrectomy. Ophthalmology 85:176, 1978.

95. Layden, WE: Pseudophakia and glaucoma. Ophthalmology 89:875, 1982.

96. Ellingson, FT: The uveitis-glaucoma-hyphema syndrome associated with the Mark-VII Choyce anterior chamber lens implant. Am Intra-Ocular Implant Soc J 4:50, 1978.

97. Keates, RH, Ehrlich, DR: "Lenses of chance" complications of anterior chamber implants. Ophthalmology 85:408, 1978.

98. Miller, D, Doane, MG: High-speed photographic evaluation of intraocular lens movements. Am J Ophthalmol 97:752, 1984.

99. Sievers, H, von Domarus, D: Foreign-body reaction against intraocular lenses. Am J Ophthalmol 97:743, 1984.

100. Hagan, JC: A comparative study of the 91Z and other anterior chamber intraocular lenses. Am Intra-Ocular Implant Soc J 10:324, 1984.

101. Liesegang, TJ, Bourne, WM, Brubaker, RF: The effect of cataract surgery on the blood-aqueous barrier. Ophthalmology 91:399, 1984.

102. Sawa, M, Sakanishi, Y, Shimizu, H: Fluorophotometric study of anterior segment barrier functions after extracapsular cataract extraction and posterior chamber intraocular lens implantation. Am J Ophthalmol 97:197, 1984.

103. Miyake, K, Asakura, M, Kobayashi, H: Effect of intraocular lens fixation of the blood-aqueous barrier. Am J Ophthalmol 98:451, 1984.

104. Percival, SPB, Das, SK: UGH syndrome after posterior chamber lens implantation. Am Intra-Ocular Implant Soc J 9:200, 1983.

105. Bene, C, Hutchins, R, Kranias, G: Cataract wound neovascularization. An often overlooked cause of vitreous hemorrhage. Ophthalmology 96:50, 1989.

106. Wiley, RG, Neville, RG, Martin, WG: Late postoperative hemorrhage following intracapsular cataract extraction with the IOLAB 91Z anterior chamber lens. Am Intra-Ocular Implant Soc J 9:466, 1983.

107. Magargal, LE, Goldberg, RE, Uram, M, et al: Recurrent microhyphema in the pseudophakic eye. Ophthalmology 90:1231, 1983.

108. Pazandak, B, Johnson, S, Kratz, R, Faulkner, GD: Recurrent intraocular hemorrhage associated with posterior chamber lens implantation. Am Intra-Ocular Implant Soc J 9:327, 1983.

109. Johnson, SH, Kratz, RP, Olson, PF: Iris transillumination defect and microhyphema syndrome. Am Intra-Ocular Implant Soc J 10:425, 1984.

110. Apple, DJ, Craythorn, JM, Olson, RJ, et al: Anterior segment complications and neovascular glaucoma following implantation of a posterior chamber intraocular lens. Ophthalmology 91:403, 1984.

111. Summers, CG, Lindstrom, RL: Ghost cell glaucoma following lens implantation. Am Intra-Ocular Implant Soc J 9:429, 1983.

112. Woodhams, JT, Lester, JC: Pigmentary dispersion glaucoma secondary to posterior chamber intra-ocular lenses. Ann Ophthalmol 16:852, 1984.

113. Huber, C: The gray iris syndrome. An iatrogenic form of pigmentary glaucoma. Arch Ophthalmol 102:397, 1984.

114. Smith, JP: Pigmentary open-angle glaucoma secondary to posterior chamber intraocular lens implantation and erosion of the iris pigment epithelium. Am Intra-Ocular Implant Soc J 11:174, 1985.

115. Caplan, MB, Brown, RH, Love, LL: Pseudophakic pigmentary glaucoma. Am J Ophthalmol 105:320, 1988.

116. Grant, WM: Open-angle glaucoma associated with vitreous filling the anterior chamber. Trans Am Ophthalmol Soc 61:196, 1963.

117. Simmons, RJ: The vitreous in glaucoma. Trans Ophthalmol Soc UK 95:422, 1975.

118. Samples, JR, Van Buskirk, EM: Open-angle glaucoma associated with vitreous humor filling the anterior chamber. Am J Ophthalmol 102:759, 1986.

119. Chandler, PA: Glaucoma from pupillary block in aphakia. Arch Ophthalmol 67:14, 1962.

120. Chandler, PA: Glaucoma in aphakia. Trans Am Acad Ophthalmol Otol 67:483, 1963.

121. Chandler, PA: Surgery of congenital cataract. Trans Am Acad Ophthalmol Otol 72:341, 1968.

122. Zauberman, H, Yassur, Y, Sachs, U: Fluorescein pupillary flow in aphakics with intact and spontaneous openings of the vitreous face. Br J Ophthalmol 61:450, 1977.

123. Boke, W, Teichmann, KD: Differential diagnosis of postoperative glaucoma following iridectomy and filtering procedures. Klin Monatsbl Augenheilkd 177:545, 1980.

124. Van Buskirk, EM: Pupillary block after intraocular lens implantation. Am J Ophthalmol 95:55, 1983.

125. Shrader, CE, Belcher, CD III, Thomas, JV, et al: Pupillary and iridovitreal block in pseudophakic eyes. Ophthalmology 91:831, 1984.

126. Moses, L: Complications of rigid anterior chamber implants. Ophthalmology 91:819, 1984.

127. Werner, D, Kaback, M: Pseudophakic pupillary-block glaucoma. Br J Ophthalmol 61:329, 1977.

128. Kielar, RA, Stambaugh, JL: Pupillary block glaucoma following intraocular lens implantation. Ophthalmic Surg 13:647, 1982.

129. Cohen, JS, Osher, RH, Weber, P, Faulkner, JD: Complications of extracapsular cataract surgery. The indications and risks of peripheral iridectomy. Ophthalmology 91:826, 1984.

130. Willis, DA, Stewart, RH, Kimbrough, RL: Pupillary block associated with posterior chamber lenses. Ophthalmic Surg 16:108, 1985.

131. Samples, JR, Bellows, AR, Rosenquist, RC, et al: Pupillary block with posterior chamber intraocular lenses. Arch Ophthalmol 105:335, 1987.

132. Forman, JS, Ritch, R, Dunn, MW, Szmyd, L: Pupillary block following posterior chamber lens implantation. Ophthalmic Laser Ther 2:85, 1987.

133. Naveh, N, Wysenbeek, Y, Solomon, A, et al: Anterior capsule adherence to iris leading to pseudophakic pupillary block. Ophthalmic Surg 22:350, 1991.

134. Schulze, RR, Copeland, JR: Posterior chamber intraocular lens implantation without peripheral iridectomy. A preliminary report. Ophthalmic Surg 13:567, 1982.

135. Simel, PF: Posterior chamber implants without iridectomy. Am Intra-Ocular Implant Soc J 8:141, 1982.

136. Van Buskirk, EM: Late onset, progressive, peripheral anterior synechiae with posterior chamber intraocular lenses. Ophthalmic Surg 18:115, 1987.

137. Chrousos, GA, Parks, MM, O'Neill, JF: Incidence of chronic glaucoma, retinal detachment and secondary membrane surgery in pediatric aphakic patients. Ophthalmology 91:1238, 1984.

138. Egbert, JE, Wright, MM, Dahlhauser, KF, et al: A prospective study of ocular hypertension and glaucoma after pediatric cataract surgery. Ophthalmology 102:1098, 1995.

139. Simon, JW, Mehta, N, Simmons, ST, et al: Glaucoma after pediatric lensectomy/vitrectomy. Ophthalmology 98:670, 1991.

140. Asrani, SG, Wilensky, JT: Glaucoma after congenital cataract surgery. Ophthalmology 102:863, 1995.

141. Vajpayee, RB, Angra, SK, Titiyal, JS, et al: Pseudophakic pupillary-block glaucoma in children. Am J Ophthalmol 111:715, 1991.

142. Barraquer, J: Zonulolisis enzymatica. Ann Med Chir 34:148, 1958.

143. Kirsch, RE: Glaucoma following cataract extraction associated with use of alpha-chymotrypsin. Arch Ophthalmol 72:612, 1964.

144. Lantz, JM, Quigley, JH: Intraocular pressure after cataract extraction: effects of alpha-chymotrypsin. Can J Ophthalmol 8:339, 1973.

145. Kirsch, RE: Further studies on glaucoma following cataract extraction associated with the use of alpha-chymotrypsin. Trans Am Acad Ophthalmol Otol 69:1011, 1965.

146. Galin, MA, Barasch, KR, Harris, LS: Enzymatic zonulolysis and intraocular pressure. Am J Ophthalmol 61:690, 1966.

147. Jocson, VL: Tonography and gonioscopy: before and after cataract extraction with alpha-chymotrypsin. Am J Ophthalmol 60:318, 1965.

148. Kalvin, NH, Hamasaki, DI, Gass, JDM: Experimental glaucoma in monkeys. I. Relationship between intraocular pressure and cupping of the optic disc and cavernous atrophy of the optic nerve. Arch Ophthalmol 76:82, 1966.

149. Lessell, S, Kuwabara, T: Experimental alpha-chymotrypsin glaucoma. Arch Ophthalmol 81:853, 1969.

150. Anderson, DR: Experimental alpha-chymotrypsin glaucoma studied by scanning electron microscopy. Am J Ophthalmol 71:470, 1971.

151. Ley, AP, Holmberg, AS, Yamashita, T: Histology of zonulolysis with alpha-chymotrypsin employing light and electron microscopy. Am J Ophthalmol 49:67, 1960.

152. Anderson, DR: Scanning electron microscopy of zonulolysis by alpha-chymotrypsin. Am J Ophthalmol 71:619, 1971.

153. Barraquer, J, Rutlan, J: Enzymatic zonulolysis and postoperative ocular hypertension. Am J Ophthalmol 63:159, 1967.

154. Gombos, GM, Oliver, M: Cataract extraction with enzymatic zonulolysis in glaucomatous eyes. Am J Ophthalmol 64:68, 1968.

155. Kirsch, RE: Dose relationship of alpha-chymotrypsin in production of glaucoma after cataract extraction. Arch Ophthalmol 75:774, 1966.

156. Terry, AC, Stark, WJ, Maumenee, AE, Fagadau, W: Neodymium-YAG for posterior capsulotomy. Am J Ophthalmol 96:716, 1983.

157. Channell, MM, Beckman, H: Intraocular pressure changes after neodymium-YAG laser posterior capsulotomy. Arch Ophthalmol 102:1024, 1984.

158. Keates, RH, Steinert, RF, Puliafito, CA, Maxwell, SK: Long-term follow-up of Nd:YAG laser posterior capsulotomy. Am Intra-Ocular Implant Soc J 10:164, 1984.

159. Kurata, F, Krupin, T, Sinclair, S, Karp, L: Progressive glaucomatous visual field loss after neodymium-YAG laser capsulotomy. Am J Ophthalmol 98:632, 1984.

160. Vine, AK: Ocular hypertension following Nd:YAG laser capsulotomy: a potentially blinding complication. Ophthalmic Surg 15:283, 1984.

161. Richter, CU, Arzeno, G, Pappas, HR, et al: Intraocular pressure elevation following Nd:YAG laser posterior capsulotomy. Ophthalmology 92:636, 1985.

162. Flohr, MJ, Robin, AL, Kelley, JS: Early complications following Q-switched neodymium:YAG laser posterior capsulotomy. Ophthalmology 92:360, 1985.

163. Stark, WJ, Worthen, D, Holladay, JT, Murray, G: Neodymium:Yag lasers. An FDA report. Ophthalmology 92:209, 1985.

164. Ruderman, JM, Mitchell, PG, Kraff, M: Pupillary block following Nd:YAG laser capsulotomy. Ophthalmic Surg 14:418, 1983.

165. Shrader, CE, Belcher, CD III, Thomas, JV, Simmons, RJ: Acute glaucoma following Nd:YAG laser membranotomy. Ophthalmic Surg 14:1015, 1983.

166. Gimbel, HV, Van Westenbrugge, JA, Sanders, DR, Raanan, MG: Effect of sulcus vs capsular fixation on YAG-induced pressure rises following posterior capsulotomy. Arch Ophthalmol 108:1126, 1990.

167. Steinert, RF, Puliafito, CA, Kumar, SR, et al: Cystoid macular edema, retinal detachment, and glaucoma after Nd:YAG laser posterior capsulotomy. Am J Ophthalmol 112:373, 1991.

168. Fourman, S, Apisson, J: Late-onset elevation in intraocular pressure after Neodymium-YAG laser posterior capsulotomy. Arch Ophthalmol 109:511, 1991.

169. Schubert, HD: Vitreoretinal changes associated with rise in intraocular pressure after Nd:YAG capsulotomy. Ophthalmic Surg 18:19, 1987.

170. Wetzel, W: Ocular aqueous humor dynamics after photodisruptive laser surgery procedures. Ophthalmic Surg 25:298, 1994.

171. Schrems, W, Glaab-Schrems, E, Kreiglstein, GK: Rises in intraocular pressure in postcataract surgery with the Neodymium-YAG laser. Klin Monatsbl Augenheilk 187:14, 1985.

172. Mitchell, PG, Blair, NP, Deutsch, TA, Hershey, JM: The effect of neodymium:YAG laser shocks on the blood-aqueous barrier. Ophthalmology 94:488, 1987.

173. Krootila, K, Oksala, O, von Dickhoff, K, et al: Ocular irritative response to YAG laser capsulotomy in rabbits: release of calcitonin gene-related peptide and effects of methysergide. Curr Eye Res 11:307, 1992.

174. Van Der Sloot, D, Stilma, JS, Boen-Tan, TN, Bezemer, PD: Prevention of IOP-rise following Nd-YAG laser capsulotomy with topical Timolol and Indomethacin. Doc Ophthalmologica 70:209, 1989.

175. Migliori, ME, Beckman, H, Channell, MM: Intraocular pressure changes after neodymium-YAG laser capsulotomy in eyes pretreated with Timolol. Arch Ophthalmol 105:473, 1987.

176. Ladas, ID, Pavlopoulos, GP, Kokolakis, SN, Theodossiadis, GP: Prophylactic use of acetazolamide to prevent intraocular pressure elevation following Nd:YAG laser posterior capsulotomy. Br J Ophthalmol 77:136, 1993.

177. Pollack, IP, Brown, RH, Crandall, AS, et al: Prevention of the rise in intraocular pressure following neodymium-YAG posterior capsulotomy using topical 1% apraclonidine. Arch Ophthalmol 106:754, 1988.

178. Silverstone, DE, Brint, SF, Olander, KW, et al: Prophylactic use of apraclonidine for intraocular pressure increase after Nd:YAG capsulotomies. Am J Ophthalmol 113:401, 1992.

179. Cullom, RD Jr, Schwartz, LW: The effect of apraclonidine on the intraocular pressure of glaucoma patients following Nd:YAG laser posterior capsulotomy. Ophthalmic Surg 24:623, 1993.

180. Rosenberg, LF, Krupin, T, Ruderman, J, et al: Apraclonidine and anterior segment laser surgery. Comparison of 0.5% versus 1.0% apraclonidine for prevention of postoperative intraocular pressure rise. Ophthalmology 102:1312, 1995.

181. Khodadoust, AA, Arkfeld, DF, Caprioli, J, Sear, ML: Ocular effect of neodymium-YAG laser. Am J Ophthalmol 98:144, 1984.

182. Drews, RC: Anterior capsulotomy with the neodymium:YAG laser: results and opinions. Am Intra-Ocular Implant Soc J 11:240, 1985.

183. McDonnell, PJ, Quigley, HA, Maumenee, AE, et al: The Honan intraocular pressure reducer. An experimental study. Arch Ophthalmol 103:422, 1985.

184. Poleski, SA, Willis, WE: Angle-supported intraocular lenses: a goniophotographic study. Ophthalmology 91:838, 1984.

185. Rowsey, JJ, Gaylor, JR: Intraocular lens disasters. Peripheral anterior synechia. Ophthalmology 87:646, 1980.

186. Bömer, TG, Lagrèze, W-DA, Funk, J: Intraocular pressure rise after phacoemulsification with posterior chamber lens implantation: effect of prophylactic medication, wound closure, and surgeon's experience. Br J Ophthalmol 79:809, 1995.

187. Hollands, RH, Drance, SM, Schulzer, M: The effect of acetylcholine on early postoperative intraocular pressure. Am J Ophthalmol 103:749, 1987.

188. West, J, Burke, J, Cunliffe, I, Longstaff, S: Prevention of acute postoperative pressure rises in glaucoma patients undergoing cataract extraction with posterior chamber lens implant. Br J Ophthalmol 76:534, 1992.

189. Ruiz, RS, Rhem, MN, Prager, TC: Effects of carbachol and acetylcholine on intraocular pressure after cataract extraction. Am J Ophthalmol 107:7, 1989.

190. Hollands, RH, Drance, SM, Schulzer, M: The effect of intracameral carbachol on intraocular pressure after cataract extraction. Am J Ophthalmol 104:225, 1987.

191. Linn, DK, Zimmerman, TJ, Nardin, GF, et al: Effect of intracameral carbachol on intraocular pressure after cataract extraction. Am J Ophthalmol 107:133, 1989.

192. Wood, TO: Effect of carbachol on postoperative intraocular pressure. J Cataract Refract Surg 14:654, 1988.

193. Hollands, RH, Drance, SM, House, PH, Schulzer, M: Control of intraocular pressure after cataract extraction. Can J Ophthalmol 25: 128, 1990.

194. Wedrich, A, Menapace, R: The effect of intracameral acetylcholine and carbachol on intraocular pressure following cataract surgery. Klin Monatsbl Augenheilkd 200:644, 1992.

195. Hayreh, SS: Anterior ischemic optic neuropathy. IV. Occurrence after cataract extraction. Arch Ophthalmol 98:1410, 1980.

196. Biedner, B, Rothkoff, L, Blumenthal, M: The effect of acetazolamide on early increased intraocular pressure after cataract extraction. Am J Ophthalmol 83:565, 1977.

197. Bloomfield, S: Failure to prevent enzyme glaucoma. A negative report. Am J Ophthalmol 64:405, 1968.

198. Packer, AJ, Fraioli, AJ, Epstein, DL: The effect of timolol and acetazolamide on transient intraocular pressure elevation following cataract extraction with alpha-chymotrypsin. Ophthalmology 88:239, 1981.

199. Obstbaum, SA, Galin, MA: The effects of timolol on cataract extraction and intraocular pressure. Am J Ophthalmol 88:1017, 1979.

200. Haimann, MH, Phelps, CD: Prophylactic timolol for the prevention of high intraocular pressure after cataract extraction. A randomized, prospective, double-blind trial. Ophthalmology 88:233, 1981.

201. Tilen, A, Leuenberger, AE: Effect of timolol and acetazolamide on intraocular hypertension after intracapsular lens extraction with alpha-chymotrypsin. Klin Monatsbl Augenheilkd 176:558, 1980.

202. Shields, MB, Braverman, SD: Timolol in the management of secondary glaucomas. Surv Ophthalmol 28:266, 1983.

203. Tomoda, T, Tuberville, AW, Wood, TO: Timolol and postoperative intraocular pressure. Am Intra-Ocular Implant Soc J 10:180, 1984.

204. Duperré, J, Grenier, B, Lemire, J, et al: Effect of timolol vs. acetazolamide on sodium hyaluronate-induced rise in intraocular pressure after cataract surgery. Can J Ophthalmol 29:182, 1994.

205. West, DR, Lischwe, TD, Thompson, VM, Ide, CH: Comparative efficacy of the β-blockers for the prevention of increased intraocular pressure after cataract extraction. Am J Ophthalmol 106:168, 1988.

206. Araie, M, Ishi, K: Effects of apraclonidine on intraocular pressure and blood-aqueous barrier permeability after phacoemulsification and intraocular lens implantation. Am J Ophthalmol 116:67, 1993.

207. Wiles, SB, MacKenzie, D, Ide, CH: Control of intraocular pressure with apraclonidine hydrochloride after cataract extraction. Am J Ophthalmol 111:184, 1991.

208. Ruiz, RS, Wilson, CA, Musgrove, KH, Prager, TC: Management of increased intraocular pressure after cataract extraction. Am J Ophthalmol 103:487, 1987.

209. Kolker, AE, Becker, B: Epinephrine maculopathy. Arch Ophthalmol 79:552, 1968.

210. Rich, WJCC: Prevention of postoperative ocular hypertension by prostaglandin inhibitors. Trans Ophthalmol Soc UK 97:268, 1977.

211. Brucker, AJ, Michels, RG, Green, WR: Pars plana vitrectomy in the management of blood-induced glaucoma with vitreous hemorrhage. Ann Ophthalmol 10:1427, 1978.

212. Theodossiadis, G, Kouris-Bairaktari, E, Velissaropoulos, P: Clinical and pathologic-anatomical results following the application of a mobile argon-laser beam in aphakic pupillary block glaucoma. Klin Monatsbl Augenheilkd 175:180, 1979.

213. Hitchings, RA: Acute aphakic pupil block glaucoma: an alternative surgical approach. Br J Ophthalmol 63:31, 1979.

214. Peyman, GA, Sanders, DR, Minatoya, H: Pars plana vitrectomy in the management of pupillary block glaucoma following irrigation and aspiration. Br J Ophthalmol 62:336, 1978.

215. Obstbaum, SA, Galin, MA, Barasch, KR, Baras, I: Laser photomydriasis in pseudophakic pupillary block. Am Intra-Ocular Implant Soc J 7:28, 1981.

216. Mackool, RJ: Closed vitrectomy and the intraocular implant. Ophthalmology 88:414, 1981.

217. Bellows, AR, Johnstone, MA: Surgical management of chronic glaucoma in aphakia. Ophthalmology 90:807, 1983.

218. Gross, RL, Feldman, RM, Spaeth, GL, et al: Surgical therapy of chronic glaucoma in aphakia and pseudophakia. Ophthalmology 95:1195, 1988.

219. Heuer, DK, Gressel, MG, Parrish, RD II, et al: Trabeculectomy in aphakic eyes. Ophthalmology 91:1045, 1984.

220. The Fluorouracil Filtering Surgery Study Group. Fluorouracil filtering surgery study one-year follow-up. Am J Ophthalmol 108:625, 1989.

221. Hampton, C, Shields, MB, Miller, KN, Blasini, M: Evaluation of a protocol for transcleral Nd:YAG cyclophotocoagulation in 100 patients. Ophthalmology 97:910, 1990.

222. Brown, SVL, Thomas, JV, Belcher, CD III, Simmons, RJ: Effect of pilocarpine in treatment of intraocular pressure elevation following neodymium:YAG laser posterior capsulotomy. Ophthalmology 92:354, 1985.

223. Bernardino, VB, Kim, JC, Smith, TR: Epithelialization of the anterior chamber after cataract extraction. Arch Ophthalmol 82:742, 1969.

224. Theobald, GD, Haas, JS: Epithelial invasion of the anterior chamber following cataract extraction. Trans Am Acad Ophthalmol Otol 52:470, 1948.

225. Weiner, MJ, Trentacoste, J, Pon, DM, Albert, DM: Epithelial downgrowth: a 30-year clinicopathological review. Br J Ophthalmol 73: 6, 1989.

226. Holliday, JN, Buller, CR, Bourne, WM: Specular microscopy and fluorophotometry in the diagnosis of epithelial downgrowth after a sutureless cataract operation. Am J Ophthalmol 116:238, 1993.

227. Eldrup-Jdrgensen, P: Epithelialization of the anterior chamber. A clinical and histopathological study of a Danish material. Acta Ophthalmol 47:328, 1969.

228. Küchle, M, Naumann, GOH: Mucogenic secondary open-angle glaucoma in diffuse epithelial ingrowth treated by block-excision. Am J Ophthalmol 111:230, 1991.

229. Sugar, A, Meyer, RF, Hood, CI: Epithelial downgrowth following penetrating keratoplasty in the aphake. Arch Ophthalmol 95:464, 1977.

230. Smith, RE, Parrett, C: Specular microscopy of epithelial downgrowth. Arch Ophthalmol 96:1222, 1978.

231. Maumenee, AE: Treatment of epithelial downgrowth and intraocular fistula following cataract extraction. Trans Am Ophthalmol Soc 62:153, 1964.

232. Calhoun, FP Jr: An aid to the clinical diagnosis of epithelial downgrowth into the anterior chamber following cataract extraction. Am J Ophthalmol 61:1055, 1966.

233. Verrey, F: Invasion epitheliale de la chambre anterieure: confirmation anatomique par l'examen cytologique de l'humeur aqueuse. Ophthalmologica 153:467, 1967.

234. Maumenee, AE, Paton, D, Morse, PH, Butner, R: Review of 40 histologically proven cases of epithelial downgrowth following cataract extraction and suggested surgical management. Am J Ophthalmol 69:598, 1970.

235. Stark, WJ, Michels, RG, Maumenee, AE, Cupples, H: Surgical management of epithelial ingrowth. Am J Ophthalmol 85:772, 1978.

236. Jensen, P, Minckler, DS, Chandler, JW: Epithelial ingrowth. Arch Ophtahl 95:837, 1977.

237. Iwamoto, T, Srinivasan, BD, DeVoe, AG: Electron microscopy of epithelial downgrowth. Ann Ophthalmol 9:1095, 1977.

238. Zavala, EY, Binder, PS: The pathologic findings of epithelial ingrowth. Arch Ophthalmol 98:2007, 1980.

239. Zagorski, Z, Shrestha, HG, Lang, GK, Naumann, GOH: Secondary glaucoma due to intraocular epithelial invasion. Klin Monatsbl Augenheilkd 193:16, 1988.

240. Terry, TL, Chisholm, JF Jr, Schonberg, AL: Studies on surface-epithelium invasion of the anterior segment of the eye. Am J Ophthalmol 22:1083, 1939.

241. Brown, SI: Treatment of advanced epithelial downgrowth. Trans Am Acad Ophthalmol Otol 77:618, 1973.

242. Brown, SI: Results of excision of advanced epithelial downgrowth. Ophthalmology 86:321, 1979.

243. Friedman, AH: Radical anterior segment surgery for epithelial invasion of the anterior chamber: report of three cases. Trans Am Acad Ophthalmol Otol 83:216, 1977.

244. Naumann, GOH, Rummelt, V: Block excision of cystic and diffuse epithelial ingrowth of the anterior chamber. Report on 32 consecutive patients. Arch Ophthalmol 110:223, 1992.

245. Loane, ME, Weinreb, RN: Glaucoma secondary to epithelial downgrowth and 5-fluorouracil. Ophthalmic Surg 21:704, 1990.

246. Fish, LA, Heuer, DK, Baerveldt, G, et al: Molteno implantation for secondary glaucomas associated with advanced epithelial ingrowth. Ophthalmology 97:557, 1990.

247. Costa, VP, Katz, LJ, Cohen, EJ, Raber, IM: Glaucoma associated with epithelial downgrowth controlled with Molteno tube shunts. Ophthalmic Surg 23:797, 1992.

248. Allen, JC: Epithelial and stromal ingrowths. Am J Ophthalmol 65:179, 1968.

249. Bettman, JW Jr: Pathology of complications of intraocular surgery. Am J Ophthalmol 68:1037, 1969.

250. Swan, KC: Fibroblastic ingrowth following cataract extraction. Arch Ophthalmol 89:445, 1973.

251. Sherrard, ES, Rycroft, PV: Retrocorneal membranes. II. Factors influencing their growth. Br J Ophthalmol 51:387, 1967.

252. Friedman, AH, Henkind, P: Corneal stromal overgrowth after cataract extraction. Br J Ophthalmol 54:528, 1970.

253. Michels, RG, Kenyon, KR, Maumenee, AE: Retrocorneal fibrous membrane. Invest Ophthalmol 11:822, 1972.

254. Ueno, H, Green, WR, Kenyon, KR, Hoover, RE: Trabecular and retrocorneal proliferation of melanocytes and secondary glaucoma. Am J Ophthalmol 88:592, 1979.

255. Karesh, JW, Nirankari, VS: Factors associated with glaucoma after penetrating keratoplasty. Am J Ophthalmol 96:160, 1983.

256. Olson, RF, Kaufman, HE: Prognostic factors of intraocular pressure after aphakic keratoplasty. Am J Ophthalmol 86:510, 1978.

257. Foulks, GN: Glaucoma associated with penetrating keratoplasty. Ophthalmology 94:871, 1987.

258. Goldberg, DB, Schanzlin, DJ, Brown, SI: Incidence of increased intraocular pressure after keratoplasty. Am J Ophthalmol 92:372, 1981.

259. Irvine, AR, Kaufman, HE: Intraocular pressure following penetrating keratoplasty. Am J Ophthalmol 68:835, 1969.

260. Brightbill, FS, Stainer, GA, Hunkeler, JD: A comparison of intracapsular and extracapsular lens extraction combined with keratoplasty. Ophthalmology 90:34, 1983.

261. Robinson, CH Jr: Indications, complications and prognosis for repeat penetrating keratoplasty. Ophthalmic Surg 10:27, 1979.

262. Heydenreich, A: Corneal regeneration and intraocular tension. Klin Monatsbl Augenheilkd 148:500, 1966.

263. Lass, JH, Pavan-Langston, D: Timolol therapy in secondary angle-closure glaucoma post penetrating keratoplasty. Ophthalmology 86:51, 1979.

264. Zimmerman, TJ, Krupin, T, Grodzki, W, Waltman, SR: The effect of suture depth on outflow facility in penetrating keratoplasty. Arch Ophthalmol 96:505, 1978.

265. Zimmerman, TJ, Waltman, SR, Sachs, U, Kaufman, HE: Intraocular pressure after aphakic penetrating keratoplasty "through-and-through" suturing. Ophthalmic Surg 10:49, 1979.

266. Nissenkorn, I, Wood, TO: Intraocular pressure following aphakic transplants. Ann Ophthalmol 15:1168, 1983.

267. Olson, RJ, Kaufman, HE: A mathematical description of causative factors and prevention of elevated intraocular pressure after keratoplasty. Invest Ophthalmol Vis Sci 16:1085, 1977.

268. Gnad, HD: Athalamia as a late complication after keratoplasty on aphakic eyes. Br J Ophthalmol 64:528, 1980.

269. Polack, FM: Graft rejection and glaucoma. Am J Ophthalmol 101:294, 1986.

270. Insler, MS, McShrerry Zatzkis, S: Pigment dispersion syndrome in pseudophakic corneal transplants. Am J Ophthalmol 102:762, 1986.

271. Schanzlin, DJ, Goldberg, DB, Brown, SI: Transplantation of congenitally opaque corneas. Ophthalmology 87:1253, 1980.

272. Yamaguchi, T, Polack, FM, Valenti, J: Electron microscopic study of epithelial downgrowth after penetrating keratoplasty. Br J Ophthalmol 65:374, 1981.

273. Olson, RJ: Aphakic keratoplasty. Determining donor tissue size to avoid elevated intraocular pressure. Arch Ophthalmol 96:2274, 1978.

274. Zimmerman, TJ, Krupin, T, Grodzki, W, et al: Size of donor corneal button and outflow facility in aphakic eyes. Ann Ophthalmol 11:809, 1979.

275. Perl, T, Charlton, KH, Binder, PS: Disparate diameter grafting. Astigmatism, intraocular pressure, and visual acuity. Ophthalmology 88:774, 1981.

276. Heidemann, DG, Sugar, A, Meyer, RF, Musch, DC: Oversized donor grafts in penetrating keratoplasty. A randomized trial. Arch Ophthalmol 103:1807, 1985.

277. Foulks, GN, Perry, HD, Dohlman, CH: Oversize corneal donor grafts in penetrating keratoplasty. Ophthalmology 86:490, 1979.

278. Zimmerman, T, Olson, R, Waltman, S, Kaufman, H: Transplant size and elevated intraocular pressure. Postkeratoplasty. Arch Ophthalmol 96:2231, 1978.

279. Bourne, WM, Davison, JA, O'Fallon, WM: The effects of oversize donor buttons on postoperative intraocular pressure and corneal curvature in aphakic penetrating keratoplasty. Ophthalmology 89:242, 1982.

280. Perry, HD, Foulks, GN: Oversize donor buttons in corneal transplantation surgery for keratoconus. Ophthalmic Surg 18:751, 1987.

281. Cohen, EJ, Kenyon, KR, Dohlman, CH: Iridoplasty for prevention of post-keratoplasty angle closure and glaucoma. Ophthalmic Surg 13:994, 1982.

282. Thoft, RA, Gordon, JM, Dohlman, CH: Glaucoma following keratoplasty. Trans Am Acad Ophthalmol Otol 78:352, 1974.

283. Wood, TO, West, C, Kaufman, HE: Control of intraocular pressure in penetrating keratoplasty. Am J Ophthalmol 74:724, 1972.

284. Olson, RJ, Kaufman, HE, Zimmerman, TJ: Effects of timolol and daranide on elevated intraocular pressure after aphakic keratoplasty. Ann Ophthalmol 11:1833, 1979.

285. Casey, TA, Gibbs, D: Complications in corneal grafting. Trans Ophthalmol Soc UK 92:517, 1972.

286. Lemp, MA, Pfister, RR, Dohlman, CG: The effect of intraocular surgery on clear corneal grafts. Am J Ophthalmol 70:719, 1970.

287. Kirkness, CM, Steele, ADMcG, Ficker, LA, Rice, NSC: Coexistent corneal disease and glaucoma managed by either drainage surgery and subsequent keratoplasty or combined drainage surgery and penetrating keratoplasty. Br J Ophthalmol 76:146, 1992.

288. McDonnell, PJ, Robin, JB, Schanzlin, DJ, et al: Molteno implant for control of glaucoma in eyes after penetrating keratoplasty. Ophthalmology 95:364, 1988.

289. Sherwood, MB, Smith, MF, Driebe, WT Jr, et al: Drainage tube implants in the treatment of glaucoma following penetrating keratoplasty. Ophthalmic Surg 24:185, 1993.

290. Binder, PS, Abel, R Jr, Kaufman, HE: Cyclocryotherapy for glaucoma after penetrating keratoplasty. Am J Ophthalmol 79:489, 1975.

291. Threlkeld, AB, Shields, MB: Noncontact transscleral Nd:YAG cyclophotocoagulation for glaucoma after penetrating keratoplasty. Am J Ophthalmol 120:569, 1995.

292. Wilensky, JT, Goldberg, MF, Alward, P: Glaucoma after pars plana vitrectomy. Trans Am Acad Ophthalmol Otol 83:114, 1977.

293. Huamonte, FU, Peyman, GA, Goldberg, MF: Complicated retinal detachment and its management with pars plana vitrectomy. Br J Ophthalmol 61:754, 1977.

294. Faulborn, J, Conway, BP, Machemer, R: Surgical complications of pars plana vitreous surgery. Ophthalmology 85:116, 1978.

295. Aaberg, TM, Van Horn, DL: Late complications of pars plana vitreous surgery. Ophthalmology 85:126, 1978.

296. Ghartey, KN, Tolentino, FI, Freeman, HM, et al: Closed vitreous surgery. XVII. Results and complications of pars plana vitrectomy. Arch Ophthalmol 98:1248, 1980.

297. Han, DP, Lewis, H, Lambrou, FH Jr, et al: Mechanisms of intraocular pressure elevation after pars plana vitrectomy. Ophthalmology 96:1357, 1989.

298. Sabates, WI, Abrams, GW, Swanson, DE, Norton, EWD: The use of intraocular gases. The results of sulfur hexafluoride gas in retinal detachment surgery. Ophthalmology 88:447, 1981.

299. Abrams, GW, Swanson, DE, Sabates, WI: The results of sulfur hexafluoride gas in vitreous surgery. Am J Ophthalmol 94:165, 1982.

300. Chang, S, Lincoff, HA, Coleman, DJ, et al: Perfluorocarbon gases in vitreous surgery. Ophthalmology 92:651, 1985.

301. Coden, DJ, Freeman, WR, Weinreb, RN: Intraocular pressure response after pneumatic retinopexy. Ophthalmic Surg 19:667, 1988.

302. Crittenden, JJ, deJuan, E Jr, Tiedeman, J: Expansion of long-acting gas bubbles for intraocular use. Principles and practice. Arch Ophthalmol 103:831, 1985.

303. Aronowitz, JD, Brubaker, RF: Effect of intraocular gas on intraocular pressure. Arch Ophthalmol 94:1191, 1976.

304. Poliner, LS, Schoch, LH: Intraocular pressure assessment in gas-filled eyes following vitrectomy. Arch Ophthalmol 105:200, 1987.

305. Simone, JN, Whitacre, MM: The effect of intraocular gas and fluid volumes on intraocular pressure. Ophthalmology 97:238, 1990.

306. Hines, MW, Jost, BF, Fogelman, KL: Oculab Tono-Pen, Goldmann applanation tonometry, and pneumatic tonometry for intraocular pressure assessment in gas-filled eyes. Am J Ophthalmol 106:174, 1988.

307. Lincoff, H, Weinberger, D, Reppucci, V, Lincoff, A: Air travel with intraocular gas. I. The mechanisms for compensation. Arch Ophthalmol 107:902, 1989.

308. Lincoff, H, Weinberger, D, Stergiu, P: Air travel with intraocular gas. II. Clinical considerations. Arch Ophthalmol 107:907, 1989.

309. Adile, SL, Peyman, GA, Greve, MDJ, et al: Postoperative chronic pressure abnormalities in the Vitreon study. Ophthalmic Surg 25:584, 1994.

310. Foster, RE, Smiddy, WS, Alfonso, EC, Parrish, RK II: Secondary glaucoma associated with retained perfluorophenanthrene. Am J Ophthalmol 118:253, 1994.

311. Lewis, H, Han, D, Williams, GA: Management of fibrin pupillary-block glaucoma after pars plana vitrectomy with intravitreal gas injection. Am J Ophthalmol 103:180, 1987.

312. Jaffe, GJ, Lewis, H, Han, DP, et al: Treatment of postvitrectomy fibrin pupillary block with tissue plasminogen activator. Am J Ophthalmol 108:170, 1989.

313. Okun, E: Intravitreal surgery utilizing liquid silicone. A long term follow-up. Tran Pac Coast Oto-Ophthalmol Soc 49:141, 1968.

314. Grey, RHB, Leaver, PK: Results of silicone oil injection in massive preretinal retraction. Trans Ophthalmol Soc UK 97:238, 1977.

315. Sugar, HS, Okamura, ID: Ocular findings six years after intravitreal silicone injection. Arch Ophthalmol 94:612, 1976.

316. Burk, LL, Shields, MB, Proia, AD, McCuen, B: Intraocular pressure following intravitreal silicone oil injection. Ophthalmic Surg 19:565, 1988.

317. de Corral, LR, Cohen, SB, Peyman, GA: Effect of intravitreal silicone oil on intraocular pressure. Ophthalmic Surg 18:446, 1987.

318. Riedel, KG, Gabel, V-P, Neubauer, L, et al: Intravitreal silicone oil injection: complications and treatment of 415 consecutive patients. Graefes Arch Clin Exp Ophthalmol 228:19, 1990.

319. Nguyen, QH, Lloyd, MA, Heuer, DK, et al: Incidence and management of glaucoma after intravitreal silicone oil injection for complicated retinal detachments. Ophthalmology 99:1520, 1992.

320. Barr, CC, Lai, MY, Lean, JS, et al: Postoperative intraocular pressure abnormalities in the silicone study. Silicone study report 4. Ophthalmology 100:1629, 1993.

321. Watzke, RC: Silicone retinopiesis for retinal detachment. A long-term clinical evaluation. Arch Ophthalmol 77:185, 1967.

322. Ando, F: Intraocular hypertension resulting from pupillary block by silicone oil. Am J Ophthalmol 99:87, 1985.

323. Zborowski-Gutman, L, Treister, G, Naveh, N, et al: Acute glaucoma following vitrectomy and silicone oil injection. Br J Ophthalmol 71:903, 1987.

324. Beekhuis, WH, Ando, F, Zivojnovic, R, et al: Basal iridectomy at 6 o'clock in the aphakic eye treated with silicone oil: Prevention of keratopathy and secondary glaucoma. Br J Ophthalmol 71: 197, 1987.

325. Lucke, K, Strobel, B, Foerster, M, Laqua, H: Secondary glaucoma after silicone oil surgery. Klin Monatsbl Augenheilkd 196:205, 1990.

326. Gao, R, Neubauer, L, Tang, S, Kampik, A: Silicone oil in the anterior chamber. Graefes Arch Clin Exp Ophthalmol 227:106, 1989.

327. Valone, J Jr, McCarthy, M: Emulsified anterior chamber silicone oil and glaucoma. Ophthalmology 101:1908, 1994.

328. Bartov, E, Huna, R, Ashkenazi, I, et al: Identification, prevention, and treatment of silicone oil pupillary block after an inferior iridectomy. Am J Ophthalmol 111:501, 1991.

329. Rentsch, FJ: Electronmicroscopical aspects of acid compartments of the ground substance and of collagen in different cases of intravitreal tissue proliferation. Der Ophthalmol 2:385, 1981.

330. Ni, C, Wang, W-J, Albert, DM, Schepens, CL: Intravitreous silicone injection. Histopathologic findings in a human eye after 12 years. Arch Ophthalmol 101:1399, 1983.

331. Laroche, L, Pavlakis, C, Saraux, H, Orcel, L: Ocular findings following intravitreal silicone injection. Arch Ophthalmol 101:1422, 1983.

332. Sebestyen, JG, Schepens, CL, Rosenthal, ML: Retinal detachment and glaucoma. I. Tonometric and gonioscopic study of 160 cases. Arch Ophthalmol 67:736, 1962.

333. Hayreh, SS, Baines, JAB: Occlusion of the vortex veins. An experimental study. Br J Ophthalmol 57:217, 1973.

334. Araie, M, Sugiura, Y, Minota, K, Akazawa, K: Effects of the encircling procedure on the aqueous flow rate in retinal detachment eyes: a fluorometric study. Br J Ophthalmol 71:510, 1987.

335. Johnson, MW, Han, DP, Hoffman, KE: The effect of scleral buckling on ocular rigidity. Ophthalmology 97:190, 1990.

336. Gardner, TW, Quillen, DA, Blankenship, GW, Marshall, WK: Intraocular pressure fluctuations during scleral buckling surgery. Ophthalmology 100:1050, 1993.

337. Yoshida, A, Hirokawa, H, Ishiko, S, Ogasawara, H: Ocular circulatory changes following scleral buckling procedures. Br J Ophthalmol 76:529, 1992.

338. Mensher, JH: Anterior chamber depth alteration after retinal photocoagulation. Arch Ophthalmol 95:113, 1977.

339. Boulton, PE: A study of the mechanism of transient myopia following extensive xenon arc photocoagulation. Trans Ophth Soc UK 93:287, 1973.

340. Blondeau, P, Pavan, PR, Phelps, CD: Acute pressure elevation following panretinal photocoagulation. Arch Ophthalmol 99:1239, 1981.

341. Schidte, SN: Changes in eye tension after panretinal xenon arc and argon laser photocoagulation in normotensive diabetic eyes. Acta Ophthalmol 60:692, 1982.

342. Kaufman, SC, Ferris, FL, III, Swartz, M, et al: Intraocular pressure following panretinal photocoagulation for diabetic retinopathy: diabetic retinopathy report no. 11. Arch Ophthalmol 105:807, 1987.

343. Tsai, JC, Lee, MB, WuDunn, D, et al: Incidence of acute intraocular pressure elevation after panretinal photocoagulation. J Glau 4: 45, 1995.

Section III

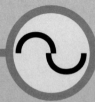

MANAGEMENT OF
GLAUCOMA

PRINCIPLES OF MEDICAL THERAPY FOR GLAUCOMA

A CLASSIFICATION OF ANTIGLAUCOMA DRUGS

The vast majority of medications that are used to control the intraocular pressure (IOP) in the management of glaucoma are administered topically in the form of eyedrops or other ocular delivery systems. The classes of topical drugs, which until recently included only autonomic agents, have grown to include carbonic anhydrase inhibitors and prostaglandins. Systemic drugs are being used with decreasing frequency as new topical agents become available, but still include carbonic anhydrase inhibitors and hyperosmotic agents.

Autonomic Agents

All the drugs in this broad category exert their pharmacologic influence by acting on the *autonomic nervous system,* which has two main subdivisions: the *cholinergic* (parasympathetic) and *adrenergic* (sympathetic) systems. These subsystems differ on the basis of (a) receptors and (b) postganglionic physiologic mediators (Fig. 24.1) (1). Receptors are located in the cell membrane and represent the sites at which both physiologic mediators and pharmacologic agents interact to produce a particular cellular response. The cell membrane is composed of lipid and protein. The actual arrangement of these components is uncertain, although the "lipid-globular protein mosaic model" theory suggests that molecules of protein are imbedded in a layer of lipid with protrusion of the globular protein on either side of the membrane (1). Although this is an oversimplification of a highly complex and poorly understood subject, it provides a conceptual basis for a discussion of drug interactions. According to this hypothesis, the extracellular side of the protein globules contain the receptors, while the intracellular side contains catalysts, which are involved in specific cellular functions in response to a physiologic mediator or drug.

Cholinergic System

It was traditionally held that only one receptor type existed in the parasympathetic nervous system, although subsequent studies suggest the possibility of more than one cholinergic receptor (2). Stimulation of the receptor(s) produces miosis and increased aqueous outflow. The mechanisms of improved outflow facility are related to contraction of the ciliary muscle in eyes with open angles and pupillary constriction in cases of pupillary-block glaucoma (3–5).

Acetylcholine is the postganglionic physiologic mediator of the cholinergic nervous system. It is produced in the postganglionic neuron, where it is stored and released when the membrane is polarized by increased Na$^+$ flux. After its release from the neuron, the mediator is rapidly inactivated by acetylcholinesterase. The short duration of this enzymatic inactivation is such that acetylcholine is not effective as a

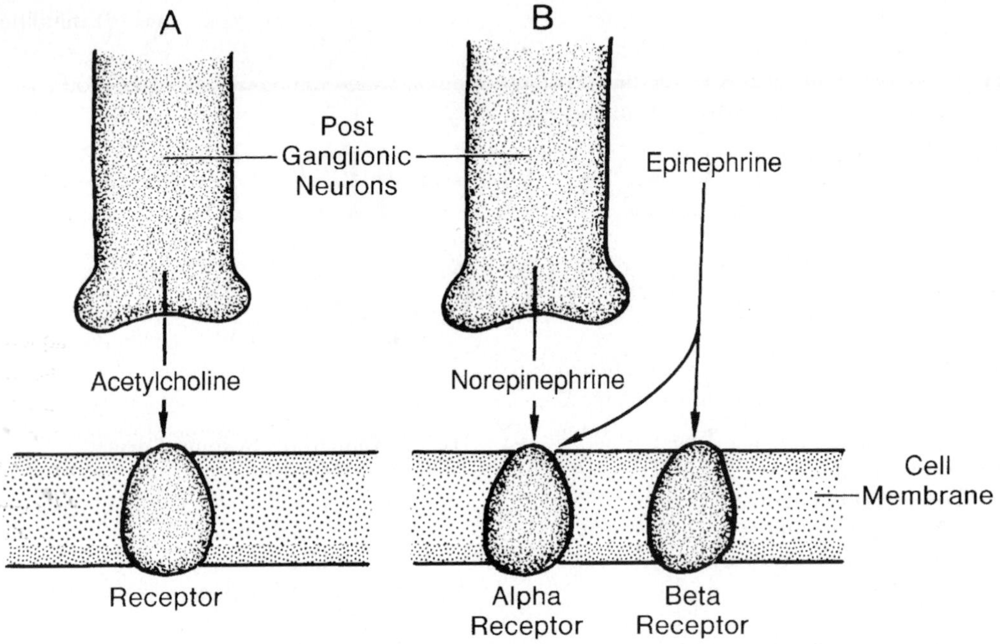

Figure 24.1. Main divisions of autonomic nervous system. **A.** Cholinergic (parasympathetic) system mediated by acetylcholine. **B.** Adrenergic (sympathetic) system, mediated by norepinephrine and epinephrine.

topical drug, although it is often injected into the anterior chamber during intraocular surgery to achieve rapid miosis.

Pharmacologic agents may either simulate or antagonize the action of the physiologic mediator. Drugs which mimic the effect of acetylcholine are referred to as *parasympathomimetics,* or *cholinergic stimulators,* or *agonists* and may act directly by stimulating the receptor or indirectly by enhancing the action of the physiologic mediator. The direct stimulator most commonly used in the treatment of glaucoma is *pilocarpine,* while an example of the indirect stimulators is *echothiophate iodide,* which enhances the action of acetylcholine by inhibiting the cholinesterases.

Drugs which block the response of acetylcholine at the receptor are called *parasympatholytics,* or *cholinergic antagonists.* This class of compounds, which includes atropine, cyclopentolate, and tropicamide, are not routinely used in the treatment of glaucoma, since the mydriasis and cycloplegia they produce may actually increase the IOP, as discussed in Chapters 9 and 10. They may, however, be used in specific situations such as glaucoma associated with active uveitis and malignant (ciliary block) glaucoma.

Adrenergic System

Two basic types of adrenergic receptors (α and β) have been identified, although subdivisions are known to exist within these categories, and it is likely that there are additional receptors that have yet to be recognized. α-*Adrenergic receptor* stimulation produces mydriasis and vasoconstriction. Two subtypes of α_2-adrenergic receptors have been identified in human nonpigmented ciliary epithelium and ciliary

muscle (6), and activation of these receptors reduces IOP by decreasing the rate of aqueous production. The β-*adrenergic receptors* have been further subdivided into β_1 and β_2 types (7). Stimulation of β_1 receptors increases cardiac contractility and lipolysis, while the β_2 subsystem is related to bronchodilatation and vasodepression. In general, stimulation of the β receptors lowers the IOP by increasing aqueous outflow facility, while inhibition of the receptors reduces aqueous production.

There are two physiologic mediators in the sympathetic nervous system, *epinephrine* and *norepinephrine,* which are often referred to as catecholamines. Epinephrine is secreted by the adrenal glands where it is produced from phenylalanine and tyrosine. This mediator stimulates both α and β receptors. Norepinephrine is the postganglionic mediator and primarily stimulates the α receptor. It is also secreted by the adrenal glands where it is made from the same amino acids as epinephrine. In the postganglionic neuron, norepinephrine is produced from tyrosine alone and stored in two pools in the axon terminal. Slow release and reuptake of the mediator constantly occur, and that which is not released is inactivated to vanilmandelic acid by monoamine oxidase. Following massive release of the mediator by nerve stimulation, 90% is recaptured by the nerve, a small amount is inactivated by catechol-o-methyltransferase and monoamine oxidase, and the remainder enters the circulation in active form (Fig. 24.2).

The pharmacologic agents within the adrenergic system, as with the cholinergic drugs, may either mimic or inhibit the action of the physiologic mediators. The *sympathomimetics,* or *adrenergic stimulators (agonists),* may act either directly or indirectly on the α receptors, the β receptors, or both. The only direct α- and β-adrenergic stimulator that is commercially available for the chronic treatment of glaucoma is the physiologic mediator *epinephrine.* An analogue of clonidine, *apraclonidine* is an α₂-stimulator that is available for treating the short-term IOP elevation associated with certain glaucoma laser procedures, as well as the chronic management of glaucoma. Another sympathomimetic, *phenylephrine,* has vasoconstrictor and pressor actions, and is commonly used to achieve pupillary dilation.

Other sympathomimetics that have been evaluated for their IOP lowering effect include the direct α stimulator and physiologic mediator, norepinephrine, and a group of indirect α stimulators, which enhance the effect of norepinephrine by (a) stimulating its release from axon terminals, (b) increasing its release in response to nerve stimulation,

(c) decreasing its reuptake, and (d) inhibiting monoamine oxidase or catechol-o-methyltransferase. Indirect β stimulators, which mimic the effect of β-adrenergic stimulation by enhancing the action of adenylate cyclase in various ways, have also been studied. In addition, another group of compounds, the adrenergic potentiators, enhance the effect of epinephrine by producing adrenergic supersensitivity.

The *sympatholytics,* or *adrenergic inhibitors (antagonists),* compete with the catecholamines for the α receptors or with epinephrine for the β receptors. β-Antagonists, or blockers, lower the IOP by reducing aqueous production. *Timolol, betaxolol, levobunolol, metipranolol,* and *carteolol* are β-blockers currently available in the United States for topical therapy in the treatment of glaucoma. α-Adrenergic antagonists produce miosis by relaxation of the iris dilator muscle, and one is commercially available (*dapiprazole*) for the reversal of mydriasis after an ocular examination.

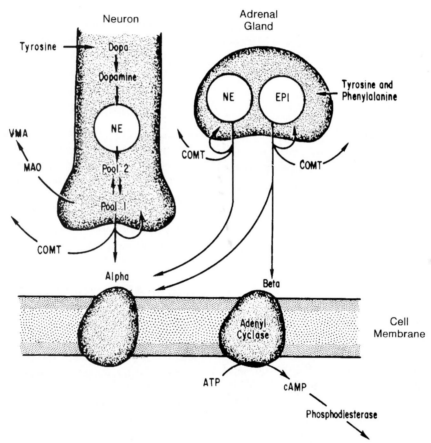

Figure 24.2. Adrenergic nervous system. Norepinephrine (NE) is produced in postganglionic neurons from tyrosine and in the adrenal glands from tyrosine and phenylalanine. It exists in two pools in the axon terminal, with a constant, slow release and reuptake or inactivation to vanilmandelic acid (VMA) by monoamine oxidase (MAO). It primarily stimulates α-adrenergic receptors, following which most is recaptured by the nerve, while the rest is inactivated by MAO or catechol-o-methyltransferase (COMT), or released in active form into the circulation. Epinephrine is produced only in the adrenal glands from tyrosine and phenylalanine and stimulates both α and β adrenergic receptors. β Stimulation activates the conversion of adenosine triphosphate (ATP) to cyclic adenosine monophosphate (cAMP) by the enzyme adenyl cyclase. Phosphodiesterase then inactivates cAMP.

Carbonic Anhydrase Inhibitors

This is the only class of systemic medications that are used on a chronic basis in the treatment of glaucoma. These agents lower the IOP by reducing aqueous production through inhibition of the enzyme, carbonic anhydrase. *Acetazolamide* is the prototype carbonic anhydrase inhibitor and may be administered either orally, intramuscularly, or intravenously. *Methazolamide* is another commonly used oral carbonic anhydrase inhibitor. More recently, the topical carbonic anhydrase inhibitor *dorzolamide* has become available for the chronic treatment of glaucoma.

Prostaglandins

This is the most recent class of drugs to be introduced for the chronic management of glaucoma. Although high concentrations of prostaglandins are associated with ocular inflammation and elevated IOP, very low concentrations reduce the pressure by increasing uveoscleral outflow. The first of these drugs to be released is *latanoprost*.

Hyperosmotic Agents

These compounds are occasionally used for the rapid reduction of severely elevated IOP on an emergency basis, or prior to some surgical procedures, although they are rarely used for prolonged periods of time. The hypotensive mechanism of these drugs is not fully understood, although it is generally felt to be through reduction of the vitreous volume. The hyperosmotics can be administered either orally, of which *glycerine* is the most common form, or intravenously, in which case *mannitol* is the most popular drug.

PHARMACOKINETICS OF TOPICAL DRUGS

Pharmacokinetics deal with the absorption, distribution, metabolism, and elimination of an administered drug (8). With regard to topical medications, the availability of the pharmacologic agent at the receptor site is influenced by (a) drug kinetics in the conjunctival cul-de-sac, (b) corneal penetration, and (c) the distribution and rate of drug elimination within the eye (9).

Drug Kinetics in the Conjunctival Cul-de-sac

Following topical instillation, a medication first mixes with the tears in the cul-de-sac. The bulk of the drug is then lost through the lacrimal drainage system, while a small amount mixes with the precorneal tear film and is absorbed by the cornea. The dilution and drainage of a pharmacologic agent and the degree to which it saturates the tear film significantly influence the bioavailability of the drug.

Dilution and Drainage

The conjunctival cul-de-sac normally contains 7–9 μL of tears and has a maximum capacity of about 30 μL (9). The drop size of commercial glaucoma medications ranges from 25.1–56.4 μL with an average of 39 μL (10). Therefore, up to one-half of the medication may spill out from the lids at the time of instillation. A large percentage of that which remains in the cul-de-sac then enters the lacrimal drainage system as a result of the pumping action created by blink movements. The loss rate in the tears is rapid, with the peak time occurring within the first few minutes after instillation. This loss not only reduces the amount of drug available for the pharmacologic effect within the eye, but also increases the potential for systemic side effects by absorption into the systemic circulation via the nasopharyngeal mucosa. The degree to which this occurs can be influenced by nasolacrimal occlusion, which is discussed later in this chapter.

Tear Film Saturation

The precorneal tear film is a stagnant fluid layer, which depends on blink movements for mixing with instilled drugs. In addition, the degree to which a drug saturates the tear film depends on the rate of drug loss in the tears and the retention time in the conjunctival cul-de-sac. The amount of precorneal tear film saturation, in turn, determines the amount of drug available for corneal penetration and subsequent transfer to the intraocular receptor sites.

CORNEAL PENETRATION (11)

It may be helpful to think of the cornea as a lipid-water-lipid sandwich in that the lipid content of the epithelium and endothelium is approximately 100-times greater than that of the stroma (12). As a result of this composition, the epithelium and endothelium are readily traversed by lipid-soluble substances (i.e., compounds in a nonionized or nonelectrolyte form), but are impermeable to water-soluble agents (ionized compounds or electrolytes). This difference in permeability characteristics creates a selective barrier, in that only drugs which can exist in both a water-soluble and lipid-soluble state are able to penetrate the intact cornea. This has been referred to as the differential solubility concept (12).

Drugs that are capable of existing in both the ionized and nonionized form include most of the weak bases, such as pilocarpine and epinephrine (12). The two forms of the drug exist in equilibrium and, as one form penetrates a particular layer of the cornea, its concentration is replenished from the other form to maintain the equilibrium (Fig. 24.3). Quater-

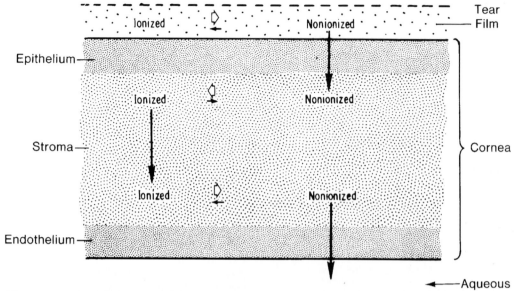

Figure 24.3. The differential solubility concept of corneal penetration. Only drugs with the potential to exist in both lipid-soluble (nonionized) and water-soluble (ionized) forms are able to penetrate the intact cornea. The two forms are in equilibrium and, as one form penetrates a particular corneal layer, its concentration is replenished from the other form to maintain the equilibrium.

nary ammonium compounds, such as echothiophate and carbachol, do not readily permeate the cornea. However, they are so potent that the small amount that does enter the eye is sufficient to produce a clinically significant antiglaucoma effect (13).

Drugs tend to concentrate in various layers of the cornea. Some of the drug may be degraded at this level, while another portion is temporarily stored in the cornea. The cornea, therefore, acts as a depot and a limiting factor for transfer of the drug to the aqueous (9, 14).

Intraocular Factors Influencing Drug Concentrations

Having penetrated the cornea, the drug must now pass through the aqueous to the appropriate structures in the anterior segment of the eye. A portion of the drug in the anterior chamber is eliminated by diffusion into the vascular system or escapes with the aqueous via the outflow system. Another percentage is bound to various ocular tissues. Both cholinergic (15, 16) and adrenergic (16) drugs appear to bind to melanin in the anterior uveal tract, which partially prevents the drug from reaching the receptor site (17–19). *In vitro* studies with synthetic melanin revealed a binding rate of 80–85% for β-blockers, compared with 40% for pilocarpine, 50% for epinephrine, and almost none for prostaglandins (20). This corresponded to *in vivo* studies, in which timolol and pilocarpine had a greater IOP-lowering effect in albino than pigmented rabbits, while prostaglandins had the same effect in both groups of animals (20). Histochemical studies show that adrenergic

nerves are located close to melanocytes (19). Some drugs, such as β-adrenergic inhibitors, are released very slowly from the pigmented uveal tissues, accounting for the longer duration of effect in pigmented eyes (9). Other drugs, including pilocarpine, are metabolized in the ocular tissues. It has also been suggested, based on studies with pilocarpine in pigmented and albino rabbits, that a larger amount of the topically applied drug may be metabolized in the cornea of eyes with more pigment (21).

That small portion of the instilled drop which escapes extraocular or intraocular elimination, tissue binding, or inactivation, may finally reach the appropriate receptor where it exerts its pharmacologic effect.

FORMULATIONS OF TOPICAL DRUGS

The pharmacokinetics of a particular drug can be greatly influenced by the manner in which it is formulated. This includes the vehicle, pH, concentration, and additives of the formulation.

Vehicles

The vehicle in which a drug is delivered effects the amount of medication available for corneal penetration by influencing the rate of drug loss in the tears, the precorneal tear film saturation, and the length of time that the drug remains in contact with the cornea (22).

Soluble Polymers

These commonly used vehicles, which include methylcellulose and polyvinyl alcohol, reduce the initial rapid drainage and prolong the drug-cornea contact time. This is presumably accomplished by increasing tear viscosity, providing solution homogeneity (uniform suspension of drug particles in solution), and reducing surface tension (23, 24). However, this has only a minimal influence on enhanced drug bioavailability in the human eye (22).

Ointments

These vehicles do significantly increase drug bioavailability by reducing loss in the tears, inhibiting dilution by the tears, providing a higher effective concentration of the drug, and increasing tissue contact time (25–27). They are limited, however, by interference with vision and aesthetic considerations.

Soluble Gels

Newer vehicles have been shown to prolong the therapeutic effect of a drug. Much of the early work with these vehicles was done with pilocarpine. One such vehicle is a soluble gel, described as a high viscosity acrylic vehicle, which reportedly delivers a 24-hour pilocarpine dose following a single, nighttime application in the cul-de-sac (28, 29). It has not yet been established whether the prolonged drug action results from an increased surge in corneal absorption or a prolongation of the drug absorption phase (22).

Emulsions and Suspensions

Another formulation that has been shown to prolong the therapeutic effect of pilocarpine is an emulsion of the drug with a polymeric material (30). The prolonged action appears to be due to both enhanced pulse entry and a prolongation of drug release from the vehicle (31). This results in a pilocarpine effect well in excess of 12 hours (32).

Drugs administered in the form of suspended particles also have enhanced availability for corneal absorption because they mix less rapidly with tears and remain in the cul-de-sac longer than those administered in solutions (13).

Liposomes

The interaction of phospholipids and water under special conditions results in concentric lipid bilayers separated by aqueous layers. These multilamellar vesicles, called liposomes, can be reduced to smaller unilamellar structures of homogenous size that are suitable for incorporation into topical medications (22). A drug will concentrate in either the lipid or aqueous layer, depending upon its solubility characteristics, resulting in enhanced corneal penetration of the drug by adsorbing to the corneal surface with direct transfer of the drug from liposomal to epithelial cell membranes (33). Temperature-sensitive liposomes, which release substances in the ocular vasculature when exposed to heat produced by an argon laser (34) or microwave (35), are also being evaluated.

Ocular Insert Devices

A variety of solid materials have been evaluated for their ability to release a drug at a sustained rate from a location on the cornea or in the conjunctival cul-de-sac. Such a sustained release has been shown to achieve the same therapeutic effect as frequent topical applications, but with significantly less medication (36).

PULSE RELEASE. In one group of insert devices, the pattern of drug release is characterized by a very high initial rate that rapidly declines because of the leaching action by the tears (22). This mode of delivery, which is also characteristic of conventional drop administration, is referred to as first order kinetics. It has the disadvantage of transient overdosing with associated side effects, followed by a prolonged period of underdosing. Included in this group of drug delivery systems are water-soluble polymer matrices (37, 38), insoluble material (39), and presoaked hydrophilic contact lenses (40, 41) and collagen corneal shields (42).

RATE-CONTROLLED RELEASE. To avoid the problems of first order delivery, a second group of inserts have been developed, which deliver the drug at a controlled rate. This is referred to as zero order kinetics since the amount of drug delivered per unit time is independent of the amount left undelivered (22). Three such systems have been evaluated: (a) *diffusional systems,* in which pilocarpine is released from between two polymeric membranes (43) (this is currently the only commercially available rate-controlled system and is discussed in the next chapter); (b) *osmotic systems,* in which the osmotic properties of a drug incorporated in a nonhydrophilic polymer matrix are used to achieve fairly constant drug delivery; and (c) *bioerodible systems,* which utilize an erodible hydrophobic matrix that does not allow leaching of the drug by the tears.

Mechanical Delivery Devices

As an alternative to the traditional drop delivery system, devices have been evaluated which mechanically transfer medication to the eye. One such device is a plastic rod with drug coated on the tip (44–46) and another is a stiffened paper strip with medication incorporated in a water-soluble polyvinyl alcohol film at the tip (47, 48). In either case, the medication dissolves in the tear film when the tip is placed in the cul-de-sac. In addition to possibly being easier to administer, these devices have the potential advantage of delivering a more appropriate volume of medication and not requiring preservatives. However, none are commercially available.

pH

As discussed before, the lipid:water solubility ratio (partition coefficient) of a compound influences corneal penetration. A greater degree of corneal penetration occurs when a higher concentration of nonionized (lipid soluble) drug exists in the instilled drop (13). The pH at which a drug is formulated influences this ratio, with weak bases (which includes most antiglaucoma preparations) being absorbed through the cornea at a higher pH, while weak acids are absorbed better at a lower pH. For example, pilocarpine penetration was shown to be better at pH 6.5–7.5 than pH 4 (49, 50), although no significant difference was noted between formulations at pH 4.1 and 5.8 (51). Solution pH also affects drug stability and patient comfort upon instillation. Fortunately, most weak bases at physiologic pH 7.4 exist predominantly in the nonionized form (13).

Concentration

Corneal penetration is enhanced by increasing the concentration of a drug up to a point. Beyond this point, the percentage of drug crossing the cornea decreases with increasing concentrations, and the greater amount of drug lost in the lacrimal drainage system increases the potential for systemic side effects. In a monkey study, topical 1% pilocarpine had a greater percentage recovered in the aqueous than 4% or 8% (52).

Additives

Certain additives that are used in commercial formulations, such as benzalkonium chloride, not only serve as a "preservative" by providing bacteriostatic activity, but also influence corneal penetration through surface wetting properties. The latter property decreases the surface tension of nonpolar drugs, allowing them to mix more readily with the precorneal tear film, leading to enhanced corneal absorption. This is particularly important with drugs that have poor corneal penetration, such as carbachol (53). Such agents, however, may also damage the corneal epithelium. Additives do not invariably prevent bacterial contamination. In seven cases of microbial keratitis, the same organism was cultured from corneal scrapings and the patient's timolol bottle (54), emphasizing the importance of proper handling of eyedrop dispensers.

Molecular Weight

Compounds with a molecular weight greater than 500 g/mole have poor corneal absorption. However, this is not a major factor since most ophthalmic drugs have a lower molecular weight (11).

Drop Size

As previously noted, the drop size of commercial glaucoma medications ranges from 25.1–56.4 μL with an average of 39 μL (10). All of these may be significantly in excess of that required for effective bioavailability. A comparison of 8- and 30-μL drop volumes of 2.5% phenylephrine in neonates and infants revealed an equivalent pupillary effect, but significantly higher plasma level with the larger drop (55).

SOME PRACTICAL ASPECTS OF MEDICAL THERAPY[a]

When to Treat

The decision of when to initiate medical therapy varies according to the type of glaucoma being treated. The general approach is to recommend therapy whenever glaucomatous damage is documented or when the degree of IOP elevation or other risk factors are such that future damage is likely. The details of this issue, as they relate to specific forms of glaucoma, were considered in Section Two.

What to Prescribe

This decision depends not only on the type of glaucoma, but also on several considerations related to the particular patient. A medication that may be effective for one form of glaucoma may be ineffective or actually counterproductive with another type. The reader must again be referred to Section Two for the details of this question as they relate to specific forms of glaucoma. In some cases, such as chronic open-angle glaucoma, several medications may be potentially effective. A prospective study of 71 open-angle glaucoma patients revealed a significant reduction in IOP with the first drug used, but not with changes to stronger drugs or combination therapy (56, 57). Therefore, in selecting the initial drug it is best to try the one which is least likely to cause significant ocular and systemic side effects. This requires careful attention to the patient's medical history and physical findings, as well as a detailed understanding of potential drug-induced side effects, which is considered in subsequent chapters of Section Three. In general, the rule-of-thumb to follow whenever prescribing medication is to use the least amount of medication that will accomplish the desired therapeutic effect with the fewest adverse reactions.

[a]Refer to Shields, MB: Color Atlas of Glaucoma. Baltimore, Williams & Wilkins, 1998, Plate III6.

How to Prescribe

It is almost always advisable to prescribe only one new drug at a time so that the efficacy of each medication can be evaluated. One exception to this rule is the patient with a markedly elevated IOP that poses an immediate threat to vision. In this emergency situation, it is usually best to advance rapidly to maximum medical therapy by starting with a combination of two or more drugs and then to gradually reduce the medication if possible after the desired pressure level is reached. Another useful practice when prescribing a new drug in the less urgent situations is to use a *uniocular trial* of therapy, in which the untreated eye serves as a control during the trial period. This allows the physician to differentiate between drug effect and spontaneous fluctuations in IOP.

Instructing the Patient

Noncompliance

Noncompliance with recommended medical therapy is a major problem in the prevention of blindness from glaucoma. Studies have shown that glaucoma, by its very nature, fosters noncompliance (58). In other words, most forms of glaucoma represent chronic diseases in which symptoms are mild or absent, treatment is prophylactic, and the consequences of stopping therapy are delayed, all of which are factors associated with poor patient compliance to medical therapy (59). As a result, even studies of compliance that are based on the patient's own estimation reveal that one-third to two-thirds of the patients miss at least one treatment per month (60–62), or use their medications incorrectly (63). Even more revealing are studies in which patient compliance is monitored by electronic devices in the medication bottle (64). Studies with these instruments have shown that 41% of the patients omitted at least 10% of their prescribed pilocarpine treatments (65) and 15% missed over half of their drops (66). Many of these patients had inadequate spacing between treatments, frequent misses at noon, and long interruptions in the use of their medication (66, 67). Traditional parameters such as the IOP, pupillary diameter, patient's report or log book, and remaining medicine in bottle, are all inadequate in distinguishing patients with low rates of compliance (68). Reducing the frequency with which a medication must be taken appears to improve compliance, but does not eliminate defaulting (69, 70). Efforts that have been shown to be effective in improving patient compliance include (a) educating the patient about the disease and its treatment, (b) tailoring the therapeutic regimen to the patient's daily schedule, (c) training in and reinforcing the instillation of eyedrops, (d) cooperating with primary care physicians, (e) alleviating side effects, and (f) improving doctor-patient relationships (58).

ABOUT THE DISEASE. It is essential for the patient to be made aware of their disease and its potential seriousness without creating undue apprehension. In other words, the patient should be told (a) that he or she has glaucoma, (b) what glaucoma is, (c) that it can lead to total, irreversible blindness, but (d) that the blindness can be prevented with proper treatment. It is not uncommon for a patient who has been on antiglaucoma medications for years to be unaware that they have glaucoma or to relate their disease to blindness, while others may live in daily fear that they will inevitably go blind. The time taken to correct these misconceptions is one of the most important measures in preventing blindness and improving the general well being of your patient.

WHY THE MEDICATION. The patient must understand that the purpose of their medication is to lower the IOP to prevent loss of vision, and that this treatment will usually not improve the present state of their visual acuity. Many patients quit using their drops because "they didn't seem to be helping."

SIDE EFFECTS. It is equally important to make the patient aware of the more common side effects that they may experience with their new drug. If the patient knows what to expect and that the symptoms may lessen with time, it will hopefully allay their apprehension when side effects do occur and prevent their premature discontinuation of the drug.

The physician should also select a drug, especially if it is the patients' first antiglaucoma medication, that has the fewest possible potential side effects. It is usually best to begin with a weaker drug, even if it is unlikely to be sufficient, to allow the patient to adjust to the use of eyedrops before going to stronger medications with more side effects.

ADMINISTRATION OF EYEDROPS. It should not be assumed that a patient knows the proper techniques for instilling eyedrops. The inability to adequately instill a drop into the eye has been identified as a major factor in the failure of medical therapy (71). When patients have been observed administering their drops, some were noted to flood their eye with an excess of medication, while others missed their eye altogether or contaminated the eyedropper by touching the lids or periocular tissue (72–74). The first step in avoiding these pitfalls is to observe the patient instill their drops in the office, since some may already have a good technique. If they do not, the following is one effective method in which the patient can be instructed: (a) pinch the lower lid or pull it forward by the lashes to create a pocket; (b) place one drop in the cul-de-sac without touching the eyedropper to ocular tissues; (c) keep the lid held forward for a few seconds while the drop settles into the cul-de-sac; (d) look down while bringing the lower lid up until it touches the eye; (e) release the lid and close the eye gently while placing gentle pressure over the lacrimal sac (Fig. 24.4) (75).

The final step of *nasolacrimal occlusion* (Fig. 24.5), when performed for 5 minutes after instillation, has been shown to significantly reduce drug loss in the tears with a marked reduction in systemic drug absorption and an in-

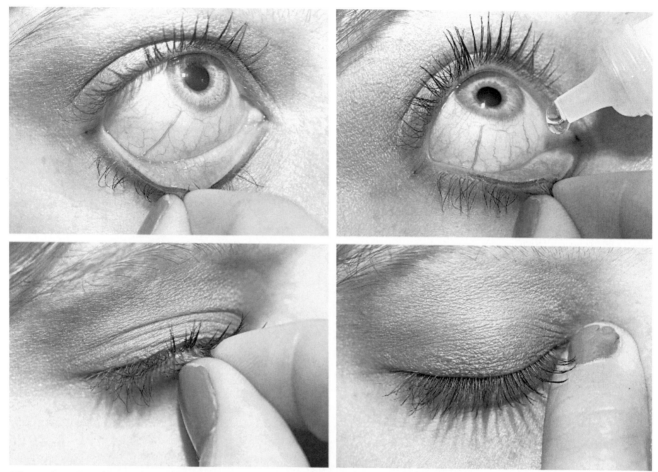

Figure 24.4. A technique for instillation of eyedrops. **A.** Pinch lower lid and pull down to create a pocket. **B.** Place one drop in pocket. **C.** Look down while bringing lower lid up to touch eye. **D.** Close eye and apply gentle pressure over lacrimal sac.

crease in anterior chamber concentration (76). However, one study of 23 normal individuals did not reveal additional IOP reduction after instillation of timolol 0.5% with either lid closure or nasolacrimal occlusion, as compared to leaving the eyes open without the occlusion (77). In addition, nasolacrimal occlusion is difficult for some patients, and gentle *eyelid closure* for 5 minutes, which minimizes lacrimal drainage by eliminating the blink movements, gave essentially the same results (76). Punctal occlusion with silicone or collagen plugs has also been evaluated, with conflicting reports as to whether this improves drug efficacy (78–80).

Some patients have difficulty keeping their eyes open during instillation of eyedrops. One study showed that instilling tropicamide 0.125% in the medial canthus with the lids closed produced a comparable mydriasis to instillation of the medication in the conventional manner (81).

THERAPEUTIC REGIMEN. It is not enough to tell the patient to use their medication two to four times each day. Some patients may fail to space their dosages properly, while others may have such difficulty establishing a daily schedule that they become poor compliers (66). In addition, if they are taking more than one drop at the same time of day, they may be instilling them so close together that they are diluting or washing each other from the cul-de-sac. The patient should be instructed to space the instillation of any two medications by at least 5–10 minutes. A patient may be on three different topical medications, which can be particularly complicated. This is especially true of the elderly, who constitute a large percentage of the glaucoma population, and whose impaired vision, limited motion, and failing memory significantly impair their ability to comply with prescribed therapy (82).

To minimize these problems, the medicine bottles should first be clearly identified. Referring to the color of the top is usually best, although large labels on the bottles may also be helpful. The patient's daily routine should then be reviewed and the times of drug instillation should be selected to correspond with specific daily activities. The best times of day are usually with meals and at bedtime for a four-time-a-day medication, and a breakfast-supper or lunch-bedtime routine for twice-daily administration. The schedule should be placed on a card, which is large enough for the patient to see and which they can keep in a convenient location (Fig. 24.6).

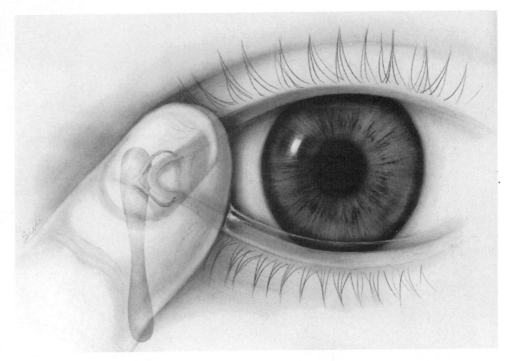

Figure 24.5. Proper placement of finger to achieve nasolacrimal occlusion. (Reproduced by permission from Zimmerman, TJ, Kooner, KS, Kandarakis, AS, Ziegler, LP: Improving the therapeutic index of topically applied ocular drugs. Arch Ophthalmol 102:551, 1984.)

name date				
drug/time	☕ **breakfast**	🍔 **lunch**	🍴🍽🍴 **supper**	🛏 **bedtime**
pilocarpine *(Green Top)*	✕	✕	✕	✕
Epifrin *(White Top)*	✕		✕	
Timoptic *(Yellow Top)*		✕		✕
Diamox *(Capsule)*	✕		✕	
DAILY DRUG REMINDER				

Figure 24.6. Example of drug schedule that can be used to instruct the patient in the use of their glaucoma medications and to serve as a reminder for the patient. (Courtesy of Sharon Brooks, RN)

Followup

Evaluation of Efficacy

It is obviously important to recheck the IOP within a few days or weeks of starting a new drug, depending on the urgency of the situation, to insure that the desired goal of pressure reduction has been achieved. This is best accomplished with the uniocular trial of therapy, as previously discussed.

When using the fellow eye as a control, however, it must be kept in mind that most antiglaucoma drops will also cause a small consensual IOP fall in the untreated eye (83).

Once a stable pressure reduction has been achieved, the patient is usually reevaluated every 3–4 months. It is a good practice to temporarily discontinue a drug once every several years to insure that it is still contributing to the reduced IOP. This is especially true if the pressure is starting to rise, which may represent the development of tolerance to a drug rather than progression of the disease. Instead of simply adding more medication, the physician should first temporarily discontinue the existing medication in one eye (one drug at a time) to insure that these are still having a significant effect on the pressure.

Patient Reinforcement

On every visit, the patient should be asked about compliance with their medication and whether they are encountering any difficulties. Noncompliance should be dealt with by reviewing the seriousness of their glaucoma and the importance of treatment and by trying to find out why they are not complying. Such circumstances may include difficult daily schedules, visual or other physical limitations, or inability to afford the medication, and each must be dealt with on an individual basis. It is also important to seek out possible side effects, which the patient may not relate to the treatment of their eyes, but which could be adversely influencing their daily life or endangering their general health.

Contact with Family Physician

It is important to keep the primary care physician informed of the patients ocular medication and to also keep a record from that physician as to the patient's additional medications or diseases so as to avoid drug interactions or the use of medications that may be contraindicated. In addition, the family physician may help in reinforcing the importance of medical compliance and in spotting side effects.

Techniques of Patient Education

The physician is ultimately responsible for the education of his or her patient and must take the time, no matter how busy the day's schedule may be, to discuss the basic aspects of the disease and its treatment when it is first diagnosed. If it has not already been done, this is the time when a good doctor-patient relationship must be established. However, the physician rarely has time to be personally involved in all aspects of patient education and should make use of other office personnel and educational materials.

The most important ancillary individual is the office nurse or technician. This person should be able to restate and expand upon what the physician has said, instruct the patient in the instillation of eyedrops, work out the therapeutic regimen, and provide the necessary reinforcement of these matters on each followup visit. That individual should also be able to answer the inevitable phone calls when patients have questions about the use of their medications or possible side effects.

Important resource materials include booklets on glaucoma, which are available from a number of health-related organizations. Videotapes have also been shown to be an effective method of patient education (84). In some centers, classes or meetings are provided for glaucoma patients to broaden their understanding of their condition. These are usually conducted by nurses, technicians, or social workers and may incorporate lectures, videotapes, question-and-answer sessions, or group discussions.

SUMMARY

Commercially available topical antiglaucoma drugs include autonomic agents, which consist of cholinergic stimulators and adrenergic stimulators and inhibitors, as well as carbonic anhydrase inhibitors and prostaglandins. Systemic drugs include carbonic anhydrase inhibitors and hyperosmotics. The pharmacokinetics of topical drugs involves interaction with the tears, corneal penetration, and intraocular factors, each of which can be influenced by the vehicle, pH, concentration, and additives of the drug formulation. In prescribing medications, important questions are when to treat, what to use, and how it should be used. To improve compliance with recommended medical therapy, the patient should be told about their disease, why they are using the medicine, how to use the drug, and what side effects to expect. It is also important to evaluate the efficacy of the therapy initially and periodically during the treatment.

REFERENCES

1. Richardson, KT: Ocular microtherapy. Membrane-controlled drug delivery. Arch Ophthalmol 93:74, 1975.
2. Bito, LZ, Merritt, SQ: Paradoxical ocular hypertensive effect of pilocarpine on echothiophate iodide-treated primate eyes. Invest Ophthalmol Vis Sci 19:371, 1980.
3. Kaufman, PL, Barany, EH: Loss of acute pilocarpine effect on outflow facility following surgical disinsertion and retrodisplacement of the ciliary muscle from the scleral spur in the cynomolgus monkey. Invest Ophthalmol 15:793, 1976.
4. Kaufman, PL, Barany, EH: Residual pilocarpine effects on outflow facility after ciliary muscle disinsertion in the cynomolgus monkey. Invest Ophthalmol 15:558, 1976.
5. Grierson, I, Lee, WR, Abraham, S: Effects of pilocarpine on the morphology of the human outflow apparatus. Br J Ophthalmol 62:302, 1978.
6. Huang, Y, Gil, DW, Vanscheeuwijck, P, et al: Localization of α_2-adrenergic receptor subtypes in the anterior segment of the human eye with selective antibodies. Invest Ophthalmol Vis Sci 36:2729, 1995.
7. Lands, AM, Arnold, A, McAuliff, JP, et al: Differentiation of receptor systems activated by sympathomimetic amines. Nature 214:597, 1967.
8. Shell, JW: Pharmacokinetics of topically applied ophthalmic drugs. Surv Ophthalmol 26:207, 1982.
9. Mishima, S: Clinical pharmacokinetics of the eye. Proctor lecture. Invest Ophthalmol Vis Sci 21:504, 1981.
10. Lederer, CM Jr, Harold, RE: Drop size of commercial glaucoma medications. Am J Ophthalmol 101:691, 1986.
11. Benson, H: Permeability of the cornea to topically applied drugs. Arch Ophthalmol 91:313, 1974.
12. Havener, WH: Ocular Pharmacology. 4th ed. St. Louis, CV Mosby, 1978, pp. 19, 429.
13. Akers, MJ: Ocular bioavailability of topically applied ophthalmic drugs. Am Pharm NS23:33, 1983.

14. Mindel, JS, Smith, H, Jacobs, M, et al: Drug reservoirs in topical therapy. Invest Ophthalmol Vis Sci 25:346, 1984.

15. Harris, LS, Galin, MA: Effect of ocular pigmentation on hypotensive response to pilocarpine. Am J Ophthalmol 72:923, 1971.

16. Melikian, HE, Lieberman, TW, Leopold, IH: Ocular pigmentation and pressure and outflow responses to pilocarpine and epinephrine. Am J Ophthalmol 72:70, 1971.

17. Lyons, JS, Krohn, DL: Pilocarpine uptake by pigmented uveal tissue. Am J Ophthalmol 75:885, 1973.

18. Newsome, DA, Stern, R: Pilocarpine adsorption by serum and ocular tissues. Am J Ophthalmol 77:918, 1974.

19. Path, PN, Jacobowitz, D: Unequal accumulation of adrenergic drugs by pigmented and nonpigmented iris. Am J Ophthalmol 78:470, 1974.

20. Nagata, A, Mishima, HK, Kiuchi, Y, et al: Binding of antiglaucomatous drugs to synthetic melanin and their hypotensive effects on pigmented and nonpigmented rabbit eyes. Jpn J Ophthalmol 37: 32, 1993.

21. Lee, VH-L, Hul, H-W, Robinson, JR: Corneal metabolism of pilocarpine in pigmented rabbits. Invest Ophthalmol Vis Sci 19: 210,1980.

22. Shell, JW: Ophthalmic drug delivery systems. Surv Ophthalmol 29:117, 1984.

23. Lemp, MA, Holly, FJ: Ophthalmic polymers as ocular wetting agents. Ann Ophthalmol 4:15, 1972.

24. Trueblood, JH, Rossomondo, RM, Carlton, WH, Wilson, LA: Corneal contact times of ophthalmic vehicles. Evaluation by microscintigraphy. Arch Ophthalmol 93:127, 1975.

25. Hardberger, R, Hanna, C, Boyd, CM: Effects of drug vehicles on ocular contact time. Arch Ophthalmol 93:42, 1975.

26. Hardberger, RE, Hanna, C, Goodart, R: Effects of drug vehicles on ocular uptake of tetracycline. Am J Ophthalmol 80:133, 1975.

27. Waltman, SR, Buerk, K, Foster, CS: Effects of ophthalmic ointments on intraocular penetration of topical fluorescein in rabbits and man. Am J Ophthalmol 78:262, 1974.

28. Mandell, AI, Stewart, RM, Kass, MA: Multiclinic evaluation of pilocarpine gel. Invest Ophthalmol Vis Sci (Suppl) 165, 1979.

29. March, WF, Stewart, RM, Mandell, AI, Bruce, LA: Duration of effect of pilocarpine gel. Arch Ophthalmol 100:1270, 1982.

30. Ticho, U, Blumenthal, M, Zonis, S, et al: Piloplex, a new long-acting pilocarpine polymer salt: a long-term study. Br J Ophthalmol 63: 45, 1979.

31. Mazor, A, Ticho, U, Rehany, U, Rose, L: Piloplex—a new long-acting polymer salt: B. Comparative study of the visual effects of pilocarpine and piloplex eyedrops. Br J Ophthalmol 63:48, 1979.

32. Klein, HZ, Lugo, M, Shields, MB, et al: A dose-response study of piloplex for duration of action. Am J Ophthalmol 99:23, 1985.

33. Schaeffer, HE, Krohn, DL: Liposomes in topical drug delivery. Invest Ophthalmol Vis Sci 21:220, 1982.

34. Zeimer, RC, Khoobehi, B, Niesman, MR, Magin, RL: A potential method for local drug and dye delivery in the ocular vasculature. Invest Ophthalmol Vis Sci 29:1179, 1988.

35. Khoobehi, B, Peyman, GA, McTurnan, WG, et al: Externally triggered release of dye and drugs from the liposomes into the eye. An in vitro and in vivo study. Ophathalmology 95:950, 1988.

36. Lerman, S, Reininger, B: Simulated sustained release pilocarpine therapy and aqueous humor dynamics. Can J Ophthalmol 6:14, 1971.

37. Maichuk, YF: Ophthalmic drug inserts. Invest Ophthalmol 14:87, 1975.

38. Katz, IM, Blackman, WM: A soluble sustained-release ophthalmic delivery unit. Am J Ophthalmol 83:728, 1977.

39. Leaders, FE, Hecht, G, VanHoose, M, Kellog, M: New polymers in drug delivery. Ann Ophthalmol 5:513, 1973.

40. Maddox, YT, Bernstein, HN: An evaluation of the bionite hydrophilic contact lens for use in a drug delivery system. Ann Ophthalmol 4: 789, 1972.

41. Hull, DS, Edelhauser, HF, Hyndiuk, RA: Ocular penetration of prednisolone and the hydrophilic contact lens. Arch Ophthalmol 92: 413, 1974.

42. Sawusch, MR, O'Brien, TP, Dick, JD, Gottsch, JD: Use of collagen corneal shields in the treatment of bacterial keratitis. Am J Ophthalmol 106:279, 1988.

43. Dohlman, CH, Pavan-Langston, D, Rose, J: A new ocular insert device for continuous constant-rate delivery of medication to the eye. Ann Ophthalmol 4:823, 1972.

44. Gwon, A, Borrmann, LR, Duzman, E, et al: Ophthalmic rods. New ocular drug delivery devices. Ophthalmology 93(S):82, 1986.

45. Alani, SD: The ophthalmic rod: a new ophthalmic drug delivery system I. Graefes Arch Clin Exp Ophthalmol 228:297, 1990.

46. Alani, SD, Hammerstein, W: The ophthalmic rod—a new drug-delivery system II. Graefes Arch Clin Exp Ophthalmol 228:302, 1990.

47. Kelly, JA, Molyneux, PD, Smith, SA, Smith, SE: Relative bioavailability of pilocarpine from a novel ophthalmic delivery system and conventional eyedrop formulations. Br J Ophthalmol 73:360, 1989.

48. Lawrenson, JG, Edgar, DF, Gudgeon, AC, et al: A comparison of the efficacy and duration of action of topically applied proxymetacaine using a novel ophthalmic delivery system versus eye drops in healthy young volunteers. Br J Ophthalmol 77:713, 1993.

49. Anderson, RA, Cowle, JB: Influence of pH on the effect of pilocarpine on aqueous dynamics. Br J Ophthalmol 52:607, 1968.

50. Ramer, RM, Gasset, AR: Ocular penetration of pilocarpine: the effect of pH on the ocular penetration of pilocarpine. Ann Ophthalmol 7: 293, 1975.

51. David, R, Goldberg, L, Luntz, MH: Influence of pH on the efficacy of pilocarpine. Br J Ophthalmol 62:318, 1978.

52. Asseff, CF, Weisman, RL, Podos, SM, Becker, B: Ocular penetration of pilocarpine in primates. Am J Ophthalmol 75:212, 1973.

53. Smolen, VF, Clevenger, JM, Williams, EJ, Bergdolt, MW: Biophasic availability of ophthalmic carbachol I: Mechanisms of cationic polymer- and surfactant-promoted miotic activity. J Pharm Sci 62:958, 1973.

54. Schein, OD, Wasson, PJ, Boruchoff, SA, Kenyon, KR: Microbial keratitis associated with contaminated ocular medications. Am J Ophthalmol 105:361, 1988.

55. Lynch, MG, Brown, RH, Goode, SM, et al: Reduction of phenylephrine drop size in infants achieves equal dilation with decreased systemic absorption. Arch Ophthalmol 105:1364, 1987.

56. Begg, IS, Cottle, RW, et al: Epidemological approach to open-angle glaucoma: 1. Control of intraocular pressure. Report of the Canadian Ocular Adverse Drug Reaction Registry Program. Can J Ophthalmol 23:273, 1988.

57. Begg, IS, Cottle, RW: Epidemiologic approach to open-angle glaucoma: 2. Survival analysis of adverse drug reactions. Report of the Canadian Ocular Adverse Drug Reaction Registry Program. Can J Ophthalmol 24:15, 1989.

58. Zimmerman, TJ, Zalta, AH: Facilitating patient compliance in glaucoma therapy. Surv Ophthalmol 28(Suppl):252, 1983.

59. Blackwell, B: Patient compliance. N Engl J Med 289:249, 1973.

60. Bloch, S, Rosenthal, AR, Friedman, L, Caldarolla, P: Patient compliance in glaucoma. Br J Ophthalmol 61:531, 1977.

61. Kass, MA, Hodapp, E, Gordon, M, et al: Patient administration of eyedrops: Part I. Interview. Ann Ophthalmol 14:775, 1982.

62. Patel, SC, Spaeth, GL: Compliance in patients prescribed eyedrops for glaucoma. Ophthalmic Surg 26:233, 1995.

63. Spaeth, GL: Visual loss in a glaucoma clinic. I. Sociological considerations. Invest Ophthalmol 9:73, 1970.

64. Kass, MA, Meltzer, DW, Gordon, M: A miniature compliance monitor for eyedrop medication. Arch Ophthalmol 102:1550, 1984.

65. Norell, SE, Granstrom, PA: Self-medication with pilocarpine among outpatients in a glaucoma clinic. Br J Ophthalmol 64:137, 1980.

66. Kass, MA, Meltzer, DW, Gordon, M, et al: Compliance with topical pilocarpine treatment. Am J Ophthalmol 101:515, 1986.

67. Granstrom, P-A: Glaucoma patients not compliant with their drug therapy: clinical and behavioural aspects. Br J Ophthalmol 66:464, 1982.

68. Kass, MA, Gordon, M, Meltzer, DW: Can ophthalmologists correctly identify patients defaulting from pilocarpine therapy? Am J Ophthalmol 101:524, 1986.

69. Kass, MA, Gordon, M, Morley, RE, et al: Compliance with topical timolol treatment. Am J Ophthalmol 103:188, 1987.

70. Cramer, JA, Mattson, RH, Prevey, ML, et al: How often is medication taken as prescribed? A novel assessment technique. JAMA 261: 3273, 1989.

71. Winfield, AJ, Jessiman, D, Williams, A, Esakowitz, L: A study of the causes of non-compliance by patients prescribed eyedrops. Br J Ophthalmol 74:477, 1990.

72. Kass, MA, Hodapp, E, Gordon, M, et al: Patient administration of eyedrops: Part II. Observation. Ann Ophthalmol 14:889, 1982.

73. Brown, MM, Brown, GC, Spaeth, GL: Improper topical self-administration of ocular medications among patients with glaucoma. Can J Ophthalmol 19:2, 1984.

74. Hosoda, M, Yamabayashi, S, Furuta, M, Tsukahara, S: Do glaucoma patients use eye drops correctly? J Glau 4:202, 1995.

75. Fraunfelder, FT: Extraocular fluid dynamics: How best to apply topical ocular medication. Trans Am Ophthalmol Soc 74:457, 1976.

76. Zimmerman, TJ, Kooner, KS, Kandarakis, AS, Ziegler, LP: Improving the therapeutic index of topically applied ocular drugs. Arch Ophthalmol 102:551, 1984.

77. Ohkawa, M, Mikami, K, Ichinohe, S, Maeda, S: Effect of eye closure and lacrimal sac compression after instillation on eyedrop efficacy. Folia Ophthalmol Jpn 41:284, 1990.

78. Huang, TC, Lee, DA: Punctal occlusion and topical medications for glaucoma. Am J Ophthalmol 107:151, 1989.

79. Gilbert, ML, Wilhelmus, KR, Osato, MS: Intracanalicular collagen implants enhance topical antibiotic bioavailability. Cornea 5:167, 1986.

80. Simel, DL, Simel, PJ: Does lacrimal duct occlusion decrease intraocular pressure in patients refractory to medical treatment for glaucoma? A randomized, sham-controlled, crossover trial. J Clin Epidemiol 41:859, 1988.

81. Loewenstein, A, Bolocinic, S, Goldstein, M, Lazar, M: Application of eye drops to the medial canthus. Graefes Arch Clin Exp Ophthalmol 232:680, 1994.

82. Polk, IJ: Drug compliance in the elderly. JAMA 248:1239, 1982.

83. Gibbens, MV: The consensual ophthalmotonic reaction. Br J Ophthalmol 72:746, 1988.

84. Rosenthal, AR, Zimmerman, JF, Tanner, J: Educating the glaucoma patient. Br J Ophthalmol 67:814, 1983.

CHOLINERGIC STIMULATORS[a]

I. Pilocarpine
   A. Mechanisms of action
      1. Ciliary muscle contraction
      2. Miosis
      3. Decreased aqueous production?
   B. Administration
      1. Ocular penetration
      2. Drug concentration
      3. Frequency of administration
      4. Delivery systems
   C. Drug interactions
   D. Side effects
      1. Systemic toxicity
      2. Ocular side effects
   E. Clinical indications

II. Dual action parasympathomimetics
   A. Carbachol
   B. Aceclidine
III. Indirect parasympathomimetics
   A. Physostigmine (eserine)
   B. Echothiophate iodide
      1. Mechanism of action
      2. Administration
      3. Side effects
      4. Clinical indications
   C. Other strong, relatively irreversible cholinesterase inhibitors

Parasympathetic

Pharmacologic agents that mimic the cholinergic effects of acetylcholine are generally referred to as *parasympathomimetics, cholinergic stimulators,* or *miotics,* the latter being due to their common action on the pupil. This was the first class of drugs to be used in the treatment of glaucoma, having been introduced in the 1870s. These compounds all have the same basic effect on aqueous humor dynamics and their primary clinical differences are in duration of action and severity of side effects.

PILOCARPINE

Pilocarpine is the most commonly used and the most extensively studied miotic. It is a direct-acting parasympathomimetic, or muscarinic agonist, although there is evidence that it may also have an indirect effect by activating choline acetyltransferase synthesis of acetylcholine (1). The following ocular effects of pilocarpine are generally representative of all the miotics.

[a]Refer to Shields, MB: Color Atlas of Glaucoma. Baltimore, Williams & Wilkins, 1998, Plates III1–2.

Mechanisms of Action

Ciliary Muscle Contraction

The principal mode of intraocular pressure (IOP) reduction by pilocarpine is *enhanced aqueous outflow.* In eyes with open anterior chamber angles, the mechanism of this action appears to be stimulation of ciliary muscle contraction. It has been demonstrated that aqueous outflow facility can be increased by accommodation (2), a posterior depression of the lens (3–5), tension on the choroid (6), or a pull on the root of the iris (7). In each of these situations, the common action appears to be traction on the scleral spur by virtue of its attachment to the ciliary musculature. The displacement of the scleral spur leads to an increased facility of aqueous outflow presumably by altering the configuration of the trabecular meshwork, Schlemm's canal, or both (Fig. 25.1). Pilocarpine and the other miotics exert a similar traction on the scleral spur by stimulating contraction of the ciliary muscle.

More direct evidence for the influence of pilocarpine-induced cyclotropia on outflow facility is the observation that disinsertion of the ciliary muscle from the scleral spur in monkeys eliminates the effect of pilocarpine on IOP and facility of outflow (8, 9). To rule out other possible mechanisms, it was

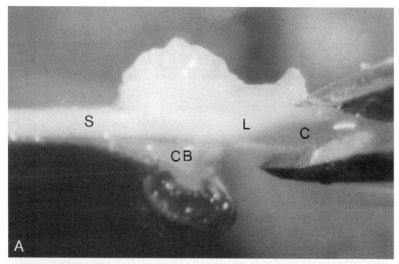

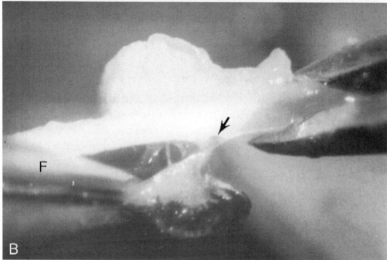

Figure 25.1. The influence of tension on the ciliary body in widening Schlemm's canal is demonstrated in a human autopsy eye. **A.** Without tension, the canal is collapsed and cannot be seen in this photo. **B.** When the ciliary body is stretched with forceps (*F*), Schlemm's canal opens (*arrow*) due to inward, posterior displacement of the scleral spur. A similar mechanism is believed to explain the improvement in outflow facility following cholinergic stimulation. Ciliary body (*CB*); sclera (*S*); limbus (*L*); cornea (*C*). (Courtesy of David G. Campbell, M.D.)

shown that the disinsertion did not alter conventional outflow (10) nor cause histologic changes in the ciliary muscle, trabecular meshwork, or Schlemm's canal (11). Histologic studies of human eyes treated with pilocarpine prior to enucleation for malignant melanoma demonstrated a posterior, internal pull on the scleral spur, with widening of the trabecular spaces, distention of the endothelial meshwork, an increase in the number of giant vacuoles, and larger, more frequent pores in the inner endothelium of Schlemm's canal (12, 13). Primate studies suggest that the greater number of giant vacuoles is a result of increased aqueous flow through the outflow system, rather than a direct action of pilocarpine on the endothelium of Schlemm's canal (14).

The contractile response of ciliary muscle to pilocarpine in monkeys diminishes with age at a rate similar to that for accommodative decline (15, 16). This aging effect does not appear to be related to alterations in choline acetyltransferase or acetylcholinesterase activity or to the affinity or number of muscarinic binding sites (17).

Ciliary ganglionectomy in monkeys produces functional denervation of the ciliary muscle, as evidenced by loss of

choline acetyltransferase activity (18) and an initial supersensitivity to pilocarpine (19). Reinnervation occurs by 6 months with return of normal accommodative response to pilocarpine (19). However, pilocarpine in these eyes has no effect on outflow facility (20), which may be related to atrophy of the ciliary muscle fibers and separation from ensheathed nerve fibers (21).

As discussed later in this chapter, topical pilocarpine and the other miotics are associated with many ocular side effects. It might be possible to separate these adverse reactions from the therapeutic effects, if they are related to different receptor subtypes. Muscarinic receptors have been shown to have five subtypes, and an M3-like muscarinic receptor subtype appears to be prominent in cultured human ciliary muscle cells (22).

Miosis

The miotic effect of pilocarpine is useful in the short-term management of certain angle-closure glaucomas. The miosis results primarily from direct stimulation of the sphincter muscle of the iris, although significant cholinergic inhibition of the dilator muscle has also been demonstrated in the bovine eye (23). Miosis improves outflow facility in eyes with angle-closure glaucomas by relieving pupillary block or by pulling peripheral iris from the anterior chamber angle. However, miosis does not appear to be related to the improvement of aqueous outflow facility in open-angle glaucomas, since total removal of the iris in monkeys did not alter the facility response to intravenous pilocarpine (24).

Decreased Aqueous Production?

There is some controversy as to whether the IOP lowering effect of pilocarpine is partially related to decreased aqueous inflow. The reduction in pressure has been reported to exceed (25) and outlast (26) the improvement in outflow facility, and pilocarpine 0.1% was shown to reduce aqueous humor formation in monkey eyes (27). Bárány (28) suggested that prolonged treatment with pilocarpine may result in subsensitivity of the ciliary muscle, with a shift in emphasis to inhibition of aqueous secretion by an unknown mechanism. Another possible explanation for a reduced outflow effect with prolonged use of pilocarpine, based on observations in primates, is an altered geometry of the chamber angle structures, leading to underperfusion of the trabecular meshwork, which stimulates the production of increased amounts of extracellular material (29).

A possible mechanism for pilocarpine-induced inhibition of aqueous production is seen in the observation that acetylcholine transiently hyperpolarizes the cell membrane potential of cultured human nonpigmented ciliary epithelial cells by an action on K^+ channels (30). There is also a suggestion from studies with rabbit iris-ciliary body tissue preparations that the cholinergic system may have a direct role in the modulation of ciliary epithelial adenylate cyclase and aqueous humor secretion (31). Conversely, fluorophotometric studies in humans revealed a stimulation of aqueous humor formation with pilocarpine, although this was too small to be of clinical significance (32).

Other Effects

It should also be noted that pilocarpine *decreases uveoscleral outflow* (33). This may have clinical significance in eyes with markedly reduced conventional outflow. As these eyes become increasingly dependent on unconventional drainage, pilocarpine may cause a paradoxic rise in IOP (34). Episcleral venous pressure does not appear to be altered by pilocarpine (25).

Administration

Ocular Penetration

The cornea is the main route by which topical pilocarpine enters the eye (35), although this tissue may also impede oc-

ular penetration. Studies differ somewhat as to the predominant portion of the cornea in which pilocarpine concentrates, with one suggesting the epithelium (36) and others the corneal stroma (37, 38). In any case, the drug is largely complexed or degraded in the cornea (39), with only a small percentage entering the anterior chamber (39–41). Selecting the optimum drug concentration, frequency of administration, and delivery system may improve the efficiency of ocular penetration.

Drug Concentration

The IOP-lowering effect of chronically-administered pilocarpine is dose-related up to a concentration of 4% (42–45). Studies differ, however, as to whether there is significant dose-response curve with single dose instillations (42, 43). Furthermore, higher concentrations of pilocarpine, such as 6%, may cause additional pressure reduction in darkly pigmented eyes (46).

Frequency of Administration

Following topical instillation in animals, the maximum concentrations of pilocarpine in the aqueous and iris were reached in approximately 20 minutes (38), and aqueous levels were gone in 4 hours (40). In studies of ocular hypertensive individuals, the maximum effect on IOP occurred within 2 hours and lasted for at least 8 hours, with a reduction in IOP of approximately 20% (43). The pressure response began to decline by the ninth hour, although there was still a 14–15% reduction at 12–15 hours after instillation (44). To insure adequate pressure control, standard pilocarpine drops have traditionally been given four times daily. It has been shown, however, that twice daily instillation of 2% pilocarpine followed by nasolacrimal occlusion gives the maximal ocular hypotensive response (47). When changing a patient to the reduced frequency, it is advisable to confirm the continued efficacy of the drug by checking the IOP 12 hours after instillation. In some emergency situations, it may be possible to improve the efficiency of pilocarpine by frequent, repeated instillations (48) or by continuous infusion (49) of dilute solutions, although such practice is rarely indicated.

Delivery Systems

A goal of any drug therapy is to achieve the desired pharmacologic effect with the least amount of medicine. Animal and human studies suggest that the volume of pilocarpine delivered by commercial droppers is significantly in excess of that needed to produce the desired response (50, 51). The result is often an initial overdosing with the associated side effects, followed by an underdosing before the next instillation. This problem can be reduced by using vehicles for drug delivery which prolong the duration of the therapeutic effectiveness, thereby decreasing the frequency of instillations and associated side effects (Table 25.1).

Table 25.1

COMMERCIAL PILOCARPINE PREPARATIONS*

Preparations	Brand Names	Concentrations (%)
Solutions		
Hydrochlorides	Akarpine	1, 2, 4
	Isopto Carpine	0.25, 0.5, 1, 2, 3, 4, 6, 8, 10
	Ocu-carpine	0.5, 1, 2, 3, 4, 6
	Pilocar	0.5, 1, 2, 3, 4, 6
	Piloptic	0.5, 1, 2, 3, 4, 6
	Pilostat	0.5, 1, 2, 3, 4, 6
	Storzine	1, 2, 4
Nitrate	Pilagan	1, 2, 4
Gel	Pilopine HS gel	4
Inserts	Ocusert Pilo-20	(20 µg/hr)
	Ocusert Pilo-40	(40 µg/hr)
Epinephrine combinations	E-Pilo-1, E-Pilo-2, etc., P₁E₁, P₂E₁, etc.	1, 2, 3, 4, 6 (+ epi. 1%)
Timolol combinations**	Timpilo Fotil	2, 4 (+ timolol 0.5%)

Other generic products may also be available.

**Not currently available in United States.*

SOLUBLE POLYMERS. Soluble polymers such as methylcellulose and polyvinyl alcohol, as discussed in Chapter 24, may increase corneal retention time and are commonly used in commercial preparations (52). However, the results of clinical studies with pilocarpine in such vehicles have been conflicting. One formulation of pilocarpine in water-soluble polymers was reported to have a prolonged duration of action with improved pressure control (53–55), although this was not confirmed by subsequent studies (56–58).

An aqueous emulsion of pilocarpine bound to a polymer vehicle (Piloplex) was shown to be more effective in twice daily administration than pilocarpine hydrochloride, four times a day (59–62). A single dose lowered the IOP in a dose-related fashion, with a duration of action of at least 14 hours (63).

PILOCARPINE GEL. The equivalent of 4% pilocarpine hydrochloride in a high-viscosity acrylic vehicle (Pilopine), when applied once daily at bedtime, has been reported to produce a significant reduction in IOP for 24 hours (64, 65). It was found to be at least as effective as pilocarpine hydrochloride drops, four times daily (66, 67), with less induced myopia and impaired nocturnal visual acuity than the drops (68). However, since the effect 12 hours after administration is greater than that at 24 hours, the physician is advised to confirm the 24-hour effect by measuring the pressure 24 hours after administration (64). A subtle, diffuse, superficial corneal haze (64) has been observed in 20–28%

of patients after prolonged use of Pilopine (69). In some patients, this persisted for 2 years after the gel was discontinued (64). The corneal haze produced no symptoms, and no long-term consequences have been reported with over a decade of use.

OILY SOLUTIONS. Oily solutions of pilocarpine have also been shown to have a greater degree and duration of effect on the pupil (70) and IOP (71) than the same drug in an aqueous solution.

OTHER VEHICLES. Other vehicles that have been shown to prolong the effect of topical pilocarpine include sodium hyaluronate (72, 73), cyanoacrylate block copolymer (73), and poly(butylcyanoacrylate) nanoparticles (74).

MEMBRANE-CONTROLLED DELIVERY SYSTEM. Pilocarpine between two polymeric membranes provides, in most patients, a constant drug release of 20 µg/hour (Ocusert P-20) or 40 µg/hour (Ocusert P-40), which is roughly comparable to 1–2% and 4% pilocarpine, respectively (75–79). The insert device is retained in the cul-de-sac (Fig. 25.2) and is effective in many patients for up to 7 days (77, 80), although both relative effectiveness (81) and duration of action (78) must be established for each patient by therapeutic trial.

This therapeutic delivery system offers distinct advantages over topical instillation of pilocarpine. The constant rate of release (zero order delivery) provides comparable pressure control with one-fifth the amount of medicine delivered by drops (75–82), which reduces side effects (75, 83, 84). Another advantage of this delivery system is that it partially

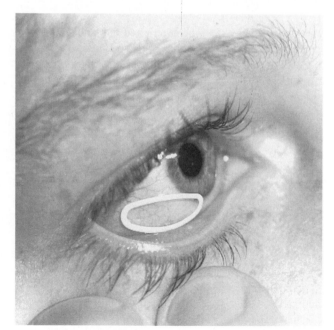

Figure 25.2. Appearance of Ocusert, a pilocarpine delivery system, in the lower cul-de-sac.

levels out the diurnal curve (85). Young patients with pigmentary glaucoma may especially benefit from Ocusert since it minimizes the pilocarpine-induced myopia, while the miotic effect may not only lower IOP, but also minimize continued pigment dispersion.

The primary disadvantages of Ocusert are occasional discomfort and retention problems (86, 87). Patients should be warned of an initial period of increased drug release following insertion of the device. This may last for 12 hours or more and it is usually advisable to change the Ocusert before bedtime and on a day when sharp vision is not essential the following morning. The patient should also be warned of occasional subsequent episodes of transient increased drug release, which has been called the "sudden leakage phenomenon" (76). Two cases of retinal detachment while using Ocusert have been reported, one of which was presumed to be related to the sudden leakage (88,89).

SOLUBLE INSERT DEVICES. Soluble insert devices impregnated with pilocarpine have been shown to provide IOP control for up to 24 hours when placed in the cul-de-sac (90, 91). A mechanical delivery device, in which pilocarpine, incorporated into a water-soluble polyvinyl alcohol film on the end of a stiffened paper strip, is placed in the lower conjunctival sac where it dissolves in the tear film, provided approximately eight-fold greater bioavailability than a conventional eyedrop formulation (92).

SOFT CONTACT LENSES. A soft contact lens that has been soaked in pilocarpine is reported to give longer corneal contact time (93, 94), greater aqueous drug levels (40, 95), and longer IOP control (96) than topically applied pilocarpine. This mode of drug delivery, however, has not been recommended for general clinic use.

INJECTIONS. It has also been reported that subconjunctival injection of 0.15–0.2 ml of 4% pilocarpine achieves a more rapid and sustained miosis than with instillation of pilocarpine drops (97). Intraocular injection of pilocarpine should be avoided since it has been shown to cause corneal edema, presumably due to the osmotic effect of the solution (98).

Drug Interactions

Other Miotics

When other miotics are administered in combination with pilocarpine, they not only fail to increase the pressure lowering effect, but may interfere with the action of pilocarpine. *Echothiophate iodide,* a potent indirect-acting parasympathomimetic, is as effective alone as in combination with pilocarpine (99). Furthermore, pretreating monkeys with echothiophate iodide or diisopropyl fluorophosphate, another potent indirect-acting parasympathomimetic, produced a reversible

subsensitivity, or insensitivity, to pilocarpine (100–104). One study showed that the administration of pilocarpine after pretreatment with echothiophate iodide paradoxically increased the IOP, while the miotic effect of pilocarpine was only partially abolished (105), supporting the concept of two or more cholinergic receptor populations. Physostigmine (eserine), a slightly weaker indirect-acting parasympathomimetic, had no additive effect on tonographic values when added to pilocarpine therapy (106).

Adrenergic Agonists

Epinephrine compounds produce additional IOP reduction when combined with pilocarpine (106, 107), and this also appears to be true for the α_2 agonist, apraclonidine. However, the effect of either combination is less than the additive effect of the two drugs. In one case report, epinephrine preparations apparently increased the induced myopia of pilocarpine Ocusert (108).

Adrenergic Antagonists

Timolol has also been shown to be partially additive with pilocarpine (109–112), which is also true of the other topical β-blockers. Studies of *fixed combinations* of pilocarpine 2–4% and timolol 0.5% given twice daily revealed a greater pressure lowering effect than either pilocarpine or timolol given alone (113–118). When changing from either pilocarpine or timolol alone in patients who were uncontrolled on the monotherapy, the additional IOP reduction with the fixed combination was approximately 3–4 mm Hg. One study showed further pressure reduction in some patients when going from the timolol 0.5%–pilocarpine 2% concentration to timolol 0.5%–pilocarpine 4% (117), while another study found no difference in the two combinations (116). Aqueous humor levels of pilocarpine 2% and timolol 0.5% in rabbits were not statistically significantly different whether the drugs were given alone or in fixed combination (119).

Two fixed combinations of timolol and pilocarpine (Timpilo and Fotil) are available in some parts of the world, and a comparison of the two revealed no significant difference in efficacy (120). A fixed combination of carteolol 2% and pilocarpine 2% has also been compared to timolol 0.5%–pilocarpine 2% with no significant difference in IOP control (121). An important clinical consideration is how the fixed combinations compare to both drugs given separately. One study revealed an equivalent efficacy (122), while another study showed a trend toward better IOP control with individual administration of the two medications (121).

Other Antiglaucoma Medications

Pilocarpine may also be used effectively in combination with carbonic anhydrase inhibitors or hyperosmotic agents.

Antibiotic and Corticosteroid Ointments

Antibiotic and corticosteroid ointments have been shown to decrease the aqueous concentration of topically applied pilocarpine in rabbits (123). Although this was felt to be due to the drug components rather than the ointment base, it is advisable, when prescribing any drop with an ointment, to instill the drop 5–10 minutes before the ointment.

Side Effects

Systemic Toxicity

Pilocarpine can produce systemic effects similar to those of muscarine (124). These include diaphoresis (perspiration), stimulation of glands, and contraction of smooth muscle. The glands involved include salivary, lacrimal, gastric, pancreatic, intestinal, and mucosa of the respiratory tract. Increased bronchial secretion may result from the pilocarpine-induced decrease in pulmonary surfactant, which is responsible for the stability of the alveoli (125). Pulmonary edema resulting from this may be fatal. Smooth muscle contraction may cause nausea, vomiting, diarrhea, and bronchospasm, the latter of which can also be fatal. Other organs in which contraction of smooth muscle may occur include the ureters, urinary bladder, gall bladder, and the capsular muscle of spleen, contraction of which may cause leukocytosis. Blood pressure and pulse may rise or fall, depending on the degree of autonomic stimulation, and high concentrations of pilocarpine may weaken myocardial contractility. Third degree atrioventricular block was reported in an elderly patient with a history of first degree atrioventricular block following seven hourly instillations of 2% pilocarpine (126). Patients with *Alzheimer's disease* have reduced levels of cholinesterase in their brain, making them more sensitive to cholinergic drugs, and progressive cognitive dysfunction has been associated with topical pilocarpine therapy (127).

Systemic toxicity is rare with the usual doses of pilocarpine used in the chronic management of glaucoma. The danger comes when large doses are given within a short period of time, as was once the practice for pupillary-block glaucoma (124). The problem is compounded by the fact that pilocarpine-induced toxicity may be confused with that of concomitant hyperosmotic therapy or of the systemic reactions to the disease itself. The antidote for systemic pilocarpine toxicity is atropine.

Ocular Side Effects

Ocular side effects are common with pilocarpine and can interfere with the patient's quality of life and compliance with recommended therapy (128).

Ciliary muscle spasm may lead to a browache, which usually subsides with continued therapy. A more debilitating effect is induced myopia, which is due to shallowing of the anterior chamber, with an axial thickening and forward shift of the lens (129–133). This is more marked in young individuals, but also occurs in presbyopes (134). Following instillation of 2% pilocarpine, the induced myopia begins in approximately 15 minutes, peaks in 45–60 minutes, and lasts for 1.5–2 hours (129, 134). A statistically significant dose-related response was found for the duration, but not the magnitude, of the effects on anterior chamber depth and lens thickness (130). As previously noted, the Ocusert delivery system for pilocarpine reduces this side effect, allowing its use in some young adult patients (75, 83, 84).

Miosis may cause dimness of vision and alterations in the visual fields as discussed in Chapter 6, especially if cataracts are present. One study of patients with chronic open-angle glaucoma showed an average deterioration in the mean defect of automated visual fields of −1.49 dB following pilocarpine-induced miosis (135). As discussed earlier in this chapter, administration of the pilocarpine gel (Pilopine) at bedtime will reduce this side effect in some patients (68). In other patients, however, the smaller pupil may actually improve visual acuity by the "pinhole" effect, and the patients may note a decline in acuity when the medication is stopped.

Retinal detachment due to the use of miotics has been suspected on the basis of circumstantial evidence, although a definite cause-and-effect relationship has not been established (136–138). These are typically rhegmatogenous detachments, and it is presumed that ciliary body contraction exerts vitreoretinal traction, which causes the retinal tears. The degree of risk appears to be related to preexisting retinal pathology (136–138), and possibly to the potency of the miotic. A vitreous hemorrhage without a detectable retinal hole or detachment has also been reported in a patient 1 day after initiating pilocarpine therapy (139). When starting a patient on any miotic, it is good practice to review their history for increased risk of retinal detachment and to perform a peripheral fundus examination. Macular holes have also been reported to develop within weeks after starting therapy with 2% pilocarpine (140, 141).

A *cataractogenic effect* of pilocarpine has been suggested from observing patients on long-term uniocular miotic therapy (142).

Corneal endothelial toxicity was dose-related in in vitro rabbit studies (143). Pilocarpine therapy was felt to be associated with allograft rejection in three postkeratoplasty patients, which the authors suggested might be related to intraocular inflammation (144). As previously noted, corneal edema may occur with intracameral injection of pilocarpine (98), which may be related to the osmotic effect of the solution.

Increased blood-aqueous barrier permeability to plasma proteins has been demonstrated clinically with a laser flare-cell meter and fluorophotometry following instillation of pilocarpine in a dose-dependent manner (145). In most patients this may not be clinically significant, although it may increase postoperative inflammation with intraocular surgery, and constitutes a relative contraindication in uveitis or rubeosis iridis.

Cicatricial pemphigoid has been reported to occur in patients on long-term topical glaucoma therapy (146, 147). In one survey of 111 patients with cicatricial pemphigoid, 29 (26%) had glaucoma (146). Most of these patients were on multiple glaucoma drops, and virtually all glaucoma medications, including pilocarpine, have been implicated. One study of 179 glaucoma patients and 420 control subjects suggested that chronic glaucoma therapy with miotic or nonmiotic agents for 3 years or longer is associated with significant foreshortening of the inferior conjunctival fornix (148). The cause-and-effect relationship of this association is uncertain, but a spectrum of drug-induced ocular pemphigoid has been proposed, ranging from a self-limiting toxic form to a progressive, immunologic form (147).

Hypersensitivity and toxic reactions may also result from the use of pilocarpine or the preservative. Allergic reactions typically involve the eyelids and conjunctiva, often with a giant papillary reaction of the superior tarsal conjunctiva, while toxic reactions will cause a follicular response in the conjunctiva (149). Many cases of pilocarpine hypersensitivity are due to the preservative, and preservative-free preparations are available.

Atypical band keratopathy (Fig. 25.3) has been observed in patients on long-term pilocarpine therapy (150, 151), but this was found to result from the preservative, phenylmercuric nitrate (152), which is no longer used.

Clinical Indications

Pilocarpine was once a first-line drug for the chronic management of open-angle glaucomas. However, its use is severely limited by the ocular side effects, and it has been largely replaced as a drug of first choice by the β-blockers and other newer topical agents. Furthermore, when compared with timolol in a 2-year trial, more patients had to discontinue the pilocarpine because of inadequate IOP control, and patients treated with pilocarpine had significantly greater visual field deterioration (153). Nevertheless, pilocarpine remains a useful second-line drug, because it usually provides additional pressure reduction when combined with any other class of antiglaucoma medication and has minimal systemic side effects. Relative contraindications to its use, in addition to intolerable side effects, include active anterior uveitis, rubeosis iridis, developmental glaucoma, and extensive obstruction of the anterior chamber angle by membranes or synechial closure. It has also been noted that the pressure-lowering effect of pilocarpine is lost after laser trabeculoplasty (154), so it may be advisable to reconfirm the efficacy by trial discontinuation of the pilocarpine approximately 1 month after the laser surgery.

DUAL ACTION PARASYMPATHOMIMETICS

The following two drugs have both a direct and indirect action on the parasympathetic nervous system (Table 25.2).

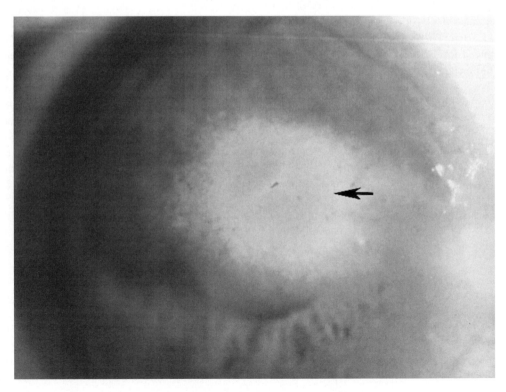

Figure 25.3. Slitlamp view of atypical band keratopathy (*arrow*) due to chronic use of pilocarpine with phenylmercuric nitrate as a preservative.

Table 25.2
OTHER COMMERCIAL MIOTIC
PREPARATIONS*

Generic Preparations	Brand Names	Concentrations (%)
Carbachol	Isopto Carbachol	0.75, 1.5, 2.25, 3
Echothiophate iodide	Phospholine Iodide	0.03, 0.06, 0.125, 0.25
Physostigmine sulfate	Eserine Sulfate	0.25
Demecarium bromide	Humorsol	0.125, 0.25
Isoflurophate	Floropryl (gel)	0.025
Intracameral injections:		
Acetylcholine chloride	Miochol	0.01 in 2 ml vial
Carbachol	Miostat	0.01 in 1.5 ml vial

Other generic products may also be available.

Carbachol

This drug produces direct motor endplate stimulation as well as an indirect parasympathomimetic effect by inhibition of acetylcholinesterase. The usual dosage of carbachol is 1.5–3.0%, three times daily. A concentration of 1.5%, instilled three times daily, was reported to have a more potent and prolonged pressure effect than 2% pilocarpine, four times a day (155). However, carbachol causes more accommodative spasm and pain than pilocarpine (133). Carbachol also has poor corneal penetration and requires an adjuvant such as benzalkonium chloride to achieve effective aqueous levels (156). In a retrospective study of 26 open-angle glaucoma patients, uncontrolled on medical therapy that included pilocarpine, changing the miotic to carbachol had a low chance of improved long-term IOP control and, in most cases, only increased the side effects (157). There are, therefore, few, if any, indications for carbachol in the chronic management of glaucoma.

N-demethylated carbachol is a synthetic tertiary nitrogen derivative of carbachol, which has a higher lipid solubility and better corneal penetration than the parent compound. It was found to be less effective than 1% pilocarpine, but also had fewer ocular and systemic side effects (158).

Intracameral carbachol, which is frequently used to achieve miosis at the end of cataract surgery, has been shown to provide better IOP control in the early postoperative period than intracameral acetylcholine (159, 160) or a placebo (balanced salt solution) (159–162). In one study, half-strength carbachol (0.005% vs. 0.01%) produced the same postoperative IOP and miosis as the full-strength, but was associated with less browache in the early postoperative period (160). Intracameral carbachol has been associated

with transient corneal swelling in rabbits (163), although a 1-year followup of cataract patients revealed no short-term or long-term adverse effects (164).

Aceclidine

This is a synthetic ester with direct motor end plate action and weak anticholinesterase activity (165, 166). The IOP lowering (166, 167) and miotic (133, 167) effects are comparable to those of pilocarpine, while aceclidine has the advantage of less accommodative spasm (133, 165, 168–170). The reason for this difference is not clear, since an in vitro study with fresh ciliary muscle strips showed no dissociation of the contractile responses to aceclidine or carbachol between the accommodation-relevant circular muscle fibers and the facility-relevant longitudinal fibers (171).

INDIRECT PARASYMPATHOMIMETICS

The pure inhibitors of acetylcholinesterase have traditionally been divided, somewhat arbitrarily, into two groups, designated "reversible" and "irreversible." Actually, none of these drugs are totally irreversible, and more precise definitions might be relatively "weaker" and "stronger" cholinesterase inhibitors, respectively (Table 25.2).

Physostigmine (Eserine)

This drug is a "weaker" cholinesterase inhibitor. It is administered as a 0.5% ointment, usually twice daily. As previously noted, it is not additive with pilocarpine (106). Furthermore, as is true of all the cholinesterase inhibitors, it causes vascular congestion, which may be a disadvantage in eyes with angle-closure glaucoma.

Echothiophate Iodide

This pharmacologic agent is a strong, relatively irreversible cholinesterase inhibitor.

Mechanism of Action

Human ocular tissue contains true cholinesterase (172), while pseudocholinesterase is found in human serum (173). In vitro and in vivo studies of cat irides indicate that true cholinesterase is the enzyme portion related to the drug-induced alteration of the iris sphincter and is the portion primarily inhibited by echothiophate iodide (174, 175). The mechanism of improved aqueous outflow facility with this drug is presumed to be the same as that previously discussed for pilocarpine. Some eyes eventually become refractory, which appears from monkey studies to be associated with structural changes in the trabecular meshwork, Schlemm's canal, and ciliary muscle that are mediated, at least in part, by an anterior segment muscarinic receptor (176).

Administration

In vitro studies indicated that echothiophate iodide has the same efficacy (maximum effect produced by a drug regardless of dose) as most of the other miotics (177). Clinical trials have shown that a concentration of 0.03% echothiophate iodide has a potency (effect produced by a particular concentration) equivalent to 1–2% pilocarpine (26), while 0.06% echothiophate iodide is comparable to 4% pilocarpine (45). No additional IOP reduction is normally achieved with concentrations of echothiophate iodide above 0.06% (45, 178), although concentrations of 0.125% or 0.25% may occasionally have additional pressure-lowering efficacy in eyes with darkly pigmented irides. Echothiophate has the advantage of a prolonged duration of action, with the maximum effect occurring in 4–6 hours and a substantial residual present after 24 hours (26), allowing it to be used on a twice daily regimen.

Side Effects

The advantage of the prolonged duration of action with echothiophate iodide therapy is significantly offset by the adverse reactions of this drug.

Systemic toxicity is related to cholinesterase depletion. Echothiophate iodide depletes both true cholinesterase, or acetylcholinesterase, which is associated with the cell wall of red blood cells, as well as pseudocholinesterase, or butyrylcholinesterase, which is a soluble form of cholinesterase found in serum. This depletion begins in the first 2 weeks of chronic therapy, peaks in 5–7 weeks, and requires several weeks to recover after discontinuing the drug (179). Pseudocholinesterase may also be depleted in newborns whose mothers received echothiophate in late pregnancy (180).

Pseudocholinesterase hydrolyzes succinylcholine, and prolonged respiratory paralysis can occur during general anesthesia if this muscle relaxant is used in a patient depleted of cholinesterase (179). Patients starting an echothiophate iodide therapy must be warned of this risk and ideally given a medical alert card to carry in their purse or wallet. Local anesthetics of the ester linkage group, such as procaine and tetracaine, are also hydrolyzed by pseudocholinesterase, and depletion of the enzyme may lead to toxic reactions to these anesthetics (181).

Topical echothiophate iodide may rarely cause the parasympathomimetic reactions of diarrhea, nausea, abdominal cramps, and malaise. A case was reported in which these symptoms developed following bilateral conjunctivodacryocystorhinostomies with Jones' tubes in a patient on long-term treatment with echothiophate iodide (182). The danger of increased systemic absorption after this operation should be considered with all topical medications.

Severe pancreatitis was reported in a patient with anticholinesterase insecticide intoxication, presumably due to increased pancreatic intraductal pressure (183). However, in a study of 44 patients on a long-term echothiophate iodide therapy for glaucoma, serum pancreatic enzyme levels were normal (184).

The antidote for echothiophate iodide toxicity is pralidoxime chloride (Protopam). This frees cholinesterase from the complex and prevents further inhibition, but does not alter the IOP lowering effect (185).

A *cataractogenic effect* has been observed with the chronic use of echothiophate for the management of glaucoma (186–188). The cataracts have been described as initially having fine anterior subcapsular vacuoles (186, 187), although nuclear and posterior subcapsular changes have also been observed (188). The side effect appears to be dose-related (188) and has not been observed in patients receiving cholinesterase inhibitor therapy for accommodative esotropia or in pesticide workers who are chronically exposed to cholinesterase inhibiting organophosphates (189).

The mechanism of echothiophate-induced cataracts is unclear. Experimental models have been produced in monkeys (190–194), which reveal swollen lens fibers, reduced protein concentration, and abnormal material in the intercellular spaces (193). One study suggested that atropine inhibits the cataractogenic effect in monkeys (195), which apparently is not related to relaxation of accommodation, since echothiophate cataracts occurred in monkeys despite retrodisplacement of the ciliary muscle (196).

OTHER OCULAR SIDE EFFECTS. A disruption of the blood-aqueous barrier may cause increased inflammation following intraocular surgery in eyes pretreated with echothiophate iodide and it is usually advisable to discontinue the drug several weeks before such surgery. Retinal detachments may be associated with miotic therapy, as discussed previously in this chapter. Iris cysts near the pupillary margin are not uncommon in children receiving echothiophate iodide for the treatment of accommodative esotropia. As previously noted, structural alterations have been observed in the iris, ciliary muscle, ciliary processes, and trabecular meshwork of monkey eyes receiving chronic topical applications of echothiophate iodide (197). Ocular pseudopemphigoid (198) and periorbital allergic contact dermatitis (199) have both been associated with the use of echothiophate iodide. Corneal epithelial toxicity with echothiophate iodide therapy is reported to be greater than with pilocarpine, but less than with carbachol (200).

Clinical Indications

Because of the significant cataractogenic effect, echothiophate iodide is usually reserved for treating open-angle glaucomas in aphakia or pseudophakia. In a retrospective study of 20 such patients, who were uncontrolled on medical therapy that included pilocarpine or carbachol, changing the miotic to echothiophate iodide restored pressure control in 60% of the patients, with half of these retaining control for the duration of the followup, which averaged 26 months (201).

Other Strong, Relatively Irreversible Cholinesterase Inhibitors

Diisopropyl Fluorophosphate

This drug is similar in action and side effects to echothiophate iodide, but produces more intense ciliary spasm and is susceptible to contamination with water.

Demecarium

This compound is also similar to the other indirect parasympathomimetics, but may be effective when echothiophate iodide has failed.

Tetraethyl Pyrophosphate

Tetraethyl pyrophosphate was found to be comparable to other strong miotics, but had the disadvantage of a considerable tendency to induce local sensitization (202, 203).

SUMMARY

The parasympathomimetics share common mechanisms of action that lead to improved aqueous outflow, either through stimulation of ciliary muscle contraction for patients with open-angle glaucoma or by the miotic effect in the treatment of angle-closure glaucoma. These drugs also share common ocular side effects, which include browache and induced myopia from ciliary muscle spasm, dimness of vision from the miosis, and a risk of retinal detachment. The most commonly used miotic is pilocarpine, which produces direct motor endplate stimulation. Another drug, carbachol, has both a direct parasympathomimetic effect, as well as an indirect action through inhibition of acetylcholinesterase, but has no clinical advantage over pilocarpine. A third group of cholinergic stimulators have only the indirect action, of which echothiophate iodide is the most commonly used. This drug has the disadvantage of a cataractogenic effect, but may be useful in aphakic and pseudophakic eyes.

REFERENCES

1. Mindel, JS, Kharlamb, AB: Alteration of acetylcholine synthesis by pilocarpine. Arch Ophthalmol 102:1546, 1984.
2. Armaly, MF, Jepson, NC: Accommodation and the dynamics of the steady-state intraocular pressure. Invest Ophthalmol 1:480, 1952.
3. Van Buskirk, EM, Grant, WM: Lens depression and aqueous outflow in enucleated primate eyes. Am J Ophthalmol 76:632, 1973.
4. Van Buskirk, EM: Changes in the facility of aqueous outflow induced by lens depression and intraocular pressure in excised human eyes. Am J Ophthalmol 82:736, 1978.
5. Van Buskirk, EM: The canine eye: lens depression and aqueous outflow. Invest Ophthalmol Vis Sci 19:789, 1980.
6. Moses, RA, Grodzki, WJ JR: Choroid tension and facility of aqueous outflow. Invest Ophthalmol Vis Sci 16:1062, 1977.
7. Cairns, JE: Goniospasis: A method designed to relieve canicular blockade in primary open-angle glaucoma. Ann Ophthalmol 8: 1417, 1976.
8. Kaufman, PL, Bárány, EH: Residual pilocarpine effects on outflow facility after ciliary muscle disinsertion in the cynomolgus monkey. Invest Ophthalmol 15:558, 1976.
9. Kaufman, PL, Bárány, EH: Loss of acute pilocarpine effect on outflow facility following surgical disinsertion and retrodisplacement of the ciliary muscle from the scleral spur in the cynomolgus monkey. Invest Ophthalmol 15:793, 1976.
10. Kaufman, PL, Bill, A, Bárány, EH: Formation and drainage of aqueous humor following iris removal and ciliary muscle disinsertion in the cynomolgus monkey. Invest Ophthalmol Vis Sci 16:226, 1977.
11. Lütjen-Drecoll, E, Kaufman, PL, Bárány, EH: Light and electron microscopy of the anterior chamber angle structures following surgical disinsertion of the ciliary muscle in the cynomolgus monkey. Invest Ophthalmol Vis Sci 16:218, 1977.
12. Grierson, I, Lee, WR, Abraham, S: Effects of pilocarpine on the morphology of the human outflow apparatus. Br J Ophthalmol 62: 302, 1978.
13. Grierson, I, Lee, WR, Moseley, H, Abraham, S: The trabecular wall of Schlemm's canal: a study of the effects of pilocarpine by scanning electron microscopy. Br J Ophthalmol 63:9, 1979.
14. Grierson, I, Lee, WR, Abraham, S: The effects of topical pilocarpine on the morphology of the outflow apparatus of the baboon (Papio cynocephalus). Invest Ophthalmol Vis Sci 18:346, 1979.
15. Lütjen-Drecoll, E, Tamm, E, Kaufman, PL: Age-related loss of morphologic responses to pilocarpine in Rhesus monkey ciliary muscle. Arch Ophthalmol 106:1591, 1988.
16. True-Gabelt, B, Crawford, K, Kaufman, PL: Outflow facility and its response to pilocarpine decline in aging rhesus monkeys. Arch Ophthalmolmol 109:879, 1991.
17. True-Gabelt, B, Kaufman, PL, Polansky, JR: Ciliary muscle muscarinic binding sites, choline acetyltransferase, and acetylcholinesterase in aging rhesus monkeys. Invest Ophthalmol Vis Sci 31:2431, 1990.
18. Erickson-Lamy, KA, Johnson, CD, True-Gabelt, B, Kaufman, PL: Ciliary muscle choline acetyltransferase and acetylcholinesterase after ciliary ganglionectomy. Exp Eye Res 51:295, 1990.
19. Erickson-Lamy, KA, Kaufman, PL: Reinnervation of primate ciliary muscle following ciliary ganglionectomy. Invest Ophthalmol Vis Sci 28:927, 1987.
20. Erickson-Lamy, KA, Kaufman, PL: Effect of cholinergic drugs on outflow facility after ciliary ganglionectomy. Invest Ophthalmol Vis Sci 29:491, 1988.
21. Rohen, JW, Eichhorn, M, Kaufman, PL, Erickson-Lamy, KA: Ciliary neuromuscular morphology in cynomolgus monkeys after ciliary ganglionectomy. Graefes Arch Clin Exp Ophthalmol 228:49, 1990.
22. Matsumoto, S, Yorio, T, DeSantis, L, Pang, I-H: Muscarinic effects on cellular functions in cultured human ciliary muscle cells. Invest Ophthalmol Vis Sci 35:3732, 1994.
23. Suzuki, R, Oso, T, Kobayashi, S: Cholinergic inhibitory response in the bovine iris dilator muscle. Invest Ophthalmol Vis Sci 24:760, 1983.
24. Kaufman, PL: Aqueous humor dynamics following total iridectomy in the cynomolgus monkey. Invest Ophthalmol Vis Sci 18:870, 1979.
25. Gaasterland, D, Kupfer, C, Ross, K: Studies of aqueous humor dynamics in man. IV. Effects of pilocarpine upon measurements in young normal volunteers. Invest Ophthalmol 14:848, 1975.
26. Barsam, PC: Comparison of the effect of pilocarpine and echothiophate on intraocular pressure and outflow facility. Am J Ophthalmol 73:742, 1972.

27. Miichi, H, Nagataki, S: Effects of pilocarpine, salbutamol, and timolol in aqueous humor formation in cynomolgus monkeys. Invest Ophthalmol Vis Sci 24:1269, 1983.

28. Bárány, EH: A pharmacologist looks at medical treatment in glaucoma—in retrospect and in prospect. Ophthalmology 86:80, 1979.

29. Lütjen-Drecoll, E, Kaufman, PL: Morphological changes in primate aqueous humor formation and drainage tissues after long-term treatment with antiglaucomatous drugs. J Glau 2:316, 1993.

30. Helbig, H, Korbmacher, C, Wohlfarth, J, et al: Effect of acetylcholine on membrane potential of cultured human nonpigmented ciliary epithelial cells. Invest Ophthalmol Vis Sci 30:890, 1989.

31. Jumblatt, JE, North, GT, Hackmiller, RC: Muscarinic cholinergic inhibition of adenylate cyclase in the rabbit iris—ciliary body and ciliary epithelium. Invest Ophthalmol Vis Sci 31:1103, 1990.

32. Nagataki, S, Brubaker, RF: Effect of pilocarpine on aqueous humor formation in human beings. Arch Ophthalmol 100:818, 1982.

33. Bill, A, Phillips, CI: Uveoscleral drainage of aqueous humour in human eyes. Exp Eye Res 12:275, 1971.

34. Bleiman, BS, Schwartz, AL: Paradoxical intraocular pressure response to pilocarpine. A proposed mechanism and treatment. Arch Ophthalmol 97:1305, 1979.

35. Doane, MB, Jensen, AD, Dohlman, CH: Penetration routes of topically applied eye medications. Am J Ophthalmol 85:383, 1978.

36. Sieg, JW, Robinson, JR: Mechanistic studies on transcorneal permeation of pilocarpine. J Pharm Sci 65:1816, 1976.

37. Van Hoose, MC, Leaders, FE: The role of the cornea in the biologic response to pilocarpine. Invest Ophthalmol 13:377, 1974.

38. Lazare, R, Horlington, M: Pilocarpine levels in the eyes of rabbits following topical application. Exp Eye Res 21:281, 1975.

39. Krohn, DL, Breitfeller, JM: Transcorneal flux of topical pilocarpine to the human aqueous. Am J Ophthalmol 87:50, 1979.

40. Asseff, CG, Weisman, RL, Podos, SM, Becker, B: Ocular penetration of pilocarpine in primates. Am J Ophthalmol 75:212, 1973.

41. Chrai, SS, Robinson, JR: Corneal permeation of topical pilocarpine nitrate in the rabbit. Am J Ophthalmol 77:735, 1974.

42. Harris, LS, Galin, MA: Dose response analysis of pilocarpine-induced ocular hypotension. Arch Ophthalmol 84:605, 2970.

43. Drance, SM, Nash, PA: The dose response of human intraocular pressure to pilocarpine. Can J Ophthalmol 6:9, 1971.

44. Drance, SM, Bensted, M, Schulzer, M: Pilocarpine and intraocular pressure. Duration of effectiveness of 4% and 8% pilocarpine instillation. Arch Ophthalmol 91:104, 1974.

45. Harris, LS: Comparison of pilocarpine and echothiophate iodide in open-angle glaucoma. Ann Ophthalmol 4:736, 1972.

46. Harris, LS, Galin, MA: Effect of ocular pigmentation of hypotensive response to pilocarpine. Am J Ophthalmol 72:923, 1971.

47. Zimmerman, TJ, Sharir, M, Nardin, GF, Fuqua, M: Therapeutic index of pilocarpine, carbachol, and timolol with nasolacrimal occlusion. Am J Ophthalmol 114:1, 1992.

48. Lerman, S, Reininger, B: Simulated sustained release pilocarpine therapy and aqueous humor dynamics. Can J Ophthalmol 6:14, 1971.

49. Birmingham, AT, Galloway, NR, Walker, DA: Intraocular pressure reduction in chronic simple glaucoma by continuous infusion of dilute pilocarpine solution. Br J Ophthalmol 63:808, 1979.

50. Patton, TF, Francoeur, M: Ocular bioavailability and systemic loss of topically applied ophthalmic drugs. Am J Ophthalmol 85:225, 2978.

51. File, RR, Patton, TF: Topically applied pilocarpine. Human pupillary response as a function of drop size. Arch Ophthalmol 98:112, 1980.

52. Shell, JW: Ophthalmic drug delivery systems. Surv Ophthalmol 29:117, 1984.

53. Barsam, PC: The most commonly used miotic—now longer acting. Ann Ophthalmol 6:809, 1974.

54. Magder, H, Boyaner, D: The use of a longer acting pilocarpine in the management of chronic simple glaucoma. Can J Ophthalmol 9:285, 1974.

55. Sherman, SE: Clinical comparison of pilocarpine preparations in heavily pigmented eyes: an evaluation of the influence of polymer vehicles on corneal penetration, drug availability, and duration of hypotensive activity. Ann Ophthalmol 9:1231, 1977.

56. Quigley, HA, Pollack, IP: Intraocular pressure control with twice-daily pilocarpine in two vehicle solutions. Ann Ophthalmol 9:427, 1977.

57. Green, K, Downs, SJ: Ocular penetration of pilocarpine in rabbits. Arch Ophthalmol 93:1165, 1975.

58. Harbin, TS Jr, Kaback, MB, Podos, SM, Becker, B: Comparative intraocular pressure effects of Adsorbocarpine and Isoptocarpine. Ann Ophthalmol 10:59, 1978.

59. Ticho, U, Blumenthal, M, Zonis, S, et al: Piloplex, a new long-acting pilocarpine polymer salt. A: long-term study. Br J Ophthalmol 63:45, 1979.

60. Mazor, Z, Ticho, U, Rehany, U, Rose, L: Piloplex, a new long-acting pilocarpine polymer salt. B: comparative study of the visual effects of pilocarpine and Piloplex eye drops. Br J Ophthalmol 63:48, 1979.

61. Ticho, U, Blumenthal, M, Zonis, S, et al: A clinical trial with Piloplex—a new long-acting pilocarpine compound: preliminary report. Ann Ophthalmol 11:555, 1979.

62. Duzman, E, Quinn, CA, Warman, A, Warman, R: One-month crossover trial comparing the intraocular pressure control of 3.4% piloplex twice daily with 2.0% pilocarpine four times daily. Acta Ophthalmol 60:613, 1982.

63. Klein, HZ, Lugo, M, Shields, MB, et al: A dose-response study of piloplex for duration of action. Am J Ophthalmol 99:23, 1985.

64. March, WF, Stewart, RM, Mandell, AI, Bruce, LA: Duration of effect of pilocarpine gel. Arch Ophthalmol 100:1270, 1982.

65. Stewart, RH, Kimbrough, RL, Smith, JP, Ward, RL: Long-acting pilocarpine gel: a dose-response in ocular hypertensive subjects. Glaucoma 6:182, 1984.

66. Goldberg, I, Ashburn, FS Jr, Kass, MA, Becker, B: Efficacy and patient acceptance of pilocarcpine gel. Am J Ophthalmol 88:843, 1979.

67. Johnson, DH, Epstein, DL, Allen, RC, et al: A one-year multicenter clinical trial of pilocarpine gel. Am J Ophthalmol 97:723, 1984.

68. Krause, K, Kuchle, JH, Baumgart, M: Comparative investigations of pilocarpine gel and pilocarpine eye drops. Klin Monatsbl Augenheilkd 187:178, 1985.

69. Johnson, DH, Keyon, KR, Epstein, DL, Van Buskirk, EM: Corneal changes during pilocarpine gel therapy. Am J Ophthalmol 101:13, 1986.

70. Smith, SA, Smith, SE, Lazare, R: An increased effect of pilocarpine on the pupil by application of the drug in oil. Br J Ophthalmol 62:314, 1978.

71. Bhojwani, SC, Jones, DK: Comparative study of aqueous and oily pilocarpine in the production of ocular hypotension. Br J Ophthalmol 65:530, 1981.

72. Camber, O, Edman, P, Gurny, R: Influence of sodium hyaluronate on the meiotic effect of pilocarpine in rabbits. Curr Eye Res 6:779, 1987.

73. Cheeks, L, Green, K, Stone, RP, Riedhammer, T: Comparative effects of pilocarpine in different vehicles on pupil diameter in albino rabbits and squirrel monkeys. Curr Eye Res 8:1251, 1989.

74. Diepold, R, Kreuter, J, Himber, J, et al: Comparison of different models for the testing of pilocarpine eyedrops using conventional eyedrops and a novel depot formulation (nanoparticles). Graefes Arch Clin Exp Ophthalmol 227:188, 1989.

75. Place, VA, Fisher, M, Herbst, S, et al: Comparative pharmacologic effects of pilocarpine administered to normal subjects by eyedrops or by ocular therapeutic systems. Am J Ophthalmol 80:706, 1975.

76. Lee, P-F, Shen, Y-T, Eberle, M: The long-acting Ocusert-pilocarpine system in the management of glaucoma. Invest Ophthalmol 14:43, 1975.

77. Quigley, HA, Pollack, IP, Harbin, TS Jr: Pilocarpine Ocuserts. Long-term clinical trials and selected pharmacodynamics. Arch Ophthalmol 93:771, 1975.

78. Armaly, MF, Rao, KR: The effect of pilocarpine Ocuset with different release rates on ocular pressure. Invest Ophthalmol 12:491, 1973.

79. Worthen, DM, Zimmerman, TJ, Wind, CA: An evaluation of the pilocarpine Ocusert. Invest Ophthalmol 13:296, 1974.

80. Drance, SM, Mitchell, DWA, Schultzer, M: The duration of action of pilocarpine Ocusert on intraocular pressure in man. Can J Ophthalmol 10:450, 1975.

81. Macoul, KL, Pavan-Langston, D: Pilocarpine Ocusert system for sustained control of ocular hypertension. Arch Ophthalmol 93:587, 1975.

82. Sendelbeck, L, Moore, D, Urquhart, J: Comparative distribution of pilocarpine in ocular tissues of the rabbit during administration by eyedro or by membrane-controlled delivery systems. Am J Ophthalmol 80:274, 1975.

83. Brown, HS, Meltzer, G, Merrill, RC, et al: Visual effects of pilocarpine in glaucoma. Comparative study of administration by eyedrops or by ocular therapeutic systems. Arch Ophthalmol 94:1716, 1976.

84. Francois, J, Goes, F, Zagorski, Z: Comparative ultrasonographic study of the effect of pilocarpine 2% and Ocusert P-20 on the eye components. Am J Ophthalmol 86:233, 1978.

85. Fruanfelder, FT, Shell, JW, Herbst, SF: Effect of pilocarpine ocular therapeutic systems on diurnal control of intraocular pressure. Ann Ophthalmol 8:1031, 1976.

86. Smith, SE, Smith, SA, Friedmann, AI, Chaston, JM: Comparison of the pupillary, refractive, and hypotensive effects of Ocusert-40 and pilocarpine eyedrops in the treatment of chronic simple glaucoma. Br J Ophthalmol 63:228, 1979.

87. Akerblom, T, Aurell, E, Cristiansson, J, et al: A multicentre study of the effect and tolerance of Ocusert P-40. Acta Ophthalmol 58:617, 1980.

88. Weseley, P, Liebmann J, Ritch, R: Rhegmatogenous retinal detachment after initiation of Ocusert therapy. Am J Ophthalmol 112:458, 1991.

89. Kalenak, JW, Zakov, ZN: Presumed sudden leakage of a pilocarpine Ocusert and rhegmatogenous retinal detachment. J Glau 3:152, 1994.

90. Bensinger, R, Shin, DH, Kass, MA, et al: Pilocarpine ocular inserts. Invest Ophthalmol 15:1008, 1976.

91. Maichuk, YF, Erichev, VP: Soluble ophthalmic drug inserts with pilocarpine: experimental and clinical study. Glaucoma 3:239, 1981.

92. Kelly, JA, Molyneux, PD, Smith, SA, Smith, SE: Relative bioavailability of pilocarpine from a novel ophthalmic delivery system and conventional eyedrop formulations. Br J Ophthalmol 73:360, 1989.

93. Krohn, DL, Breitfeller, JM: Quantitation of pilocarpine flux enhancement across isolated rabbit cornea by hydrogel polymer lenses. Invest Ophthalmol 14:152, 1975.

94. Ruben, M, Watkins, R: Pilocarpine dispensation for the soft hydrophilic contact lens. Br J Ophthalmol 59:455, 1975.

95. Ramer, RM, Gasset, AR: Ocular penetration of pilocarpine: the effect of hydrophilic soft contact lenses on the ocular penetration of pilocarpine. Ann Ophthalmol 6:1325, 1974.

96. Podos, SM, Becker, B, Asseff, C, Hartstein, J: Pilocarpine therapy with soft contact lenses. Am J Ophthalmol 73:336, 1972.

97. Mehta, HK: Subconjunctival injection of pilocarpine. Trans Ophthalmol Soc UK 96:184, 1976.

98. Jay, JL, MacDonald, M: Effects of intraocular miotics on cultured bovine corneal endothelium. Br J Ophthalmol 62:815, 1978.

99. Kini, MM, Dahl, AA, Roberts, CR, et al: Echothiophate, pilocarpine, and open-angle glaucoma. Arch Ophthalmol 89:190, 1973.

100. Kaufman, PL, Bárány, EH: Subsensitivity to pilocarpine in primate ciliary muscle following topical anticholinesterase treatment. Invest Ophthalmol 14:302, 1975.

101. Kaufman, PL, Bárány, EH: Subsensitivity to pilocarpine of the aqueous outflow system in monkey eyes after topical anticholinesterase treatment. Am J Ophthalmol 82:883, 1976.

102. Kaufman, PL: Anticholinesterase-induced cholinergic subsensitivity in primate accommodative mechanism. Am J Ophthalmol 85:622, 1978.

103. Bito, LZ, Baroody, RA: Gradual changes in the sensitivity of rhesus monkey eyes to miotics and the dependence of these changes on the regimen of topical cholinesterase inhibitor treatment. Invest Ophthalmol Vis Sci 18:794, 1979.

104. Erickson-Lamy, KA, Polansky, JR, Kaufman, PL, Zlock, DM: Cholinergic drugs alter ciliary muscle response and receptor content. Invest Ophthalmol Vis Sci 28:375, 1987.

105. Bito, LZ, Mirritt, SQ: Paradoxical ocular hypertensive effect of pilocarpine on echothiophate iodide-treated primate eyes. Invest Ophthalmol Vis Sci 19:371, 1980.

106. Kronfeld, PC: The efficacy of combinations of ocular hypotensive drugs. A tonographic approach. Arch Ophthalmol 78:140, 1967.

107. Harris, LS, Mittag, TW, Galin, MA: Aqueous dynamics of pilocarpine-treated eyes. The influence of topically applied epinephrine. Arch Ophthalmol 86:1, 1971.

108. Duffey, RJ, Ferguson, JG: Interaction of dipivefrin and epinephrine with the pilocarpine ocular therapeutic system (Ocusert). Arch Ophthalmol 104:1135, 1986.

109. Keates, EU: Evaluation of timolol maleate combination therapy in chronic open-angle glaucoma. Am J Ophthalmol 88:565, 1979.

110. Smith, RJ, Nagasubramanian, S, Watkins, R, Poinoosawmy, D: Addition of timolol maleate to routine medical therapy. A clinical trial. Br J Ophthalmol 64:779, 1980.

111. Nielsen, NV, Eriksen, JS: Timolol in maintenance treatment of ocular hypertenson and glaucoma. Acta Ophthalmol 57:1070, 1979.

112. Kass, MA: Efficacy of combining timolol with other antiglaucoma medications. Surv Ophthalmol 28:274, 1983.

113. Airaksinen, PJ, Valkonen, R, Stenborg, T, et al: A double-masked study of timolol and pilocarpine combined. Am J Ophthalmol 104:587, 1987.

114. Maclure, GM, Vogel, R, Sturm, A, Binkowitz, B: Effect on the 24-hour diurnal curve of intraocular pressure of a fixed ratio combination of timolol 0.5% and pilocarpine 2% in patients with COAG not controlled on timolol 0.5%. Br J Ophthalmol 73:827, 1989.

115. Lofors, KT, Hovding G, Viksmoen, L, et al: Twelve-hour IOP control obtained by a single dose of timolol/pilocarpine combination eye drops. Acta Ophthalmol 68:323, 1990.

116. Sturm, A, Vogel, R, Binkowitz, B, et al: A fixed combination of timolol and pilocarpine: double-masked comparisons with timolol and with pilocarpine. J Glau 1:7, 1992.

117. Puustjarvi, TJ, Repo, LP: Timolol-pilocarpine fixed-ratio combinations in the treatment of chronic open angle glaucoma. A controlled multicenter study of 48 weeks. Arch Ophthalmol 110:1725, 1992.

118. Zadok, D, Geyer, O, Zadok, J, et al: Combined timolol and pilocarpine vs pilocarpine alone and timolol alone in the treatment of glaucoma. Am J Ophthalmol 117:728, 1994.

119. Ellis, PP, Wu, P-Y, Riegel, M: Aqueous humor pilocarpine and timolol levels after instillation of the single drug or in combination. Invest Ophthalmol Vis Sci 32:520, 1991.

120. Uusitalol, RJ, Palkama, A: Efficacy and safety of timolol/pilocarpine combination drops in glaucoma patients. Acta Ophthalmol 72:496, 1994.

121. Demailly, P, Allaire, C, Bron, V, Trinquand, C: Effectiveness and tolerance of β- blocker/pilocarpine combination eye drops in primary open-angle glaucoma and high intraocular pressure. J Glau 4:235, 1995.

122. Söderström, MB, Wallin, Ö, Granström, P-A, Thorburn, W: Timolol-pilocarpine combined vs timolol and pilocarpine given separately. Am J Ophthalmol 107:465, 1989.

123. Ellis, PP, Riegel, M: Influence of ophthalmic ointments on the penetration of pilocarpine drops. J Ocul Pharmacol 5:119, 1989.

124. Greco, JJ, Kelman, CD: Systemic pilocarpine toxicity in the treatment of angle closure glaucoma. Ann Ophthalmol 5:57, 1973.

125. Curti, PC, Renovanz, H-D: The effect of unintentional overdoses of pilocarpine on pulmonary surfactant in mice. Klin Monatsbl Augenheilkd 179:113, 1981.

126. Littman, L, Kempler, P, Rhola, M, Fenyvesi, T: Severe symptomatic atrioventricular block induced by pilocarpine eye drops. Arch Intern Med 147:586, 1987.

127. Reyes, PF, Dwyer, BA, Schwartzman, RJ, Sacchetti, T: Mental status changes induced by eye drops in dementia of the Alzheimer type. J Neurol Neurosurg Psychiatry 50:113, 1987.

128. Granstrom, PA, Norell, S: Visual ability and drug regimen: Relation to compliance with glaucoma therapy. Acta Ophthalmol 61:206, 1983.

129. Abramson, DH, Coleman, DJ, Forbes, M, Franzen, LA: Pilocarpine. Effect on the anterior chamber and lens thickness. Arch Ophthalmol 87:615, 1972.

130. Abramson, DH, Chang, S, Coleman, DJ, Smith, ME: Pilocarpine-induced lens changes. An ultrasonic biometric evaluation of dose response. Arch Ophthalmol 92:464, 1974.

131. Abramson, DH, Chang, S, Coleman, DJ: Pilocarpine therapy in glaucoma. Effects on anterior chamber depth and lens thickness in patients receiving long-term therapy. Arch Ophthalmol 94:914, 1976.

132. Pooinoosawmy, D, Nagasubramanian, S, Brown, NAP: Effect of pilocarpine on visual acuity and on the dimensions of the cornea and anterior chamber. Br J Ophthalmol 60:676, 1976.

133. Francois, J, Goes, F: Ultrasonographic study of the effect of different miotics on the eye components. Ophthalmologica 175:328, 1977.

134. Abramson, DH, Franzen, LA, Coleman, DJ: Pilocarpine in the presbyope. Demonstration of an effect on the anterior chamber and lens thickness. Arch Ophthalmol 89:100, 1973.

135. Webster, AR, Luff, AJ, Canning, CR, Elkington, AR: The effect of pilocarpine on the glaucomatous visual field. Br J Ophthalmol 77:721, 1993.

136. Pape, LG, Forbes, M: Retinal detachment and miotic therapy. Am J Ophthalmol 85:558, 1978.

137. Beasley, H, Fraunfelder, FT: Retinal detachments and topical ocular miotics. Ophthalmology 86:95, 1979.

138. Alpar, JJ: Miotics and retinal detachment: A survey and case report. Ann Ophthalmol 11:395, 1979.

139. Schuman, JS, Hersh, P, Kylstra, J: Vitreous hemorrhage associated with pilocarpine. Am J Ophthalmol 108:333, 1989.

140. Garlikov, RS, Chenoweth, RG: Macular hole following topical pilocarpine. Ann Ophthalmol 7:1313, 1975.

141. Benedict, WL, Shami, M: Impending macular hole associated with topical pilocarpine. Am J Ophthalmolmol 114:765, 1992.

142. Levene, RZ: Uniocular miotic therapy. Trans Am Acad Ophthalmol Otol 79:376, 1975.

143. Coles, WH: Pilocarpine toxicity. Effects on the rabbit corneal endothelium. Arch Ophthalmol 93:36, 1975.

144. Massry, GG, Assil, KK: Pilocarpine-associated allograft rejection in postkeratoplasty patients. Cornea 14:202, 1995.

145. Mori, M, Araie, M, Sakurai, M, Oshika, T: Effects of pilocarpine and tropicamide on blood-aqueous barrier permeability in man. Invest Ophthalmol Vis Sci 33:416, 1992.

146. Tauber, J, Melamed, S, Foster, CS: Glaucoma in patients with ocular cicatricial pemphigoid. Ophthalmology 96:33, 1989.

147. Fiore, PM, Jacobs, IH, Goldbert, DB: Drug-induced pemphigoid. A spectrum of diseases. Arch Ophthalmol 105:1660, 1987.

148. Schwab, IR, Linberg, JV, Gioia, VM, et al: Foreshortening of the inferior conjunctival fornix associated with chronic glaucoma medications. Ophthalmology 99:197, 1992.

149. Jackson, WB: Differentiating conjunctivitis of diverse origins. Surv Ophthalmol 38(Suppl):91, 1993.

150. Kennedy, RE, Roca, PD, Landers, PH: Atypical band keratopathy in glaucomatous patients. Am J Ophthalmol 72:917, 1971.

151. Brazier, DJ, Hitchings, RA: Atypical band keratopathy following long-term pilocarpine treatment. Br J Ophthalmol 73:294, 1989.

152. Kennedy, RE, Roca, PD, Platt, DS: Further observations on atypical band keratopathy in glaucoma patients. Trans Am Ophthalmol Soc 72:107, 1974.

153. Vogel, R, Crick, RP, Mills, KB, et al: Effect of timolol versus pilocarpine on visual field progression in patients with primary open-angle glaucoma. Ophthalmology 99:1505, 1992.

154. Quaranta, L, Ripandelli, G, Manni, GL, Bucci, MG: Hypotensive effect of pilocarpine after argon laser trabeculoplasty. J Glau 1:233, 1992.

155. O'Brein, CS, Swan, KD: Carbaminoylcholine chloride in the treatment of glaucoma simplex. Arch Ophthalmol 27:253, 1942.

156. Smolen, VF, Clevenger, JM, Williams, EJ, Bergdolt, MW: Biophasic availability of ophthalmic carbachol I: mechanisms of cationic polymer- and surfactant-promoted miotic activity. J Pharm Sci 62:958, 1973.

157. Reichert, RW, Shields, MB, Stewart, WC: Intraocular pressure response to replacing pilocarpine with carbachol. Am J Ophthalmol 106:747, 1988.

158. Hung, PT, Hsieh, JW, Chiou, GCY: Ocular hypotensive effects of N-demethylated carbachol on open angle glaucoma. Arch Ophthalmol 100:262, 1982.

159. Ruiz, RS, Rhem, MN, Prager, TC: Effects of carbachol and acetylcholine on intraocular pressure after cataract extraction. Am J Ophthalmol 107:7, 1989.

160. Hollands, RH, Drance, SM, House, PH, Schulzer, M: Control of intraocular pressure after cataract extraction. Can J Ophthalmol 25:128, 1990.

161. Linn, DK, Zimmerman, TJ, Nardin, GF, et al: Effect of intracameral carbachol on intraocular pressure after cataract extraction. Am J Ophthalmol 107:133, 1989.

162. Wood, TO: Effect of carbachol on postoperative intraocular pressure. J Cataract Refract Surg 14:654, 1988.

163. Birnbaum, DB, Hull, DS, Green, K, Frey, NP: Effect of carbachol on rabbit corneal endothelium. Arch Ophthalmol 105:253, 1987.

164. Zimmerman, TJ, Dukar, U, Nardin, GF, et al: Carbachol dose response. Am J Ophthalmol 108:456, 1989.

165. Fechner, PU, Teichmann, KD, Weyrauch, W: Accommodative effects of aceclidine in the treatment of glaucoma. Am J Ophthalmol 79:104, 1975.

166. Drance, SM, Fairclough, M, Schulzer, M: Dose response of human intraocular pressure to aceclidine. Arch Ophthalmol 88:394, 1972.

167. Riegel, D, Leydhecker, W: Experiences with aceclidine in the treatment of simple glaucoma. Klin Monatsbl Augenheilkd 151:882, 1967.

168. Fechner, PU: Avoiding spasm of accommodation in the treatment of young glaucoma patients. Klin Monatsbl Augenheilkd 158:112, 1971.

169. Pilz, A, Lommatzsch, P, Ulrich, W-D: Experimentelle und klinsche Untersuchungen mit Aceclidin (Glaucostat). Ophthalmologica 168:376, 1974.

170. Erickson-Lamy, K, Schroeder, A: Dissociation between the effect of aceclidine on outflow facility and accommodation. Exp Eye Res 50:143, 1990.

171. Poyer, JF, Kaufman, PL, Flügel, C: Age does not affect contractile responses of the isolated rhesus monkey ciliary muscle to muscarinic agonists. Curr Eye Res 12:413, 1993.

172. Leopold, IH, Furman, M: Cholinesterase isoenzymes in human ocular tissue homogenates. Am J Ophthalmol 72:460, 1971.

173. Juul, P: Human plasma cholinesterase isoenzymes. Clin Chim Acta 19:205, 1968.

174. Harris, LS, Shimyno, M, Mittag, TW: Cholinesterases and contractility of cat irides. Effect of echothiophate iodide. Arch Ophthalmol 89:49, 1973.

175. Harris, LS, Shimmyo, M, Mittag, TW: Effects of echothiophate on cholinesterases in cat irides. Arch Ophthalmol 91:57, 1974.

176. Lütjen-Drecoll, E, Kaufman, PL: Biomechanics of echothiophate-induced anatomic changes in monkey aqueous outflow system. Graefes Arch Clin Exp Ophthalmol 224:564, 1986.

177. Harris, LS, Shimmyo, M, Hughes, J: Dose-response of cholinergic agonists on cat irides. Arch Ophthalmol 91:299, 1974.

178. Harris, LS: Dose-response analysis of echothiophate iodide. Arch Ophthalmol 86:502, 1971.

179. Ellis, PP, Esterdahl, M: Echothiophate iodide therapy in children. Effect upon blood cholinersterase levels. Arch Ophthalmol 77:598, 1967.

180. Birks, DA, Prior, VJ, Silk, E, Whittaker, M: Echothiophate iodide treatment of glaucoma in pregnancy. Arch Ophthalmol 79:283, 1968.

181. Ellis, PP, Littlejohn, K: Effects of topical anticholinesterases on procaine hydrolysis. Am J Ophthalmol 77:71, 1974.

182. Wood, JR, Anderson, RL, Edwards, JJ: Phospholine iodide toxicity and Jones' tubes. Ophthalmology 87:346, 1980.

183. Dressel, TD, Goodale, RL, Arneson, MA, Borner, JW: Pancreatitis as a complication of anticholinesterase insecticide intoxication. Ann Surg 189:199, 1979.

184. Friberg, TR, Thomas, JV, Dressel, TD: Serum cholinesterase, serum lipase, and serum amylase levels during long-term echothiophate iodide therapy. Am J Ophthalmol 91:530, 1981.

185. Lipson, ML, Holmes, JH, Ellis, PP: Oral administration of pralidoxime chloride in echothiophate iodide therapy. Arch Ophthalmol 82:830, 1969.

186. Axelsson, U, Holmberg, Å: The frequency of cataract after miotic therapy. Acta Ophthalmol 44:421, 1966.

187. Axelsson, U: Studies on echothiophate (phospholine iodide) and paraoxon (mintacol) with regard to cataractogenic effect. Acta Ophthalmol Suppl 102, 1969.

188. Thoft, RA: Incidence of lens changes in patients treated with echothiophate iodide. Arch Ophthalmol 80:317, 1968.

189. Pietsch, RL, Bobo, CB, Finklea, JF, Vallotton, WW: Lens opacities and organophosphate cholinesterase-inhibiting agents. Am J Ophthalmol 73:236, 1973.

190. Kaufman, PL, Axelsson, U: Induction of subcapsular cataracts in aniridic vervet monkeys by echothiophate. Invest Ophthalmol 14:863, 1975.

191. Kaufman, PL, Axelsson, U, Bárány, E: Induction of subcapsular cataracts in cynomolgus monkeys by echothiophate. Arch Ophthalmol 95:499, 1977.

192. Albrecht, M, Bárány, E: Early lens changes in Macaca fascicularis monkeys under topical treatment with echothiophate or carbachol studied by slit-image photography. Invest Ophthalmol Vis Sci 18L179, 1979.

193. Philipson, B, Kaufman, PL, Fagerholm, P, et al: Echothiophate cataracts in monkeys. Electron microscopy and microradiography. Arch Ophthalmol 97:340, 1979.

194. Michon, J Jr, Kinoshita, JH: Experimental miotic cataract. II. Permeability, cation transport, and intermediary metabolism. Arch Ophthalmol 79:611, 1968.

195. Kaufman, PL, Axelsson, U, Bárány, EH: Atropine inhibition of echothiophate cataractogenesis in monkeys. Arch Ophthalmol 95:1262, 1977.

196. Kaufman, PL, Erickson, KA, Neider, MW: Echothiophate iodide cataracts in monkeys. Occurrence despite loss of accommodation induced by retrodisplacement of ciliary muscle. Arch Ophthalmol 101:125, 1983.

197. Lütjen-Drecoll, E, Kaufman, PL: Echothiophate-induced structural alterations in the anterior chamber angle of the cynomolgus monkey. Invest Ophthalmol Vis Sci 18:918, 1979.

198. Patten, JT, Cavanagh, HD, Allansmith, MR: Induced ocular pseudophemigoid. Am J Ophthalmol 82:272, 1976.

199. Mathias, CGT, Maibach, HI, Irvine, A, Adler, W: Allergic contact dermatitis to echothiophate iodide and phenylephrine. Arch Ophthalmol 97:286, 1979.

200. Krejci, L, Harrison, R: Antiglaucoma drug effects on corneal epithelium. A comparative study in tissue culture. Arch Ophthalmol 84:766, 1970.

201. Reichert, RW, Shields, MB: Intraocular pressure response to the replacement of pilocarpine or carbachol with echothiophate. Graefes Arch Clin Exp Ophthalmol 229:252, 1991.

202. Grant, WM: Miotic and antiglaucomatous activity of tetraethyl pyrophosphate in human eyes. Arch Ophthalmol 39:579, 1948.

203. Grant, WM: Additional experiences with tetraethyl pyrophosphate in treatment of glaucoma. Arch Ophthalmol 44:362, 1950.

Chapter 26

ADRENERGIC STIMULATORS[a]

[handwritten notes: Sympathetic / Parasympathetic / Epinephrine / Acetylcholine / Adrenergic / Cholinergic / Dilates / Constricts]

EPINEPHRINE

This direct-acting sympathomimetic stimulates both α- and β-adrenergic receptors and is a standard topical drug for the chronic management of open-angle forms of glaucoma.

Mechanisms of Action

Theories regarding the mechanism of IOP reduction in response to epinephrine therapy have changed considerably in recent years. Early observations suggested that the primary action was decreased aqueous production (1–5). It was subsequently noted, however, that an improvement in aqueous outflow facility occurred after prolonged use of epinephrine (6, 7). Still more recent studies have revealed that increased outflow is an early and predominant feature of epinephrine-

induced pressure reduction (8–14), and that aqueous production is actually increased during one phase of the drug response (15–17).

Sears and Neufeld (18–20) have proposed a unified concept for the action of epinephrine on aqueous humor dynamics, which consists of the following three phases.

Phase One: Decreased Aqueous Production

Within minutes after instillation of epinephrine, aqueous inflow is reduced, presumably due to the α-adrenergic effect of vasoconstriction, which reduces the ultrafiltration of plasma into the stroma of the ciliary processes. Vascular casting studies in rabbits have shown that α-adrenergic stimulation is associated with constriction of sphincter-like structures in the vessel lumen just as the ciliary process arterioles branch from the major arterial circle of the iris, with downstream luminal narrowing and poor ciliary process capillary filling (21). Topical epinephrine in monkeys (22) and retrobulbar injections in rabbits (23) have both been

[a]Refer to Shields, MB: Color Atlas of Glaucoma. Baltimore, Williams & Wilkins, 1998, Plates III3–4.

shown to significantly reduce blood flow in the iris and ciliary body. This α-adrenergic effect on aqueous production, however, is transient and not of sufficient magnitude to significantly influence IOP (20).

Phase Two: Early Increase in Outflow Facility

This phase overlaps with the first and has two components. The first portion is actually a part of phase one and is believed to be an early, moderate-sized α-adrenergic effect on true outflow facility (20). The second component occurs hours after administration, when the vasoconstrictor and mydriatic effects are gone, and lasts for several hours. Fluorophotometric and tonographic studies in normal (15–17) and ocular hypertensive (17) human eyes suggest that IOP reduction for at least the first several hours after topical instillation of epinephrine is associated with improved facility of outflow.

The mechanism of improved outflow is uncertain. Tonographic studies performed in conjunction with fluorophotometry suggest that epinephrine may increase the rate of outflow via the uveoscleral pathway (15, 17). Studies in rabbits and humans have shown that either systemic or topical indomethacin, a cyclooxygenase inhibitor, can inhibit the epinephrine-induced reduction of IOP, increased facility of outflow, and disruption of the blood-aqueous barrier, suggesting that endogenous production of prostaglandins may be associated with the hypotensive mechanism of topically applied epinephrine (24–26). The mechanism of improved outflow does not appear to be mediated by the iris or ciliary body, since epinephrine and norepinephrine-induced increased facility of outflow in monkey eyes was not influenced by removal of the iris or total disinsertion of the ciliary muscle (27, 28). The increase in outflow facility associated with topical epinephrine was blocked by timolol in an in vitro human eye perfusion model (29), and by timolol, but not betaxolol, in monkeys (30). These findings suggest that the effect is mediated by β_2-adrenergic receptors, probably through stimulation of cyclic adenosine monophosphate (cAMP) synthesis, since the latter has been shown to mediate increased outflow facility in primates (31). Tissue culture studies, however, suggest that the action of epinephrine on human trabecular endothelium is mediated through both α- and β-adrenergic receptors and intimately involves the cytoskeletal system of the cells (32). Cytochalasin B, which increases outflow facility by disrupting actin filaments in trabecular endothelial cells, has been shown to potentiate the facility-increasing effect of epinephrine (33), and phalloidin, a peptide that inhibits actin filament depolymerization, was shown to partially inhibit the facility-increasing action of epinephrine (32). These findings suggest that epinephrine may increase outflow facility by altering endothelial cell shape through depolymerization of actin filaments in the cells.

During phase two, fluorophotometric and tonographic studies in normotensive (15–17) and ocular hypertensive (17) human volunteers have revealed a slight increase in aqueous humor formation for at least the first several hours after topical epinephrine administration. Chronic administration of epinephrine 2% twice daily for 2 weeks, however, showed no measurable effect on either the rate of aqueous flow or the circadian rhythm of aqueous flow (35), although intravenous epinephrine in normal human volunteers increased aqueous flow by 27% (36). The effect of epinephrine on aqueous production does not appear to be influenced by thymoxamine, an α-adrenergic antagonist (37). Pretreatment with timolol, a β-adrenergic antagonist (38), as well as sympathetic denervation secondary to third neuron Horner's syndrome (39), were both associated with a decrease in aqueous humor flow in response to the administration of epinephrine. It may be, therefore, that epinephrine increases aqueous formation during phase two by stimulating β-adrenergic receptors, but that the drug cannot maintain a sustained effect on aqueous flow.

Phase Three: Late Increase in Outflow Facility

This phase is believed to occur weeks to months after continued administration of epinephrine. The mechanism is uncertain, but may be related to glycosaminoglycans' metabolism in the trabecular meshwork (18, 20). This is consistent with the observation that epinephrine activates lysosomal hyaluronidase in the rabbit iris (40). Other possible causes of the long-term effect include supersensitivity to topical epinephrine, which has been noted with chronic use of the drug (41), or the gradual release of the agent from pigment-binding sites.

Administration

Concentrations

Studies have shown that the pressure lowering effect of epinephrine is proportional to the concentration of free base (or active form of the drug) within the range of 0.25% to 1% (18), and that 2% may have some additional efficacy over the 1% concentration (5). It has also been shown that topical epinephrine may be an effective ocular hypotensive drug in concentrations as low as 0.06% (42). Standard commercial preparations are available in concentrations of 0.5%, 1%, and 2%.

Frequency of Administration

Twice daily instillation provides a continuous pressure lowering effect in most cases. However, a question which needs further study is whether more frequent administration, e.g., four times daily, might maximize the early effect of decreased aqueous production.

Standard Formulations

Standard commercial preparations are available in three salt forms: hydrochloride, borate, and bitartrate (Table 26.1). No

Table 26.1.

COMMERCIAL ADRENERGIC STIMULATORS*

Generic Preparations	*Brand Names*	*Concentrations (%)*
Epinephrine HCl	Epifrin	0.25, 0.5, 1, 2
	Glaucon	0.5, 1, 2
Epinephryl borate	Epinal	0.25, 0.5, 1
	Eppy/N	0.5, 1, 2
Epinephrine bitartrate	Epitrate	2 (1.1 free base)
Dipivefrin HCl	Propine	0.1
Pilocarpine/ epinephrine	E-Pilo-1, E-Pilo-2, etc., P_1E_2, P_2E_1, etc.	1, 2, 3, 4, 6(pilo) + 1(epi)
Apraclonidine HCl	Iopidine	0.5, 1
Brimonidine tartrate	Alphagan	0.2

Other generic epinephrine products may also be available.

significant difference has been found in the pressure lowering efficacy of these three preparations (10), although the drugs may differ slightly with regard to side effects.

EPINEPHRINE HYDROCHLORIDE. Epinephrine hydrochloride has the advantage of stability and is available in all three concentrations (0.5%, 1%, and 2%) of the free base. It has the disadvantage of irritation upon instillation because of a low pH of approximately 3.5.

EPINEPHRYL BORATE. Epinephryl borate is a complex of boric acid and epinephrine and causes less irritation due to a higher pH of 7.4 (43). It is also available in 0.5%, 1%, and 2% concentrations of free base.

EPINEPHRINE BITARTRATE. Epinephrine bitartrate also has the disadvantage of irritation with instillation due to a low pH. In addition, the stated concentration of some commercial preparations is higher than the free base of epinephrine. This salt form has been tested in rabbits in a polymeric matrix, which releases the drug osmotically at a rate of 1–4 µg of free base per hour over a 12-hour period (44). This form of drug delivery provided IOP control equivalent to that of the drug in drop form, but with considerably less total medication and without reducing the tear film pH.

Dipivefrin

Dipivefrin, or dipivalyl epinephrine (DPE), is a modification of epinephrine in which two pivalic acid groups are added to the parent drug (45–47). The new compound is significantly more lipophilic than epinephrine, which increases the corneal penetration by 17-fold (48). In addition, dipivefrin is a prodrug, which is a drug that undergoes biotransformation before exhibiting its pharmacologic effect. The compound is hydrolyzed to epinephrine after absorption into the eye (49), with the majority of the hydrolysis occurring in the cornea

(50). The enzymatic conversion of dipivefrin by esterases releases the pivalic acid, which is not metabolized in the eye, but is rapidly eliminated without apparent sequestration in ocular tissues (51). Preliminary rabbit studies suggested that echothiophate iodide inhibits the hydrolysis of dipivefrin (52), consistent with the in vitro observation that echothiophate is a competitive, reversible inhibitor of the soluble corneal dipivefrin esterases (53). However, subsequent studies indicated that the lack of hypotensive effect with dipivefrin in rabbits is due to an ocular hypertensive response to echothiophate (54), that cholinesterase inhibitors do not effect the conversion of dipivefrin to epinephrine (55), and that the combination of dipivefrin and echothiophate is an effective form of therapy in humans (56). It has also been shown that instillation of dipivefrin in rabbits for 4 weeks does not alter esterase activity or dipivefrin hydrolysis, suggesting the potential for prolonged efficacy of the drug (57). As with other forms of epinephrine, dipivefrin reduces ciliary body blood flow in human eyes (58).

Clinical trials indicate that the pressure lowering effect of 0.1% dipivefrin is somewhere between that of 1% and 2% epinephrine (59–62), and is comparable to betaxolol 0.5% (63). Dipivefrin has the advantage over standard epinephrine formulations of less systemic toxicity, especially with regard to the cardiovascular side effects (64). Advantages with regard to ocular toxicity include less burning and irritation with instillation (65), and the elimination of hydrophilic contact lens discoloration (66). However, external ocular toxicity, including large bulbar conjunctival follicles, may occur with prolonged use of dipivefrin (67–70). Once the drug is converted to epinephrine within the eye, it presumably has the same intraocular complications as other forms of epinephrine.

Adrenergic Supersensitivity

Another method for enhancing the effect of epinephrine is to increase the sensitivity of ocular tissues to the drug. Agents that have been evaluated for this purpose include 6-hydroxydopamine, guanethidine, and glucocorticoids.

6-HYDROXYDOPAMINE. This compound produces a "chemical sympathectomy" by causing temporary degeneration of axon terminals (71–74). The result is a transient increase in outflow facility due to an initial release of norepinephrine, and a more sustained effect on IOP reduction when given with epinephrine therapy by enhancing the action of the exogenous epinephrine. A similar effect has been demonstrated in rabbits with α-methyl-para-tyrosine, an inhibitor of norepinephrine synthesis (75). These drugs produce both an α- and β-adrenergic supersensitivity, although the latter appears to be the predominant effect with 6-hydroxydopamine (71–73).

Clinical trials of 6-hydroxydopamine-enhanced epinephrine therapy showed a significant IOP reduction in most patients (76). However, this never gained clinical acceptance, in part due to the practical disadvantage that 6-hydroxydopamine must be administered by subconjunctival injection or iontophoresis at weekly to monthly intervals (77, 78). Furthermore, both 6-hydroxydopamine and α-methyl-para-tyrosine cause a subsensitivity to cholinergic drugs in rabbits (75).

GUANETHIDINE. This drug is a postganglionic adrenergic antagonist which creates an adrenergic supersensitivity by depleting stores of catecholamines (79). It may lower the IOP when given alone, presumably by an effect on both aqueous production and outflow (80), but is particularly effective when used in combination with epinephrine (81, 82). Clinical trials with such a combined drop, which is available in some parts of the world, revealed significant, sustained reductions in IOP (83–91). The IOP lowering effect is reportedly equal to or better than epinephrine alone (91, 92), pilocarpine (92), or timolol (93). However, one study revealed a biphasic response in which a phase of elevated IOP occurred due to increased aqueous production (94). Furthermore, guanethidine is reported to cause soreness, conjunctival hyperemia, corneal epithelial changes, lid edema, and ptosis in some patients (95). The effect of ptosis by topical guanethidine has actually been used to treat thyrotoxic lid retraction (79). However, the combination drops are said to be generally well-tolerated (83–89), and the side effects can be reduced by using lower concentrations of guanethidine, although this also reduces the pressure-lowering efficacy (96).

GLUCOCORTICOIDS. These agents enhance the sensitivity to catecholamines in various tissues. In a clinical trial of ocular hypertensive patients, pretreatment with three applications of dexamethasone 0.01% significantly increased the IOP-lowering effect of epinephrine 0.1% (97).

Drug Interactions

Miotics and Carbonic Anhydrase Inhibitors

When an epinephrine compound and a miotic are given in combination therapy, the reduction in IOP is usually significantly greater than the effect of either drug given alone. This fact is utilized in some commercial preparations which combine epinephrine and pilocarpine in a single formulation. Epinephrine also provides additional IOP reduction in most cases when added to carbonic anhydrase inhibitor therapy. Furthermore, the combination of epinephrine, a miotic, and a carbonic anhydrase inhibitor may be an effective regimen when any two of the three drugs alone is insufficient.

β-Adrenergic Inhibitors

The interaction between epinephrine and β-adrenergic blockers is less clear-cut than with the drugs noted earlier. Since epinephrine stimulates and β-blockers inhibit β-adrenergic receptors, it might be anticipated that one drug would interfere with the action of the other. Clinical studies suggest that this does occur to a degree, although some ad-

ditive effect on IOP may be achieved with simultaneous use of the two drugs (98–100).

When timolol, a nonselective β-adrenergic inhibitor, is given to eyes pretreated with epinephrine, there is a significant additional pressure reduction for the first few weeks, after which the pressure lowering effect of the combined regimen is only slightly greater than with timolol alone (101–105). When the reverse sequence is followed, and epinephrine therapy is added to eyes already receiving timolol, an additional reduction in IOP is usually small or absent (101–107). Continued therapy with either epinephrine (108, 109) or dipivefrin (104, 107, 110), in combination with timolol, provides a small additional IOP reduction in most patients in the magnitude of 1–3 mm Hg over that achieved with timolol alone. A mixture of epinephrine and timolol has also been shown to lower the IOP significantly more than either drug alone (111). One study suggested that the combined effect might be enhanced by separating the administration of the two drugs by several hours rather than several minutes (108). However, a subsequent study revealed no difference between these two treatment plans (112). Pretreatment with topical epinephrine has also been shown to decrease the systemic concentration of timolol (113), suggesting that it may be best to give the epinephrine first when using both drugs within a short time period of each other.

Based on the above observations, Thomas and Epstein (101) postulated a model for the influence of the adrenergic system on aqueous humor dynamics. As previously discussed, stimulation of β-adrenergic receptors in the inflow system appears to increase aqueous production. Assuming that this system has a "resting tone," inhibition by a β-blocker would reduce aqueous production, as well as block the influence of epinephrine on inflow. Stimulation of β-adrenergic receptors in the outflow system is believed to increase aqueous outflow, as supported by tonographic and fluorophotometric studies (15–17). This system presumably has no resting tone, since timolol therapy alone does not alter outflow. Timolol does, however, block the effect of epinephrine on outflow, which most likely explains the minimal additional effect of adding epinephrine to timolol therapy.

Studies with betaxolol, a cardioselective, β_1-adrenergic inhibitor, support the concept that the effect of epinephrine on aqueous outflow is mediated through β_2-adrenergic receptors, since the addition of either epinephrine hydrochloride (114) or dipivefrin (115) to betaxolol has a greater additional pressure lowering effect than the addition of either drug to timolol. In clinical practice, therefore, adding an epinephrine compound as a second drug will usually have a greater additional IOP-lowering effect when the first drug is betaxolol, rather than a nonselective β-blocker, such as timolol. However, since betaxolol alone has less pressure-lowering efficacy than the nonselective agents, the net effect of epinephrine with either β-blocker is essentially the same.

Studies have also shown that the ocular hypotensive effect of topical epinephrine is reduced by treatment with oral timolol (116), as well as oral or topical indomethacin, a cyclooxygenase inhibitor (24–26).

Side Effects

Side effects are common with the topical administration of standard epinephrine preparations. It may be helpful to think of these in three categories: systemic, extraocular, and intraocular.

Systemic Toxicity

These adverse reactions include elevated blood pressure, tachycardia, arrhythmias, headaches, tremor, nervousness, and anxiety. As previously noted, dipivefrin is not converted to active epinephrine until it enters the eye and is, therefore, associated with fewer systemic effects than the standard forms of epinephrine. The systemic absorption is 55–65% of the topically applied dose for both forms of epinephrine (117), which may be substantially reduced by performing nasolacrimal occlusion.

Extraocular Reactions

Side effects involving the lids and external portion of the eye constitute the most common adverse reactions encountered with topical epinephrine therapy.

BURNING. Burning on instillation is practically universal with the hydrochloride and bitartrate preparations, but may be minimized with the use of epinephryl borate or dipivefrin.

REACTIVE HYPEREMIA. Reactive hyperemia occurs with all forms of epinephrine, although maybe somewhat less with dipivefrin. The patient often fails to associate this with use of the drug, since the initial vasoconstrictive effect of epinephrine tends to whiten the conjunctiva, and the hyperemia appears later (Fig. 26.1).

ADRENOCHROME PIGMENTATION. Oxidation and polymerization of epinephrine converts the drug to adrenochrome, a pigment of the melanin family, which may be deposited in several ocular structures. In the lower palpebral conjunctiva, it forms small, round deposits, which are usually asymptomatic (118) (Fig. 26.2), while deposits in the upper conjunctiva tend to be branching or "staghorn" in shape (Fig. 26.3) and may abrade the cornea (119–121). When IOP elevation and bullous keratopathy are present, adrenochrome may deposit in the superficial cornea, producing a so-called "black cornea" (Fig. 26.4) (122–128). Adrenochrome may also deposit in the lacrimal sac (129) or nasolacrimal duct (130, 131). It has been reported to stain a senile scleral plaque, giving the appearance of a malignant melanoma (132). It may also discolor soft contact lenses (133, 134), which, as previously noted, is reported to not occur with dipivefrin (66).

MISCELLANEOUS. Other less common extraocular reactions include tearing, photophobia, blurred vision, epidermalization of the lacrimal punctum (135), and madarosis (loss of eyelashes) (136). An association with ocular pemphigoid has been suggested (137, 138), although a clear cause-and-effect relationship has not been established. In an evaluation of 17 glaucoma patients with ocular cicatricial pemphigoid, eight were receiving dipivefrin, although each patient was on one or more other topical glaucoma medication (139). True allergic reactions with topical epinephrine are not com-

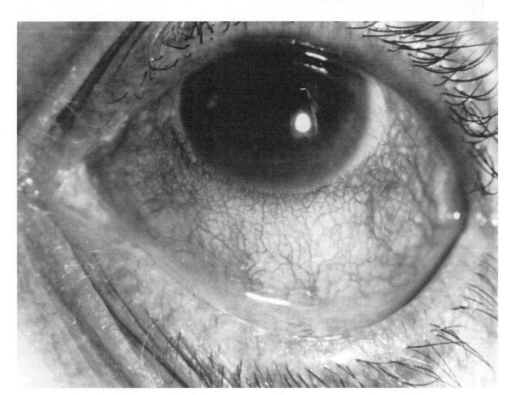

Figure 26.1. Diffuse conjunctival reactive hyperemia as a complication of chronic topical epinephrine therapy. (Reprinted by permission from Bigger JF: Norepinephrine therapy in patients allergic to or intolerant of epinephrine. Ann Ophthalmol 11:183, 1979.)

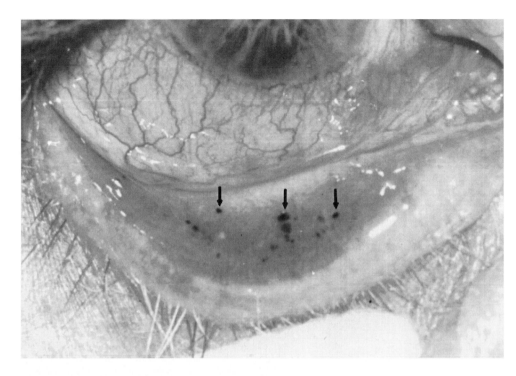

Figure 26.2. Adrenochrome deposits *(arrows)* of the lower palpebral conjunctiva in patient on chronic topical epinephrine therapy showing small, round configuration, which is typical of this location. (Reprinted by permission from Cashwell, LF, Shields, MB, Reed, JW: Adrenochrome pigmentation. Arch Ophthalmol 95:514, 1977.)

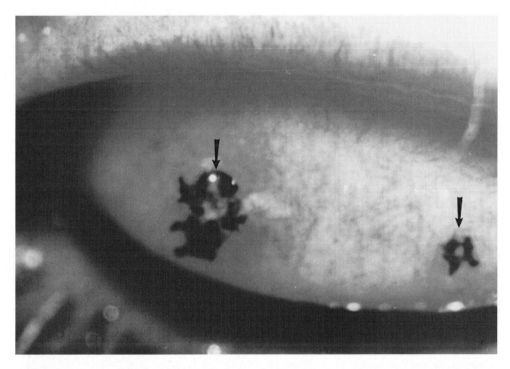

Figure 26.3. "Staghorn"-shaped adrenochrome deposits *(arrows)* of the upper palpebral conjunctiva due to chronic topical epinephrine, typical of the complication in this location. (Reprinted by permission from Cashwell, LF, Shields, MB, Reed, JW: Adrenochrome pigmentation. Arch Ophthalmol 95:514, 1977.)

mon. As previously noted, however, the prolonged use of dipivefrin may be associated with external ocular toxicity, including large bulbar conjunctival follicles (67–70).

Intraocular Reactions

While less common than the extraocular side effects, the intraocular reactions generally have more serious consequences. With regard to dipivefrin, it should be anticipated

that the intraocular reactions will be the same as with other forms of epinephrine, since it becomes the active drug after entering the eye.

MYDRIASIS. Mydriasis is a standard, although somewhat variable, response to epinephrine. It is usually of no consequence, but may precipitate angle-closure glaucoma in the predisposed eye, and is clearly contraindicated in such cases before an iridotomy has been performed.

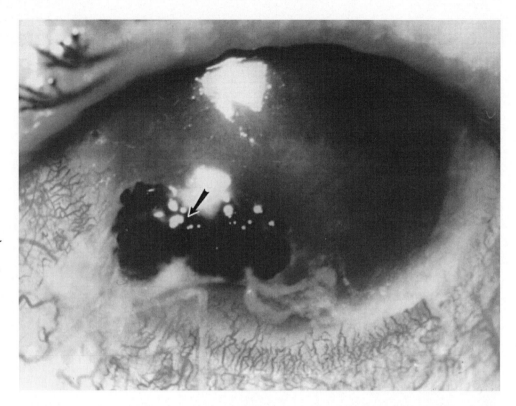

Figure 26.4. "Black cornea" adrenochrome deposition (*arrow*) in patient with bullous keratopathy and chronic topical epinephrine therapy. (Reprinted by permission from Cashwell, LF, Shields, MB, Reed, JW: Adreno-chrome pigmentation. Arch Ophthalmol 95:514, 1977, and courtesy of David Donaldson, M.D.)

EPINEPHRINE MACULOPATHY. Epinephrine maculopathy is a form of cystoid macular edema, which occurs in some apha-kic eyes receiving topical epinephrine (140, 141). A fluores-cein angiographic study of 128 consecutive eyes revealed macular edema in 28% of those receiving epinephrine and in 13% of those not on the drug (142). The pathogenesis of ep-inephrine maculopathy may be related to the epinephrine-induced synthesis of prostaglandins (143), which leads to a disruption of the blood-ocular barrier (25, 144). Epinephrine maculopathy is usually reversible, at least with early dis-continuation of the drug, and is probably dose related.

CORNEAL ENDOTHELIAL DAMAGE. Corneal endothelial dam-age has been observed with intracameral injection of epi-nephrine 1:1000 in rabbit (145, 146) and monkey (145) eyes, but not with a 1:5000 concentration (145). Decreased endothelial cell counts have also been reported in glaucoma patients after prolonged use of topical epinephrine (147).

OCULAR HYPOXIA. It has been suggested that epinephrine might reduce optic nerve head perfusion by causing vasoconstriction of the adrenergically-innervated vessels behind the lamina cribrosa, and that this might be a particularly serious problem in the unprotected fellow eye during uniocular treatment with epinephrine (148). Topical epinephrine 2% was shown to in-crease macular blood flow 2 hours after instillation in normal volunteers, using the blue-field simulation technique (149). The lens appears to serve as a barrier to posterior diffusion of ep-inephrine, since aphakic eyes, following topical epinephrine therapy, have significantly more labeled epinephrine in the choroid and, to a lesser degree, in the retina and optic nerve,

than phakic eyes (150). Aphakic eyes also have an attenuated epinephrine effect in the anterior segment with a potentiation of vasoconstriction in the posterior pole (151). It has also been shown that topical epinephrine causes a decrease in anterior chamber PO_2 (152), which might have clinical significance in some situations such as neovascular glaucoma.

Clinical Indications

With the advent of newer topical antiglaucoma drugs, there has been a decline in the use of epinephrine compounds. Be-cause of reduced ocular and systemic side effects, dipivefrin is the most commonly used form of epinephrine. It is rarely used as a first-line drug, but may be a useful second drug, especially in combination with miotics and carbonic anhy-drase inhibitors. Nasolacrimal occlusion may reduce the sys-temic side effects of topical epinephrine, although it does not appear to enhance the pressure-lowering efficacy, except possibly with lower doses, such as 0.5% (153). Relative con-traindications to the use of epinephrine include eyes with po-tentially occludable angles and with aphakia or pseudo-phakia, due to the risk of epinephrine maculopathy.

APRACLONIDINE

Apraclonidine, or para-aminoclonidine, is a para-amino de-rivative of clonidine, an α_2-adrenergic agonist that is used clinically as a potent systemic antihypertensive agent. Topical apraclonidine hydrochloride is available in a 1% concentra-tion for the treatment of short-term IOP elevation, especially in association with anterior segment laser procedures, and in a 0.5% preparation for the chronic management of glaucoma.

Parent Compound (Clonidine)

Clonidine is believed to exert its systemic hypotensive effect by activation of central α_2- adrenergic receptors and reduction of sympathetic outflow from the brain. It has also been shown to lower the IOP following systemic or topical administration (154–157). The mechanism of pressure reduction, as suggested by fluorophotometric studies in human eyes, is reduced aqueous production (158), which may be due to constriction of afferent vessels in the ciliary processes (159). The clinical value of clonidine as an ocular hypotensive agent is limited by the fact that it penetrates the blood-brain barrier, even with topical administration, occasionally causing significant systemic hypotensive episodes. Topical clonidine 0.125% was shown to reduce ocular perfusion pressure by a decrease in systemic blood pressure, as well as a local perfusion pressure-reducing effect (160).

Mechanisms of Action

Apraclonidine has the advantage over clonidine of minimal blood-brain barrier penetration, thereby reducing the cardiovascular side effects (161). As with clonidine, fluorophotometric studies suggest that apraclonidine lowers the IOP by reducing aqueous production (162, 163) with little, if any, effect on blood-aqueous barrier permeability (162). In one clinical trial, there was also a suggestion that apraclonidine may increase outflow facility and reduce episcleral venous pressure (163). Apraclonidine was found to increase prostaglandin levels in the aqueous humor of rabbits, and flurbiprofen, an inhibitor of prostaglandin synthesis, blocked the ocular hypotensive effect of the drug in monkeys (164). These findings suggested that apraclonidine might increase outflow facility by an effect on uveoscleral outflow, although studies of normal volunteers (165, 166) and ocular hypertensive and glaucoma patients (167) showed no significant influence of flurbiprofen on the IOP-lowering effect of apraclonidine.

Efficacy Studies

Studies with 1% apraclonidine indicate that a single dose lowers the mean IOP a maximum of 37% (168), and that this is maintained for at least 1 month of twice daily therapy (169). Apraclonidine 0.25% and 0.5% given twice daily for 1 week were equally effective, with an average IOP reduction of 27%, which was significantly more than that achieved with a 0.125% concentration (170). A comparison of 0.5% and 1% apraclonidine showed no significant difference in pressure lowering efficacy in either normotensive or ocular

hypertensive subjects (171). No significant contralateral IOP effect was seen with 0.25% or 0.5% apraclonidine (161).

In a double-masked, randomized, 90-day clinical trial of open-angle glaucoma patients, apraclonidine 0.25% and 0.5%, both given three times daily, reduced the IOP an average of 3.6 mm Hg and 5.4 mm Hg, respectively, compared to 5.0 mm Hg with timolol 0.5% twice daily (172). Apraclonidine also had a similar effect to β-adrenergic antagonists on daytime aqueous flow, with an average reduction of 30% (173). Unlike timolol, however, which does not effect aqueous flow during sleep, apraclonidine caused a 27% reduction of the spontaneous nocturnal rate (173).

Side Effects

Systemic side effects that have been identified with topical apraclonidine include a transient dry nose or dry mouth, which was reported by 30–50% of patients (169, 170). Several studies have confirmed the lack of effect of apraclonidine on blood pressure and pulse (161, 168–171). However, a case of near syncope and chest tightness ten minutes after receiving 1 drop of apraclonidine 1% has been reported (174).

The most significant ocular side effect with apraclonidine is a follicular conjunctivitis with or without contact dermatitis. Of 64 patients on long-term therapy with the 1% concentration, 48% developed an allergic reaction (175). It has also been reported with lower doses of 0.125% and 0.25% (176). In the long-term study, the mean latency period for developing the reaction was 4.7 months, and those without a local reaction after 10 months can apparently tolerate the drug indefinitely (175). Other ocular side effects that have been reported with apraclonidine include eyelid retraction, mydriasis, and conjunctival blanching (168, 170). A significant decrease in conjunctival oxygen tension has been observed 1 and 3 hours after instillation of apraclonidine 1% (177), although the clinical significance of this has yet to be established.

Clinical Indications

The main value of apraclonidine appears to be the ability to minimize short-term IOP elevations. In rabbits treated with laser irradiation of the iris, apraclonidine prevented the IOP rise and significantly reduced the aqueous protein elevation, but did not affect the increase in prostaglandins (178). In clinical studies, apraclonidine has been shown to be highly effective in minimizing the transient IOP rise following several anterior segment laser procedures, including trabeculoplasty (179–181), iridotomy (179, 181–183), and capsulotomy (183–186). The protocol initially studied called for 1 drop of 1% apraclonidine 1 hour before the laser procedure and a second drop immediately after the operation, although a single drop of 1% or 0.5% immediately after the surgery has a similar effect (180, 186). Apraclonidine has also been reported to be useful in treating acute angle closure glaucoma (187) and in controlling the postoperative IOP spike following phaco-emulsification and intraocular lens implantation (188) and combined extracapsular cataract extraction and trabeculectomy (189). In addition to controlling the postoperative IOP, apraclonidine also significantly reduced the aqueous flare after phacoemulsification, presumably by reducing the blood-aqueous barrier permeability (188). It has also been reported that apraclonidine has clinical value in controlling the IOP rise in open-angle glaucoma patients after dilatation with tropicamide (190).

Apraclonidine 0.5% can also be used in the chronic management of glaucoma. Although the recommended frequency is three times daily, it is effective in many patients with twice daily use. Several studies have shown significant additional IOP reduction when apraclonidine is added to long-term therapy with timolol (191–195) and other nonselective β-blockers (192). The benefit is less significant when apraclonidine is added to maximally tolerated medical therapy for glaucoma, although most studies indicate slight additional IOP reduction in many patients (196–198), which is limited by tachyphylaxis (196) and the high incidence of allergic reactions (175).

BRIMONIDINE

Brimonidine tartrate is a selective α_2-adrenergic agonist. The topical 0.2% concentration has been shown to be comparable to timolol 0.5% and greater than betaxol 0.25% in IOP-lowering efficacy (199). The mechanism of pressure reduction appears to be a decrease in aqueous flow and an increase in uveoscleral outflow, with no significant effect on conventional outflow or episcleral venous pressure (200). Single-dose administration of brimonidine 0.2% produced a slight reduction in systolic blood pressure at rest and during recovery from exercise, but had no significant effect on mean respiratory rate or forced expiratory volume (199).

As with apraclonidine, brimonidine has been shown to be useful in controlling the IOP rise after anterior segment laser surgery. In two vehicle-controlled, multicenter trials involving a total of 480 patients undergoing 360% argon laser trabeculoplasty, brimonidine 0.5% provided effective postoperative pressure control, whether it was given before, after, or before and after the procedure (201, 202).

INVESTIGATIONAL α-ADRENERGIC AGONISTS

Other α_2 Agonists

Dexmedetomidine, the dextroisomer of the α_2-adrenergic agonist medetomidine, has been shown to lower the IOP in rabbits, with a significant contralateral effect (203). Two other investigational α_2-adrenergic agonists, UL 14304–18 and B-HT 920, also produced bilateral pressure reduction when administered unilaterally in monkeys, which appeared to be related to reduced aqueous production (204).

Norepinephrine

The postganglionic physiologic mediator of the adrenergic nervous system, norepinephrine, has limited potential for clinical usefulness because of instability. However, newer, more stable preparations have led to a reevaluation of the drug. Concentrations of 2–4%, given twice daily, significantly lowered the IOP, presumably by an α-induced increase in outflow facility, without causing β-induced side effects such as tachycardia (205, 206). Rabbit studies revealed an early mydriasis and rise in IOP (207, 208) before the pressure reduction occurs (207).

The ocular effects of norepinephrine can be potentiated by bilateral cervical ganglionectomy (208), monoamine oxidase inhibitors (pargyline or pheniprazone) (209), or protriptyline, which potentiates adrenergic activity by blocking catecholamine uptake into postganglionic neurons (210). A prodrug, norepinephrine dipivalylate, has been shown to produce a significant and prolonged dose-related reduction of IOP in human subjects (211). Norepinephrine is also limited by adaptation, or the development of subsensitivity, which was suppressed in rabbit eyes by treatment with flurbiprofen, an inhibitor of prostaglandin synthesis (212).

Pargyline

The monoamine oxidase inhibitor, pargyline, is an indirect α-adrenergic stimulator, used in the treatment of systemic hypertension (213). It has been shown to lower the IOP in rabbits by decreasing aqueous production (213, 214), provided the adrenergic nervous system is intact (215). Topical pargyline 0.5% significantly lowered the pressure in open-angle glaucoma patients, without affecting the pupil (216).

INVESTIGATIONAL β-ADRENERGIC AGONISTS

Isoproterenol

Isoproterenol is a direct β-adrenergic agonist. The racemic form, DL-isoproterenol, reduces IOP in humans, but causes tachycardia with palpitation and weakness, which is an L-isomer effect (217, 218). D-isoproterenol also reduces the IOP in rabbits (218, 219), without causing tachycardia, vasoconstriction, or mydriasis (218). However, D-isoproterenol does not appear to have the same pressure effect in human eyes (219). The mechanism of IOP reduction is unknown, but is apparently unrelated to aqueous production (220).

Forskolin

This diterpene derivative of the plant, Coleus forskohlii, stimulates adenylate cyclase activity, without interacting with cell surface receptors, to increase intracellular levels of cyclic AMP (221). This in turn may enhance norepinephrine release at intraocular synapses (222). Forskolin has been shown to lower IOP in rabbits, monkeys, and humans (221, 223, 224). Tolerance developed by the third day in monkeys (223), but was not seen after 15 days with rabbits (221). According to several studies, the mechanism of IOP lowering is reduced aqueous production (221, 223, 225, 226), which may be related to an increase in the permeability of the blood-aqueous barrier (227). However, a fluorophotometric study in normal volunteers revealed no statistically significant effect of forskolin on aqueous production during the day or night (228). Forskolin has a specific affinity for melanin granules, which may delay the onset but prolong the duration of the ocular hypotensive effect (229).

Cholera Toxin

Cholera toxin, a specific, irreversible activator of adenylate cyclase, stimulates cyclic AMP production in the anterior uvea (230, 231) and scleral-trabecular ring (231) in rabbits, with a subsequent reduction in IOP. The mechanism of pressure lowering is uncertain, with one study indicating decreased aqueous flow (230), while another suggested increased outflow facility (231). Ultracytochemistry studies suggest the cell-surface receptors that mediate the action on aqueous production are likely located in the apical plasma membranes of the ciliary epithelium (232). Fine structural studies of rabbit ciliary processes after treatment with cholera toxin revealed capillary dilatation and stromal edema with no significant damage to the epithelial layers (233).

Terbutaline

This selective β_2-adrenergic stimulator is used in the treatment of bronchial asthma, and has been shown to inhibit induced IOP elevation in rabbits (234). The IOP effect is less than that of timolol or pilocarpine, but more than that of epinephrine or clonidine (234). Tolerance develops after a few days, which is prevented by concomitant treatment with diclofenac, a potent nonsteroidal anti-inflammatory drug (235). Ibuterol, a prodrug of terbutaline, was significantly more efficacious than the parent compound in rabbit studies (236).

Salbutamol

Salbutamol is another selective β_2-adrenergic agonist. It has been shown to lower IOP in human eyes, associated with an increase in both the rate of aqueous production and tonographic facility of outflow (237). The latter was calculated to be due to an increase in uveoscleral outflow.

Pirbuterol

This active sympathomimetic bronchodilator has a high affinity for β_2-adrenergic receptors and has been shown to lower IOP in rabbits, presumably by activating adenylate cyclase (238).

INVESTIGATIONAL NONSPECIFIC ADRENERGIC AGENTS

Vanadate

Topical administration of 1% vanadate lowered the IOP in rabbits, associated with a significant decrease in aqueous humor flow (239, 240). Possible mechanisms of reduced flow are inhibition of ciliary epithelium (Na^+K^+) ATPase or stimulation of adenylate cyclase (241). However, the anterior uveal content of vanadate at the time of IOP reduction was too small for these actions, and other cellular mechanisms are considered likely (242).

Nylidrin

The nonspecific adrenergic agent, nylidrin hydrochloride, lowered IOP in rabbits and monkeys, apparently by increasing uveoscleral outflow (243). Although purported to be a sympathomimetic amine, it has a complex mode of action, which may include a partial agonist action on β_1-adrenergic receptors but an antagonist action on β_2-receptors (238).

SUMMARY

Epinephrine is the only α- and β-adrenergic stimulator commercially available for the chronic treatment of glaucoma. It lowers IOP through a complex system that primarily involves improved aqueous outflow. Side effects occur in three categories: systemic (e.g., elevated blood pressure, tachycardia, and tremor), extraocular (e.g., irritation, reactive hyperemia, and adrenochrome pigmentation), and intraocular (e.g., mydriasis and cystoid macular edema in aphakia). These adverse reactions, especially the systemic and extraocular, can be reduced by use of the epinephrine prodrug, dipivefrin. Apraclonidine and brimonidine are α_2-adrenergic agonists that are useful in controlling short-term pressure elevations, especially in association with certain laser procedures, as well as the long-term management of glaucoma, although the latter is limited by a high incidence of allergic reactions. Other adrenergic stimulators that have been investigated for the treatment of glaucoma include α-adrenergic agonists such as norepinephrine, β-adrenergic agonists, including isoproterenol and forskolin, and nonspecific adrenergic agents.

REFERENCES

1. Goldmann, H: L'origine de l'hypertension oculaire dans le glaucome primitif. Ann Ocul (Paris) 184:1086, 1951.
2. Weekers, R, Prijot, E, Gustin, J: Recent advances and future prospects in the medical treatment of ocular hypertension. Br J Ophthalmol 38:742, 1954.
3. Weekers, R, Delmarcelle, Y, Gustin, J: Treatment of ocular hypertension by adrenalin and diverse sympathomimetic amines. Am J Ophthalmol 40:666, 1955.
4. Becker, B, Ley, AP: Epinephrine and acetazolamide in the therapy of the chronic glaucomas. Am J Ophthalmol 45:639, 1958.
5. Garner, LL, Johnstone, WW, Ballintine, EJ, Carroll, ME: Effect of 2% levo-rotary epinephrine on the intraocular pressure of the glaucomatous eye. Arch Ophthalmol 62:230, 1959.
6. Becker, B, Pettit, TH, Gay, AJ: Topical epinephrine therapy of open-angle glaucoma. Arch Ophthalmol 66:219, 1961.
7. Ballintine, EJ, Garner, LL: Improvement of the coefficient of outflow in glaucomatous eyes. Prolonged local treatment with epinephrine. Arch Ophthalmol 66:314, 1961.
8. Kronfeld, PC: Dose-effect relationships as an aid in the evaluation of ocular hypotensive drugs. Invest Ophthalmol 3:258, 1964.
9. Krill, AE, Newell, FW, Novak, M: Early and long-term effects of levo-epinephrine on ocular tension and outflow. Am J Ophthalmol 59:833, 1965.
10. Criswick, VG, Drance, SM: Comparative study of four different epinephrine salts on intraocular pressure. Arch Ophthalmol 75:768, 1966.
11. Richards, JSF, Drance, SM: The effect of 2% epinephrine on aqueous dynamics in the human eye. Can J Ophthalmol 2:259, 1967.
12. Kronfeld, PC: Early effects of single and repeated doses of L-epinephrine in man. Am J Ophthalmol 72:1058, 1971.
13. Vannas, S, Linkova, M: Adrenalin therapy in glaucoma. Acta Ophthalmolmologica XX Meeting of Nordic Ophthalmologists 1971, p. 39.
14. Green, K, Padgett, D: Effect of various drugs on pseudofacility and aqueous humor formation in the rabbit eye. Exp Eye Res 28:239, 1979.
15. Townsend, DJ, Brubaker, RF: Immediate effect of epinephrine on aqueous formation in the normal human eye as measured by fluorophotometry. Invest Ophthalmol Vis Sci 19:256, 1980.
16. Nagataki, S, Brubaker, RF: Early effect of epinephrine on aqueous formation in the normal human eye. Ophthalmology 88:278, 1981.
17. Schenker, HI, Yablonski, ME, Podos, SM, Linder, L: Fluorophotometric study of epinephrine and timolol in human subjects. Arch Ophthalmol 99:1212, 1981.
18. Sears, ML: The mechanism of action of adrenergic drugs in glaucoma. Invest Ophthalmol 5:115, 1966.
19. Sears, ML, Neufeld, AH: Adrenergic modulation of the outflow of aqueous humor. Invest Ophthalmol 14:83, 1975.
20. Sears, ML: Autonomic nervous system: adrenergic agonists. In Handbook of Experimental Pharmacology. Vol. 69. Sears, ML, ed. Berlin, Springer-Verlag, 1984.
21. Van Buskirk, EM: The ciliary vasculature and its perturbation with drugs and surgery. Trans Am Ophthalmol Soc 86:794, 1988.
22. Alm, A: The effect of topical L-epinephrine on regional ocular blood flow in monkeys. Invest Ophthalmol Vis Sci 19:487, 1980.
23. Jay, WM, Aziz, MZ, Green, K: Further studies on the effect of retrobulbar epinephrine injection on ocular and optic nerve blood flow. Curr Eye Res 5:63, 1986.
24. Camras, CB, Feldman, SG, Podos, SM, et al: Inhibition of the epinephrine-induced reduction of intraocular pressure by systemic indomethacin in humans. Am J Ophthalmol 100:169, 1985.
25. Miyake, K, Miyake, Y, Kuratomi, R: Long-term effects of topically applied epinephrine on the blood-ocular barrier in humans. Arch Ophthalmol 105:1360, 1987.
26. Anderson, L, Wilson, WS: Inhibition by indomethacin of the increased facility of outflow induced by adrenaline. Exp Eye Res 50:119, 1990.
27. Kaufman, PL, Bárány, EH: Adrenergic drug effects on aqueous outflow facility following ciliary muscle retrodisplacement in the cynomolgus monkey. Invest Ophthalmol Vis Sci 20:644, 1981.
28. Kaufman, PL: Epinephrine, norepinephrine, and isoproterenol dose-outflow facility response relationships in cynomolgus monkey eyes with and without ciliary muscle retrodisplacement. Acta Ophthalmol 64:356, 1986.
29. Erickson-Lamy, KA, Nathanson, JA: Epinephrine increases facility of outflow and cyclic AMP content in the human eye in vitro. Invest Ophthalmol Vis Sci 33:2672, 1992.
30. Robinson, JC, Kaufman, PL: Effects and interactions of epinephrine, norepinephrine, timolol, and betaxolol on outflow facility in the cynomolgus monkey. Am J Ophthalmol 109:189, 1990.
31. Neufeld, AH, Sears, ML: Adenosine 3′, 5′-monophosphate analogue increases the outflow facility of the primate eye. Invest Ophthalmol 14:688, 1975.
32. Tripathi, BJ, Tripathi, RC: Effect of epinephrine in vitro on the morphology, phagocytosis, and mitotic activity of human trabecular endothelium. Exp Eye Res 39:731, 1984.
33. Robinson, JC, Kaufman, PL: Cytochalasin B potentiates epinephrine's outflow facility-increasing effect. Invest Ophthalmol Vis Sci 32:1614, 1991.
34. Robinson, JC, Kaufman, PL: Phalloidin inhibits epinephrine's and cytochalasin B's facilitation of aqueous outflow. Arch Ophthalmol 112:1610, 1994.
35. Schneider, TL, Brubaker, RF: Effect of chronic epinephrine on aqueous humor flow during the day and during sleep in normal healthy subjects. Invest Ophthalmol Vis Sci 32:2507, 1991.
36. Kacere, RD, Dolan, JW, Brubaker, RF: Intravenous epinephrine stimulates aqueous formation in the human eye. Invest Ophthalmol Vis Sci 33:2861, 1992.
37. Lee, DA, Brubaker, RF, Nagataki, S: Acute effect of thymoxamine on aqueous humor formation in the epinephrine-treated normal eye as measured by fluorophotometry. Invest Ophthalmol Vis Sci 24:165, 1983.
38. Higgins, RG, Brubaker, RF: Acute effect of epinephrine on aqueous humor formation in the timolol-treated normal eye as measured by fluorophotometry. Invest Ophthalmol Vis Sci 19:420, 1980.
39. Wentworth, WO, Brubaker, RF: Aqueous humor dynamics in a series of patients with third neuron Horner's syndrome. Am J Ophthalmol 92:407, 1981.
40. Hayasaka, S, Sears, M: Effects of epinephrine, indomethacin, acetylsalicylic acid, dexamethasone, and cyclic AMP on the in vitro activity of lysosomal hyaluronidase from the rabbit iris. Invest Ophthalmol Vis Sci 17:1109, 1978.
41. Flach, AJ, Kramer, SG: Supersensitivity to topical epinephrine after long-term epinephrine therapy. Arch Ophthalmol 98:482, 1980.
42. Harris, LS, Galin, MA, Lerner, R: The influence of low dose L-epinephrine on intraocular pressure. Ann Ophthalmol 2:253, 1970.
43. Vaughan, D, Shaffer, R, Riegelman, S: A new stabilized form of epinephrine for the treatment of open-angle glaucoma. Arch Ophthalmol 66:232, 1961.
44. Birss, SA, Longwell, A, Heckbert, S, Keller, N: Ocular hypotensive efficacy of topical epinephrine in normotensive and hypertensive rabbits: continuous drug delivery vs. eyedrops. Ann Ophthalmol 10:1045, 1978.

45. Kaback, MB, Podos, SM, Hargin, TS Jr, et al: The effects of dipivalyl epinephrine on the eye. Am J Ophthalmol 81:768, 1976.
46. Bigger, JF: Dipivefrin and glaucoma. Perspect Ophthalmol 4:87, 1980.
47. Adamek, R: New perspectives in glaucoma therapy with epinephrine and epinephrine derivatives. Klin Monatsbl Augenheilkd 176:978, 1980.
48. Mandell, AI, Stentz, F, Kitabchi, AE: Dipivalyl epinephrine: a new pro-drug in the treatment of glaucoma. Ophthalmology 85:268, 1978.
49. Wei, C-P, Anderson, JA, Leopold, I: Ocular absorption and metabolism of topically applied epinephrine and dipivalyl ester of epinephrine. Invest Ophthalmol Vis Sci 17:315, 1978.
50. Anderson, JA, Davis, WL, Wei, C-P: Site of ocular hydrolysis of a prodrug, dipivefrin, and a comparison of its ocular metabolism with that of the parent compound, epinephrine. Invest Ophthalmol Vis Sci 19:817, 1980.
51. Tamaru, RD, Davis, WL, Anderson, JA: Comparison of ocular disposition of free pivalic acid and pivalic acid esterified in dipivefrin. Arch Ophthalmol 101:1127, 1983.
52. Abramovsky, I, Mindel, JS: Dipivefrin and echothiophate. Contraindications to combined use. Arch Ophthalmol 97:1937, 1979.
53. Anderson, JA, Richman, JB, Mindel, JS: Effects of echothiophate on enzymatic hydrolysis of dipivefrin. Arch Ophthalmol 102:913, 1984.
54. Mindel, JS, Koenigsberg, AM, Kharlamb, AB, et al: The effect of echothiophate on the biphasic response of rabbit ocular pressure to dipivefrin. Arch Ophthalmol 100:147, 1982.
55. Mindel, JS, Cohen, G, Barker, LA, Lewis, DE: Enzymatic and nonenzymatic hydrolysis of D, L-dipivefrin. Arch Ophthalmol 102:457, 1984.
56. Mindel, JS, Yablonski, ME, Tavitian, HO, et al: Dipivefrin and echothiophate. Efficacy of combined use in human beings. Arch Ophthalmol 99:1583, 1981.
57. Nakamura, M, Shirasawa, E, Hikida, M: No changes in rabbit corneal esterase activities with dipivefrine by hydrochloride instillation for 4 weeks. Graefes Arch Clin Exp Ophthalmol 231:551, 1993.
58. Michelson, G, Groh, MJM: Dipivefrin reduces blood flow in the ciliary body in humans. Ophthalmology 101:659, 1994.
59. Kass, MA, Mandell, AI, Goldberg, I, et al: Dipivefrin and epinephrine treatment of elevated intraocular pressure. A comparative study. Arch Ophthalmol 97:1865, 1979.
60. Kohn, AN, Moss, AP, Hargett, NA, et al: Clinical comparison of dipivalyl epinephrine and epinephrine in the the treatment of glaucoma. Am J Ophthalmol 87:196, 1979.
61. Bischoff, P: Clinical studies conducted with a new epinephrine derivative for the treatment of glaucoma (dipivalyl epinephrine). Klin Monatsbl Augenheilkd 172:565, 1978.
62. Krieglstein, GK, Leydhecker, W: The dose-response relationships of dipivalyl epinephrine in open-angle glaucoma. Graefes Arch Clin Exp Ophthalmol 205:141, 1978.
63. Albracht, DC, LeBlanc, RP, Cruz, AM, et al: A double-masked comparison of betaxolol and dipivefrin for the treatment of increased intraocular pressure. Am J Ophthalmol 116:307, 1993.
64. Kerr, CR, Hass, I, Drance, SM, et al: Cardiovascular effects of epinephrine and dipivalyl epinephrine applied topically to the eye in patients with glaucoma. Br J Ophthalmol 66:109, 1982.
65. Yablonski, ME, Shin, DH, Kolker, AE, et al: Dipivefrin use in patients with intolerance to topically applied epinephrine. Arch Ophthalmol 95:2157, 1977.
66. Newton, MJ, Nesburn, AB: Lack of hydrophilic lens discoloration in patients using dipivalyl epinephrine for glaucoma. Am J Ophthalmol 87:193, 1979.
67. Theodore, JA, Leibowitz, HM: External ocular toxicity of dipivalyl epinephrine. Am J Ophthalmol 88:1013, 1979.
68. Wandel, T, Spinak, M: Toxicity of dipivalyl epinephrine. Ophthalmology 88:259, 1981.
69. Liesegang, TJ: Bulbar conjunctival follicles associated with dipivefrin therapy. Ophthalmology 92:228, 1985.
70. Coleiro, JA, Sigurdsson, H, Lockyer, JA: Follicular conjunctivitis on dipivefrin therapy for glaucoma. Eye 2:440, 1988.
71. Holland, MG: Treatment of glaucoma by chemical sympathectomy with 6-hydroxydopamine. Trans Am Acad Ophthalmol Otol 76:437, 1972.
72. Holland, MG, Wei, C-P: Epinephrine dose-response characteristics of glaucomatous human eyes following chemical sympathectomy with 6-hydroxydopamine. Ann Ophthalmol 5:633, 1973.
73. Holland, MG, Wei, C-P: Chemical sympathectomy in glaucoma therapy: an investigation of alpha and beta adrenergic supersensitivity. Ann Ophthalmol 5:783, 1973.
74. Diamond, JG: 6-Hydroxydopamine in treatment of open-angle glaucoma. Arch Ophthalmol 94:41, 1976.
75. Colasanti, BK, Trotter, RR: Responsiveness of the rabbit eye to adrenergic and cholinergic agonists after treatment with 6-hydroxydopamine or alpha-methyl-para-tyrosine: Part II—Intraocular pressure changes. Ann Ophthalmol 10:1209, 1978.
76. Talusan, E, Schwartz, B, Mandell, AI, et al: 6-Hydroxydopamine in the treatment of open-angle glaucoma. Am J Ophthalmol 92:792, 1981.
77. Kitazawa, Y, Nose, H, Horie, T: Chemical sympathectomy with 6-hydroxydopamine in the treatment of primary open-angle glaucoma. Am J Ophthalmol 79:98, 1975.
78. Watanabe, H, Levene, RZ, Bernstein, MR: 6-Hydroxydopamine therapy in glaucoma. Trans Am Acad Ophthalmol Otol 83:69, 1977.
79. Sneddon, JM, Turner, P: The interactions of local guanethidine and sympathomimetic amines in the human eye. Arch Ophthalmol 81:622, 1969.
80. Bonomi, L, Di Comite, P: Outflow facility after guanethidine sulfate administration. Arch Ophthalmol 78:337, 1967.
81. Crombie, AL: Adrenergic supersensitization as a therapeutic tool in glaucoma. Trans Ophthalmol Soc UK 94:570, 1974.
82. Jones, DEP, Norton, DA, Harvey, J, Davies, DJG: Effect of adrenaline and guanethidine in reducing intraocular pressure in rabbits' eyes. Br J Ophthalmol 59:304, 1975.
83. Nagasubramanian, S, Tripathi, RC, Poinoosawmy, D, Gloster, J: Low concentration guanethidine and adrenaline therapy of glaucoma. A preliminary report. Trans Ophthalmol Soc UK 96:179, 1976.
84. Mills, KB, Ridgway, AEA: A double-blind comparison of guanethidine-and-adrenaline drops with 1% adrenaline alone in chronic simple glaucoma. Br J Ophthalmol 62:320, 1978.
85. Hoyng, PhFJ, Dake, CL: The combination of guanethidine 3% and adrenaline 0.5% in 1 eyedrop (GA) in glaucoma treatment. Br J Ophthalmol 63:56, 1979.
86. Romano, J, Patterson, G: Evaluation of a 5% guanethidine and 0.5% adrenaline mixture (Ganda 5.05) and of a 3% guanethidine and 0.5% adrenaline mixture (Ganda 3.05) in the treatment of open-angle glaucoma. Br J Ophthalmol 63:52, 1979.
87. Jones, DEP, Norton, DA, Davies, DJG: Control of glaucoma by reduced dosage guanethidine-adrenaline formulation. Br J Ophthalmol 63:813, 1979.
88. Hoyng, PhFJ, Dake, CL: Maintenance therapy of glaucoma patients with guanethidine (3%) and adrenaline (0.5%) once daily. Graefes Arch Clin Exp Ophthalmol 214:269, 1980.
89. Van Husen, H: A combination of 1% guanethidine and 0.2% epinephrine in drop form to lower IOP in open angle glaucoma. Klin Monatsbl Augenheilkd 177:622, 1980.
90. Murray, A, Glover, D, Hitchings, R: Low-dose combined guanethidine 1% and adrenaline 0.5% in the treatment of chronic simple glaucoma: a prospective study. Br J Ophthalmol 65:533, 1981.
91. Hitchings, RA, Glover, D: Adrenaline 1% combined with guanethidine 1% versus adrenaline 1%: a randomised prospective double-blind cross-over study. Br J Ophthalmol 66:247, 1982.
92. Romano, JH, Nagasubramanian, S, Poinoosawmy, D: Double-masked cross-over comparison of Ganda 1.02 (guanethidine 1% and adrenaline 0.2% mixture) with gutt. adrenaline 1% (Simplene 1%) and with pilocarpine 1% (Sno-Pilo 1%). Br J Ophthalmol 65:50, 1981.

93. Heilmann, K: Course of intraocular pressure during long-term treatment with a combination of guanethidine and epinephrine. Klin Monatsbl Augenheilkd 183:17, 1983.

94. Hoyng, PhFJ, Dake, CL: The aqueous humor dynamics and the biphasic response in intraocular pressure induced by guanethidine and adrenaline in the glaucomatous eye. Graefes Arch Clin Exp Ophthalmol 214:263, 1980.

95. Gloster, J: Guanethidine and glaucoma. Trans Ophthalmol Soc UK 94:573, 1974.

96. Urner-Bloch, U, Aeschlimann, JE, Gloor, BP: Treatment of chronic simple glaucoma with an adrenaline/guanethidine combination at three different dosages (comparative double-blind study). Graefes Arch Clin Exp Ophthalmol 213:175, 1980.

97. Bealka, N, Schwartz, B: Enhanced ocular hypotensive response to epinephrine with prior dexamethasone treatment. Arch Ophthalmol 109:346, 1991.

98. Keates, EU: Evaluation of timolol maleate combination therapy in chronic open-angle glaucoma. Am J Ophthalmol 88:565, 1979.

99. Smith, RJ, Nagasubramanian, S, Watkins, R, Poinoosawmy, D: Addition of timolol maleate to routine medical therapy: a clinical trial. Br J Ophthalmol 64:779, 1980.

100. Nielsen, NV, Eriksen, JS: Timolol in maintenance treatment of ocular hypertension and glaucoma. Acta Ophthalmol 57:1070, 1979.

101. Thomas, JV, Epstein, DL: Timolol and epinephrine in primary open angle glaucoma. Transient additive effect. Arch Ophthalmol 99:91, 1981.

102. Thomas, JV, Epstein, DL: Study of the additive effect of timolol and epinephrine in lowering intraocular pressure. Br J Ophthalmol 65:596, 1981.

103. Goldberg, I, Ashburn, FS Jr, Palmberg, PF, et al: Timolol and epinephrine. A clinical study of ocular interactions. Arch Ophthalmol 98:484, 1980.

104. Keates, EC, Stone, RA: Safety and effectiveness of concomitant administration of dipivefrin and timolol maleate. Am J Ophthalmol 91:243, 1981.

105. Ohrstrom, A, Pandolfi, M: Regulation of intraocular pressure and pupil size by beta-blockers and epinephrine. Arch Ophthalmol 98:2182, 1980.

106. Ohrstrom, A, Kattstrom, O: Interaction of timolol and adrenaline. Br J Ophthalmol 65:53, 1981.

107. Knupp, JA, Shields, MB, Mandell, AI, et al: Combined timolol and epinephrine therapy for open angle glaucoma. Surv Ophthalmol 28(Suppl):280, 1983.

108. Cyrlin, MS, Thomas, JV, Epstein, DL: Additive effect of epinephrine to timolol therapy in primary open angle glaucoma. Arch Ophthalmol 100:414, 1982.

109. Korey, MS, Hodapp, E, Kass, MA, et al: Timolol and epinephrine. Long-term evaluation of concurrent administration. Arch Ophthalmol 100:742, 1982.

110. Ober, M, Scharrer, A: The effect of timolol and dipivalyl-epinephrine in the treatment of the elevated intraocular pressure. Graefes Arch Clin Exp Ophthalmol 213:273, 1980.

111. Drance, SM, Douglas, GR, Wijsman, KJ, Schulzer, M: Adrenergic and adrenolytic effects on intraocular pressure. Graefes Arch Clin Exp Ophthalmol 229:50, 1991.

112. Tsoy, EA, Meekins, BB, Shields, MB: Comparison of two treatment schedules for combined timolol and dipivefrin therapy. Am J Ophthalmol 102:320, 1986.

113. Urtti, A, Kyyronen, K: Ophthalmic epinephrine, phenylephrine, and pilocarpine affect the systemic absorption of ocularly applied timolol. J Ocul Pharmacol Ther 5:127, 1989.

114. Allen, RC, Epstein, DL: Additive effect of betaxolol and epinephrine in primary open angle glaucoma. Arch Ophthalmol 104:1178, 1986.

115. Weinreb, RN, Ritch, R, Kushner, FH: Effect of adding betaxolol to dipivefrin therapy. Am J Ophthalmol 101:196, 1986.

116. Ohrstrom, A: Dose response of oral timolol combined with adrenaline. Br J Ophthalmol 66:242, 1982.

117. Anderson, JA: Systemic absorption of topical ocularly applied epinephrine and dipivefrin. Arch Ophthalmol 98:350, 1980.

118. Corwin, ME, Spencer, WH: Conjunctival melanin depositions. A side-effect of topical epinephrine therapy. Arch Ophthalmol 69:73, 1963.

119. Veirs, ER, McGrew, JC: Ocular complications from topical epinephrine therapy of glaucoma. EENT Monthly 42:46, 1963.

120. Cashwell, LF, Shields, MB, Reed, JW: Adrenochrome pigmentation. Arch Ophthalmol 95:514, 1977.

121. Pardos, GJ, Krachmer, JH, Mannis, MJ: Persistent corneal erosion secondary to tarsal adrenochrome deposit. Am J Ophthalmol 90:870, 1980.

122. Reinecke, RD, Kuwabara, T: Corneal deposits secondary to topical epinephrine. Arch Ophthalmol 70:170, 1963.

123. Krejci, L, Harrison, R: Corneal pigment deposits from topically administered epinephrine. Experimental production. Arch Ophthalmol 82:836, 1969.

124. Green, WR, Kaufer, GJ, Dubroff, S: Black cornea. A complication of topical use of epinephrine. Ophthalmologica 154:88, 1967.

125. Cleasby, G, Donaldson, DD: Epinephrine pigmentation of the cornea. Arch Ophthalmol 78:74, 1967.

126. Madge, GE, Geeraets, WJ, Guerry, DP III: Black cornea secondary to topical epinephrine. Am J Ophthalmol 71:402, 1971.

127. McCarthy, RW, LeBlanc, R: A "black cornea" secondary to topical epinephrine. Can J Ophthalmol 11:336, 1976.

128. Kaiser, PK, Pineda, R, Albert, DM, Shore, JW: "Black cornea" after long-term epinephrine use. Arch Ophthalmol 110:1273, 1992.

129. Barishak, R, Romano, A, Stein, R: Obstruction of lacrimal sac caused by topical epinephrine. Ophthalmologica 159:373, 1969.

130. Spaeth, GL: Nasolacrimal duct obstruction caused by topical epinephrine. Arch Ophthalmol 77:355, 1967.

131. Bradbury, JA, Rennie, IG, Parsons, MA: Adrenaline dacryolith: detection by ultrasound examination of the nasolacrimal duct. Br J Ophthalmol 72:935, 1988.

132. Soong, HK, McKenney, MJ, Wolter, JR: Adrenochrome staining of senile plaque resembling malignant melanoma. Am J Ophthalmol 101:380, 1986.

133. Sugar, J: Adrenochrome pigmentation of hydrophilic lenses. Arch Ophthalmol 91:11, 1974.

134. Miller, D, Brooks, SM, Mobilia, E: Adrenochrome staining of soft contact lenses. Ann Ophthalmol 8:65, 1976.

135. Romano, A, Barishak, R, Stein, R: Obstruction of lacrimal puncta caused by topical epinephrine. Ophthalmologica 166:301, 1973.

136. Kass, MA, Stamper, RL, Becker, B: Madarosis in chronic epinephrine therapy. Arch Ophthalmol 88:429, 1972.

137. Kristensen, EB, Norn, MS: Benign mucous membrane pemphigoid. 1. Secretion of mucus and tears. Acta Ophthalmol 52:266, 1974.

138. Fiore, PM, Jacobs, IH, Goldberg, DB: Drug-induced pemphigoid. A spectrum of diseases. Arch Ophthalmol 105:1660, 1987.

139. Tauber, J, Melamed, S, Foster, CS: Glaucoma in patients with ocular cicatricial pemphigoid. Ophthalmology 96:33, 1989.

140. Kolker, AE, Becker, B: Epinephrine maculopathy. Arch Ophthalmol 79:552, 1968.

141. Michels, RG, Maumenee, AE: Cystoid macular edema associated with topically applied epinephrine in aphakic eyes. Am J Ophthalmol 80:379, 1975.

142. Thomas, JV, Gragoudas, ES, Blair, NP, Lapus, JV: Correlation of epinephrine use and macular edema in aphakic glaucomatous eyes. Arch Ophthalmol 96:625, 1978.

143. Miyake, K, Shirasawa, E, Hikita, M, et al: Synthesis of prostaglandin E in rabbit eyes with topically applied epinephrine. Invest Ophthalmol Vis Sci 29:332, 1988.

144. Miyake, K, Kayazawa, F, Manabe, R, Miyake, Y: Indomethacin and the epinephrine-induced breakdown of the blood-ocular barrier in rabbits. Invest Ophthalmol Vis Sci 28:482, 1987.

145. Hull, DS, Chemotti, T, Edelhauser, HF, et al: Effect of epinephrine on the corneal endothelium. Am J Ophthalmol 79:245, 1975.

146. Edelhauser, HF, Hyndiuk, RA, Zeeb, A, Schultz, RO: Corneal edema and the intraocular use of epinephrine. Am J Ophthalmol 93:327, 1982.

147. Waltman, SR, Yarian, D, Hart, W Jr, Becker, B: Corneal endothelial changes with long-term topical epinephrine therapy. Arch Ophthalmol 95:1357, 1977.

148. Kramer, SG: Considerations on epinephrine therapy in glaucoma. Ann Ophthalmol 10:1077, 1978.

149. Robinson, F, Chen, S, Petrig, BL, et al: The acute effect of topical epinephrine on macular blood flow in humans. Invest Ophthalmol Vis Sci 33:18, 1992.

150. Kramer, SG: Epinephrine distribution after topical administration to phakic and aphakic eyes. Trans Am Ophthalmol Soc 78:947, 1980.

151. Morgan, TR, Mirate, DJ, Bowman, K, Green, K: Topical epinephrine and regional ocular blood flow in aphakic eyes of rabbits. Arch Ophthalmol 101:112, 1983.

152. Stefansson, E, Robinson, D, Wolbarsht, ML, et al: Effect of epinephrine on PO$_2$ in anterior chamber. Arch Ophthalmol 101:636, 1983.

153. Zimmerman, TJ, Sharir, M, Nardin, GF, Fuqua, M: Therapeutic index of epinephrine and dipivefrin with nasolacrimal occlusion. Am J Ophthalmol 114:8, 1992.

154. Harrison, R, Kaufmann, CS: Clonidine. Effects of a topically administered solution on intraocular pressure and blood pressure in open-angle glaucoma. Arch Ophthalmol 95:1368, 1977.

155. Hodapp, E, Kolker, AE, Kass, MA, et al: The effect of topical clonidine on intraocular pressure. Arch Ophthalmol 99:1208, 1981.

156. Petursson, G, Cole, R, Hanna, C: Treatment of glaucoma using minidrops of clonidine. Arch Ophthalmol 102:1180, 1984.

157. Krieglstein, GK, Langham, ME, Leydhecker, W: The peripheral and central neural actions of clonidine in normal and glaucomatous eyes. Invest Ophthalmol Vis Sci 17:149, 1978.

158. Lee, DA, Topper, JE, Brubaker, RF: Effect of clonidine on aqueous humor flow in normal human eyes. Exp Eye Res 38:239, 1984.

159. Macri, FJ, Cevario, SJ: Clonidine. Effects on aqueous humor formation and intraocular pressure. Arch Ophthalmol 96:2111, 1978.

160. Marquardt, R, Pillunat, LE, Stodtmeister, R: Ocular hemodynamics following local application of clonidine. Klin Monatsbl Augenheilkd 193:637, 1988.

161. Coleman, AL, Robin, AL, Pollack, IP, et al: Cardiovascular and intraocular pressure effects and plasma concentrations of apraclonidine. Arch Ophthalmol 108:1264, 1990.

162. Gharagozloo, NZ, Relf, SJ, Brubaker, RF: Aqueous flow is reduced by the alpha-adrenergic agonist, apraclonidine hydrochloride (ALO 2145). Ophthalmology 95:1217, 1988.

163. Toris, CB, Tafoya, ME, Camras, CB, Yablonski, ME: Effects of apraclonidine on aqueous humor dynamics in human eyes. Ophthalmology 102:456, 1995.

164. Wang, R-F, Camras, CB, Podos, SM, et al: The role of prostaglandins in the para-aminoclonidine-induced reduction of intraocular pressure. Trans Am Ophthalmol Soc 87:94, 1989.

165. Sulewski, ME, Robin, AL, Cummings, HL, Arkin, LM: Effects of topical flurbiprofen on the intraocular pressure lowering effects of apraclonidine and timolol. Arch Ophthalmol 109:807, 1991.

166. McCannel, C, Koskela, T, Brubaker, RF: Topical flurbiprofen pretreatment does not block apraclonidine's effect on aqueous flow in humans. Arch Ophthalmolmol 109:810, 1991.

167. Siegel, MJ, Camras, CB, Lustgarten, JS, Popos, SM: Effect of flurbiprofen on the reduction of intraocular pressure after administration of 1% apraclonidine in patients with glaucoma. Arch Ophthalmol 110:598, 1992.

168. Robin, AL: Short-term effects of unilateral 1% apraclonidine therapy. Arch Ophthalmol 106:912, 1988.

169. Abrams, DA, Robin, AL, Pollack, IP, et al: The safety and efficacy of topical 1% ALO 2145 (p-aminoclonidine hydrochloride) in normal volunteers. Arch Ophthalmol 105:1205, 1987.

170. Jampel, HD, Robin, AL, Quigley, HA, Pollack, IP: Apraclonidine. A one-week dose-response study. Arch Ophthalmol 106:1069, 1988.

171. Abrams, DA, Robin, AL, Crandall, AS, et al: A limited comparison of apraclonidine's dose response in subjects with normal or increased intraocular pressure. Am J Ophthalmol 108:230, 1989.

172. Nagasubramanian, S, Hitchings, RA, Demailly, P, et al: Comparison of apraclonidine and timolol in chronic open-angle glaucoma. A three-month study. Ophthalmology 100:1318, 1993.

173. Koskela, T, Brubaker, RF: Apraclonidine and timolol. Combined effects in previously untreated normal subjects. Arch Ophthalmol 109:804, 1991.

174. King, MH, Richards, DW: Near syncope and chest tightness after administration of apraclonidine before argon laser iridotomy. Am J Ophthalmol 110:308, 1990.

175. Butler, P, Mannschreck, M, Lin, S, et al: Clinical experience with the long-term use of 1% apraclonidine. Arch Ophthalmol 113:293, 1995.

176. Wilkerson, M, Lewis, RA, Shields, MB: Follicular conjunctivitis associated with apraclonidine. Am J Ophthalmol 111:105, 1991.

177. Serdahl, CL, Galustian, J, Lewis, RA: The effects of apraclonidine on conjunctival oxygen tension. Arch Ophthalmol 107:1777, 1989.

178. Sugiyama, K, Kitazawa, Y, Kawai, K: Apraclonidine effects on ocular responses to YAG laser irradiation to the rabbit iris. Invest Ophthalmol Vis Sci 31:708, 1990.

179. Brown, RH, Stewart, RH, Lynch, MG, et al: ALO 2145 reduces the intraocular pressure elevation after anterior segment laser surgery. Ophthalmology 95:378, 1988.

180. Holmwood, PC, Chase, RD, Krupin, T, et al: Apraclonidine and argon laser trabeculoplasty. Am J Ophthalmol 114:19, 1992.

181. Krupin, T, Stank, T, Feitl, ME: Apraclonidine pretreatment decreases the acute intraocular pressure rise after laser trabeculoplasty or iridotomy. J Glau 1:79, 1992.

182. Kitazawa, Y, Taniguchi, T, Sugiyama, K: Use of apraclonidine to reduce acute intraocular pressure rise following Q-switched Nd:YAG laser iridotomy. Ophthalmic Surg 20:49, 1989.

183. Sridharrao, B, Badrinath, SS: Efficacy and safety of apraclonidine in patients undergoing anterior segment laser surgery. Br J Ophthalmol 73:884, 1989.

184. Pollack, IP, Brown, RH, Crandall, AS, et al: Prevention of the rise in intraocular pressure following neodymium-YAG posterior capsulotomy using topical 1% apraclonidine. Arch Ophthalmol 106:754, 1988.

185. Silverstone, DE, Brint, SF, Olander, KW, et al: Prophylactic use of apraclonidine for intraocular pressure increase after Nd:YAG capsulotomies. Am J Ophthalmol 113:401, 1992.

186. Cullom RD Jr, Schwartz, LW: The effect of apraclonidine on the intraocular pressure of glaucoma patients following Nd:YAG laser posterior capsulotomy. Ophthalmic Surg 24:623, 1993.

187. Krawitz, PL, Podos, SM: Use of apraclonidine in the treatment of acute angle closure glaucoma. Arch Ophthalmol 108:1208, 1990.

188. Araie, M, Ishi, K: Effects of apraclonidine on intraocular pressure and blood-aqueous barrier permeability after phacoemulsification and intraocular lens implantation. Am J Ophthalmol 116:67, 1993.

189. Robin, AL: Effect of topical apraclonidine on the frequency of intraocular pressure elevations after combined extracapsular cataract extraction and trabeculectomy. Ophthalmology 100:628, 1993.

190. Hill, RA, Minckler, DS, Lee, M, et al: Apraclonidine prophylaxis for postcycloplegic intraocular pressure spikes. Ophthalmology 98:1083, 1991.

191. Morrison, JC, Robin, AL: Adjunctive glaucoma therapy. A comparison of apraclonidine to dipivefrin when added to timolol maleate. Ophthalmology 96:3, 1989.

192. Yaldo, MK, Shin, DH, Parrow, KA, et al: Additive effect of 1% apraclonidine hydrochloride to nonselective β-blockers. Ophthalmology 98:1075, 1991.

193. Gharagozloo, NZ, Brubaker, RF: Effect of apraclonidine in long-term timolol users. Ophthalmology 98:1543, 1991.

194. Blasini, M, Shields, MB: Apraclonidine hydrochloride as an adjunct to timolol maleate therapy. J Glau 1:148, 1992.

195. Stewart, WC, Ritch, R, Shin, DH, et al: The efficacy of apraclonidine as an adjunct to timolol therapy. Arch Ophthalmol 113:287, 1995.

196. Lish, AJ, Camras, CB, Podos, SM: Effect of apraclonidine on intraocular pressure in glaucoma patients receiving maximally tolerated medications. J Glau 1:19, 1992.

197. Cardakli, UF, Smythe, BA, Eisele, JR, et al: Effect of chronic apraclonidine treatment on intraocular pressure in advanced glaucoma. J Glau 2:271, 1993.

198. Robin, AL, Ritch, R, Shin, DH, et al: Short-term efficacy of apraclonidine hydrochloride added to maximum-tolerated medical therapy for glaucoma. Am J Ophthalmol 120:423, 1995.

199. Nordlund, JR, Pasquale, LR, Robin, AL, et al: The cardiovascular, pulmonary, and ocular hypotensive effects of 0.2% brimonidine. Arch Ophthalmol 113:77, 1995.

200. Toris, CB, Gleason, ML, Camras, CB, Yablonski, ME: Effects of brimonidine on aqueous humor dynamics in human eyes. Arch Ophthalmol 113:1514, 1995.

201. Barnebey, HS, Robin, AL, Zimmerman, TJ, et al: The efficacy of brimonidine in decreasing elevations in intraocular pressure after laser trabeculoplasty. Ophthalmology 100:1083, 1993.

202. David, R, Spaeth, GL, Clevenger, CE, et al: Brimonidine in the prevention of intraocular pressure elevation following argon laser trabeculoplasty. Arch Ophthalmol 111:1387, 1993.

203. Vartiainen, J, MacDonald, E, Urtti, A, et al: Dexmedetomidine-induced ocular hypotension in rabbits with normal or elevated intraocular pressures. Invest Ophthalmol Vis Sci 33:2019, 1992.

204. Serle, JB, Steidl, S, Wang, R-F, et al: Selective α_2-adrenergic agonists B-HT 920 and UK14304–18. Effects on aqueous humor dynamics in monkeys. Arch Ophthalmol 109:1158, 1991.

205. Pollack, IP, Rossi, H: Norepinephrine in treatment of ocular hypertension and glaucoma. Arch Ophthalmol 93:173, 1975.

206. Pollack, IP: Effect of L-norepinephrine and adrenergic potentiators on the aqueous humor dynamics of man. Am J Ophthalmol 76:641, 1973.

207. Potter, DE, Rowland, JM: Adrenergic drugs and intraocular pressure: Effects of selective beta-adrenergic agonists. Exp Eye Res 27:615, 1978.

208. Waitzman, MB, Woods, WD, Cheek, WV: Effects of prostaglandins and norepinephrine on ocular pressure and pupil size in rabbits following bilateral cervical ganglionectomy. Invest Ophthalmol Vis Sci 18:52, 1979.

209. Colasanti, BK, Bárány, EH: Potentiation of the mydriatic effect of norepinephrine in the rabbit after monoamine oxidase inhibition. Invest Ophthalmol Vis Sci 18:200, 1979.

210. Kitazawa, Y: Topical adrenergic potentiators in primary open-angle glaucoma. Am J Ophthalmol 74:588, 1972.

211. Stewart, RH, Kimbrough, RL, Martin, PA, et al: Norepinephrine dipivalylate dose-response in ocular hypertensive subjects. Ann Ophthalmol 13:1279, 1981.

212. Duffin, RM, Christensen, RE, Bergamini, MVW: Suppression of adrenergic adaptation in the eye with a prostaglandin synthesis inhibitor. Invest Ophthalmol Vis Sci 21:756, 1981.

213. Zeller, EA, Shoch, D, Cooperman, SG, Schnipper, RI: Enzymology of the refractory media of the eye. IX. On the role of monoamine oxidase in the regulation of aqueous humor dynamics of the rabbit eye. Invest Ophthalmol 6:618, 1967.

214. Zeller, EA, Shoch, D, Czerner, TB, et al: Enzymology of the refractory media of the eye. X. Effects of topically administered bradykinin, amine releasers, and pargyline on aqueous humor dynamics. Invest Ophthalmol 10:274, 1971.

215. Bausher, LP: Identification of A and B forms of monoamine oxidase in the iris-ciliary body, superior cervical ganglion, and pineal gland of albino rabbits. Invest Ophthalmol 15:529, 1976.

216. Mehra, KS, Roy, PN, Singh, R: Pargyline drops in glaucoma. Arch Ophthalmol 92:453, 1974.

217. Ross, RA, Drance, SM: Effects of topically applied isoproterenol on aqueous dynamics in man. Arch Ophthalmol 83:39, 1970.

218. Seidehamel, RJ, Dungan, KW, Hickey, TE: Specific hypotensive and antihypertensive ocular effects of D-isoproterenol in rabbits. Am J Ophthalmol 79:1018, 1975.

219. Kass, MA, Reid, TW, Neufeld, AH, et al: The effect of D-isoproterenol on intraocular pressure of the rabbit, monkey, and man. Invest Ophthalmol 15:113, 1976.

220. Brubaker, RF, Gaasterland, D: The effect of isoproterenol on aqueous humor formation in humans. Invest Ophthalmol Vis Sci 25:357, 1984.

221. Caprioli, J, Sears, M, Bausher, L, et al: Forskolin lowers intraocular pressure by reducing aqueous inflow. Invest Ophthalmol Vis Sci 25:268, 1984.

222. Jumblatt, JE, North, GT: Potentiation of sympathetic neurosecretion by forskolin and cyclic AMP in the rabbit iris-ciliary body. Curr Eye Res 5:495, 1986.

223. Lee, P-Y, Podos, SM, Mittag, T, Severin, C: Effect of topically applied forskolin on aqueous humor dynamics in cynomolgus monkey. Invest Ophthalmol Vis Sci 25:1206, 1984.

224. Badian, M, Dabrowski, J, Grigoleit, H-G, et al: Effect of forskolin-eyedrops on the intraocular pressure of healthy male subjects. Klin Monatsbl Augenheilkd 185:522, 1984.

225. Caprioli, J, Sears, M: Combined effect of forskolin and acetazolamide on intraocular pressure and aqueous flow in rabbit eyes. Exp Eye Res 39:47, 1984.

226. Burstein, NL, Sears, ML, Mead, A: Aqueous flow in human eyes is reduced by forskolin, a potent adenylate cyclase activator. Exp Eye Res 39:745, 1984.

227. Bartels, SP, Lee, SR, Neufeld, AH: The effects of forskolin on cyclic AMP, intraocular pressure and aqueous humor formation in rabbits. Curr Eye Res 6:307, 1987.

228. Brubaker, RF, Carlson, KH, Kullerstrand, LJ, McLaren, JW: Topical forskolin (Colforsin) and aqueous flow in humans. Arch Ophthalmol 105:637, 1987.

229. Shibata, T, Mishima, H, Kurokawa, T: Ocular pigmentation and intraocular pressure response to forskolin. Curr Eye Res 7:667, 1988.

230. Gregory, D, Sears, M, Bausher, L, et al: Intraocular pressure and aqueous flow are decreased by cholera toxin. Invest Ophthalmol Vis Sci 20:371, 1981.

231. Bartels, SP, Roth, HO, Neufeld, AH: Effects of intravitreal cholera toxin on adenosine 3', 5'-monophosphate, intraocular pressure, and outflow facility in rabbits. Invest Ophthalmol Vis Sci 20:410, 1981.

232. Mishima, H, Sears, M, Bausher, L, Gregory, D: Ultracytochemistry of cholera-toxin binding sites in ciliary processes. Cell Tissue Res 223:241, 1982.

233. Mishima, H, Bausher, L, Sears, M, et al: Fine structural studies of ciliary processes after treatment with cholera toxin or its B subunit. Graefes Arch Clin Exp Ophthalmol 219:272, 1982.

234. Bonomi, L, Perfetti, S, Bellucci, R, Massa, F: Effects of terbutaline on experimentally induced ocular hypertension in the rabbit. Glaucoma 4:134, 1982.

235. Bonomi, L, Perfetti, S, Bellucci, R, et al: Prevention by diclofenac of the subsensitivity to the IOP-lowering effect of terbutaline. Glaucoma 6:241, 1984.

236. Bonomi, L, Perfetti, S, Bellucci, R, et al: Intraocular pressure lowering effect of ibuterol in the rabbit. Glaucoma 6:216, 1984.

237. Coakes, RL, Siah, PB: Effects of adrenergic drugs on aqueous humour dynamics in the normal human eye. I. Salbutamol. Br J Ophthalmol 68:393, 1984.

238. Mittag, TW, Tormay, A, Messenger, M, Podos, SM: Ocular hypotension in the rabbit. Receptor mechanisms of pirbuterol and nylidrin. Invest Ophthalmol Vis Sci 26:163, 1985.

239. Krupin, T, Becker, B, Podos, SM: Topical vanadate lowers intraocular pressure in rabbits. Invest Ophthalmol Vis Sci 19:1360, 1980.

240. Podos, SM, Lee, P-Y, Severin, C, Mittag, T: The effect of vanadate on aqueous humor dynamics in cynomolgus monkeys. Invest Ophthalmol Vis Sci 25:359, 1984.

241. Becker, B: Vanadate and aqueous humor dynamics. Invest Ophthalmol Vis Sci 19:1156, 1980.

242. Mittag, TW, Serle, JB, Podos, SM, et al: Vanadate effects on ocular pressure, (Na^+K^+) ATPase and adenylate cyclase in rabbit eyes. Invest Ophthalmol Vis Sci 25:1335, 1984.

243. Sobel, L, Serle, JB, Podos, SM, et al: Topical nylidrin and aqueous humor dynamics in rabbits and monkeys. Arch Ophthalmol 101:1281, 1983.

Chapter 27

ADRENERGIC INHIBITORS

β-ADRENERGIC INHIBITORS

Early Experience

β-Adrenergic inhibitors or antagonists, or "β-blockers" as they are commonly called, are the most frequently used class of drugs for the treatment of glaucoma. The first commercially available β-blocker was *propranolol,* which was introduced in 1967 for the treatment of cardiac arrhythmias, angina pectoris, and systemic hypertension. The drug was also found to reduce intraocular pressure (IOP) when given orally (1–5), topically (6, 7), or intravenously (8).

Early experience with β-adrenergic antagonists, however, revealed adverse reactions that limited the usefulness of many of these compounds as topical antiglaucoma agents. Propranolol, as well as several other β-blockers, were found to cause corneal anesthesia, due to membrane stabilizing activity (6), and to reduce tear production (9). The latter side effect was a particular problem with *practolol,* another systemic β-blocking agent, which caused a severe dry eye syndrome in some patients, possibly through an immunologic mechanism (10). The practolol response was occasionally associated with subconjunctival fibrosis, corneal ulcers, and a skin rash (10–12). Other β-blockers were found to have carcinogenicity in test animals (13).

Timolol

Timolol maleate is a nonselective, β_1- and β_2-adrenergic antagonist. It was found in preliminary trials to have none of the adverse reactions described above for some β-blockers (14, 15).

Efficacy Studies

Rabbit studies revealed an IOP lowering effect in both the treated (16, 17) and the fellow untreated eye (17). Single doses in human volunteers effectively lowered the IOP in normotensive individuals (14), as well as patients with chronic open-angle glaucoma (18, 19), and a small hypotensive effect was again noted in the fellow, untreated eye (20). Short-term, multiple-dose trials with open-angle glaucoma patients demonstrated a sustained reduction in IOP (21–24).

Comparative studies showed the IOP lowering efficacy of timolol to be greater than that of epinephrine (22, 25) and equal to or slightly weaker than various concentrations of combined epinephrine and guanethidine (26). When compared with pilocarpine, timolol had an equivalent or slightly greater IOP lowering effect (27–31). In a more recent study, timolol twice daily was compared with pilocarpine four times daily with advancing doses, as required,

413

of 0.25–0.5% and 2–4%, respectively (32). The study included 189 chronic open-angle glaucoma patients who were followed for 2 years with automated visual fields every 4 months. More patients receiving pilocarpine discontinued the study because of inadequate IOP control, and patients receiving pilocarpine had significantly greater visual field deterioration. In another comparative study, echothiophate iodide was preferred over timolol in the treatment of glaucoma in aphakia (33).

Mechanisms of Action

Tonographic (34, 35) and fluorophotometric (36–38) studies in humans, as well as research with cats (39) and monkeys (40, 41), all indicate that timolol lowers the IOP primarily, if not exclusively, by reducing aqueous humor production. This effect is not seen in sleeping human subjects, during which time the aqueous flow is normally less than half the daytime flow rate (38, 42). The carbonic anhydrase inhibitor, acetazolamide, does lower aqueous flow in sleeping humans (42). The reason for this difference is not clear, although it appears that different mechanisms mediate the effects of sleep, timolol, and acetazolamide on aqueous production. The absence of endogenous epinephrine in patients with bilateral adrenalectomies does not influence the circadian rhythm of aqueous flow nor the daytime effect of timolol on the flow (43), while timolol does lower aqueous flow at night in humans receiving systemic epinephrine (44). Primate studies have demonstrated a topical timolol effect on aqueous flow in the fellow, untreated eye, the degree of which is dose-related (41).

The influence of timolol on inflow presumably represents a direct action on the ciliary processes, either on the nonpigmented epithelium to decrease secretion or on local capillary perfusion to reduce ultrafiltration (45, 46). The possibility of a direct action by β-adrenergic agents on the formation of aqueous humor is supported by the identification of β-adrenergic receptors (47), predominantly of the β_2 subtype (48–52), in both animal (47, 49–51) and human (48, 52) ciliary processes.

To explain the mechanism by which an adrenergic antagonist might reduce aqueous production, it is necessary to postulate a physiologic, sympathetic "resting tone" in the ciliary process receptors that are associated with the formation of aqueous humor (45, 46). Animal studies have supported the concept that adrenergic innervation participates in the IOP lowering action of timolol (53), although this was not substantiated in a human study in which sympathetic denervation from postganglionic Horner's syndrome effected neither flow nor pressure (54). The possibility that tone could arise from catecholamines brought to the tissue by the circulation was not supported by the previously cited study in which the absence of adrenally derived epinephrine did not influence aqueous flow (43).

The influence of timolol on aqueous humor formation may be related to inhibition of catecholamine-stimulated synthesis of cyclic AMP, which has been demonstrated in rabbit studies (55). Although the duration of this effect is shorter than that of the IOP reduction, it may be that pigment binding of the drug provides a slow-release depot, which helps maintain the concentration of timolol for a prolonged effect (56).

It does not appear that timolol significantly influences the blood-aqueous barrier. Simultaneous bilateral fluorescein angiography of the iris revealed no effect of timolol on dye leakage (57). Topical application of timolol is associated with a significant increase in aqueous humor protein (58), although the normal ratio of albumin to IgG (59) and of the different molecular weight classes of protein (60) are not altered, suggesting that this finding is a result of reduced aqueous humor flow and not a change in permeability of the blood-aqueous barrier. It also appears that the timolol mechanism is not prostaglandin-mediated, since it is not altered by concurrent therapy with either indomethacin (61) or flurbiprofen (62).

There is some evidence that timolol may reduce aqueous humor formation by a mechanism other than β-adrenergic blockade. In a study with rabbit eyes, there was a suggestion that timolol might act as a dopaminergic antagonist to lower blood flow to the ciliary body (63). However, metoclopramide, a dopamine-2 antagonist, did not affect the ocular hypotensive action of timolol in normal human volunteers (64).

Most studies indicate that timolol has little, if any, influence on outflow facility (34, 35). A theoretic explanation for this is that, unlike the system related to aqueous inflow, there may be no sympathetic resting tone associated with aqueous outflow. This assumption may not be entirely correct, however, since topical timolol was associated with a small myopic shift in one human study, suggesting that sympathetic innervation is involved in the resting tone of the ciliary muscle (65). In addition, some tonographic studies have shown a small increase in outflow (66), and β-adrenergic receptors, primarily of the β_2 subtype, have been demonstrated in human trabecular meshwork (67, 68). A histologic study of the outflow apparatus in human eyes, treated with timolol before enucleation for malignant melanoma, revealed no morphologic changes suggestive of a pressure lowering action by the drug (69). However, the trabecular meshwork in primates after long-term timolol therapy revealed degeneration of the trabecular cells, partial destruction of the beams, rarefaction of the meshwork, and disconnection of the trabecular lamellae from the ciliary muscle fibers (70).

Administration

CONCENTRATIONS. Timolol maleate is commercially available in 0.25% and 0.5% concentrations (Table 27.1). Recently, timolol hemihydrate became available in 0.25% and 0.5% concentrations. Early experience with chronic open-angle glaucoma patients indicated that the maximum IOP lowering effect of timolol maleate is achieved with the 0.5% concentration (14, 18). In other studies, however, the

Table 27.1.
COMMERCIAL TOPICAL β-BLOCKERS

Generic Preparations	*Brand Names*	*Concentrations (%)*
Timolol maleate*	Timoptic	0.25, 0.5
	Timoptic XE	0.25, 0.5
Timolol hemi-hydrate*	Betimol	0.25, 0.5
Betaxolol HCl	Betoptic	0.5
	Betoptic S**	0.25
Levobunolol HCl*	Betagan	0.25, 0.5
	AkBeta	0.25, 0.5
Carteolol HCl	Ocupress	1.0
Metipranolol HCl	OptiPranolol	0.3

*Other generic products may be available for timolol and levobunolol.

**Suspension.

0.25% concentration was equally or more efficacious than the 0.5%, although the latter provided a somewhat longer duration of action (71, 72). One investigation revealed that adequate IOP control could be achieved in over half the patients with 0.1% timolol (73), and another showed that even a 0.008% concentration had a definite but minimal ocular hypotensive effect (74). Dose-response studies of aqueous humor formation in primates showed that a dose of timolol as small as 2.5 μg can suppress aqueous flow by a statistically significant 20%, suggesting that standard clinical doses may be excessive (75). Nevertheless, individuals with darker irides appear to require higher concentrations of timolol (76). In one study, timolol had a significant ocular hypotensive effect 1 hour after instillation in patients with blue irides, but no effect in brown-eyed patients, which probably relates to early pigment binding (77).

FREQUENCY OF ADMINISTRATION. Good corneal penetration of timolol has been demonstrated in rabbit (78) and human (79, 80) eyes, with peak aqueous humor concentrations in human eyes occurring within 1–2 hours. The IOP-lowering effect peaks approximately 2 hours after administration (14, 18) and lasts for at least 24 hours (19). The optimum frequency of administration in most cases is twice daily, although once-a-day treatment has been shown to be adequate in many cases (81, 82). One study found no significant difference whether timolol 0.5% was given in the morning or evening (83), while another study suggested that instillation at 12 PM may optimize the ratio of ocular to systemic absorption (84). Timolol in a gel vehicle was found to elicit a 1–2 mm Hg greater efficacy than the solution during 24 hours after instillation (85). When timolol is discontinued following long-term therapy, aqueous flow does not increase significantly until the fourth day and the IOP effect may still be seen 14 days later (86). This may be due, at least in part, to concentration of the drug in melanotic tissues, with slow

release. In rabbits receiving topical timolol for 42 days, the drug was still present in pigmented ocular tissues 42 days after withdrawal of the drug (87).

Long-term Efficacy

Numerous long-term studies have confirmed the continued efficacy of chronic timolol therapy for many patients (88–95). In a significant number of cases, however, the pressure responsiveness to timolol will decrease with continued administration. This occurs in two phases, which Boger (96) called the "short-term 'escape' and long-term 'drift.'"

SHORT-TERM "ESCAPE". Many patients will experience a dramatic reduction in IOP with the initiation of timolol therapy. However, the pressure nearly always rises during the next few days to finally plateau at a maintenance level (27, 97–99). The 1-hour IOP response to timolol does not predict which patients will have a significant loss of responsiveness 3–4 weeks later (99). It has been demonstrated that the number of β-receptors in ocular tissues increases during the first few days of timolol therapy (100), which may explain this "escape" phenomenon. In any case, it is good clinical practice to wait approximately 1 month after initiating timolol to determine the efficacy of therapy.

LONG-TERM "DRIFT". Once the IOP has leveled off following the initiation of timolol therapy, control will be maintained in most cases. Some patients, however, will have a slow decline in pressure response to timolol, usually beginning 3 months to a year after starting treatment (66, 88–95). Fluorophotometric studies indicate that aqueous flow is higher in most patients following 1 year of timolol therapy as compared to the value 1 week after initiating treatment (101). Some patients will regain responsiveness to timolol after a "washout" period. In one study of 39 eyes showing a long-term drift with timolol 0.5%, 23 eyes received dipivefrin (a prodrug of epinephrine) during a 30- or 60-day "timolol holiday," and the remainder received artificial tears in place of the timolol (102). When the timolol was reinstituted, the dipivefrin-treated group had a mean IOP decrease of 8.2 mm Hg, compared to 3.9 in the nondipivefrin-treated group, and the response to timolol was more prolonged in eyes treated for 60 days with dipivefrin. Based on this observation, a treatment strategy of "pulsatile therapy," in which timolol 0.5% is given for 6 months, alternating with dipivefrin for 2 months, was studied and shown to minimize long-term drift as compared to continuous use of timolol (103).

Drug Interactions

Long-term, multiple-drug studies have shown that timolol will cause additional lowering of IOP in many cases when added to maximum tolerable antiglaucoma therapy (104–106). However, when instituting combination or multiple drug therapy, the possibility of changes in ocular and systemic absorption must be considered. In a rabbit study, adding pilocarpine or epinephrine to timolol reduced the intraocular timolol concentrations, while epinephrine also reduced the systemic absorption of timolol by about 50% (107).

In clinical practice, the combined effect of timolol and a *miotic* (108–111) is, for most patients, significantly greater than the effect of either medication alone, although less than the arithmetic sum of the effects of the individual drugs. As discussed in Chapter 25, a *combined timolol 0.5% and pilocarpine 2–4% (TP2 and TP4)* formulation, administered twice daily, provides IOP reduction that is equivalent to timolol and pilocarpine when given separately two and three times daily, respectively (112). The effect of the fixed combination is significantly greater than either drug given alone (113–117), and aqueous levels in rabbits are the same with the combined or separate administration (118). One study showed no difference in the efficacy of TP2 and TP4 (116), while another revealed that some patients, uncontrolled on TP2, may receive additional IOP reduction with the higher concentration (119).

The combination of timolol and an *epinephrine* compound has less clinical value. This subject was reviewed in the previous chapter, with the conclusion that, while a statistically significant additional pressure reduction may occur when one drug is added to the other (120), the amount of this reduction is usually very small, with considerable variation from one patient to the next (121, 122). Therefore, the efficacy in each individual case must be confirmed by a uniocular therapeutic trial before chronic therapy with this combination of drugs is prescribed. Combined therapy with timolol and an epinephrine-guanethidine formulation was shown to have greater IOP-lowering efficacy than the epinephrine-guanethidine combination or timolol alone (123).

As noted in Chapter 26, the α_2-adrenergic agonist *apraclonidine* appears to have a somewhat better additional effect when added to timolol than is the case with epinephrine or its derivatives. The oral *carbonic anhydrase inhibitors* have been shown to be especially effective as a second drug with timolol (108, 110, 124–127), and early experience suggests that this is also true for the topical agent *dorzolamide*. In addition, the topical prostaglandin *latanoprost* appears to be effective in conjunction with timolol therapy. The latter two combinations are discussed in the next two chapters.

Another important clinical question is the efficacy and safety of combined topical timolol and *oral β-blockers*. In general, topical timolol will produce additional IOP reduction, without altering pulse or blood pressure, in patients pretreated with oral timolol (128, 129), propranolol (130), alprenolol (131), or metoprolol (131), although the IOP-lowering efficacy of topical β-blockers appears to diminish with increasing dosages of the oral β-blocker (130, 131).

Side Effects

As previously noted, early clinical experience suggested that adverse ocular and systemic reactions are unusually low

with topical timolol therapy. Specifically, the drug does not affect the pupillary size (132) nor accommodation, and rarely causes burning or conjunctival hyperemia. However, continued experience has disclosed side effects, some of which can have serious consequences.

OCULAR TOXICITY. Ocular toxicity is uncommon with timolol therapy, although allergic and toxic reactions have been reported. Ocular cicatricial pemphigoid has been reported in patients receiving topical timolol (133, 134). In most of these cases, the patient was also receiving additional glaucoma medications, although a small number were being treated with timolol alone when the pemphigoid was diagnosed. Burning and conjunctival hyperemia may occasionally occur and are frequently associated with superficial punctate keratopathy and corneal anesthesia (135–139). Timolol does not affect corneal sensation in most patients, although a small subgroup may have markedly diminished corneal sensitivity (138, 139). Chronic therapy with timolol has been shown to damage the ocular surface, especially the mucus layer of the tear film (140). Corneal epithelial erosions were reported in two patients wearing gas permeable contact lenses soon after starting topical timolol therapy, and the combination of timolol and a contact lens in rabbits caused marked alterations in corneal epithelium and endothelium (141).

Some animal studies have suggested that topical timolol inhibits corneal epithelial wound healing (142, 143), although another study of timolol and several other β-blockers in a rabbit model, suggest that β-blockers have no deleterious effect on corneal epithelial wound healing and may actually accelerate wound closure (144). Eight patients were described in which the combination of epithelial defects and topical steroid and β-blocker therapy led to a precipitation of calcium phosphate deposits in the superficial stroma (145). One rabbit study showed ultrastructural corneal endothelial changes following topical timolol therapy for 1 month (143), although most human and animal investigations have revealed no toxicity of topical timolol therapy to the corneal endothelium (146–148). Tissue culture studies with human Tenon's fibroblasts suggests that β-blockers do not stimulate cell proliferation directly, but may do so by chronic inflammation from the irritating effects of the antiglaucoma medications and/or their preservatives (149). This may have implications regarding the success of glaucoma filtering surgery.

Tear production may be reduced in some cases, although this is usually of no consequence unless the patient has low baseline tear flow (150–154). Reduced central visual acuity has been noted in some patients on timolol therapy (135–137). In some cases this may be due to a change in the refractive error or the pupillary diameter associated with discontinuation of miotic therapy, while the cause in other patients is not clear.

A potentially serious ocular effect that has been the focus of considerable investigation is the influence of β-blockers on ocular blood flow. If the drug reduces vascular perfusion of the optic nerve head, this may cancel the benefit of reduced IOP. The preliminary results, however, have been conflicting, which may relate to the different study techniques and the uncertainty of what they are actually measuring. A rabbit study using injected microspheres indicated that both nonselective and cardioselective β-blockers decrease ocular blood flow (155). However, high-resolution Doppler ultrasonography suggested that timolol improves flow velocity of the central retinal artery in normal and diabetic individuals (156, 157), while other studies suggest that timolol has no significant effect on either the choroidal vasculature in normal subjects (158) or retinal hemodynamics in normal-tension glaucoma patients (159).

SYSTEMIC TOXICITY. Systemic toxicity has been reported more often than ocular reactions and constitutes the more significant adverse effects of topical timolol therapy.

IMPROVING THE THERAPEUTIC INDEX. Measurable plasma levels of timolol are present within 8 minutes or less of topical application (160), and punctal occlusion after instillation of the drug, as described in Chapter 24, collapses the dose-response curve and extends the duration of action (161), while significantly reducing plasma timolol levels (162), which may help to minimize the systemic side effects. Coadministration with phenylephrine and the use of a viscous vehicle have also been shown to improve the eye:plasma peak timolol concentrations (163, 164). As mentioned earlier, instillation at 12 PM was shown to optimize the ratio of ocular to systemic absorption, possibly relating to the circadian rhythm of drug absorption into the eye and bloodstream (84).

CARDIOVASCULAR. Blockade of β_1 adrenergic receptors slows the pulse rate and weakens myocardial contractility. In most healthy patients, these effects are of no consequence. However, a potential for serious complications exists in patients with preexisting conditions such as sinus bradycardia, greater than first-degree heart block, and congestive heart failure. Topical timolol therapy has been associated with severe bradycardia, arrhythmias, heart failure, and syncope (135–137, 165–167).

Even healthy individuals may be at risk under certain circumstances, such as the stress of surgery (168) or heavy exercise (169, 170). In the latter situation, timolol has been shown to affect maximal heart rate and time to exhaustion (169, 170). The induced bradycardia may also be more pronounced when timolol is used concomitantly with other drugs, such as quinidine (171) or the calcium antagonist, verapamil (172).

RESPIRATORY. Blockade of β_2-adrenergic receptors produces contraction of bronchial smooth muscle, which may cause bronchospasm and airway obstruction, especially in asthmatics (135, 137, 165, 167, 173–176) or any patient with bronchospasm requiring xanthines or inhaled steroids (177). Thirteen cases of death in status asthmaticus following initiation of timolol therapy had been reported to the National

Registry of Drug-Induced Ocular Side Effects by 1984 (176). Dyspnea (165, 178) and apneic spells (179) have also been reported. These may be more common in young children, and caution must be taken by nursing mothers, since high levels of timolol were found in the milk of a mother receiving topical timolol (180).

CENTRAL NERVOUS SYSTEM. Central nervous system effects may be the most common class of systemic reactions to timolol therapy and include depression, anxiety, confusion, dysarthria, hallucinations, lightheadedness, drowsiness, weakness, fatigue, tranquilization, dissociative behavior, disorientation, and emotional lability (135–137, 165, 181). However, one study of patients receiving oral β-blockers did not find a correlation with depression after correcting for confounding variables (182).

CHOLESTEROL LEVELS. Oral β-blockers are known to adversely alter plasma lipid profiles, and 0.5% topical timolol twice daily for 2 months, without nasolacrimal occlusion, has been shown to decrease plasma high-density lipoprotein (HDL) cholesterol levels of a magnitude that has been estimated to increase the risk of coronary artery disease by 21% (183). Another study found no significant adverse effects of topical timolol on serum lipoprotein levels (184), although the sample size was small in a heterogenous patient population with no controls. The issue of β-blockers on cholesterol is considered further in this chapter under the discussion of *carteolol.*

OTHER SYSTEMIC REACTIONS. Other systemic reactions that have been reported in association with timolol therapy include gastrointestinal distress (nausea, diarrhea, and cramping) (135, 137, 165), dermatologic disorders (maculopapular rash, alopecia, and hives) (137, 165, 185), and sexual impotence (135, 136). Since these observations were made in a predominantly elderly population, it is difficult to confirm a cause-and-effect relationship in all cases. Of greater concern with timolol therapy, however, is the exacerbation of myasthenia gravis (186, 187) and the altered response to hypoglycemic episodes in diabetic patients, which may mask the awareness of the attack (188).

Clinical Indications

Although timolol was originally evaluated and approved for the treatment of chronic open-angle glaucoma, it has subsequently been found to lower the IOP in essentially all forms of glaucoma (189, 190). Since it lowers the IOP by reducing aqueous production and does not alter the pupil, it is helpful in situations in which conventional aqueous outflow cannot be improved medically and in which miosis or mydriasis are not desirable. Timolol is reported to help control glaucoma in aphakia during the early postoperative period (191–194) as well as in chronic cases (66, 190, 195). The drug has also been found to control angle-closure glaucoma after penetrating keratoplasty (196), and following an iridectomy for angle-closure glaucoma when the pressure elevation persisted postoperatively (197).

Timolol therapy in children is not always successful, but is often useful. The incidence of side effects in the pediatric group are similar to those in the adult population, although experience with the very young is still limited and extreme caution must be exercised (198–201).

Another possible indication that has been evaluated for timolol is IOP reduction in ocular hypertensives to prevent the development of glaucomatous damage. In one study, timolol therapy was found to be significantly protective against visual field and optic nerve head damage (202), while another study showed that timolol lowered the IOP approximately 5 mm Hg below that of an untreated control group, but did not alter the pressure curve over time (203) nor the differential light sensitivity in tested meridia (204).

Betaxolol

The foregoing discussion regarding the mechanisms, side effects, and clinical indications of timolol generally applies to the other topical β-blockers that are used in the management of glaucoma. There are, however, some notable exceptions, which are considered in the remainder of this chapter. The most striking differences are seen between the nonselective and cardioselective β-blockers.

Betaxolol hydrochloride is a cardioselective, $β_1$-adrenergic antagonist. While its action appears to be predominantly on the $β_1$-receptors, receptor occupancy studies of human aqueous from betaxolol-treated eyes suggest a role of $β_2$-receptor blockade (205). In any case, the mechanism of ocular hypotension appears to be the same as that for timolol, with reduction of aqueous humor production, but no effect on outflow resistance or pupillary diameter (206).

Efficacy

In preliminary clinical trials, betaxolol provided a significant reduction in IOP when evaluated alone (207) or in comparison with a placebo (208–210). When compared with timolol at 0.25% and 0.5% concentrations, the magnitude of IOP reduction in most studies is slightly less with betaxolol, and there may be a greater need for adjunctive therapy than with timolol (211–214). In one study of 153 glaucoma patients who were controlled on timolol, the half who were switched to betaxolol, in a masked and random fashion, had a significant increase in IOP (215). However, when betaxolol 0.5% and timolol 0.5%, both given twice daily, were compared in long-term, parallel trials of 18–30 months in open-angle glaucoma patients, the timolol group had better IOP levels, but the betaxolol group had a more favorable course regarding retinal sensitivity as measured by static automated perimetry (216–218). The possible explanation for this is discussed later under side effects. In a 3-month comparative trial of betaxolol 0.5% and dipivefrin 0.1%, IOP reductions were similar, with mean decreases of 4.1 mm Hg and 3.5 mm Hg, respectively (219).

Drug Interactions

As with other β-blockers, betaxolol usually provides significant additional IOP reduction when added to miotic or carbonic anhydrase inhibitor therapy (220). The interaction with epinephrine compounds, however, may differ somewhat from that of timolol and other nonselective β-blockers. In both monkey (221) and human (222) studies, adding epinephrine to established betaxolol therapy was associated with a significant additional lowering of IOP and a significant increase in the outflow facility, which was not seen when adding epinephrine to timolol-treated eyes. In addition, adding betaxolol in open-angle glaucoma patients already on dipivefrin therapy resulted in a mean additional IOP reduction of 3.6 mm Hg at 4 weeks (223). The additive effect of epinephrine compounds when used in conjunction with betaxolol may represent a $β_2$ effect on outflow, which is blocked by nonselective β-blockers, but less so by cardioselective $β_1$-antagonists. However, since the nonselective β-blockers have a greater IOP lowering effect than betaxolol, when either is used alone, the net effect of combined therapy with epinephrine and either a nonselective or cardioselective β-blocker is often the same.

Side Effects

OCULAR. Betaxolol is similar to the other topical β-blockers in having a low incidence of ocular side effects, although the original formulation with a 0.5% concentration caused more burning with instillation than the other commercial β-blockers (211). However, a newer ophthalmic delivery vehicle with 0.25% betaxolol, formulated as a suspension, has the same IOP-lowering efficacy as the 0.5% preparation with significantly less discomfort (224). As with other β-blockers, betaxolol may reduce corneal sensitivity in a small number of patients (139). One case of aphakic cystoid macular edema has been reported associated with betaxolol therapy (225), and three cases have been described of periocular cutaneous pigmentary changes, which returned to normal after discontinuation of topical betaxolol (226).

SYSTEMIC. With regard to adverse systemic reactions, the primary advantage of betaxolol over timolol is the absent or reduced $β_2$-adrenergic inhibition, which minimizes the risk of respiratory side effects. The drug does not cause a decrease in airflow in most patients with proven airway disease (227–231), although exceptions to this have been reported (231–234), and caution must still be exercised in these patients. While oral administration of the $β_1$-blocker has been reported to significantly inhibit exercise tachycardia (235), this is less common with topical betaxolol therapy (236, 237), and may be less than with topical timolol (236). Cardiovascular side effects have been reported with topical betaxolol therapy, including arrhythmia (232), bradycardia (232), sinus arrest (238), and decompensation of congestive heart failure (239), although these reactions, again, may be less than with nonselective β-blockers. With regard to central nervous system side effects, there may also be less of a risk for this with betaxolol than with timolol therapy (240), although such complications have been reported in association with betaxolol therapy (241).

The reduction in β_1-related systemic side effects, and possibly the apparently better protection of visual function with topical betaxolol as compared to nonselective β-blockers, may relate to the difference in aqueous and plasma concentrations between the two classes of drugs. When betaxolol 0.5% or timolol 0.25% were given prior to cataract surgery, the plasma concentrations of betaxolol were lower than those of timolol, while the aqueous levels were twice as high for betaxolol as for timolol (242). In a similar study design, β_1-receptor and β_2-receptor occupancy by aqueous samples was absent 65% and 80%, respectively, for timolol, compared to less than 20% and negligible, respectively, for betaxolol (243). In another study, timolol and carteolol (also a nonselective β-blocker) blocked both the β_1 and β_2 effects of isoproterenol, while betaxolol had minimal influence on either receptor effect (244). The latter investigators suggest that the low rate of systemic diffusion with betaxolol may relate to the high lipophilic and protein-binding properties, which favor a high level of local diffusion and a fixation to lacrimal proteins before the drug reaches the general circulation, where it binds to plasma proteins, leaving only a small amount to circulate freely (244).

Whatever the explanation for the difference in systemic levels of nonselective and cardioselective β-blockers proves to be, one of the effects may be an influence on blood flow. Neither timolol nor betaxolol lowered peripheral blood flow as determined by laser-Doppler measurements at a fingertip, but betaxolol caused a significant increase in flow as compared to no treatment (245). In a study of normal-tension glaucoma patients, color Doppler imaging of orbital vessels showed an increase in end-diastolic velocity and a decrease in resistance index with betaxolol, but not with timolol (246). However, when the two drugs were evaluated in rabbits with an intraluminal microvascular corrosion casting technique, neither produced an observable vasomotor effect (247). Whether β-blockers do significantly influence ocular blood flow, and whether there is a significant difference between nonselective and cardioselective agents, and whether this difference explains the relative effects of timolol and betaxolol on visual function (if that observation is, in fact, real) are important questions, the answers of which await further study.

Clinical Indications

Betaxolol is clearly the β-blocker of choice in patients with asthma or other bronchospastic pulmonary disorders, although even it must be used with caution in those patients. Because it also appears to have a reduction in other systemic side effects, as compared to nonselective β-blockers, it is a reasonable first choice when initiating β-blocker therapy in most patients. However, because it also has slightly less oc-

ular hypotensive effect than the nonselective agents, it may be reasonable to switch to one of the latter drugs, if betaxolol does not provide adequate IOP control.

Levobunolol

Levobunolol (L-bunolol) is an analog of propranolol with potent nonselective β_1- and β_2-adrenergic antagonism. It presumably has the same mechanism of IOP reduction as timolol, although one tonographic study suggested that it may also increase aqueous outflow (248). In preliminary short-term studies, the onset of an ocular hypotensive effect occurred within the first hour after instillation, peaked at 3 hours, and lasted up to 24 hours (249). Concentrations of 0.3% and 0.6% levobunolol provided significant IOP reductions up to 4 hours, while the effect of 1% and 2% concentrations persisted at 12 hours (250). However, in a 3-month comparison with the vehicle, 0.5% and 1% concentrations of levobunolol produced similar average pressure reductions (251). Levobunolol is commercially available in original and generic preparations in concentrations of 0.25% and 0.5% (Table 27.1).

In comparative short-term and long-term clinical studies, levobunolol in various concentrations was equivalent to timolol with regard to ocular hypotensive efficacy and side effects when the two drugs were administered twice daily (249, 252–261). It was also shown to be equivalent to the nonselective β-blocker metipranolol (262), but had significantly greater pressure-lowering efficacy than betaxolol in a 3-month study (263).

Levobunolol is effective with once-daily administration in a high percentage of patients (264), with once-daily instillation of the 0.5% concentration providing similar IOP control to twice-daily use of the same drug (265), and the 0.25% concentration given once-daily providing adequate control in many cases (266). When compared in 0.5% concentrations, once-daily levobunolol or timolol provided IOP control in 72% and 64% of patients, respectively (267). In a comparison of 0.25% concentrations of levobunolol and timolol given once daily, however, the overall mean decrease in IOP was the same (268). In commercial bottles, a drop of the original levobunolol is significantly larger than that of timolol, which appears to be due to both the dispensing system and the increased viscosity of levobunolol (269). However, the drop size does not appear to influence the efficacy or safety of the drug (270).

Levobunolol has been found to be effective in controlling the early postoperative IOP rise following extracapsular cataract extraction (271, 272), and laser posterior capsulotomy (272). It has also been shown to provide additional IOP reduction when added to dipivefrin, with efficacy and safety comparable to concomitant timolol and dipivefrin therapy (273).

As with other β-blockers, levobunolol lowers the pulse rate at rest and during exercise, as compared to a placebo (274).

When compared with betaxolol, there was no significant difference in pulse or blood pressure at rest, but levobunolol was associated with significantly lower values during exercise (275). With regard to ocular blood flow, neither levobunolol, betaxolol, nor carteolol influenced perimacular hemodynamics as determined by blue field entoptic simulation in normal volunteers, which the authors felt suggests normal autoregulation (276). In a placebo-controlled study, levobunolol caused increased ocular pulsatile flow in normal and glaucomatous eyes, the implication of which is unclear (277).

Since levobunolol is equivalent to timolol with regard to IOP-lowering efficacy and safety, the clinical indications are essentially the same as those noted previously for timolol.

Carteolol

Carteolol is a nonselective β-adrenergic antagonist with *intrinsic sympathomimetic activity*. The latter feature produces an early, transient adrenergic agonist response that is not found in the other commercially available topical β-blockers. Studies with systemic β-blockers indicate that intrinsic sympathomimetic activity does not interfere with the therapeutic benefits of β-blockers (278), and it was anticipated that this activity in carteolol might partially protect against the adverse reactions of β-adrenergic-stimulation.

In a vehicle-controlled trial, carteolol 1% and 2% produced mean IOP reductions of 23% and 26%, respectively (279). When compared with timolol, the ocular hypotensive efficacy and duration of action were comparable in most studies (280–284), although one trial showed that timolol 0.5% caused a significantly greater reduction in IOP at 12 hours after instillation than did carteolol 2% (285). Another study indicated that 1% and 2% concentrations of carteolol have comparable pressure lowering efficacy (286). Carteolol has also been studied as a fixed combination with pilocarpine. Various combinations of carteolol 1% and 2% with pilocarpine 2% and 4% and timolol 0.5% with pilocarpine 2% and 4% gave mean IOP reductions of 24–40% (279, 287). However, either carteolol or timolol in combination with pilocarpine was slightly less effective than when the two drugs were given separately (287).

In most studies comparing carteolol and timolol, there was no significant difference in the effects on pulse or blood pressure (280–284). Carteolol has been shown, however, to cause less ocular irritation than timolol in the first few minutes after instillation (281, 282). The influence of carteolol on ocular blood flow is unclear (as is true of all β-blockers). One study revealed a significant drop in ciliary systolic perfusion pressure, which was not seen with timolol or betaxolol (288), while another study showed a significant increase in ocular pulsatile blood flow with carteolol, but not with timolol (289). Yet another study showed that carteolol, as compared to a placebo, had no significant effect on human retinal circulation with regard to changes in vessel diameter, maximum erythrocyte velocity, and volumetric blood flow

rate (290). In a 1-year comparative trial of carteolol and timolol, the visual fields did not change significantly in either group (291).

While the intrinsic sympathomimetic activity of carteolol does not appear to protect against cardiovascular effects such as reduced pulse and blood pressure, there is evidence that it may decrease the cardiovascular risks associated with cholesterol abnormalities. As noted earlier in this chapter, topical therapy with timolol 0.5% twice daily was shown to lower plasma HDL cholesterol levels to a degree that increased the risk of myocardial infarction by 21% (183). A comparative trial of carteolol 1% and timolol 0.5% in 58 healthy, normolipidemic adult men confirmed the earlier findings with regard to timolol and showed significantly less effect of carteolol on HDL (292). Carteolol therapy was associated with a 3.3% decrease in HDL and a 4% increase in total cholesterol/HDL ratio, compared to 8% and 10%, respectively, with timolol. These values extrapolate to an increased myocardial infarction risk of 6.6% and 17% for carteolol and timolol, respectively. While the implications of these findings are not clear for glaucoma populations, it seems prudent to consider carteolol when prescribing β-blockers in patients with cholesterol abnormalities or other risks for myocardial infarction. It also underscores the importance of recommending nasolacrimal occlusion for all patients using topical β-blockers.

Metipranolol

Metipranolol is a nonselective β-blocker that has been shown in a placebo-controlled trial to significantly lower the IOP by reducing the rate of aqueous flow with no effect on outflow (293). Comparative studies have shown that it is comparable to timolol (294, 295) and levobunolol (262) with regard to efficacy and safety. One study showed metipranolol to be effective in controlling IOP elevation after cataract surgery (296). A fixed combination of metipranolol 0.1% and pilocarpine 2% was found to have better IOP-lowering efficacy than either drug used alone (297). Metipranolol is commercially available in a 0.3% concentration (Table 27.1).

Although most studies have shown a safety profile for metipranolol that is comparable to other nonselective β-blockers (262, 294, 295), one study suggested an improved therapeutic index relative to timolol with regard to exercise-induced tachycardia (298). However, another revealed more bronchoconstriction in asthmatic patients with metipranolol than with timolol or carteolol (299). As with other topical β-blockers, metipranolol may cause a brief corneal anesthesia in some patients (300). The most troublesome ocular reaction that has been reported with metipranolol, however, is a *granulomatous anterior uveitis*, characterized by mutton-fat keratitic precipitates, flare and cells, and IOP elevation. In the United Kingdom, 15 cases were described in one report with reference to 51 more cases from other parts of the country (301). Seven patients, rechallenged with metipranolol, all developed an adverse reaction within 14 days (302), and the drug was withdrawn from clinical use in the UK. A retrospective study of 1306 patients treated with metipranolol in Germany revealed a low risk of uveitis associated with the medication, and it was assumed that the problem was related to the unique formulation used in the UK (303). However, three cases have been reported in the United States (304, 305), one of which recurred when inadvertently rechallenged (305).

Other Topical β-Blockers

The following β-blockers have also been evaluated for their ocular hypotensive effect. None are available in the United States for topical therapy at the time of this publication. However, several are available in oral form for treatment of cardiovascular and other systemic disorders, which may also influence the IOP and the effect of the topical β-blocker (Table 27.2).

D-Timolol

Previous reference to timolol in this chapter has been to L-timolol (or the S-enantiomer), which is the stereoisomer form of the drug currently used in the treatment of glaucoma. More recent research with D-timolol (the R-enantiomer) reveals that this is a significantly less potent β-adrenergic antagonist with regard to both IOP reduction and systemic effects (306–308). It does, however, have some beneficial ocular hypotensive effect and may prove to have clinical value due to the reduction in systemic side effects (307, 308).

Atenolol

Atenolol is a selective β_1-adrenergic antagonist with no intrinsic sympathomimetic or membrane-stabilizing properties (309, 310). Oral atenolol (25–100 mg) provided significant IOP reduction when compared to a placebo (311, 312), and an oral dose of 50 mg had a better pressure lowering effect than 40 mg of propranolol (313) or 500 mg of acetazolamide (314). Topical administration of 2% atenolol was comparable to 2% pilocarpine (315), and 4% atenolol was more effective than 1% epinephrine (316). However, a long-term study showed that the initial pressure control gradually wore off in some patients (317).

Metoprolol

Metoprolol is a cardioselective β_1-adrenergic antagonist which, like betaxolol, has been shown to reduce IOP without the adverse respiratory side effects of the nonselective β-blockers (318, 319). Significant aqueous humor concentrations are achieved with oral administration (320), and prolonged ocular hypotensive action has been demonstrated with

both oral administration of 100-mg tablets or topical instillation of 1–5% metoprolol (318). The topical administration is well-tolerated except for transient burning, and the ocular hypotensive effect persists in most cases, except for an early, partial loss of the initial pressure reduction (321, 322). Metoprolol 3% was similar to pilocarpine 2–4% in lowering IOP in one study (323), and was roughly equivalent to the ocular hypotensive effect of timolol in another evaluation (324).

Pindolol

Pindolol is a potent β-adrenergic antagonist with an intrinsic sympathomimetic effect, and is reported to provide a good ocular hypotensive effect (325–327). Pindolol 0.5–1% has been shown to provide prolonged IOP reduction without significant ocular or systemic side effects (326, 327), although reports are conflicting regarding the influence of pindolol on corneal anesthesia (325, 328). Comparisons with timolol revealed no significant differences in the ocular hypotensive action of the two drugs (329–331).

Nadolol

Nadolol is a nonselective β-blocker with no intrinsic sympathomimetic action. Oral administration of nadolol 10–80 mg daily has been shown to cause a significant, dose-related reduction in IOP (332). A significant IOP lowering for 24 hours was achieved with 40 mg once daily (333) and with 10 or 20 mg twice daily (334). Nadolol 20 mg daily was equivalent to topical timolol 0.25% twice daily (335, 336), and nadolol 40 or 80 mg daily had a comparable ocular hypotensive effective to timolol 0.5% twice daily (336). However, the oral medication caused a significantly greater reduction in heart rate (332, 335, 336) and blood pressure (332, 335). Topical preparations also produce a significant dose-dependent IOP reduction, which lasts more than 9 hours with the higher concentrations of 1–2% (337). When compared to the ocular hypotensive effect of timolol,

Table 27.2.
COMMERCIAL ORAL β-BLOCKERS*

Generic Preparations	Brand Names	With Diuretic Antihypertensive
Acebutolol HCl	Sectral	
Atenolol	Tenormin	Tenoretic
Carteolol	Cartrol	
Labetalol HCl	Normodyne	Normozide
Metoprolol tartrate	Lopressor	Lopressor HCT
Nadolol	Corgard	Corzide
Penbutolol sulfate	Levatol	
Pindolol	Visken	
Propranolol HCl	Inderal	Inderide
Timolol Maleate	Blocadren	Timolide

*Other generic products may also be available

however, nadolol is much less effective with continued use (338). This may be due to poor corneal penetration, and the prodrug analogue of nadolol, diacetyl nadolol, was found to be as effective as timolol in lowering the IOP up to 8 hours with less efficacy thereafter (339). However, diacetyl nadolol 2% had a lower incidence of tolerance than timolol 0.5% during a 3-month study (340).

Befunolol

Befunolol 0.25% and 0.5% was reported to provide good IOP reduction during a 3-month study (341), with no significant diminution of effect during a 1-year follow-up (342). In a preliminary study, changing from timolol 0.5% to befunolol 0.5% therapy was associated with a significant additional decrease in IOP (343).

Penbutolol

Penbutolol (344) has also been evaluated as a topical antiglaucoma agent, with encouraging preliminary results, and it is likely that additional β-adrenergic inhibitors will continue to appear as research continues with this important class of drugs.

α-ADRENERGIC INHIBITORS

Thymoxamine

Thymoxamine hydrochloride competes with norepinephrine for α-adrenergic receptors. As a result, it produces miosis by inhibiting the dilator muscle of the iris without influencing the ciliary muscle-induced facility of aqueous outflow (345). It also has no effect on the rate of aqueous humor formation, IOP, or anterior chamber volume (346). This provides the following potential clinical applications for the drug.

Reversal of Mydriasis

Thymoxamine 0.1% can reverse the mydriatic effect of phenylephrine 2.5% within 1 hour in most patients (347), and of ephedrine 0.5%, but not when the latter is combined with homatropine 0.5% (348). Because it does not cause shallowing of the anterior chamber or ciliary spasm, it provides safe, rapid reversal of the effects of an adrenergic mydriatic drug. Intraocular administration of 0.2–0.5 ml of thymoxamine 0.01% or 0.02% was effective in reversing phenylephrine- or epinephrine-induced mydriasis in cataract surgery and other intraocular procedures with no corneal endothelial damage (349).

Management of Angle-Closure Glaucoma

Thymoxamine has the advantages of (a) causing miosis despite pressure-induced ischemia of the iris sphincter and

(b) not increasing the posterior vector force of the iris, which might aggravate the pupillary block. In a study of patients with acute angle-closure glaucoma, 0.5% thymoxamine was administered every minute for five times and then every 15 minutes for 2–3 hours. The attacks were broken in all cases, except those with peripheral anterior synechiae or prolonged angle closure (350).

Differentiating Angle-Closure Glaucoma from Open-Angle Glaucoma with Narrow Angles

Since thymoxamine produces miosis without effecting the ciliary muscle-controlled facility of outflow, it will break an angle-closure attack, but have no effect on open-angle glaucoma (351). It has been demonstrated that this property of thymoxamine can be used as a diagnostic adjunct to gonioscopy in distinguishing between angle-closure glaucoma and open-angle glaucoma with narrow angles (352).

Management of Pigmentary Glaucoma

One theory for the mechanism of pigment dispersion in pigmentary glaucoma, as discussed in Section Two, is contact between the iris pigment epithelium and packets of lens zonules. It has been suggested that miosis without cyclotropia, as produced by thymoxamine, theoretically provides an effective means of minimizing this effect (353).

Management of Eyelid Retraction

Thymoxamine 0.5% causes a substantial narrowing of the palpebral fissure in many patients with eyelid retraction, especially cases secondary to thyroid disease, and it has been suggested that this may have value in the diagnosis of thyroid eye disease and possibly in the medical treatment of eyelid retraction (354).

Dapiprazole

This α-adrenergic antagonist is similar in action to thymoxamine and is commercially available for the reversal of mydriasis after an ocular examination. It was evaluated in human volunteers and found to produce miosis and IOP reduction (355). Higher concentrations of 1–2% caused transient conjunctival hyperemia and ptosis, while lower doses of 0.25% had loss of effectiveness with time.

Bunazosin

This selective α_1-adrenergic antagonist significantly lowered IOP in normal volunteers in single doses of 0.025–0.2% and was effective for 1 week at 0.1% (356). In a placebo-controlled trial with bunazosin 0.3%, significant IOP reduction lasted more than 10 hours (357). The mechanism of IOP reduction is presumed to be increased uveoscleral outflow, since it does not influence aqueous production, conventional outflow, or episcleral venous pressure (356). It also does not alter blood-aqueous barrier permeability (356) or pulsatile ocular blood flow (357), but does cause miosis, ptosis, and conjunctival hyperemia (357).

Prazosin

This postsynaptic α-adrenergic antagonist is used as an oral medication to lower blood pressure and produce peripheral vasodilatation. Rabbit studies have shown that topical administration of 0.001–0.1% prazosin causes a dose-related lowering of IOP by reducing aqueous humor formation (358, 359).

Corynanthine

This selective α_1-adrenergic antagonist produced IOP reduction in animals without altering conventional outflow facility or the rate of aqueous humor flow (360). As with bunazosin, it was postulated that the mechanism of pressure reduction might be an increase in uveoscleral outflow. In a clinical trial, a single dose of corynanthine 1% had no IOP-lowering effect, while 2% and 5% concentrations did lower the IOP, although a 3-week study with the 2% did not reveal a sustained pressure reduction (361).

α- AND β-ADRENERGIC INHIBITORS

Labetalol

This is a combined α- and β-adrenergic blocking agent, which has been shown to produce a significant, dose-related IOP reduction in rabbits (362–364), although it has a poor ocular hypotensive effect in human eyes (364, 365).

SUMMARY

β-Adrenergic inhibitors lower the IOP by reducing aqueous production. The drugs in this class differ primarily with regard to IOP lowering efficacy and relative ocular and systemic side effects. Timolol, a potent β_1- and β_2-adrenergic antagonist, has a profound ocular hypotensive action with few ocular side effects, but a potential for serious systemic adverse reactions, especially on the cardiovascular (β_1) and pulmonary (β_2) systems. Betaxolol, a cardioselective β_1-blocker, is slightly less effective than timolol in lowering IOP, but has the advantage of reduced side effects, especially with the pulmonary system. Levobunolol, carteolol, and metipranolol are nonselective β-adrenergic inhibitors that are similar to timolol in ocular hypotensive efficacy and incidence of side effects, with the exception of carteolol, which contains intrinsic sympathomimetic activity that may reduce the β-blocker effect on high-density lipoprotein cholesterol. Many other β-blockers are also being evaluated for the treatment of glaucoma. α-Adrenergic antagonists produce miosis by inhibiting the dilator muscle of the iris. Some of these drugs, such as thymoxamine, have no direct effect on aqueous humor dynamics, while others, such as bunazosin, also have some ocular hypotensive action.

REFERENCES

1. Wettrell, K, Pandolfi, M: Effect of oral administration of various beta-blocking agents on the intraocular pressure in healthy volunteers. Exp Eye Res 21:451, 1975.
2. Pandolfi, M, Ohrstrom, A: Treatment of ocular hypertension with oral beta-adrenergic blocking agents. Acta Ophthalmol 52:464, 1974.
3. Wettrell, K, Pandolfi, M: Early dose response analysis of ocular hypotensive effects of propranolol in patients with ocular hypertension. Br J Ophthalmol 60:680, 1976.
4. Wettrell, K, Pandolfi, M: Propranolol vs acetazolamide. A long-term double-masked study of the effect on intraocular pressure and blood pressure. Arch Ophthalmol 97:280, 1979.
5. Ohrstrom, A, Pandolfi, M: Long-term treatment of glaucoma with systemic propranolol. Am J Ophthalmol 86:340, 1978.
6. Musini, A, Fabbri, B, Bergamaschi, M, et al: Comparison of the effect of propranolol, lignocaine, and other drugs on normal and raised intraocular pressure in man. Am J Ophthalmol 72:773, 1971.
7. Maerte, HJ, Merkle, W: Long-term treatment of glaucoma with propranolol ophthalmic solution. Klin Monatsbl Augenheilkd 177:437, 1980.
8. Takats, I, Szilvassy, I, Kerek, A: Intraocular pressure and circulation of aqueous humour in rabbit eyes following intravenous administration of propranolol (Inderal). Graefes Arch Clin Exp Ophthalmol 185:331, 1972.
9. Cubey, RB, Taylor, SH: Ocular reaction to propranolol and resolution on continued treatment with a different beta-blocking drug. Br Med J 4:327, 1975.
10. Garner, A, Rahi, AHS: Practolol and ocular toxicity. Antibodies in serum and tears. Br J Ophthalmol 60:684, 1976.
11. Rahi, AHS, Chapman, CM, Garner, A, Wright, P: Pathology of practolol-induced ocular toxicity. Br J Ophthalmol 60:312, 1976.
12. Skegg, DCG, Doll, R: Frequency of eye complaints and rashes among patients receiving practolol and propranolol. Lancet 2:475, 1977.
13. Status report on beta-blockers. FDA Drug Bull 8:13, 1978.
14. Katz, IM, Hubbard, WA, Getson, AJ, Gould, AL: Intraocular pressure decrease in normal volunteers following timolol ophthalmic solution. Invest Ophthalmol 15:489, 1976.
15. Zimmerman, TJ: Timolol maleate-a new glaucoma medication? Invest Ophthalmol Vis Sci 16:687, 1977.
16. Vareilles, P, Silverstone, D, Plazonnet, B, et al: Comparison of the effects of timolol and other adrenergic agents on intraocular pressure in the rabbit. Invest Ophthalmol Vis Sci 16:987, 1977.
17. Radius, RL, Diamond, GR, Pollack, IP, Langham, ME: Timolol. A new drug for management of chronic simple glaucoma. Arch Ophthalmol 96:1003, 1978.
18. Zimmerman, TJ, Kaufman, HE: Timolol. A beta-adrenergic blocking agent for the treatment of glaucoma. Arch Ophthalmol 95:601, 1977.
19. Zimmerman, TJ, Kaufman, HE: Timolol: Dose response and duration of action. Arch Ophthalmol 95:605, 1977.
20. Spinelli, D, Montanari, P, Vigasio, F, Cormanni, V: Effects of timolol maleate on untreated contralateral eye. J Fr Ophthalmol 5:153, 1982.

21. Ritch, R, Hargett, NA, Podos, SM: The effect of 1.5% timolol maleate on intraocular pressure. Acta Ophthalmol 56:6, 1978.

22. Moss, AP, Ritch, R, Hargett, NA, et al: A comparison of the effects of timolol and epinephrine on intraocular pressure. Am J Ophthalmol 86:489, 1978.

23. Zimmerman, TJ, Kass, MA, Yablonski, ME, Becker, B: Timolol maleate. Efficacy and safety. Arch Ophthalmol 97:656, 1979.

24. LeBlanc, RP, Krip, G: Timolol—Canadian multicenter study. Ophthalmology 88:244, 1981.

25. Sonntag, JR, Brindley, GO, Shields, MB, et al: Timolol and epinephrine. Comparison of efficacy and side effects. Arch Ophthalmol 97:273, 1979.

26. Hoyng, PFJ, Verbey, NLJ: Timolol vs guanethidine-epinephrine formulations in the treatment of glaucoma. An open clinical trial. Arch Ophthalmol 102:1788, 1984.

27. Boger, WP III, Steinert, RF, Puliafito, CA, Pavan-Langston, D: Clinical trial comparing timolol ophthalmic solution to pilocarpine in open-angle glaucoma. Am J Ophthalmol 86:8, 1978.

28. Hass, I, Drance, SM: Comparison between pilocarpine and timolol on diurnal pressures in open-angle glaucoma. Arch Ophthalmol 98:480, 1980.

29. Merte, HJ, Merkle, W: Experiences in a double-blind study with different concentrations of timolol and pilocarpine. Klin Monatsbl Augenheilkd 177:443, 1980.

30. Calissendorff, B, Maren, N, Wettrell, K, Ostberg, A: Timolol versus pilocarpine separately or combined with acetazolamide—effects on intraocular pressure. Acta Ophthalmol 58:624, 1980.

31. Merté, H-J, Merkle, W: Experiences in a double-blind study with different concentrations of timolol and pilocarpine. Klin Monatsbl Augenheilkd 177:443, 1980.

32. Vogel, R, Crick, RP, Mills, KB, et al: Effect of Timolol versus pilocarpine on visual field progression in patients with primary open-angle glaucoma. Ophthalmology 99:1505, 1992.

33. Christakis, C, Mangouritsas, N: Comparative studies of the pressure-lowering effect of timolol and phospholine iodide. Klin Monatsbl Augenheilkd 179:197, 1981.

34. Zimmerman, TJ, Harbin, R, Pett, M, Kaufman, HE: Timolol and facility of outflow. Invest Ophthalmol Vis Sci 16:623, 1977.

35. Sonntag, JR, Brindley, GO, Shields, MB: Effect of timolol therapy on outflow facility. Invest Ophthalmol Vis Sci 17:293, 1978.

36. Coakes, RL, Brubaker, RF: The mechanism of timolol in lowering intraocular pressure in the normal eye. Arch Ophthalmol 96:2045, 1978.

37. Yablonski, ME, Zimmerman, TJ, Waltman, SR, Becker, B: A fluorophotometric study of the effect of topical timolol on aqueous humor dynamics. Exp Eye Res 27:135, 1978.

38. Topper, JE, Brubaker, RF: Effects of timolol, epinephrine, and acetazolamide on aqueous flow during sleep. Invest Ophthalmol Vis Sci 26:1315, 1985.

39. Liu, HK, Chiou, GCY, Garg, LC: Ocular hypotensive effects of timolol in cat eyes. Arch Ophthalmol 98:1467, 1980.

40. Miichi, H, Nagataki, S: Effects of pilocarpine, salbutamol, and timolol on aqueous humor formation in cynomolgus monkeys. Invest Ophthalmol Vis Sci 24:1269, 1983.

41. Bartels, SP: Aqueous humor flow measured with fluorophotometry in timolol-treated primates. Invest Ophthalmol Vis Sci 29:1498, 1988.

42. McCannel, CA, Heinrich, SR, Brubaker, RF: Acetazolamide but not timolol lowers aqueous humor flow in sleeping humans. Graefes Arch Clin Exp Ophthalmol 230:518, 1992.

43. Maus, TL, Young, WF Jr, Brubaker, RF: Aqueous flow in humans after adrenalectomy. Invest Ophthalmol Vis Sci 35:3325, 1994.

44. Rettig, ES, Larsson, L-I, Brubaker, RF: The effect of topical timolol on epinephrine-stimulated aqueous humor flow in sleeping humans. Invest Ophthalmol Vis Sci 35:554, 1994.

45. Neufeld, AH: Experimental studies on the mechanism of action of timolol. Surv Ophthalmol 23:363, 1979.

46. Neufeld, AH, Bartels, SP, Liu, JHK: Laboratory and clinical studies on the mechanism of action of timolol. Surv Ophthalmol 28:286, 1983.

47. Bromberg, BB, Gregory, DS, Sears, ML: Beta-adrenergic receptors in ciliary processes of the rabbit. Invest Ophthalmol Vis Sci 19:203, 1980.

48. Nathanson, JA: Human ciliary process adrenergic receptor: pharmacological characterization. Invest Ophthalmol Vis Sci 21:798, 1981.

49. Trope, GE, Clark, B: Beta adrenergic receptors in pigmented ciliary processes. Br J Ophthalmol 66:788, 1982.

50. Trope, GE, Clark, B: Binding potencies of two new β_2 specific blockers to beta receptors in the ciliary processes and the possible relevance of these drugs to intraocular pressure control. Br J Ophthalmol 68:245, 1984.

51. Schmitt, CJ, Gross, DM, Share, NN: Beta-adrenergic receptor subtypes in iris-ciliary body of rabbits. Graefes Arch Clin Exp Ophthalmol 221:167, 1984.

52. Wax, MB, Molinoff, PB: Distribution and properties of β-adrenergic receptors in human iris-ciliary body. Invest Ophthalmol Vis Sci 28:420, 1987.

53. Liu, JHK, Bartels, SP, Neufeld, AH: Effects of timolol on intraocular pressure following ocular adrenergic denervation. Cur Eye Res 3:1113, 1984.

54. Wentworth, WO, Brubaker, RF: Aqueous humor dynamics in a series of patients with third neuron Horner's syndrome. Am J Ophthalmol 92:407, 1981.

55. Bartels, SP, Roth, O, Jumblatt, MM, Neufeld, AH: Pharmacological effects of topical timolol in the rabbit eye. Invest Ophthalmol Vis Sci 19:1189, 1980.

56. Bartels, SP, Liu, JHK, Neufeld, AH: Decreased beta-adrenergic responsiveness in cornea and iris-ciliary body following topical timolol or epinephrine in albino and pigmented rabbits. Invest Ophthalmol Vis Sci 24:718, 1983.

57. Airaksinen, PJ, Alanko, HI: Vascular effects on timolol and pilocarpine in the iris. A simultaneous bilateral fluorescein angiographic study. Acta Ophthalmol 61:195, 1983.

58. Beardsley, TL, Shields, MB: Effect of timolol on aqueous humor protein concentration in humans. Am J Ophthalmol 95:448, 1983.

59. Stur, M, Grabner, G, Dorda, W, Zehetbauer, G: The effect of timolol on the concentrations of albumin and IgG in the aqueous humor of the human eye. Am J Ophthalmol 96:726, 1983.

60. Stur, M, Grabner, G, Huber-Spitzy, V, et al: Effect of timolol on aqueous humor protein concentration in the human eye. Arch Ophthalmol 104:899, 1986.

61. Goldberg, HS, Feldman, F, Cohen, MM, Clark, L: Effect of topical indomethacin and timolol maleate on intraocular pressure in normal subjects. Am J Ophthalmol 99:576, 1985.

62. Sulewski, ME, Robin, AL, Cummings, HL, Arkin, LM: Effects of topical flurbiprofen on the intraocular pressure lowering effects of apraclonidine and timolol. Arch Ophthalmol 109:807, 1991.

63. Wantenabe, K, Chiou, GCY: Action mechanism of timolol to lower the intraocular pressure in rabbits. Ophthalmic Res 15:160, 1983.

64. Mekki, QA, Turner, P: Dopamine-2 receptor blockade does not affect the ocular hypotensive action of timolol. Br J Ophthalmol 72:598, 1988.

65. Gilmartin, B, Hogan, RE, Thompson, SM: The effect of timolol maleate on tonic accommodation, tonic vergence, and pupil diameter. Invest Ophthalmol Vis Sci 25:763, 1984.

66. Lin, L-L, Galin, MA, Ostbaum, SA, Katz, I: Longterm timolol therapy. Surv Ophthalmol 23:377, 1979.

67. Wax, MB, Molinoff, PB, Alvarado, J, Polansky, J: Characterization of β-adrenergic receptors in cultured human trabecular cells and in human trabecular meshwork. Invest Ophthalmol Vis Sci 30:51, 1989.

68. Jampel, HD, Lynch, MG, Brown, RH, et al: β-Adrenergic receptors in human trabecular meshwork. Identification and autoradiographic localization. Invest Ophthalmol Vis Sci 28:772, 1987.

69. McMenamin, PG, Lee, WR, Grierson, I, Grindle, FCJ: Giant vacuoles in the lining endothelium of the human Schelmm's canal after topical timolol maleate. Invest Ophthalmol Vis Sci 24:339, 1983.

70. Lütjen-Drecoll, E, Kaufman, PL: Morphological changes in primate aqueous humor formation and drainage tissues after long-term treatment with antiglaucomatous drugs. J Glau 2:316, 1993.

71. Collignon-Brach, J, Weekers, R: Timolol. Etude clinique. J Fr Ophthalmol 2:603, 1979.

72. Mills, KB: Blind randomised non-crossover long-term trial comparing topical timolol 0.25% with timolol 0.5% in the treatment of simple chronic glaucoma. Br J Ophthalmol 67:216, 1983.

73. Dausch, D, Schad, K: Are 0.1% timolol-maleate eyedrops suitable for treating chronic glaucoma? Klin Monatsbl Augenheilkd 180:141, 1982.

74. Mottow-Lippa, LS, Lippa, EA, Naidoff, MA, et al: 0.008% timolol ophthalmic solution. A minimal-effect dose in a normal volunteer model. Arch Ophthalmol 108:61, 1990.

75. Robinson, JC, Kaufman, PL: Dose-dependent suppression of aqueous humor formation by timolol in the cynomolgus monkey. J Glau 2:251, 1993.

76. Katz, IM, Berger, ET: Effects of iris pigmentation on response of ocular pressure to timolol. Surv Ophthalmol 23:395, 1979.

77. Salminen, L, Imre, G, Huupponen, R: The effect of ocular pigmentation on intraocular pressure response to timolol. Acta Ophthalmol Suppl 63:15, 1985.

78. Schmitt, CJ, Lotti, VJ, LeDouarec, JC: Penetration of timolol into the rabbit eye. Measurements after ocular instillation and intravenous injection. Arch Ophthalmol 98:547, 1980.

79. Phillips, CI, Bartholomew, RS, Kazi, G, et al: Penetration of timolol eye drops into human aqueous humour. Br J Ophthalmol 65:593, 1981.

80. Phillips, CI, Bartholomew, RS, Levy, AM, et al: Penetration of timolol eye drops into human aqueous humour: The first hour. Br J Ophthalmol 69:217, 1985.

81. Soll, DB: Evaluation of timolol in chronic open-angle glaucoma. Once a day vs twice a day. Arch Ophthalmol 98:2178, 1980.

82. Yalon, M, Urinowsky, E, Rothkoff, L, et al: Frequency of timolol administration. Am J Ophthalmol 92:526, 1981.

83. Letchinger, SL, Frohlichstein, D, Glieser, DK, et al: Can the concentration of timolol or the frequency of its administration be reduced? Ophthalmology 100:1259, 1993.

84. Ohdo, S, Grass, GM, Lee, VHL: Improving the ocular to systemic ratio of topical timolol by varying the dosing time. Invest Ophthalmol Vis Sci 32:2790, 1991.

85. Laurence, J, Holder, D, Vogel, R, et al: A double-masked, placebo-controlled evaluation of timolol in a gel vehicle. J Glau 2:177, 1993.

86. Schlecht, LP, Brubaker, RF: The effects of withdrawal of timolol in chronically treated glaucoma patients. Ophthalmology 95:1212, 1988.

87. Trope, GE, Menon, IA, Liu, GS, et al: Ocular timolol levels after drug withdrawal: an experimental model. Can J Ophthalmol 29:217, 1994.

88. Krieglstein, GK: A follow-up study on the intraocular pressure response of timolol eye drops. Klin Monatsbl Augenheilkd 175:627, 1979.

89. Merte, HJ, Merkle, W: Results of long-term treatment of glaucoma with timolol ophthalmic solution. Klin Monatsbl Augenheilkd 177:562, 1980.

90. Steinert, RF, Thomas, JV, Boger, WP III: Long-term drift and continued efficacy after multiyear timolol therapy. Arch Ophthalmol 99:100, 1981.

91. Plan, Ch, Boulmier, A: Long-term treatment of chronic glaucoma with timolol drops: results after four years. J Fr Ophthalmol 4:751, 1981.

92. Airaksinen, PJ, Valle, O, Takki, KK, Klemetti, A: Timolol treatment of chronic open-angle glaucoma and ocular hypertension. A 2.5-year multicenter study. Graefes Arch Clin Exp Ophthalmol 219:68, 1982.

93. Blika, S, Saunte, E: Timolol maleate in the treatment of glaucoma simplex and glaucoma capsulare. A three-year followup study. Acta Ophthalmol 60:967, 1982.

94. Maclure, GM: Chronic open angle glaucoma treated with timolol. A four-year study. Trans Ophthalmol Soc UK 103:78, 1983.

95. LeBlanc, RP, Saheb, NE, Krip, G: Timolol: Long-term Canadian multicentre study. Can J Ophthalmol 20:128, 1985.

96. Boger, WP III: Shortterm "escape" and longterm "drift." The dissipation effects of the beta adrenergic blocking agents. Surv Ophthalmol 28:235, 1983.

97. Boger, WP III, Puliafito, CA, Steinert, RF, Langston, DP: Long-term experience with timolol ophthalmic solution in patients with open-angle glaucoma. Ophthalmology 85:259, 1978.

98. Oksala, A, Salminen, L: Tachyphylaxis in timolol therapy for chronic glaucoma. Klin Monatsbl Augenheilkd 177:451, 1980.

99. Krupin, T, Singer, PR, Perlmutter, J, et al: One-hour intraocular pressure response to timolol. Lack of correlation with long-term response. Arch Ophthalmol 99:840, 1981.

100. Neufeld, AH, Zawistowski, KA, Page, ED, Bromberg, BB: Influences on the density of beta-adrenergic receptors in the cornea and iris-ciliary body of the rabbit. Invest Ophthalmol Vis Sci 17:1069, 1978.

101. Brubaker, RF, Nagataki, S, Bourne, WM: Effect of chronically administered timolol on aqueous humor flow in patients with glaucoma. Ophthalmology 89:280, 1982.

102. Gandolfi, SA: Restoring sensitivity to timolol after long-term drift in primary open-angle glaucoma. Invest Ophthalmol Vis Sci 31:354, 1990.

103. Gandolfi, SA, Vecchi, M: Serial administration of adrenergic antagonist and agonist ("pulsatile therapy") reduces the incidence of long-term drift to timolol in humans. Invest Ophthalmol Vis Sci 37:684, 1996.

104. Ashburn, FS Jr, Gillespie, JE, Kass, MA, Becker, B: Timolol plus maximum tolerated antiglaucoma therapy: a one-year follow-up study. Surv Ophthalmol 23:389, 1979.

105. Sonty, S, Schwartz, B: The additive effect of timolol on open angle glaucoma patients on maximal medical therapy. Surv Ophthalmol 23:381, 1979.

106. Zimmerman, TJ, Gillespie, JE, Kass, MA, et al: Timolol plus maximum-tolerated antiglaucoma therapy. Arch Ophthalmol 97:278, 1979.

107. Luo, AM, Sasaki, H, Lee, VHL: Ocular drug interactions involving topically applied timolol in the pigmented rabbit. Curr Eye Res 10:231, 1991.

108. Keates, EU: Evaluation of timolol maleate combination therapy in chronic open-angle glaucoma. Am J Ophthalmol 88:565, 1979.

109. Smith, RJ, Nagasubramanian, S, Watkins, R, Poinoosawmy, D: Addition of timolol maleate to routine medical therapy. A clinical trial. Br J Ophthalmol 64:779, 1980.

110. Nielsen, NV, Eriksen, JS: Timolol in maintenance treatment of ocular hypertension and glaucoma. Acta Ophthalmol 57:1070, 1979.

111. Kass, MA: Efficacy of combining timolol with other antiglaucoma medications. Surv Ophthalmol 28:274, 1983.

112. Söderström, MB, Wallin, Ö, Granström, P-A, Thorburn, W: Timolol-pilocarpine combined vs timolol and pilocarpine given separately. Am J Ophthalmol 107:465, 1989.

113. Schnarr, K-D, Merte, H-J: Effectivity and tolerance of an active substance combination of timolol and pilocarpine—a pilot study. Klin Monatsbl Augenheilkd 191:436, 1987.

114. Maclure, GM, Vogel, R, Sturm, A, Binkowitz, B: Effect on the 24-hour diurnal curve of intraocular pressure of a fixed ratio combination of timolol 0.5% and pilocarpine 2% in patients with COAG not controlled on timolol 0.5%. Br J Ophthalmol 73:827, 1989.

115. Airaksinen, PJ, Valkonen, R, Stenborg, T, et al: A double-masked study of timolol and pilocarpine combined. Am J Ophthalmol 104:587, 1987.

116. Sturm, A, Vogel, R, Binkowitz, B, et al: A fixed combination of timolol and pilocarpine: double-masked comparisons with timolol and with pilocarpine. J Glau 1:7, 1992.

117. Zadok, D, Geyer, O, Zadok, J, et al: Combined timolol and pilocarpine vs pilocarpine alone and timolol alone in the treatment of glaucoma. Am J Ophthalmol 117:728, 1994.

118. Ellis, PP, Wu, P-Y, Riegel, M: Aqueous humor pilocarpine and timolol levels after instillation of the single drug on in combination. Invest Ophthalmol Vis Sci 32:520, 1991.

119. Puustjärvi, TJ, Repo, LP, et al: Timolol-pilocarpine fixed-ratio combinations in the treatment of chronic open angle glaucoma. Arch Ophthalmol 110:1725, 1992.

120. Drance, SM, Douglas, GR, Wijsman, KJ, Schulzer, M: Adrenergic and adrenolytic effects on intraocular pressure. Graefes Arch Clin Exp Ophthalmol 229:50, 1991.

121. Alexander, DW, Berson, FG, Epstein, DL: A clinical trial of timolol and epinephrine in the treatment of primary open-angle glaucoma. Ophthalmology 95:247, 1988.

122. Tsoy, EA, Meekins, BB, Shields, MB: Comparison of two treatment schedules for combined timolol and dipivefrin therapy. Am J Ophthalmol 102:320, 1986.

123. Pfeiffer, N, Grehn, F: Treatment of primary open-angle glaucoma by a combination of timolol 0.5% and epinephrine 0.5% plus guanethidine 3%. Klin Monatsbl Augenheilkd 194:161, 1989.

124. Scharrer, A, Ober, M: Timolol and acetazolamide in the treatment of increased intraocular pressure. Graefes Arch Clin Exp Ophthalmol 212:129, 1979.

125. Berson, FG, Epstein, DL: Separate and combined effects of timolol maleate and acetazolamide in open-angle glaucoma. Am J Ophthalmol 92:788, 1981.

126. Dailey, RA, Brubaker, RF, Bourne, WM: The effects of timolol maleate and acetazolamide on the rate of aqueous formation in normal human subjects. Am J Ophthalmol 93:232, 1982.

127. Kass, MA, Korey, M, Gordon, M, Becker, B: Timolol and acetazolamide. A study of concurrent administration. Arch Ophthalmol 100:941, 1982.

128. Batchelor, ED, O'Day, DM, Shand, DG, Wood, AJ: Interaction of topical and oral timolol in glaucoma. Ophthalmology 86:60, 1979.

129. Maren, N, Alvan, G, Calissendorff, BM, et al: Additive intraocular pressure reducing effect of topical timolol during systemic beta-blockade. Acta Ophthalmol 60:16, 1982.

130. Blondeau, P, Coté, M, Tétrault, L: Effect of timolol eye drops in subjects receiving systemic propranolol therapy. Can J Ophthalmol 18:18, 1983.

131. Gross, FJ, Schuman, JS: Reduced ocular hypotensive effect of topical β-blockers in glaucoma patients receiving oral β-blockers. J Glau 1:174, 1992.

132. Johnson, SH, Brubaker, RF, Trautman, JC: Absence of an effect of timolol on the pupil. Invest Ophthalmol Vis Sci 17:924, 1978.

133. Tauber, J, Melamed, S, Foster, CS: Glaucoma in patients with ocular cicatricial pemphigoid. Ophthalmology 96:33, 1989.

134. Fiore, PM, Jacobs, IH, Goldberg, DB: Drug-induced pemphigoid. A spectrum of diseases. Arch Ophthalmol 105:1660, 1987.

135. McMahon, CD, Shaffer, RN, Hoskins, HD Jr, Hetherington, J Jr: Adverse effects experienced by patients taking timolol. Am J Ophthalmol 88:736, 1979.

136. Wilson, RP, Spaeth, GL, Poryzees, E: The place of timolol in the practice of ophthalmology. Ophthalmology 87:451, 1980.

137. Van Buskirk, EM: Adverse reactions from timolol administration. Ophthalmology 87:447, 1980.

138. Van Buskirk, EM: Corneal anesthesia after timolol maleate therapy. Am J Ophthalmol 88:739, 1979.

139. Weissman, SS, Asbell, PA: Effects of topical timolol (0.5%) and betaxolol (0.5%) on corneal sensitivity. Br J Ophthalmol 74:409, 1990.

140. Herreras, JM, Pastor, JC, Calonge, M, Asensio, VM: Ocular surface alteration after long-term treatment with an antiglaucomatous drug. Ophthalmology 99:1082, 1992.

141. Arthur, BW, Hay, GJ, Wasan, SM, Willis, WE: Ultrastructural effects of topical timolol on the rabbit cornea. Outcome alone and in conjunction with a gas permeable contact lens. Arch Ophthalmol 101:1607, 1983.

142. Nork, TM, Holly, FJ, Hayes, J, et al: Timolol inhibits corneal epithelial wound healing in rabbits and monkeys. Arch Ophthalmol 102:1224, 1984.

143. Liu, GS, Basu, PK, Trope, GE: Ultrastructural changes of the rabbit corneal epithelium and endothelium after timoptic treatment. Graefes Arch Clin Exp Ophthalmol 225:325, 1987.

144. Reidy, JJ, Zarzour, J, Thompson, HW, Beuerman, RW: Effect of topical β blockers on corneal epithelial wound healing in the rabbit. Br J Ophthalmol 78:377, 1994.

145. Huige, WMM, Beekhuis, WH, Rijneveld, WJ, et al: Unusual deposits in the superficial corneal stroma following combined use of topical corticosteroid and beta-blocking medication. Doc Ophthalmol 78:169, 1991.

146. Brubaker, RF, Coakes, RL, Bourne, WM: Effect of timolol on the permeability of corneal endothelium. Ophthalmology 86:108, 1979.

147. Staatz, WD, Radius, RL, Van Horn, DL, Schultz, RO: Effects of timolol on bovine corneal endothelial cultures. Arch Ophthalmol 99:660, 1981.

148. Alanko, HI, Airaksinen, PJ: Effects of topical timolol on corneal endothelial cell morphology in vivo. Am J Ophthalmol 96:615, 1983.

149. Williams, DE, Nguyen, KD, Shapourifar-Tehrani, S, et al: Effects of timolol, betaxolol, and levobunolol on human Tenon's fibroblasts in tissue culture. Invest Ophthalmol Vis Sci 33:2233, 1992.

150. Nielsen, NV, Eriksen, JS: Timolol. Transitory manifestations of dry eyes in long-term treatment. Acta Ophthalmol 57:418, 1979.

151. Bonomi, L, Zavarise, G, Noya, E, Michieletto, S: Effects of timolol maleate on tear flow in human eyes. Graefes Arch Clin Exp Ophthalmol 213:19, 1980.

152. Coakes, RL, Mackie, IA, Seal, DV: Effects of long-term treatment with timolol on lacrimal gland function. Br J Ophthalmol 65:603, 1981.

153. Kuppens, EVMJ, Stolwijk, TR, de Keizer, RJW, van Best, JA: Basal tear turnover and topical timolol in glaucoma patients and healthy controls by fluorophotometry. Invest Ophthalmol Vis Sci 33:3442, 1992.

154. Göbbels, M, Mönks, T, Spitznas, M: Effect of topical 0.5% timolol on tear flow in patients with primary open-angle glaucoma as assessed by fluorophotometry. Ger J Ophthalmol 2:241, 1993.

155. Chiou, GCY, Chen, YJ: Effects of antiglaucoma drugs on ocular blood flow in ocular hypertensive rabbits. J Ocular Pharmacol Ther 9:13, 1993.

156. Steigerwalt, RD Jr, Belcaro, G, Cesarone, MR, et al: Doppler ultrasonography of the central retinal artery in normals treated with topical timolol. Eye 7:403, 1993.

157. Steigerwalt, RD Jr, Belcaro, G, Cesarone, MR, et al: Doppler ultrasonography of the central retinal artery in patients with diabetes and vascular disease treated with topical timolol. Eye 9:495, 1995.

158. Grajewski, AL, Ferrari-Dileo, G, Feuer, WJ, Anderson, DR: Beta-adrenergic responsiveness of choroidal vasculature. Ophthalmology 98:989, 1991.

159. Truckenbrodt, C, Klein, S, Vilser, W: Does timolol influence the retinal hemodynamics in patients with normal-pressure glaucoma? Ophthalmology 89:452, 1992.

160. Kaila, T, Salminen, L, Huupponen, R: Systemic absorption of topically applied ocular timolol. J Ocul Pharmacol Ther 1:79, 1985.

161. Zimmerman, TJ, Sharir, M, Nardin, GF, Fuqua, M: Therapeutic index of pilocarpine, carbachol, and timolol with nasolacrimal occlusion. Am J Ophthalmol 114:1, 1992.

162. Passo, MS, Palmer, EA, Van Buskirk, EM: Plasma Timolol in glaucoma patients. Ophthalmology 91:1361, 1984.

163. Kyyrönen, K, Urtti, A: Improved ocular: systemic absorption ratio of timolol by viscous vehicle and phenylephrine. Invest Ophthalmol Vis Sci 31:1827, 1990.

164. Järvinen, K, Urtti, A: Cardiac effects of different eyedrop preparations of timolol in rabbits. Curr Eye Res 11:469, 1992.

165. Fraunfelder, FT: Interim report: National Registry of possible drug-induced ocular side effects. Ophthalmology 87:87, 1980.

166. Flammer, J, Barth, D: Cardiovascular effects of local timolol therapy. Klin Monatsbl Augenheilkd 176:561, 1980.

167. Nelson, WL, Fraunfelder, FT, Sills, JM, et al: Adverse respiratory and cardiovascular events attributed to timolol ophthalmic solution, 1978–1985. Am J Ophthalmol 102:606, 1986.

168. Caprioli, J, Sears, ML: Caution on the preoperative use of topical timolol. Am J Ophthalmol 95:561, 1983.

169. Doyle, WJ, Weber, PA, Meeks, RH: Effect of topical timolol maleate on exercise performance. Arch Ophthalmol 102:1517, 1984.

170. Leier, CV, Baker, ND, Weber, PA: Cardiovascular effects of ophthalmic timolol. Ann Intern Med 104:197, 1986.

171. Dinai, Y, Sharir, M, Naveh, N, Halkin, H: Bradycardia induced by interaction between quinidine and ophthalmic timolol. Ann Intern Med 103:890, 1985.

172. Pringle, SD, MacEwen, CJ: Severe bradycardia due to interaction of timolol eye drops and verapamil. Br Med J 294:155, 1987.

173. Jones, FL Jr, Ekberg, NL: Exacerbation of asthma by timolol. N Engl J Med 301:270, 1979.

174. Holtmann, HW, Holle, JP, Glanzer, K: Alteration of bronchial flow resistance due to timolol 0.25% in bronchial asthma. Klin Monatsbl Augenheilkd 176:441, 1980.

175. Schoene, RB, Martin, TR, Charan, NB, French, CL: Timolol-induced bronchospasm in asthmatic bronchitis. JAMA 245:1460, 1981.

176. Van Buskirk, EM, Fraunfelder, FT: Ocular beta-blockers and systemic effects. Am J Ophthalmol 98:623, 1984.

177. Avorn, J, Glynn, RJ, Gurwitz, JH, et al: Adverse pulmonary effects of topical β blockers used in the treatment of glaucoma. J Glau 2: 158, 1993.

178. Burnstine, RA, Felton, JL, Ginther, WH: Cardiorespiratory reaction to timolol maleate in a pediatric patient: A case report. Ann Ophthalmol 14:905, 1982.

179. Olson, RJ, Bromberg, BB, Zimmerman, TJ: Apneic spells associated with timolol therapy in a neonate. Am J Ophthalmol 88:120, 1979.

180. Lustgarten, JS, Podos, SM: Topical timolol and the nursing mother. Arch Ophthalmol 101:1381, 1983.

181. Coyle, JT: Timoptic and depression. J Ocul Ther Surg Nov-Dec: 311, 1983.

182. Bright, RA, Everitt, DE: Beta-blockers and depression. Evidence against an association. JAMA 267:1783, 1992.

183. Coleman, AL, Diehl, DLC, Jampel, HD, et al: Topical timolol decreases plasma high-density lipoprotein cholesterol level. Arch Ophthalmol 108:1260, 1990.

184. West, J, Longstaff, S: Topical timolol and serum lipoproteins. Br J Ophthalmol 74:663, 1990.

185. Fraunfelder, FT, Meyer, SM, Menacker, SJ: Alopecia possibly secondary to topical ophthalmic β-blockers. JAMA 263:1493, 1990.

186. Shaivitz, SA: Timolol and myasthenia gravis. JAMA 252:1611, 1979.

187. Coppeto, JR: Timolol-associated myasthenia gravis. Am J Ophthalmol 98:244, 1984.

188. Velde, TM, Kaiser, FE: Ophthalmic timolol treatment causing altered hypoglycemic response in a diabetic patient. Arch Intern Med 143:1627, 1983.

189. Wilson, RP, Kanal, N, Spaeth, GL: Timolol: Its effectiveness in different types of glaucoma. Ophthalmology 86:43, 1979.

190. Zimmerman, TJ, Canale, P: Timolol—further observations. Ophthalmology 86:166, 1979.

191. Obstbaum, SA, Galin, MA: The effects of timolol on cataract extraction and intraocular pressure. Am J Ophthalmol 88:1017, 1979.

192. Haimann, MH, Phelps, CD: Prophylactic timolol for the prevention of high intraocular pressure after cataract extraction. A randomized, prospective, double-blind trial. Ophthalmology 88:233, 1981.

193. Sierpinski-Bart, J, Neumann, E: Timolol in early ocular hypertension following cataract extraction. Glaucoma 3:234, 1981.

194. Shields, MB, Braverman, SD: Timolol in the management of secondary glaucomas. Surv Ophthalmol 28:266, 1983.

195. Steinbach, P-D: Pressure-lowering effect of timolol in various forms of glaucoma. Klin Monatsbl Augenheilkd 176:844, 1980.

196. Lass, JH, Pavan-Langston, D: Timolol therapy in secondary angle-closure glaucoma post penetrating keratoplasty. Ophthalmology 86:51, 1979.

197. Phillips, CI: Timolol in operated closed-angle glaucoma. Br J Ophthalmol 64:240, 1980.

198. McMahon, CD, Hetherington, J Jr, Hoskins, HD Jr, Shaffer, RN: Timolol and pediatric glaucomas. Ophthalmology 88:249, 1981.

199. Boger, WP III, Walton, DS: Timolol in uncontrolled childhood glaucomas. Ophthalmology 88:253, 1981.

200. Zimmerman, TJ, Kooner, KS, Morgan, KS: Safety and efficacy of timolol in pediatric glaucoma. Surv Ophthalmol 28:262, 1983.

201. Hoskins, HD Jr, Hetherington, J Jr, Magee, SD, et al: Clinical experience with timolol in childhood glaucoma. Arch Ophthalmol 103:1163, 1985.

202. Epstein, DL, Krug, JH Jr, Hertzmark, E, et al: A long-term clinical trial of timolol therapy versus no treatment in the management of glaucoma suspects. Ophthalmology 96:1460, 1989.

203. Chauhan, BC, Drance, SM, Douglas, GR: The time-course of intraocular pressue in timolol-treated and untreated glaucoma suspects. Am J Ophthalmol 107:471, 1989.

204. Chauhan, BC, Drance, SM, Douglas, GR: The effect of long-term intraocular pressure reduction on the differential light sensitivity in glaucoma suspects. Invest Ophthalmol Vis Sci 29:1478, 1988.

205. Vuori, M-L, Kaila, T, Iisalo, E, Saari, JM: Concentrations and antagonist activity of topically applied betaxolol in aqueous humour. Acta Ophthalmol 71:677, 1993.

206. Reiss, GR, Brubaker, RF: The mechanism of betaxolol, a new ocular hypotensive agent. Ophthalmology 90:1369, 1983.

207. Berrospi, R, Leibowitz, HM: Betaxolol. A new β-adrenergic blocking agent for treatment of glaucoma. Arch Ophthalmol 100: 943, 1982.

208. Radius, RL: Use of betaxolol in the reduction of elevated intraocular pressure. Arch Ophthalmol 101:898, 1983.

209. Caldwell, DR, Salisbury, CR, Guzek, JP: Effects of topical betaxolol in ocular hypertensive patients. Arch Ophthalmol 102:539, 1984.

210. Feghali, JG, Kaufman, PL: Decreased intraocular pressure in the hypertensive human eye with betaxolol, a β₁-adrenergic antagonist. Am J Ophthalmol 100:777, 1985.

211. Berry, DP, Van Buskirk, EM, Shields, MB: Betaxolol and timolol. A comparison of efficacy and side effects. Arch Ophthalmol 102: 42, 1984.

212. Stewart, RH, Kimbrough, RL, Ward, RL: Betaxolol vs timolol. A six-month double-blind comparison. Arch Ophthalmol 104:46, 1986.

213. Allen, RC, Hertzmark, E, Walker, AM, Epstein, DL: A double-masked comparison of betaxolol vs timolol in the treatment of open-angle glaucoma. Am J Ophthalmol 101:535, 1986.

214. Nyman, K: Intraocular pressure reduction with topically administered pilocarpine, timolol and betaxolol in normal tension glaucoma. Acta Ophthalmol 71:686, 1993.

215. Vogel, R, Tipping, R, Kulaga, SF Jr, et al: Changing therapy from timolol to betaxolol. Effect on intraocular pressure in selected patients with glaucoma. Arch Ophthalmol 107:1303, 1989.

216. Messmer, C, Flammer, J, Stümpfig, D: Influence of betaxolol and timolol on the visual fields of patients with glaucoma. Am J Ophthalmol 112:678, 1991.

217. Kaiser, HJ, Flammer, J, Messmer, C, et al: Thirty-month visual field follow-up of glaucoma patients treated with β-blockers. J Glau 1: 153, 1992.

218. Collignon-Brach, J: Long-term effect of ophthalmic β-adrenoceptor antagonists on intraocular pressure and retinal sensitivity in primary open-angle glaucoma. Curr Eye Res 11:1, 1992.

219. Albracht, DC, LeBlanc, RP, Cruz, AM, et al: A double-masked comparison of betaxolol and dipivefrin for the treatment of increased intraocular pressure. Am J Ophthalmol 116:307, 1993.

220. Smith, JP, Weeks, RH, Newland, EF, Ward, RL: Betaxolol and acetazolamide. Combined ocular hypotensive effect. Arch Ophthalmol 102:1794, 1984.

221. Robinson, JC, Kaufman, PL: Effects and interactions of epinephrine, norepinephrine, timolol, and betaxolol on outflow facility in the cynomolgus monkey. Am J Ophthalmol 109:189, 1990.

222. Allen, RC, Epstein, DL: Additive effect of betaxolol and epinephrine in primary open angle glaucoma. Arch Ophthalmol 104:1178, 1986.

223. Weinreb, RN, Ritch, R, Kushner, FH: Effect of adding betaxolol to dipivefrin therapy. Am J Ophthalmol 101:196, 1986.

224. Weinreb, RN, Caldwell, DR, Goode, SM, et al: A double-masked three-month comparison between 0.25% betaxolol suspension and 0.5% betaxolol ophthalmic solution. Am J Ophthalmol 110:189,1990.

225. Hesse, RJ, Swan, JL II: Aphakic cystoid macular edema secondary to betaxolol therapy. Ophthalmic Surg 19:562, 1988.

226. Arnoult, L, Bowman, ZL, Kimbrough, RL, Stewart, RH: Periocular cutaneous pigmentary changes associated with topical betaxolol. J Glau 4:263, 1995.

227. Schoene, RB, Abuan, T, Ward, RL, Beasley, CH: Effects of topical betaxolol, timolol, and placebo on pulmonary function in asthmatic bronchitis. Am J Ophthalmol 97:86, 1984.

228. Van Buskirk, EM, Weinreb, RN, Berry, DP, et al: Betaxolol in patients with glaucoma and asthma. Am J Ophthalmol 101:531, 1986.

229. Ofner, S, Smith, TJ: Betaxolol in chronic obstructive pulmonary disease. J Ocular Pharmacol Ther 3:171, 1987.

230. Bleckmann, H, Dorow, P: Treatment of patients with glaucoma and obstructive airway diseases with betaxolol and placebo eye drops. Klin Monatsbl Augenheilkd 191:199, 1987.

231. Weinreb, RN, Van Buskirk, EM, Cherniack, R, Drake, MM: Long-term betaxolol therapy in glaucoma patients with pulmonary disease. Am J Ophthalmol 106:162, 1988.

232. Nelson, WL, Kuritsky, JN: Early postmarketing surveillance of betaxolol hydrochloride, September 1985-September 1986. Am J Ophthalmol 103:592, 1987.

233. Roholt, PC: Betaxolol and restrictive airway disease. Arch Ophthalmol 105:1172, 1987.

234. Harris, LS, Greenstein, SH, Bloom, AF: Respiratory difficulties with betaxolol. Am J Ophthalmol 102:274, 1986.

235. Cadigan, PJ, London, DR, Pentecost, BL, et al: Cardiovascular effects of single oral doses of the new beta-adrenoceptor blocking agent betaxolol (SL 75212) in healthy volunteers. Br J Clin Pharmacol 9:569, 1980.

236. Atkins, JM, Pugh, BR Jr, Timewell, RM: Cardiovascular effects of topical beta-blockers during exercise. Am J Ophthalmol 99: 173, 1985.

237. Dickstein, K, Hapnes, R, Aarsland, T, et al: Comparison of topical timolol vs betaxolol on cardiopulmonary exercise performance in healthy volunteers. Acta Ophthalmol 66:463, 1988.

238. Zabel, RW, MacDonald, IM: Sinus arrest associated with betaxolol ophthalmic drops. Am J Ophthalmol 104:431, 1987.

239. Ball, S: Congestive heart failure from betaxolol. Arch Ophthalmol 105:320, 1987.

240. Lynch, MG, Whitson, JT, Brown, RH, et al: Topical β-blocker therapy and central nervous system side effects. A preliminary study comparing betaxolol and timolol. Arch Ophthalmol 106:908, 1988.

241. Orlando, RG: Clinical depression associated with betaxolol. Am J Ophthalmol 102:275, 1986.

242. Vuori, M-L, Ali-Melkkila, T, Kaila, T, et al: Plasma and aqueous humour concentrations and systemic effects of topical betaxolol and timolol in man. Acta Ophthalmol 71:201, 1993.

243. Vuori, M-L, Ali-Melkkila, T, Kaila, T, et al: β_1- and β_2-antagonist activity of topically applied betaxolol and timolol in the systemic circulation. Acta Ophthalmol 71:682, 1993.

244. LeJeunne, C, Munera, Y, Hugues, F-C: Systemic effects of three β-blocker eyedrops: Comparison in healthy volunteers of β_1- and β_2-adrenoceptor inhibition. Clin Pharmacol Ther 47:578, 1990.

245. Graf-Grauwiller, T, Stümpfig, D, Flammer, J: Do beta-blockers cause vasospasm? Ophthalmologica 206:45, 1993.

246. Harris, A, Spaeth, GL, Sergott, RC, Katz, LJ, Cantor, LB, Martin, BJ: Retrobulbar arterial hemodynamic effects of betaxolol and timolol in normal-tension glaucoma. Am J Ophthalmol 120:168, 1995.

247. Orgül, S, Mansberger, S, Bacon, DR, Van Buskirk, EM, Cioffi, GA: Optic nerve vasomotor effects of topical beta-adrenergic antagonists in rabbits. Am J Ophthalmol 120:441, 1995.

248. Calugaru, M: The effect of topically applied levobunolol on the trabecular outflow of aqueous humor in open-angle glaucoma. Klin Monatsbl Augenheilkd 194:164, 1989.

249. Duzman, E, Ober, M, Scharrer, A, Leopold, IH: A clinical evaluation of the effects of topically applied levobunolol and timolol on increased intraocular pressure. Am J Ophthalmol 94:318, 1982.

250. Partamian, LG, Kass, MA, Gordon, M: A dose-response study of the effect of levobunolol on ocular hypertension. Am J Ophthalmol 95:229, 1983.

251. Bensinger, RE, Keates, EU, Gofman, JD, et al: Levobunolol. A three-month efficacy study in the treatment of glaucoma and ocular hypertension. Arch Ophthalmol 103:375, 1985.

252. Cinotti, A, Cinotti, D, Grant, W, et al: Levobunolol vs timolol for open-angle glaucoma and ocular hypertension. Am J Ophthalmol 99:11, 1985.

253. Long, D, Zimmerman, T, Spaeth, G, et al: Minimum concentration of levobunolol required to control intraocular pressure in patients with primary open-angle glaucoma or ocular hypertension. Am J Ophthalmol 99:18, 1985.

254. Berson, FG, Cohen, HB, Foerster, RJ, et al: Levobunolol compared with timolol for the long-term control of elevated intraocular pressure. Arch Ophthalmol 103:379, 1985.

255. Stryz, JR, Merte, HJ: A one-year comparison of 0.5% and 1.0% levobunolol with 0.5% timolol eye drops in the treatment of open-angle glaucoma. Klin Monatsbl Augenheilkd 187:537, 1985.

256. Freyler, H, Novack, GD, Menapace, R, et al: Comparison of ocular hypotensive efficacy and safety of levobunolol and timolol. Klin Monatsbl Augenheilkd 193:257, 1988.

257. Boozman, FW III, Carriker, R, Foerster, R, et al: Long-term evaluation of 0.25% levobunolol and timolol for therapy for elevated intraocular pressure. Arch Ophthalmol 106:614, 1988.

258. Berson, FG, Cinotti, A, Cohen, H, et al: Levobunolol. A beta-adrenoceptor antagonist effective in the long-term treatment of glaucoma. Ophthalmology 92:1271, 1985.

259. Geyer, O, Lazar, M, Novack, GD, et al: Levobunolol compared with timolol: a four-year study. Br J Ophthalmol 72:892, 1988.

260. The Levobunolol Study Group: Levobunolol. A four-year study of efficacy and safety in glaucoma treatment. Ophthalmology 96: 642, 1989.

261. Beehler, CC, Stewart, WC, MacDonald, DK, et al: A comparison of the ocular hypotensive efficacy of twice-daily 0.25% levobunolol to 0.5% timolol in patients previously treated with 0.5% timolol. J Glau 1:237:1992.

262. Krieglstein, GK, Novack, GD, Voepel, E, et al: Levobunolol and metipranolol: comparative ocular hypotensive efficacy, safety, and comfort. Br J Ophthalmol 71:250, 1987.

263. Long, DA, Johns, GE, Mullen, RS, et al: Levobunolol and betaxolol. A double-masked controlled comparison of efficacy and safety in patients with elevated intraocular pressure. Ophthalmology 95: 735, 1988.

264. Rakofsky, SI, Melamed, S, Cohen, JS, et al: A comparison of the ocular hypotensive efficacy of once-daily and twice-daily levobunolol treatment. Ophthalmology 96:8, 1989.

265. Derick, RJ, Robin, AL, Tielsch, J, et al: Once-daily versus twice-daily levobunolol (0.5%) therapy. A crossover study. Ophthalmology 99:424, 1992.

266. Wandel, T, Fishman, D, Novack, GD, et al: Ocular hypotensive efficacy of 0.25% levobunolol instilled once daily. Ophthalmology 95:252, 1988.

267. Wandel, T, Charap, AD, Lewis, RA, et al: Glaucoma treatment with once-daily levobunolol. Am J Ophthalmol 101:298, 1986.

268. Silverstone, D, Zimmerman, T, Choplin, N, et al: Evaluation of once-daily levobunolol 0.25% and timolol 0.25% therapy for increased intraocular pressure. Am J Ophthalmol 112:56, 1991.

269. Schwartz, JS, Christensen, RE, Lee, DA: Comparison of timolol maleate and levobunolol: Doses and volume per bottle. Arch Ophthalmol 107:17, 1989.

270. Charap, AD, Shin, DH, Petursson, G, et al: Effect of varying drop size on the efficacy and safety of a topical beta blocker. Ann Ophthalmol 21:351, 1989.

271. West, DR, Lischwe, D, Thompson, VM, Ide, CH: Comparative efficacy of the β-blockers for the prevention of increased intraocular pressure after cataract extraction. Am J Ophthalmol 106:168, 1988.

272. Silverstone, DE, Novack, GD, Kelley, EP, Chen, KS: Prophylactic treatment of intraocular pressure elevations after neodymium:YAG laser posterior capsulotomies and extracapsular cataract extractions with levobunolol. Ophthalmology 95:713, 1988.

273. Allen, RC, Robin, AL, Long, D, et al: A combination of levobunolol and dipivefrin for the treatment of glaucoma. Arch Ophthalmol 106:904, 1988.

274. Weiser, BA, Feldman, F, Ananthanarayan, CR, et al: Cardiovascular effects of levobunolol eyedrops in healthy subjects. Can J Ophthalmol 26:211, 1991.

275. Lewis, SE, Controlled comparison of the cardiovascular effects of levobunolol 0.25% ophthalmic solution and betaxolol 0.25% ophthalmic suspension. J Glau 3:308, 1994.

276. Harris, A, Shoemaker, JA, Burgoyne, J, et al: Acute effect of topical β-adrenergic antagonists on normal perimacular hemodynamics. J Glau 4:36, 1995.

277. Bosem, ME, Lusky, M, Weinreb, RN: Short-term effects of levobunolol on ocular pulsatile flow. Am J Ophthalmol 114:280, 1992.

278. Frishman, WH, Kostis, J: The significance of intrinsic sympathomimetic activity in beta-adrenoceptor blocking drugs. Cardiovasc Rev Rep 3:503, 1982.

279. Keates, EU, Friedland, BR, Stewart, RH, et al: Carteolol hydrochloride: controlled evaluations of its ocular hypotensive efficacy relative to its vehicle, and, in combination with pilocarpine, relative to timolol. J Glau 3:315–322, 1994.

280. Kitazawa, Y, Azuma, I, Takase, M: Evaluation of the effect of carteolol eyedrops for primary open-angle glaucoma and ocular hypertension. Igaku No Ayumi 127:859, 1983.

281. Negishi, C, Kanai, A, Nakajima, A, et al: Ocular effects of β-blocking agent carteolol on healthy volunteers and glaucoma patients. Jpn J Ophthalmol 25:464, 1981.

282. Scoville, B, Mueller, B, White, BG, Krieglstein, GK: A double-masked comparison of carteolol and timolol in ocular hypertension. Am J Ophthalmol 105:150, 1988.

283. Brazier, DJ, Smith, SE: Ocular and cardiovascular response to topical carteolol 2% and timolol 0.5% in healthy volunteers. Br J Ophthalmol 72:101, 1988.

284. Stewart, WC, Shields, MB, Allen, RC, et al: A three-month comparison of 1% and 2% Carteolol and 0.5% timolol in open-angle glaucoma. Graefes Arch Clin Exp Ophthalmol 229:258, 1991.

285. Duff, GR, Newcombe, RG: The 12-hour control of intraocular pressure on carteolol 2% twice daily. Br J Ophthalmol 72:890, 1988.

286. Duff, GR: A double-masked crossover study comparing the effects of carteolol 1% and 2% on intra-ocular pressure. Acta Ophthalmol 65:618, 1987.

287. Demailly, P, Allaire, C, Bron, V, Trinquand, C: Effectiveness and tolerance of β-blocker/pilocarpine combination eye drops in primary open-angle glaucoma and high intraocular pressure. J Glau 4:235, 1995.

288. Pillunat, L, Stodtmeister, R: Effect of different antiglaucomatous drugs on ocular perfusion pressures. J Ocular Pharmacol Ther 4:231, 1988.

289. Yamazaki, S, Baba, H, Tokoro, T: Effects of timolol and cartiolol on ocular pulsatile blood flow. Acta Soc Ophthalmol Jpn 96:973, 1992.

290. Grunwald, JE, Delehanty, J: Effect of topical carteolol on the normal human retinal circulation. Invest Ophthalmol Vis Sci 33:1853, 1992.

291. Flammer, J, Kitazawa, Y, Bonomi, L, et al: Influence of carteolol and timolol in IOP and visual fields in glaucoma: a multi-center, double-masked, prospective study. Eur J Ophthalmol 2:169, 1992.

292. Freedman, SF, Freedman, NJ, Shields, MB, et al: Effects of ocular carteolol and timolol on plasma high-density lipoprotein cholesterol level. Am J Ophthalmol 116:600, 1993.

293. Serle, JB, Lustgarten, JS, Podos, SM: A clinical trial of metipranolol, a noncardioselective beta-adrenergic antagonist, in ocular hypertension. Am J Ophthalmol 112:302, 1991.

294. Kruse, W: Metipranolol—a new beta-receptor blocking agent. Klin Monatsbl Augenheilkd 182:582, 1983.

295. Merte, HJ, Stryz, JR, Mertz, M: Comparative studies on initial pressure reduction using metipranolol 0.3% and timolol 0.25% in eyes with open-angle glaucoma. Klin Monatsbl Augenheilkd 182:286, 1983.

296. Schmitz Valckenberg, P: The use of metipranolol to prevent elevation of intraocular pressure after cataract extraction. Klin Monatsbl Augenheilkd 182:150, 1983.

297. Scharrer, A, Ober, M: Fixed combination of metipranolol 0.1% and pilocarpine 2% compared with the individual drugs in glaucoma therapy. A controlled, randomized clinical study for intraindividual comparison of efficacy and tolerance. Klin Monatsbl Augenheilkd 189:450, 1986.

298. Lyden, M, Applebaum, HJ: Effect of ophthalmic metipranolol and timolol on exercise-induced tachycardia. J Glau 4:124, 1995.

299. Le Jeunne, CL, Hughues, FC, Dufier, JL, et al: Bronchial and cardiovascular effects of ocular topical β-antagonists in asthmatic subjects: comparison of timolol, carteolol, and metipranolol. J Clin Pharmacol 29:97, 1989.

300. Draeger, J, Schneider, B, Winter, R: The local anesthetic action of metipranolol as compared to timolol. Klin Monatsbl Augenheilkd 182:210, 1983.

301. Akingbehin, T, Villada, JR: Metipranolol-associated granulomatous anterior uveitis. Br J Ophthalmol 75:519, 1991.

302. Akingbehin, T, Villada, JR, Walley, T: Metipranolol-induced adverse reactions: I. The rechallenge study. Eye 6:277, 1992.

303. Kessler, C, Christ, T: Incidence of uveitis in glaucoma patients using metipranolol. J Glau 2:166, 1993.

304. Schultz, JS, Hoenig, JA, Charles H: Possible bilateral anterior uveitis secondary to metipranolol (OptiPranolol) therapy. Arch Ophthalmol 111:1606, 1993.

305. Melles, RB, Wong, IG: Metipranolol-associated granulomatous iritis. Am J Ophthalmol 118:712, 1994.

306. Liu, JHK, Bartels, SP, Neufeld, AH: Effects of L- and D-timolol on cyclic AMP synthesis and intraocular pressure in water-loaded, albino and pigmented rabbits. Invest Ophthalmol Vis Sci 24:1276, 1983.

307. Keates, EU, Stone, R: The effect of D-timolol on intraocular pressure in patients with ocular hypertension. Am J Ophthalmol 98:73, 1984.

308. Share, NN, Lotti, VJ, Gautheron, P, et al: R-Enantiomer of timolol: a potential selective ocular antihypertensive agent. Graefes Arch Clin Exp Ophthalmol 221:234, 1984.

309. Wettrell, K, Pandolfi, M: Effect of topical atenolol on intraocular pressure. Br J Ophthalmol 61:334, 1977.

310. Elliot, MJ, Cullen, PM, Phillips, CI: Ocular hypotensive effect of atenolol (Tenormin, ICI). A new beta-adrenergic blocker. Br J Ophthalmol 59:296, 1975.

311. Stenkula, E, Wettrell, K: A dose-response study of oral atenolol administered once daily in patients with raised intra-ocular pressure. Graefes Arch Clin Exp Ophthalmol 218:96, 1982.

312. Tutton, MK, Smith, RJH: Comparison of ocular hypotensive effects of 3 dosages of oral atenolol. Br J Ophthalmol 67:664, 1983.

313. MacDonald, MJ, Cullen, PM, Phillips, CI: Atenolol versus propranolol. A comparison of ocular hypotensive effect of an oral dose. Br J Ophthalmol 60:789, 1976.

314. MacDonald, MJ, Gore, SM, Cullen, PM, Phillips, CI: Comparison of ocular hypotensive effects of acetazolamide and atenolol. Br J Ophthalmol 61:345, 1977.

315. Wettrell, K, Wilke, K, Pandolfi, M: Topical atenolol versus pilocarpine: a double-blind study of the effect on ocular tension. Br J Ophthalmol 62:292, 1978.

316. Phillips, CI, Gore, SM, Gunn, PM: Atenolol versus adrenaline eye drops and an evaluation of these two combined. Br J Ophthalmol 62:296, 1978.

317. Brenkman, RF: Long-term hypotensive effect of atenolol 4% eyedrops. Br J Ophthalmol 62:287, 1978.

318. Alm, A, Wickstrom, CP: Effects of systemic and topical administration of metoprolol on intraocular pressure in healthy subjects. Acta Ophthalmol 58:740, 1980.

319. Urner-Bloch, U, Bucheli, J, Elta, H, et al: Clinical trials of various glaucoma drugs acting on the adrenergic system. Klin Monatsbl Augenheilkd 176:555, 1980.

320. Calissendorff, B: Aqueous humour concentration of metoprolol after oral administration. Acta Ophthalmol 65:721, 1987.

321. Bucheli, J, Aeschlimann, J, Gloor, B: The influence of metoprolol eye drops on intraocular pressure. Klin Monatsbl Augenheilkd 177: 146, 1980.

322. Krieglstein, GK: The long-term ocular and systemic effects of topically applied metoprolol tartrate in glaucoma and ocular hypertension. Acta Ophthalmol 59:15, 1981.

323. Nielsen, PG, Ahrendt, N, Buhl, H, Byrn, E: Metoprolol eyedrops 3%, a short-term comparison with pilocarpine and a five-month follow-up study. Acta Ophthalmol 60:347, 1982.

324. Collignon-Brach, J, Weekers, R: Comparative clinical study of metoprolol and timolol. J Fr Ophthalmol 4:275, 1981.

325. Bonomi, L, Steindler, P: Effect of pindolol on intraocular pressure. Br J Ophthalmol 59:301, 1975.

326. Dausch, D, Gorlich, W, Honegger, H: Is pindolol suitable for the treatment of glaucoma? Klin Monatsbl Augenheilkd 184:536, 1984.

327. Smith, RJH, Blamires, T, Nagasubramanian, S, et al: Addition of pindolol to routine medical therapy: a clinical trial. Br J Ophthalmol 66:102, 1982.

328. Huuppone, R, Salminen, L: Transient corneal anaesthesia after topical pindolol in rabbits. Acta Ophthalmol 63:19, 1985.

329. Andréasson, S, Møller Jensen, K: Effect of pindolol on intraocular pressure in glaucoma: Pilot study and a randomised comparison with timolol. Br J Ophthalmol 67:228, 1983.

330. Dausch, D, Gorlich, W, Honegger, H: Clinical suitability of pindolol eye drops for the treatment of chronic open-angle glaucoma. Klin Monatsbl Augenheilkd 184:539, 1984.

331. Flammer, J, Robert, Y, Gloor, B: Influence of pindolol and timolol treatment on the visual fields of glaucoma patients. J Ocul Pharmacol Ther 2:305, 1986.

332. Williamson, J, Atta, HR, Kennedy, PA, Muir, JG: Effect of orally administered nadolol on the intraocular pressure in normal volunteers. Br J Ophthalmol 69:38, 1985.

333. Rennie, IG, Smerdon, DL: The effect of a once-daily oral dose of nadolol on intraocular pressure in normal volunteers. Am J Ophthalmol 100:445, 1985.

334. Duff, GR: The effect of twice daily nadolol on intraocular pressure. Am J Ophthalmol 104:343, 1987.

335. Duff, GR, Watt, AH, Graham, PA: A comparison of the effects of oral nadolol and topical timolol on intraocular pressure, blood pressure, and heart rate. Br J Ophthalmol 71:698, 1987.

336. Williamson, J, Young, JDH, Atta, H, et al: Comparative efficacy of orally and topically administered β blockers for chronic simple glaucoma. Br J Ophthalmol 69:41, 1985.

337. Krieglstein, GK: Nadolol eye drops in glaucoma and ocular hypertension: a controlled clinical study of dose response and duration of action. Graefes Arch Clin Exp Ophthalmol 217:309, 1981.

338. Krieglstein, GK, Mohamed, J: The comparative multiple-dose intraocular pressure responses of nadolol and timolol in glaucoma and ocular hypertension. Acta Ophthalmol 60:284, 1982.

339. Duzman, E, Chen, C-C, Anderson, J, et al: Diacetyl derivative of nadolol. I. Ocular pharmacology and short-term ocular hypotensive effect in glaucomatous eyes. Arch Ophthalmol 100:1916, 1982.

340. Duzman, E, Rosen, N, Lazar, M: Diacetyl nadolol: 3-month ocular hypotensive effect in glaucomatous eyes. Br J Ophthalmol 67:668, 1983.

341. Merte, HJ, Stryz, JR: Initial experience with the beta-blocker befunolol in the treatment of open angle glaucoma. Klin Monatsbl Augenheilkd 184:55, 1984.

342. Merte, HJ, Stryz, JR: Further experience with the β-blocker befunolol in treatment of open-angle glaucoma over a period of one year. Klin Monatsbl Augenheilkd 184:316, 1984.

343. Tanaka, Y, Nakaya, H, Yamada, Y, Nakamura, Y: Therapeutic results obtained in patients with glaucoma with alteration from 0.5% timolol eye solution to 0.5% befunolol eye solution. Folia Ophthalmol Jpn 36:741, 1985.

344. Krieglstein, GK, Gramer, E, Leydhecker, W: The ocular responses of oral administration of penbutolol in the glaucomatous patient. Acta Ophthalmol 58:608, 1980.

345. Wand, M, Grant, WM: Thymoxamine hydrochloride: an alpha-adrenergic blocker. Surv Ophthalmol 25:75, 1980.

346. Lee, DA, Brubaker, RF, Nagataki, S: Effect of thymoxamine on aqueous humor formation in the normal human eye as measured by fluorophotometry. Invest Ophthalmol Vis Sci 21:805, 1981.

347. Relf, SJ, Ghargozloo, NZ, Skuta, GL, et al: Thymoxamine reverses phenylephrine-induced mydriasis. Am J Ophthalmol 106: 251, 1988.

348. Small, S, Stewart-Jones, JH, Turner, P: Influence of thymoxamine on changes in pupil diameter and accommodation produced by homatropine and ephedrine. Br J Ophthalmol 60:132, 1978.

349. Grehn, F, Fleig, T, Schwarzmüller, E: Thymoxamine: A miotic for intraocular use. Graefes Arch Clin Exp Ophthalmol 224:174, 1986.

350. Halasa, AH, Rutkowski, PC: Thymoxamine therapy for angle-closure glaucoma. Arch Ophthalmol 90:177, 1973.

351. Wand, M, Grant, WM: Thymoxamine hydrochloride: effects on the facility of outflow and intraocular pressure. Invest Ophthalmol 15:400, 1976.

352. Wand, M, Grant, WM: Thymoxamine test: differentiating angle-closure glaucoma from open-angle glaucoma with narrow angles. Arch Ophthalmol 96:1009, 1978.

353. Campbell, DG: Pigmentary dispersion and glaucoma. A new theory. Arch Ophthalmol 97:1667, 1979.

354. Dixon, RS, Anderson, RL, Hatt, MU: The use of thymoxamine in eyelid retraction. Arch Ophthalmol 97:2147, 1979.

355. Iuglio, N: Ocular effects of topical application of dapiprazole in man. Glaucoma 6:110, 1984.

356. Oshika, T, Araie, M, Sugiyama, T, et al: Effect of bunazosin hydrochloride on intraocular pressure and aqueous humor dynamics in normotensive human eyes. Arch Ophthalmol 109:1569, 1991.

357. Trew, DR, Wright, LA, Smith, SE: Ocular responses in healthy subjects to topical bunazosin 0.3%—an α_1-adrenoceptor antagonist. Br J Ophthalmol 75:411–1991.

358. Smith, BR, Murray, DL, Leopold, IH: Influence of topically applied prazosin on the intraocular pressure of experimental animals. Arch Ophthalmol 97:1933, 1979.

359. Krupin, T, Feitl, M, Becker, B: Effect of prazosin on aqueous humor dynamics in rabbits. Arch Ophthalmol 98:1639, 1980.

360. Serle, JB, Stein, AJ, Podos, SM, Severin, CH: Corynanthine and aqueous humor dynamics in rabbits and monkeys. Arch Ophthalmol 102:1385, 1984.

361. Serle, JB, Podos, SM, Lustgarten, JS, et al: The effect of corynanthine on intraocular pressure in clinical trials. Ophthalmology 92:977, 1985.

362. Leopold, IH, Murray, DL: Ocular hypotensive action of labetalol. Am J Ophthalmol 88:427, 1979.

363. Murray, DL, Podos, SM, Wei, C-P, Leopold, IH: Ocular effects in normal rabbits of topically applied labetalol. A combined α- and β-adrenergic antagonist. Arch Ophthalmol 97:723, 1979.

364. Bonomi, L, Perfetti, S, Bellucci, R, et al: Ocular hypotensive action of labetalol in rabbit and human eyes. Graefes Arch Clin Exp Ophthalmol 217:175, 1981.

365. Krieglstein, GK, Kontic, D: Nadolol and labetalol. Comparative efficacy of two beta-blocking agents in glaucoma. Graefes Arch Clin Exp Ophthalmol 216:313, 1981

CARBONIC ANHYDRASE INHIBITORS

The carbonic anhydrase inhibitors are presently the only class of drugs that are commonly used as systemically-administered agents in chronic glaucoma therapy. With the recent introduction of topical carbonic anhydrase inhibitors, this class of drugs has assumed an increasingly important role in the management of glaucoma.

The prototype, acetazolamide, was introduced as an ocular hypotensive drug in 1954 (1), and most of our basic understanding of the carbonic anhydrase inhibitors comes from experience with this compound. Other commercially available members of this drug class include the oral agents, methazolamide, dichlorphenamide, and ethoxyzolamide, and the topical agent, dorzolamide. The carbonic anhydrase inhibitors all share the same basic mechanisms of action. Side effects with the oral compounds essentially differ only in degree, while those with the topical drugs are significantly less. We will first consider these common aspects of the carbonic anhydrase inhibitors before discussing unique features of the individual oral and topical compounds.

MECHANISMS OF ACTION

Carbonic Anhydrase

Carbonic anhydrase (CA) is an enzyme that is responsible for the catalytic hydration of CO_2 and dehydration of H_2CO_3:

$$CO_2 + H_2O \underset{CA}{\rightleftarrows} H_2CO_3 \rightleftarrows HCO_3^- + H^+$$

The enzyme exists in several isoenzyme forms throughout the body, but in the ciliary processes of human eyes it is almost purely CA II (formerly called type C) (2–4). Histochemical studies of animal and human eyes have revealed carbonic anhydrase in the pigmented and nonpigmented epithelium of the ciliary body, most prominently in the basal and lateral membranes (5, 6). Clear-cut regional differences have been observed in the nonpigmented ciliary epithelium of human and monkey eyes, which coincide with morphologic indicators of secretory activity (6). Theories as to how carbonic anhydrase relates to aqueous production were discussed in Chapter 3. The most likely explanation is that it helps to maintain a pH that is optimum for the enzymes involved in ion transport.

Carbonic Anhydrase Inhibition

The carbonic anhydrase inhibitors belong to the sulfonamide class of drugs. They have an active moiety, which is identical to carbonic acid and complimentary to carbonic anhydrase, that interferes with the function of the enzyme. The failure of acetazolamide to decrease intraocular pressure (IOP) in patients with carbonic anhydrase type II deficiency suggests that it is this isozyme that the drug inhibits (7).

The carbonic anhydrase inhibitors lower IOP by reducing aqueous humor formation. Fluorophotometric studies indicate that acetazolamide decreases aqueous flow during the day in the human eye by 21% (8) to 27% (9). Unlike the nonselective β-adrenergic inhibitor timolol, which has no statistically significant effect on the flow rate in sleeping subjects, acetazolamide has been shown to reduce the already low nocturnal flow rate by an additional 24% (8). When added to timolol, which alone reduced daytime flow by 33%, the combination of the two aqueous suppressants reduced the flow rate by 44% (9). Oral acetazolamide increases aqueous protein concentration, the measurement of which has been used to monitor the time change of its effect on aqueous flow rate. Using this technique, a maximum reduction in flow rate of 40 ± 11% was calculated at 1.75 hours after administration of the drug (10). The mechanism by which a reduction in aqueous production is accomplished is uncertain, but the following theories have been considered.

Ion Transport

Ion transport associated with secretion of aqueous humor may be altered by the inhibition of carbonic anhydrase, possibly by creation of a local acid environment (11). The principal ion that appears to be effected by carbonic anhydrase inhibitors differs according to the animal model being studied (11–13) and has not been established in human eyes.

Metabolic Acidosis

Metabolic acidosis is known to reduce IOP and has been proposed as the mechanism of action for oral carbonic anhydrase inhibitors (14). However, studies have shown that the ocular hypotensive effect of these drugs is neither time-related to the metabolic acidosis (15) nor dependent upon alterations of pH in the blood (16–18) or aqueous (18). Nevertheless, strong oral carbonic anhydrase inhibitors, which do create a metabolic acidosis, may exert an additional pressure lowering effect by this mechanism.

Blood Flow

It has been suggested that the acetazolamide-induced acidosis may improve visual function in glaucoma patients by increasing blood flow to the optic nerve, since visual field improvement has been documented following administration of the drug, independent of a change in perfusion pressure (19). Acetazolamide was shown to significantly influence flow velocity in the middle cerebral artery of the brain, although it had less effect on the ophthalmic and central retinal arteries (20), and a study with the blue-field simulation technique revealed no significant effect of acetazolamide on macular leukocyte velocity, or presumably on blood flow (21). Furthermore, although acetazolamide was shown to reduce the venous pressure of the cat eye, which paralleled the IOP fall (22), ocular blood flow does not appear to be involved in the pressure lowering action of this drug (23).

Other Observations

An *adrenergic effect* of carbonic anhydrase inhibitors has also been considered since the action of acetazolamide in dogs was found to be altered by adrenalectomy or adrenergic-blocking agents (24). The *diuretic effect* of the carbonic anhydrase inhibitors is not a factor in the reduction of IOP (25, 26). Whole-blood levels of zinc, a component of carbonic anhydrase, are increased in patients receiving carbonic anhydrase inhibitors, suggesting that the drug induces synthesis of the enzyme (27).

Other Applications of Carbonic Anhydrase Inhibitors

Carbonic anhydrase has also been demonstrated in the *retina* (4) and appears to be related to fluid movement from the retina toward the choroid (28). Acetazolamide has been shown to increase the rate of subretinal fluid absorption in experimental retinal detachment (28, 29) and to increase the adhesion between retina and pigment epithelium (30). It may also be effective in the treatment of macular edema in patients with retinal pigment epithelial cell disease (31–33) and chronic iridocyclitis (34), although not macular edema associated with primary retinal vascular diseases (31).

ADMINISTRATION

Routes of Delivery

It was once believed that the carbonic anhydrase inhibitors were only effective when given orally, intramuscularly, or intravenously. While these routes of delivery, especially the oral, are still used in clinical practice, more recent research has disclosed that some carbonic anhydrase inhibitors are also effective when delivered topically.

Dose-Response Curve

The dose-response curve for carbonic anhydrase inhibitors is very restricted in that aqueous production is not significantly reduced until more than 90% of the carbonic anhydrase activity is inhibited (35). For this reason, it is important that the drug not be used in inadequate doses (36). However, it may be that some of the systemic dosages in common use exceed that required for maximum benefit, which is considered in the discussion of the individual carbonic anhydrase inhibitors.

Distribution and Metabolism

Carbonic anhydrase inhibitors are not distributed randomly throughout the body fluids, but have a preferential affinity for certain tissues, including the iris and ciliary processes (37). The drugs are not metabolized, but are excreted unchanged in the urine.

SIDE EFFECTS

Ocular Side Effects

The only ocular reaction that has been clearly identified with the systemic administration of carbonic anhydrase inhibitors is an idiosyncratic, transient *myopia,* which is a sulfonamide-related reaction (38). Ultrasonography of a patient with induced myopia associated with sulfonamide therapy revealed shallowing of the anterior chamber without thickening of the lens, suggesting that ciliary body edema might cause forward movement of the lens-iris diaphragm (39). A case of bilateral transient myopia, angle-closure glaucoma, and choroidal detachment was described following oral administration of acetazolamide 500 mg prior to cataract surgery (40). The mechanism of angle closure was felt to be forward shift of the lens-iris diaphragm due to the choroidal detachment, rather than a change in lens thickness, since one eye was pseudophakic. The patient had asymptomatic exposure to the drug before the first cataract procedure, which is typical of ocular idiosyncratic reactions to acetazolamide.

Topical carbonic anhydrase inhibitors have minimal ocular adverse reactions, primarily associated with irritation immediately after instillation and occasional hypersensitivity reactions. The topical agents are considered in more detail later in this chapter.

Systemic Side Effects

Systemic side effects are common with oral carbonic anhydrase inhibitor therapy, frequently necessitating discontinuation of these drugs, while they are rare with topical therapy. *Paresthesias* of the fingers, toes, and around the mouth is a common side effect, and *urinary frequency* from the diuretic action is experienced by nearly all patients initially. However, both of these effects are usually transient and of no serious consequence.

Serum Electrolyte Imbalances

Serum electrolyte imbalances may create more debilitating problems.

Metabolic acidosis, associated with bicarbonate depletion, occurs with the higher dosages of carbonic anhydrase inhibitors and should be avoided in patients with hepatic insufficiency, renal failure, adrenocortical insufficiency, hyperchloremic acidosis, depressed sodium or potassium levels, or severe pulmonary obstruction (41). The risk in patients with liver disease was reemphasized in a case report of a patient with cirrhosis who developed hepatic encephalopathy due to

ammonia intoxication within days after starting acetazolamide therapy (42). The risk of metabolic acidosis with carbonic anhydrase inhibitor therapy is especially common among elderly patients (43).

A *symptom complex* of malaise, fatigue, weight loss, anorexia, depression, and decreased libido is not uncommon in patients on oral carbonic anhydrase inhibitor therapy (44, 45). It has been correlated with the degree of metabolic acidosis, and preliminary experience suggests that treatment with sodium bicarbonate (44) or sodium acetate (46) may help to minimize this situation. It has also been reported that combined therapy with a carbonic anhydrase inhibitor and aspirin may cause serious acid-base imbalance and salicylate intoxication (47).

Potassium depletion may occur during the initial phase of carbonic anhydrase inhibitor therapy, due to increased urinary excretion, especially if diuresis is brisk, and is the apparent explanation for the frequent paresthesias. However, this is normally transient (48) and does not lead to significant hypokalemia unless it is given concomitantly with chlorothiazide diuretics, digitalis, corticosteroids, or ACTH, or in patients with hepatic cirrhosis. Potassium supplement is only indicated when significant hypokalemia is documented (49). Hyperkalemic and hyperchloremic metabolic acidosis has also been described in an elderly patient on carbonic anhydrase inhibitor therapy for glaucoma, which was felt to be due to transcellular movement of potassium and limited potassium secretion due to mild renal failure (50).

Serum sodium and chloride may also be transiently reduced, the latter occurring primarily with dichlorphenamide.

Gastrointestinal Symptoms

Gastrointestinal symptoms are also very common and include vague abdominal discomfort, a peculiar metallic taste, nausea, and diarrhea. These symptoms do not appear to be related to any serum chemical change, and the cause is unknown. Taking the medication with meals may help to reduce the symptoms in some cases (44).

Sulfonamide-Related Reactions

The following side effects are common to the sulfonamide group of drugs, and constitute the most serious adverse reactions related to carbonic anhydrase inhibitor therapy.

Renal calculi formation has been shown to be increased in patients receiving acetazolamide (51). The precise mechanism is unknown, but there may be an association with reduced excretion of urinary citrate (52) or magnesium (38), since both are believed to help keep calcium salts in solution. An alkaline urine is also known to predispose to precipitation of calcium salts, and this has been proposed as the mechanism of urolithiasis associated with carbonic anhydrase inhibitor therapy (53, 54). However, it has been shown that the urinary pH returns to pretreatment levels once the initial acetazolamide-induced bicarbonate diuresis subsides (55), and some patients with renal stones during acetazolamide therapy may actually have an acidic urine (56). Renal colic may also be associated with carbonic anhydrase inhibitor therapy and may rarely be accompanied by hematuria or anuria (57).

Blood dyscrasias are rare, but thrombocytopenia, agranulocytosis, aplastic anemia, and neutropenia have been reported with acetazolamide or methazolamide therapy (58–62). The National Registry of Drug-induced Ocular Side Effects received 79 case reports, as of 1985, of suspected hematologic reactions to oral carbonic anhydrase inhibitor therapy, of which 26 were fatal (61). The authors of that report recommended that, in addition to warning the patient to report a persistent sore throat, fever, fatigue, pallor, easy bruising, epistaxis, purpura, or jaundice, a complete blood count should be obtained before initiating therapy and every 6 months thereafter. The latter recommendation led to considerable controversy within the ophthalmic community. A survey revealed that the vast majority of ophthalmologists who responded do not routinely monitor blood counts of patients on carbonic anhydrase inhibitor therapy, and the authors of that report suggested that routine blood monitoring is of questionable value because of the idiosyncratic, nondose-related nature of the dyscrasias and the variability of their onset (62).

There is clearly a division of opinion on this issue, although an editorial on the subject provided a well-balanced perspective (63). The authors began by noting that agranulocytosis and thrombocytopenia are nearly always acute in onset with initial clinical features of acute bacterial infection and bleeding, respectively. They cannot be predicted by monitoring blood cell counts, and are completely reversible upon cessation of the drug. Aplastic anemia, on the other hand, typically has a delayed, insidious onset and is frequently fatal. Most cases occur within less than 6 months of initiating therapy, and some patients have been known to recover after stopping the drug. To be most effective, blood cell counts (hematocrit, white blood cell count, and platelet count) should be obtained initially and every two months for the first 6 months. It is estimated, however, that this would cost approximately $1,500,000 for each life saved from aplastic anemia. The authors concluded that "a physician should not be regarded as negligent if he or she does not routinely monitor blood cell counts" but that "a physician who does so cannot be accused of thoughtlessly squandering health resources" (63).

Other sulfonamide-related side effects include exfoliative dermatitis, hypersensitive nephropathy, and the previously discussed acute myopia (38). Methazolamide therapy has been associated with maculopapular and urticarial types of skin eruptions (64), as well as Stevens-Johnson syndrome (65).

Other Adverse Reactions

Other adverse reactions that have been reported in association with oral carbonic anhydrase inhibitor therapy include elevated blood uric acid (38), hirsutism (66), and a transient (30 minutes) elevation of cerebral blood flow and cerebrospinal fluid pressure (38). Teratogenic effects have been observed in rats (67) and in one human case, although the mother was also on the anticholinergic, dicyclomine, during weeks 8–12 of pregnancy (68). Caution during pregnancy is advised. It has also been noted that an oral hypoglycemic agent, acetohexamide, has been inadvertently substituted for acetazolamide because of the similar names (69, 70).

The adverse reactions noted earlier for systemic carbonic anhydrase inhibitors appear to be more frequent and debilitating in the older age population, with patients 40 years of age or less having a significantly higher incidence of long-term tolerance (71). Measures that may help to reduce the side effects, as previously noted, include supplemental alkali therapy and taking the medication with meals. It has also been noted that some patients who cannot tolerate one form of oral carbonic anhydrase inhibitor will do better with another agent or with a lower dose of the drug (72). Undoubtedly the most significant advance in reducing the systemic side effects of the carbonic anhydrase inhibitors has been the introduction of the topical agents, which is discussed later in this chapter.

SYSTEMIC CARBONIC ANHYDRASE INHIBITORS (TABLE 28.1)

Acetazolamide

As previously noted, acetazolamide is the prototype of the carbonic anhydrase inhibitors, and most of the preceding information in this chapter was based on experience with this drug.

Table 28.1.
COMMERCIAL CARBONIC
ANHYDRASE INHIBITORS*

Generic Preparations	*Brand Names*	*Strengths*
Oral		
Acetazolamide	Diamox, tablets	125, 250 mg
	Diamox sequels	500 mg
	Diamox, parenteral	500 mg/vial
Methazolamide	Neptazane	25, 50 mg
	Glauctabs	25, 50 mg
	MZM	25, 50 mg
Dichlorphenamide	Daranide	50 mg
Topical		
Dorzolamide	Trusopt	2%

Other generic products may also be available.

Administration

The traditional oral dosage for long-term therapy in adults is 250 mg tablets every 6 hours or 500 mg sustained-release capsules twice a day. However, a single-dose study showed that 63 mg gave the maximum effect on the IOP (73). In the same study, 250 mg gave a slightly longer duration of action, but 500 mg had no advantage. However, in a study of open-angle glaucoma patients, uncontrolled on maximum topical therapy, there was a consistent, positive dose response to acetazolamide 125-, 250-, and 500-mg tablets and acetazolamide 500- and 1000-mg sustained-release capsules (74). A daily 500-mg sustained-release capsule was shown to provide a substantial pressure-lowering effect for at least 23 hours, although one capsule twice a day was more effective than the daily dose in controlling the pressure (75). Twice daily 500-mg sustained-release capsules is equivalent to one 250-mg tablet every 6 hours (75, 76). The analgesic, diflunisal 500 mg twice daily, has been shown to increase total plasma concentrations and the IOP-lowering effect of acetazolamide, when the two drugs are given concomitantly (77). The recommended dose of acetazolamide for children is 5–10 mg/Kg of body weight every 4–6 hours (78).

In tablet form, the ocular hypotensive effect peaks in 2 hours and lasts up to 6 hours, while that of the capsule peaks in 8 hours and persists beyond 12 hours. For more rapid action, the drug may be given intravenously, which provides a peak effect in 15 minutes and a duration of 4 hours. A useful routine for emergency situations, such as acute angle-closure glaucoma, is to give 250 mg intramuscularly and 250 mg intravenously.

Metabolic acidosis is greater with intravenous injections of acetazolamide than with oral administration (14). The acidosis associated with chronic oral therapy is such, however, that the reduced serum carbon dioxide level is said to be a useful indicator of compliance with acetazolamide therapy (79). An oral drug delivery system has been investigated, which releases acetazolamide at a rate of 15 mg/hour and is reported to cause fewer side effects (80).

Advantages

The main advantage of acetazolamide over the other oral carbonic anhydrase inhibitors is that more is known about the drug by virtue of larger laboratory and clinical experience. In one study, acetazolamide sustained-release capsules, given twice daily, were found in a crossover, randomized study to be better tolerated than four times daily dosages of methazolamide 50 mg (which was the next best tolerated), ethoxyzolamide 125 mg, acetazolamide 250 mg, or dichlorphenamide 50 mg (81). However, another study found acetazolamide 250 mg twice daily and the 500-mg sustained-release formulation at bedtime to be comparable in efficiency and in frequency and severity of side effects (82). Generic acetazolamide tablets are commercially available and have been shown to be comparable to the brand-name acetazolamide in IOP reduction and blood levels of the drug, while providing a significant cost savings (83).

Methazolamide

Administration

Although methazolamide has been recommended in dosages of up to 100 mg three times daily (78), studies suggest that considerably less is needed in most cases to provide the desired therapeutic effect (84–87). A dose of 25 mg twice daily was found to produce significant IOP reduction without metabolic acidosis (84, 85). Studies differ as to whether higher doses of methazolamide produce additional pressure reduction (85, 86), but a 500-mg sustained release capsule of acetazolamide was shown to have a greater ocular hypotensive effect than either 25 or 50 mg of methazolamide (86). A suggested regimen for the titrated use of carbonic anhydrase inhibitor therapy is to begin with methazolamide 25 mg twice a day, advancing to 50 mg of methazolamide twice daily if necessary, and finally to the acetazolamide 500-mg sustained-release capsule twice a day as required to achieve the desired effect (88).

Advantages

The main advantage of methazolamide is that the drug can be used in smaller dosages, which causes fewer side effects. This is due to low protein binding, which allows the drug to diffuse more readily into tissue and thereby be more active on a weight basis in reducing aqueous production (84, 85). It also has a significantly longer plasma half-life than acetazolamide. In addition, there is evidence that methazolamide causes significantly less renal side effects (52, 89) although renal stone formation during methazolamide therapy has been reported (90, 91).

Dichlorphenamide

The recommended dosage of this carbonic anhydrase inhibitor is 25–100 mg three times a day. Its greater potency is probably due to a double molecular configuration resembling carbonic acid. The drug causes less metabolic acidosis, due to increased chloride excretion, but often has sustained diuresis with chronic use (78).

Ethoxyzolamide

This carbonic anhydrase inhibitor is given in a dosage of 125 mg every 6 hours and is similar in action and side effects to acetazolamide (78).

TOPICAL CARBONIC ANHYDRASE INHIBITORS[a]

Early Experience

With the numerous and significant side effects associated with oral and parenteral administration of carbonic anhydrase inhibitors, there was an obvious need for topical forms of these drugs that concentrate the effect in the eye and reduce adverse system reactions. Early experience with acetazolamide revealed no ocular hypotensive effect when given topically or subconjunctivally (26). This was initially felt to indicate that an effect on carbonic anhydrase in the blood was necessary for the action of carbonic anhydrase inhibitors on aqueous humor formation. It was subsequently learned, however, that limited ocular penetration, which resulted in an insufficient amount of drug reaching the ciliary body, was the primary explanation for the poor topical response in the early studies. This observation led to a considerable amount of investigation into new vehicles and forms of carbonic anhydrase inhibitors to enhance the topical delivery of these drugs.

In rabbit studies, topical administration of acetazolamide was shown to blunt a water-induced ocular hypertensive response (92, 93) and both acetazolamide and methazolamide, delivered topically by high-water-content soft contact lenses, produced significant IOP reduction in albino rabbits (94). In vitro studies of human and rabbit cornea revealed similar permeability to methazolamide and ethoxyzolamide, although in vivo studies showed that topical methazolamide produced markedly higher aqueous concentrations in rabbit than in human eyes (95). This discrepancy was thought possibly to be due to a relatively greater blinking rate and tear turnover and a lower corneal/conjunctival area in humans. In any case, it further emphasized the need for new forms of carbonic anhydrase inhibitors for topical delivery.

Evaluation of New Compounds

Newer carbonic anhydrase inhibitors, which combine certain elements of water- and lipid-solubility to enhance corneal penetration, were shown to effectively lower aqueous production and IOP in rabbits. Examples of such drugs included *trifluoromethazolamide,* a halogenated derivative of methazolamide (96), *6-hydroxyethoxyzolamide,* an analogue of ethoxyzolamide (97), and L-645,151, which is also structurally related to ethoxyzolamide (98). The latter drug was limited by hypersensitivity reaction and never tried clinically (99). Clinical experience with another ethoxyzolamide analogue, *aminozolamide* gel, revealed a significant

lowering of IOP (100), which lasted about 8 hours but was associated with a high incidence of bulbar injection and follicular conjunctivitis (101).

A considerable amount of research was performed with the topical carbonic anhydrase inhibitor, *MK-927,* the hydrochloride salt of an amino-substituted heteroaromatic sulfonamide. Topical MK-927 was shown to lower the IOP in normotensive rabbits (102) and glaucomatous monkeys (103). The concentration of the drug reaching the ciliary processes of rabbit eyes was similar to that of parenteral sulfonamides, indicating that inhibition of carbonic anhydrase exceeds 99% (104). Increasing the ionization of MK-927 was found to increase the ocular hypotensive activity by sequestering the drug in the cornea, leading to prolonged drug delivery and activity (105). Three drops of MK-927 2% administered within 70 minutes produced significant IOP reduction in both normal volunteers (106) and patients with chronic open-angle glaucoma or ocular hypertension (107), with no contralateral effect in either group. A single dose of MK-927 2% in open-angle glaucoma patients and ocular hypertensives gave a peak mean IOP reduction of 10.5 mm Hg at 4.5 hours postdose (108). Dose response studies indicated that MK-927 0.125% and 0.5% had little or no effect on IOP, while a 1% concentration produced a significantly greater pressure reduction than a placebo for up to 6 hours, and the 2% preparation caused further lowering of IOP with a duration of 8 hours (109–111). However, even MK-927 2% had less ocular hypotensive activity than systemic agents such as methazolamide, which may relate to the additional effect of metabolic acidosis with the oral compounds (109), and there was considerable variability in peak response to single doses within individual patients (110).

The search for a better topical carbonic anhydrase inhibitor led to the evaluation of *sezolamide* (MK-417), the pharmacologically more active S-enantiomer of MK-927. When sezolamide 1.8% and MK-927 2% were compared in glaucoma patients, both were well-tolerated with mild burning and tearing, but no effect on pupil size or other side effects (112). Sezolamide, however, was found to have slightly greater IOP-lowering activity than MK-927 (112, 113).

Dorzolamide

This analogue of MK-927 (previously designated L-671,152 or MK-507) was found to be superior to either MK-927 or sezolamide, and was approved in the United States in 1995 for the chronic management of glaucoma.

Laboratory Research

Dorzolamide has been shown to be a more potent inhibitor of human erythrocyte CAII than MK-927 and to have a greater and more prolonged effect in rabbit and monkey studies (114, 115). As with other carbonic anhydrase inhibitors it lowers the IOP by reducing aqueous humor flow (116).

Clinical Trials

In a 4-week safety and efficacy study, dorzolamide 2% three times daily showed peak IOP activity 2 hours after administration, with an average IOP reduction on day 29 of 18.4% (117). In that study, CA II activity in red blood cells decreased 21% and the mean corneal thickness increased slightly. When compared with sezolamide 1.8% in two clinical trials with open-angle glaucoma patients or ocular hypertensives, dorzolamide 2% gave slightly better peak mean IOP reductions of 22.1% and 26.2%, compared to 21.3% and 22.5% with sezolamide, although the differences were not statistically significant (118–119). In an open-label study, dorzolamide 1% reduced the IOP 16.7–24.1% at 2 hours after administration and 12.9–17.5% at 8 hours, which was consistent for the 52-week trial (120).

Clinical Indications

Dorzolamide is commercially available in a 2% formulation, and the recommended dosage is three times daily. When compared to timolol 0.5% and betaxolol 0.5%, both given twice daily, in a 1-year trial, the mean percent IOP reduction with dorzolamide was 23%, compared to 25% and 21% with timolol and betaxolol, respectively (121). When compared with pilocarpine four times daily as a second drug in patients not controlled on timolol 0.5%, dorzolamide gave comparable additional IOP reduction, but was preferred by patients 7 to 1 because of reduced side effects (122).

Dorzolamide has minimal ocular side effects, which primarily include irritation and occasional hypersensitivity reaction. The influence on corneal thickness has not yet been confirmed, and no clinically significant corneal problems have been reported. The main advantage of dorzolamide is the marked reduction in systemic side effects associated with the oral agents. However, mild systemic reactions may occur in some patients, and the risk of idiosyncratic blood dyscrasias has yet to be established.

SUMMARY

Carbonic anhydrase inhibitors lower IOP by reducing aqueous production, probably through an alteration in ion transport associated with secretion of aqueous humor. The numerous systemic side effects of oral carbonic anhydrase inhibitors include diuresis, paresthesias, malaise, anorexia, serum electrolyte imbalances, gastrointestinal upset, renal calculi, and blood dyscrasias. The oral drugs in this class, which differ primarily only in degree of side effects, include acetazolamide, methazolamide, dichlorphenamide, and ethoxyzolamide. The topical carbonic anhydrase, dorzolamide, has the significant advantage of rare systemic side effects.

REFERENCES

1. Becker, B: Decrease in intraocular pressure in man by a carbonic anhydrase inhibitor, Diamox. Am J Ophthalmol 37:13, 1954.
2. Dobbs, PC, Epstein, DL, Anderson, PF: Identification of isoenzyme C as the principal carbonic anhydrase in human ciliary processes. Invest Ophthalmol Vis Sci 18:867, 1979.
3. Wistrand, PJ, Garg, LC: Evidence of a high-activity C type of carbonic anhydrase in human ciliary processes. Invest Ophthalmol Vis Sci 18:802, 1979.
4. Wistrand, PJ, Schenholm, M, Lönnerholm, G: Carbonic anhydrase isoenzymes CA I and CA II in the human eye. Invest Ophthalmol Vis Sci 27:419, 1986.
5. Lutgen-Drecoll, E, Lönnerholm, G: Carbonic anhydrase distribution in the rabbit eye by light and electron microscopy. Invest Ophthalmol Vis Sci 21:782, 1981.
6. Lutjen-Drecoll, E, Lönnerholm, G, Eichhorn, M: Carbonic anhydrase distribution in the human and monkey eye by light and electron microscopy. Graefes Arch Clin Exp Ophthalmol 220:285, 1983.
7. Krupin, T, Sly, WS, Whyte, MP, Dodgson, SJ: Failure of acetazolamide to decrease intraocular pressure in patients with carbonic anhydrase II deficiency. Am J Ophthalmol 99:396, 1985.
8. McCannel, CA, Heinrich, SR, Brubaker, RF: Acetazolamide but not timolol lowers aqueous humor flow in sleeping humans. Graefes Arch Clin Exp Ophthalmol 230:518, 1992.
9. Dailey, RA, Brubaker, RF, Bourne, WM: The effects of timolol maleate and acetazolamide on the rate of aqueous formation in normal human subjects. Am J Ophthalmol 93:232, 1982.
10. Oshika, T, Araie, M: Time course of changes in aqueous protein concentration flow rate after oral acetazolamide. Invest Ophthalmol Vis Sci 31:527, 1990.
11. Berggren, L: Direct observation of secretory pumping in vitro of the rabbit eye ciliary processes. Influence of ion milieu and carbonic anhydrase inhibition. Invest Ophthalmol 3:266, 1964.
12. Maren, TH: The rates of movement of Na+, Cl-, and HCO3- from plasma to posterior chamber: effect of acetazolamide and relation to the treatment of glaucoma. Invest Ophthalmol 15:356, 1976.
13. Holland, MG, Gipson, CC: Chloride ion transport in the isolated ciliary body. Invest Ophthalmol 9:20, 1970.
14. Bietti, G, Virno, M, Pecori-Giraldi, J, Pellegrino, N: Acetazolamide, metabolic acidosis, and intraocular pressure. Am J Ophthalmol 80:360, 1975.
15. Soser, M, Ogriseg, M, Kessler, B, Zirm, H: New findings concerning changes in intraocular pressure and blood acidosis after peroral application of acetazolamide. Klin Monatsbl Augenheilkd 176:88, 1980.
16. Benedikt, O, Zirm, M, Harnoncourt, K: Relations between metabolic acidosis and intraocular pressure after inhibition of carbonic anhydrase with acetazolamide. Graefes Arch Clin Exp Ophthalmol 190:247, 1974.
17. Friedman, Zvi, Krupin, T, Becker, B: Ocular and systemic effects of acetazolamide in nephrectomized rabbits. Invest Ophthalmol Vis Sci 23:209, 1982.
18. Mehra, KS: Relationship of pH of aqueous and blood with acetazolamide. Ann Ophthalmol 11:63, 1979.
19. Flammer, J, Drance, SM: Effect of acetazolamide on the differential threshold. Arch Ophthalmol 101:1378, 1983.
20. Harris, A, Tippke, S, Sievers, C, et al: Acetazolamide and CO2: acute effects on cerebral and retrobulbar hemodynamics. J Glau 5:39, 1996.
21. Grunwald, JE, Zinn, H: The acute effect of oral acetazolamide on macular blood flow. Invest Ophthalmolmol Vis Sci 33:504, 1992.
22. Macri, FJ: Acetazolamide and the venous pressure of the eye. Arch Ophthalmol 63:953, 1960.
23. Bill, A: Effects of acetazolamide and carotid occlusion on the ocular blood flow in unanesthetized rabbits. Invest Ophthalmol 13:954, 1974.

24. Thomas, RP, Riley, MW: Acetazolamide and ocular tension. Notes concerning the mechanism of action. Am J Ophthalmol 60:241, 1965.

25. Peczon, JD, Grant, WM: Diuretic drugs in glaucoma. Am J Ophthalmol 66:680, 1968.

26. Becker, B: The mechanism of the fall in intraocular pressure induced by the carbonic anhydrase inhibitor, Diamox. Am J Ophthalmol 39:177, 1955.

27. Walker, AM, Arrigg, C, Hertzmark, E, Epstein, DL: Carbonic anhydrase inhibitors induce elevations in human whole-blood zinc levels. Arch Ophthalmol 102:1785, 1984.

28. Tsuboi, S, Pederson, J: Experimental retinal detachment: X. Effect of acetazolamide on vitreous fluorescein disappearance. Arch Ophthalmol 103:1557, 1985.

29. Marmor, MF, Negi, A: Pharmacologic modifications of subretinal fluid absorption in the rabbit eye. Arch Ophthalmol 104:1674, 1986.

30. Marmor, MF, Maack, T: Enhancement of retinal adhesion and subretinal fluid resorption by acetazolamide. Invest Ophthalmol Vis Sci 23:121, 1982.

31. Cox, SN, Hay, E, Bird, AC: Treatment of chronic macular edema with acetazolamide. Arch Ophthalmol 106:1190, 1988.

32. Fishman, GA, Gilbert, LD, Fiscella, RG, et al: Acetazolamide for treatment of chronic macular edema in retinitis pigmentosa. Arch Ophthalmol 107:1445, 1989.

33. Chen, JC, Fitzke, FW, Bird, AC: Long-term effect of acetazolamide in a patient with retinitis pigmentosa. Invest Ophthalmol Vis Sci 31:1914, 1990.

34. Farber, MD, Lam, S, Tessler, HH, et al: Reduction of macular oedema by acetazolamide in patients with chronic iridocyclitis: a randomised prospective crossover study. Br J Ophthalmol 78:4, 1994.

35. Friedenwald, JS: Current studies on acetazoleamide (Diamox) and aqueous humor flow. Am J Ophthalmol 40:139, 1955.

36. Becker, B: Misuse of acetazolamide. Am J Ophthalmol 43:799, 1957.

37. Goren, SB, Newell, FW, O'Toole, JJ: The localization of Diamox-S[35] in the rabbit eye. Am J Ophthalmol 51:87, 1961.

38. Grant, WM: Antiglaucoma drugs: problems with carbonic anhydrase inhibitors. In: Symposium on Ocular Therapy. Volume 6. Leopold, IH, ed. St. Louis, CV Mosby, 1972, p. 19.

39. Bovino, JA, Marcus, DF: The mechanism of transient myopia induced by sulfonamide therapy. Am J Ophthalmol 94:99, 1982.

40. Fan, JT, Johnson, DH, Burk, RR: Transient myopia, angle-closure glaucoma, and choroidal detachment after oral acetazolamide. Am J Ophthalmol 115:813, 1993.

41. Block, ER, Rostand, RA: Carbonic anhydrase inhibition in glaucoma: hazard or benefit for the chronic lunger? Surv Ophthalmol 23:169, 1978.

42. Margo, CE: Acetazolamide and advanced liver disease. Am J Ophthalmol 101:611, 1986.

43. Heller, I, Halevy, J, Cohen, S, Theodor, E: Significant metabolic acidosis induced by acetazolamide: not a rare complication. Arch Intern Med 145:1815, 1985.

44. Epstein, DL, Grant, WM: Carbonic anhydrase inhibitor side effects. Serum chemical analysis. Arch Ophthalmol 95:1378, 1977.

45. Wallace, TR, Fraunfelder, FT, Petursson, GJ, Epstein, DL: Decreased libido—a side effect of carbonic anhydrase inhibitor. Ann Ophthalmol 11:1563, 1979.

46. Arrigg, CA, Epstein, DL, Giovanoni, R, Grant, WM: The influence of supplemental sodium acetate on carbonic anhydrase inhibitor-induced side effects. Arch Ophthalmol 99:1969, 1981.

47. Anderson, CJ, Kaufman, PL, Sturm, RJ: Toxicity of combined therapy with carbonic anhydrase inhibitors and aspirin. Am J Ophthalmol 86:516, 1978.

48. Spaeth, GL: Potassium, acetazolamide, and intraocular pressure. Arch Ophthalmol 78:578, 1967.

49. Critchlow, AS, Freeborn, SF, Roddie, RA: Potassium supplements during treatment of glaucoma with acetazolamide. Br Med J 289:21, 1984.

50. Wakabayashi, Y: Hyperkalaemia induced by carbonic anhydrase inhibitor. Br J Ophthalmol 75:176, 1991.

51. Kass, MA, Kolker, AE, Gordon, M, et al: Acetazolamide and urolithiasis. Ophthalmology 88:261, 1981.

52. Constant, MA, Becker, B: The effect of carbonic anhydrase inhibitors on urinary excretion of citrate by humans. Am J Ophthalmol 49:929, 1960.

53. Simpson, DP: Effect of acetazolamide on citrate excretion in the dog. Am J Physiol 206:883, 1964.

54. Kondo, T, Sakaue, E, Koyama, S, et al: Urolithiasis during treatment of carbonic anhydrase inhibitors. Folia Ophthalmol Jpn 19:576, 1968.

55. Parfitt, AM: Acetazolamide and renal stone formation. Lancet 2:153, 1970.

56. Persky, L, Chambers, D, Potts, A: Calculus formation and ureteral colic following acetazolamide (Diamox) therapy. JAMA 161:1625, 1956.

57. Charron, RC, Feldman, F: Acetazolamide therapy with renal complications. Can J Ophthalmol 9:282, 1974.

58. Wisch, N, Fischbein, FI, Siegel, R, et al: Aplastic anemia resulting from the use of carbonic anhydrase inhibitors. Am J Ophthalmol 75:130, 1973.

59. Gangitano, JL, Foster, SH, Contro, RM: Nonfatal methazolamide-induced aplastic anemia. Am J Ophthalmol 86:138, 1978.

60. Werblin, TP, Pollack, IP, Liss, RA: Blood dyscrasias in patients using methazolamide (Neptazane) for glaucoma. Ophthalmology 87:350, 1980.

61. Fraundfelder, FT, Meyer, SM, Bagby, GC, Jr, Dreis, MW: Hematologic reactions to carbonic anhydrase inhibitors. Am J Ophthalmol 100:79, 1985.

62. Mogk, LG, Cyrlin, MN: Blood dyscrasias and carbonic anhydrase inhibitors. Ophthalmology 95:768, 1988.

63. Zimran, A, Beutler, E: Can the risk of acetazolamide-induced aplastic anemia be decreased by periodic monitoring of blood cell counts? Am J Ophthalmol 104:654, 1987.

64. Gandham, SB, Spaeth, GL, De Leonardo, M, Costa, VP: Methazolamide-induced skin eruptions. Arch Ophthalmol 111:370, 1993.

65. Flach, AJ, Smith, RE, Fraunfelder, FT: Stevens-Johnson syndrome associated with methazolamide treatment reported in two Japanese-American women. Ophthalmology 102:1677, 1995.

66. Weiss, IS: Hirsutism after chronic administration of acetazolamide. Am J Ophthalmol 78:327, 1974.

67. Maren, TH: Teratology and carbonic anhydrase inhibition. Arch Ophthalmol 85:1, 1971.

68. Worsham, GF, Beckman, EN, Mitchell, EH: Sacrococcygeal teratoma in a neonate. JAMA 240:251, 1978.

69. Hargett, NA, Ritch, R, Mardirossian, J, et al: Inadvertent substitution of acetohexamide for acetazolamide. Am J Ophthalmol 84:580, 1977.

70. Rutzen, AR, Weiss, JS: Substitution of acetohexamide for acetazolamide. Am J Ophthalmol 116:379, 1993.

71. Shrader, CE, Thomas, JV, Simmons, RJ: Relationship of patient age and tolerance to carbonic anhydrase inhibitors. Am J Ophthalmol 96:730, 1983.

72. Lichter, PR: Reducing side effects of carbonic anhydrase inhibitors. Ophthalmology 88:266, 1981.

73. Friedland, BR, Mallonee, J, Anderson, DR: Short-term dose response characteristics of acetazolamide in man. Arch Ophthalmol 95:1809, 1977.

74. Lichter, PR, Musch, DC, Medzihradsky, F, Standardi, CL: Intraocular pressure effects of carbonic anhydrase inhibitors in primary open-angle glaucoma. Am J Ophthalmol 107:11, 1989.

75. Berson, FG, Epstein, DL, Grant, WM, et al: Acetazolamide dosage forms in the treatment of glaucoma. Arch Ophthalmol 98:1051, 1980.

76. Joyce, PW, Mills, KB, Richardson, T, Mawer, GE: Equivalence of conventional and sustained release oral dosage formulations of acetazolamide in primary open angle glaucoma. Br J Clin Pharmacol 27:597, 1989.

77. Yablonski, ME, Maren, TH, Hayashi, M, et al: Enhancement of the ocular hypotensive effect of acetazolamide by diflunisal. Am J Ophthalmol 106:332, 1988.

78. Havener, WH: Ocular Pharmacology. 4th ed. St. Louis, CV Mosby, 1978, p. 475.

79. Alward, PD, Wilensky, JT: Determination of acetazolamide compliance in patients with glaucoma. Arch Ophthalmol 99:1973, 1981.

80. Theeuwes, F, Bayne, W, McGuire, J: Gastrointestinal therapeutic system for acetazolamide. Efficacy and side effects. Arch Ophthalmol 96:2219, 1978.

81. Lichter, PR, Newman, LP, Wheeler, NC, Beall, OV: Patient tolerance to carbonic anhydrase inhibitors. Am J Ophthalmol 85:495, 1978.

82. Joyce, PW, Mills, KB: Comparison of the effect of acetazolamide tablets and sustets on diurnal intraocular pressure in patients with chronic simple glaucoma. Br J Ophthalmol 74:413, 1990.

83. Ellis, PP, Price, PK, Kelmenson, R, Rendi, MA: Effectiveness of generic acetazolamide. Arch Ophthalmol 100:1920, 1982.

84. Maren, TH, Haywood, JR, Chapman, SK, Zimmerman, TJ: The pharmacology of methazolamide in relation to the treatment of glaucoma. Invest Ophthalmol Vis Sci 16:730, 1977.

85. Stone, RA, Zimmerman, TJ, Shin, DH, et al: Low-dose methazolamide and intraocular pressure. Am J Ophthalmol 83:674, 1977.

86. Dahlen, K, Epstein, DL, Grant, WM, et al: A repeated dose-response study of methazolamide in glaucoma. Arch Ophthalmol 96:2214, 1978.

87. Merkle, W: Effect of methazolamide on the intraocular pressure of patients with open-angle glaucoma. Klin Monatsbl Augenheilkd 176:181, 1980.

88. Zimmerman, TJ: Acetazolamide and methazolamide. Ann Ophthalmol 10:509, 1978.

89. Becker, B: Use of methazolamide (Neptazane) in the therapy of glaucoma. Comparison with acetazolamide (Diamox). Am J Ophthalmol 49:1307, 1960.

90. Ellis, PP: Urinary calculi with methazolamide therapy. Doc Ophthalmol 34:137, 1973.

91. Shields, MB, Simmons, RJ: Urinary calculus during methazolamide therapy. Am J Ophthalmol 81:622, 1976.

92. Stein, A, Pinke, R, Krupin, T, et al: The effect of topically administered carbonic anhydrase inhibitors on aqueous humor dynamics in rabbits. Am J Ophthalmol 95:222, 1983.

93. Flach, AJ, Peterson, JS, Seligmann, KA: Local ocular hypotensive effect of topically applied acetazolamide. Am J Ophthalmol 98:66, 1984.

94. Friedman, Z, Allen, RC, Raph, SM: Topical acetazolamide and methazolamide delivered by contact lenses. Arch Ophthalmol 103:963, 1985.

95. Edelhauser, HF, Maren, TH: Permeability of human cornea and sclera to sulfonamide carbonic anhydrase inhibitors. Arch Ophthalmol 106:1110, 1988.

96. Bar-Ilan, A, Pessah, NI, Maren, TH: The effects of carbonic anhydrase inhibitors on aqueous humor chemistry and dynamics. Invest Ophthalmol Vis Sci 25:1198, 1984.

97. Lewis, RA, Schoenwald, RD, Eller, MG, et al: Ethoxzolamide analogue gel. A topical carbonic anhydrase inhibitor. Arch Ophthalmol 102:1821, 1984.

98. Bar-Ilan, A, Pessah, NI, Maren, TH: Ocular penetration and hypotensive activity of the topically applied carbonic anhydrase inhibitor L-645,151. J Ocul Pharmacol Ther 2:109, 1986.

99. Maren, TH: The development of topical carbonic anhydrase inhibitors. J Glau 4:49, 1995.

100. Lewis, RA, Schoenwald, RD, Barfknecht, CF, Phelps, CD: Aminozolamide gel. A trial of a topical carbonic anhydrase inhibitor in ocular hypertension. Arch Ophthalmol 104:842, 1986.

101. Kalina, PH, Shetlar, DJ, Lewis, RA, et al: 6-amino-2-benzothiazolesulfonamide. The effect of a topical carbonic anhydrase inhibitor on aqueous humor formation in the normal human eye. Ophthalmology 95:772, 1988.

102. Sugrue, MF, Gautheron, P, Grove, J, et al: MK-927: a topically effective ocular hypotensive carbonic anhydrase (CA) inhibitor in rabbits. Invest Ophthalmol Vis Sci 29(Suppl):81, 1988.

103. Wang, RF, Serle, JB, Podos, SM, Sugrue, MF: The effect of MK-927, a topical carbonic anhydrase inhibitor, on IOP in glaucomatous monkeys. Curr Eye Res 9:163, 1990.

104. Maren, TH, Bar-Ilan, A, Conroy, CW, Brechue, WF: Chemical and pharmacological properties of MK-927, a sulfonamide carbonic anhydrase inhibitor that lowers intraocular pressure by the topical route. Exp Eye Res 50:27, 1990.

105. Brechur, WF, Maren, TH: pH and drug ionization affects ocular pressure lowering of topical carbonic anhydrase inhibitors. Invest Ophthalmol Vis Sci 34:2581, 1993.

106. Lippa, EA, von Denffer, HA, Hofmann, HM, Brunner-Ferber, FL: Local tolerance and activity of MK-927, a novel topical carbonic anhydrase inhibitor. Arch Ophthalmol 106:1694, 1988.

107. Bron, AM, Lippa, EA, Hofmann, HM, et al: MK-927: a topically effective carbonic anhydrase inhibitor in patients. Arch Ophthalmol 107:1143, 1989.

108. Pfeiffer, N, Hennekes, R, Lippa, EA, et al: A single dose of the topical carbonic anhydrase inhibitor MK-927 decreases IOP in patients. Br J Ophthalmol 74:405, 1990.

109. Higginbotham, EJ, Kass, MA, Lippa, EA, et al: MK-927: a topical carbonic anhydrase inhibitor. Dose response and duration of action. Arch Ophthalmol 108:65, 1990.

110. Serle, JB, Lustgarten, JS, Lippa, EA, et al: MK-927, a topical carbonic anhydrase inhibitor. Dose response and reproducibility. Arch Ophthalmol 108:838, 1990.

111. Lippa, EA, Aasved, H, Airaksinen, PJ, et al: Multiple-dose, dose-response relationship for the topical carbonic anhydrase inhibitor MK-927. Arch Ophthalmol 109:46, 1991.

112. Pfeiffer, B, Gerling, J, Lippa, EA, et al: Comparative tolerability of topical carbonic anhydrase inhibitor MK-927 and its S-enantiomer MK-417. Graefes Arch Clin Exp Ophthalmol 229:111, 1991.

113. Bron, A, Lippa, EA, Gunning, F, et al: Multiple-dose efficacy comparison of the two topical carbonic anhydrase inhibitors sezolamide and MK-927. Arch Ophthalmol 109:50, 1991.

114. Sugrue, MF, Mallorga, P, Schwam, H, et al: A comparison of L-671,152 and MK-927, two topically effective ocular hypotensive carbonic anhydrase inhibitors, in experimental animals. Curr Eye Res 9:607, 1990.

115. Wang, R-F, Serle, JB, Podos, SM, Sugrue, MF: The ocular hypotensive effect of the topical carbonic anhydrase inhibitor L-671,152 in glaucomatous monkeys. Arch Ophthalmol 108:511, 1990.

116. Wang, R-F, Serle, JB, Podos, SM, Sugrue, MF: MK-507 (L-671,152), a topically active carbonic anhydrase inhibitor, reduces aqueous humor production in monkeys. Arch Ophthalmol 109:1297, 1991.

117. Wilkerson, M, Cyrlin, M, Lippa, EA, et al: Four-week safety and efficacy study of dorzolamide, a novel, active topical carbonic anhydrase inhibitor. Arch Ophthalmol 111:1343, 1993.

118. Lippa, EA, Schuman, JS, Higginbotham, EJ, et al: MK-507 versus sezolamide. Comparative efficacy of two topically active carbonic anhydrase inhibitors. Ophthalmology 98:308, 1991.

119. Gunning, FP, Greve, EL, Bron, AM, et al: Two topical carbonic anhydrase inhibitors sezolamide and dorzolamide in Gelrite vehicle: a multiple-dose efficacy study. Graefes Arch Clin Exp Ophthalmol 231:384, 1993.

120. The MK-507 Clinical Study Group: Long-term glaucoma treatment with MK-507, dorzolamide, a topical carbonic anhydrase inhibitor. J Glau 4:6, 1995.

121. Strahlman, E, Tipping, R, Vogel, R, et al: A double-masked, randomized 1-year study comparing dorzolamide (Trusopt), timolol, and betaxolol. Arch Ophthalmol 113:1009, 1995.

122. Laibovitz, R, Strahlman, ER, Barber, BL, Strohmaier, KM: Comparison of quality of life and patient preference of dorzolamide and pilocarpine as adjunctive therapy to timolol in the treatment of glaucoma. J Glau 4:306, 1995.

Chapter 29

PROSTAGLANDINS

I. Prostaglandins

II. Latanoprost

I. Prostaglandins
II. Latanoprost
  A. Initial studies
  B. Mechanisms of action

C. Clinical efficacy
D. Drug interactions
E. Side effects
III. Other investigational prostaglandins

Prostaglandins (PGs) are ubiquitous local hormones that represent part of the family of arachidonic acid derivatives, or *eicosanoids*. In most tissues of the body, release of arachidonic acid results in the complex *arachidonic acid cascade*, in which a cyclooxygenase pathway leads to the synthesis of stable PGs and labile products such as thromboxane A$_2$ and prostacyclin, while a lipoxygenase pathway leads to the production of leukotrienes. There are several types of PGs, which are designated as A, B, D, E, and F, with numerous subsets. Prostaglandins and other eicosanoids are produced in small amounts in conjunction with physiologic processes and in larger amounts in association with pathologic events. The latter includes ocular inflammation and hypertension, which were the focus of early PG research. Subsequent studies, however, indicated that smaller amounts of PGs actually moderate the inflammatory response and lower the intraocular pressure (IOP), which led to the investigation of these agents for the medical management of glaucoma (1, 2).

LATANOPROST

Initial Studies

In rabbit studies, the topical application of 25–200 µg of PGs caused an initial rise in IOP, followed by pressure reduction for 15–20 hours, whereas a 5-µg dose produced ocular hypotension without an initial pressure rise (3). Daily or twice daily administration of various PGs was shown to maintain a sustained IOP reduction in rabbits, cats, and monkeys (4–9). Other arachidonic acid metabolites were also shown to lower the IOP in rabbits (10, 11). In preliminary human studies, topical application of the tromethamine salt of prostaglandin type F$_{2\alpha}$ (PGF$_{2\alpha}$) produced significant dose-related IOP reduction in normotensive volunteers, but was associated with ocular irritation, conjunctival hyperemia, and headaches (12, 13). However, the lipid-soluble es-

ter of PGF$_{2\alpha}$, which has better corneal penetration and can be used in lower doses than the salt, also had a significant dose-related ocular hypotensive effect in both normal volunteers (14, 15) and open-angle glaucoma patients (16) without serious side effects. These observations stimulated a continuation of extensive laboratory and clinical research that led to the development of the first practical prostaglandin for the treatment of glaucoma, the PGF$_{2\alpha}$ analogue prodrug, PGF$_{2\alpha}$ isopropyl ester, which is also designated as PhXA41 or latanoprost (Xalatan). It was approved by the FDA in 1996.

Mechanisms of Action

Studies of human autopsy eyes revealed high levels of specific binding sites for both PGF$_{2\alpha}$ and PGE$_{2\alpha}$ in areas of the ciliary muscles and iris sphincter muscle, suggesting that PGs could modulate uveoscleral outflow by binding to receptors in the ciliary muscles (17). In most animal and human studies, the ocular hypotensive effect of PGs did not appear to be explained by reduced aqueous production, reduced episcleral venous pressure, or increased conventional aqueous outflow (14, 18–22). Although one study in human eyes suggested that improved conventional outflow might contribute to the hypotensive effect (23), the bulk of the evidence supports the hypothesis that the primary, if not exclusive, mechanism of IOP reduction by PGs is *improved uveoscleral outflow*.

The precise mechanism by which PGs improve uveoscleral outflow is unclear, although two possible mechanisms that have been studied are relaxation of the ciliary muscle (24) and loss of extracellular material from among the ciliary muscle bundles (25). Support for the former possibility includes the observation that pilocarpine, which causes contraction of the ciliary muscle and is known to reduce uveoscleral outflow, antagonized the PGF$_{2\alpha}$-induced ocular hypotension in monkeys (24). In vitro studies of ciliary muscle response to

440

$PGF_{2\alpha}$ have been conflicting. Prostaglandin $F_{2\alpha}$ consistently relaxed carbachol-precontracted fresh ciliary muscle strips from monkey eyes (26), while calcium efflux studies of cultured human ciliary smooth muscle cells suggests that $PGF_{2\alpha}$ may actually cause contraction of the cells (27). Physiologic studies in monkeys suggests a dual action of $PGF_{2\alpha}$ on the ciliary muscle, involving a short-onset, long-lasting relaxation and narrowing of the muscle fiber bundles and a slowly developing, shorter-duration dissolution of the intermuscular connective tissue (28).

Adrenergic antagonists were reported to block the PG-induced increase in total outflow facility (29), although the addition of topical $PGF_{2\alpha}$ to open-angle glaucoma patients uncontrolled on timolol alone led to further significant IOP reduction (30). Neither indomethacin nor sympathectomy altered the ocular hypertensive effect of PGs, suggesting that the mechanism does not involve de novo synthesis of prostaglandin or release of endogenous norepinephrine (3).

Clinical Efficacy

Latanoprost has undergone extensive clinical trials, primarily in the concentration of 0.006%, for efficacy, drug interactions, and side effects. In an in-hospital (to insure compliance), placebo-controlled study of 15 glaucoma patients, latanoprost or placebo was given once daily at 9 PM, and pressures were measured the following day at 8 AM and 8 PM (31). The IOP reduction in the treated eyes was 20–30% on the first morning, and this did not become attenuated during the 23 hours after treatment. There may be some additional effect during the first few weeks in that a 2-week, placebo-controlled trial of latanoprost, either once or twice daily, in ocular hypertensives, gave a 28–36% IOP reduction, with once daily being at least as effective as twice daily (32). However, the effect may subsequently decline before stabilizing. In a 1-month study of ocular hypertensives and glaucoma patients, an early IOP reduction of 31–38% with twice-daily administration declined during the first 2 weeks and then leveled off at approximately 20% (33).

The 0.006% concentration represents 60 µg/ml. In a dose-response study, a single administration of 25, 50, and 100 µg/ml in ocular hypertensives and open-angle glaucoma patients gave mean IOP reductions 8 hours after treatment of 3.4, 4.9, and 5.9 mm Hg, respectively (34). However, continued therapy again appears to influence the IOP response. In the 1-month study noted above, 35, 60, and 115 µg/ml showed only a weak dose-response relationship even on the second day of treatment (33).

Latanoprost 0.005%, given once daily, has been compared to timolol 0.5% twice daily in several 6-month trials of ocular hypertensive and glaucoma patients. Three such studies included a total of 829 volunteers (35–37). In one of these trials, the diurnal IOP reduction at 6 months was 27% with timolol, 31% with latanoprost applied in the morning, and 35% with latanoprost in the evening (35). The efficacy of the evening latanoprost was statistically superior to timolol or morning latanoprost. In the other two comparative trials, latanoprost was given only in the evening, with one study reporting 6-month diurnal IOP reductions of 32.7% and 33.7% for timolol and latanoprost, respectively (36), while the other described 6-month IOP reductions of 4.9 ± 2.9 mm Hg and 6.7 ± 3.4 mm Hg for timolol and latanoprost, respectively (37). The latter difference was statistically significant.

Drug Interactions

As noted previously, the addition of latanoprost to open-angle glaucoma patients uncontrolled on timolol alone led to further significant IOP reduction (30). Subsequent studies have confirmed this earlier observation. When latanoprost twice daily was added in open-angle glaucoma patients who were uncontrolled on timolol 0.5% twice daily, there was a significant further reduction of IOP at 4 hours, which was maintained throughout the 1-week study, with a mean additional IOP reduction of 6–9 mm Hg on the last day and 12 hours after the final dose (38). In another study of ocular hypertensives or open-angle glaucoma patients, either timolol or latanoprost alone twice daily for 1 week gave IOP reductions of 24% and 31%, respectively, while adding latanoprost to timolol or timolol to latanoprost gave further IOP reductions of 13% and 14%, respectively (39). Another study showed that once daily administration of latanoprost in the combined therapy was again at least as effective, and probably superior, to twice daily (40). In that study, with baseline IOPs of 24.8–24.9 mm Hg on timolol twice daily alone, the average daytime pressures at 4 and 12 weeks after treatment were 16.8 and 15.7 mm Hg, respectively, on latanoprost once daily in the evening, and 18.1 and 18.0 mm Hg, respectively, on latanoprost twice daily. It has also been shown that, unlike timolol, latanoprost lowers the IOP at night as well as during the day, providing uniform around-the-clock IOP reduction when administered once daily either alone or in combination with timolol (41).

The interaction of latanoprost with pilocarpine is less clear than that with timolol. As previously noted, pilocarpine antagonized the $PGF_{2\alpha}$-induced ocular hypotension in monkeys (24). This is not surprising, since pilocarpine causes contraction of the ciliary muscle and reduction of uveoscleral outflow, in contrast to latanoprost, which is believed to lower IOP by improving uveoscleral outflow, possibly through relaxation of the ciliary muscle. This is consistent with an ultrasound biomicroscopic study of 36 healthy young Japanese subjects, which showed that pilocarpine 2% increased the ciliary body thickness by 8.3%, while latanoprost 0.005% decreased the thickness by 3.3% (42). However, in a clinical trial of 20 ocular hypertensive patients who were initially treated with either pilocarpine 2% three times daily or latanoprost 0.005% twice daily, the IOP reduction at the end of 1 week was 14.3% on pilocarpine alone and 23.4% on latanoprost alone (43). When pilocarpine was then added to latanoprost, the additional IOP reduction was 7.4%, compared with 14.2% when latanoprost was added to pilocarpine.

Side Effects

The intraocular inflammatory effects of aqueous cell and flare and miosis, which result from the administration of large doses of PGs, were not seen in animal or human eyes in the doses associated with the ocular hypotensive response (4–9, 12–16, 44, 45). Furthermore, the absorptive transport systems of the ciliary processes appear to prevent topically applied PGs and other eicosanoids from causing retinal toxicity (1). Extraocular irritation has been more of a problem in human studies with the salt of $PGF_{2\alpha}$ (12, 13), although, as previously noted, this is significantly reduced by using the lipid-soluble ester of the compound (14–16). In the clinical trials with latanoprost, the most commonly reported ocular reaction was mild conjunctival hyperemia, which tended to become less pronounced with continued use (31–37). Mild-to-moderate ocular irritation was reported with higher concentrations, but not with the 0.006% (33). In the 6-month trials, some patients had episodes of mild punctate corneal epithelial erosions (35, 36). The most significant side effect of latanoprost was increased pigmentation of the iris (35–37). This was seen in 10% of the patients in one study, but only occurred in eyes with mixed green-brown or blue/gray-brown iris color (35).

With regard to systemic side effects, the amount of PG entering the circulation from the low doses of its ester that is required to lower the IOP is a small fraction of the amount of endogenous PGs that are normally released from virtually all tissues of the body (2). No significant systemic reactions were reported with latanoprost in any of the clinical trials (31–37).

OTHER INVESTIGATIONAL PROSTAGLANDINS

Several other prostaglandins or their analogues are under investigation for use in the management of glaucoma. *PhXA34* is an analogue of $PFG_{2\alpha}$-isopropyl ester, or latanoprost, which was initially felt to improve the effect/side effect relationship as compared to the parent compound. In single dose trials, 1, 3, and 10 μg of PhXA34 reduced the IOP in normal volunteers by about 2, 3, and 4 mm Hg, respectively, after 6–10 hours (46), while 0.3, 1, 3, and 10 μg also had a dose-related IOP reduction in ocular hyper-

tensives of 11–35% (47). In a 1-week trial of 10 μg of PhXA34 once daily in normal subjects, the mean IOP was below 9 mm Hg at 12 hours and associated with mild ocular discomfort and some hyperemia (46). A 6-day study of 0.003% (1-μg) and 0.01% (3-μg) concentrations of PhXA34, given twice daily to 29 ocular hypertensives, revealed a significant dose-dependent IOP reduction, with conjunctival hyperemia only occurring with the higher concentration (48). When a single administration of 1 μg of PhXA34 or latanoprost was evaluated in 54 healthy Japanese volunteers, latanoprost appeared to be at least 1.5 times more active than PhXA34 (49).

Prostaglandin D2 (PGD_2) and its analogue, BW245C, appear to have a different mechanism of IOP reduction than the prostaglandins discussed earlier. In rabbit studies, the main hypotensive mechanism was reduced aqueous production (50). There is a wide range of prostanoid receptor subtypes, which are named according to the natural prostaglandin that has modest selectivity for the receptor. In the case of PGD_2, stimulation of the DP-receptor suppresses aqueous production, but has no effect in normotensive monkeys on uveoscleral outflow (51). An evaluation of PGD_2 analogues with membrane fractions of rabbit iris-ciliary body complex suggests that the effect on aqueous flow is related to stimulation of adenylate cyclase activity (52). Preliminary evidence suggested that the ocular hypotensive effect of PGD_2 might be separated from the inflammatory effect on the conjunctiva by using a selective DP-receptor agonist (53). However, single-dose studies of PGD_2 and BW245C in normotensive human volunteers revealed weak IOP efficacy at low doses and significant side effects of conjunctival hyperemia, itching, and foreign-body and mild burning sensations at higher concentrations (54).

Prostaglandin E_2 (PGE_2) has been shown to have relatively selective binding sites (possibly a single class of binding sites) in bovine iris-ciliary body membrane preparations (55). In a study with precontracted cat ciliary smooth muscle, PGE_2 produced significantly more potent ciliary muscle relaxation than either PGD_2 or $PGF_{2\alpha}$ (56).

SUMMARY

Prostaglandins are ubiquitous local hormones that produce ocular inflammation and hypertension in large concentrations, but moderate inflammation and reduce IOP in smaller amounts. Natural prostaglandins and their analogues have been evaluated for the management of glaucoma. Latanoprost, an analogue of prostaglandin $F_2\alpha$, reduces IOP by improving uveoscleral outflow and is a potent ocular antihypertensive agent when given once daily, with minimal ocular and virtually no systemic side effects. Other prostaglandins, each of which is relatively selective for specific prostanoid receptor subtypes, are also being evaluated for the treatment of glaucoma.

REFERENCES

1. Bito, LZ: Prostaglandins and other eicosanoids: their ocular transport, pharmacokinetics, and therapeutic effects. Trans Ophthalmol Soc UK 105:162, 1986.

2. Bito, LZ: Prostaglandins. Old concepts and new perspectives [Editorial]. Arch Ophthalmol 105:1036, 1987.

3. Camras, CB, Bito, LZ, Eakins, KE: Reduction of intraocular pressure by prostaglandins applied topically to the eyes of conscious rabbits. Invest Ophthalmol Vis Sci 16:1125, 1977.

4. Stern, FA, Bito, LZ: Comparison of the hypotensive and other ocular effects of prostaglandins E_2 and $F_{2\alpha}$ on cat and rhesus monkey eyes. Invest Ophthalmol Vis Sci 22:588, 1982.

5. Bito, LZ, Draga, A, Blanco, J, Camras, CB: Long-term maintenance of reduced intraocular pressure by daily or twice daily topical application of prostaglandins to cat or rhesus monkey eyes. Invest Ophthalmol Vis Sci 24:312, 1983.

6. Bito, LZ, Srinivasan, BD, Baroody, RA, Schubert, H: Noninvasive observations on eyes of cats after long-term maintenance of reduced intraocular pressure by topical application of prostaglandin E_2. Invest Ophthalmol Vis Sci 24:376, 1983.

7. Camras, CB, Podos, SM, Rosenthal, JS, et al: Multiple dosing of prostaglandin $F_{2\alpha}$ or epinephrine on cynomolgus monkey eyes. I. Aqueous humor dynamics. Invest Ophthalmol Vis Sci 28:463, 1987.

8. Kulkarni, PS, Srinivasan, BD: Prostaglandins E_3 and D_3 lower intraocular pressure. Invest Ophthalmol Vis Sci 26:1178, 1985.

9. Wong, R-F, Camras, CB, Lee, P-Y, et al: Effects of prostaglandins $F_{2\alpha}$, A_2, and their esters in glaucomatous monkey eyes. Invest Ophthalmol Vis Sci 31:2466, 1990.

10. Hoyng, PFJ, de Jong, N: Iloprost, a stable prostacyclin analog, reduces intraocular pressure. Invest Ophthalmol Vis Sci 28:470, 1987.

11. Masferrer, JL, Dunn, MW, Schwartzman, ML: 12(R)-hydroxyeicosatetraenoic acid, an endogenous corneal arachidonate metabolite, lowers intraocular pressure in rabbits. Invest Ophthalmol Vis Sci 31:535, 1990.

12. Giuffre, G: The effects of prostaglandin $F_{2\alpha}$ in the human eye. Graefes Arch Clin Exp Ophthalmol 222:139, 1985.

13. Lee, P-Y, Shao, H, Xu, L, Qu, C-K: The effect of prostaglandin $F_{2\alpha}$ on intraocular pressure in normotensive human subjects. Invest Ophthalmol Vis Sci 29:1474, 1988.

14. Kerstetter, JR, Brubaker, RF, Wilson, SE, Kullerstrand, LJ: Prostaglandin $F_{2\alpha}$-1-isopropyl ester lowers intraocular pressure without decreasing aqueous humor flow. Am J Ophthalmol 105:30, 1988.

15. Villumsen, J, Alm, A: Prostaglandin $F_{2\alpha}$-isopropyl ester eye drops: effects in normal human eyes. Br J Ophthalmol 73:419, 1989.

16. Villumsen, J, Alm, A, Söderström, M: Prostaglandin $F_{2\alpha}$-isopropyl ester eye drops: effect on intraocular pressure in open-angle glaucoma. Br J Ophthalmol 73:975, 1989.

17. Matsuo, T, Cynader, MS: Localisation of prostaglandin $F_{2\alpha}$ and E_2 binding sites in the human eye. Br J Ophthalmol 76:210, 1992.

18. Lee, P-Y, Podos, SM, Severin, C: Effect of prostaglandin $F_{2\alpha}$ on aqueous humor dynamics of rabbit, cat, and monkey. Invest Ophthalmol Vis Sci 25:1087, 1984.

19. Moses, RA, Parkison, G, Snower, DP: Prostaglandin E_2 effect on the facility of outflow in the rabbit eye. Ann Ophthalmol 13:721, 1981.

20. Crawford, K. Kaufman, PL, Gabelt, B'AT: Effects of topical $PGF_{2\alpha}$ on aqueous humor dynamics in cynomolgus monkeys. Curr Eye Res 6:1035, 1987.

21. Hayashi, M, Yablonski, ME, Bito, LZ: Eicosanoids as a new class of ocular hypotensive agents. 2. Comparison of the apparent mechanism of the ocular hypotensive effects of A and F type prostaglandins. Invest Ophthalmol Vis Sci 28:1639, 1987.

22. Toris, CB, Camras, CB, Yablonski, ME: Effects of PhXA41, a new prostaglandin $F_{2\alpha}$ on aqueous humor dynamics in human eyes. Ophthalmology 100:1297, 1993.

23. Ziai, N, Dolan, JW, Kacere, RD, Brubaker, RF: The effects on aqueous dynamics of PhXA41, a new prostaglandin $F_{2\alpha}$ analogue, after topical application in normal and ocular hypertensive human eyes. Arch Ophthalmol 111:1351, 1993.

24. Crawford, K, Kaufman, PL: Pilocarpine antagonizes prostaglandin $F_{2\alpha}$-induced ocular hypotension in monkeys. Evidence for enhancement of uveoscleral outflow by prostaglandin $F_{2\alpha}$. Arch Ophthalmol 105:1112, 1987.

25. Luetjen-Drecoll, E, Tamm, E: Morphological study of the anterior segment of cynomolgus monkey eyes following treatment with prostaglandin $F_{2\alpha}$. Exp Eye Res 47:761, 1988.

26. Poyer, JF, Millar, C, Kaufman, PL: Prostaglandin $F_{2\alpha}$ effects on isolated rhesus monkey ciliary muscle. Invest Ophthalmol Vis Sci 36:2461, 1995.

27. Weinreb, RN, Kim, D-M, Lindsey, JD: Propagation of ciliary smooth muscle cells in vitro and effects of prostaglandin $F_{2\alpha}$ on calcium efflux. Invest Ophthalmol Vis Sci 33:2679, 1992.

28. Crawford, KS, Kaufman, PL: Dose-related effects of prostaglandin $F_{2\alpha}$ isopropyl ester on intraocular pressure, refraction, and pupil diameter in monkeys. Invest Ophthalmol Vis Sci 32:510, 1991.

29. Green, K, Kim, K: Interaction of adrenergic antagonists with prostaglandin E_2 and tetrahydrocannabinol in the eye. Invest Ophthalmol 15:102, 1976.

30. Villumsen, J, Alm, A: The effect of adding prostaglandin $F_{2\alpha}$-isopropyl ester to timolol in patients with open angle glaucoma. Arch Ophthalmol 108:1102, 1990.

31. Rácz, P, Ruzsonyi, MR, Nagy, ZT, Bito, LZ: Maintained intraocular pressure reduction with once-a-day application of a new prostaglandin $F_{2\alpha}$ analogue (PhXA41). An in-hospital, placebo-controlled study. Arch Ophthalmol 111:657, 1993.

32. Nagasubramanian, S, Sheth, GP, Hitchings, RA, Stjernschantz, J: Intraocular pressure-reducing effect of PhXA41 in ocular hypertension. Comparison of dose regimens. Ophthalmology 100:1305, 1993.

33. Alm, A, Villumsen, J, Törnquist, P, et al: Intraocular pressure-reducing effect of PhXA41 in patients with increased eye pressure. A one-month study. Ophthalmology 100:1312, 1993.

34. Hotehama, Y, Mishima, HK, Kitazawa, Y, Masuda, K: Ocular hypotensive effect of PhXA41 in patients with ocular hypertension or primary open-angle glaucoma. Jpn J Ophthalmol 37:270, 1993.

35. Alm, A, Stjernschantz, J, et al: Effects on intraocular pressure and side effects of 0.005% latanoprost applied once daily, evening or morning. A comparison with timolol. Ophthalmology 102:1743, 1995.

36. Watson, P, Stjernschantz, J, et al: A six-month, randomized, double-masked study comparing latanoprost with timolol in open-angle glaucoma and ocular hypertension. Ophthalmology 103:126, 1996.

37. Camras, CB: Comparison of latanoprost and timolol in patients with ocular hypertension and glaucoma. A six-month masked, multicenter trial in the United States. Ophthalmology 103:138, 1996.

38. Lee, P-Y, Shao, H, Camras, CB, Podos, SM: Additivity of prostaglandin $F_{2\alpha}$-1-isopropyl ester to timolol in glaucoma patients. Ophthalmology 98:1079, 1991.

39. Rulo, AH, Greve, EL, Hoyng, PF: Additive effect of latanoprost, a prostaglandin $F_{2\alpha}$ analogue, and timolol in patients with elevated intraocular pressure. Br J Ophthalmol 78:899, 1994.

40. Alm, A, Widengård, I, Kjellgren, D, et al: Latanoprost administered once daily caused a maintained reduction of intraocular pressure in glaucoma patients treated concomitantly with timolol. Br J Ophthalmol 79:12, 1995.

41. Rácz, P, Ruzsonyi, MR, Nagy, ZT, et al: Around-the-clock intraocular pressure reduction with once-daily application of latanoprost by itself or in combination with timolol. Arch Ophthalmol 114:268, 1996.

42. Mishima, HK, Shoge, K, Takamatsu, M, et al: Ultrasound biomicroscopic study of ciliary body thickness after topical application of pharmacologic agents. Am J Ophthalmol 121:319, 1996.

43. Friström, B, Nilsson, SEG: Interaction of PhXA41, a new prostaglandin analogue, with pilocarpine. A study on patients with elevated intraocular pressure. Arch Ophthalmol 111:662, 1993.

44. Camras, CB, Bhuyan, KC, Podos, SM, et al: Multiple dosing of prostaglandin $F_{2\alpha}$ or epinephrine on cynomolgus monkey eyes. II. Slit-lamp biomicroscopy, aqueous humor analysis, and fluorescein angiography. Invest Ophthalmol Vis Sci 28:921, 1987.

45. Camras, CB, Friedman, AH, Rodrigues, MM, et al: Multiple dosing of prostaglandin $F_{2\alpha}$ or epinephrine on cynomolgus monkey eyes. III. Histopathology. Invest Ophthalmol Vis Sci 29:1428, 1988.

46. Alm, A, Villumsen, J: PhXA34, a new potent ocular hypotensive drug. A study on dose-response relationship and on aqueous humor dynamics in healthy volunteers. Arch Ophthalmol 109:1564, 1991.

47. Villumsen, J, Alm, A: PhXA34-a prostaglandin $F_{2\alpha}$ analogue. Effect on intraocular pressure in patients with ocular hypertension. Br J Ophthalmol 76:214, 1992.

48. Camras, CB, Schumer, RA, Marsk, A, et al: Intraocular pressure reduction with PhXA34, a new prostaglandin analogue, in patients with ocular hypertension. Arch Ophthalmol 110:1733, 1992.

49. Hotehama, Y, Mishima, HK: Clinical efficacy of PhXA34 and PhXA41, two novel prostaglandin $F_{2\alpha}$-isopropyl ester analogues for glaucoma treatment. Jpn J Ophthalmol 37:259, 1993.

50. Goh, Y, Araie, M, Nakajima, M, et al: Effect of topical prostaglandin D_2 on the aqueous humor dynamics in rabbits. Graefes Arch Clin Exp Ophthalmol 227:476, 1989.

51. Crawford, KS, Kaufman, PL, Hubbard, WC, Woodward, DF: The DP-receptor agonist SQ27986 raises but does not lower intraocular pressure in ocular normotensive monkeys. J Glau 1:94, 1992.

52. Goh, Y, Nakajima, M: Stimulatory effects of prostaglandin D_2 analogues on adenylate cyclase in rabbit iris-ciliary body membrane fractions. Exp Eye Res 51:585, 1990.

53. Woodward, DF, Hawley, SB, Williams, LS, et al: Studies on the ocular pharmacology of prostaglandin D_2. Invest Ophthalmol Vis Sci 31: 138, 1990.

54. Nakajima, M, Goh, Y, Izuma, I, Hayaishi, O: Effects of prostaglandin D_2 and its analogue, BW245C, on intraocular pressure in humans. Graefes Arch Clin Exp Ophthalmol 229:411, 1991.

55. Bhattacherjee, P, Csukas, S, Paterson, CA: Prostaglandin E_2 binding sites in bovine iris-ciliary body. Invest Ophthalmol Vis Sci 31: 1109, 1990.

56. Chen, J, Woodward, DF: Prostanoid-induced relaxation of precontracted cat ciliary muscle is mediated by EP_2 and DP receptors. Invest Ophthalmol Vis Sci 33:3195, 1992.

Chapter 30

HYPEROSMOTICS

I. Mechanisms of action
    A. Reduced vitreous volume
    B. Hypothalamic-neural theory
    C. Altered ciliary epithelium
II. Side effects
III. Specific hyperosmotic agents
    A. Oral agents
        1. Glycerol
        2. Isosorbide
        3. Other oral agents

B. Intravenous agents
    1. Mannitol
    2. Urea
    3. Other intravenous agents

The drugs discussed in this chapter represent another class of compounds that may be administered systemically (orally or intravenously) for the control of elevated intraocular pressure (IOP). Unlike the carbonic anhydrase inhibitors, however, the use of these medications is generally limited to short-term, emergency situations such as acute angle-closure glaucoma or other glaucomas with dangerously high pressures. With the advent of new topical drugs such as α_2-adrenergic agonists for short-term IOP control, the hyperosmotics are being used less commonly, but still have an occasional role in the management of glaucoma. Another clinical use for hyperosmotic agents is the reduction of vitreous volume as a prophylactic measure prior to some intraocular surgical procedures. The mechanisms of action and the side effects of the drugs within this class of compounds are similar, with some notable exceptions, and these features are discussed collectively before considering specific aspects of the individual agents.

MECHANISMS OF ACTION

Reduced Vitreous Volume

As noted earlier, one action of the hyperosmotic agents is reduction of vitreous volume. It is this effect that is generally believed to be responsible for lowering the IOP. This concept is supported by rabbit studies, which demonstrated a reduction in vitreous body weight of approximately 3–4% with various hyperosmotic agents (1). The mechanism of vitreous shrinkage is commonly considered to result from an osmotic gradient between the blood and ocular tissues, which initially pulls fluid from the eye.

With time, a variable amount of the hyperosmotic agent may enter the eye, depending upon the permeability of the blood-ocular barriers to the drug and the size of the drug molecules. As the compound is cleared from the systemic circulation, there may be a reversal of the osmotic gradient in some cases, resulting in a transient rise in IOP.

Hypothalamic-Neural Theory

Some studies have shown that changes in IOP and serum osmolarity do not always correlate (2–5), and it may be that additional factors are involved in the ocular hypotensive effect of hyperosmotics. One alternative theory is that osmotic agents (both hyperosmotics and hypo-osmotics) influence the IOP through the central nervous system.

It has been observed that human eyes with optic nerve lesions do not manifest the usual elevation in IOP after water drinking (6). Unilateral optic nerve transection in rabbits and monkeys also was associated with a reduced ocular hypertensive response to hypo-osmotics, as well as a diminished IOP lowering effect with hyperosmotic agents (2, 7, 8). These observations raised the possibility that the influence of osmotic agents on the IOP is mediated through the optic nerve (2, 6–8).

Additional studies suggested that the central nervous system effect of osmotic agents on IOP might originate in the hypothalamus. Phenobarbital, which has a depressant effect on the hypothalamus, lowers the IOP in rabbits, presumably by inhibition of aqueous humor formation, and this action was shown to be reduced by optic nerve transection (9). Furthermore, pretreatment with phenobarbital prevented the ocular hypotensive response to hyperosmotic agents in rabbits with intact optic nerves (10). In addition, the injection of osmotic agents into the third ventricle of rabbits altered the IOP without effecting serum osmolarity, and this effect was eliminated by optic nerve transection (11). Bilateral lesions in the supraoptic nuclei (an area of the hypothalamus near the optic tracts which is known to be related to water balance) abolished the IOP response to hypo-osmotics in rabbits (12).

The above observations are felt to support the theory that osmotic agents exert their influence on IOP through the central nervous system, possible originating in the hypothalamus and mediated by efferent fibers in the optic nerve (2, 6, 7, 8, 10). The exact mechanism of pressure reduction is uncertain, although preliminary evidence suggests a decrease in aqueous production (10).

Other reported studies, however, have challenged the hypothalamic-neural theory. Ventriculocisternal perfusion of a hypo-osmotic solution in rabbits did not influence the IOP (13), nor did unilateral optic nerve transection in rabbits alter the IOP response to osmotic agents (14, 15). An alternative explanation that has been proposed for the diminished IOP response to osmotic agents in eyes with optic atrophy is that an associated reduction in the retinal vasculature decreases the available route of fluid movement from the eye (14). There is clearly a need for further investigation of this question.

Altered Ciliary Epithelium

It has been observed in monkey studies that intra-arterial injections of hyperosmotic agents cause a breakdown of the blood-aqueous barrier associated with destruction of the non-pigmented ciliary epithelium (16–19). However, similar changes do not occur following intravenous administration (16, 17), and it is unlikely that this is part of the ocular hypotensive effect associated with clinical hyperosmotic therapy. It has been reported, however, that therapeutic doses of intravenous mannitol (discussed later in this chapter) caused increased aqueous flare in humans, which may be related to osmotic stress on the blood-aqueous barrier (20).

SIDE EFFECTS

Side effects with hyperosmotic therapy are common and can be serious (21), or even fatal (22, 23). The magnitude of these adverse reactions varies with the specific agent and mode of administration.

Nausea and Vomiting

Nausea and vomiting are frequently encountered, especially with the oral (liquid) agents, presumably due to the heavy sweet taste. This is transient and usually of no consequence, but can be a problem if the vomiting occurs during surgery or leads to loss of the medication. The nausea can be minimized by serving the medication with ice and a tart flavoring.

Diuresis

Diuresis is a standard response to hyperosmotic therapy and is particularly a problem with the use of intravenous agents. In some cases, massive diuresis during surgery may necessitate the use of an indwelling catheter.

Other Reactions

Other reactions that may occur with all hyperosmotics, but which are worse with intravenous agents, include headache, backache, giddiness, diarrhea, confusion and disorientation (21), chills and fever, cardiovascular overload, intracranial hemorrhage (22), pulmonary edema, acidemia, and renal insufficiency (23).

SPECIFIC HYPEROSMOTIC AGENTS (TABLE 30.1)

Oral Agents

Glycerol

Glycerol, or glycerine, is administered as a liquid in a dosage of 1–1.5 g/kg of body weight of a 50% solution (24, 25). The ocular hypotensive effect occurs within 10 minutes of administration, peaks in 30 minutes, and lasts for approximately 5 hours (24, 25). Glycerol is distributed throughout the extracellular body fluids and has poor ocular penetration, which enhances the osmotic gradient effect and allows effective repeated administrations (24). In addition, the drug is metabolized, which causes less diuresis and increased safety. However, the caloric content of 4.32 kcal/g (25) and the osmotic diuresis with resultant dehydration can cause problems with repeated administration in diabetics (26).

Isosorbide

Isosorbide is another oral hyperosmotic agent, which became commercially available in 1980. Numerous studies have con-

Table 30.1.
COMMERCIAL HYPEROSMOTIC AGENTS*

Generic Preparations	Brand Names	Concentrations (%)
Oral agents		
Glycerine	Glyrol	75
	Osmoglyn	50
Isosorbide	Ismotic	45
Intravenous agents		
Mannitol	Osmitrol	5, 10, 15, 20
Urea	Ureaphil	40 g/150 ml

Other generic products may also be available.

firmed the ocular hypotensive efficacy of this agent (27–32). The drug has an advantage over glycerol in that 95% is excreted unchanged in the urine (27), which eliminates the caloric problem (28). Other side effects are also reported to be less with isosorbide than with other hyperosmotics (27–31). The recommended dosage is 1.5 g/kg of body weight of a 50% solution, which produces a peak ocular hypotensive effect in 1–3 hours and lasts for 3–5 hours (31). As in the case of glycerol, it may also be given in repeated doses. It should be noted that isosorbide dinitrate (Isordil), an organic nitrate used in the treatment of angina pectoris, has a similar name and care must be taken to avoid confusing these two drugs (33).

Other Oral Drugs

Other oral drugs that have been found to be effective as hyperosmotic agents in lowering the IOP include glycine (34), sodium lactate (35), propylene glycol (36), and ethyl alcohol, although the latter is only effective in large doses (37).

Intravenous Agents

These drugs generally produce a greater ocular hypotensive effect than oral hyperosmotics. They may be indicated when the oral agents are felt to be insufficient or when they cannot be taken for reasons such as nausea.

Mannitol

Mannitol is reported to have an equivalent (38) or greater (39) ocular hypotensive effect than urea, and is said to be more efficacious than glycerol (39). In one study, intravenous mannitol and oral isosorbide produced equivalent pressure reduction at 30 and 60 minutes, although mannitol was more effective in maintaining the reduction (27). The drug is distributed in the extracellular fluid compartments and has poor ocular penetration (24). As previously noted, intravenous mannitol has been shown to increase aqueous flare in humans (20), which may have implications regarding increased postoperative inflammation.

Although it is rapidly excreted unmetabolized in the urine, the transient rise in blood volume requires caution in patients with poor cardiac output. In general, side effects are infrequent, but may include headache, angina-like chest pain (38) and an anaphylactic reaction (41). Death has been reported in a patient who developed pulmonary edema, acidemia, and anuria following mannitol therapy, and special caution is advised in patients with compromised renal function (23).

A dosage of 2 g/kg of body weight of a 20% solution, given intravenously in 30 minutes, has been suggested (24). It may be, however, that significantly lower doses are equally effective. In one study of patients prior to cataract surgery, 100 ml of 20% mannitol, given over 20 minutes had the same effect on magnitude of IOP reduction and deepen-

ing of the anterior chamber as 200 ml of the same solution, although the latter had a more rapid and sustained ocular hypotensive effect (41). The onset of action is in 20–60 minutes, and the duration varies from 2–6 hours (24, 38, 41).

Urea

Urea may be slightly less effective than mannitol because it diffuses more freely throughout the body water and eventually penetrates into the eye (24). In addition, urea has the significant disadvantage of causing tissue necrosis if it extravasates during intravenous administration (21). Death from a subdural hematoma has occurred following urea administration for systemic hypertension (22).

Glycerol (42–44) and glycerol with sorbitol (43, 44) have also been given intravenously, and preliminary experience suggests that these may prove to have value as intravenous hyperosmotic agents.

SUMMARY

The systemic administration of a hyperosmotic agent is occasionally used as a short-term or emergency method of lowering the IOP. The ocular hypotensive mechanism is not fully understood, but probably relates primarily to a reduction in vitreous volume. Side effects can be serious and include nausea and vomiting, diuresis, headache, disorientation, and cardiovascular overload. Specific hyperosmotic agents may be given orally, such as glycerol and isosorbide, or intravenously, which includes mannitol and urea.

REFERENCES

1. Robbins, R, Galin, MA: Effect of osmotic agents on the vitreous body. Arch Ophthalmol 82:694, 1969.
2. Podos, SM, Krupin, T, Becker, B: Effect of small-dose hyperosmotic injections on intraocular pressure of small aminals and man when optic nerves are transected and intact. Am J Ophthalmol 71:898, 1971.
3. Ramsell, JT, Ellis, PP, Paterson, CA: Intraocular pressure changes during hemodialysis. Am J Ophthalmol 72:926, 1971.
4. Olsen, T, Schmitz, O, Hansen, HE: Influence of hemodialysis on corneal thickness and intraocular pressure. Klin Monatsbl Aguenheilkd 181:25, 1982.
5. Goldberg, DB, Mannarino, AP, Greco, JA: Intraocular pressure and ocular pain during hemodialysis. J Ocul Ther Surg 3:246, 1984.
6. Riise, D, Simonsen, SE: Intraocular pressure in unilateral optic nerve lesion. Acta Ophthalmol 47:750, 1969.
7. Krupin, T, Podos, SM, Becker, B: Effect of optic nerve transection on osmotic alterations of intraocular pressure. Am J Ophthalmol 70:214, 1970.
8. Krupin, T, Podos, SM, Lehman, RAW, Becker, B: Effects of optic nerve transection on intraocular pressure in monkeys. Arch Ophthalmol 84:668, 1970.
9. Becker, B, Krupin, T, Podos, SM: Phenobarbital and aqueous humor dynamics: effect in rabbits with intact and transected optic nerves. Am J Ophthalmol 70:686, 1970.
10. Podos, SM, Krupin, T, Becker, B: Mechanism of intraocular pressure response after optic nerve transection. Am J Ophthalmol 72:79, 1971.

11. Krupin, T, Podos, SM, Becker, B: Alteration of intraocular pressure after third ventricle injections of osmotic agents. Am J Ophthalmol 76:948, 1973.

12. Cox, CE, Fitzgerald, CR, King, RL: A preliminary report on the supraoptic nucleus and control of intraocular pressure. Invest Ophthalmol 14;26, 1975.

13. Liu, JHK, Neufeld, AH: Study of central regulation of intraocular pressure using ventriculocisternal perfusion. Invest Ophthalmol Vis Sci 26:136, 1985.

14. Serafano, DM, Brubaker, RF: Intraocular pressure after optic nerve transection. Invest Ophthalmol Vis Sci 17:68, 1978.

15. Lam, K-W, Shihab, Z, Fu, Y-A, Lee, P-F: The effect of optic nerve transection upon the hypotensive action of ascorbate and mannitol. Ann Ophthalmol 12:1102, 1980.

16. Laties, AM, Rapoport, S: The blood-ocular barriers under osmotic stress. Studies on the freeze-dried eye. Arch Ophthalmol 94:1086, 1976.

17. Shabo, AL, Maxwell, DS, Kreiger, AE: Structural alterations in the ciliary process and the blood-aqueous barrier of the monkey after systemic urea injections. Am J Ophthalmol 81:162, 1976.

18. Okisaka, S, Kuwabara, T, Rapoport, SI: Effect of hyperosmotic agents on the ciliary epithelium and trabecular meshwork. Invest Ophthalmol 15:617, 1976.

19. Gaasterland, DE, Barranger, JA, Rapoport, SI, et al: Long-term ocular effects of osmotic modification of the blood-brain barrier in monkeys. I. Clinical examinations; aqueous ascorbate and protein. Invest Ophthalmol Vis Sci 24:153, 1983.

20. Miyake, K, Miyake, Y, Maekubo, K: Increased aqueous flare as a result of a therapeutic dose of mannitol in humans. Graefes Arch Clin Exp Ophthalmol 230:115, 1992.

21. Tarter, RC, Linn, JC Jr: A clinical study of the use of intravenous urea in glaucoma. Am J Ophthalmol 52:323, 1961.

22. Marshall, S, Hinman, F Jr: Subdural hematoma following administration of urea for diagnosis of hypertension. JAMA 182:813, 1962.

23. Grabie, MT, Gipstein, RM, Adams, DA, Hepner, GW: Contraindications for mannitol in aphakic glaucoma. Am J Ophthalmol 91:265, 1981.

24. Havener, WH: Ocular Pharmacology. 4th ed. St. Louis, CV Mosby, 1978, p. 440.

25. Virno, M, Cantore, P, Bietti, C, Bucci, MG: Oral glycerol in ophthalmology. A valuable new method for the reduction of intraocular pressure. Am J Ophthalmol 55:1133, 1963.

26. Oakley, DE, Ellis, PP: Glycerol and hyperosmolar nonketotic coma. Am J Ophthalmol 81:469, 1976.

27. Barry, KG, Khoury, AH, Brooks, MH: Mannitol and isosorbide. Sequential effects on intraocular pressure, serum osmolality, sodium, and solids in normal subjects. Arch Ophthalmol 81:695, 1969.

28. Krupin, T, Kolker, AE, Becker, B: A comparison of isosorbide and glycerol for cataract surgery. Am J Ophthalmol 69:737, 1970.

29. Wisznia, KI, Lazar, M, Leopold, IH: Oral isosorbide and intraocular pressure. Am J Ophthalmol 70:630, 1970.

30. Mehra, KS, Singh, R, Char, JN, Rajyashree, K: Lowering of intraocular tension. Effects of isosorbide and glycerin. Arch Ophthalmol 85:167, 1971.

31. Mehra, KS, Singh, R: Lowering of intraocular pressure by isosorbide. Effects of different doses of drug. Arch Ophthalmol 86:623, 1971.

32. Wood, TO, Waltman, SR, West, C, Kaufman, HE: Effect of isosorbide on intraocular pressure after penetrating keratoplasty. Am J Ophthalmol 75:221, 1973.

33. Buckley, EG, Shields, MB: Isosorbide and isorbide dinitrate. Am J Ophthalmol 89:457, 1980.

34. Fox, SL, Kranta, JC Jr: The use of glycine in the reduction of intraocular pressure. EENT Monthly 51:469, 1972.

35. Chiang, TS, Stocks, SA, Jones, C, Thomas, RP: The ocular hypotensive effect of sodium lactate in rabbits. Arch Ophthalmol 86:566, 1971.

36. Bietti, G: Recent experimental, clinical, and therapeutic research on the problems of intraocular pressure and glaucoma. Am J Ophthalmol 73:475, 1972.

37. Obstbaum, SA, Podos, SM, Kolker, AE: Low-dose oral alcohol and intraocular pressure. Am J Ophthalmol 76:926, 1973.

38. Smith, EW, Drance, SM: Reduction of human intraocular pressure with intravenous mannitol. Arch Ophthalmol 68:734, 1962.

39. Vucicevic, AM, Tark, E III, Ahmad, S: Echographic studies of osmotic agents. Ann Ophthalmol 11:1331, 1979.

40. Spaeth, GL, Spaeth, EB, Spaeth, PG, Lucier, AC: Anaphylactic reaction to mannitol. Arch Ophthalmol 78:583, 1967.

41. O'Keeffe, M, Nabil, M: The use of mannitol in intraocular surgery. Ophthalmic Surg 14:55, 1983.

42. Holtmann, HW: Experiences with glycerin infusions for intra-ocular pressure-lowering. Klin Monatsbl Augenheilkd 161:322, 1972.

43. Masiakowski, J, Warchalowska, D, Orlowski, WJ: Effect of osmotic agents on intraocular pressure. I. Survey of pharmacological possibilities. Klin Oczna 43:365, 1973.

44. Bartkowska-Orlowska, M, Orlowski, WJ, Warchalowska, D, Masiakowski, J: Effect of osmotic agents on intraocular pressure. II. Intravenous administration of glycerol and glycerol with sorbitol under experimental conditions. Klin Oczna 43:371, 1973.

OTHER INVESTIGATIONAL ANTIGLAUCOMA DRUGS

The classes of drugs discussed in the preceding five chapters provide effective intraocular pressure (IOP) control for the majority of glaucoma patients. However, because of intolerable side effects and lack of efficacy in some cases, these drugs are not always able to prevent progressive glaucomatous damage. There is a need, therefore, to continue the search for new and better antiglaucoma medications. Much of this work is presently being done with new forms of drugs from the classes that were discussed in the previous chapters. In addition, research continues with the following groups of drugs.

CANNABINOIDS

In 1971, Hepler and Frank (1) reported that smoking a marihuana cigarette caused a significant reduction in the IOP. It was subsequently shown in animal and human studies that several derivatives of *tetrahydrocannabinol* (THC), the primary class of active ingredients in marihuana, effectively lowered the IOP when given orally (2–6), or intravenously (7–10), while the reported effects of topical cannabinoids were conflicting (2, 11–17). These observations stimulated the search for cannabinoids that would be suitable for the long-term management of glaucoma. To date, these studies have yielded the following data.

Mechanism of Action

It was once thought that smoking marihuana might lower the IOP indirectly by the drug-induced relaxation effect (18). Extensive animal studies, however, confirmed a direct ocular hypotensive effect. The local effect may be primarily due to vasodilatation of the efferent vessels in the anterior uvea, which reduces the ultrafiltration pressure for aqueous humor formation (10, 19, 20). This action was reported to be inhibited by ganglionectomy (9, 21), β-adrenergic blockers (21), or vasodilators (22). Biochemical studies in rabbits suggested that the ocular hypotensive mechanism of marihuana-derived material is not mediated through adenylate cyclase, ATPase or substance P, but may possibly be due to modification of the surface membrane glycoprotein residues on the ciliary epithelium (23).

The IOP reduction was also found to be associated with increased facility of outflow (9, 10, 19), which was shown to be blocked by ganglionectomy (9, 21) or α-adrenergic antagonists (20, 21). In another study, however, surgical removal of all autonomic input in cats did not alter the ocular hypotensive effect of Δ^9-THC (24). The cannabinoids were also shown to stimulate monoamine oxidase activity, which could possibly be related to the influence of these compounds on the IOP (25). Other reported actions associated with cannabinoid therapy included increased aqueous protein (10) and antagonism of the in vivo ocular production of prostaglandin from arachidonic acid (26). Δ^9-THC produced ocular hypotension and miosis in rabbits when given intravenously, but not when administered into the cerebral ventricles, suggesting that the action of cannabinoids on IOP does not originate in the central nervous system (27).

Side Effects

Although marihuana and many of the cannabinoids are known to be highly effective in lowering the IOP, the numerous side effects of all the compounds thus far tested in humans seriously limit their general usefulness in the long-term management of glaucoma (4, 28, 29). The best known of these adverse reactions is the altered mental status, which has been observed during trial therapy with inhalation of marihuana (30) and with oral administration of THC derivatives (4, 5). Heavy marihuana use (median of 29 days in preceding 30 days) among college students, as compared to light use (median of 1 day in last 30), was associated with residual neuropsychologic effects even after a day of supervised abstinence from the drug (31).

Ocular side effects associated with marihuana inhalation include conjunctival hyperemia, a slight miosis, and reduced tear production (28, 29, 32, 33). Individuals who had used marihuana chronically for 10 years or more, but had abstained for at least 3 hours prior to testing, had increased basal lacrimation, decreased dark adaptation, decreased color-match limits, decreased Snellen acuity, and slightly increased IOP as compared to matched nonuser controls (34).

From the standpoint of controlling glaucoma, the most disturbing adverse reaction is systemic hypotension, which has been observed with oral (4, 5) and intravenous (8) cannabinoids, as well as marihuana inhalation (30). If the drop in blood pressure is associated with reduced perfusion of the optic nerve head, the cannabinoids could be lowering the IOP without protecting against progressive glaucomatous optic atrophy (4, 35). Even with topical administration, systemic hypotension may be a problem. Animal studies suggest that topical cannabinoid therapy reduces the IOP by a systemic mechanism (13), and trials with glaucoma patients revealed occasional systemic hypotension (14).

Before a cannabinoid can be recommended for the management of glaucoma, one must be found that dissociates the ocular and systemic side effects from the ocular hypotensive action. To date, no such pharmacologic agent has been found. With the promise of so many other classes of drugs for the chronic management of glaucoma, as discussed in this and preceding chapters, there has been a marked decline in research with cannabinoids for glaucoma. However, the potential for its use still remains, if the criteria can be met for an appropriate antiglaucoma agent.

ETHACRYNIC ACID

Ethacrynic acid is a sulfhydryl-reactive diuretic that has been shown to increase aqueous outflow when perfused into the anterior chamber of living monkey eyes and enucleated calf eyes (36). Intracameral injections of concentrations ranging from 0.5 to 7.5 mmol/L in living monkeys provided no reliable reduction in IOP with concentrations less than 3.0 mmol/L, while concentrations above 3.75 mmol/L caused an increasing incidence and severity of corneal edema (37). Within the 3.0–3.75 mmol/L range, the maximal mean IOP reduction occurred after 6 hours, with the experimental IOP decreasing 2.9 mm Hg.

The mechanism of increased aqueous outflow with ethacrynic acid is uncertain, but appears to be related to alterations in the trabecular meshwork cells. When anterior segments of human donor eyes were perfused with the drug, neither toxic effects nor a morphologic correlate of the facility increase were observed with 0.01 mmol/L, while separations between trabecular cells and breaks between inner-wall cells were observed at 0.1 mmol/L, and focal areas of cell swelling and necrosis were noted at 0.25 mmol/L (38). Cell cultures derived from trabecular meshworks of human and bovine eyes revealed reversible alteration in cell shape when exposed to ethacrynic acid at concentrations up to 0.4 mmol/L, with coincident changes in the staining pattern of major cytoskeletal components including actin, α-actinin, vinculin, and vimentin (39). In the same study, taxol (which stabilizes microtubule structure) blocked the ethacrynic acid-induced changes in tubulin. It may be, therefore, that ethacrynic acid increases the outflow facility by alterations in the cytoskeleton of outflow pathway cells (39).

Two limitations to the clinical application of ethacrynic acid in the management of glaucoma are poor corneal penetration and toxic effects, especially on the cornea and trabecular meshwork. While intracameral ethacrynic acid lowered the IOP in normotensive monkeys 1–3 mm Hg for up to 48 hours, topical application induced no change in IOP (40). However, when ethacrynic acid in ointment was applied to normotensive monkeys for 5 days, the difference in IOP between drug- and placebo-treated eyes at 0, 1, and 3 hours after the last treatment was −2.8, −1.7 and −3.7 mm Hg, respectively, with a 40 ± 15% increase in outflow facility (41).

A study of toxicity and outflow effects on human trabecular meshwork in perfusion organ culture revealed increased facility of outflow of at least 40%, but with dose-related histologic effects on the trabecular cells that included nuclear chromatin clumping, cellular swelling, cytoplasmic membrane disruption and cell necrosis, with no recovery or reversal of these changes (42). In an attempt to increase this low therapeutic index, the effects of various thiol adducts of ethacrynic acid on outflow facility were explored in enucleated calf eyes, and a dose response effect was demonstrated with ethacrynic acid-cysteine (43). When ethacrynic acid-cysteine was given topically to rabbits and monkeys, it lowered the IOP with less corneal edema than was seen with topical ethacrynic acid, and the corneal side effects were even further reduced by pretreatment with topical acetylcysteine (44).

When ethacrynic acid was injected intracamerally in five eyes of five patients with advanced glaucoma, a reduction in IOP from 9 to 31 mm Hg was observed 3–5 hours after treatment and lasted for 3 days (45). These and other observations stimulated a multicenter, randomized, double-masked, placebo-controlled trial in which ethacrynic acid or placebo were administered intracamerally at the end of cataract surgery in patients with coexisting glaucoma. No statistically significant difference was noted in the postoperative intraocular pressure course between the two groups (89).

While ethacrynic acid may not prove to be suitable for the management of glaucoma, experience gained from the related research suggests the potential usefulness of drugs that improve aqueous outflow by altering trabecular meshwork cell shape, possibly through action on the cytoskeleton.

VASOACTIVE PEPTIDES

Several biologically active peptides (combinations of two or more amino acids, which provide information exchange between cells in various forms such as hormones or neurotransmitters) have been found in abundance in the anterior ocular segments of various animal species. They appear to have a wide range of actions on aqueous humor dynamics. *Vasoactive intestinal peptide,* for example, which has specific receptors in rabbit ciliary processes (46), has been shown to enhance aqueous humor flow following intravenous or intracameral administration in monkeys (47). Other peptides, some of which are discussed later, have a biphasic action on the IOP. With most of these agents, however, there is a prominent ocular hypotensive component, which has stimulated the study for vasoactive peptides that might be suitable for the treatment of glaucoma.

Endothelins

Endothelins are a group of vasoconstrictor polypeptides that were first isolated from porcine aortic endothelial cells. Three endothelin genes, designated ET-1, ET-2, and ET-3, have been isolated in the human genome, and two distinct types of endothelin receptors, designated ETA and ETB, have been cloned. High concentrations of ET-1 and ET-3 have been demonstrated in the iris and ciliary body of rabbit eyes (48).

Intraocular injections of endothelins in animals have produced variable effects on aqueous humor dynamics and IOP, with most studies showing a significant ocular hypotensive component. When ET-1 was injected intravitreally in rabbit eyes, there was a biphasic IOP response, with an initial rise in 1–2 hours followed by a reduction for more

than 96 hours (49). The later response was associated with a 58% decrease in aqueous formation and a 94% increase in total outflow facility, but no significant effect on uveoscleral outflow. In another rabbit study, however, the injection of ET-1 or ET-3 into the anterior vitreous produced an IOP reduction of 43% and 45%, respectively, which was not due to increased aqueous outflow and was not prevented by indomethacin (48). The IOP reduction in rabbits appears to be mediated, at least in part, through the ETB receptors, since sarafotoxin S6c, a selective ETB agonist, reduces IOP in rabbits in a dose-dependent fashion (50).

Studies in other animal species support a role for endothelin in impaired outflow facility. Experiments with cultured bovine trabecular meshwork cells suggests that ET-1 may be involved in the regulation of aqueous humor dynamics by changing intracellular calcium and pH in meshwork cells (51). Intracameral injections of ET-1 in living monkey eyes increased outflow facility 22–71%, which was felt to be mediated, at least in part, through an action on the ciliary muscle (52).

Atrial Natriuretic Peptides

Atrial natriuretic peptides (ANP) are a group of polypeptides synthesized by cardiac atrial myocytes. They have been shown to reduce IOP and aqueous flow in rabbits and monkeys, which may be mediated by activation of guanylate cyclase and an increase in cyclic guanosine monophosphate (cGMP) (53). A cGMP analogue, 8-bomoguanosine 3':5'-cyclic monophosphate (Br cGMP), has been shown to decrease aqueous formation and increase aqueous outflow when injected intracamerally or intravitreally in monkeys (54), and to reduce IOP when administered topically in rabbits (55, 6), which was not associated with a significant change in tonographic outflow facility (56).

Candoxatril, which increases endogenous ANP by inhibiting neutral endopeptidase, has been shown to significantly lower IOP in a placebo-controlled trial of human patients, which correlated with an increase in endogenous ANP (57).

Neuropeptide Y

Neuropeptide Y, which is also abundant in ciliary processes, has been shown in rabbit studies to modulate adenylate cyclase in iris dilator muscle, ciliary body, and ciliary epithelium (58–60).

OTHER INVESTIGATIONAL ANTIHYPERTENSIVE AGENTS

A wide variety of additional agents have been evaluated for their influence on aqueous humor dynamics as potential

IOP-lowering drugs in the management of glaucoma. The following is only a partial list of these agents.

Dopaminergic Agents

Dopaminergic agents produce a variety of aqueous humor dynamics responses because they not only act on five different dopamine receptors, but also on adrenoreceptors (61). *Haloperidol,* a dopaminergic antagonist that is used as an antipsychotic, was reported to be equivalent or superior to timolol in suppressing artificially elevated IOP in rabbits (62, 63). The mechanism of action was felt to be reduction of aqueous humor production by the lowering of blood flow to the ciliary body.

Bromocriptine is an ergot derivative that is used in the treatment of hyperprolactinemia, acromegaly, and Parkinson's disease. It is a dopamine-2 receptor agonist and a dopamine-1 and α-adrenoreceptor antagonist. It has been shown to reduce IOP following oral administration in normal volunteers (64, 65) and glaucoma patients (65), which is associated with a significant increase in outflow facility (65). This action appears to be related to stimulation of dopamine-2 receptors, since it is blocked by metoclopramide, a specific dopamine-2 antagonist (64).

Glucocorticoid Agents

Glucocorticoid receptors are common to all cells including those of the trabecular meshwork, although different types of cells respond to glucocortoids in a variety of ways (61). As discussed in Chapter 20, corticosteroids tend to increase the IOP in a certain percentage of individuals, and some drugs may block this action. *Tetrahydrocortisol,* for example, is a metabolite of cortisol, which was shown to lower the dexamethasone-induced ocular hypertension in rabbits (66). *Mifepristone* is a specific glucocorticoid receptor antagonist, which lowers IOP in rabbits, possibly by blocking the glucocorticoid receptor-mediated effects in ocular tissues (67).

Spironolactone

Spironolactone, a synthetic steroidal aldosterone antagonist with potassium-sparing diuretic-antihypertensive activity, produced significant IOP reduction in glaucoma patients, which persisted 2 weeks after termination of the treatment (68).

Antazoline

Antazoline is an antihistamine of the ethylenediamine class that has been shown to lower the IOP following topical administration in rabbits, apparently by decreasing aqueous production (69).

Angiotensin Converting Enzyme Inhibitor

Angiotensin converting enzyme inhibitor in a topical formulation has been shown to lower the IOP in dogs and humans with ocular hypertension or open-angle glaucoma (70).

Organic Nitrates

Organic nitrates such as intravenous nitroglycerin or oral isosorbide dinitrate have been reported to lower IOP in glaucoma and nonglaucoma patients (71).

Melatonin

Melatonin, a hormone produced by the pineal gland with a well-characterized circadian rhythm, was shown to lower the IOP in normal volunteers (72).

Calcium Channel Blockers

Calcium channel blockers produce vasodilation by inhibiting the entrance of calcium ions into vascular smooth muscle cells and are used in the management of coronary heart disease. They have been shown to have ocular hypotensive activity (73), which lasted up to 10 hours in human volunteers (74). These drugs may also protect the optic nerve head by improving vascular perfusion, which is discussed later.

Tetracycline Derivatives

Demeclocycline, tetracycline, and other tetracycline derivatives were shown to lower the IOP in rabbits, which appears to be related to reduced aqueous humor production (75).

Acepromazine

Acepromazine, an analogue of chlorpromazine that is used as a tranquilizer in veterinary medicine, had no effect on IOP when given topically to normotensive rabbits, but reduced the pressure for at least 32 hours in rabbits with chronic IOP elevation produced by argon laser applications to the trabecular meshwork (76).

DIRECT OPTIC NERVE HEAD PROTECTORS

All of the drugs previously discussed indirectly protect the optic nerve head from progressive glaucomatous atrophy by lowering the IOP. An alternative approach is to administer medications that directly protect the nerve head from the effects of the elevated pressure or, as in some cases of normal-tension glaucoma in which elevated IOP may not be a significant factor, to protect the nerve from other mechanisms of glaucomatous optic neuropathy.

Early Studies

In 1948, McGuire (77) reported the use of bishydroxy-coumarin (Dicumarol) to protect the optic nerve head by improving vascular perfusion. However, other investigators could not confirm his findings (78). Subsequently, diphenyl-hydantoin (Dilantin) (79) and phosphatide complexes (80) were also reported to directly protect the optic nerve head from progressive glaucomatous damage in preliminary studies. Although none of these observations were ever confirmed, continued research has disclosed newer pharmacologic approaches that may eventually yield effective direct optic nerve head protection.

Calcium Channel Blockers

As noted earlier in this chapter, calcium channel blockers may not only have some ocular hypotensive effect in human subjects (73, 74), but may also help to protect the optic nerve head, especially in normal-tension glaucoma, by improving ocular blood flow. Intravenous *nicardine* in monkeys caused an early decrease in optic nerve head blood flow, followed by a slow rise to finally exceed the initial value 80 minutes after injection, but then fell again with additional infusion of the drug (81). The main cause of this phenomenon was believed to be a decrease in systemic blood flow despite a significant decrease in mean arterial pressure (82).

A single oral dose of *nimodipine* in normal-tension glaucoma patients and control subjects was shown to improve contrast sensitivity (83). In a 6-month, uncontrolled trial, 6 of 25 normal-tension glaucoma patients receiving *nifedipine* showed constant, sustained visual field improvement during the course of the study (84). In another study of normal-tension glaucoma patients who received either nifedipine, acetazolamide, or no therapy, however, no statistically significant difference was seen in progression of optic nerve head damage (85). In yet a third study, 56 patients with normal-tension glaucoma or chronic open-angle glaucoma who were receiving a calcium channel blocker for nonophthalmic reasons (e.g., cardiac disease or systemic hypertension) were compared to similar groups not receiving such medication for a mean observation period of 3.4 years (86). In the normal-tension group, visual field progression was seen in 2 of 18 eyes (11%) receiving calcium channel blockers, compared to 10 of 18 eyes (56%) of the controls, while no marked difference was seen in the open-angle group.

Other Potential Direct Protectors

Other vasodilators may also prove to have value in preventing glaucomatous optic atrophy. Several dopamine antagonists, for example, in addition to lowering the IOP in rabbits, have been shown to increase the ocular pulsatile blood flow (87). A review of other potential optic nerve head protectors included nitric oxide, free-radical scavengers and antioxidants, inhibitors of excitotoxins, and nerve regeneration and growth factors (88). This is clearly a wide open and extremely important field for continued research in the medical management of glaucoma.

SUMMARY

In addition to continued research with the drug groups discussed in the preceding chapters, other classes of compounds are also being studied for possible use in the treatment of glaucoma. Cannabinoids effectively lower the IOP by an uncertain mechanism, although the lack of a drug form that dissociates this action from the systemic side effects has limited the usefulness of these agents. Ethacrynic acid effectively improves aqueous outflow, but is limited by poor corneal penetration and was not effective when given intracamerally in a clinical trial. Preliminary experience with several additional classes of drugs, including vasoactive peptides, offers promise for new ocular hypotensive agents. In addition, drugs are being studied that may directly protect the optic nerve from the effects of elevated IOP or from pressure-independent mechanisms of glaucomatous optic neuropathy.

REFERENCES

1. Hepler, RS, Frank, IR: Marihuana smoking and intraocular pressure. JAMA 217:1392, 1971.
2. Green, K, Kim, K: Acute dose response of intraocular pressure to topical and oral cannabinoids. Proc Soc Exp Biol Med 154:228, 1977.
3. Newell, FW, Stark, P, Jay, WM, Schanzlin, DJ: Nabilone: a pressure-reducing synthetic benzopyran in open-angle glaucoma. Ophthalmology 86:156, 1979.
4. Tiedeman, JS, Shields, MB, Weber, PA, et al: Effect of synthetic cannabinoids on elevated intraocular pressure. Ophthalmology 88:270, 1981.
5. Merritt, JC, McKinnon, S, Armstrong, JR, et al: Oral delta⁹-tetrahydrocannabinol in heterogeneous glaucomas. Ann Ophthalmol 12:947, 1980.
6. Weber, PA, Bianchine, JR, Howes, JF: Nabitan hydrochloride: ocular hypotensive effect in normal human volunteers. Glaucoma 3:163, 1981.
7. Purnell, WD, Gregg, JM: Delta⁹-tetrahydrocannabinol, euphoria and intraocular pressure in man. Ann Ophthalmol 7:921, 1975.
8. Cooler, P, Gregg, JM: Effect of delta⁹-tetrahydrocannabinol on intraocular pressure in humans. So Med J 70:951, 1977.
9. Green, K, Kim, K: Mediation of ocular tetrahydrocannabinol effects by adrenergic nervous system. Exp Eye Res 23:443, 1976.
10. Green, K, Pederson, JE: Effect of delta¹-tetrahydrocannabinol on aqueous dynamics and ciliary body permeability in the rabbit. Exp Eye Res 15:499, 1973.

11. Green, K, Kim, K, Wynn, H, Shimp, RG: Intraocular pressure, organ weights and the chronic use of cannabinoid derivatives in rabbits for one year. Exp Eye Res 25:465, 1977.

12. Green, K, Bigger, JF, Kim, K, Bowman, K: Cannabinoid penetration and chronic effects in the eye. Exp Eye Res 24:197, 1977.

13. Merritt, JC, Peiffer, RL, McKinnon, SM, et al: Topical delta^9-tetrahydrocannabinol on intraocular pressure in dogs. Glaucoma 3:13, 1981.

14. Merritt, JC, Olsen, JL, Armstrong, JR, McKinnon, SM: Topical delta^9-tetrahydrocannabinol in hypertensive glaucomas. J Pharm Pharmacol 33:40, 1981.

15. Merritt, JG, Whitaker, R, Page, CJ, et al: Topical delta^8-tetrahydrocannabinol as a potential glaucoma agent. Glaucoma 4:253, 1982.

16. Green, K, Roth, M: Ocular effects of topical administration delta^9-tetrahydrocannabinol in man. Arch Ophthalmol 100:265, 1982.

17. Jay, WM, Green, K: Multiple-drop study of topically applied 1% delta^9-tetrahydrocannabinol in human eyes. Arch Ophthalmol 101:591, 1983.

18. Flom, MC, Adams, AJ, Jones, RT: Marijuana smoking and reduced pressure in human eyes: drug action or epiphenomenon? Invest Ophthalmol 14:52, 1975.

19. Green, K, Wynn, H, Padgett, D: Effects of delta^9-tetrahydrocannabinol on ocular blood flow and aqueous humor formation. Exp Eye Res 26:65, 1978.

20. Green, K, Kim, K: Interaction of adrenergic antagonists with prostaglandin E$_2$ and tetrahydrocannabinol in the eye. Invest Ophthalmol 15:102, 1976.

21. Green, K, Bigger, JF, Kim, K, Bowman, K: Cannabinoid action on the eye as mediated through the central nervous system and local adrenergic activity. Exp Eye Res 24:189, 1977.

22. Green, K, Kim, K: Papaverine and verapamil interaction with prostaglandin E$_2$ and delta^9-tetrahydrocannabinol in the eye. Exp Eye Res 24:207, 1977.

23. Green, K, Cheeks, K, Mittag, T, et al: Marihuana-derived material: biochemical studies of the ocular responses. Curr Eye Res 4:631, 1985.

24. Colasanti, BK, Powell, SR: Effect of delta^9-tetrahydrocannabinol on intraocular pressure after removal of autonomic input. J Ocul Pharm 1:47, 1985.

25. Gawienowski, AM, Chatterjee, D, Anderson, PJ, et al: Effect of delta^9-tetrahydrocannabinol on monoamine oxidase activity in bovine eye tissues, in vitro. Invest Ophthalmol Vis Sci 22:482, 1982.

26. Green, K, Podos, SM: Anatagonism of arachidonic acid-induced ocular effects by delta^1-tetrahydrocannabinol. Invest Ophthalmol 13:422, 1974.

27. Liu, JHK, Dacus, AC: Central nervous system and peripheral mechanisms in ocular hypotensive effect of cannabinoids. Arch Ophthalmol 105:245, 1987.

28. Green, K: Marihuana and the eye. Invest Ophthalmol 14:261, 1975.

29. Green, K, Roth, M: Marijuana in the medical management of glaucoma. Perspect Ophthalmol 4:101, 1980.

30. Merritt, JC, Crawford, WJ, Alexander, PC, et al: Effect of marihuana on intraocular and blood pressure in glaucoma. Ophthalmology 87:222, 1980.

31. Pope, HG Jr, Yurgelun-Todd, D: The residual cognitive effects of heavy marijuana use in college students. JAMA 275:521, 1996.

32. Hepler, RS, Frank, IM, Ungerleider, JT: Pupillary constriction after marijuana smoking. Am J Ophthalmol 74:1185, 1972.

33. Brown, B, Adams, AJ, Haegerstrom-Portnoy, G, et al: Pupil size after use of marijuana and alcohol. Am J Ophthalmol 83:350, 1977.

34. Dawson, WW, Jimenez-Antillon, CF, Perez, JM, Zeskind, JA: Marijuana and vision—after ten years' use in Costa Rica. Invest Ophthalmol Vis Sci 16:689, 1977.

35. Gaasterland, DE: Efficacy in glaucoma treatment—the potential of marijuana. Ann Ophthalmol 12:448, 1980.

36. Epstein, DL, Freddo, TF, Bassett-Chu, S, et al: Influence of ethacrynic acid on outflow facility in the monkey and calf eye. Invest Ophthalmol Vis Sci 28:2067, 1987.

37. Tingey, DP, Ozment, RR, Schroeder, A, Epstein, DL: The effect of intracameral ethacrynic acid on the intraocular pressure of living monkeys. Am J Ophthalmol 113:706, 1992.

38. Liang, L-L, Epstein, DL, deKater, AW, et al: Ethacrynic acid increases facility of outflow in the human eye in vitro. Arch Ophthalmol 110:106, 1992.

39. Erickson-Lamy, K, Schroeder, A, Epstein, DL: Ethacrynic acid induces reversible shape and cytoskeletal changes in cultured cells. Invest Ophthalmol Vis Sci 33:2631, 1992.

40. Croft, MA, Hubbard, WC, Kaufman, PL: Effect of ethacrynic acid on aqueous outflow dynamics in monkeys. Invest Ophthalmol Vis Sci 35:1167, 1994.

41. Croft, MA, Kaufman, PL: Effect of daily topical ethacrynic acid on aqueous humor dynamics in monkeys. Curr Eye Res 14:777, 1995.

42. Johnson, DH, Tschumper, RC: Ethacrynic acid: outflow effects and toxicity in human trabecular meshwork in perfusion organ culture. Curr Eye Res 12:385, 1993.

43. Epstein, DL, Hooshmand, LB, Epstein, MPM: Thiol adducts of ethacrynic acid increase outflow facility in enucleated calf eyes. Curr Eye Res 11:253, 1992.

44. Tingey, DP, Schroeder, A, Epstein, MPM, Epstein, DL: Effects of topical ethacrynic acid adducts on intraocular pressure in rabbits and monkeys. Arch Ophthalmol 110:699, 1992.

45. Melamed, S, Kotas-Neumann, R, Barak, A, Epstein, DL: The effect of intracamerally injected ethacrynic acid on intraocular pressure in patients with glaucoma. Am J Ophthalmol 113:508, 1992.

46. Horio, B, Law, NM, Rosenzweig, SA: Characterization of vasoactive intestinal peptide receptors in rabbit ciliary processes. Invest Ophthalmol Vis Sci 36:192, 1995.

47. Nilsson, SFE, Mäepea, O, Samuelsson, M, Bill, A: Effects of timolol on terbutaline- and VIP-stimulated aqueous humor flow in the cynomolgus monkey. Curr Eye Res 9:863, 1990.

48. MacCumber, MW, Jampel, HD, Snyder, SH: Ocular effects of the endothelins. Abundant peptides in the eye. Arch Ophthalmol 109:705, 1991.

49. Taniguchi, T, Okada, K, Haque, MSR, et al: Effects of endothelin-1 on intraocular pressure and aqueous humor dynamics in the rabbit eye. Curr Eye Res 13:461, 1994.

50. Haque, MSR, Taniguchi, T, Sugiyama, K, et al: The ocular hypotensive effect of the ETB receptor selective agonist, sarafotoxin S6c, in rabbits. Invest Ophthalmol Vis Sci 36:804, 1995.

51. Kohmoto, H, Matsumoto, S, Serizawa, T: Effects of endothelin-1 on [Ca^{2+}]$_i$ and pH$_i$ in trabecular meshwork cells. Curr Eye Res 13:197, 1994.

52. Erickson-Lamy, K, Korbmacher, C, Schuman, JS, Nathanson, JA: Effect of endothelin on outflow facility and accommodation in the monkey eye in vivo. Invest Ophthalmol Vis Sci 32:492, 1991.

53. Nathanson, JA: Atriopeptin-activated guanylate cyclase in the anterior segment. Identification, localization, and effects of atriopeptins on IOP. Invest Ophthalmol Vis Sci 28:1357, 1987.

54. Kee, C, Kaufman, PL, Gabelt, B'AT: Effect of 8-Br cGMP on aqueous humor dynamics in monkeys. Invest Ophthalmol Vis Sci 35:2769, 1994.

55. Stein, PJ, Clack, JW: Topical application of a cyclic GMP analog lowers IOP in normal and ocular hypertensive rabbits. Invest Ophthalmol Vis Sci 35:2765, 1994.

56. Becker, B: Topical 8-bromo-cyclic GMP lowers intraocular pressure in rabbits. Invest Ophthalmol Vis Sci 31:1647, 1990.

57. Wolfensberger, TJ, Singer, DRJ, Freegard, T, et al: Evidence for a new role of natriuretic peptides: control of intraocular pressure. Br J Ophthalmol 78:446, 1994.

58. Cepelík, J, Hynie, S: Inhibitory effects of neuropeptide Y on adenylate cyclase of rabbit ciliary processes. Curr Eye Res 9:121, 1990.

59. Piccone, M, Littzi, J, Krupin, T, et al: Effects of neuropeptide Y on the isolated rabbit iris dilator muscle. Invest Ophthalmol Vis Sci 29:330, 1988.

60. Jumblatt, JE, Gooch, JM: Neuropeptide Y modulates adenylate cyclase in the rabbit iris ciliary body and ciliary epithelium. Exp Eye Res 51:229, 1990.

61. Tripathi, RC, Yang, C, Tripathi, BJ, Borisuth, NSC: Role of receptors in the trabecular meshwork of the eye as targeted to the development of antiglaucoma therapy. Drug Dev Res 27:191, 1992.

62. Chiou, GCY: Ocular hypotensive actions of haloperidol, a dopaminergic antagonist. Arch Ophthalmol 102:143, 1984.

63. Chiou, GCY: Treatment of ocular hypertension and glaucoma with dopamine antagonists. Ophthal Res 16:129, 1984.

64. Mekki, QA, Turner, P: Stimulation of dopamine receptors (type 2) lowers human intraocular pressure. Br J Ophthalmol 69:909, 1985.

65. Costagliola, C, Carella, C, Amato, G, et al: Effect of oral bromocriptine administration on intraocular pressure in normotensive and glaucomatous human subjects. J Glau 4:386, 1995.

66. Southren, AL, I'Hommedieu, D, Gordon, GG, Weinstein, BI: Intraocular hypotensive effect of a topically applied cortisol metabolite: 3α, 5β-tetrahydrocortisol. Invest Ophthalmol Vis Sci 28:901, 1987.

67. Munden, PM, Schmidt, TJ: Mifepristone blocks specific glucocorticoid receptor binding in rabbit iris-ciliary body. Arch Ophthalmol 110:703, 1992.

68. Witzmann, R: The effect of spironolactone on intraocular pressure in glaucoma patients. Klin Monatsbl Augenheilkd 176:445, 1980.

69. Krupin, T, Silverstein, B, Feitl, M, et al: The effect of H1-blocking antihistamines on intraocular pressure in rabbits. Ophthalmology 87:1167, 1980.

70. Constad, WH, Fiore, P, Samson, C, Cinotti, AA: Use of an angiotensin converting enzyme inhibitor in ocular hypertension and primary open-angle glaucoma. Am J Ophthalmol 105:674, 1988.

71. Wizemann, A, Wizemann, V: The use of organic nitrates to lower intraocular pressure in outpatient and surgical treatment. Klin Monatsbl Augenheilkd 177:292, 1980.

72. Samples, JR, Krause, G, Lewy, AJ: Effect of melatonin on intraocular pressure. Curr Eye Res 7:649, 1988.

73. Monica, ML, Hesse, RJ, Messerli, FH: The effect of a calcium-channel blocking agent on intraocular pressure. Am J Ophthalmol 96:814, 1983.

74. Abelson, MB, Gilbert, CM, Smith, LM: Sustained reduction of intraocular pressure in humans with the calcium channel blocker verapamil. Am J Ophthalmol 105:155, 1988.

75. Wallace, I, Krupin, T, Stone, RA, Moolchandani, J: The ocular hypotensive effects of demeclocycline, tetracycline and other tetracycline derivatives. Invest Ophthalmol Vis Sci 30:1594, 1989.

76. Hayreh, SS, Kardon, RH, McAllister, DL, Fleury, PJ: Acepromazine. Effects on intraocular pressure. Arch Ophthalmol 109:119, 1991.

77. McGuire, WP: The effect of dicumarol on the visual fields in glaucoma. A preliminary report. Trans Am Ophthalmol Soc 84:96, 1948.

78. Shields, MB, Wadsworth, JAC: An evaluation of anticoagulation in glaucoma therapy. Ann Ophthalmol 9:1115, 1977.

79. Becker, B, Stamper, RL, Asseff, C, Podos, SM: Effect of diphenylhydantoin on glaucomatous field loss: a preliminary report. Trans Am Acad Ophthalmol Otol 76:412, 1972.

80. Hruby, K, Weiss, H: Therapeutic utilization of phosphatide complexes in ophthalmology. Ophthalmol Digest June 9, 1976.

81. Noguchi, S, Kimura, Y, Nitta, A, et al: Blood flow in the optic nerve-head following intravenous administration of calcium antagonist. Acta Soc Ophthalmol Jpn 96:967, 1992.

82. Harino, S, Riva, CE, Petrig, BL: Intravenous nicardipine in cats increases optic nerve head but not retinal blood flow. Invest Ophthalmol Vis Sci 33:2885, 1992.

83. Bose, S, Pilz, JR, Breton, ME: Nimodipine, a centrally active calcium antagonist, exerts a beneficial effect on contrast sensitivity in patients with normal-tension glaucoma and in control subjects. Ophthalmology 102:1236, 1995.

84. Kitazawa, Y, Shirai, H, Go, FJ: The effect of calcium antagonist on visual field in low tension glaucoma. Graefes Arch Clin Exp Ophthalmol 227:408, 1989.

85. Lumme, P, Tuulonen, A, Airaksinen, PJ, Alanko, HI: Neuroretinal rim area in low tension glaucoma. Effect of nifedipine and acetazolamide compared to no treatment. Acta Ophthalmol 69:293, 1991.

86. Netland, PA, Chaturvedi, N, Dreyer, EB: Calcium channel blockers in the management of low-tension and open-angle glaucoma. Am J Ophthalmol 115:608, 1993.

87. Hong, S-J, Chiou, GCY: Effects of dopamine agonists and antagonists on pulsatile blood flow of ocular hypertensive rabbits. J Ocular Pharmacol Ther 9:117, 1993.

88. Schumer, RA, Podos, SM: The nerve of glaucoma! Arch Ophthalmol 112:37, 1994.

89. Arthur Neufeld, PhD, personal communication.

Chapter 32

ANATOMIC PRINCIPLES OF GLAUCOMA SURGERY

All laser and incisional surgical procedures for glaucoma are designed to reduce the intraocular pressure (IOP) by either increasing the rate of aqueous humor outflow or reducing aqueous production. The involved anatomy, therefore, is the anterior ocular structures related to aqueous outflow and the portions of the ciliary body associated with aqueous inflow. To properly perform any of the operations that make up the armamentarium of glaucoma surgery, the surgeon must be familiar with both the internal and external aspects of these structures. In this chapter, we consider these portions of the ocular anatomy as they relate to glaucoma surgery.

AN OVERVIEW OF THE ANATOMY

The structures involved in aqueous humor dynamics, i.e., aqueous production and aqueous outflow, are in immediate proximity to each other in the periphery of the anterior ocular segment. The interrelationship between these structures was considered in Chapter 2 with a stepwise construction of a schematic model that may be summarized as follows.

At the junction between the cornea and the sclera is the transitional zone of connective tissue known as the *limbus*. On the inner surface of the limbus, extending for 360°, is a depression, referred to as the scleral sulcus. The anterior margin of this sulcus slopes gradually into the peripheral cornea, while the posterior margin contains a lip of connective tissue called the *scleral spur*. This spur might be thought of as the dividing point between the structures of aqueous outflow anteriorly and those of aqueous production posteriorly. The *trabecular meshwork* attaches, in part, to the anterior side of the scleral spur and extends forward to blend into the sloping anterior wall of the scleral sulcus, which converts the sulcus into *Schlemm's canal*. The bulk of aqueous humor in the anterior chamber flows through the trabecular meshwork to Schlemm's canal, from whence it leaves the eye via intrascleral channels and episcleral veins.

The *ciliary body* attaches to the posterior portion of the scleral spur. This is actually the only firm attachment of the ciliary body, with the remaining surfaces between the sclera and the ciliary body creating a potential space, referred to as the supraciliary space. The *ciliary processes,* the actual site of aqueous production, occupy the innermost and anterior-most portion of the ciliary body. The *iris* inserts into the ciliary body just anterior to the ciliary processes. Consequently, a peripheral iridectomy, as performed during glaucoma filtering surgery, will often allow visualization of two to four ciliary processes. The insertion of the iris is usually such that a portion of the anterior ciliary body remains gonioscopically visible between the iris root and scleral spur. This is referred to as the ciliary body band. The remainder of the trabecular meshwork, i.e., that which does not attach to the scleral spur, attaches to this band and to the peripheral iris.

INTERNAL ANATOMY (FIG. 32.1)

Ciliary Body

Most of the ciliary body is located posterior to the iris and cannot be directly visualized except in unusual circumstances, such as with marked iris retraction or absence of

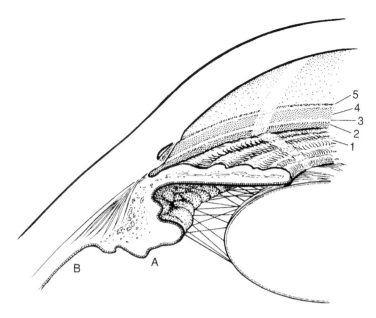

Figure 32.1. Internal anatomy. The ciliary body is located just posterior to the iris and is divided into the pars plicata (A) and the pars plana (B). The remaining internal structures can be seen by gonioscopy and include 1. iris, 2. ciliary body band, 3. scleral spur, 4. trabecular meshwork, and 5. Schwalbe's line.

portions of the iris. The anterior 2–3 mm of the ciliary body, the *pars plicata,* is thicker than the posterior portion and contains the radial ridges of the ciliary processes. The latter are the site of aqueous production and the target of cyclodestructive procedures. In those unusual circumstances in which they can be visualized directly (cycloscopy), direct treatment with laser transpupillary cyclophotocoagulation may be possible. In most cases, however, an indirect, transscleral route must be used for the cyclodestructive element, requiring the use of external landmarks, which is discussed later in this chapter. The posterior 4 mm of the ciliary body is the thinner *pars plana,* which must also be approached by using external landmarks.

Gonioscopic Anatomy

The following structures in the anterior chamber can be visualized by gonioscopic examination and are involved in a number of laser and incisional glaucoma surgical procedures.

Iris

The iris is the posterior-most structure of the anterior chamber angle. It is helpful to remember that the peripheral portion of the iris is thinner than the more central iris, which makes it, among other reasons, the preferred site for a laser iridotomy. Other anatomic considerations related to optimum laser iridotomy sites are iris crypts, or thinner areas of stroma which may be easier to penetrate. In addition, areas of increased pigmentation, such as iris freckles, may improve the absorption of laser energy in lightly pigmented eyes when using argon laser.

Ciliary Body Band

The ciliary body band is located just anterior to the root of the iris and typically has a dark gray or brown appearance by gonioscopic examination. The width of this band will vary considerably from one patient to the next, with myopes often having a wide band and hyperopes a narrow band. Care must be taken to avoid confusing this pigmented band with the trabecular meshwork in patients with lightly pigmented meshwork, especially when interpreting the depth of the anterior chamber angle. It is also important to avoid this error during laser trabeculoplasty. The patient will usually let the surgeon know when the latter mistake is made, since the ciliary body contains nerve endings and is sensitive to the application of laser energy.

Scleral Spur

The scleral spur is seen gonioscopically as a sharp, white line just anterior to the ciliary body band. In some patients, however, the visualization of the spur may be obscured to variable degrees by iris processes or heavy pigment dispersion. This was the principal site of surgery with a cyclodialysis procedure (an operation rarely used today), in which the ciliary body was separated from the scleral spur. In the early stages of neovascular glaucoma, new vessels may be seen extending across the scleral spur from the iris and ciliary body to the trabecular meshwork. The vessels can be obliterated at this site with laser applications in a procedure called goniophotocoagulation, which is also rarely used today.

Trabecular Meshwork

Just anterior to the scleral spur is the functional portion of the trabecular meshwork, i.e., that portion adjacent to

Schlemm's canal, through which the aqueous humor flows. This portion of the meshwork is demarcated gonioscopically by the presence of variable amounts of pigment. Since this pigment is carried to the meshwork from uveal tissue by the aqueous humor flow, it will typically be light in young individuals and will vary considerably among individuals later in life according to the amount of pigment dispersion. In some patients, especially with pathologic states such as the pigment dispersion syndrome and exfoliation syndrome, the meshwork will be extremely heavily pigmented. In other individuals, the meshwork may be so lightly pigmented that it is hard to see, which can lead to the incorrect diagnosis of a narrow, potentially occludable anterior chamber angle. In some of these cases, blood reflux into Schlemm's canal or iris processes, which typically extend to the meshwork, may help identify this structure.

It is this pigmented portion of the trabecular meshwork to which the laser energy should be applied during laser trabeculoplasty. It should be kept in mind, however, that there is another less pigmented portion of the meshwork just anterior to the functional, pigmented portion. In performing laser trabeculoplasty, it has been found that overlapping the laser beam between the pigmented and nonpigmented portions of the meshwork, i.e., along the anterior border of the pigmented portion, may help to reduce the complications of transient postoperative IOP rise and peripheral anterior synechia formation.

Schwalbe's Line

Schwalbe's line is the anterior-most structure in the anterior chamber angle and represents the junction between the nonpigmented portion of the trabecular meshwork and the peripheral cornea. In most individuals, a portion of this junction is represented by a small ridge. This is an important landmark when performing a goniotomy, since the internal incision in that operation is made just posterior to Schwalbe's line. The structure may be difficult to visualize gonioscopically, unless there has been a moderate degree of pigment dispersion, in which case there may be a buildup of pigment along the anterior side of the ridge, especially inferiorly. Care must be taken to avoid confusing this pigmented line with the trabecular meshwork when performing laser trabeculoplasty. In other cases in which there is minimal pigmentation, it is often helpful to establish the location of Schwalbe's line gonioscopically to help in determining the depth of the peripheral anterior chamber. A fine beam of light from the slitlamp can be seen reflecting from both the anterior and posterior surfaces of the peripheral cornea. As the clear portion of the peripheral cornea approaches Schwalbe's line, it is replaced externally by opaque limbal tissue, which causes the two beams to converge at Schwalbe's line, providing a useful way for determining the location of this structure.

EXTERNAL ANATOMY (FIG. 32.2)

Anterior Limbus

On the external surface of the eye, the anterior boundary of the limbus is defined as the termination of Bowman's membrane, which is approximately 0.5 mm anterior to the insertion of the conjunctiva and Tenon's capsule. This has been referred to as the *corneolimbal junction,* or the apparent or anterior limbus. It is important to note that the conjunctiva inserts more anteriorly in the superior and inferior quadrants. Consequently, the limbus will be wider in these quadrants, ranging between 1 and 1.5 mm, and will gradually taper to the narrowest width in the nasal and temporal quadrants, where the range is between 0.3 and 0.5 mm (1). In performing glaucoma filtering surgery, some surgeons choose to take advantage of the wider areas of the limbus by placing the surgical site at the 12 o'clock position. When performing surgery that involves the ciliary body, such as a cyclodestructive procedure or a pars plana incision, it is also important to remember that these structures will be slightly more posterior in relation to the apparent limbus in the superior and inferior quadrants.

Conjunctiva and Tenon's Capsule

The conjunctiva and Tenon's capsule cover the limbus. The adhesions between conjunctiva and Tenon's capsule are moderately firm, so that sharp dissection is usually required when dissecting between these two structures, as is done in some techniques of preparing the conjunctival flap for glaucoma filtering surgery. The adhesions between Tenon's capsule and the underlying limbus and sclera is less firm, and these structures can often be separated with blunt dissection. However, Tenon's capsule is firmly attached to the connective tissue of the limbus approximately 0.5 mm posterior to the insertion of the conjunctiva, which creates a potential space between the anterior conjunctiva/Tenon's capsule tissue and the limbal connective tissue. If the surgeon wishes to obtain maximum exposure of the limbus when preparing a limbus-based conjunctival flap, it is necessary to dissect this adherence between Tenon's capsule and the limbal tissue. It may be preferable, however, especially when performing filtering surgery with an adjunctive antimetabolite, to leave this adhesion intact to avoid creating a filtering bleb that is too thin at the limbus.

Posterior Limbus

When the conjunctiva and Tenon's capsule have been reflected, the posterior boundary of the limbus can now be seen. This has been referred to as the *sclerolimbal junction*

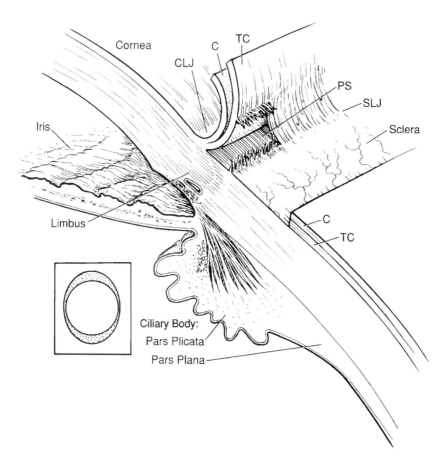

Figure 32.2. External anatomy. On the external surface, the limbus is bounded posteriorly by the sclerolimbal junction (SLJ) and anteriorly by the corneolimbal junction (CLJ). The width of the limbus varies from a maximum superiorly to a minimum on the sides *(inset)* due to the relative insertion of the conjunctiva (C). Tenon's capsule *(TC)* is firmly attached to limbal connective tissue approximately 0.5 mm behind the conjunctival insertion, creating a potential space *(PS)*. Cyclodestructive procedures should be placed over the pars plicata, usually 1.0–1.5 mm posterior to the corneolimbal junction, while a posterior sclerotomy should be made through the pars plana, approximately 3–4 mm posterior to the corneolimbal junction.

or the surgical or posterior limbus. It is identified as the junction of the opaque, white sclera posteriorly and the translucent, bluish-gray limbus anteriorly. This boundary of the limbus is more useful than the anterior limbus in glaucoma surgery because it helps to identify the location of the deeper structures of the anterior chamber angle. The scleral spur, for example, is located just posterior to the sclerolimbal junction and Schlemm's canal, therefore, would be found just anterior to this landmark. In performing a trabeculotomy ab externo, a radial, scratch incision across the sclerolimbal junction should reveal Schlemm's canal in the posterior portion of the gray zone. When performing a trabeculectomy, a circumferential incision beneath the partial-thickness scleral flap at the corneolimbal junction will enter the anterior chamber just in front of the trabecular meshwork. By extending the dissection posteriorly with radial incisions to the sclerolimbal junction, a flap of deep-limbal tissue will be created that can be reflected to expose the anterior chamber angle structures and can be excised along the scleral spur. If the latter incision is mistakenly made more posteriorly, the ciliary body may be damaged, resulting in brisk bleeding. A fistula that is too posterior is also at risk of being obstructed by uveal tissue. Hence the importance of correctly identifying the external landmarks during glaucoma filtering surgery.

The anterior ciliary arteries enter the ciliary body behind the scleral spur in locations corresponding to the positions of the rectus muscle tendons. These vessels should be avoided, when possible, during surgery, to minimize excessive bleeding. Since the ciliary body cannot usually be visualized internally, external landmarks must be used when performing surgical procedures associated with these structures. In performing cyclodestructive procedures, which involve the pars plicata, it was once suggested that the destructive element, e.g., the cryoprobe, should be placed 2–3 mm behind the corneolimbal junction, allowing for the previously discussed variation in this landmark (1). This location in most eyes, however, will result in entry into the eye that is posterior to the pars plicata. This may not have been significant with the earlier cyclodestructive procedures in which the area of tissue destruction was so broad. With transscleral laser cyclophotocoagulation, however, the zone of tissue destruction is more precise, and a placement of the laser beam 1.5 mm behind the corneolimbal junction superiorly and inferiorly and 1.0 mm temporally and nasally is most likely to reach the pars plicata. When making a pars plana incision, as during a posterior sclerotomy for malignant glaucoma or when draining a suprachoroidal detachment or hemorrhage, the incision should be made 3–4 mm behind the corneolimbal junction.

SUMMARY

Laser and incisional surgical procedures for glaucoma are directed at the anatomic structures associated with aqueous inflow, i.e., the ciliary body, and aqueous outflow, which includes the iris and the trabecular meshwork and related outflow pathways. For successful glaucoma surgery, it is necessary to be familiar with these structures by direct internal visualization through slitlamp and gonioscopic examination, as well as by their relationship to the external aspects of the limbal connective tissue and the overlying conjunctiva and Tenon's capsule.

REFERENCE

1. Sugar, HS: Surgical anatomy for glaucoma. Surv Ophthalmol 13: 143, 1968.

PRINCIPLES OF LASER SURGERY FOR GLAUCOMA

The introduction of laser therapy has undoubtedly been the most significant advance in the surgical treatment of glaucoma during the second half of the 20th century, and there is promise of ever increasing technologic advances and surgical applications as we approach the 21st century. The concept of using light energy to alter the structure of intraocular tissues, however, actually preceded the development of laser technology. Meyer-Schwickerath (1), beginning in the late 1940s, pioneered this field of ocular surgery, first using focused sunlight and later the xenon-arc photocoagulator. Although the latter technique proved useful for certain retinal disorders, xenon-arc photocoagulation for the treatment of glaucoma never gained clinical acceptance.

In 1960, Maiman (2) described the first laser, which used a ruby crystal. However, it was not until the development of the continuous-wave argon laser, near the end of that decade, that the virtual explosion of laser applications for ocular diseases began. After several years of investigative work in the early 1970s, clinicians began applying laser energy to treat various forms of glaucoma, and today it is the most commonly used mode of glaucoma surgery.

In this chapter, we briefly review the physical and biologic aspects of laser therapy. The application of these principles to the treatment of specific forms of glaucoma is considered in subsequent chapters.

BASIC PRINCIPLES OF LASERS (3–6)

Albert Einstein speculated that atoms, under certain conditions, could absorb light or other radiation and then be stimulated to emit the borrowed energy. His theory formed the basis of *Light Amplification by Stimulated Emission of Radiation* (laser).

When atoms absorb energy, called "pumping," they are "excited" from a lower to a higher energy level. If more atoms are in the excited than in the unexcited state, "population inversion" is said to exist. Under such circumstances, photons with an energy equal to the difference between the two levels of excitation have an enhanced probability of stimulating the atoms to decay back to their lower energy level by emitting photons, a process called "stimulated emission." The emitted photons stimulate the emission of more photons, leading to a chain reaction.

If this system is enclosed between two mirrors, the photons will bounce back and forth, creating multiple stimulated emissions of light or "light amplification." The mirrors are said to form a "cavity" which, in addition to amplifying the light, creates a parallel beam and acts as a resonator to limit the number of wavelengths. When the light amplification is sufficient, some photons are allowed to leave the cavity in the form of a laser beam (Fig. 33.1).

The laser beam can be delivered as a "continuous-wave" or in a "pulsed mode." In the latter situation, the energy is concentrated and delivered in a very short period of time, which can be accomplished in one of two ways. With one technique, called "Q-switching," light is not allowed to travel back and forth in the cavity until maximum population inversion is reached. This is accomplished with either an electronic shutter or misalignment of the mirrors. When the shutter is opened or the mirrors are aligned, stimulated emission and light amplification occur suddenly, and the energy is released in a pulse of a few to tens of nanoseconds.

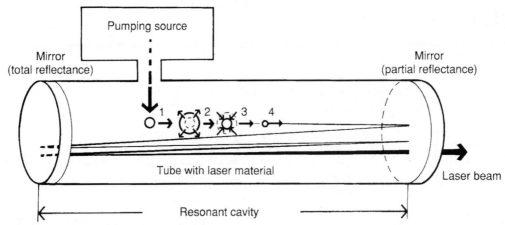

Figure 33.1. Schematic of laser system. Laser material is placed in a tube between two mirrors. When an energy source is pumped into the tube, atoms in the laser material *(1)* are excited to a higher energy level *(2)*. In the excited state, atoms have an enhanced probability of being stimulated by photons to decay back to the lower energy level *(3)* by emitting photons *(4)*. The emitted photons bounce between the mirrors, stimulating other excited atoms, until sufficient light amplification is achieved, at which time the light is allowed to leave the cavity as a laser beam.

In the other form of pulsed delivery, called "mode-locking," the energy is also released after achieving maximum population inversion, but different modes of light are synchronized, creating peaks of energy, which are emitted in tens of nanoseconds as a chain of pulses, each of which lasts a few tens of picoseconds. To provide some appreciation for the brevity of these exposures, it has been noted that the ratio between the duration of a Q-switched laser pulse and a conventional continuous-wave argon laser exposure is roughly the same as the ratio between the argon exposure and a human lifetime (7)!

PROPERTIES OF LASER ENERGY

Light emitted by a laser differs from normal "white" light in several ways.

Coherence

Unlike the photons in a light bulb, which are emitted randomly, the resonator effect of the laser cavity causes the photons to be synchronized or coherent, i.e., in phase with each other in time and space.

Collimation

Since light amplification occurs only for photons that are aligned with the mirrors, a nearly parallel beam is produced, as opposed to the diverging beam of an incandescent lamp. Although limited divergence occurs with all laser beams, it is minimal enough that a small focal spot can be created when the light is delivered through an optical system.

Monochromacy

Since the photons are emitted due to the release of energy between two defined levels of the atom, the resulting light has a narrow range of wavelengths.

High Intensity

The light amplification of a laser can produce a beam with significantly more intensity than that of the sun.

LASER-INDUCED TISSUE INTERACTIONS

The tissue effects produced by laser surgery are of three types: thermal, ionizing, and photochemical (8).

Thermal Effects

In this situation, the absorption of laser energy by the target tissue produces temperatures high enough to induce chemical changes that can cause local inflammation and scarring *(photocoagulation)* or to vaporize intracellular and extracellular fluids, creating an incision in the tissue *(photovaporization)*. Factors influencing the laser thermal effect include (a) wavelength of the incident light, (b) duration of exposure, and (c) amount of light energy per area of exposure. Melanin, the pigment of most target tissues in glaucoma laser surgery, has a peak absorption in the blue-green portion of the visible spectrum. Therefore, lasers with wavelengths between 400 and 600 nm are most useful for these procedures, and the *argon laser* is the prototype photocoagulator.

The heat generated by the absorption of laser energy is dissipated by the surrounding tissue. A short exposure time and a high energy level/area reduce heat conduction, which causes tissue temperatures to reach the critical boiling point, producing gas bubbles with tissue disruption and photovaporization through a microexplosion. This reaction can be used to create holes in ocular tissues, as with laser iridotomy. At lower energy levels, photocoagulation may produce contraction of collagen, which is the mechanism of pupilloplasty and iridoplasty, and possibly of laser trabeculoplasty.

Ionizing Effects

If very intense laser energy is focused into a very small area for a very short period of time, a reaction occurs that is independent of pigment absorption and is referred to as *photodisruption*. An instantaneous electric field is generated, which literally strips electrons from target atoms, producing a gaseous state called "plasma" (7). As ionized atoms of a plasma recombine with free electrons, photons with a wide range of energies are emitted, producing a spark of incoherent white light. Associated shock and pressure waves create additional mechanical damage to target tissues, resulting in a reaction that can disrupt both pigmented and nonpigmented structures. Thermal effects are also involved in the mechanism of photodisruption (9).

The *neodymium:YAG laser* is the most commonly used photodisruptor. The pulse may be Q-switched or mode-locked, both of which have been shown to produce the same size of rupture in polyethylene membranes (9). The main clinical use has been for the disruption, or cutting, of relatively transparent anterior segment structures, most notably the posterior lens capsule. In glaucoma surgery, the primary application of the Q-switched neodymium:YAG laser is the creation of iridotomies. Neodymium:YAG lasers can also be used in a pulsed thermal or continuous-wave mode for transscleral cyclophotocoagulation.

Photochemical Effects

The target tissue in this laser-induced effect is volatilized (vaporized) by short-pulsed ultraviolet radiation *(photoablation)*. Some tissues, such as tumors, can be photosensitized with hematoporphyrin or other photosensitizing agent and selectively destroyed with laser energy of a specific wavelength *(photodynamic therapy* or *photoradiation)*.

LASER DELIVERY SYSTEMS

Most laser units utilize a slitlamp biomicroscope, in which a system of fiberoptics and/or mirrors in an articulated arm direct the laser beam from the laser tube, through the slitlamp, and into the patient's eye (Fig. 33.2). Various types of contact lenses are normally used during laser surgery with slitlamp

delivery. Some contain mirrors to direct the laser beam into the anterior chamber angle, while others incorporate convex lenses to concentrate the light energy on the iris. Other laser delivery systems utilize contact probes attached to the fiberoptics, which allows application of laser energy to the ocular tissues either by external placement of the probe on the eye or by aiming directly at internal ocular structures with the probe tip in the eye.

For lasers within the visual spectrum, an aiming beam of attenuated laser energy can be used to allow positioning and focusing of the laser beam on the target tissue. For lasers with wavelengths outside the visual spectrum, an additional laser such as the helium-neon is used as the aiming beam. A foot pedal or finger trigger is used to release the full laser energy, producing the tissue alteration. The variables on the control units of most laser systems include spot size (usually expressed in microns), exposure duration (expressed in tenths of seconds, milliseconds, microseconds, or nanoseconds), and energy (joules or millijoules) or power (watts or milliwatts). Energy in joules equals power in watts times duration in seconds.

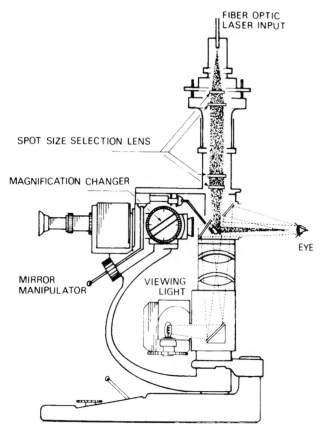

Figure 33.2. Schematic of slitlamp delivery system for ophthalmic lasers. Laser light enters the slitlamp through a fiberoptic or system of mirrors and is reflected by mirrors in the slitlamp into the patient's eye. (Reprinted with permission from Sliney D, Wolbarsht M: Safety with lasers and other optical sources. A comprehensive handbook. New York, Plenum Press, 1980.)

SPECIFIC LASERS FOR GLAUCOMA SURGERY

Lasers differ primarily according to the medium in which the atoms exist that produce the stimulated emission of photons. The lasers used most commonly for glaucoma surgery are argon, neodymium:YAG, and semiconductor diode, although experience with many other lasers has also been reported.

Argon Lasers

The medium in these instruments is argon gas, which is pumped by an electrical discharge. The wavelengths are in the blue (488-nm) and green (514-nm) portions of the visible spectrum which is optimum for absorption by melanin. Most argon lasers operate in the continuous-wave mode and have maximum power levels of 2–6 watts. Units are also available, however, which produce pulses of approximately 100 microseconds with powers of 20–50 watts. The latter instruments achieve full power only as needed, which reduces heat buildup and improves energy efficiency.

Neodymium:YAG Lasers

In these instruments, the neodymium atoms are embedded in a crystal of yttrium-aluminum-garnet (YAG) and are pumped by a xenon flash lamp. The laser wavelength is in the near infrared (1064-nm) range, although it can be made a visible light emitter by frequency doubling or an ultraviolet emitter by frequency tripling (8). Neodymium:YAG lasers can be operated in the continuous-wave mode to provide a photocoagulation effect, but are more commonly used with pulsed delivery, using either Q-switching or mode-locking, to allow photodisruption.

Semiconductor Diode Lasers

Two light-emitting diodes are used in this system to produce a wavelength in the near infrared spectrum (800–820 nm). Solid state construction allows compact size, durability, and low maintenance. The wavelength between that of the argon and neodymium:YAG lasers provides better scleral penetration than the argon and better absorption by melanin than the neodymium:YAG lasers, making it potentially useful for transscleral cyclophotocoagulation. Diode lasers can also be operated in the red range of the visible spectrum (640 nm) in which case they are used as an aiming beam.

Other Lasers

Many new lasers are being developed and evaluated for ocular surgery. Among these are the *dye lasers* which are capable of producing monochromatic wavelengths at rela-
tively high output powers through a large range of the visible spectrum. This allows the selection of a wavelength that would be most highly absorbed by the target tissue, thereby minimizing the transmittal of laser energy through the ocular media (10). *Carbon dioxide lasers* in the infrared spectrum (10,600 nm) have been used in the continuous-wave mode to cut tissue by vaporization with very little coagulation necrosis, while *excimer lasers* in the ultraviolet range (193 and 248 nm) are being evaluated in the pulsed mode to cut tissue with no visible necrosis. The *ruby laser* in the visible spectrum (694 nm) can produce photoablation with high-energy pulses, and the *krypton laser* in the yellow-red wavelength can be used for photocoagulation. The *helium-neon laser* in the red wavelength is, as previously noted, used as an aiming beam in many laser systems that operate at nonvisible wavelengths (8).

LASER SAFETY

The properties of laser energy, while providing an ideal tool for the surgical manipulation of tissues, also pose serious hazards, including electric shock, direct laser burns, explosions, and fires. Probably the most common and serious health hazard, however, is accidental exposure of the retina, either directly or from reflected laser light.

The following classification of lasers is generally accepted regarding hazards (11):

Class I. Do not emit hazardous levels.
Class II. Visible-light lasers that are safe for momentary viewing, but should not be stared into continuously. An example is the aiming beam of ophthalmic lasers.
Class III. Unsafe for even momentary viewing, requiring procedural controls and safety equipment.
Class IV. Also pose a significant fire and skin hazard. Most therapeutic laser beams used in ocular surgery are in this class.

During glaucoma laser surgery, the patient has the greatest risk of injury from accidental exposure of the retina or lens. Techniques for avoiding these complications during specific laser procedure are discussed in subsequent chapters. The risk to the corneal endothelium has been evaluated with specular microscopy 1 year after laser trabeculoplasty or iridotomy, which showed a significant increase in cell size in one study (12), but no statistically significant changes in another study (13).

The surgeon is theoretically protected during each exposure of therapeutic laser energy in most slitlamp delivery systems by a filter which is built into the system. There has been recent evidence, however, that subtle, but definite, alterations in color vision can be seen in ophthalmic laser surgeons who are exposed chronically to argon blue light (14–17). Since there is no apparent clinical advantage to blue-green wavelengths in ophthalmic surgery, it is advisable to use green-only whenever possible.

Aside from the patient and surgeon, the individuals at greatest risk of retinal burns are other personnel in the laser room during the treatment whose eyes may be exposed to reflected laser light. One study with argon lasers and various contact lenses indicated that a hazard can exist for a bystander at the side of the slitlamp who is exposed to unattenuated back reflections of the treatment beam within 1 m of the contact lens (18). To minimize this hazard, only antireflective coated contact lenses should be used, ancillary personnel should wear protective goggles or look away from the laser when it is in use, and access to the laser room should be limited to necessary individuals during the treatment.

SUMMARY

Lasers operate on the principle that excited atoms can be stimulated to emit photons, resulting in a markedly amplified light that possesses the unique properties of coherence, collimation, monochromacy, and high intensity. The nature of this light allows precise alteration of tissues by thermal effects (photocoagulation and photovaporization), ionizing effects (photodisruption), and photochemical effects (photoablation and photodynamic therapy or photoradiation). These tissue interactions, especially the photocoagulation and photodisruption, are used in a wide variety of glaucoma surgical procedures.

REFERENCES

1. Meyer-Schwickerath, G: Light coagulation (translated by Drance, SM). St. Louis, CV Mosby, 1960.
2. Maiman, TH: Stimulated optical radiation in ruby. Nature 187: 493, 1960.
3. L'Esperance, FA Jr: Ophthalmic lasers. Photocoagulation, photoradiation, and surgery. 2nd ed. St. Louis, CV Mosby, 1983.
4. Belcher, CD, Thomas, JV, Simmons, RJ: Photocoagulation in glaucoma and anterior segment disease. Baltimore, Williams and Wilkins, 1984.
5. Schwartz, L, Spaeth, G, Brown, G: Laser therapy of the anterior segment. A practical approach. Thorofare, NJ, Slack Inc., 1984.
6. Peyman, GA, Raichand, M, Zeimer, RC: Ocular effects of various laser wavelengths. Surv Ophthalmol 28:391, 1984.
7. Mainster, MA, Sliney, DH, Belcher, CD III, Buzney, SM: Laser photodisruptors. Damage mechanisms, instrument design and safety. Ophthalmology 90:973, 1983.
8. Council on Scientific Affairs: Lasers in medicine and surgery. JAMA 256:900, 1986.
9. Vogel, A, Hentschel, W, Holzfuss, J, Lauterborn, W: Cavitation bubble dynamics and acoustic transient generation in ocular surgery with pulsed neodymium:YAG lasers. Ophthalmology 93:1259, 1986.
10. L'Esperance, FA, Jr: Clinical photocoagulation with the organic dye laser. A preliminary communication. Arch Ophthalmol 103:1312, 1985.
11. Sliney, D, Wolbarsht, M: Safety with lasers and other optical sources. A comprehensive handbook. New York, Plenum Press, 1980.
12. Hong, C. Kitazawa, Y, Tanishima, T: Influence of argon laser treatment of glaucoma on corneal endothelium. Jpn J Ophthalmol 27:567, 1983.
13. Thoming, C, Van Buskirk, EM, Samples, JR: The corneal endothelium after laser therapy for glaucoma. Am J Ophthalmol 103:518, 1987.
14. Arden, GB, Gündüz, K, Perry, S: Colour vision testing with a computer graphics system. Clin Vis Sci 2:303, 1988.
15. Gündüz, K, Arden, GB: Changes in colour contrast sensitivity associated with operating argon lasers. Br J Ophthalmol 73:241, 1989.
16. Berninger, TA, Canning, CR, Gündüz, K, et al: Using argon laser blue light reduces ophthalmologists' color contrast sensitivity. Argon blue and surgeons' vision. Arch Ophthalmol 107:1453, 1989.
17. Arden, GB, Berninger, T, Hogg, CR, Perry, S: A survey of color discrimination in German ophthalmologists. Changes associated with the use of lasers and operating microscopes. Ophthalmology 98:567, 1991.
18. Sliney, DH, Mainster, MA: Potential laser hazards to the clinician during photocoagulation. Am J Ophthalmol 103:758, 1987.

Chapter 34

PRINCIPLES OF INCISIONAL SURGERY

I. Wound healing
   A. Clot phase
   B. Proliferative phase
   C. Granulation phase
   D. Collagen phase
II. Anesthesia
   A. Local anesthesia
      1. Retrobulbar
      2. Peribulbar
      3. Sub-Tenon's
   B. Adjuncts to local anesthesia

III. Basic techniques and instrumentation
   A. Lid separation
   B. Traction sutures
   C. Hemostasis
   D. Tissue handling
   E. Suturing

A division between laser surgery for glaucoma and the more traditional glaucoma operations is becoming more and more artificial. The latter surgical category was originally distinguished by the term "conventional surgery," although laser techniques have now become the more conventional forms of surgery for glaucoma, prompting the need to reconsider our terminology. "Invasive surgery" is not a satisfactory alternative, since invading the eye with a laser beam can cause just as much tissue alteration as invading it with a knife. The term "incisional surgery," as used in this text, is not fully satisfactory either, since some of the newer laser procedures include incisional techniques. The fact is that, as laser technology continues to expand, the day will undoubtedly come when all glaucoma surgery will include laser instruments. For these reasons, the chapters which follow combine laser and incisional procedures under general surgical categories, and this chapter, while it pertains primarily to incisional techniques, actually relates to both disciplines of glaucoma surgery.

WOUND HEALING

The incision of any tissue is followed by a complex process that attempts to heal the wound. The desire in most operations is to achieve complete, strong wound healing. For the glaucoma surgeon who is performing a filtering procedure, however, excessive wound healing can be a detriment, leading to failure of the operation. In this chapter, we consider some general aspects of wound healing, while specifics related to filtering surgery and measures to prevent excessive scarring are discussed in Chapter 37.

It may help to think of the complex, and only partially understood, process of wound healing in four phases: (a) clot phase; (b) proliferative phase; (c) granulation phase; (d) collagen phase.

Clot Phase

Almost immediately after a tissue incision, blood vessels constrict and leak blood cells and plasma proteins, which include fibrinogen, fibronectin, and plasminogen. Under the influence of certain tissue factors, these blood elements clot to form a gel-like fibrin-fibronectin matrix (1).

Proliferative Phase

Inflammatory cells, including monocytes and macrophages, along with fibroblasts and new capillaries, migrate into the clot. In a rabbit model of filtering surgery, fibroblasts were seen to migrate from episcleral tissue, epimysium of the superior rectus, and subconjunctival connective tissue (2), and in a monkey model they were proliferating along the walls of the limbal fistula by day 6 (3). Using the incorporation of tritiated thymidine as a marker of cell division to study the time course of cellular proliferation following filtering surgery in monkeys,

466

incorporation was detected as early as 24 hours postoperatively, peaked in 5 days, and returned to baseline by day 11 (4).

Granulation Phase

As the fibrin-fibronectin clot is degraded by inflammatory cells, the fibroblasts begin to synthesize fibronectin, interstitial collagens, and glycosaminoglycans to form young fibrovascular connective tissue, or granulation tissue (1). In the rabbit model, granulation tissue was seen in the fistula by the third day (2), while in the monkey model it was lining the fistula by at least day 10 (3).

Collagen Phase

Procollagen is synthesized intracellularly by fibroblasts and is then secreted into the extracellular spaces where it undergoes biochemical transformation into tropocollagen. The tropocollagen molecules aggregate into immature soluble collagen fibrils, which then undergo cross-linking to form mature collagen. Blood vessels are eventually partially reabsorbed and fibroblasts largely disappear, leaving a dense collagenous scar with scattered fibroblasts and blood vessels (1).

ANESTHESIA

While most laser procedures require only topical anesthesia, incisional surgery, and some glaucoma laser operations, require local anesthesia. Some surgeons prefer general anesthesia, although this is usually reserved for children or adults in whom cooperation or other considerations do not permit surgery under local anesthesia.

Local Anesthesia

Commonly used injectable anesthetics include *lidocaine, bupivacaine,* and *mepivacaine.* When compared on the basis of induced lid akinesia, these three agents were found to be similar with regard to onset (less that 6 minutes) and depth of anesthesia, while bupivacaine had the longest duration of effect (up to 6 hours, compared to 90 minutes for mepivacaine and 15–30 minutes for lidocaine) (5). In an evaluation of combined agents, 0.5% bupivacaine, 2% lidocaine, and 1:100,000 epinephrine were more effective in producing lid and globe akinesia than bupivacaine alone or the two anesthetics without epinephrine (6). Bupivacaine alone was slower in producing anesthesia, but was more effective in producing akinesia than the two anesthetics combined without epinephrine. The three combinations were similar with regard to frequency of pain during a 30-minute operation and the need for analgesia 6 hours postoperatively.

Epinephrine may enhance the effect of local anesthetics, presumably by minimizing systemic spread from the injection site by its vasoconstrictive action. However, it may also impose an additional risk in glaucomatous eyes by reducing vascular perfusion to an already compromised optic nerve head. Another supplement to local anesthesia that does appear to be safe and effective is *hyaluronidase,* which serves to improve local tissue spread within the injection site by breaking down the connective tissue ground substances.

While *retrobulbar* and *orbicularis anesthesia* are traditionally given as separate injections, it has been shown that the retrobulbar injection alone provides adequate facial akinesia in the vast majority of cases (7), and this has also been my experience. For the retrobulbar injection, an Atkinson needle has the advantages of being short and blunt, both of which help avoid retrobulbar hemorrhage. An injection of 3–5 cc of a 50–50 mixture of 0.75% bupivacaine and 2–4% lidocaine with hyaluronidase usually provides adequate anesthesia and akinesia. Firm pressure to the globe for 30 seconds after the injection may also help to minimize retrobulbar hemorrhage by tamponading any small bleeding vessel.

Some surgeons prefer to avoid the risks associated with retrobulbar anesthesia by using *peribulbar* (transconjunctival injection near the equator of the glove without entering the muscle cone) or *sub-Tenon's* (more anterior placement near the surgical site) anesthesia. The latter may be the safest of these approaches in glaucoma patients, since both retrobulbar and peribulbar injections can cause significant IOP elevations. In a study of 104 eyes with and without glaucoma, receiving either retrobulbar or peribulbar anesthesia for intraocular surgery, the 40 eyes with glaucoma had higher and more persistent increases in IOP (8). One minute postinjection, the IOP was 10 mm Hg or more above baseline in 35% of the glaucomatous eyes and 20 mm Hg or more in 10%. The mean IOP elevation after 5 minutes was greater with retrobulbar anesthesia, although ocular compression significantly lowered the IOP at 5 minutes.

A reported technique for sub-Tenon's anesthesia involves injection of lidocaine 2% over the superior, medial and lateral rectus muscles in conjunction with a lid block and standard sedative (9). In a randomized trial comparing this approach with retrobulbar anesthesia, the sub-Tenon's anesthesia required a smaller volume of local anesthetic, less additional anesthesia, and less postoperative analgesia (9).

Adjuncts to Local Anesthesia

Although general anesthesia is not commonly used in glaucoma surgery, it is advisable to routinely utilize the assistance of an anesthesiologist or anesthetist to monitor the patient's vital signs and to provide adjunctive medications as required. The latter may include short-acting analgesics such as fentanyl citrate, and short-acting central nervous system depressants such as midazolam HCl, for sedation. In addition, ultrashort-acting barbiturate anesthetics such as methohexital sodium (Brevitol) can be administered intravenously to provide a few minutes of sleep while the retrobulbar injection is being given.

BASIC TECHNIQUES AND INSTRUMENTATION

Lid Separation

Good exposure of the surgical field is critical to a successful glaucoma operation. This begins with the selection of an appropriate lid speculum. There is a wide range of instrument designs, each with certain advantages and disadvantages. A desirable speculum, however, is one that not only separates the lids, but also lifts them from the globe, and allows the surgeon to adjust the degree of lid separation. One design has been described, which provides these features, as well as a longer arm for the inferior cul de sac, which turns the eye down without the need for a traction suture (10).

Traction Sutures

Since most glaucoma surgery is performed in the superior quadrants, the next step toward good exposure is to rotate the eye down, which is usually accomplished with a traction (or bridle) suture. A traditional technique is the *superior rectus traction suture,* in which a 4–0 silk suture is passed transconjunctivally beneath the muscles and then attached to the head of the surgical drape with a clamp (Fig. 34.1). Potential complications with this approach include subconjunctival hemorrhage, conjunctival defects, scleral perforation, patient discomfort, and postoperative ptosis. A *corneal traction suture,* in which a 6–0 or 7–0 silk suture on a cutting needle is passed through approximately

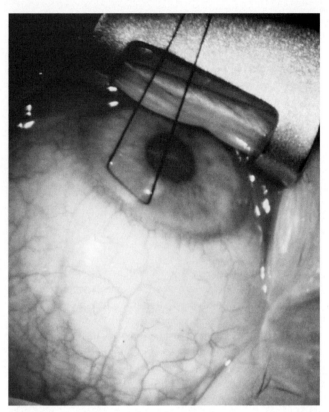

Figure 34.2. Eye rotated down by corneal traction suture and attached to surgical drape over cheek.

three-fourths thickness, superior, peripheral cornea and attached to the drape over the cheek (Fig. 34.2), provides good exposure while eliminating the foregoing complications (11, 12). However, it can distort the cornea and anterior chamber when the eye is soft.

Hemostasis

As noted earlier in this chapter, bleeding is the first step in the wound healing process, which can lead to excessive, detrimental scarring especially in glaucoma filtering surgery. It is desirable, therefore, in all surgical procedures to minimize bleeding. This is first done, of course, by trying to avoid large vessels, such as the anterior ciliary arteries near the insertions of the rectus muscles. When bleeding does occur, it should be continuously flushed from the surgical site with a gentle stream of balanced salt solution. Small bleeders may eventually close spontaneously, although most require cauterization. An ideal cautery unit for glaucoma surgery is a small diameter, tapered, blunt, bipolar cautery instrument (Fig. 34.3) (13). This will provide adequate cauterization of episcleral bleeders without excessive tissue charring or tissue contraction, and can also be used at lower energy levels to cauterize intraocular bleeding as from the ciliary body or iris.

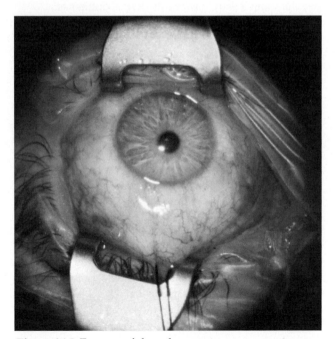

Figure 34.1. Eye rotated down by superior rectus traction suture and attached to head of surgical drape.

Tissue Handling

Most glaucoma surgery is performed on the extraocular tissues of the anterior ocular segment. Gentle handling of these tissues is essential to avoid tearing the conjunctiva or cutting more tissue than necessary, which can also increase the risks of excessive scarring. When possible, it is best to grasp Tenon's capsule and avoid direct instrument contact with the conjunctiva. When it is necessary to grasp the conjunctiva, it should be done with smooth-tipped forceps to avoid piercing or tearing the conjunctiva. When dissecting conjunctiva, it is best to use a blunt dissecting instrument when possible, and cut tissue with scissors or a blade only when necessary. Details regarding specific instruments for the various surgical procedures are provided in the following chapters that deal with those operations.

Suturing

To minimize excessive inflammatory reaction and subsequent scarring, it is important to select suture material with the least tendency to induce tissue reaction. For corneoscleral suturing, 9–0 or 10–0 nylon on a fine, cutting needle may be the most satisfactory. For the conjunctiva, however, polyglycolic acid or polyglactin sutures are nearly as nonreactive as nylon and have the advantage of biodegradation. It is also important to use a needle that will not tear or leave a large hole in the conjunctiva. Fine, tapered, noncutting needles are available on the fine, biodegradable sutures, and are excellent for all conjunctival work.

SUMMARY

The wound healing process following the incision of a tissue includes clot formation, cellular proliferation, granulation tissue formation, and the synthesis and maturation of collagen. Most incisional glaucoma surgery is performed under local anesthesia, with agents such as lidocaine and bupivacaine. Epinephrine, as a supplement, is usually avoided due to the risk to the optic nerve head, although hyaluronidase may be useful as a tissue spreading factor. Basic techniques and instrumentation for incisional glaucoma surgery include attention to good surgical exposure with an appropriate lid speculum and traction suture, adequate hemostasis, gentle wound handling, and the proper suture and needle for wound closure.

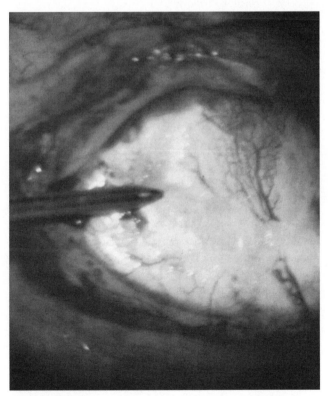

Figure 34.3. **Cauterization of sclera with tapered, blunt tip, bipolar cautery instrument.**

REFERENCES

1. Skuta, GL, Parrish, RK, II: Wound healing in glaucoma filtering surgery. Surv Ophthalmol 32:149, 1987.
2. Miller, MH, Grierson, I, Unger, WI, Hitchings, RA: Wound healing in an animal model of glaucoma fistulizing surgery in the rabbit. Ophthalmic Surg 20:350, 1989.
3. Desjardins, DC, Parrish, RK, II, Folberg, R, et al: Wound healing after filtering surgery in owl monkeys. Arch Ophthalmol 104:1835, 1986.
4. Jampel, HD, McGuigan, LJB, Dunkelberger, GR, et al: Cellular proliferation after experimental glaucoma filtration surgery. Arch Ophthalmol 106:89, 1988.
5. Parrish, RK, II, Spaeth, GL, Poryzees, EM, Hargens, CW: Evaluation of local anesthetic agents using a new force-sensitive lid speculum. Ophthalmic Surg 14:575, 1983.
6. Vettese, T, Breslin, CW: Retrobulbar anesthesia for cataract surgery: comparison of bupivacaine and bupivacaine/lidocaine combinations. Can J Ophthalmol 20:131, 1985.
7. Martin, SR, Baker, SS, Muenzler, WS: Retrobulbar anesthesia and orbicularis akinesia. Ophthalmic Surg 17:232, 1986.
8. O'Donoghue, E, Batterbury, M, Lavy, T: Effect on intraocular pressure of local anaesthesia in eyes undergoing intraocular surgery. Br J Ophthalmol 78:605, 1994.
9. Buys, YV, Trope, GE: Prospective study of sub-Tenon's versus retrobulbar anesthesia for inpatient and day-surgery trabeculectomy. Ophthalmology 100:1585, 1993.
10. Yamabayashi, S, Tsukahara, S: New lid speculum for glaucoma filtering surgery. Ophthalmic Surg 25:128, 1994.
11. Conklin, JD, Goins, KM, Smith, TJ: Corneal traction suture in trabeculectomy. Ophthalmic Surg 22:494, 1991.
12. Cohen, SW: Corneal traction suture. Ophthalmic Surg 19:371, 1988.
13. Shields, MB: Evaluation of a tapered, blunt, bipolar cautery tip for trabeculectomy. Ophthalmic Surg 25:54, 1994.

SURGERY OF THE ANTERIOR CHAMBER ANGLE

In this chapter, we consider the laser and incisional operations that are designed to reduce the intraocular pressure (IOP) through increased aqueous outflow by treating specific structures within the anterior chamber angle. Filtration procedures and drainage implant devices, which involve not only the anterior chamber angle but also limbal and external ocular tissues, are considered separately in Chapters 37 and 38, respectively.

LASER TRABECULOPLASTY[a]

Historical Background

In 1961, Zweng and Flocks (1) introduced the concept of applying light energy to the anterior chamber angle for the treatment of glaucoma. Using the xenon-arc photocoagulator of Meyer-Schwickerath, they selectively coagulated the fil-

tration angles of cats, dogs, and monkeys and reported subsequent lowering of the IOP. Histopathologic examination of the treated tissue revealed fragmentation of the trabecular lamellae, atrophy of ciliary muscle, and destruction of ciliary processes. Little more was said about this technique, however, until over a decade later, when several investigators revived the concept by utilizing the light energy of the laser. Yet another decade of investigative work would elapse before the operation would achieve widespread clinical popularity.

In the early 1970s, reports began to appear from several parts of the world, most notably from Krasnov (2) in Russia, Hager (3) in Germany, Demailly and associates (4) in France, and Worthen and Wickham (5) in the United States, regarding attempts to improve aqueous outflow by creating holes in the trabecular meshwork with laser energy. Although trabecular

[a]Refer to M.B. Shields: Color Atlas of Glaucoma. Baltimore: Williams & Wilkins, 1998, Plate III7.

perforations were achieved, they eventually closed in most cases due to fibrosis, and IOP reduction was usually temporary. The value of laser treatment to the trabecular meshwork came under further question when, in 1975, Gaasterland and Kupfer (6) reported that experimental glaucoma could be produced by applying argon laser energy to the meshwork of rhesus monkeys. The following year, however, Ticho and Zauberman (7) noted that long-term reduction in IOP occurred in some patients despite the lack of permanent trabecular openings. This led to a new concept in laser trabecular therapy in which lower energy levels were used to photocoagulate, rather than to penetrate, portions of the meshwork. In 1979, Wise and Witter (8) described the first successful protocol of what has become known as laser trabeculoplasty. Their preliminary work was corroborated in 1981 (9–11), and in less than 5 years laser trabeculoplasty became the most commonly performed operation for glaucoma.

Theories of Mechanism

Tonographic studies indicate that laser trabeculoplasty reduces IOP by improving the facility of outflow (12–16), while fluorophotometric investigations show no significant influence on aqueous production (14, 17, 18). Although fluorescein leakage into the anterior chamber, suggesting a breakdown in the blood-aqueous barrier, is seen during the first week after trabeculoplasty, it is gone within 1 month and does not seem to be a factor in the long-term effect of this procedure (19).

The mechanism of improved aqueous outflow facility by laser trabeculoplasty is uncertain. Wise and Witter (8) originally postulated that the thermal energy produced by pigment absorption of laser light caused shrinkage of collagen in the trabecular lamellae. They felt that the subsequent shortening of the treated meshwork might enlarge existing spaces between two treatment sites or expand Schlemm's canal by pulling the meshwork centrally. Laboratory studies have provided partial support for this theory, but have also suggested alternative or additional mechanisms of action.

Light and electron microscopic and immunohistochemical evaluations of trabecular meshwork from normal and glaucomatous human eyes, obtained hours to weeks after trabeculoplasty, revealed disruption of trabecular beams, fibrinous material, and necrosis of occasional cells, followed by shrinkage of the collagenous components of the meshwork (20–22) and accumulation of fibronectin in the aqueous drainage channels (22). Surviving endothelial cells near the laser lesions showed phagocytic and migratory activity (21). Specimens obtained several months after therapy had partial or total occlusion of intertrabecular spaces by a monocellular layer (20–22). These observations were felt to support the theories of heat-induced stretching of collagen in the trabecular lamellae and fibronectin-mediated attachment of beams supporting an adhesive tightening of the trabecular components (22).

Studies with monkeys have provided similar observations to those noted in humans, with some additional insight into the mechanism of laser trabeculoplasty. Within the first few hours there is disruption of the trabecular beams and coagulative necrosis with accumulation of debris in the juxtacanalicular region (23). As with the human eyes, surviving trabecular endothelial cells are noted to have increased phagocytic activity with removal of tissue debris (23) and increased cell division (24). By 1 month, the treated regions are flat with collapsed beams and are covered with corneal endothelium (25). The latter is more likely to occur when the laser energy is applied to the anterior portion of the trabecular meshwork (26). Perfusion with ferritin shows lack of flow through the treated meshwork, with diversion of flow through the adjacent non-lasered meshwork, which becomes structurally altered to compensate for the overload of flow (27). It has also been suggested that concomitant collagen degeneration and loss of trabecular cells may widen the intertrabecular spaces with improved outflow (28). However, light and electron microscopic studies of the trabecular meshwork and the inner wall of Schlemm's canal 3–17 months after 360° trabeculoplasty in monkeys revealed no significant difference from untreated eyes (29). Whether the human eye has similar reparative capacity is unclear, but this and other studies suggest that alternative or additional mechanisms to the mechanical theory must account for the long-term benefit of laser trabeculoplasty.

Studies of human autopsy eyes treated with laser trabeculoplasty revealed a significant reduction in the trabecular cell density and an increase in radioactive sulfate incorporation into the extracellular matrix of lasered eyes (30). The latter findings have also been reported with human trabecular tissue treated with trabeculoplasty prior to trabeculectomy and subsequently studied with radioactive leucine (22), and in cat eyes that were studied in vivo with radioactive thymidine following trabeculoplasty (31, 32). Studies with a human corneoscleral explant organ culture system indicate that laser trabeculoplasty causes an early trabecular endothelial cell division in the anterior meshwork, with migration of the new cells to repopulate the burn sites over the next few weeks (33, 34). It has been postulated that laser trabeculoplasty eliminates some trabecular cells, which may stimulate the remaining cells to produce a different composition of extracellular matrix with less outflow-obstructing properties (30–32).

While the precise mechanism of laser trabeculoplasty remains only partially understood, it appears to include, as postulated by Van Buskirk (35), a complex interaction of mechanical, cellular, and biochemical properties.

Basic Techniques

Instrumentation

The original, and still most commonly used, laser unit for trabeculoplasty is the continuous-wave argon laser. It has traditionally been operated in the blue-green, biochromatic wavelength spectrum (454.5–528.7 nm). When compared with the use of green, monochromatic laser light (514.5 nm), no differences were noted in the postoperative IOP course or incidence of complications (36, 37). As noted in Chapter 33, however, there is a suggestion that green-only argon light may be safer for the surgeon with regard to an influence on color vision. Alternative laser units for trabeculoplasty are discussed later in this chapter under "Variations in Technique."

A contact lens with a mirror for visualization of the anterior chamber angle (gonioprism) is used in trabeculoplasty. As with all contact lenses for laser application, it should have an antireflection coating on the front surface. A standard Goldmann-type three-mirror lens, in which one mirror is inclined at 59° for gonioscopy, or a single-mirror gonioscopy lens can be used. Both, however, have the slight disadvantage of requiring rotation of the lens to view all quadrants of the anterior chamber angle. This objection can be eliminated by use of the Thorpe four-mirror gonioscopy lens, in which all mirrors are inclined at 62°, or the Ritch trabeculoplasty laser lens, in which two mirrors are inclined at 59° for viewing the inferior quadrants and two at 64° for the superior angle (Fig. 35.1) (38, 39). In the latter lens, a 17-diopter planoconvex button lens over two mirrors provides ×1.4 magnification, reducing a 50-μm laser spot to 35 μm, which may be particularly useful, since a 50-μm spot size with most argon lasers produces a burn in excess of 70 μm (40).

Gonioscopic Considerations

Successful laser trabeculoplasty requires accurate identification and treatment of the trabecular meshwork. The surgeon

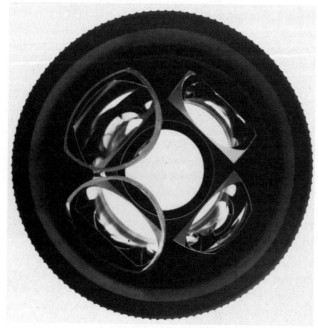

Figure 35.1. Ritch trabeculoplasty laser lens. (Reprinted with permission from Ritch, R: A new lens for argon laser trabeculoplasty. Ophthalmic Surg 16:331, 1985.)

must, therefore, have a detailed knowledge of the anterior chamber angle anatomy and its many variations. The basic aspects of this subject were covered in Chapters 3 and 32, and we now consider some additional features that are pertinent to laser trabeculoplasty.

Two variations of the anterior chamber angle that may interfere with accurate laser application to the trabecular meshwork are (a) the degree of pigmentation, and (b) the width of the chamber angle. With regard to pigmentation, some angles are so diffusely pigmented from the ciliary body band to Schwalbe's line that the exact location of the meshwork is obscured (Fig. 35.2). This is usually most marked in the inferior quadrants, and a careful inspection of all quadrants before starting treatment will usually disclose the position of the meshwork in some areas, which can then be used as a guide in locating the meshwork in the remainder of the angle. At the opposite extreme, the trabecular meshwork in some angles is so lightly pigmented that it is hard to see (Fig. 35.3). In some cases, iris processes, which normally extend to the meshwork, may be a useful indicator. Identification of the ciliary body band or Schwalbe's line may also help determine the relative position of the meshwork.

A narrow anterior chamber angle can lead to improper placement of the laser burns or may prohibit performing trabeculoplasty. If visualization of the meshwork is obscured by peripheral iris, a heavily pigmented Schwalbe's line may be mistaken for the meshwork. Rotating the contact lens in relation to the eye, by asking the patient to look in the direction of the mirror being used, will often provide a deeper view into the angle, enhancing visualization of the meshwork. Care must be taken with this maneuver, however, not to distort the size and shape of the aiming beam. If positioning of the contact lens is not sufficient to expose the meshwork, it may be possible to deepen the chamber angle by applying low energy laser burns to the peripheral iris, a technique called iridoplasty, or gonioplasty, that is discussed in Chapter 36. If the angle is still too narrow, a laser iridotomy, also discussed in the next chapter, should be performed, and the trabeculoplasty should be done at a later date.

Original Protocol

The original protocol of Wise and Witter (8) has remained the standard approach to laser trabeculoplasty, against which variations in technique have been evaluated. A ×25 magnification in the slitlamp delivery system usually provides an optimum balance between detail and field of view. Argon laser settings of 0.1-second duration exposure and 50-μm beam diameter have remained constant through most variations in protocol. One study compared durations of 0.2–0.1 seconds and found no advantage to the former (41). The most commonly used power levels range between 700 and 1500 mW, with an average of 1000 mW. One study evaluated powers ranging from 100 mW to

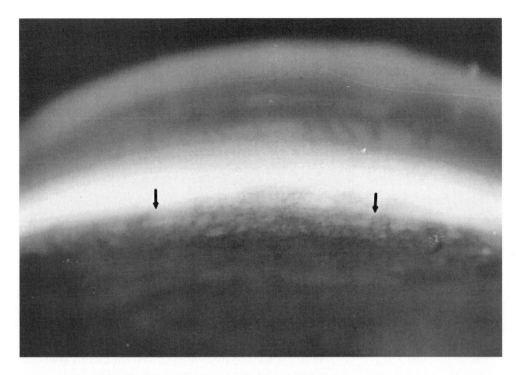

Figure 35.2. Gonioscopic view of wide open anterior chamber angle in which heavy pigmentation interferes with precise location of the trabecular meshwork *(arrow)*.

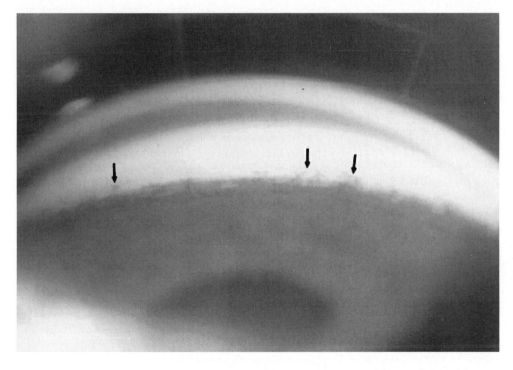

Figure 35.3. Gonioscopic view of wide open anterior chamber angle in which scant pigmentation hampers identification of trabecular meshwork. In this case, iris processes *(arrows)* help determine the position of the meshwork.

1000 mW and found that powers of more than 500 mW gave the maximum success rates (42). The power should be adjusted to produce a depigmentation spot or a small gas bubble at the treatment site (Fig. 35.4). This response is influenced by the amount of pigment in the trabecular meshwork. With a heavily pigmented meshwork, a lower power level may be sufficient, while lightly pigmented meshworks require higher levels.

Originally, laser burns were applied onto or immediately posterior to the pigmented band of the trabecular meshwork, with approximately 100 applications evenly spaced around the full 360° of the meshwork (8). Complications associated with this basic protocol, however, led to variations in technique. We first consider the complications and how they are managed and then the variations in technique that have been used to minimize the complications.

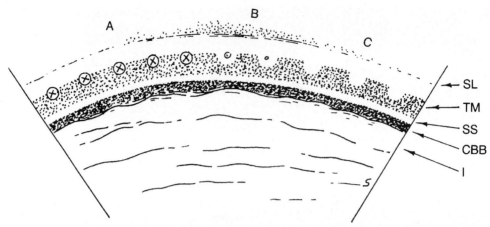

Figure 35.4. Placement of laser burns *(A)* along anterior portion of trabecular meshwork *(TM)*. Desired visual result is depigmentation of the treatment site *(B, C)* and/or a small gas bubble *(B)*. Schwalbe's line *(SL)*, scleral spur *(SS)*, ciliary body band *(CBB)*, iris *(I)*.

Complications and Postoperative Management

Transient IOP elevation in the immediate postoperative period is the most serious early complication of laser trabeculoplasty (43–48). In most cases, the pressure rise is mild and lasts less than 24 hours, causing no long-term problems. In some patients, however, the elevation is marked and sustained and can lead to further loss of vision, especially in eyes with advanced visual field loss before trabeculoplasty. The IOP rise occurs within 2 hours after treatment in most cases, although some eyes may not develop an increase until 4–7 hours after therapy (46, 47). Postoperative management, therefore, should include a pressure check within the first few hours after the procedure. Patients who have a significant early postoperative pressure rise or who have advanced glaucomatous damage should also be seen the following day. However, a pressure rise on the first postoperative day is uncommon, with only 4.2% having a rise greater than 3 mm Hg in one study, and it is considered reasonable to see the other, lower risk patients again in 2–3 weeks (49).

The main patient characteristic associated with the transient pressure rise is meshwork pigmentation (48). Two patients with exfoliation syndrome had a delayed IOP rise during the first postlaser month, associated with inflammatory precipitates on the trabecular meshwork (50). It should also be noted that eyes with active inflammation are at a high risk of marked IOP rise after laser trabeculoplasty, and the operation is contraindicated in these eyes.

Histopathologic studies suggest that the mechanism of posttrabeculoplasty pressure rise is an inflammatory reaction, with fibrinous material and tissue debris in the meshwork (20, 23, 51, 52).

Iritis is a common early posttrabeculoplasty complication. In one study, using a laser flare-cell meter, 49% of 71 eyes showed significant inflammation, which peaked 2 days after the treatment (53). The inflammation was significantly more frequent in eyes with exfoliation syndrome or pigmentary glaucoma than in those with chronic open-angle glaucoma. The postoperative iritis is usually mild and transient and easily controlled with a brief postoperative course of topical corticosteroids. A typical protocol for postoperative management includes prednisolone 1%, or fluorometholone 0.1%, or equivalent four times daily for 5 days. The topical nonsteroidal anti-inflammatory drug diclofenac 0.1% has also been reported to effectively control the inflammation after argon laser trabeculoplasty (54).

The formation of *peripheral anterior synechiae* is also a common complication of trabeculoplasty (55). These are typically small and tented, corresponding to the location of the laser applications. *Alterations of corneal endothelium* after laser trabeculoplasty may include a significant increase in cell size (56), although another study showed no statistically significant changes (57).

The most serious late posttrabeculoplasty complication is, at the present time, more theoretic than real. Histopathologic studies, as previously described, show changes in the trabecular meshwork, including an endothelial layer over the inner surface (Fig. 35.5), which could eventually lead to an increase in resistance to aqueous outflow (20, 21, 25, 26). Whether the glaucoma in eyes treated with laser trabeculoplasty will one day become more difficult to control due to these structural changes remains a matter of concern. To date, however, with more than 15 years of extensive clinical experience, there is no evidence of this potential complication. Nevertheless, there is undoubtedly a limit to the amount of laser trabeculoplasty that an eye can tolerate, as is discussed later in this chapter with regard to repeat procedures. There has also been concern that laser trabeculoplasty might interfere with the success rate of subsequent filtering surgery, although this did not appear to be the case in one study (58).

Variations in Technique

Alternative Protocols with Argon Laser

The parameter evaluated most extensively has been the total number of laser applications and the amount of trabecular meshwork that is treated. Applying 25 burns to 90% of the meshwork appears to be less effective than protocols with larger amounts of treatment (59, 60). However, the application of 50 burns to either 180° or 360° was found to have a similar effect on IOP reduction as treatment of 100 burns to 360° of the meshwork (60–62). In one such study, the eyes receiving 50 applications over 180° or 360° had a lower probability of requiring subsequent filtering surgery than those receiving 100 applications over 360° (63). A two-stage protocol, in which treatment of the full 360° circumference is divided into two sessions 1 month apart, gave the same reduction in IOP as the full treatment in one session (64). With this technique, most of the pressure reduction is achieved with the first stage of therapy, although some patients may have minimal benefit from stage one, and yet a substantial pressure reduction after the second stage of therapy (65). The main advantage of the lower number of laser applications during a single session is a reduction in the transient IOP rise during the immediate postoperative period (43, 44, 60–62, 64–66). In one study, however, the frequency and magnitude of postlaser IOP increase was the same in groups receiving 360° treatment in one or two stages (67). The long-term outcome does not appear to be influenced by which quadrants are treated first. One study randomized patients into initial inferior versus superior halves and found no significant difference (68).

Another variation from the basic protocol that appears to minimize the complication of early posttreatment pressure rise is the placement of the laser applications along the anterior portion of the pigmented meshwork (Fig. 35.6) (60, 62, 66). An anterior placement of the laser burns also reduces the complication of peripheral anterior synechiae formation (55, 69). It may, however, increase the potential complication of cellular proliferation from the corneal endothelium over the trabecular meshwork (26).

Alternative Lasers

In addition to the variations in the basic protocol with the argon laser, several other laser wavelengths have been evaluated for laser trabeculoplasty. A *krypton* laser, with red (647.1 nm) or yellow (568.2 nm) wavelengths, was effective in preliminary trials of laser trabeculoplasty (70), although one comparative study showed the argon laser to be significantly more effective (37). Preliminary experience with the *neodymium:YAG* laser (1064 nm) in the thermal mode revealed tissue responses in monkey eyes that were similar but deeper into the meshwork than those produced by argon laser (28). Tonographic studies in a clinical trial revealed increased outflow correlating with the fall in IOP (16). In a study of 106 eyes of 57 patients, treated with 50 applications of neodymium:YAG laser over 180°, using a 100-μm spot size, 200–400 msec, and 9 W of power, the cumulative success rate (22 mm Hg or less) was 71.5% at 2 years (71).

Semiconductor diode lasers (810 nm) have been evaluated more recently for laser trabeculoplasty. These units have the advantages of solid-state construction, with increased durability and less maintenance requirements than

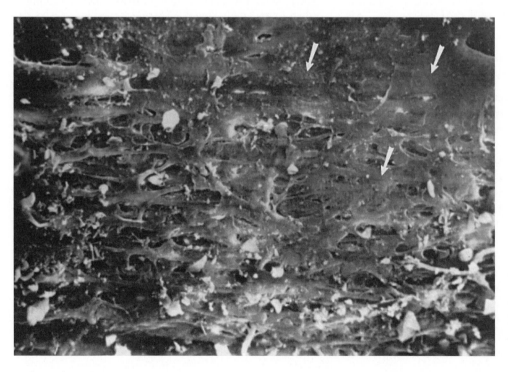

Figure 35.5. Scanning electron microscopic view of trabeculectomy specimen from eye with failed argon laser trabeculoplasty showing endothelial growth over portions of the intertrabecular spaces *(arrows)*.

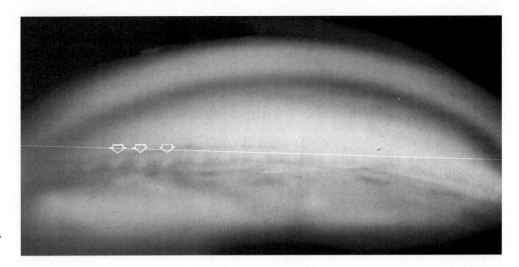

Figure 35.6. Gonioscopic view of depigmentation sites *(arrows)* along anterior margin of trabecular meshwork immediately after argon laser trabeculoplasty.

most other lasers, and compact, portable size with attachments for standard slitlamps. Typical settings for trabeculoplasty are 75–100-μm spot size, 0.1–0.2-second duration, and 750–1200 mW of power, with otherwise the same basic protocol as with argon laser trabeculoplasty. Ultrastructural studies of cadaver eyes (72) and one eye treated prior to enucleation for malignant melanoma (73) revealed similar alterations in the trabecular meshwork with diode and argon lasers, as previously described. Uncontrolled pilot studies revealed mean IOP reductions of 10.2 mm Hg 2 weeks after diode laser trabeculoplasty, 9.55 mm Hg at 6 months (74), 8.42 mm Hg at 1 year, and 7.9 mm Hg at 2 years (75). Comparative trials with argon laser trabeculoplasty revealed no significant differences in IOP response at 2 months (76) or 1 year (77), but did reveal significantly less disruption of the blood-aqueous barrier with the diode laser (76). There was also less postoperative pain and peripheral anterior synechiae in eyes treated with the diode laser (76).

Pharmacologic Control of Pressure Rise

One drop of 4% pilocarpine immediately after the procedure was shown to be effective in minimizing the IOP rise (78). Subsequently, however, topical application of the α_2-adrenergic agonist *apraclonidine* 1%, 1 hour before and immediately after laser trabeculoplasty, was shown to have a marked effect on minimizing the postoperative pressure rise (79). When compared to pilocarpine 4%, timolol 0.5%, dipivefrin 0.1%, or acetazolamide 250 mg, each given 1 hour before and immediately after trabeculoplasty, only 3% of apraclonidine-treated eyes had IOP rises greater than 5 mm Hg, in contrast to 33%, 32%, 38%, and 39%, respectively, with the other treatments (80). One study found that adding pilocarpine to apraclonidine therapy further reduced the incidence of postoperative pressure rise (81). It has also been shown that a single drop of apraclonidine 15 minutes before (82) or immediately after (83) the laser treatment is as effective as the two doses, and that apraclonidine 0.5% is as effective as 1% (84). This has now become a standard part of

laser trabeculoplasty for most surgeons. So profound is the benefit of apraclonidine that treatment in two sessions of 180° each may no longer be necessary to avoid the transient IOP rise. In one study, 360° trabeculoplasty with perioperative apraclonidine had the same early postoperative IOP course as the 180° treatment without apraclonidine (85).

Another α_2-adrenergic agonist, brimonidine 0.5%, has also been shown to effectively control the postlaser pressure rise when given either before or after the treatment (86, 87). Acetazolamide was also shown to reduce the IOP rise following laser trabeculoplasty in one study (88), although, as previously noted, it is less effective than apraclonidine (80). Neither corticosteroids (89) nor the prostaglandin synthetase inhibitors indomethacin (90–92) or flurbiprofen (93), significantly influenced the postoperative IOP. One study actually showed that patients receiving topical indomethacin had higher pressures after 1 month than those receiving a placebo (91). Prostaglandin synthetase inhibitors also appear to have no influence on the postoperative iritis (90, 94).

Results

Short-term Intraocular Pressure Control

Most reports show that useful IOP reduction is achieved in approximately 85% of eyes treated with laser trabeculoplasty (8–11, 13, 43, 95). Some eyes may have a pressure drop within the first few hours after treatment, although days or weeks are usually required to achieve the full response to trabeculoplasty, with further pressure reduction rarely occurring beyond 1 month. The magnitude of the final pressure reduction averages 6–9 mm Hg, which is usually not sufficient to allow discontinuation of all medical therapy, although the medication can occasionally be reduced or eliminated (96). One study has suggested that pilocarpine is no longer able to induce a further decrease in IOP after trabeculoplasty (97), and it is probably advisable to reevaluate the efficacy of any miotic approximately 1 month after the laser treatment.

FACTORS INFLUENCING INTRAOCULAR PRESSURE RESPONSE. Many factors influence the IOP response to laser trabeculoplasty. Eyes with higher *pretreatment pressures* tend to have a greater fall in IOP (98). Despite this fact, a pretreatment pressure above 30 mm Hg has been associated with a higher frequency of failures (95, 99), while eyes with pressures in the normal range may obtain useful pressure reduction after trabeculoplasty (100–102).

Another significant factor is the *type of glaucoma*. A particularly favorable response is obtained with chronic open-angle glaucoma, exfoliation syndrome, and pigmentary glaucoma (12, 95, 98, 99, 103–106). Success in the latter two conditions is most likely related to the favorable influence of increased trabecular meshwork pigmentation (107). In pigmentary glaucoma, younger patients appear to have a more sustained pressure reduction than older patients with the same condition (105, 106). Other forms of glaucoma that respond to laser trabeculoplasty, although less well than those noted above, include open-angle glaucoma in aphakia or pseudophakia (108) and angle-closure glaucoma after an iridotomy (103). While eyes that have had multiple operations generally do not do well with trabeculoplasty (104), those with a single failed trabeculectomy may obtain useful pressure reduction after the laser therapy (109). Other forms of glaucoma that do not respond well to laser trabeculoplasty include glaucoma associated with uveitis, angle recession glaucoma, and congenital or juvenile glaucoma (103, 104, 110).

Some investigators feel that young *age* has an unfavorable influence on the results of laser trabeculoplasty (95, 111), although no effect of age was seen in another study (99). As previously noted, young patients with pigmentary glaucoma appear to do better than older patients with the same condition (105, 106). Black versus white race does not appear to influence the results of laser trabeculoplasty (112).

Long-term Intraocular Pressure Control

A major question regarding the results of laser trabeculoplasty is how long the IOP reduction will last. While a high percentage of patients will show an initial favorable reduction in IOP, the majority of patients will gradually lose this effect (113–120). Failure is most common in the first year, with reported rates of 19–23%, and thereafter failure occurs at a rate of 5–9% per year (118, 120). As a result, it can be anticipated that approximately half of the patients will have lost the benefit of the initial trabeculoplasty by 5 years and two-thirds within 10 years following the surgery.

REPEAT TRABECULOPLASTY. If a successful IOP reduction is never achieved following 360° laser trabeculoplasty, further laser therapy is generally not felt to be indicated. However, if an initial good response to treatment, lasting for approximately a year or more, is followed by a return to higher pressures, there may be value in repeating the surgery. Most studies have shown a much lower success rate with repeat trabeculoplasty than with the initial treatment, in the range of one-third to one-half (119, 121–127). In one long-term study, success rates were 35% at 6 months, 21% at 12 months, 11% at 24 months, and 5% at 48 months (127). Some studies have noted a higher incidence of transient pressure rise following repeat laser trabeculoplasty (121, 122, 127), and it is probably advisable to perform these in two stages of 180° each.

Indications

Laser trabeculoplasty may be indicated in the treatment of those forms of open-angle glaucoma in which favorable responses have been reported, including chronic open-angle glaucoma, the exfoliation syndrome, pigmentary glaucoma, and glaucoma in aphakia or pseudophakia. During the first decade of experience with laser trabeculoplasty, the procedure was used as a supplement to maximum tolerable medical therapy and studies have shown it to be effective in this regard (43, 128). The rationale for this approach was based not only on the risk of early postoperative complications, especially the transient pressure rise, but also on the concern that eyes treated with laser trabeculoplasty might eventually become more difficult to control than if they had been left on medical therapy. The histopathologic studies showing proliferation of a cellular layer over the trabecular meshwork have given reason to seriously consider this theoretic complication (20, 21, 25, 26). Nevertheless, short-term (128–133) and long-term (134–136) studies of laser trabeculoplasty for open-angle glaucoma suggest that the procedure may be safe and effective as initial treatment for glaucoma. In a multicenter, clinical trial (the Glaucoma Laser Trial), 271 patients with newly diagnosed chronic open-angle glaucoma were randomized into initial argon laser trabeculoplasty in one eye and timolol 0.5% in the other eye, with the same stepped regimen of additional medical therapy in either eye as required (135). During the first 2 years of followup, the laser-treated eyes had a slightly lower mean IOP of 1–2 mm Hg, although over half of these eyes eventually required the addition of one or more medications. In a followup study of 203 of these patients, with a mean duration of 7 years, eyes initially treated with laser trabeculoplasty had 1.2 mm Hg greater reduction in IOP, 0.6-dB greater improvement in visual field, and slightly less optic nerve head deterioration (136). Although these findings suggest that initial treatment with argon laser trabeculoplasty is at least as efficacious as initial treatment with topical medication, the latter approach is still more commonly practical in North America. A survey of American Glaucoma Society members indicated that 2.3% usually employ initial trabeculoplasty, while 84.5% will usually try combinations of two or more medications before recommending laser trabeculoplasty (137).

TRABECULOTOMY[b]

The basic principle of this operation is the creation of an opening in the trabecular meshwork to establish direct communication between the anterior chamber and Schlemm's canal. It is generally performed with incisional surgical techniques, although laser techniques are also being evaluated.

Incisional Trabeculotomy

In 1960, Burian (138) and Smith (139) independently described techniques for incising the trabecular meshwork from an ab externo approach. The procedure was modified by Harms and Dannheim (140), who reported success in

[b]Refer to M.B. Shields: Color Atlas of Glaucoma. Baltimore: Williams & Wilkins, 1998, Plates III8–10.

adults as well as children, although the primary application of trabeculotomy has been with the management of childhood glaucomas.

Basic Technique (Fig. 35.7)

The following technique, described by McPherson (141), encompasses aspects of the procedures developed by Allen and Burian (142) and Harms and Dannheim (140).

A conjunctival flap is prepared in the same manner as used for filtering surgery (Chapter 37), and a 2 × 4 mm limbus-based, partial-thickness scleral flap is dissected. A radial incision is made across the sclerolimbal junction until Schlemm's canal is entered. To confirm the identity of the canal, a nylon suture may be threaded into one of the cut ends and observed gonioscopically to insure that the suture is in the canal. Alternatively, the exposed portion of the suture may be bent anteriorly or posteriorly, noting whether it

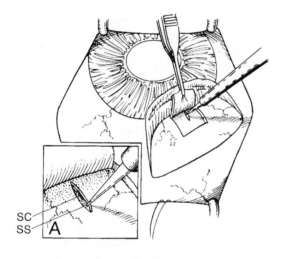

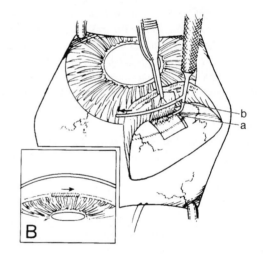

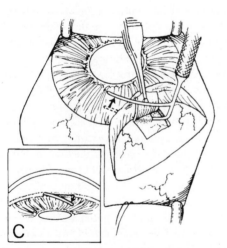

Figure 35.7. Trabeculotomy. **A.** Beneath a partial-thickness scleral flap, a radial incision is made across the sclerolimbal junction until Schlemm's canal *(SC)* is identified just anterior to the circumferential fibers of scleral spur *(SS)*. **B.** The internal arm *(a)* of a trabeculotome is threaded into Schlemm's canal, using the external, parallel arm *(b)* as a guide; inset shows the gonioscopic appearance of the internal arm as it moves through the canal *(arrow)*. **C.** The trabeculotome is rotated *(arrows)* causing the internal arm to tear through the trabecular meshwork into the anterior chamber.

returns to a position parallel to the canal when released. Failure to do so suggests that a false passage may have been created into the anterior chamber or supraciliary space.

One arm of a McPherson trabeculotome is threaded into Schlemm's canal, using the other, parallel arm, as a guide. The trabeculotome is then rotated so that the arm within the canal tears through trabecular meshwork into the anterior chamber. The same procedure is then performed on the other side of the radial incision.

The scleral and conjunctival flaps are closed in the same manner as for filtering procedures. Postoperative care includes the use of topical antibiotics and steroids. A low dose of pilocarpine may also be useful by keeping the cut edges of trabecular meshwork separated, and the pupil can be dilated once daily with phenylephrine to avoid posterior synechiae.

Variations

SUTURE TRABECULOTOMY. In the technique originally described by Smith (139), a nylon suture was threaded into Schlemm's canal for over one-third of the circumference, and the two exposed ends were pulled taut, causing the suture to rupture through the trabecular meshwork into the anterior chamber. In subsequent modifications, the canal is threaded for 360° with either a continuous suture or two that are threaded between incisions 180° apart, and a 360° trabeculotomy is performed (143). In one study, this technique was successful in 13 of 15 children with congenital glaucoma (143).

COMBINED TRABECULOTOMY-TRABECULECTOMY. If Schlemm's canal cannot be located with certainty, which is not uncommon in highly buphthalmic eyes, it is possible to convert the procedure to a trabeculectomy by removing a block of deep limbal tissue beneath the scleral flap. In addition, the two procedures can be combined by first performing the trabeculotomy and then creating the fistula beneath the scleral flap. In some situations, such as the Sturge-Weber syndrome in which the exact mechanism of the glaucoma is uncertain (see Chapter 18), the combined procedure may offer the best chance of success (144). A similar combined technique has been suggested for late onset congenital glaucoma in which a 2 × 2 mm block of tissue beneath the scleral flap is excised, but without penetrating the trabecular meshwork (145). This procedure was reported to be successful in all of seven eyes, five of which had diffuse filtering blebs. Combined trabeculotomy-trabeculectomy was compared to primary trabeculectomy alone in children with congenital glaucoma, and the cumulative chance of success at 24 months was 93.5% and 72%, respectively (146).

ELECTROCAUTERY. Electrocautery has been utilized in modified trabeculotomies by insulating all sides of the probe except that exposed to the trabecular meshwork (147–149). By burning an opening in the meshwork, it is felt that fibrotic closure of the severed edges is avoided. Success has been reported with this technique in patients with chronic open-angle glaucoma, as well as congenital glaucoma (149). A similar

approach has also been described in which electric discharges are used to create holes in the trabecular meshwork (150).

MISCELLANEOUS VARIATIONS. Other experimental types of trabeculotomy utilize aqueous veins to localize Schlemm's canal by threading a probe through a large vein and into the canal (151) or by forcing air into a vein, which causes multiple ruptures in the meshwork (152). An instrument has also been developed, the trabeculectome, which excises a strip of trabecular meshwork as it is pulled along the anterior chamber angle by a probe in Schlemm's canal (153).

Complications

If Schlemm's canal is not properly identified, a false passage may be created either into the anterior chamber or the supraciliary space. The latter may result in the creation of a cyclodialysis and possible hyphema. If Schlemm's canal cannot be identified, the procedure can be converted to a trabeculectomy. When the probe is rotated into the anterior chamber, it may strip Descemet's membrane if it is too far anterior, or damage the iris or lens if it is too far posterior. As with all intraocular glaucoma procedures, postoperative bleeding and infection are potential complications.

Laser Trabeculotomy (Trabeculopuncture)

As noted at the outset of this chapter, the earliest efforts to treat glaucoma by the application of laser energy to the trabecular meshwork were attempts to create holes through the trabecular meshwork into Schlemm's canal (2–5, 7). This approach lost popularity due to early failures and to the subsequent enthusiasm for laser trabeculoplasty, although advances in the technology of pulsed lasers have led to a reevaluation of laser trabeculotomy, or trabeculopuncture.

In laboratory studies with monkeys, the Q-switched ruby laser did not produce persistent penetration to Schlemm's canal (154). With Q-switched neodymium:YAG lasers, holes were created in the trabecular meshwork, but were soon sealed by proliferation of corneal endothelium and scar tissue (155, 156). Laboratory studies with human ocular tissue have shown that pulsed neodymium:YAG lasers at energy levels between 3 and 6 mJ can produce discrete lesions into Schlemm's canal with minimal damage to adjacent structures (157, 158). In human autopsy eyes, energy levels of 30 mJ produced openings in the trabecular meshwork of approximately 100 μm in diameter (159). A similar technique was used in four human eyes treated within 18 hours of enucleation, which produced irregular craters of 150–300 μm in the meshwork, with denuding of endothelial cells and deposition of debris in the adjacent trabecular and corneal tissues (160).

Preliminary clinical experience with laser trabeculotomy has provided variable results. In one series of eight eyes of six patients with juvenile glaucoma, pressure control was achieved in six eyes (75%) with a mean followup of 6 months (161). The most effective technique in this study was to make two confluent trabeculotomies of 1 clock hour each in extent. Another study of 69 eyes of 61 patients with open-angle glaucoma, however, had a success rate of only 46% 1 year after treatment (162). Nd:YAG laser trabeculopuncture may have value in patients with angle-recession glaucoma. In one series, the probability of success at 1 year was calculated at 90%, compared to 27% with argon laser trabeculoplasty (163). In another study, however, the success rate at a mean of 12 months was only 41.7% with Nd:YAG laser trabeculopuncture (164).

GONIOTOMY[c]

In 1938, Barkan (165) described an operation for congenital glaucoma in which an incision in the anterior chamber angle was felt to reduce obstruction to aqueous outflow caused by a membrane across the trabecular meshwork. Although the presence of a true membrane has never been established, the operation is effective in a high percentage of cases, presumably by incising whatever abnormal tissue is responsible for the outflow obstruction. This operation differs primarily from trabeculotomy in that only a portion of the internal trabecular tissue is incised. It is still preferred by many pediatric glaucoma surgeons. Subsequent modifications of the basic technique may also be useful for other forms of glaucoma in both children and adults.

Basic Technique (Fig. 35.8) (165)

The procedure can be performed with a binocular head loupe, although the operating microscope provides better visualization (166). The patient's head is rotated away from the side of the surgery and the operative eye is slightly abducted. A surgical goniolens is then placed over the nasal cornea, leaving 2–3 mm of temporal cornea exposed for the knife entry. Fixation of the globe is essential, and this can be accomplished with locking forceps held by an assistant.

The goniotomy knife penetrates the cornea 1 mm anterior to the limbus at 10 o'clock in the right eye or 4 o'clock in the left eye. The blade is passed across the anterior chamber to a point in the chamber angle 180% from the entry site. The shaft of the knife is tapered to maintain a water tight seal. Numerous modifications of Barkan's goniotomy knife have been described, including attached fiber optics for intraocular illumination (167). A 23- or 25-gauge needle can also be used as the knife, and this has been attached to a syringe containing sodium hyaluronic acid (168) or to a flexible endoscope, which allows observation of the anterior chamber angle on a videoscreen (169).

Using the tip of the goniotomy blade, the angle tissue is incised posterior to Schwalbe's line for approximately one-third of the angle circumference. The intent is to incise only

<hr />

[c]Refer to M.B. Shields: Color Atlas of Glaucoma. Baltimore: Williams & Wilkins, 1998, Plates III8–10.

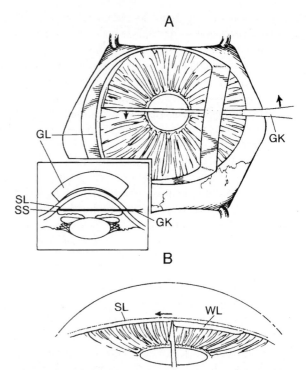

Figure 35.8. Goniotomy. **A.** With a surgical goniolens (*GL*) positioned on the cornea, a goniotomy knife (*GK*) is inserted through peripheral cornea and passed across the anterior chamber to the angle in the opposite quadrant. **B.** Under direct gonioscopic visualization, angle tissue is excised between Schwalbe's line (*SL*) and scleral spur (*SS*) for approximately one-third of the chamber angle circumference. This creates a white line (*WL*) as the cut edge of tissue retracts from the incision. *Arrows* indicate the direction of knife movement during incision of angle tissue.

the abnormal layer of tissue in front of the trabecular meshwork, and this is best judged by observing a white line develop as the cut edge of tissue retracts posteriorly and sclera is seen through intact trabecular meshwork.

The knife is then withdrawn, taking care not to injure adjacent ocular structures, and the anterior chamber is deepened with air or a balanced salt solution. In one study of seven infants treated with two simultaneous goniotomies in one eye and a single goniotomy in the fellow eye, no significant differences were noted in the results (170). If bilateral surgery is needed, it has been suggested that both procedures can be done at the same operation (171), although these should be done with different sets of instruments. Postoperative management consists of topical antibiotics, a miotic, and topical steroids.

Complications

Intraoperative Complications

Placement of the incision is critical in performing a goniotomy. If the incision is too posterior, bleeding from the ciliary body may occur, while an incision that is too anterior will have no effect. Iridodialysis or cyclodialysis may also be inadvertently created during a goniotomy procedure (171).

Shallowing or loss of the anterior chamber during the operation prevents adequate visualization of the angle and increases the risk of damage to ocular structures. If this occurs, the knife should be withdrawn and the chamber should be deepened with balanced salt solution or sodium hyaluronate through the entry site.

As with any operation under general anesthesia, the risks of the anesthesia must also be considered. In a series of 401 goniotomies under general anesthesia, the most serious complication was cardiopulmonary arrest, which occurred in 1.8% (171).

Postoperative Complications

A moderate hyphema is common after goniotomy, but rarely leads to serious sequelae. In 401 goniotomies, postoperative bleeding was reported in 0.6%, but useful vision was lost in only one case (171). Postoperative infection is rare.

Permanent visual impairment following surgery for glaucoma in children may be on an anatomic basis, but is more often due to amblyopia and large refractive errors (172). An important aspect of the postoperative management is to anticipate these causes of reduced vision and treat them appropriately.

Variations in Techniques

Goniopuncture

Scheie (173, 174) described a form of goniotomy which incorporated a filtering procedure and was designed primarily for children in whom standard goniotomies had failed. In this procedure, saline is first injected beneath Tenon's capsule near the inferior limbus to create a bleb. The blade of a Scheie needle-knife is then passed through the peripheral cornea just below the horizontal plane and diagonally across the anterior chamber to the inferior angle. The trabecular meshwork and limbal tissue are penetrated with the tip of the blade until it is visible in the sub-Tenon's bleb. The knife is then removed and the anterior chamber is deepened with saline.

Goniodiathermy

A disadvantage of goniopuncture is that the limbal incision tends to scar closed. To avoid this, a technique was developed in which an intraocular diathermy probe is introduced into the goniopuncture tract to cause a gaping of the wound edges. Preliminary experience in rabbits was felt to be encouraging (175).

Direct Goniotomy

When corneal clouding prevents visualization for standard goniotomy, it has been suggested that the goniotomy might be performed directly through a 60° limbal incision (176). However, most surgeons prefer a trabeculotomy in these cases.

Trabeculodialysis

In this modification of the goniotomy technique, the trabecular meshwork is scraped from the scleral sulcus with the flat side of a goniotomy blade (177). This technique is especially useful in *glaucoma associated with inflammation,* presumably because the trabecular tissue is friable and easily scraped away in these cases (177–179). A histologic study has shown that this operation works by establishing a communication between the anterior chamber and Schlemm's canal (179). In one series of 23 children or young adults with glaucoma associated with anterior uveitis, trabeculodialysis controlled the IOP in 60% of the cases (180), while a similar series of 22 patients had an IOP less than 21 mm Hg in 56% with a mean followup of 52 months. (181).

Laser Goniotomy

By applying laser energy with a neodymium:YAG laser anterior to the insertion of the iris in patients with developmental glaucomas, it was possible to separate the iris tissue from the trabecular band. This technique improved the IOP control in seven of eight eyes with juvenile glaucoma (182). In another study of 10 children with bilateral, symmetric congenital glaucoma, one eye was treated with incisional goniotomy under general anesthesia and the other with laser goniotomy under chloral hydrate sedation, with similar pressure results (183).

Results and Comparison of Trabeculotomy and Goniotomy

Glaucoma in Childhood

Opinions differ regarding the procedure of choice for the management of congenital glaucoma. Many pediatric glaucoma surgeons prefer the time-honored goniotomy, utilizing trabeculotomy only in cases with marked corneal clouding or after repeated goniotomy failures. Reported success with goniotomy ranges from approximately 80% to 90%, although in one-third to one-half of the eyes, the procedure must be repeated one or more times (184–187). A less favorable outcome is usually seen when the disease is detected either at birth or later in childhood, or if there is a very high IOP or marked buphthalmos.

Other surgeons prefer trabeculotomy as the initial procedure for most cases of congenital glaucoma. The reported success rates with this operation are basically the same as with goniotomy, although it may be that fewer repeat procedures are required with trabeculotomy than with goniotomy (184, 188–194). The same factors appear to influence the outcome of trabeculotomies as were noted above for goniotomy.

Advocates of goniotomy point out that it is anatomically more precise, with less surgical trauma to adjacent tissues (195), while those who prefer trabeculotomy as a primary procedure note that it is not dependent on a clear cornea (196). Since childhood glaucoma surgery is not performed frequently by most surgeons, there is an advantage in having one procedure that can be used for all cases. In addition, with the trabeculotomy technique it is possible to determine whether or not Schlemm's canal is present and to convert immediately to a filtering procedure if necessary. In the final analysis, however, the two surgical approaches appear to provide equally good results in the hands of experienced surgeons (197).

Glaucoma in Juveniles and Adults

While trabeculotomy and goniotomy are used primarily for glaucomas in childhood, some success has been reported with trabeculotomy in juveniles and adults. In a series of 16 eyes of 11 patients with juvenile open-angle glaucoma, ranging in age between 10 and 45 years, trabeculotomy maintained an IOP of 21 mm Hg or less in 88% during a mean followup of 7 years (198). In a retrospective study of 227 adults with chronic open-angle glaucoma and 65 with the exfoliation syndrome, the final success probability at 5 years after trabeculotomy was 56% and 73.5%, respectively (199). When 79 adults with chronic open-angle glaucoma were randomly assigned to either trabeculotomy or trabeculectomy with adjunctive mitomycin C, the probability of success at 1 year was 86% and 84%, respectively, and the only significant difference was less frequent complications in the trabeculotomy group (200).

CYCLODIALYSIS

Cyclodialysis, as an operation for glaucoma, was described by Heine (201) in 1905. It has been employed as an alternative to filtering surgery, especially in aphakic eyes or in combination with cataract extraction. The procedure has lost popularity in recent years, however, due to unpredictable results and newer, alternative surgical techniques.

Theories of Mechanism

Cyclodialysis involves the separation of the ciliary body from the scleral spur, which creates a direct communication between the anterior chamber and the suprachoroidal space. Most studies suggested that this lowers the IOP by an increase in pressure-dependent uveoscleral outflow (202–206).

It was also proposed, however, that reduced aqueous production, due to an alteration in the ciliary body anatomy, is the principal mode of ocular hypotension (207, 208). It may be that both mechanisms are involved in a successful cyclodialysis procedure. This was suggested by an intraocular manometric study of a glaucoma patient before and after cyclodialysis, which revealed both improved outflow and reduced aqueous production (209).

Basic Technique (201, 210)

An incision is made through conjunctiva and Tenon's capsule approximately 8 mm from the corneolimbal junction, usually in a superior quadrant between the insertions of two rectus muscles. A 3–4 mm full-thickness scleral incision, 4–6 mm from the anatomic limbus, is then made parallel to the limbus.

A cyclodialysis spatula is inserted through the scleral incision and into the supraciliary space. Staying close to the inner scleral surface, the spatula is advanced until the tip enters the anterior chamber. Lateral movements of the spatula tip are then made to either side of the entry point to separate about one-third of the ciliary body from the scleral spur (Fig. 35.9). After withdrawal of the spatula, only the conjunctiva is closed.

Variations

Variations of Basic Technique

An alternative technique is to create the cyclodialysis with multiple forward thrusts of the spatula, by which up to

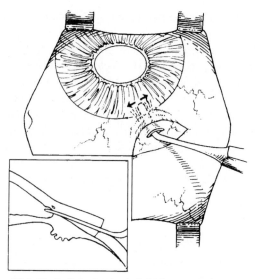

Figure 35.9. Cyclodialysis. A cyclodialysis spatula is passed through a full-thickness scleral incision and the suprachoroidal space until it enters the anterior chamber. With lateral movements of the spatula tip (*arrows*), approximately one-third of the ciliary body is separated from the scleral spur.

one-half of the ciliary body can be disinserted (211). The injection of air (212, 213) or sodium hyaluronate (214) into the anterior chamber has been advocated as a means of holding the cleft open during the early postoperative period. Modifications of the cyclodialysis spatula have also been reported (215, 216).

IMPLANTS. Implants (or setons) of various material have been inserted into the cyclodialysis cleft to keep it open (217–220), although no evidence of lasting success has been provided for any of these techniques.

IRIDOCYCLORETRACTION. Krasnov (221) described a technique for the treatment of chronic angle-closure glaucoma in which two or three scleral pedicles are folded forward into a cyclodialysis cleft to keep the angle open. A modification of this technique, using a single scleral pedicle, was designed to maintain a patent cyclodialysis cleft in aphakic eyes (222). Reports concerning the usefulness of the latter procedure are conflicting (222, 223). In another modification, called "filtering iridocycloretraction," two limbal-based scleral strips are inserted into the anterior chamber and supraciliary space in eyes with chronic angle-closure glaucoma to widen the anterior chamber angle and maintain communication between both the subconjunctival and suprachoroidal spaces (224).

LASER CYCLODIALYSIS. A cyclodialysis technique has been evaluated in monkey eyes in which an argon laser beam is directed between the ciliary body band and root of the iris (225). A subsequent clinical trial of 52 eyes in 36 patients with open-angle glaucoma revealed a success rate of 73% after a 1-year followup (226).

Postoperative Management

Postoperative management includes topical antibiotics and corticosteroids. In addition, the use of a miotic has been recommended to keep the cyclodialysis cleft open through traction on the longitudinal ciliary muscle (202).

Complications (210, 211)

Operative Complications

Hemorrhage is a frequent complication during a cyclodialysis procedure. The risk may be minimized by making a more anterior scleral incision, avoiding anterior ciliary arteries, and keeping the cyclodialysis spatula close to the sclera to avoid perforating the ciliary body. When brisk bleeding does occur, it can usually be stopped by placing a large air bubble in the anterior chamber for several minutes. *Improper position of the spatula* can cause several complications. If the cyclodialysis spatula is too far anterior as it enters the anterior chamber, it may strip Descemet's membrane or oth-

erwise damage the cornea. A position that is too posterior may tear the ciliary body or iris, injure the lens, or rupture the hyaloid face and possibly cause vitreous loss. At any time after surgery, there may be a sudden, marked rise in IOP, which is felt to be due to closure of the cyclodialysis cleft. This can be prevented or reversed in some cases with the use of miotics.

Hypotony

This is a common postoperative complication of cyclodialysis. With the infrequent use of this operation in the management of glaucoma, however, the primary clinical interest in cyclodialysis in recent years has been in techniques to treat the inadvertent cyclodialysis that may result from injury or surgical trauma with subsequent hypotony. Penetrating cyclodiathermy or cyclocryotherapy to "wall off" the cleft may correct the problem, but the results are highly unpredictable. The application of argon laser energy into the cyclodialysis cleft has been reported to successfully close the cleft in some cases (227, 228). Successful laser settings include 0.1–0.2 seconds, 50–100 μm, 300–700 mW. In especially difficult cases, powers of 2–3 W have been used (228). The latter technique usually requires retrobulbar anesthesia, while topical anesthesia is typically sufficient for the lower power settings. Contiguous laser burns are applied to all exposed scleral and uveal surfaces of the cleft for approximately 50 burns. Successful closure of a cyclodialysis cleft with sutures has also been described (229, 230), and may be the procedure of choice when the argon laser therapy has failed.

GONIOSYNECHIALYSIS

Campbell and Vela (231) reported successful preliminary experience with a procedure for synechial angle-closure glaucoma. The technique involves deepening the anterior chamber with sodium hyaluronate and separating the synechiae from the trabecular meshwork with an irrigating cyclodialysis spatula under direct gonioscopic visualization (Fig. 35.10). The procedure has also been employed during penetrating keratoplasty, using a dental mirror to visualize the anterior chamber angle (232). The primary value of the procedure is felt to be for patients in whom the synechiae have not been present for a prolonged period of time. In one study of 15 patients with synechial angle-closure glaucoma, goniosynechialysis alone (five cases) or in combination with other surgical procedures (10 cases) was associated with a reduction in mean IOP from 40 mm Hg to 14 mm Hg (233). In a series of 70 eyes with angle-closure glaucoma that did not respond to laser or incisional iridectomy, goniosynechialysis maintained an IOP below 20 mm Hg in 87% of aphakic eyes, but only 42% of phakic eyes (234). It has also been reported that successful

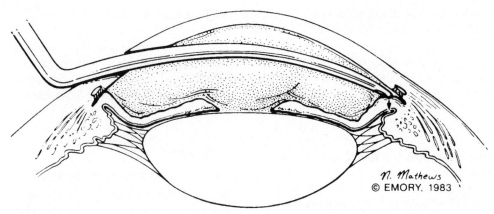

Figure 35.10. Goniosynechialysis. After deepening the anterior chamber with sodium hyaluronate, an irrigating cyclodialysis spatula is used to separate synechiae from the trabecular meshwork with an anterior to posterior movement. (Reprinted with permission from Campbell, DG, Vela, A: Modern goniosynechialysis for the treatment of synechial angle-closure glaucoma. Ophthalmology 91:1052, 1984.)

goniosynechialysis was achieved in 5 of 7 patients with a Q-switched neodymium:YAG laser (235).

GONIOPHOTOCOAGULATION

Simmons and associates (236, 237) described a form of laser treatment for use in the early, open-angle stages of neovascular glaucoma. The purpose of the procedure is to eliminate new vessels in the anterior chamber angle by direct laser photocoagulation. The technique involves the application of argon laser energy to the vessels as they cross the scleral spur to arborize on the trabecular meshwork. The customary laser settings are 0.2 seconds, 150 μm, and power sufficient to blanch and constrict the vessels (usually 100–800 mW) (237).

This technique is rarely used today, but when used it is most effective in the preglaucoma, or rubeosis, stage of the disease to prevent progression of angle neovascularization with subsequent angle closure and intractable glaucoma. It has been used in conjunction with panretinal photocoagulation, especially when the latter was not successful, or when the retinal therapy was not possible or advisable. In the more advanced, florid open-angle stage of neovascular glaucoma, however, goniophotocoagulation must be used with caution, since it may cause hemorrhage or accelerated closure of the anterior chamber angle.

TRABECULAR ASPIRATION

An irrigation-aspiration device has been described for the removal of pigment and exfoliation material from the trabecular meshwork in eyes with glaucoma associated with the exfoliation syndrome. Its use has been reported in 12 eyes prior to cataract extraction (238) and in 12 as a primary surgical procedure (239), with significant IOP reduction in both groups.

SUMMARY

Laser trabeculoplasty involves the application of evenly spaced photocoagulation burns to all or part of the trabecular meshwork. In the majority of cases, this leads to lowering of IOP through improvement of aqueous outflow by mechanisms that are not fully understood. The most serious known complication is an early, transient rise in ocular tension. A significant number of patients lose the ocular hypotensive effect with time, and repeated trabeculoplasty is less effective than the initial procedure.

Incisional trabeculotomy is an ab externo procedure in which trabecular meshwork is incised to establish communication between the anterior chamber and Schlemm's canal. Laser trabeculotomy is being evaluated as an alternative approach in which meshwork is punctured ab interno with pulsed laser energy. Goniotomy is an ab interno procedure in which abnormal tissue in the anterior chamber angle is incised. Incisional trabeculotomy and goniotomy are the primary surgical procedures for childhood glaucomas, although variations of the basic trabeculotomy technique may be useful for some types of glaucoma in juveniles and adults.

Cyclodialysis, which involves the separation of the ciliary body from the scleral spur, was once used to treat glaucoma, but the primary clinical interest today is treatment of inadvertent cyclodialyses with hypotony. Other reported surgical procedures of the anterior chamber angle include goniosynechialysis for synechial angle-closure glaucoma, goniophotocoagulation for neovascular glaucoma, and trabecular aspiration for the exfoliation syndrome.

REFERENCES

1. Zweng, HC, Flocks, M: Experimental photocoagulation of the anterior chamber angle. A prelimary report. Am J Ophthalmol 52:163, 1961.
2. Krasnov, MM: Laser puncture of the anterior chamber angle in glaucoma. Vestn Oftalmol 3:27, 1972.

3. Hager, H: Besondere mikrochirurgische Eingriffe. II. Erste Erfahrungen mit der Argon-laser-gerat 800. Klin Monatsbl Augenheilkd 163:437, 1973.

4. Demailly, P, Haut, J, Bonnet-Boutier, M: Trabeculotomie au laser a l'argon (note preliminaire). Bull Soc Ophthalmol Fr 73:259, 1973.

5. Worthen, DM, Wickham, MG: Argon laser trabeculotomy. Trans Am Acad Ophthalmol Otol 78:371, 1974.

6. Gaasterland, D, Kupfer, C: Experimental glaucoma in the rhesus monkey. Invest Ophthalmol 14:455, 1975.

7. Ticho, U, Zauberman, H: Argon laser application to angle structures in the glaucomas. Arch Ophthalmol 94:61, 1976.

8. Wise, JB, Witter, SL: Argon laser therapy for open-angle glaucoma. A pilot study. Arch Ophthalmol 97:319, 1979.

9. Wise, JB: Long-term control of adult open angle glaucoma by argon laser treatment. Ophthalmology 88:197, 1981.

10. Schwartz, AL, Whitten, ME, Bleiman, B, Martin, D: Argon laser trabecular surgery in uncontrolled phakic open angle glaucoma. Ophthalmology 88:203, 1981.

11. Wilensky, JT, Jampol, LM: Laser therapy for open angle glaucoma. Ophthalmology 88:213, 1981.

12. Pohjanpelto, P: Argon laser treatment of the anterior chamber angle for increased intraocular pressure. Acta Ophthalmol 59:211, 1981.

13. Lichter, PR: Argon laser trabeculoplasty. Trans Am Ophthalmol Soc 80:288, 1982.

14. Brubaker, RF, Liesegang, TJ: Effect of trabecular photocoagulation on the aqueous humor dynamics of the human eye. Am J Ophthalmol 96:139, 1983.

15. Merte, H-J, Denffer, H, Hirsch, B: Tonographic findings following argon laser trabeculoplasty. Klin Monatsbl Augenheilkd 186:220, 1985.

16. Schrems, W, Sold, J, Krieglstein, GK, Leydhecker, W: Tonographic response of laser trabeculoplasty in chronic glaucoma. Klin Monatsbl Augenheilkd 187:170, 1985.

17. Araie, M, Yamamoto, T, Shirato, S, Kitazawa, Y: Effects of laser trabeculoplasty on the human aqueous humor dynamics: a fluorophotometric study. Ann Ophthalmol 16:540, 1984.

18. Yablonski, ME, Cook, DJ, Gray, J: A fluorophotometric study of the effect of argon laser trabeculoplasty on aqueous humor dynamics. Am J Ophthalmol 99:579, 1985.

19. Feller, DB, Weinreb, RN: Breakdown and reestablishment of blood-aqueous barrier with laser trabeculoplasty. Arch Ophthalmol 102:537, 1984.

20. Rodrigues, MM, Spaeth, GL, Donohoo, P: Electron microscopy of argon laser therapy in phakic open-angle glaucoma. Ophthalmology 89:198, 1982.

21. Alexander, RA, Grierson, I, Church, WH: The effect of argon laser trabeculoplasty upon the normal human trabecular meshwork. Graefes Arch Clin Exp Ophthalmol 227:72, 1989.

22. Babizhayev, MA, Brodskaya, MW, Mamedov, NG, Batmanov, YY: Clinical, structural and molecular phototherapy effects of laser irradiation on the trabecular meshwork of human glaucomatous eyes. Graefes Arch Clin Exp Ophthalmol 228:90, 1990.

23. Melamed, S, Pei, J, Epstein, DL: Short-term effect of argon laser trabeculoplasty in monkeys. Arch Ophthalmol 103:1546, 1985.

24. Dueker, DK, Norberg, M, Johnson, DH, et al: Stimulation of cell division by argon and Nd:YAG laser trabeculoplasty in cynomolgus monkeys. Invest Ophthalmol Vis Sci 31:115, 1990.

25. Melamed, S, Pei, J, Epstein, DL: Delayed response to argon laser trabeculoplasty in monkeys. Morphological and morphometric analysis. Arch Ophthalmol 104:1078, 1986.

26. van der Zypen, E, Fankhauser, F: Ultrastructural changes of the trabecular meshwork of the monkey (Macaca speciosa) following irradiation with argon laser light. Graefes Arch Clin Exp Ophthalmol 221:249, 1984.

27. Melamed, S, Epstein, DL: Alterations of aqueous humour outflow following argon laser trabeculoplasty in monkeys. Br J Ophthalmol 71:776, 1987.

28. Van der Zypen, E, Fankhauser, F, England, C, Kwasniewska, S: Morphology of the trabecular meshwork within monkey (Macaca speciosa) eyes after irradiation with the free-running Nd:YAG laser. Ophthalmology 94:171, 1987.

29. Kee, C, Pickett, JP, Dueker, DK, Kaufman, PL: Argon laser trabeculoplasty and pilocarpine effects on outflow facility in the cynomolgus monkey. J Glau 4:334, 1995.

30. Van Buskirk, EM, Pond, V, Rosenquist, RC, Acott, TS: Argon laser trabeculoplasty. Studies of mechanism of action. Ophthalmology 91:1005, 1984.

31. Kimpel, MW, Johnson, DH: Factors influencing in vivo trabecular cell replication as determined by ^{3}H-thymidine labelling; an autoradiographic study in cats. Curr Eye Res 11:297, 1992.

32. Bylsma, SS, Samples, JR, Acott, TS, et al: DNA replication in the cat trabecular meshwork after laser trabeculoplasty in vivo. J Glau 3:36, 1994.

33. Bylsma, SS, Samples, JR, Acott, TS, Van Buskirk, EM: Trabecular cell division after argon laser trabeculoplasty. Arch Ophthalmol 106:544, 1988.

34. Acott, TS, Samples, JR, Bradley, JMB, et al: Trabecular repopulation by anterior trabecular meshwork cells after laser trabeculoplasty. Am J Ophthalmol 107:1, 1989.

35. Van Buskirk, EM: Pathophysiology of laser trabeculoplasty. Surv Ophthalmol 33:264, 1989.

36. Smith, J: Argon laser trabeculoplasty: Comparison of bichromatic and monochromatic wavelengths. Ophthalmology 91:355, 1984.

37. Makabe, R: Comparison of krypton and argon laser trabeculoplasty. Klin Monatsbl Augenheilkd 189:118, 1986.

38. Dieckert, JP, Mainster, MA, Ho, PC: Contact lenses for laser applications. Ophthalmology Instru Book Suppl 55, 1983.

39. Ritch, R: A new lens for argon laser trabeculoplasty. Ophthalmic Surg 16:331, 1985.

40. Wise, JB: Errors in laser spot size in laser trabeculoplasty. Ophthalmology 91:186, 1984.

41. Blondeau, P, Roberge, JF, Asselin, Y: Long-term results of low power, long duration laser trabeculoplasty. Am J Ophthalmol 104:339, 1987.

42. Rouhiainen, H, Terasvirta, M: The laser power needed for optimum results in argon laser trabeculoplasty. Acta Ophthalmol 64:254, 1986.

43. Thomas, JV, Simmons, RJ, Belcher, CD III: Argon laser trabeculoplasty in the presurgical glaucoma patient. Ophthalmology 89:187, 1982.

44. Weinreb, RN, Ruderman, J, Juster, R, Zweig, K: Immediate intraocular pressure response to argon laser trabeculoplasty. Am J Ophthalmol 95:279, 1983.

45. Hoskins, HD Jr, Hetherington, J Jr, Minckler, DS, et al: Complications of laser trabeculoplasty. Ophthalmology 90:796, 1983.

46. Krupin, T, Kolker, AE, Kass, MA, Becker, B: Intraocular pressure the day of argon laser trabeculoplsty in primary open-angle glaucoma. Ophthalmology 91:361, 1984.

47. Frucht, J, Bishara, S, Ticho, U: Early intraocular pressure resposne following laser trabeculoplasty. Br J Ophthalmol 69:771, 1985.

48. Glaucoma Laser Trial Research Group: The glaucoma laser trial. 1. Acute effects of argon laser trabeculoplasty on intraocular pressure. Arch Ophthalmol 107:1135, 1989.

49. Mittra, RA, Allingham, RR, Shields, MB: Follow-up of argon laser trabeculoplasty: is a day-one postoperative IOP check necessary? Ophthalmic Surg Lasers 26:410, 1995.

50. Fiore, PM, Melamed, S, Epstein, DL: Trabecular precipitates and elevated intraocular pressure following argon laser trabeculoplasty. Ophthalmic Surg 20:697, 1989.

51. Greenidge, KC, Rodrigues, MM, Spaeth, GL, et al: Acute intraocular pressure elevation after argon laser trabeculoplasty and iridectomy: a clinicopathologic study. Ophthalmic Surg 15:105, 1984.

52. Koss, MC, March, WF, Nordquist, RE, Gherezghiher, T: Acute intraocular pressure elevation produced by argon laser trabeculoplasty in the cynomolgus monkey. Arch Ophthalmol 102:1699, 1984.

53. Mermoud, A, Pittet, N, Herbort, CP: Inflammation patterns after laser trabeculoplasty measured with the laser flare meter. Arch Ophthalmol 110:368, 1992.

54. Herbort, CP, Mermoud, A, Schnyder, C, Pittet, N: Anti-inflammatory effect of diclofenac drops after argon laser trabeculoplasty. Arch Ophthalmol 111:481, 1993.

55. Rouhiainen, HJ, Teräsvirta, ME, Tuovinen, EJ: Peripheral anterior synechiae formation after trabeculoplasty. Arch Ophthalmol 106:189, 1988.

56. Hong, C, Kitazawa, Y, Tanishima, T: Influence of argon laser treatment of glaucoma on corneal endothelium. Jpn J Ophthalmol 27:567, 1983.

57. Traverso, C, Cohen, EJ, Groden, LR, et al: Central corneal endothelial cell density after argon laser trabeculoplasty. Arch Ophthalmol 102:1322, 1984.

58. Schoenlebe, DB, Bellows, AR, Hutchinson, BT: Failed laser trabeculoplasty requiring surgery in open-angle glaucoma. Ophthalmic Surg 18:796, 1987.

59. Wilensky, JT, Weinreb, RN: Low-dose trabeculoplasty. Am J Ophthalmol 95:423, 1983.

60. Schwartz, LW, Spaeth, GL, Traverso, C, Greenidge, KC: Variation of techniques on the results of argon laser trabeculoplasty. Ophthalmology 90:781, 1983.

61. Weinreb, RN, Ruderman, J, Juster, R, Wilensky, JT: Influence of the number of laser burns administered on the early results of argon laser trabeculoplasty. Am J Ophthalmol 95:287, 1983.

62. Lustgarten, J, Podos, SM, Ritch, R, et al: Laser trabeculoplasty. A prospective study of treatment variables. Arch Ophthalmol 102:517, 1984.

63. Grayson, DK, Ritch, R, Camras, C, et al: Influence of treatment protocol on the long-term efficacy of argon laser trabeculoplasty. J Glau 2:7, 1993.

64. Heijl, A: One- and two-session laser trabeculoplasty. A randomized, prospective study. Acta Ophthalmol 62:715, 1984.

65. Klein, HZ, Shields, MB, Earnest, JT: Two-stage argon laser trabeculoplasty in open-angle glaucoma. Am J Ophthalmol 99:392, 1985.

66. Kitazawa, Y, Yamamoto, T, Shirato, S, Eguchi, S: Argon laser trabeculoplasty: Methods and results. Klin Monatsbl Augenheilkd 184:274, 1984.

67. Elsas, T, Johnsen, H, Brevik, TA: The immediate pressure response to primary laser trabeculoplasty—a comparison of one- and two-stage treatment. Acta Ophthalmol 67:664, 1989.

68. Grayson, D, Chi, T, Liebmann, J, Ritch, R: Initial argon laser trabeculoplasty to the inferior vs. superior half of trabecular meshwork. Arch Ophthalmol 112:446, 1994.

69. Traverso, CE, Greenidge, KC, Spaeth, GL: Formation of peripheral anterior synechiae following argon laser trabeculoplasty. A prospective study to determine relationship to position of laser burns. Arch Ophthalmol 102:861, 1984.

70. Spurny, RC, Lederer, CM Jr: Krypton laser trabeculoplasty. A clinical report. Arch Ophthalmol 102:1626, 1984.

71. Kwasniewska, S, Fankhauser, F, Larsen, SE, Cruz-Orive, LM: The efficacy of cw Nd:YAG laser trabeculoplasty. Ophthalmic Surg 24:304, 1993.

72. McMillan, TA, Stewart, WC, Legler, UFC, et al: Comparison of diode and argon laser trabeculoplasty in cadaver eyes. Invest Ophthalmol Vis Sci 35:706, 1994.

73. McHugh, D, Marshall, J, Ffytche, TJ, et al: Ultrastructural changes of human trabecular meshwork after photocoagulation with a diode laser. Invest Ophthalmol Vis Sci 33:2664, 1992.

74. McHugh, D, Marshall, J, Ffytche, TJ, et al: Diode laser trabeculoplasty (DLT) for primary open-angle glaucoma and ocular hypertension. Br J Ophthalmol 74:743, 1990.

75. Moriarty, AP, McHugh, JDA, Ffytche, TJ, et al: Long-term follow-up of diode laser trabeculoplasty for primary open-angle glaucoma and ocular hypertension. Ophthalmology 100:1614, 1993.

76. Moriarty, AP, McHugh, JDA, Spalton, DJ, et al: Comparison of the anterior chamber inflammatory response to diode and argon laser trabeculoplasty using a laser flare meter. Ophthalmology 100:1263, 1993.

77. Brancato, R, Carassa, R, Trabucchi, G: Diode laser compared with argon laser for trabeculoplasty. Am J Ophthalmol 112:50, 1991.

78. Ofner, S, Samples, JR, Van Buskirk, EM: Pilocarpine and the increase in intraocular pressure after trabeculoplasty. Am J Ophthalmol 97:647, 1984.

79. Robin, AL, Pollack, IP, House, B, Enger, C: Effects of ALO 2145 on intraocular pressure following argon laser trabeculoplasty. Arch Ophthalmol 105:646, 1987.

80. Robin, AL: Argon laser trabeculoplasty medical therapy to prevent the intraocular pressure rise associated with argon laser trabeculoplasty. Ophthalmic Surg 22:31, 1991.

81. Dapling, RB, Cunliffe, IA, Longstaff, S: Influence of apraclonidine and pilocarpine alone and in combination on post laser trabeculoplasty pressure rise. Br J Ophthalmol 78:30, 1994.

82. Birt, CM, Shin, DH, Reed, SY, et al: One vs. two doses of 1.0% apraclonidine for prophylaxis of intraocular pressure spike after argon laser trabeculoplasty. Can J Ophthalmol 30:266, 1995.

83. Holmwood, PC, Chase, RD, Krupin, T, et al: Apraclonidine and argon laser trabeculoplasty. Am J Ophthalmol 114:19, 1992.

84. Rosenberg, LF, Krupin, T, Ruderman, J, et al: Apraclonidine and anterior segment laser surgery. Comparison of 0.5% versus 1.0% apraclonidine for prevention of postoperative intraocular pressure rise. Ophthalmology 102:1312, 1995.

85. Allf, BE, Shields, MB: Early intraocular pressure response to laser trabeculoplasty 180° without apraclonidine versus 360° with apraclonidine. Ophthalmic Surg 22:539, 1991.

86. David, R, Spaeth, GL, Clevenger, CE, et al: Brimonidine in the prevention of intraocular pressure elevation following argon laser trabeculoplasty. Arch Ophthalmol 111:1387, 1993.

87. The Brimonidine-ALT Study Group: Effect of brimonidine 0.5% on intraocular pressure spikes following 360° argon laser trabeculoplasty. Ophthalmic Surg Lasers 26:404, 1995.

88. Metcalfe, TW, Etchells, DE: Prevention of the immediate intraocular pressure rise following argon laser trabeculoplasty. Br J Ophthalmol 73:612, 1989.

89. Ruderman, JM, Zweig, KO, Wilensky, JT, Weinreb, RN: Effects of corticosteroid pretreatment on argon laser trabeculoplasty. Am J Ophthalmol 96:84, 1983.

90. Pappas, HR, Berry, DP, Partamian, L, et al: Topical indomethacin therapy before argon laser trabeculoplasty. Am J Ophthalmol 99:571, 1985.

91. Gelfand, YA, Wolpert, W: Effects of topical indomethacin pretreatment on argon laser trabeculoplasty: A randomised, double-masked study on black South Africans. Br J Ophthalmol 69:668, 1985.

92. Tuulonen, A: The effect of topical indomethacin on acute pressure elevation of laser trabeculoplasty in capsular glaucoma. Acta Ophthalmol 63:245, 1985.

93. Weinreb, RN, Robin, AL, Baerveldt, G, et al: Flurbiprofen pretreatment in argon laser trabeculoplasty for primary open-angle glaucoma. Arch Ophthalmol 102:1629, 1984.

94. Hotchkiss, ML, Robin, AL, Pollack, IP, Quigley, HA: Nonsteroidal anti-inflammatory agents after argon laser trabeculoplasty. A trial with flurbiprofen and indomethacin. Ophthalmology 91:969, 1984.

95. Forbes, M, Bansal, RK: Argon laser goniophotocoagulation of the trabecular meshwork in open-angle glaucoma. Trans Am Ophthalmol Soc 76:257, 1981.

96. Pollack, IP, Robin, AL, Sax, H: The effect of argon laser trabeculoplasty on the medical control of primary open-angle glaucoma. Ophthalmology 90:785, 1983.

97. Quaranta, L, Ripandelli, G, Manni, GL, Bucci, MG: Hypotensive effect of pilocarpine after argon laser trabeculoplasty. J Glau 1:233, 1992.

98. Brooks, AMV, Gillies, WE: Do any factors predict a favourable response to laser trabeculoplasty? Aus J Ophthal 12:149, 1984.

99. Tuulonen, AN, Airaksinen, J, Kuulasmaa, K: Factors influencing the outcome of laser trabeculoplasty. Am J Ophthalmol 99:388, 1985.

100. Strasser, G, Stelzer, R: Laser trabeculoplasty in low-tension glaucoma. Klin Monatsbl Augenheilkd 183:507, 1983.

101. Schwartz, AL, Perman, KI, Whitten, M: Argon laser trabeculoplasty in progressive low-tension glaucoma. Ann Ophthalmol 16:560, 1984.

102. Sharpe, ED, Simmons, RJ: Argon laser trabeculoplasty as a means of decreasing intraocular pressure from "normal" levels in glaucomatous eyes. Am J Ophthalmol 99:704, 1985.

103. Robin, AL, Pollack IP: Argon laser trabeculoplasty in secondary forms of open-angle glaucoma. Arch Ophthalmol 101:382, 1983.

104. Lieberman, MF, Hoskins, HD Jr, Hetherington, J Jr: Laser trabeculoplasty and the glaucomas. Ophthalmology 90:790, 1983.

105. Lunde, MW: Argon laser trabeculoplasty in pigmentary dispersion syndrome with glaucoma. Am J Ophthalmol 96:721, 1983.

106. Ritch, R, Liebmann, J, Robin, A, et al: Argon laser trabeculoplasty in pigmentary glaucoma. Ophthalmology 100:909, 1993.

107. Rouhiaine, HJ, Teräsvirta, ME, Tuovinen, EJ: The effect of some treatment variables on the results of trabeculoplasty. Arch Ophthalmol 106:611, 1988.

108. Dreyer, EB, Gorla, M: Laser trabeculoplasty in the pseudophakic patient. J Glau 2:313, 1993.

109. Fellman, RL, Starita, RJ, Spaeth, GL, Poryzees, EM: Argon laser trabeculoplasty following failed trabeculectomy. Ophthalmic Surg 15:195, 1984.

110. Wilensky, JT, Weinreb, RN: Early and late failures of argon laser trabecuolplasty. Arch Ophthalmol 101:895, 1983.

111. Safran, MJ, Robin, AL, Pollack, IP: Argon laser trabeculoplasty in younger patients with primary open-angle glaucoma. Am J Ophthalmol 97:292, 1984.

112. Krupin, T, Patkin, R, Kurata, FK, et al: Argon laser trabeculoplasty in black and white patients with primary open-angle glaucoma. Ophthalmology 93:811, 1986.

113. Grinich, NP, Van Buskirk, EM, Samples, JR: Three-year efficacy of argon laser trabeculoplasty. Ophthalmology 94:858, 1987.

114. Schwartz, AL, Kopelman, J: Four-year experience with argon laser trabecular surgery in uncontrolled open-angle glaucoma. Ophthalmology 90:771, 1983.

115. Tuulonen, A, Niva, A-K, Alanko, HI: A controlled five-year follow-up study of laser trabeculoplasty as primary therapy for open-angle glaucoma. Am J Ophthalmol 104:334, 1987.

116. Shingleton, BJ, Richter, CU, Bellows, AR, et al: Long-term efficacy of argon laser trabeculoplasty. Ophthalmology 94:1513, 1987.

117. Ticho, U, Nesher, R: Laser trabeculoplasty in glaucoma. Ten-year evaluation. Arch Ophthalmol 107:844, 1989.

118. Spaeth, GL, Baez, KA: Argon laser trabeculoplasty controls one-third of cases of progressive, uncontrolled, open angle glaucoma for 5 years. Arch Ophthalmol 110:491, 1992.

119. Spiegel, D, Wegscheider, E, Lung, O-E: Argon laser trabeculoplasty: long-term follow-up of at least 5 years. Ger J Ophthalmol 1:156, 1992.

120. Shingleton, BJ, Richter, CU, Dharma, SK, et al: Long-term efficacy of argon laser trabeculoplasty. A 10-year follow-up study. Ophthalmology 100:1324, 1993.

121. Starita, RJ, Fellman, RL, Spaeth, GL, Poryzees, E: The effect of repeating full-circumference argon laser trabeculoplasty. Ophthalmic Surg 15:41, 1984.

122. Brown, SVL, Thomas, JV, Simmons, RJ: Laser trabeculoplasty retreatment. Am J Ophthalmol 99:8, 1985.

123. Richter, CU, Shingleton, BJ, Bellows, AR, et al: Retreatment with argon laser trabeculoplasty. Ophthalmology 94:1085, 1987.

124. Messner, D, Siegel, LI, Kass, MA, et al: Repeat argon laser trabeculoplasty. Am J Ophthalmol 103:113, 1987.

125. Grayson, DK, Camras, CB, Podos, SM, Lustgarten, JS: Long-term reduction of intraocular pressure after repeat argon laser trabeculoplasty. Am J Ophthalmol 106:312, 1988.

126. Weber, PA, Burton, GD, Epitropoulos, AT: Laser trabeculoplasty retreatment. Ophthalmic Surg 20:702, 1989.

127. Feldman, RM, Katz, LJ, Spaeth, GL, et al: Long-term efficacy of repeat argon laser trabeculoplasty. Ophthalmology 98:1061, 1991.

128. Sherwood, MB, Lattimer, J, Hitchings, RA: Laser trabeculoplasty as supplementary treatment for primary open angle glaucoma. Br J Ophthalmol 71:188, 1987.

129. Thomas, JV, El-Mofty, A, Hamdy, EE, Simmons, RJ: Argon laser trabeculoplasty as initial therapy for glaucoma. Arch Ophthalmol 102:702, 1984.

130. Rosenthal, AR, Chaudhuri, PR, Chiapella, AP: Laser trabeculoplasty primary therapy in open-angle glaucoma. A preliminary report. Arch Ophthalmol 102:699, 1984.

131. Migdal, C, Hitchings, R: Primary therapy for chronic simple glaucoma. The role of argon laser trabeculoplasty. Trans Ophthalmol Soc UK 104:62, 1984.

132. Tuulonen, A, Koponen, J, Alanko, HI, Airaksinen, PJ: Laser trabeculoplasty versus medication treatment as primary therapy for glaucoma. Acta Ophthalmol 67:275, 1989.

133. Odberg, T: Primary argon laser trabeculoplasty after pretreatment with timolol. A safe and economic therapy of early glaucoma. Acta Ophthalmol 68:317, 1990.

134. Elsås, T, Johnsen, H: Long-term efficacy of primary laser trabeculoplasty. Br J Ophthalmol 75:34, 1991.

135. The Glaucoma Laser Trial Research Group. The glaucoma laser trial (GLT). 2. Results of argon laser trabeculoplasty versus topical medicines. Ophthalmology 97:1403, 1990.

136. Glaucoma Laser Trial Research Group: The glaucoma laser trial (GLT) and glaucoma laser trial follow-up study: 7. Results. Am J Ophthalmol 120:718, 1995.

137. Schwartz, AL: Argon laser trabeculoplasty in glaucoma: what's happening (survey of results of American Glaucoma Society members). J Glau 2:329, 1993.

138. Burian, HM: A case of Marfan's syndrome with bilateral glaucoma. With description of a new type of operation for developmental glaucoma (trabeculotomy ab externo). Am J Ophthalmol 50:1187, 1960.

139. Smith, R: A new technique for opening the canal of Schlemm. Preliminary report. Br J Ophthalmol 44:370, 1960.

140. Harms, H, Dannheim, R: Trabeculotomy results and problems. In: MacKensen, C, ed. Microsurgery in Glaucoma. Karger, Gasel, 1970, p. 121.

141. McPherson, SD Jr: Results of external trabeculotomy. Am J Ophthalmol 76:918, 1973.

142. Allen, L, Burian, HM: Trabeculotomy ab externo. Am J Ophthalmol 53:19, 1962.

143. Beck, AD, Lynch, MG: 360% trabeculotomy for primary congenital glaucoma. Arch Ophthalmol 113:1200, 1995.

144. Board, RJ, Shields, MB: Combined trabecultomy-trabeculectomy for the management of glaucoma associated with Sturge-Weber syndrome. Ophthalmic Surg 12:813, 1981.

145. Rothkoff, L, Blumenthal, M, Biedner, B: Trabeculotomy in late onset congenital glaucoma. Br J Ophthalmol 63:38, 1979.

146. Elder, MJ: Combined trabeculotomy-trabeculectomy compared with primary trabeculectomy for congenital glaucoma. Br J Ophthalmol 78:745, 1994.

147. Moses, RA: Electrocautery puncture of the trabecular meshwork in enucleated human eyes. Am J Ophthalmol 72:1094, 1971.

148. Maselli, E, Sirellini, M, Pruneri, F, Galantino, G: Diathermotrabeculotomy ab externo. A new technique for opening the canal of Schlemm. Br J Ophthalmol 59:516, 1975.

149. Maselli, E, Galantino, G, Pruneri, F, Sirellini, M: Diathermotrabeculotomy ab externo: indications and long-term results. Br J Ophthalmol 61:675, 1977.

150. Hager, H, Hauck, W, Heppke, G, Hoffmann, F, Resewitz, E-P: Experimental principles of trabecular-electro-puncture (TEP). Graefes Arch Clin Exp Ophthalmol 185:95, 1972.

151. Bonnet, M, Schiffer, H-P: On trabeculotomy ab externo. Localisation of the canal of Schlemm by passing a catheter through an aqueous vein. Klin Monatsbl Augenheilkd 161:563, 1972.

152. Jocson, VL: Air trabeculotomy. Am J Ophthalmol 79:107, 1975.

153. Skjaerpe, F: Selective trabeculectomy. A report of a new surgical method for open angle glaucoma. Acta Ophthalmol 61:714, 1983.

154. Gaasterland, DE, Bonney, CH III, Rodrigues, MM, Kuwabara, T: Long-term effects of Q-switched ruby laser on monkey anterior chamber angle. Invest Ophthalmol Vis Sci 26:129, 1985.

155. Van der Zypen, E, Fankhauser, F: The ultrastructural features of laser trabeculopuncture and cyclodialysis. Ophthalmologica 179:189, 1979.

156. Melamed, S, Pei, J, Puliafito, CA, Epstein, DL: Q-switched neodymium-YAG laser trabeculopuncture in monkeys. Arch Ophthalmol 103:129, 1985.

157. Dutton, GN, Cameron, SA, Allan, D, Thomas, R: Parameters for neodymium-YAG laser trabeculotomy: an in-vitro study. Br J Ophthalmol 71:782, 1987.

158. Dutton, GN, Allan, D, Cameron, SA: Pulsed neodymium-YAG laser trabeculotomy: energy requirements and replicability. Br J Ophthalmol 73:177, 1989.

159. Venkatesh, S, Lee, WR, Guthrie, S, et al: An in-vitro morphological study of Q-switched neodymium:YAG laser trabeculotomy. Br J Ophthalmol 70:89, 1986.

160. Lee, WR, Dutton, GN, Cameron, SA: Short-pulsed neodymium:YAG laser trabeculotomy. An in vivo morphological study in the human eye. Invest Ophthalmol Vis Sci 29:1698, 1988.

161. Melamed, S, Latina, MA, Epstein, DL: Neodymium:YAG laser trabeculopuncture in juvenile open-angle glaucoma. Ophthalmology 94:163, 1987.

162. Del Priore, LV, Robin, AL, Pollack, IP: Long-term follow-up of neodymium:YAG laser angle surgery for open-angle glaucoma. Ophthalmology 95:277, 1988.

163. Fukuchi, T, Iwata, K, Sawaguchi, S, et al: Nd:YAG laser trabeculopuncture (YLT) for glaucoma with traumatic angle recession. Graefes Arch Clin Exp Ophthalmol 231:571, 1993.

164. Melamed, S, Ashkenazi, I, Gutman, I, Blumenthal, M: Nd:YAG laser trabeculopuncture in angle-recession glaucoma. Ophthalmic Surg 23:31, 1992.

165. Barkan, O: Technic of goniotomy. Arch Ophthalmol 19:217, 1938.

166. Draeger, J: New microsurgical techniques to improve chamber angle surgery. Glaucoma 2:403, 1980.

167. Amoils, SP, Simmons, RJ: Goniotomy with intraocular illumination. A preliminary report. Arch Ophthalmol 80:488, 1968.

168. Hodapp, E, Heuer, DK: A simple technique for goniotomy. Am J Ophthalmol 102:537, 1986.

169. Joos, KM, Alward, WLM, Folberg, R: Experimental endoscopic goniotomy. A potential treatment for primary infantile glaucoma. Ophthalmology 100:1066, 1993.

170. Catalano, RA, King, RA, Calhoun, JH, Sargent, RA: One versus two simultaneous goniotomies as the initial surgical procedure for primary infantile glaucoma. J Pediatr Ophthalmol Strabismus 26:9, 1989.

171. Litinsky, SM, Shaffer, RN, Hetherington, J, Hoskins, HD: Operative complications of goniotomy. Trans Am Acad Ophthalmol Otol 83:78, 1977.

172. Biglan, AW, Hiles, DA: The visual results following infantile glaucoma surgery. J Pediatr Ophthalmol Strabismus 16:377, 1979.

173. Scheie, HG: Goniopuncture—a new filtering operation for glaucoma. Arch Ophthalmol 44:761, 1950.

174. Scheie, HG: Goniopuncture: an evaluation after eleven years. Arch Ophthalmol 65:38, 1961.

175. Kozart, DM, Cameron, JD: Goniodiathermy: experimental studies on ab interno filtration. Ann Ophthalmol 10:1597, 1978.

176. Fernandez, JL, Galin, MA: Technique of direct goniotomy. Arch Ophthalmol 90:305, 1973.

177. Haas, J: Goniotomy in aphakia. In: Welsh, R, ed. The second report on cataract surgery. Miami, Miami Educational Press, 1971, p. 551.

178. Hoskins, HD, Hetherington, J Jr, Shaffer, RN: Surgical management of the inflammatory glaucomas. Perspect Ophthalmol 1:173, 1977.

179. Herschler, J, Davis, B: Modified goniotomy for inflammatory glaucoma. Histologic evidence for the mechanism of pressure reduction. Arch Ophthalmol 98:684, 1980.

180. Kanski, JJ, McAllister, JA: Trabeculodialysis for inflammatory glaucoma in children and young adults. Ophthalmology 92:927, 1985.

181. Williams, RD, Hoskins, HD, Shaffer, RN: Trabeculodialysis for inflammatory glaucoma: a review of 25 cases. Ophthalmic Surg 23:36, 1992.

182. Yumita, A, Shirato, S, Yamamoto, T, Kitazawa, Y: Goniotomy with Q-switched ND-YAG laser in juvenile developmental glaucoma: a preliminary report. Jpn J Ophthalmol 28:349, 1984.

183. Senft, SH, Tomey, KF, Traverso, CE: Neodymium-YAG laser goniotomy vs. surgical goniotomy. A preliminary study in paired eyes. Arch Ophthalmol 107:1773, 1989.

184. Promesberger, H, Busse, H, Mewe, L: Findings and surgical therapy in congenital glaucoma. Klin Monatsbl Augenheilkd 176:186, 1980.

185. Broughton, WL, Parks, MM: An analysis of treatment of congenital glaucoma by goniotomy. Am J Ophthalmol 91:566, 1981.

186. Draeger, J, Wirt, H, Von Domarus, D: Long-term results after goniotomy. Klin Monatsbl Augenheilkd 180:264, 1982.

187. Francois, J, Van Oye, R, Mendoza, A, De Sutter, E: Goniotomy for congenital glaucoma. J Fr Ophthalmol 5:661, 1982.

188. McPherson, SD Jr, McFarland, D: External trabeculotomy for developmental glaucoma. Ophthalmology 87:302, 1980.

189. Luntz, MH, Livingston, DG: Trabeculotomy ab externo and trabeculectomy in congenital and adult-onset glaucoma. Am J Ophthalmol 83:174, 1977.

190. Gregersen, E, Kessing, SVV: Congenital glaucoma before and after the introduction of microsurgery. Results of "macrosurgery" 1943–1963 and of microsurgery (trabeculotomy/ectomy) 1970–1974. Acta Ophthalmol 55:422, 1977.

191. Luntz, MH: Congenital, infantile, and juvenile glaucoma. Ophthalmology 86:793, 1979.

192. Dannheim, R, Haas, H: Visual acuity and intraocular pressure after surgery in congenital glaucoma. Klin Monatsbl Augenheilkd 177:296, 1980.

193. Quigley, HA: Childhood glaucoma. Results with trabeculotomy and study of reversible cupping. Ophthalmology 89:219, 1982.

194. McPherson, SD Jr, Berry, DP: Goniotomy vs. external trabeculotomy for developmental glaucoma. Am J Ophthalmol 95:427, 1983.

195. Hoskins, HD Jr, Shaffer, RN, Hetherington, J: Goniotomy vs. trabeculotomy. J Pediatr Ophthalmol Strabismus 21:153, 1984.

196. Luntz, MH: The advantages of trabeculotomy over goniotomy. J Pediatr Ophthalmol Strabismus 2:150, 1984.

197. Anderson, DR: Trabeculotomy compared to goniotomy for glaucoma in children. Ophthalmology 90:805, 1983.

198. Kjer, B, Kessing, SV: Trabeculotomy in juvenile primary open-angle glaucoma. Ophthalmic Surg 24:663, 1993.

199. Tanihara, H, Negi, A, Akimoto, M, et al: Surgical effects of trabeculotomy ab externo on adult eyes with primary open angle glaucoma and pseudoexfoliation syndrome. Arch Ophthalmol 111:1653, 1993.

200. Chihara, E, Nishida, A, Kodo, M, et al: Trabeculotomy ab externo: an alternative treatment in adult patients with primary open-angle glaucoma. Ophthalmic Surg 24:735, 1993.

201. Heine, L: Die Cyklodialyse, eine neue Glaucomoperation. Deutsche Med Wehnschr 31:825, 1905.

202. Barkan, O: Cyclodialysis: Its mode of action. Histologic observations in a case of glaucoma in which both eyes were successfully treated by cyclodialysis. Arch Ophthalmol 43:793, 1950.

203. Bill, A: The routes for bulk drainage of aqueous humour in rabbits with and without cyclodialysis. Doc Ophthalmol 20:157, 1966.

204. Pederson, JE, Gaasterland, DE, MacLellan, HM: Experimental ciliochoroidal detachment. Effect on intraocular pressure and aqueous humor flow. Arch Ophthalmol 97:536, 1979.

205. Suguro, K, Toris, CB, Pederson, JE: Uveoscleral outflow following cyclodialysis in the monkey eye using a fluorescent tracer. Invest Ophthalmol Vis Sci 26:810, 1985.

206. Toris, CB, Pederson, JE: Effect of intraocular pressure on uveoscleral outflow following cyclodialysis in the monkey eye. Invest Ophthalmol Vis Sci 26:1745, 1985.

207. Auricchio, G: Considerations on mechanism of action of cyclodialysis. Boll Ocul 35:401, 1956.

208. Chandler, PA, Maumenee, AE: A major cause of hypotony. Trans Am Acad Ophthalmol Otol 52:563, 1961.

209. Gills, JP Jr, Paterson, CA, Paterson, ME: Action of cyclodialysis utilizing an implant studied by manometry in a human eye. Exp Eye Res 6:75, 1967.

210. Ascher, KW: Some details of the technique of cyclodialysis. Am J Ophthalmol 50:1207, 1960.

211. O'Brien, CS, Weih, J: Cyclodialysis. Arch Ophthalmol 42:606, 1949.

212. Haisten, MW, Guyton, JS: Cyclodialysis with air injection: Technique and results in ninety-four consecutive operations. Arch Ophthalmol 590:507, 1958.

213. Miller, RD, Nisbet, RM: Cyclodialysis with air injection in black patients. Ophthalmic Surg 12:92, 1981.

214. Alpar, JJ: Sodium hyaluronate (Healon) in cyclodialysis. CLAO J 11:201, 1985.

215. Simmons, RJ, Kimbrough, RL: A modified cyclodialysis spatula. Ophthalmic Surg 10:67, 1979.

216. Cohen, SW, Banko, W, Nath, S: A fiber-optics cyclodialysis spatula. Ophthalmic Surg 10:74, 1979.

217. Gills, JP: Cyclodialysis implants in human eyes. Am J Ophthalmol 61:841, 1966.

218. Streeten, BW, Belkowitz, M: Experimental hypotony with silastic. Arch Ophthalmol 78:503, 1967.

219. Richards, RD: Long-term results of gonioplasty. Am J Ophthalmol 70:715, 1970.

220. Portney, GL: Silicone elastomer implantation cyclodialysis. A negative report. Arch Ophthalmol 89:10, 1973.

221. Krasnov, MM: Iridocyclo-retraction in narrow-angle glaucoma. Br J Ophthalmol 55:389, 1971.

222. Aviner, Z: Modified Krasnov's iridocycloretraction for aphakic glaucoma. Ann Ophthalmol 7:859, 1975.

223. Sugar, HS: Experiences with some modifications of cyclodialysis for aphakic glaucoma. Ann Ophthalmol 9:1045, 1977.

224. Nesterov, AP, Kolesnikova, LN: Filtering iridocycloretraction in chronic closed-angle glaucoma. Am J Ophthalmol 99:340, 1985.

225. Mizukawa, A: Histopathological study on argon laser cyclodialysis of cynomolgus monkey eyes. Folia Ophthalmol Jpn 35:526, 1984.

226. Mizukawa, A, Okisaka, S, Taketani, P: Argon laser cyclodialysis for open angle glaucoma. Folia Ophthalmol Jpn 36:750, 1985.

227. Partamian, LG: Treatment of a cyclodialysis cleft with argon laser photocoagulation in a patient with a shallow anterior chamber. Am J Ophthalmol 99:5, 1985.

228. Ormerod, LD, Baerveldt, G, Sunalp, MA, Riekhof, FT: Management of the hypotonous cyclodialysis cleft. Ophthalmology 98:1384, 1991.

229. Best, W, Hartwig, H: Traumatic cyclodialysis and its treatment. Klin Monatsbl Augenheilkd 170:917, 1977.

230. Tate, GW Jr, Lynn, JR: A new technique for the surgical repair of cyclodialysis induced hypotony. Ann Ophthalmol 10:1261, 1978.

231. Campbell, DG, Vela, A: Modern goniosynechialysis for the treatment of synechial angle-closure glaucoma. Ophthalmology 91:1052, 1984.

232. Weiss, JS, Waring, GO, III: Dental mirror for goniosynechialysis during penetrating keratoplasty. Am J Ophthalmol 100:331, 1985.

233. Shingleton, BJ, Chang, MA, Bellows, AR, Thomas, JV: Surgical goniosynechialysis for angle-closure glaucoma. Ophthalmology 97:551, 1990.

234. Tanihara, H, Nishiwaki, K, Nagata, M: Surgical results and complications of goniosynechialysis. Graefes Arch Clin Exp Ophthalmol 230:309, 1992.

235. Senn, P, Kopp, B: Nd:YAG laser goniosynechiolysis in angle-closure glaucoma. Klin Monatsbl Augenheilkd 196:210, 1990.

236. Simmons, RJ, Dueker, DK, Kimbrough, RL, Aiello, LM: Goniophotocoagulation for neovascular glaucoma. Trans Am Acad Ophthalmol Otol 83:80, 1977.

237. Simmons, RJ, Deppermann, SR, Dueker, DK: The role of goniophotocoagulation in neovascularization of the anterior chamber angle. Ophthalmology 87:79, 1980.

238. Jacobi, PC, Krieglstein, GK: Trabecular aspiration: clinical results of a new surgical approach to improve trabecular facility in glaucoma capsulare. Ophthalmic Surg 25:641, 1994.

239. Jacobi, PC, Krieglstein, GK: Trabecular aspiration. A new mode to treat pseudoexfoliation glaucoma. Invest Ophthalmol Vis Sci 36:2270, 1995.

SURGERY OF THE IRIS

LASER IRIDOTOMY[a]

Historical Background

In 1956, Meyer-Schwickerath (1) first reported the use of light energy to create a hole in the iris. Using the xenon-arc photocoagulator, he and others found that a peripheral iridotomy could be produced, but that the amount of heat required damaged the cornea and lens (1, 2). With the introduction of lasers in the 1960s, investigation of this treatment modality continued, primarily with ruby lasers (3–7). However, as with laser trabeculoplasty, it was not until the advent of argon laser technology in the 1970s that laser iridotomy became clinically practical. By the mid-1970s, several reports of successful argon laser iridotomy appeared in the literature (8–11), and by the end of that decade, laser iridotomy had replaced incisional iridectomy as the surgical procedure of choice for angle-closure glaucomas. During the 1980s, continued study of laser iridotomy techniques led to the popular use of the neodymium:YAG (Nd:YAG) laser for this operation.

[a]Refer to M.B. Shields: Color Atlas of Glaucoma. Baltimore: Williams & Wilkins, 1998, Plates III11–12.

Techniques

Instrumentation

Several different types of *lasers* and surgical techniques can be used to create an iridotomy. The unit most commonly used in the early days of laser surgery was the continuous-wave argon laser (8–17). Other lasers were also shown to be effective for creating iridotomies, including the pulsed argon laser (13, 16, 18, 19) and the krypton laser (20). However, the pulsed Nd:YAG laser subsequently gained popularity (21–28) and today is the most commonly used unit for creating laser iridotomies. A portable Nd:YAG laser has been shown to be effective for use in remote geographic areas (29). Newer lasers are also being evaluated for performing iridotomies. These units and the relative merits of the argon versus Nd:YAG laser iridotomies are considered later in this chapter.

A *contact lens* is helpful in performing a laser iridotomy, since it (a) keeps the lids separated, (b) minimizes corneal epithelial burns by acting as a heat sink, and (c) provides some control of eye movement. In addition, convex-surfaced contact lenses have been designed to increase the power density on the iris (30–32). The most commonly used is the Abraham iridotomy lens, which has a +66-diopter planoconvex button bonded to the front surface of the contact lens (Fig. 36.1) (30). This lens doubles the laser beam diameter at the level of the cornea, while reducing it to approximately one-half the original size on the iris, which reduces the power density at the cornea to one-fourth the original level and increases it on the iris by a factor of four. Another contact lens, the Wise iridotomy-sphincterotomy lens, has a +103-diopter optical button decentered 2.5 mm, which further reduces the iris focal spot and increases the energy density (32). These principles have their greatest application with the argon laser, although the same contact lenses are also useful with the Nd:YAG laser.

With all lasers and contact lenses, a high magnification, e.g., ×40, should be used in the slitlamp delivery system.

Preoperative Medication

Topical *pilocarpine* should be instilled prior to the procedure to maximally thin and stretch the peripheral iris. If the patient presents with an acute attack of angle-closure glaucoma, it is best to break the attack medically if possible and maintain the patient on medication to allow clearing of any corneal edema and to facilitate constriction of the pupil. If significant iritis persists after breaking the attack, it may be advisable to use topical steroids for 24–48 hours before proceeding with the laser surgery. However, if the attack does not respond to medical therapy, laser iridotomy (or iridoplasty, or pupilloplasty, as discussed later in this chapter) may be effective in breaking the attack (33).

In nearly all cases, only *topical anesthesia,* such as proparacaine 0.5%, is required. Only rarely is a retrobulbar injection needed for a patient with nystagmus or who is uncooperative. It has become a standard practice among most surgeons to also use topical *apraclonidine* to reduce the risk of a postoperative intraocular pressure (IOP) rise. In the original studies, apraclonidine 1% was instilled 45–60 min-

utes before and immediately after the procedure (34, 35), although it has also been shown that a single postoperative drop of apraclonidine 0.5% is as effective as the 1% concentration in preventing IOP elevation (36).

Selecting the Treatment Site

Any quadrant of the iris can be used to create the laser iridotomy, although the superior iris is preferable in most cases, since it places the iridotomy beneath the upper lid. The 12 o'clock position is usually avoided, since gas bubbles may collect in that area, especially with argon laser iridotomy, and interfere with completion of the procedure. The superior-nasal quadrant has the advantage of directing the laser beam toward the nasal periphery of the retina. One exception to the selection of a superior iris quadrant is the patient with silicone oil in an aphakic eye, in which case the iridotomy should be placed inferiorly to avoid blockage by the oil which rises to the top of the eye.

Whichever quadrant is used, the slitlamp should always be positioned so the laser beam is directed away from the macula. The iridotomy is usually placed between the middle and peripheral thirds of the iris. However, if this is not feasible, due to peripheral corneal haze or close proximity between peripheral iris and cornea, a more central location can be used, as long as it is peripheral to the sphincter muscle.

There are several features of the iris that may facilitate creation of the iridotomy. An area of thin iris or a large crypt is usually easier to penetrate. In lightly pigmented eyes, a local area of increased pigmentation, such as a freckle, may improve absorption of argon laser energy. In addition, the radially arranged white collagen strands in the stroma can be very difficult to penetrate, especially with argon laser, and it is helpful to select a treatment site where two strands are more widely separated (Fig. 36.2) (37).

Techniques with Continuous-wave Argon Laser

Several basic techniques have been advocated for producing iridotomies with the continuous-wave argon laser. The "hump" technique involves first creating a localized elevation of the iris with a large diameter, low energy burn, and then penetrating the hump with small, intense burns (38). In the "drumhead" technique, large diameter, low energy burns are placed around the intended treatment site to put the iris on stretch, and that area is then penetrated with small, high energy burns (14, 39). A third, and probably most commonly used, approach goes directly to penetrating burns (13, 16, 17). The latter technique may be modified by using multiple short-duration burns (40, 41). None of these approaches, however, is ideal for all situations, and it is best to tailor the iridotomy technique primarily according to the color of the iris. For irides of any color, the argon laser settings are first selected for the iris stroma and then adjusted for the pigment epithelium.

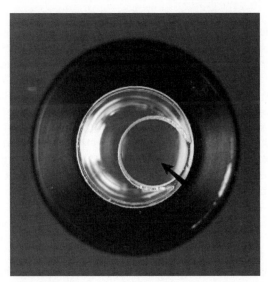

Figure 36.1. **Abraham contact lens with planoconvex button (*arrow*) bonded to front surface for laser iridotomy.**

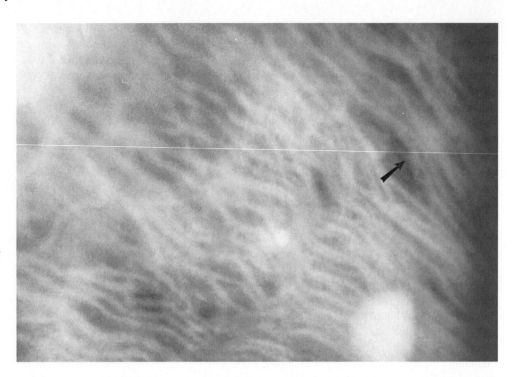

Figure 36.2. Slitlamp view of light blue iris showing white collagen strands which are difficult to penetrate with argon laser energy and should be avoided when possible by selecting an area where they are separated *(arrow).*

MEDIUM BROWN IRIS. This is the easiest iris to penetrate with continuous-wave argon laser, and the following method represents one technique in these patients. Protocols for irides of other color are modifications of this basic technique.

Argon laser settings of 0.1–0.2-second duration, 50-μm spot size, and 700–1500 (average, 1000) mW are initially used to create a crater in the iris stroma. The first few applications may produce gas bubbles, which will usually float up away from the treatment site (Fig. 36.3). If the bubble does not move, it can be dislodged by going through it with the next laser application or by placing the beam adjacent to the bubble. A cluster of several, contiguous burns are used to produce a stromal crater of approximately 500 μm in diameter. Additional laser applications are then placed in the bed of the crater until the pigment epithelial layer is reached, as evidenced by a cloud of pigment (Fig. 36.4).

When most of the stroma in the crater has been eliminated and only pigment epithelium remains, the laser intensity should be reduced to clean away the remaining tissue. Typical settings for this stage of the procedure are 100 μm and 500–700 mW, or 50 μm and 200–600 mW, with a duration of 0.1–0.2 seconds. Higher intensity burns at this stage of the treatment may dislodge adjacent pigment epithelium, creating a so-called "cascade phenomenon," which causes further obstruction of the iridotomy. These same settings can be used for irides of other color, since the pigment epithelial layer is similar in all eyes.

This two-stage technique for argon laser iridotomy in the medium brown iris normally takes 30–60 laser applications to create a patent iridotomy.

DARK BROWN IRIS. A laser iridotomy is more difficult to achieve in these eyes, partially because of the thick, dense stroma. Standard initial settings, as described earlier, often produce a black char in the stromal crater, making the site resistant to further penetration. One way to minimize this complication and achieve a patent iridotomy in the dark brown iris is to use multiple, short-duration burns, called the "chipping" technique (38, 40, 42). The important feature of this modification is the short exposure time of 0.02–0.05 seconds, with standard settings of 50 μm and 700–1500 mW. With this approach, minute fragments of stroma are "chipped away," often requiring 200–300 applications to penetrate the stroma. Once the pigment epithelial layer is reached, the settings should be changed to the lower intensity level, as described for the medium brown iris, to complete the procedure.

BLUE IRIS. These eyes can also be difficult with argon laser iridotomy because the lightly pigmented stroma does not absorb laser light sufficiently to produce a burn through this portion of the iris. The pigment epithelium near the treatment site may be dislodged, leaving intact stroma that is impermeable to aqueous flow. Some surgeons prefer a two-stage approach, in which settings of 500 μm and 200–300 mW are first used to create a local tan-colored area of increased stromal density, followed by penetration burns of 50 μm, 500–700 mW, and 0.1 second to create a full-thickness hole in the stroma (43). Others have suggested a direct approach, using settings of 50 μm, 1000–1500 mW, and a prolonged duration of 0.5 seconds, which will usually burn a hole through the stroma in two to three applications (37, 42). With either technique, the settings should then be changed to those described for the medium brown iris to penetrate or remove the remaining pigment epithelium from the iridotomy site.

Techniques with Neodymium:YAG Laser

As previously noted, this is now the most commonly used technique for laser iridotomy. The extremely high energy levels and short exposure times of these lasers electro-mechanically disrupt tissue, independent of pigment absorption and the thermal effect. As a result, they are particularly useful in creating iridotomies in light blue irides, but are effective in all eyes. The technique usually involves simultaneous perforation of the iris stroma and pigment epithelium with energy levels in the range of 5–15 mJ (21–28). The pulse duration is fixed for each instrument, in the range of 12 nanoseconds, but the number of pulses per burst can be adjusted in most units, with surgeons generally preferring one to three pulses per burst. The spot size is also fixed, although some units provide a choice between a single focal point or multiple focal points, with the latter creating a larger lesion. Since the wavelength of the Nd:YAG laser is beyond the visible spectrum, a helium-neon or diode laser beam is typically used for focusing on the iris. With instruments that allow a selected separation between the focal points of the two laser beams, the setting should be such that they are coincident when performing a laser iridotomy.

The standard technique utilizes the same criteria as for argon laser iridotomy in selecting the iris site, although it is often possible to place the iridotomy more peripherally with the Nd:YAG laser. The latter is desirable, among other reasons, to avoid injuring the lens. When selecting the treatment site, attention should be given to avoiding any apparent iris vessels, since these are more likely to bleed with Nd:YAG than with argon laser surgery. It is often possible to create a patent iridotomy with a single laser application, and rarely are more than two or three required, especially in blue or light brown eyes. However, the iridotomy may be smaller than those produced with an argon laser (Fig. 36.5). Cases have

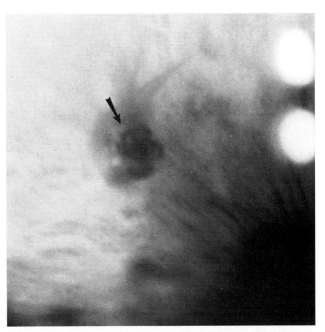

Figure 36.4. Pigment cloud (*arrow*) released from pigment epithelium when it has been perforated during creation of laser iridotomy.

been reported of acute angle closure glaucoma in eyes with patent, but small, Nd:YAG laser iridotomies, and it has been suggested that an iridotomy should be at least 150–200 μm in diameter (44). The iridotomy may change in shape and position and occasionally in area after dilatation (45), and it is good practice to make it large enough initially, but also to check it after dilatation. If there is doubt regarding the size of the iridotomy during the procedure and it is difficult to enlarge it, it is advisable to create more than one iridotomy.

Several variations in technique have been described. One utilizes both the argon and Nd:YAG lasers by first creating a stromal crater with short-duration argon laser burns and then penetrating the iris with low energy, single pulse Nd:YAG applications (46–48). This has an advantage of minimizing bleeding by first coagulating iris vessels. It is especially useful in eyes with thick, dark iris stroma, in which the Nd:YAG laser energy may cause considerable disruption and dispersion of stromal tissue before penetrating the iris. Another technique involves multiple, low energy (1.0–1.7 mJ) applications in a line across the radial iris fibers to create an iridotomy of larger, more controllable size, which was felt to be safer than a similar approach with the argon laser or the standard higher energy Nd:YAG technique (49, 50). Iridotomies have also been created experimentally with the transscleral application of longer duration, thermal Nd:YAG laser burns via a fiber optic system (51).

Techniques with Other Lasers

PULSED ARGON LASER. This instrument emits laser energy in a chain of very short pulses, rather than in a continuous wave, which vaporizes the absorbing tissue with minimal

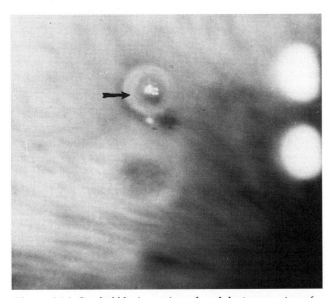

Figure 36.3. Gas bubble (*arrow*) produced during creation of argon laser iridotomy.

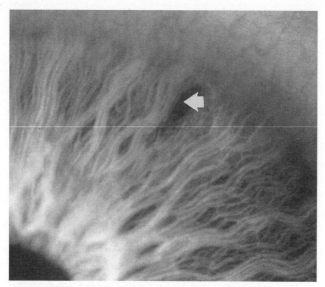

Figure 36.5. Typical appearance of peripheral iridotomy created with a neodymium:YAG laser.

heat loss and destruction to the surrounding area. These features provide some advantage over continuous-wave argon lasers for producing iridotomies in that more energy is used in penetrating the iris, with less distortion and disruption of surrounding tissue (18).

The basic technique is similar to that for continuous-wave argon laser iridotomy, with the straight or chipping method being used in most cases. The settings, however, differ considerably for the pulsed argon laser unit. The perforating mode is employed, and the power setting is 20–25 W. The usual parameters are 50 μm, 0.2 seconds, and 300 pulses/second, adjusted according to tissue response (the individual pulse is fixed at 128 microseconds). With these settings, the number of exposures to achieve an iridotomy varies from 2 to 250, depending on the type of iris (18).

NEODYMIUM:YTTRIUM LITHIUM FLUORIDE (ND:YLF) LASER. This 1053-nm laser can create iridotomies of precise size and shape with minimal thermal damage to surrounding tissue because of low energy per pulse levels, with a short pulse duration in picoseconds, and a high repetition rate. Optimal settings, established in a series of cadaver eyes, included a rectangular cutting pattern of 0.3 × 0.3 mm, 500-μm cutting depth, 50-μm spot separation, 200–400 pulses per second (52). Preliminary clinical experience reveals that iridotomies with well-defined margins and size can be created with minimal complications (52, 53).

SEMICONDUCTOR DIODE LASER. As noted in previous chapters, the semiconductor diode laser has several distinct advantages over other lasers, including the small, portable size, the solid-state construction, which provides durability and relatively low maintenance requirements, and the need for only a standard electric outlet and no water cooling. With a wavelength of approximately 805 nm and operation in the

continuous-wave mode, the mechanism of iridotomy is like that of the argon laser, i.e., absorption by melanin, resulting in photocoagulation, rather than the electromechanical disruption of the Nd:YAG and Nd:YLF lasers. In rabbit studies and preliminary clinical trials, the settings and the clinical and histopathologic results were all similar to those noted in this chapter for the argon laser (54–56).

OTHER LASERS. As noted previously, the krypton laser was found to be effective in creating iridotomies (20). A Q-switched ruby laser was also found in monkey studies to be suitable for producing iridotomies (57), and dye lasers have been used clinically to create iridotomies with a single pulse (58).

Comparison of Argon and Neodymium:YAG Laser Iridotomies

Histologic studies have shown that iridotomies created with an argon laser have more extensive early edema and tissue destruction at the margins of the treatment site (18, 19), as compared to that with Nd:YAG laser, in which the lesions are more circumscribed with limited tissue alterations at the margins (26, 28). However, freeze-frame analysis of high speed cinematography in ox eyes showed particles traveling over 8 mm from the Nd:YAG treatment site at speeds in excess of 20 km/h (27), and the shock waves affected the trabecular meshwork and corneal endothelium of monkey eyes when the Nd:YAG application was within 0.8 mm of the limbus (59).

Argon and Nd:YAG laser iridotomies were compared in human autopsy eyes using a high-magnification video recording system that allowed real-time observation of the posterior iris during the laser procedures (60). With argon laser iridotomy, there was a gradual mounding up of iris pigment epithelium with each successive energy application before final penetration. In contrast, Nd:YAG laser iridotomy caused a complete disruption and dispersal of the pigment epithelium with a single pulse of energy. These observations may explain the tendency for argon laser iridotomies to become obstructed with pigment epithelium, which is rarely seen with Nd:YAG laser iridotomies.

In clinical comparisons of the two surgical approaches, the Nd:YAG laser iridotomies had the disadvantage of frequent bleeding, although this usually stops spontaneously or by applying pressure to the eye with the contact lens, and rarely leads to significant complications (23, 24, 61, 62). Disadvantages of argon laser iridotomy, on the other hand, include more iritis, pupillary distortion and late closure of the iridotomy. In one study of 33 eyes in which an iridotomy could not be created with the argon laser, a patent iridotomy was achieved in all eyes with the Nd:YAG laser in single sessions (63). Neodymium:YAG laser iridotomies, in general, require considerably fewer total applications with a marked reduction in total energy delivery as compared to argon laser iridotomies.

Prevention and Management of Complications

As with laser trabeculoplasty, a transient IOP rise and a mild anterior uveitis are common early postoperative complications. Other potential complications include closure of the iridotomy, corneal damage, hyphema, cataract formation, retinal burns, malignant glaucoma, and monocular blurring.

Transient Intraocular Pressure Rise

This is one of the most common serious complications in the early period after either argon (64) or Nd:YAG (65) laser iridotomies. The IOP rise is caused by a reduction in outflow facility, with an actual decrease in aqueous production (66). A biphasic IOP response has been seen in rabbits, in which the initial pressure rise of 0.5–2 hours is followed by a prolonged IOP reduction of 6–24 hours (67). Studies in rabbits also suggest that this pressure response is related to a release of prostaglandin (67–69) and prostaglandin-like substances (70) into the aqueous with a breakdown in the blood-aqueous barrier and an accumulation of blood plasma and fibrin in the anterior chamber angle (69, 71–73). A histopathologic study in monkey eyes revealed a rapid accumulation of particulate debris in the angle (74), which may also contribute to the transient pressure elevation.

Clinically, the risk of a transient IOP rise was found in one study to be related to the total energy delivered, but not to the presence of chronic angle-closure glaucoma (65), while another study found no correlation with total laser energy, but did find that the preoperative outflow facility was directly related to the maximum postoperative IOP elevation (66). As previously noted, 1 drop of apraclonidine 0.5–1% either 1 hour before and/or immediately after the laser surgery has a profound effect on minimizing this complication (34–36).

Anterior Uveitis

Some degree of transient iritis occurs after laser iridotomy in all eyes, which is associated with the blood-aqueous barrier breakdown noted in animal studies (69, 71–73). Topical steroids for the first 3–5 postoperative days are sufficient to control this mild complication in the majority of cases. In rare cases, however, an eye may have a marked inflammation, sometimes occurring days or weeks after the procedure, and hypopyon (75, 76) and granulomatous endophthalmitis (76) have been reported following laser iridotomy. The latter complication was associated with several large tears in the anterior lens capsule of a blind eye with a mature cataract (76). A case of prolonged iritis with transient cystoid macular edema has also been described (77), and two cases have been reported in which postoperative inflammation and long-term miotic therapy were felt to be responsible for occlusion of the pupil with a pigmented pseudomembrane (78).

Closure of Iridotomy

The iridotomy may close during the first few weeks, especially with argon laser iridotomy, due to accumulation of pigment granules and debris. It is advisable, therefore, to continue pilocarpine for the first 4–6 postoperative weeks. If the iridotomy remains patent, it is usually safe to stop the miotic after this time, unless needed to control a chronic pressure elevation. It has been suggested that a mydriatic provocative test should be employed after stopping the miotic to confirm the functional reliability of the iridotomy (17). Late closure is rare with Nd:YAG laser iridotomies. In one series of 200 cases, the two late closures were both in eyes with preexisting chronic uveitis (79).

As discussed earlier in this chapter, the minimum diameter of a laser iridotomy that is needed to prevent further attacks of angle-closure glaucoma has yet to be determined and probably differs from one patient to the next. Cases have been reported in which angle closure recurred despite patent, but small iridotomies and, as previously noted, a minimum diameter of 150–200 μm has been recommended (44, 80). In some eyes following argon laser surgery, the laser iridotomy will spontaneously enlarge over months or years (81), although this should not be relied upon in borderline situations, in which case the opening should be further enlarged.

Patency of the iridotomy is best confirmed by visualizing anterior lens capsule or vitreous face through the opening (Fig. 36.6). Transillumination can also be used, although this is sometimes misleading, especially with a blue iris, in which dislodged pigment epithelium can produce a transillumination defect despite an intact overlying stroma, which is impermeable to aqueous flow.

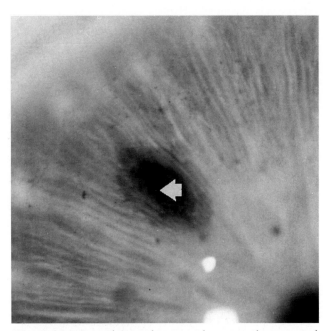

Figure 36.6. Argon laser iridotomy with patency demonstrated by visualization of anterior lens capsule *(arrow).*

Corneal Damage

Focal epithelial and endothelial burns of the cornea are not uncommon when larger amounts of laser energy are used, although these usually heal quickly with no apparent sequelae. In monkey eyes, laser iridotomy was not associated with significant endothelial cell damage (82). In several prospective clinical trials, pachymetry has revealed no significant difference in corneal thickness before and after laser iridotomy (83–85). Specular microscopic studies have been less conclusive, however, with some showing no significant difference in endothelial cell count (83, 84), while others have revealed a slight reduction in cell density (85, 86) or an increase in cell size (87). Generalized corneal decompensation has been reported in several series, nearly all of which involved argon laser iridotomy (88–91). This often begins with focal corneal edema overlying the iridotomy site, followed by generalized corneal decompensation which may not appear until months to years after the laser surgery. These cases frequently require penetrating keratoplasty, histology of which typically reveals abnormalities characteristic of Fuchs' dystrophy (89, 91). Factors that may predispose to this complication include episodes of angle closure glaucoma with pressure elevations and inflammation, cornea guttata, diabetes, and high total laser energy (88–91).

Hyphema

As previously noted, a small amount of bleeding from the iridotomy site is common following Nd:YAG laser iridotomy, but is rarely of serious consequence (21–25). Persistent bleeding from the treatment site can usually be stopped by applying pressure to the eye with the contact lens for a few seconds to a minute. Hyphemas are uncommon after argon laser iridotomies, but may occur (92, 93), especially in eyes with rubeosis iridis or uveitis.

Cataract Formation

Focal anterior lens opacities are common beneath an iridotomy produced with argon laser energy (23, 25, 94). Most of these are nonprogressive, although reduced visual acuity due to cataract progression has been documented (94). The rate of progression is similar to that following incisional surgical iridectomy (17), and a clear cause-and-effect relationship between either surgical approach and cataracts has not been established. Lens changes are much less common with Nd:YAG laser iridotomies (23–25), although capsular damage (95) with rare cataract formation (96) has been reported. In two rabbit studies, no lens damage was seen with either argon or Nd:YAG laser iridotomies, even when additional laser applications were placed through patent iridotomies (97, 98). A monkey study, however, suggested a threshold for lens damage with Nd:YAG laser iridotomy, with no damage at 6 mJ or less and one to two pulses per

burst, but local damage with higher energies or three pulses per burst (99).

Retinal Burns

Most visual function studies have shown no adverse effect from argon laser iridotomy (100), and the same is presumably true for Nd:YAG laser iridotomy. One study, however, did reveal static perimetric and fluorescein angiographic evidence of focal retinal damage in the quadrant of treatment 6 months after argon laser iridotomy (101). Retinal damage is best minimized by always aiming the laser beam toward peripheral retina. Failure to do so may result in serious retinal burns, and acute, permanent loss of vision has been reported due to inadvertent foveal photocoagulation during laser iridotomy (102). The risk is also reduced but not eliminated by the use of an Abraham lens (103). One case of temporary bilateral serous choroidal and nonrhegmatogenous retinal detachment following Nd:YAG laser iridotomy has also been reported (104).

Malignant Glaucoma

Cases of possible malignant glaucoma have also been reported following laser iridotomy for acute or chronic angle-closure glaucoma (105, 106), one of which was a simultaneous bilateral case 4 weeks after bilateral laser iridotomy (107).

Monocular Blurring

If the iridotomy is not fully covered by the upper lid, the patient may complain of monocular blurring or other visual symptoms (108). Care must be taken, therefore, in selecting the proper surgical site for the laser iridotomy.

INCISIONAL IRIDECTOMY

Laser Iridotomy Versus Incisional Iridectomy

The incisional surgical iridectomy is one of the safest, most effective operations for glaucoma. For the laser iridotomy to replace it as the procedure of choice, therefore, significant advantages had to be demonstrated. Long-term followup studies have shown that laser iridotomies are comparable to the incisional procedures in terms of efficacy and safety (17, 109–111). In addition, the laser approach has the advantages of (a) being a clinic or office procedure, (b) eliminating the need for retrobulbar anesthesia, (c) reducing surgical complications, such as wound leak, hyphema, and endophthalmitis, (d) shortening postoperative recovery time, and (e) lowering costs. These advantages have led to a significant increase in the annual rate of laser iridotomies as compared to incisional iridectomies before the laser was in common use, which is felt to represent an improvement in the quality of care (112).

For the reasons noted above, laser iridotomy has become the procedure of choice for most cases of angle-closure glaucoma. There are situations, however, when the incisional approach is still required. Some patients are not able to sit at the slitlamp or are unable to cooperate sufficiently for laser therapy. At other times, the cornea may be too cloudy or the iris may be too close to the cornea to allow laser iridotomy. There is also the rare case in which a patent iridotomy cannot be achieved with laser treatment, or in which the opening repeatedly closes postoperatively. The latter is particularly common in eyes with marked uveitis. For these reasons, the surgeon must still be familiar with the time honored procedure of incisional iridectomy.

Techniques

Peripheral Iridectomy

BASIC TECHNIQUE (FIG. 36.7). In the technique described by Chandler (113), a small conjunctival flap is prepared in one of the superior quadrants with either a fornix or limbus base. A 3–4-mm incision is made into the anterior chamber, beginning approximately 1–1.5 mm behind the corneolimbal junction.

If the iris prolapses, it is lifted up with iris forceps and a small section is excised using iris scissors that are held parallel to the limbus. If the iris does not spontaneously come through the limbal opening, a slight pressure on the posterior margin of the incision may cause the prolapse. Factors that may prevent the peripheral iris from prolapsing through

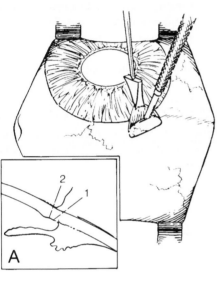
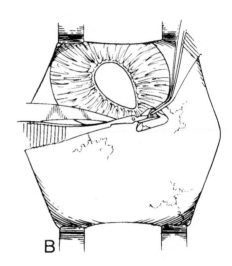
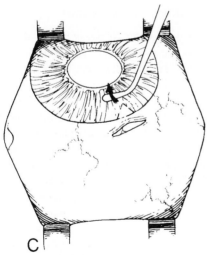

Figure 36.7. Peripheral iridectomy **A.** Incision into anterior chamber may be placed *(1)* behind the corneolimbal junction or *(2)* in peripheral cornea (note the slant of each incision). **B.** Peripheral iris is grasped with forceps and excised with iris scissors. **C.** Remaining iris is reposited by a gentle stroking action across the cornea *(arrow)*.

the limbal incision include (a) inaccurate placement of the incision, (b) a hypotonus eye, (c) peripheral anterior synechiae, (d) a hole elsewhere in the iris, and (e) ciliary-iridial processes (attachments between the posterior, peripheral iris and the ciliary body).

When iris prolapse cannot be achieved, the iris is grasped with forceps and brought up through the incision to make the iridectomy. The iris is then reposited by a gentle stroking action across the cornea in a direction away from the incision, using a blunt instrument such as a muscle hook.

In closing the wound, a single suture may be placed through both the limbal wound and conjunctiva if a fornix-based flap was used. With a limbus-based flap, closure of the conjunctiva alone may be sufficient, if the limbal incision was beveled slightly to achieve spontaneous apposition.

MODIFICATIONS. Some surgeons prefer to make the incision into the anterior chamber through *clear cornea* adjacent to the corneolimbal junction (114–116). The main advantage is that the undamaged conjunctiva remains available for future filtering surgery if required. The incision is usually placed perpendicular to the limbus in order to reach peripheral iris (Fig. 36.7), and suture closure is generally necessary. However, some surgeons feel suturing is not essential (114), especially if the incision is beveled posteriorly (116).

Another modification of the peripheral iridectomy is *transfixation,* in which the anterior chamber is entered at the limbus with a narrow cataract knife. The blade is then passed across the anterior segment of the eye, piercing first the peripheral iris and then iris near the sphincter muscle. This approach has been favored by some surgeons for the management of iris bombé in an inflamed eye, in the hope that it would reduce the danger of hemorrhage. However, one study showed that a conventional peripheral iridectomy does not have a greater incidence of bleeding (117). The nonincisional laser approach is now generally preferable to either of these techniques for this situation.

Sector Iridectomy

There are some situations in which a sector iridectomy may have advantages over a peripheral iridectomy. Such situations include (a) the need for a larger optical opening, (b) to minimize total posterior synechiae, and (c) to provide a better view of the fundus when retinal disease is suspected. In the technique described by King and Wadsworth (118), a larger limbal incision than for the peripheral iridectomy is required so that the iris can be grasped within 1–2 mm of the pupillary margin and brought well out through the wound. A radial cut is then made across the iris at one side of the exposed portion, the iris is torn at its root, and a second incision is made across the other side of the exposed tissue. This creates a truly basal iridectomy. An alternative approach is to grasp midperipheral iris, withdraw it until the pupillary margin is exposed, and excise the tissue with a single cut.

Prevention and Management of Complications

Intraoperative Complications

HEMORRHAGE. Cut edges of the iris normally do not bleed. However, hemorrhage may occur, especially if inflammation or neovascularization is present. To minimize bleeding in the latter situations, the use of bipolar cauterization of the iris surface before cutting the iridectomy has been suggested (119, 120). Brisk bleeding is especially likely to occur if the ciliary body is inadvertently cut. Hemorrhage from either iris or ciliary body can usually be stopped by placing a large air bubble in the anterior chamber for several minutes.

INCOMPLETE IRIDECTOMY. It is possible to cut only the stroma of the iris, leaving intact pigment epithelium, which prevents a successful operation. This complication should be avoided at the time of surgery by checking the iridectomy specimen for the presence of the dark pigment epithelium and by noting transillumination through the iridectomy if there is any doubt as to its patency. If the complication is discovered postoperatively, it is best managed by penetrating the epithelial layer with the argon laser (121). Low energy settings of 300–400 mW, with a 100-μm spot size and a 0.1-second duration of exposure, is sufficient in most cases, and the pigment epithelium is usually eliminated with a few applications.

INJURY TO THE LENS. Injury to the lens or disruption of the lens zonules with possible dislocation of the lens and vitreous loss should be avoided by gentle surgical manipulation. Intralenticular hemorrhage has also been reported as a rare complication of iridectomy (122).

Postoperative Complications

ELEVATED INTRAOCULAR PRESSURE. If the central anterior chamber is flat and the IOP is elevated, *malignant (ciliary block) glaucoma* should be considered. Fortunately, this is an uncommon complication, with only one such case encountered in one series of 155 eyes (123). However, the consequences can be devastating, and the management of this situation was discussed in Chapter 23. An incomplete iridectomy is another cause of high pressure and a flat anterior chamber, with the distinguishing feature from malignant glaucoma being more central anterior chamber depth with a bombé configuration of the iris. This situation can be managed as described above with the argon laser. A formed anterior chamber and patent iridectomy with an elevated pressure suggests that chronic obstruction of the trabecular meshwork may be present. The latter should initially be managed with antiglaucoma medications, although laser trabeculoplasty or a filtering procedure may be required if medical therapy is inadequate.

HYPHEMAS. Hyphemas should be handled conservatively with elevation of the head and limited activity.

CATARACTS. The frequency with which peripheral iridectomies lead to cataract formation is somewhat controversial. However, several studies indicate that some degree of lenticular opacity occurs in up to half of the cases with an acute angle-closure glaucoma attack and in one-third of the eyes treated prophylactically (123–127). The mechanism of this complication is uncertain, although the frequency increases with age.

ENDOPHTHALMITIS. As with any intraocular procedure, infection is a potential complication.

LASER PERIPHERAL IRIDOPLASTY (GONIOPLASTY)

There are occasions in which a laser iridotomy is difficult to create due to persistent edema of the cornea. There are other times in which a patent iridotomy may fail to relieve angle closure, as with a microphthalmic or nanophthalmic eye, the swelling or forward rotation of the ciliary body, or the presence of peripheral anterior synechiae. In each of these situations, it may be possible to open the anterior chamber angle by applying low energy argon laser contraction burns to the peripheral iris. The procedure has been referred to as laser peripheral iridoplasty, gonioplasty, or peripheral iris retraction.

Mechanisms of Action

The mechanism of action is a tightening of the peripheral iris, which pulls it posteriorly from the trabecular meshwork. The histopathology of both eyes, treated with peripheral iridoplasty 16 days before the patient's death, revealed contraction furrow formation, proliferation of fibroblast-like cells, collagen deposition on the iris surface, denaturation of stromal collagen, and coagulative necrosis of blood vessels within the anterior two-thirds of the iris stroma (128). These findings are believed to suggest that the immediate, short-term mechanism of peripheral iridoplasty is heat shrinkage of collagen, while the long-term effects may be related to contraction of a fibroblastic membrane. The observation of coagulative necrosis of iris blood vessels also provides a note of caution that overtreatment may lead to iris necrosis.

Techniques

Suggested argon laser settings for peripheral iridoplasty vary considerably, with ranges of 50–500 μm spot size, 0.5-second duration, and 150–1000 mW of power (33, 129–131). In general, however, a laser application of rela-

tively large area, long duration, and low power is preferable, and reasonable initial settings are 200 μm, 0.2 seconds, and 400 mW. The power or duration should be increased if no contraction is produced, but reduced if pigment liberation is produced by the laser application. The recommended number of applications also varies. Approximately 10–15 burns are usually applied to peripheral iris in each quadrant, and additional applications can be placed in a row adjacent to the first burns if necessary (Fig. 36.8). It is usually advisable to treat no more than 180° of angle in a single session.

The most commonly used technique for applying the laser burns is with a Goldmann three-mirror or single-mirror goniolens, which causes the laser beam to strike the iris tangentially. It is important with this technique to insure that a portion of the laser beam does not strike exposed angle structures. An alternative is to apply the laser burns directly through peripheral cornea, which is usually best done through the flat surface of a laser contact lens. When using this technique, the spot size should be larger and the power lower than with the tangential approach, since the direct approach creates smaller burns with higher energy per unit area.

Indications

As noted earlier, peripheral iridoplasty may be useful in opening a functionally closed anterior chamber angle, as with pupillary block glaucoma, when corneal edema prevents adequate laser energy delivery to create an iridotomy (33). In other cases, a patent iridotomy may fail to relieve the angle closure because of "crowding" of the angle, as with a small, microphthalmic or nanophthalmic (132) eye, an eye with plateau iris, iris cysts, or forward rotation of the ciliary body due to various mechanisms, including retinal

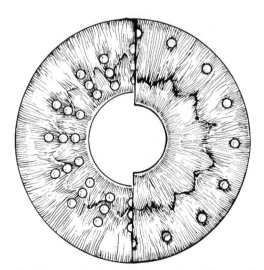

Figure 36.8. Laser peripheral iridoplasty (*right*) deepens the anterior chamber angle with low-energy contraction burns to the peripheral iris, while laser pupilloplasty (*left*) dilates the pupil with low-energy contraction burns to the more central iris.

detachment surgery (133). Laser peripheral iridoplasty has been shown to be successful in opening the anterior chamber angle in many of these cases. Another reason for failure of a patent iridotomy is the presence of extensive peripheral anterior synechiae. It has been reported that gonioplasty can open the angle in some of these cases if the laser energy is applied to the base of the synechiae (129, 130). The success rate is higher if the duration of synechial closure is short, and it has been suggested that gonioscopy should be performed immediately after an iridotomy for pupillary block glaucoma and gonioplasty should be performed for any synechial closure (129). However, success has also been reported after several years of synechial closure (130). Another reported indication for gonioplasty is to open areas of persistent or recurrent synechial closure after incisional goniosynechialysis (131). In addition, peripheral iridoplasty can be used to deepen the anterior chamber angle to facilitate laser trabeculoplasty.

Complications

Peripheral iridoplasty may be complicated by further elevation of the IOP. This is usually transient, but may be chronic if the outflow structures are further compromised by the laser applications. A mild, transient iritis is a consistent finding and should be treated with several days of topical steroids. Other potential complications include corneal endothelial burns, distortion of the pupil, and focal iris atrophy.

LASER PUPILLOPLASTY

Laser pupilloplasty is a technique by which the pupil can be partially dilated by applying contraction burns near the pupillary portion of the iris. Suggested argon laser settings are 200–500 μm, 0.2–0.5 seconds, and 200–500 mW (33). Several rows of laser energy are applied to the sphincter portion of the iris, starting at the pupillary border and working peripherally. One technique is to use a smaller spot size near the pupillary border and then enlarge the spot size for more peripheral burns. The contraction of stroma with each application tents the pupil in the direction of the treatment site. Radial rows of contraction burns can be applied for 360° to create symmetric pupillary dilatation, or in one quadrant to create focal dilatation (Fig. 36.8).

One indication for laser pupilloplasty is as another alternative treatment for pupillary block when a laser iridotomy is not possible, as with a cloudy cornea. It is an especially useful technique for pupillary block glaucoma in aphakia or pseudophakia (134–136). By peaking the pupil in one quadrant, the iris may be retracted away from an area of vitreous contact or beyond a point of apposition with the intraocular lens implant, thereby reestablishing communication between the anterior and posterior chambers. This usually only works when the amount of lens-iris contact is minimal, since the degree of pupillary retraction is small. When pupilloplasty is not effective in these cases, combined therapy with peripheral iridoplasty may be effective (33).

Pupilloplasty may also be used to dilate a chronically constricted pupil, although the amount of dilatation is usually small and often temporary. The procedure in this situation may be complicated by a significant IOP rise. Transient iritis is also a consistent complication and should be treated with several days of topical steroids.

OTHER LASER PROCEDURES FOR THE IRIS[b]

Iris Sphincterotomy

A technique has been described in which the pupil can be enlarged, reshaped, or repositioned by making a linear cut across the iris with an argon laser set at 0.01–0.05 seconds, 50 μm, and 1.5 W, allowing the intrinsic tension of the iris to spread the cut apart (137).

Iridolenticular Synechialysis

In eyes with posterior synechiae due to uveitis, it has been reported that a Q-switched Nd:YAG laser can be used to break to iris-lens adhesions (138). Laser settings were 1 mJ and a single burst per pulse, and care was taken to apply the energy only to the iris near the synechiae, staying away from the lens.

SUMMARY

Laser iridotomies have become the procedure of choice for the surgical management of angle-closure glaucomas and can be achieved with either continuous-wave or pulsed lasers. Techniques vary with the type of laser and the color of the iris. Complications include transient IOP elevation, uveitis, and burns of the cornea, lens, or retina. There are some situations in which laser iridotomies are not possible to achieve, in which case incisional iridectomies are still required. Laser energy can also be used to treat certain types of angle-closure glaucoma by mechanically flattening the peripheral iris (iridoplasty or gonioplasty) or dilating the pupil (pupilloplasty). Sphincterotomy and iridolenticular synechialysis are yet other reported iris procedures that can be performed with lasers.

---

[b]Refer to M.B. Shields: Color Atlas of Glaucoma. Baltimore: Williams & Wilkins, 1998, Plate III13.

REFERENCES

1. Meyer-Schwickerath, G: Erfahrungen mit der Lichtokoagulation der Netzhaut und der Iris. Doc Ophthalmol 10:91, 1956.
2. Hogan, MF, Schwartz, A: Experimental photocoagulation of the iris of guinea pigs. Am J Ophthalmol 49:629, 1960.
3. Flocks, M, Zweng, HC: Laser coagulation of ocular tissues. Arch Ophthalmol 72:604, 1964.
4. Snyder, WB: Laser coagulation of the anterior segment. Arch Ophthalmol 77:93, 1967.
5. Hallman, VL, Perkins, ES, Watts, GK, et al: Laser iradiation of the anterior segment of the eye. I. Rabbit eyes. Exp Eye Res 7:481, 1968.
6. Hallman, VL, Perkins, ES, Watts, GK, et al: Laser irradiation of the anterior segment of the eye. II. Monkey eyes. Exp Eye Res 8:1, 1969.
7. Perkins, ES: Laser iridotomy for secondary glaucoma. Trans Ophthalmol Soc UK 91:777, 1971.
8. Khuri, CH: Argon laser iridectomies. Am J Ophthalmol 76:490, 1973.
9. L'Esperance, FA Jr, James, WA Jr: Argon laser photocoagulation of iris abnormalities. Trans Am Acad Ophthalmol Otol 79:321, 1975.
10. Abraham, RK, Miller, GL: Outpatient argon laser iridectomy for angle closure glaucoma: a two-year study. Trans Am Acad Ophthalmol Otol 79:529, 1975.
11. Anderson, DR, Forster, RK, Lewis, ML: Laser iridotomy for aphakic pupillary block. Arch Ophthalmol 93:343, 1975.
12. Pollack, IP, Patz, A: Argon laser iridotomy: an experimental and clinical study. Ophthalmic Surg 7:22, 1976.
13. Pollack, IP: Use of argon laser energy to produce iridotomies. Trans Am Ophthalmol Soc 87:674, 1979.
14. Podos, SM, Kels, BD, Moss, AP, et al: Continuous-wave argon laser iridectomy in angle-closure glaucoma. Am J Ophthalmol 88:836, 1979.
15. Yassur, Y, Melamed, S, Cohen, S, Ben-Sira, I: Laser iridotomy in closed-angle glaucoma. Arch Ophthalmol 97:1920, 1979.
16. Pollack, IP: Use of argon laser energy to produce iridotomies. Ophthalmic Surg 11:506, 1980.
17. Quigley, HA: Long-term follow-up of laser iridotomy. Ophthalmology 88:218, 1981.
18. Schwartz, LW, Rodrigues, MM, Spaeth, GL, et al: Argon laser iridotomy in the treatment of patients with primary angle-closure or pupillary block glaucoma: a clinicopathologic study. Ophthalmology 85:294, 1978.
19. Rodrigues, MM, Streeten, B, Spaeth, GL, Schwartz, LW: Argon laser iridotomy or primary angle closure or pupillary block glaucoma. Arch Ophthalmol 96:2222, 1978.
20. Yassur, Y, David, R, Rosenblatt, I, Marmour, U: Iridotomy with red krypton laser. Br J Ophthalmol 70:295, 1986.
21. Latina, MA, Puliafito, CA, Steinert, RR, Epstein, DL: Experimental iridotomy with the Q-switched neodymium-YAG laser. Arch Ophthalmol 102:1211, 1984.
22. Klapper, RM: Q-switched neodymium:YAG laser iridotomy. Ophthalmology 91:1017, 1984.
23. Robin, AL, Pollack IP: A comparison of neodymium:YAG and argon laser iridotomies. Ophthalmology 91:1011, 1984.
24. McAllister, JA, Schwartz, LW, Moster, M, Spaeth, GL: Laser peripheral iridectomy comparing Q-switched neodymium YAG with argon. Trans Ophthalmol Soc UK 104:67, 1984.
25. Pollack, IP, Robin, AL, Dragon, DM, et al: Use of the neodymium:YAG laser to create iridotomies in monkeys and humans. Trans Am Ophthalmol Soc 82:307, 1984.
26. Rodrigues, MM, Spaeth, GL, Moster, M, et al: Histopathology of neodymium:YAG laser iridectomy in humans. Ophthalmology 92:1696, 1985.
27. Vernon, SA, Cheng, H: Freeze frame analysis on high speed cinematography of Nd/YAG laser explosions in ocular tissues. Br J Ophthalmol 70:321, 1986.
28. Goldberg, MF, Tso, MOM, Mirolovich, M: Histopathological characteristics of neodymium-YAG laser irodotomy in the human eye. Br J Ophthalmol 71:623, 1987.
29. Robin, AL, Arkell, S, Gilbert, SM, et al: Q-switched neodymium-YAG laser iridotomy. A field trial with a portable laser system. Arch Ophthalmol 104:526, 1986.
30. Abraham, RK: Protocol for single-session argon laser iridectomy for angle-closure glaucoma. Int Ophthalmol Clin 21:145, 1981.
31. Schirmer, KE: Argon laser surgery of the iris, optimized by contact lenses. Arch Ophthalmol 101:1130, 1983.
32. Wise, JB, Munnerlyn, CR, Erickson, PJ: A high-efficiency laser iridotomy-sphincterotomy lens. Am J Ophthalmol 101:546, 1986.
33. Ritch, R: Argon laser treatment for medically unresponsive attacks of angle-closure glaucoma. Am J Ophthalmol 94:197, 1982.
34. Robin, AL, Pollack, IP, deFaller, JM: Effects of topical ALO 2145 (p-aminoclonidine hydrochloride) on the acute intraocular pressure rise after argon laser iridotomy. Arch Ophthalmol 105:1208, 1987.
35. Krupin, T, Stank, T, Feitl, ME: Apraclonidine pretreatment decreases the acute intraocular pressure rise after laser trabeculoplasty or iridotomy. J Glau 1:79, 1992.
36. Rosenberg, LF, Krupin, T, Ruderman, J, et al: Apraclonidine and anterior segment laser surgery. Comparison of 0.5% versus 1.0% apraclonidine for prevention of postoperative intraocular pressure rise. Ophthalmology 102:1312, 1995.
37. Hoskins, HD, Migliazzo, CV: Laser iridectomy—a technique for blue irises. Ophthalmic Surg 15:488, 1984.
38. Abraham, RK: Procedure for outpatient argon laser iridectomies for angle closure glauocma. Int Ophthalmol Clin 16:1, 1976.
39. Harrad, RA, Stannard, KP, Shilling, JS: Argon laser iridotomy. Br J Ophthalmol 69:368, 1985.
40. Yamamoto, T, Shirato, S, Kitazawa, Y: Argon laser iridotomy in angle-closure glaucoma: a comparison of two methods. Jpn J Ophthalmol 26:387, 1982.
41. Mandelkorn, RM, Mendelsohn, AD, Olander, KW, Zimmerman, TJ: Short exposure times in argon laser iridotomy. Ophthalmic Surg 12:805, 1981.
42. Kolker, AE: Techniques of argon laser iridectomy. Trans Am Ophthalmol Soc 82:303, 1984.
43. Stetz, D, Smith, H Jr, Ritch, R: A simplified technique for laser iridectomy in blue irides. Am J Ophthalmol 96:249, 1983.
44. Fleck, BW: How large must an iridotomy be? Br J Ophthalmol 74:583, 1990.
45. Fleck, BW, Fairley, E, Wright, E: A photometric study of the effect of pupil dilatation on Nd:YAG laser iridotomy area. Br J Ophthalmol 76:678, 1992.
46. Damerow, A, Utermann, D: Combined thermal-photodisruptive iridotomy with the argon and Nd:YAG laser. Klin Monatsbl Augenheilkd 195:61, 1989.
47. Goins, K, Schmeisser, E, Smith, T: Argon laser pretreatment in Nd:YAG iridotomy. Ophthalmic Surg 21:497, 1990.
48. Ho, T, Fan, R: Sequential argon-YAG laser iridotomies in dark irides. Br J Ophthalmol 76:329, 1992.
49. Wise, JB: Large iridotomies by the linear incision technique using the neodymium:YAG laser at low energy levels. A study using cynomolgus monkeys. Ophthalmology 94:82, 1987.
50. Wise, JB: Low-energy linear-incision neodymium:YAG laser iridotomy versus linear-incision argon laser iridotomy. A prospective clinical investigation. Ophthalmology 94:1531, 1987.
51. Rol, P, Kwasniewska, S, van der Zypen, E, Fankhauser, F: Transscleral iridotomy using a neodymium:YAG laser operated both with standard equipment and an optical fiber system—a preliminary report: Part 1—optical system and biomicroscopic results. Ophthalmic Surg 18:176, 1987.
52. Oram, O, Gross, RL, Severin, TD, et al: Picosecond neodymium: yttrium lithium fluoride (Nd:YLF) laser peripheral iridotomy. Am J Ophthalmol 119:408, 1995.

53. Frangie, JP, Park, SB, Aquavella, SV: Peripheral iridotomy using Nd:YLF laser. Ophthalmic Surg 23:220, 1992.

54. Jacobson, JJ, Schuman, JS, El Koumy, H, Puliafito, CA: Diode laser peripheral iridectomy. Int Ophthalmol Clin 30:120, 1990.

55. Emoto, I, Okisaka, S, Nakajima, A: Diode laser iridotomy in rabbit and human eyes. Am J Ophthalmol 113:321, 1992.

56. Schuman, JS, Puliafito, CA, Jacobson, JJ: Semiconductor diode laser peripheral iridotomy. Arch Ophthalmol 108:1207, 1990.

57. Bonney, CH, Gassterland, DE: Low-energy, Q-switched ruby laser iridotomies in Macaca mulatta. Invest Ophthalmol Vis Sci 18:278, 1979.

58. Bass, MS, Cleary, CV, Perkins, ES, Wheeler, CB: Single treatment laser iridotomy. Br J Ophthalmol 63:29, 1979.

59. Richardson, TM, Brown, SV, Thomas, JV, Simmons, RJ: Shock-wave effect on anterior segment structures following experimental neodymium:YAG laser iridectomy. Ophthalmology 92:1387, 1985.

60. Prum, BE, Jr, Shields, SR, Shields, MB, et al: In vitro videographic comparison of argon and Nd:YAG laser iridotomy. Am J Ophthalmol 111:589, 1991.

61. Moster, MR, Schwartz, LW, Spaeth, GL, et al: Laser iridectomy: a controlled study comparing argon and neodymium:YAG. Ophthalmology 93:20, 1986.

62. Del Priore, LV, Robin, AL, Pollack, IP: Neodymium:YAG and argon laser iridotomy. Long-term follow-up in a prospective, randomized clinical trial. Ophthalmology 95:1207, 1988.

63. Robin, AL, Pollack, IP: Q-switched neodymium-YAG laser iridotomy in patients in whom the argon laser fails. Arch Ophthalmol 104:531, 1986.

64. Krupin, T, Stone, RA, Cohen, BH, et al: Acute intraocular pressure response to argon laser iridotomy. Ophthalmology 92:922, 1985.

65. Taniguchi, T, Rho, SH, Gotoh, Y, Kitazawa, Y: Intraocular pressure rise following Q-switched neodymium:YAG laser iridotomy. Ophthalmol Laser Ther 2:99, 1987.

66. Wetzel, W: Ocular aqueous humor dynamics after photodisruptive laser surgery procedures. Ophthalmic Surg 25:298, 1994.

67. Sugiyama, K, Kitazawa, Y, Kawai, K, Enya, T: Biphasic intraocular pressure response to Q-switched Nd:YAG laser irradiation of the iris and the apparent mediatory role of prostaglandins. Exp Eye Res 51:531, 1990.

68. Gailitis, R, Peyman, GA, Pulido, J, et al: Prostaglandin release following Nd:YAG iridotomy in rabbits. Ophthalmic Surg 17:467, 1986.

69. Joo, C-K, Kim, J-H: Prostaglandin E in rabbit aqueous humor after Nd-YAG laser photodisruption of iris and the effect of topical indomethacin pretreatment. Invest Ophthalmol Vis Sci 33:1685, 1992.

70. Weinreb, RN, Weaver, D, Mitchell, MD: Prostanoids in rabbit aqueous humor: effect of laser photocoagulation of the iris. Invest Ophthalmol Vis Sci 26:1087, 1985.

71. Sanders, DR, Joondeph, B, Hutchins, R, et al: Studies on the blood-aqueous barrier after argon laser photocoagulation of the iris. Ophthalmology 90:169, 1983.

72. Schrems, W, van Dorp, HP, Wendel, M, Krieglstein, GK: The effect of YAG laser iridotomy on the blood aqueous barrier in the rabbit. Graefes Arch Clin Exp Ophthalmol 221:179, 1984.

73. Tawara, A, Inomata, H: Histological study on transient ocular hypertension after laser iridotomy in rabbits. Graefes Arch Clin Exp Ophthalmol 225:114, 1987.

74. Robin, AL, Pollack, IP, Quigley, HA, et al: Histologic studies of angle structures after laser iridotomy in primates. Arch Ophthalmol 100:1665, 1982.

75. Cohen, JS, Bibler, L, Tucker, D: Hypopyon following laser iridotomy. Ophthalmic Surg 15:604, 1984.

76. Margo, CE, Lessner, A, Goldey, SH, Sherwood, M: Lens-induced endophthalmitis after Nd:YAG laser iridotomy. Am J Ophthalmol 113:97, 1992.

77. Choplin, NT, Bene, CH: Cystoid macular edema following laser iridotomy. Ann Ophthalmol 15:172, 1983.

78. Geyer, O, Mayron, Y, Rothkoff, L, Lazar, M: Pigmented pupillary pseudomembranes as a complication of argon laser iridotomy. Ophthalmic Surg 22:162, 1991.

79. Schwartz, LW, Moster, MR, Spaeth, GL, et al: Neodymium-YAG laser iridectomies in glaucoma associated with closed or occludable angles. Am J Ophthalmol 102:41, 1986.

80. Brainard, JO, Landers, JH, Shock, JP: Recurrent angle closure glaucoma following a patent 75-micron laser iridotomy: a case report. Ophthalmic Surg 13:1030, 1982.

81. Sachs, SW, Schwartz, B: Enlargement of laser iridotomies over time. Br J Ophthalmol 68:570, 1984.

82. Hirst, LW, Robin, AL, Sherman, S, et al: Corneal endothelial changes after argon-laser iridotomy and panretinal photocoagulation. Am J Ophthalmol 93:473, 1982.

83. Smith, J, Whitted, P: Corneal endothelial changes after argon laser iridotomy. Am J Ophthalmol 98:153, 1984.

84. Panek, WC, Lee, DA, Christensen, RE: Effects of argon laser iridotomy on the corneal endothelium. Am J Ophthalmol 105:395, 1988.

85. Panek, WC, Lee, DA, Christensen, RE: The effects of Nd:YAG laser iridotomy on the corneal endothelium. Am J Ophthalmol 111:505, 1991.

86. Marraffa, M, Marchini, G, Pagliarusco, A, et al: Ultrasound biomicroscopy and corneal endothelium in Nd:YAG-laser iridotomy. Ophthalmic Surg Lasers 26:519, 1995.

87. Hong, C, Kitazawa, Y, Tanishima, T: Influence of argon laser treatment of glaucoma on corneal endothelium. Jpn J Ophthalmol 27:567, 1983.

88. Schwartz, AL, Martin, NF, Weber, PA: Corneal decompensation after argon laser iridectomy. Arch Ophthalmol 106:1572, 1988.

89. Zabel, RW, MacDonald, IM, Mintsioulis, G: Corneal endothelial decompensation after argon laser iridotomy. Can J Ophthalmol 26:367, 1991.

90. Jeng, S, Lee, J-S, Huang, SCM: Corneal decompensation after argon laser iridectomy—a delayed complication. Ophthalmic Surg 22:565, 1991.

91. Wilhelmus, KR: Corneal edema following argon laser iridotomy. Ophthalmic Surg 23:533, 1992.

92. Hodes, BL, Bentivegna, JF, Weyer, NJ: Hyphema complicating laser iridotomy. Arch Ophthalmol 100:924, 1982.

93. Rubin, L, Arnett, J, Ritch, R: Delayed hyphema after argon laser iridectomy. Ophthalmic Surg 15:852, 1984.

94. Yamamoti, T, Shirato, S, Kitazawa, Y: Treatment of primary angle-closure glaucoma by argon laser iridotomy: a long-term follow-up. Jpn J Ophthalmol 29:1, 1985.

95. Welch, DB, Apple, DJ, Mendelsohn, AD, et al: Lens injury following iridotomy with a Q-switched neodymium-YAG laser. Arch Ophthalmol 104:123, 1986.

96. Berger, CM, Lee, DA, Christensen, RE: Anterior lens capsule perforation and zonular rupture after Nd:YAG laser iridotomy. Am J Ophthalmol 107:674, 1989.

97. Seedor, JA, Greenidge, KC, Dunn, MW: Neodymium:YAG laser iridectomy and acute cataract formation in the rabbit. Ophthalmic Surg 17:478, 1986.

98. Higginbotham, EJ, Ogura, Y: Lens clarity after argon and neodymium:YAG laser iridotomy in the rabbit. Arch Ophthalmol 105:540, 1987.

99. Gaasterland, DE, Rodrigues, MM, Thomas, G: Threshold for lens damage during Q-switched Nd:YAG laser iridectomy. A study of rhesus monkey eyes. Ophthalmology 92:1616, 1985.

100. Anderson, DR, Knighton, RW, Feuer, WJ: Evaluation of phototoxic retinal damage after argon laser iridotomy. Am J Ophthalmol 107:398, 1989.

101. Karmon, G, Savir, H: Retinal damage after argon laser iridotomy. Am J Ophthalmol 101:554, 1986.

102. Berger, BB: Foveal photocoagulation from laser iridotomy. Ophthalmology 91:1029, 1984.

103. Bongard, B, Pederson, JE: Retinal burns from experimental laser iridotomy. Ophthalmic Surg 16:42, 1985.

104. Karjalainen, K, Laatikainen, L, Raitta, C: Bilateral nonrhegmatogenous retinal detachment following neodymium:YAG laser iridotomies. Arch Ophthalmol 104:1134, 1986.

105. Brooks, AMV, Harper, CA, Gillies, WE: Occurrence of malignant glaucoma after laser iridotomy. Br J Ophthalmol 73:617, 1989.

106. Robinson, A, Prialnic, M, Deutsch, D, Savir, H: The onset of malignant glaucoma after prophylactic laser iridotomy. Am J Ophthalmol 110:95, 1990.

107. Aminlari, A, Sassani, JW: Simultaneous bilateral malignant glaucoma following laser iridotomy. Graefes Arch Clin Exp Ophthalmol 231:12, 1993.

108. Murphy, PH, Trope, GE: Monocular blurring. A complication of YAG laser iridotomy. Ophthalmology 98:1539, 1991.

109. Robin, A, Pollack IP: Argon laser peripheral iridotomies in the treatment of primary angle closure glaucoma. Long-term follow-up. Arch Ophthalmol 100:919, 1982.

110. Go, F-J, Yamamoto, T, Kitazawa, Y: Argon laser irodotomy and surgical iridectomy in treatment of primary angle-closure glaucoma. Jpn J Ophthalmol 28:36, 1984.

111. Salmon, JF: Long-term intraocular pressure control after Nd:YAG laser iridotomy in chronic angle-closure glaucoma. J Glau 2:291, 1993.

112. Rivera, AH, Brown, RH, Anderson, DR: Laser iridotomy vs. surgical iridectomy. Have the indications changed? Arch Ophthalmol 103:1350, 1985.

113. Chandler, PA: Peripheral iridectomy. Arch Ophthalmol 72:804, 1964.

114. Weene, LE: Self-sealing incision for peripheral iridectomy. Ophthalmic Surg 9:64, 1978.

115. Freeman, LB, Ridgway, AEA: Peripheral iridectomy via a corneal section: a follow-up study. Ophthalmic Surg 10:53, 1979.

116. Ahmad, N: Transcorneal peripheral iridectomy. Ophthalmic Surg 11:124, 1980.

117. Curran, RE: Surgical management of iris bombé. Arch Ophthalmol 90:464, 1973.

118. King, JH, Wadsworth, JAC: An atlas of ophthalmic surgery, second edition. Philadelphia, JB Lippincott, 1970, p. 416.

119. Kass, MA, Hersh, SB, Albert, DM: Experimental iridectomy with bipolar microcautery. Am J Ophthalmol 81:451, 1976.

120. Hersh, SB, Kass, MA: Iridectomy in rubeosis iridis. Ophthalmic Surg 7:19, 1976.

121. Tessler, HH, Peyman, GA, Huamonte, F, Menachof, I: Argon laser iridotomy in incomplete peripheral iridectomy. Am J Ophthalmol 79:1051, 1975.

122. Feibel, RM, Bigger, JF, Smith, ME: Intralenticular hemorrhage following iridectomy. Arch Ophthalmol 87:36, 1972.

123. Go, F-J, Kitazawa, Y: Complications of peripheral iridectomy in primary angle-closure glaucoma. Jpn J Ophthalmol 25:222, 1981.

124. Sugar, HS: Cataract formation and refractive changes after surgery for angle-closure glaucoma. Am J Ophthalmol 69:747, 1970.

125. Floman, N, Berson, D, Landau, L: Peripheral iridectomy in closed angle glaucoma—late complications. Br J Ophthalmol 61:101, 1977.

126. Godel, V, Regenbogen, L: Cataractogenic factors in patients with primary angle-closure glaucoma after peripheral iridectomy. Am J Ophthalmol 83:180, 1977.

127. Krupin, T, Mitchell, KB, Johnson, MF, Becker, B: The long-term effects of iridectomy for primary acute angle-closure glaucoma. Am J Ophthalmol 86:506, 1978.

128. Sassani, JW, Ritch, R, McCormick, S, et al: Histopathology of argon laser peripheral iridoplasty. Ophthalmic Surg 24:740, 1993.

129. Weiss, HS, Shingleton, BJ, Goode, SM, et al: Argon laser gonioplasty in the treatment of angle-closure glaucoma. Am J Ophthalmol 114:14, 1992.

130. Wand, M: Argon laser gonioplasty for synechial angle closure. Arch Ophthalmol 110:363, 1992.

131. Tanihara, H, Nagata, M: Argon-laser gonioplasty following goniosynechialysis. Graefes Arch Clin Exp Ophthalmol 229:505, 1991.

132. Kimbrough, RL, Trempe, CS, Brockhurst, RJ, Simmons, RJ: Angle-closure glaucoma in nanophthalmos. Am J Ophthalmol 88:572, 1979.

133. Burton, TC, Folk, JC: Laser iris retraction for angle-closure glaucoma after retinal detachment surgery. Ophthalmology 95:742, 1988.

134. Patti, JC, Cinotti, AA: Iris photocoagulation therapy of aphakic pupillary block. Arch Ophthalmol 93:347, 1975.

135. Theodossiadis, G: A new argon-laser-approach for the management of aphakic pupillary block. Klin Monatsbl Augenheilk 169:153, 1976.

136. Theodossiadis, GP: Pupilloplasty in aphakic and pseudophakic pupillary block glaucoma. Trans Ophthalmol Soc UK 104:137, 1985.

137. Wise, JB: Iris sphincterotomy, iridotomy, and synechiotomy by linear incision with the argon laser. Ophthalmology 92:641, 1985.

138. Kumar, H, Ahuja, S, Garg, SP: Neodymium:YAG laser iridolenticular synechiolysis in uveitis. Ophthalmic Surg 25:288, 1994.

FILTERING SURGERY

The incisional operation most frequently used for chronic forms of glaucoma, especially in adults, is commonly referred to as a filtering procedure. Although a number of variations for this surgical procedure have been described, all filtering operations share the same basic mechanism of action and general surgical principles. We first consider these aspects and then discuss specific filtration techniques and potential complications.

MECHANISMS OF ACTION

Drainage Fistula

The basic mechanism of all filtering procedures is the creation of an opening, or *fistula,* at the limbus, which allows aqueous humor to drain from the anterior chamber, thereby circumventing the pathologic obstruction to outflow. The aqueous flows directly or indirectly into subconjunctival spaces and is then removed by one or more routes.

Filtering Bleb

Most, but not all, successful glaucoma filtering procedures are characterized by an elevation of the conjunctiva at the surgical site, which is commonly referred to as a *filtering bleb.* The clinical appearance of these blebs varies considerably with regard to diameter, elevation, and vascularity. The blebs which are most often associated with good intraocular pressure (IOP) control are avascular with numerous microcysts in the epithelium and are either low and diffuse or more circumscribed and elevated (Fig. 37.1) (1, 2).

The histologic appearance of both functioning and failed filtering blebs consists of normal epithelium with no encircling-type junctions between the cells that would limit fluid flow (2). The subepithelial connective tissue correlates better with bleb status, in that functioning blebs have loosely arranged tissue with histologically clear spaces, while the failed blebs have dense collagenous connective tissue (2).

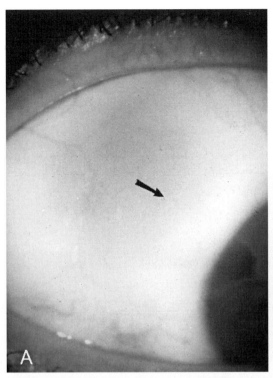 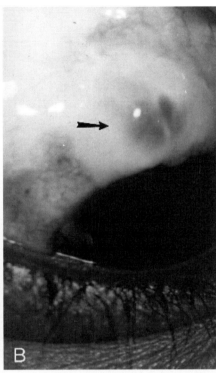

Figure 37.1. Types of functioning filtering blebs *(arrows)*. **A.** Low, diffuse bleb. **B.** Discrete, elevated bleb. Note that both are avascular.

Routes of Aqueous Drainage

Studies have suggested that aqueous in the filtering bleb usually filters through the conjunctiva (3) and mixes with the tear film (4, 5), or is absorbed by vascular (3) or perivascular (6) conjunctival tissue. Less commonly a filtering procedure may be associated with IOP control in the absence of an apparent filtering bleb. This is more common when the fistula is covered by a partial-thickness scleral flap (trabeculectomy), and suggested mechanisms of aqueous drainage in these cases include flow through (a) lymphatic vessels near the scarred margins of the surgical area, (b) atypical, newly incorporated aqueous veins, and (c) normal aqueous veins (3, 6).

GENERAL FEATURES OF FILTERING SURGERY

The various types of filtering surgery differ primarily according to the method used to create the drainage fistula. The other aspects of the operation, as well as the postoperative care, are basically the same for all filtering procedures and will be discussed first before considering specific fistulizing techniques.

Traction Sutures

Good surgical exposure is critical to the successful outcome of a filtering procedure. In most cases, this requires the use of a traction suture. The two most common techniques are (a) a superior rectus traction suture and (b) a clear cornea traction suture. With the former technique, the globe is rotated down, and the superior

rectus muscle is grasped with forceps, through conjunctiva, 10–15 mm behind the limbus. A 4–0 silk suture is then passed through conjunctiva and around the muscle beneath the tips of the forceps, and the suture is attached to the head of the surgical drape. With the clear cornea technique, a 6–0 silk suture is passed to a corneal depth of approximately ¾ thickness, 1 mm from the limbus with a bite width of 4–5 mm, and is then attached to the drape over the cheek. The rectus suture has the potential disadvantages of a subconjunctival hemorrhage or a hole in the conjunctiva that may leak postoperatively, while the corneal suture may distort the cornea and anterior chamber during the surgery.

Limbal Stab Incision

Some surgeons make a beveled incision into the anterior chamber at the limbus, usually in the inferior-temporal quadrant, as a route for injecting fluid at the end of the procedure. This can be done with a tapered, pointed knife, with the cutting edge facing the anterior chamber angle. The tip of the blade is rotated toward the angle during the withdrawal, to widen the inner portion of the incision (Fig. 37.2). This can be done at the outset of the procedure. If antifibrosis agents (discussed later in this chapter) are to be used, however, it may be best to wait until after that step of the operation, to avoid a route for potential entry of the drug into the anterior chamber.

Preparation of the Conjunctival Flap

Preparation of the conjunctival flap is a critical step in all filtering procedures, since the most common cause of failure is

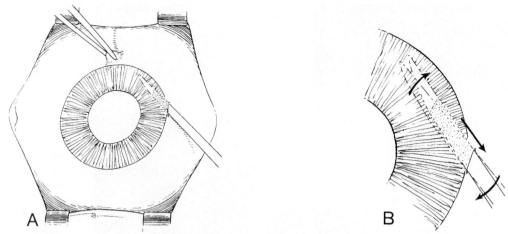

Figure 37.2. Limbal stab incision. **A.** Entry at limbus with cutting edge of blade facing the anterior chamber angle. **B.** Rotation of knife tip toward the angle during withdrawal.

scarring of the filtering bleb. While techniques differ among surgeons, all agree that meticulous detail with minimal tissue damage and bleeding is essential.

Position of the Flap

Some surgeons elect to make the flap at the 12 o'clock position to take advantage of the wider limbus in this area. Others prefer one of the superior quadrants, leaving the adjacent quadrant available for future surgery if required. The inferior quadrant has been used in cases of previous failed filtering surgery or when other ocular surgery has resulted in scarring of conjunctiva in the superior quadrants (7). However, the latter technique is associated with an increased risk of endophthalmitis and should usually be avoided.

Limbus- Versus Fornix-Based Flap

Conjunctival flaps for glaucoma filtering surgery have traditionally been limbus-based, i.e., with the initial incision in the fornix (Fig. 37.3), although some surgeons prefer a fornix-based flap, particularly in association with a trabeculectomy (8–10). Several studies have been described which compared limbus- and fornix-based conjunctival flaps in association with trabeculectomy and have all reported comparable success rates (10–15). However, one investigative team found slightly better postoperative IOP control with the limbus-based flap (13), while others found better pressure control (10) and more diffuse blebs with the fornix-based flaps. Surgeons differ on this aspect of filtering surgery, with some preferring the relative ease and improved surgical exposure of the fornix-based flap, while others prefer the tighter wound closure that may be achieved with the limbus-based flaps. One circumstance in which a fornix-based conjunctival flap is especially useful is when such a flap was used previously, as during cataract surgery, leaving a band of scar tissue at the limbus. It is difficult in these cases to dissect a limbus-based flap sufficiently anteriorly without creating holes in the conjunctiva. A preferable alternative is to excise the band of scar tissue and pull the new edge of the conjunctival flap down to peripheral cornea.

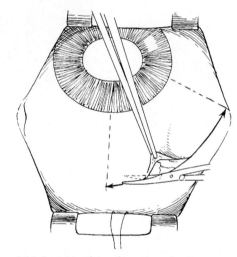

Figure 37.3. Incision through conjunctiva in preparation of a limbus-based conjunctival flap.

Management of Tenon's Capsule

There is also some controversy regarding the value of removing all or a portion of Tenon's capsule in the area of the conjunctival flap. Two studies revealed no difference in postoperative IOP control between eyes with excision of the capsular tissue as compared to those in which it was left partially or totally intact (16, 17). For this reason, many surgeons routinely preserve Tenon's capsule by dissecting between the capsule and episclera when preparing the conjunctival flap. This may be especially important when using adjunctive antifibrosis agents, to avoid excessively thin or leaking filtering blebs in the late postoperative course. Others, however, will excise variable portions of Tenon's capsule when it appears to be unusually thick, as in young patients. This can be accomplished by dissecting between the conjunctiva and Tenon's capsule and then excising the capsule from the episclera (Fig. 37.4).

An alternative approach is to dissect Tenon's capsule from underlying episclera, strip a portion of the capsule from the conjunctiva with gentle traction, and then excise the exposed portion of capsular tissue (Fig. 37.5). With all techniques, blunt dissection is used whenever possible to avoid bleeding, and sharp dissection is used when required. Gentle handling of the conjunctiva is essential at all times, and nontoothed conjunctival forceps are preferable to avoid tearing the conjunctiva.

Fistulizing Procedure

During the fistulizing procedure, it is important to keep the conjunctival flap moist and to minimize handling of the tissue. This can be conveniently accomplished by reflecting the flap over the cornea with a moist Gelfoam sponge (Fig. 37.6). A surgical sponge can also be used to gently retract the flap.

Use of Viscoelastic Agents

The injection of a viscoelastic agent, e.g., *sodium hyaluronate,* into the anterior chamber at the completion of the filtering procedure was not found in most studies to reduce the incidence of postoperative flat anterior chambers (18, 19). However, Wand (20, 21) showed that injecting the agent through a paracentesis incision at the outset of a trabeculectomy procedure was associated with a lower incidence of this complication, presumably by avoiding intraoperative hypotony and the subsequent suprachoroidal effusion that may initiate the cascade of events leading to the condition. Others have supported his findings and noted that the technique also tends to minimize intraoperative bleeding (22) and postoperative corneal endothelial cell loss (23). Complications include iris prolapse during surgery (21), and a higher early

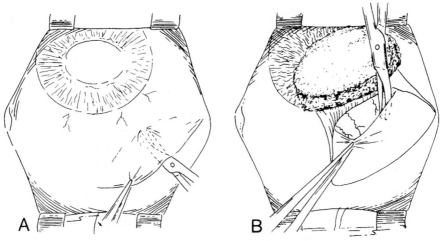

Figure 37.4. Total Tenonectomy. **A.** Blunt and sharp dissection between conjunctiva and Tenon's capsule, observing closure of blades through the conjunctiva to avoid creating a buttonhole. **B.** Dissection of Tenon's capsule from episclera, beginning with incision near limbus and extending back to site of initial conjunctival incision where the capsule is excised.

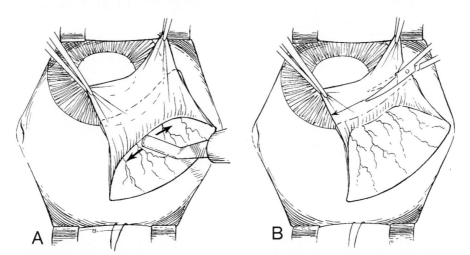

Figure 37.5. Partial Tenonectomy. **A.** Blunt dissection of Tenon's capsule from episclera. **B.** Excision of the portion of Tenon's capsule that can be stripped from conjunctiva. (Reprinted by permission from Shields, MB: Trabeculectomy vs. full-thickness filtering operation for control of glaucoma. Ophthalmic Surg 11:498, 1980.)

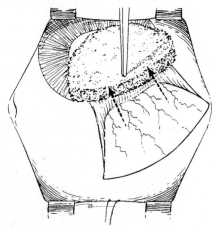

Figure 37.6. Retraction of conjunctival flap over cornea with moist Gelfoam sponge. (Reprinted by permission from Shields, MB: Trabeculectomy vs. full-thickness filtering operation for control of glaucoma. Ophthalmic Surg 11:498, 1980.)

postoperative IOP (23), for which Wand has recommended, respectively, the preoperative use of pilocarpine 2% and a slightly less tight closure of the scleral flap (21).

Peripheral Iridectomy

A peripheral iridectomy is a routine part of all standard filtering procedures, and is usually made after the fistula has been prepared (24). However, if the iris prolapses into the limbal wound, it is generally best to make the iridectomy and then complete the fistula. A large iridectomy is desirable to avoid obstruction of the fistula by the peripheral iris. The technique for the incisional peripheral iridectomy was discussed in the previous chapter.

Closure of the Conjunctival Flap

Tight wound closure is also a critical aspect of any filtering procedure, since a leaking wound may lead to a persistently flat anterior chamber and failure of the filtering bleb to develop properly. A fine suture, such as 10–0 nylon, or absorbable polyglycolic acid, or polyglactin, on a tapered, wire needle is desirable since it minimizes leakage at the suture sites, as well as excessive tissue reaction. For closure of a limbus-based flap, a running suture with close bites provides the tightest closure (Fig. 37.7). When Tenon's capsule has been preserved, a double running closure, first of the capsular tissue and then conjunctiva, increases the chances of tight wound closure. This is especially important when adjunctive antifibrosis agents are used.

A running suture can also be placed along the limbus for fornix-based flaps, especially if a small edge of conjunctiva is retained adjacent to the limbus (25). Various techniques have been described for placing a running mattress suture at the limbus, which provides tight wound closure and is especially useful when adjunctive antifibrosis agents are used

(25, 26). In other situations, surgeons find it adequate to use a single, interrupted suture at either end of the flap, which pulls the conjunctiva tightly over peripheral cornea (9).

Injection of Fluid

If a limbal stab incision was made at the outset, as previously described, a balanced salt solution is injected into the anterior chamber via that incision at two stages during the completion of the procedure. The first of these is after suturing the scleral flap in a trabeculectomy to insure appropriate flow around the flap. The anterior chamber should deepen and the eye should become slightly firm before fluid begins to flow around the flap edges. If the flow is too brisk, and the chamber collapses, more sutures should be added. Conversely, sutures may need to be loosened if the eye remains too firm. The second stage of fluid injection is after closure of the conjunctival flap (Fig. 37.8). This should deepen the anterior chamber and create a sustained elevation of the conjunctival flap, thereby demonstrating patency of the fistula and watertight closure of the conjunctival incision.

Postoperative Management

Topical mydriatic-cycloplegic and antibiotic therapy should be used routinely for the first 2–3 weeks. In addition, most surgeons prefer to use a topical corticosteroid to reduce scar formation of the filtering bleb. Other drugs which may reduce scarring of the filtering bleb will be discussed later in this chapter under "Wound Healing and Antifibrosis Therapy."

FISTULIZING TECHNIQUES

There are two basic types of fistulas: (a) those which extend through the full thickness of the limbal tissue and (b) those

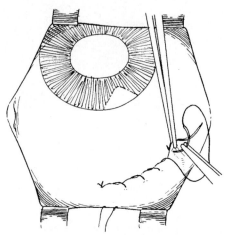

Figure 37.7. Closure of conjunctival flap with running suture. (Reprinted by permission from Shields, MB: Trabeculectomy vs. full-thickness filtering operation for control of glaucoma. Ophthalmic Surg 11:498, 1980.)

which are covered by a partial-thickness scleral flap. During the first half of the 20th century, the former technique was used exclusively. The concept of a guarded fistula (trabeculectomy) began to gain popularity in the 1970s. The relative merits of these two basic surgical approaches are discussed at the end of this chapter. With the advent of adjunctive antifibrosis agents, however, the full-thickness procedures no longer have any significant advantage over the trabeculectomy and are rarely used today. We therefore consider first the trabeculectomy techniques and then review the full-thickness procedures that were once commonly used.

Partial-Thickness Fistulas (Trabeculectomy)[a]

The standard full-thickness filtering procedures were often complicated by excessive aqueous filtration, which led to a high incidence of prolonged flat anterior chambers, associated with corneal decompensation, synechiae formation, and cataracts. In addition, the filtering blebs often became very thin and were prone to rupture, creating the danger of endophthalmitis. One way to minimize these complications is to place a partial-thickness scleral flap over the fistula. This concept was suggested by Sugar (27) in 1961, but was popularized by the 1968 report of Cairns (28). Both authors referred to the technique as a *trabeculectomy,* and it has become the standard technique for filtering surgery.

Theories of Mechanism (Fig. 37.9)

It was originally thought that aqueous might flow into the cut ends of Schlemm's canal (28). Subsequent studies, how-

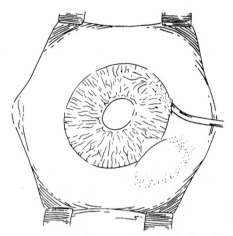

Figure 37.8. Injection of balanced salt solution into anterior chamber, with elevation of conjunctival flap.

[a]Refer to M.B. Shields: Color Atlas of Glaucoma. Baltimore: Williams & Wilkins, 1998, Plates III14–23.

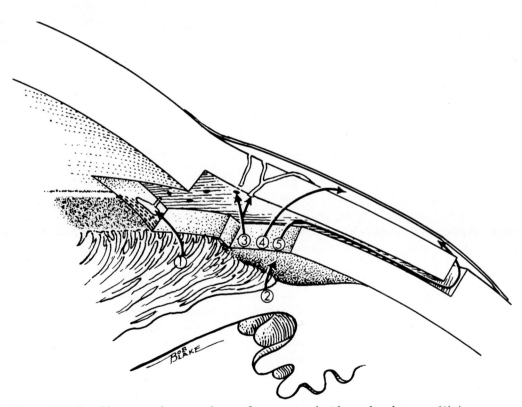

Figure 37.9. Possible routes of aqueous humor flow associated with a trabeculectomy: *(1)* Aqueous flow into cut ends of Schlemm's canal (rare); *(2)* Cyclodialysis (if tissue is dissected posterior to scleral spur); *(3)* Filtration through outlet channels in scleral flap; *(4)* Filtration through connective tissue substance of scleral flap; *(5)* Filtration around the margins of the scleral flap.

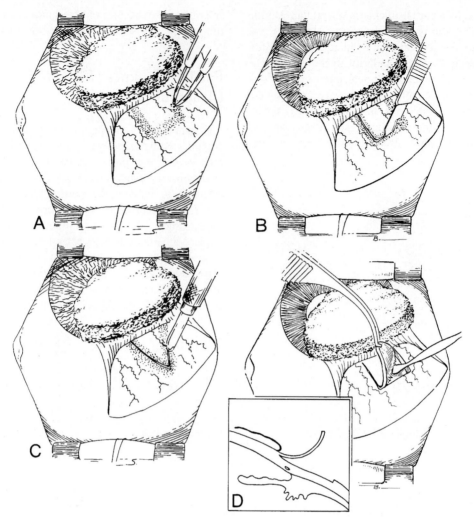

Figure 37.10. Trabeculectomy. **A.** Cauterization of area intended for margins of scleral flap.
B. Margins of scleral flap outlined by partial-thickness incisions. **C.** Triangular scleral flap
as an alternative technique. **D.** Dissection of scleral flap.

ever, showed fibrotic closure of the canal at its cut ends in
monkey (29) and human (30) eyes, and the presence of
Schlemm's canal in the "trabeculectomy" specimen did not
correlate with the outcome of the procedure (31–33). Furthermore, the majority of successful cases have a filtering
bleb (34), and the amount of fluorescein-stained aqueous in
the filtration area correlates with the success of the procedure (35), indicating that external filtration is the principal
mode of IOP reduction.

Whether the route of external filtration is primarily
through or around the partial-thickness scleral flap has also
been a matter of controversy. The outer layers of limbus and
anterior sclera do not differ ultrastructurally from the inner
layers in a way that might predispose to increased passage
of aqueous (36). Nevertheless, perfusion studies of human
autopsy eyes, in which a trabeculectomy was created and the
margins of the scleral flap were sealed with adhesive, did
show a significant flow through the scleral flap (37). However, fluorescein angiographic studies of eyes with successful trabeculectomies showed the primary route of external

filtration to be around the margins of the scleral flap (38). It
may be, therefore, that external filtration occurs by either
route, depending on how tightly the scleral flap is sutured or
how thin the flap is prepared. Other possible mechanisms of
IOP reduction by trabeculectomy include cyclodialysis (29)
or aqueous outflow through newly developed aqueous veins,
lymphatic vessels, or normal aqueous veins (39, 40).

Basic Trabeculectomy Technique (Fig. 37.10)

The margins of a 5 × 5-mm scleral flap, adjacent to the corneolimbal junction, are outlined first with light cautery and
then with partial-thickness scleral incisions. A lamellar flap,
hinged at the limbus, is then dissected forward until at least
1 mm of the bluish-gray zone is exposed. It is difficult to
precisely determine the relative thickness of the scleral flap,
but in general it should be one-half to two-thirds sclera
thickness.

The fistula is begun by first entering the anterior chamber with a knife just behind the hinge of the scleral flap, and

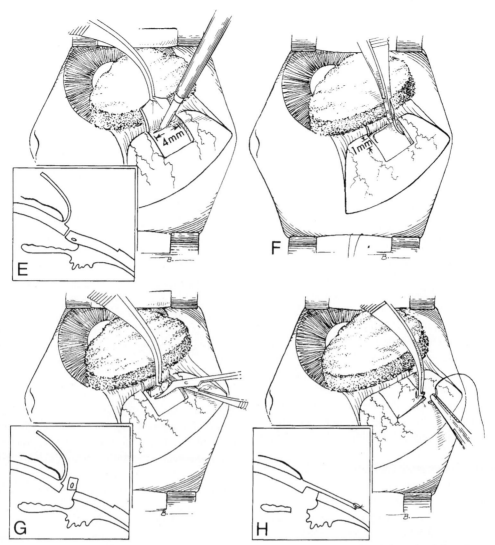

Figure 37.10. (cont'd) **E.** Anterior chamber entered just behind the hinge of the scleral flap. **F.** Completion of anterior and lateral margins of deep limbal incision with scissors. **G.** Flap of deep limbal tissue excised by cutting along scleral spur. **H.** Approximation of scleral flap. (Portions reprinted by permission from Shields, MB: Trabeculectomy vs. full-thickness filtering operation for control of glaucoma. Ophthalmic Surg 11:498, 1980.)

then widening the incision with the knife or scissors to approximately 4 mm. Radial incisions are then extended posteriorly on either end of the initial incision for 1 mm, leaving a 0.5-mm lip of sclera between the fistula and margins of the scleral flap on both sides. A 1 × 4-mm block of tissue is then reflected until the angle structures can be visualized, and the tissue is excised with scissors along the scleral spur.

After making a peripheral iridectomy, the scleral flap is then approximated with 10–0 nylon sutures. Some surgeons prefer to approximate the flap loosely with two sutures at the posterior corners to promote filtration around the margins of the scleral flap, while others use additional sutures for tighter closure to avoid the complications of hypotony and a flat anterior chamber. In one study of 339 trabeculectomies, the incidence of a shallow or flat anterior chamber was sig-

nificantly less when the flap was closed with seven to nine sutures as compared to two to six sutures (41). Tight closure is especially important when using adjunctive antifibrosis agents, since these eyes are much more prone to excessive filtration and hypotony. Most surgeons today prefer to achieve tight scleral wound closure, with the plan to lyse sutures postoperatively with an argon or diode laser, if necessary (42). An alternative to laser suture lysis is the use of releasable sutures, which can be removed, as required, at the slitlamp. Several effective techniques for releasable sutures have been described (43–47). As noted earlier in this chapter, the scleral flap can be tested for adequate flow resistance, before closing the conjunctival flap, by injecting balanced salt solution into the anterior chamber via a paracentesis.

Modifications in Technique

The numerous variations of the guarded filtering procedure that have been reported primarily involve modifications in the scleral flap or in the fistulizing technique.

VARIATIONS IN THE SCLERAL FLAP. Rather than making a square flap, some surgeons prefer a triangular (48, 49) or semicircular (50) shape. There is no apparent advantage of one shape over another with regard to long-term success. Some surgeons attempt to influence the degree of postoperative filtration by modifying the scleral flap. It has been suggested, for example, that the thickness of the flap correlates with the final IOP, in that thinner flaps provide greater filtration and lower pressures (51). Other variations in surgical technique have included attempts to enhance filtration around the flap by applying light cautery to the lateral margins (38), omitting all sutures for the scleral flap (52), or excising the distal 2 mm of the flap (52). These techniques, however, predated the era of antifibrosis agents and should be avoided when such adjunctive therapy is used.

Another variation in creating the scleral flap involves the scleral tunnel technique, as used with phacoemulsification (53). The sides of the tunnel are then incised with scissors to create the flap. Yet another technique avoids the scleral flap altogether by approaching the limbus from a partial-thickness corneal flap (54, 55). This has the potential advantage of eliminating conjunctival dissection.

VARIATIONS IN THE FISTULIZING TECHNIQUE. Watson (56, 57) modified Cairn's basic technique by starting the dissection of the tissue block posteriorly over ciliary body, separating it from the underlying structure, and excising it at Schwalbe's line. Other techniques that have been used to create the fistula beneath a scleral flap include trephinations (50, 58, 59), sclerectomies (60–62), thermal sclerostomies (63–65), and sclerostomies with a carbon dioxide laser (66).

Krasnov (67) described a procedure, called *sinusotomy*, in which a strip of sclera is excised to expose a portion of Schlemm's canal. It is not clear whether the benefit of this operation is from relieving obstruction of the scleral outlet channels or from relieving the collapse of Schlemm's canal (68, 69), or whether it is just another filtration technique. A similar technique called *nonpenetrating trabeculectomy* carries the subscleral dissection of deep limbal tissue down to Schlemm's canal, but leaves the trabecular meshwork intact (70). This is felt to be especially advantageous in aphakic eyes, and is also reported to have less postoperative complications than a standard trabeculectomy in the phakic eye (71). The technique has been modified by using the neodymium:YAG laser postoperatively to perforate the meshwork at the surgical site (72, 73).

MODIFICATIONS FOR NEOVASCULAR GLAUCOMA. As discussed in Chapter 16, intraocular surgery in eyes with neo-

vascular glaucoma is often complicated by intraoperative hyphema. One trabeculectomy variation to minimize this risk includes excision of a large trabecular segment, partial nonpenetrating cyclodiathermy in the scleral bed, and partial ablation of abnormal iris vessels with a wide sector iridectomy (74). Another technique utilizes bipolar cautery to directly treat vessels in the anterior chamber angle and the ciliary processes in the area of the filtering surgery (75). The carbon dioxide laser is felt by some surgeons to be particularly useful for creating the fistula in eyes with neovascular glaucoma, since it also cauterizes any neovascular tissue in the corneoscleral angle (76). Another surgical approach for this disorder is a pars plana filtering procedure combined with a lensectomy and vitrectomy. This was only successful in 50% of the eyes in one series (77), although success rates with other techniques are not much better when dealing with neovascular glaucoma. Drainage implant devices have also been used for this disorder and are discussed in the next chapter. The optimum approach to filtering surgery in eyes with neovascular glaucoma, however, is to precede it with panretinal photocoagulation, whenever possible, which will often reduce the rubeosis irides sufficiently to allow a standard trabeculectomy to be performed.

MODIFICATIONS FOR GLAUCOMA IN APHAKIA. The fornix-based conjunctival flap, as previously discussed (8–11), is particularly useful in eyes that have had previous intraocular surgery, especially when a fornix-based conjunctival flap was used during the cataract procedure. The conjunctiva in these eyes is usually tightly scarred down to episclera near the limbus, making preparation of a limbus-based flap difficult. When using a fornix-based flap, it is probably best to suture the lateral margins of the scleral flap to promote drainage posteriorly. An anterior vitrectomy may also be required if loose vitreous is in the anterior chamber or presents at the iridectomy site. As previously noted, nonpenetrating trabeculectomy has also been advocated for glaucoma in aphakia (70).

Wound Healing and Antifibrosis Agents[b]

The most common cause of failure in glaucoma filtering surgery is scarring of the filtering bleb (78). The increased amount of collagen in the failed blebs suggests that proliferation of fibroblasts with the associated production of collagen and glycosaminoglycans is important in the response to filtering surgery (2). However, as discussed in Chapter 34, wound healing is a complex process with several phases, and it is likely that bleb failure in filtering surgery involves many of these factors, as well as certain unique characteristics of the glaucomatous eye.

[b]Refer to M.B. Shields: Color Atlas of Glaucoma. Baltimore: Williams & Wilkins, 1998, Plate III17.

Influence of Aqueous Humor on Wound Healing

Aqueous humor normally slows or fails to support the growth of conjunctival fibroblasts in tissue culture (79–81). A possible explanation is that aqueous contains an inhibitory factor for fibroblast proliferation. Cell culture studies have shown that the high concentration of *ascorbic acid,* normally present in aqueous humor, is cytotoxic to dividing human Tenon's capsule fibroblasts, which may contribute to the development of a successful filtering bleb (82). Aqueous humor also contains a wide variety of *growth factors* which maintain the normal function of ocular tissues in health and have a significant role in abnormal states and wound healing (83). *Transforming growth factor-β,* a potent modulator of tissue repair, has been identified in human aqueous and may play a role in the healing process following glaucoma filtering surgery (84).

Contrary to the influence of primary aqueous humor, aqueous obtained shortly after intraocular surgery (81) or mixed with 20% desiccated embryo extract (85) does promote proliferation of fibroblasts. Secondary aqueous humor has also been shown to stimulate the proliferation of cultured corneal endothelial cells (86). In addition, aqueous humor has chemoattractant activity for ocular fibroblasts, and this activity is significantly greater in eyes that have previously failed glaucoma surgery (87). It may be, therefore, that components of normal aqueous humor, as well as alterations in some glaucoma patients, variably influence both success and failure of the filtering bleb.

Other Factors Influencing Wound Healing

Numerous studies have suggested that both young age and black race adversely influence the outcomes of glaucoma filtering surgery. The explanation for these observations is not clear. Histologic studies of conjunctival specimens obtained prior to trabeculectomy in patients with chronic open-angle glaucoma showed no significant influence of age or black versus white race on conjunctival factors that might relate to surgical outcome (88, 89). A more significant influence may be *chronic topical glaucoma medical therapy* prior to trabeculectomy. Some studies have identified long-term topical combination therapy as a risk factor for failure of trabeculectomy (90, 91), although one study that compared success rates before and after the introduction of topical β-blockers did not indicate that the preoperative use of topical medication influenced the outcome of surgery (92). Histologic studies of conjunctiva from patients following chronic topical glaucoma medical therapy revealed a significant degree of subclinical inflammation (93, 94), although one study could only correlate the number of goblet cells with successful outcomes (95). Conjunctival impression cytology correlated significant degrees of metaplasia with the number of glaucoma medications used (96), while a tissue culture study of human Tenon's capsule fibroblasts showed no tendency of adrenergic drugs to stimulate fibroblast proliferation (97). One clinical study, however, indicated that stopping topical adrenergic therapy and adding topical corticosteroids 1 month before surgery was associated with a decrease in the number of conjunctival fibroblasts and inflammatory cells and an improvement in the success rate of trabeculectomy (98).

Antifibrosis Agents

CORTICOSTEROIDS. Considerable attention has been given to measures, primarily in the form of drugs, that may prevent bleb failure by modulating the wound healing process. The first of these to be used clinically were the corticosteroids. Tissue culture studies of human Tenon's capsule fibroblasts have shown that both corticosteroids and nonsteroidal anti-inflammatory drugs inhibit cell attachment and proliferation (99). A rabbit study showed that topical dexamethasone prolongs the duration of a functioning filtering bleb (100), and clinical investigations have confirmed the efficacy of topical corticosteroids, although no additional benefit was achieved with systemic steroids (101–103). It has also been suggested that subconjunctival triamcinolone before filtering surgery may improve the success rate (104). In one prospective, placebo-controlled, randomized trial, the nonsteroidal anti-inflammatory drug, flurbiprofen, provided no apparent benefit following trabeculectomy surgery (105). Despite the benefit of corticosteroids, the incidence of bleb failure remains high with certain types of glaucoma, e.g., glaucomas in aphakia and pseudophakia and neovascular glaucoma, which has prompted the search for additional agents to modify wound healing.

5-FLUOROURACIL. 5-Fluorouracil (5-FU) was the first drug to be studied extensively as an adjunct to corticosteroids in the control of wound healing following trabeculectomy. This pyrimidine analogue antimetabolite, which blocks DNA synthesis through the inhibition of thymidylate synthesis, has been shown to inhibit fibroblast proliferation in cell cultures (106, 107). The subconjunctival injection of 5-FU after filtering surgery significantly improved bleb formation in monkeys (108) and improved the rate of success in difficult clinical cases (109, 110). A subsequent multicenter, randomized clinical trial of 213 patients with glaucoma in aphakia or pseudophakia or a previous failed filter in a phakic eye confirmed the ability of 5-FU to improve the success rate of filtering surgery in these high risk cases (111, 112). However, the protocol required twice daily subconjunctival injections of 5 mg 5-FU for 7 days and then once daily for 7 more days. In addition, significant complications included conjunctival wound leaks and corneal epithelial defects in the early postoperative course (111), as well as an increased risk of late-onset bleb leakage (112). Efforts have been made, therefore, to find lower effective doses, alternative delivery systems, and alternative agents.

Success has been reported with daily injections of 5 mg 5-FU for 7–14 days (113–115), which probably represents the most common range of dosages in current use. In one study of 263 patients with open-angle glaucoma, "secondary" glaucoma, or refractory glaucoma, the average total dose of 5-FU was 36.5, 36.0, and 49.5, respectively, and the probability of IOP control below 16 mm Hg with 5-year followup was 77.9%, 66.8%, and 26.9%, respectively (115). Adjunctive 5-FU has also been shown to increase the success rate of trabeculectomy in eyes undergoing initial filtering surgery (116), in young patients under 40 years of age (117, 118), as well as infants (119), and in patients requiring extremely low IOPs (120). However, the complication rate is higher than in trabeculectomy without 5-FU, and caution is advised, especially with initial surgery (112). There is a high risk of long-term failure in patients with neovascular glaucoma (121). The treatment is believed to be most effective if started prophylactically on the first postoperative day, although success has been reported with starting 3–15 days postoperatively when signs of impending bleb failure are noted (122, 123).

With regard to *alternative delivery systems,* topical 5-FU delayed bleb scarring in animal models, but had too much corneal toxicity (124). Iontophoresis was also effective in rabbits (125), but has questionable clinical application. Subconjunctival implants that provide a controlled release of 5-FU have also been evaluated. Collagen implants were not felt to be suitable because they incited a granulomatous inflammatory reaction in primates (126), and rabbits (127), although less so in guinea pigs (127). Bioerodible polymers produced less inflammation and looked promising in preliminary studies (128–130). Liposomes may also prolong the subconjunctival drug availability (131, 132). Several clinical trials have shown that 5-FU is also beneficial when used intraoperatively, usually on a surgical sponge soaked in 25–50 mg/ml of the drug and applied to the surgical site for 5 minutes (133–136).

MITOMYCIN-C. Mitomycin-C was reported by Chen (137) in 1983 to enhance the IOP lowering efficacy of trabeculectomy when applied intraoperatively in eyes at high risk of surgical failure. Mitomycin-C (MMC) is an antineoplastic antibiotic isolated from *Streptomyces caespitosus.* Tissue culture studies of human Tenon's capsule fibroblasts revealed almost complete *inhibition of fibroblast proliferation* (138), the degree of which correlated with the outcome of filtering surgery (139). When compared to 5-FU, the effect on rabbit fibroblast proliferation was much more prolonged with MMC (140) and 5-FU was toxic to cultured mouse fibroblasts while sparing bovine vascular endothelial cells, whereas MMC was cytotoxic for both cell types (141). Intraoperative application of MMC in rabbits significantly prolonged bleb duration following glaucoma filtering surgery (142).

Subsequent clinical trials supported the benefit of MMC as an adjunct to trabeculectomy (143), and randomized comparisons with postoperative subconjunctival 5-FU consistently showed intraoperative MMC to have superior IOP-lowering efficacy following trabeculectomy (144–147). MMC has been shown to enhance the success rate of tra-

beculectomy for refractory glaucoma in black patients (148), in glaucoma associated with uveitis (149), congenital and developmental glaucomas (150), normal-tension glaucoma (151), and in primary, uncomplicated trabeculectomies (152–154). However, extreme care must be exercised with the use of adjunctive MMC, especially in the primary, uncomplicated cases, because of the significant incidence of serious complications.

Although adjunctive MMC is less likely to cause the postoperative complications that are typically associated with 5-FU, such as corneal epithelial toxicity and wound leaks (144–147), it is associated with other complications that can be even more serious. The most significant of these is *hypotony maculopathy,* in which prolonged IOP reduction is associated with disc edema, vascular tortuosity, and chorioretinal folds in the macular area, with marked reduction in visual acuity (155). The main cause of the hypotony is excessive filtration, and histologic studies of excised overfiltering blebs have revealed an irregular epithelium and a largely acellular subepithelium of loosely arranged connective tissue (156–158). However, another mechanism of hypotony may be aqueous hyposecretion, since one enucleated human eye revealed disruption of the ciliary body epithelium beneath the site of MMC application (158), which has also been seen in a rabbit model (159), while a monkey study revealed suppression of aqueous humor flow (160). Other potential complications, as suggested by animal studies, include anterior chamber reaction and corneal endothelial toxicity if the MMC gets inside the eye (161, 162). The management of these complications is discussed later in this chapter under "Prevention and Management of Complications." However, the following modifications in technique may minimize the complications.

In early protocols, a sponge soaked in MMC 0.5 mg/ml was applied to the subconjunctival tissues for 5 minutes. Subsequent attempts to reduce the risk of hypotony have included reduced concentrations and exposure times (156, 163). It has also been suggested that titration of exposure time according to each patient's risk of excessive fibrosis may enhance the balance between successful IOP control and incidence of complications (156). However, the optimum protocol has yet to be established. A variety of sponges have been advocated as vehicles for the MMC, including Merocel and various microsurgical sponges, and it may be that manipulating the size or shape of the sponge can influence the effect of the MMC (164–166). One study suggested that placing the sponge beneath the scleral flap, rather than over intact episclera, may improve the success rate without increasing complications (167). It has also been shown in rabbits that irrigating the ocular tissues with balanced salt solution after removal of the sponge substantially reduces intraocular diffusion of MMC (168).

ALTERNATIVE AGENTS. Alternative agents that have been evaluated as antiproliferative drugs include cytosine arabinoside (169–171), bleomycin (169), rapamycin (172), doxorubicin (106), daunorubicin (173), 5-fluorouridine

5'-monophosphate (131), 5-fluoroorotate (132), heparin (174), taxol (175), cytochalasin-B (175), colchicine (175), immunotoxins (176), and interferon-α-2b (177, 178). Beta irradiation was also shown to inhibit fibroblast proliferation in tissue culture (179, 180) and to delay wound healing in rabbits (181). Beta irradiation was not found to be effective in a preliminary clinical trial in improving the results of trabeculectomies (182), although a study of patients aged 18 years or less with congenital glaucoma suggested a beneficial effect on the prognosis of trabeculectomy (183). In addition to drugs that influence fibroblast proliferation, agents have also been evaluated that will alter other phases of the wound healing process. For example, tissue plasminogen activator, which causes localized fibrinolysis (184–186), γ-interferon (187–189) and calcium ionophores (190), which inhibit collagen biosynthesis, and β-aminoproprionitrile (191, 192) and D-penicillamine (100, 191), which inhibit cross-linking of collagen, have shown promise in in vitro and in vivo studies. In the future, it is likely that combinations of agents will be administered according to the various phases of the wound healing process in an effort to prevent bleb failure.

Earlier Full-Thickness Fistulas

The original type of limbal fistula, which has been largely replaced by trabeculectomy with or without adjunctive antifibrosis agents, involves creation of a direct opening through the full thickness of the limbal tissue. The fistula may be created by a variety of techniques.

Sclerectomy

In 1906, LaGrange (193) described a technique in which a full-thickness limbal incision was made, and a piece of tissue was then excised from the anterior lip of the wound to create a limbal fistula. Holth (194) modified this procedure 3 years later by performing the sclerectomy with a punch. Subsequent surgical variations included excision of tissue from both the anterior and posterior lips of the circumferential incision (195, 196) or from the lateral lip of a radial incision (197). However, the sclerectomy technique that became most popular in the mid-20th century was the *posterior lip sclerectomy* as described by Iliff and Haas (198).

TECHNIQUE (FIG. 37.11). A scratch incision is begun just behind the insertion of the conjunctival flap in an area of sclera that has been lightly cauterized. The incision is beveled inward at an angle of approximately 75% to the limbal surface and is continued until the anterior chamber is entered. Scissors are then used to widen the incision to about 5 mm.

A sclerectomy punch, such as a 1.5-mm Holth punch, is used to excise full-thickness limbal tissue from the posterior lip of the incision, creating a fistula of approximately 1×3 mm. Care must be taken to avoid cutting into the ciliary body, which can lead to significant bleeding.

MODIFICATIONS. This technique may be modified slightly by applying light cautery to the posterior margins of the sclerectomy, which further enlarges the fistula and may help to inhibit postoperative scarring (199). Sclerectomy punches have also been modified. One popular instrument is the Gass sclerectomy punch, which is a guillotine-type punch designed to excise a 1.5-mm semicircle of tissue (200). The latter instrument has been further modified by rotating the opening of the punch 45° away from the handle to facilitate better visualization under the operating microscope (201).

Trephination

In 1909, Elliot (202) and Fergus (203) both described a glaucoma filtering procedure in which the fistula was created with a small trephine placed just behind the corneolimbal junction. Elliot (204) later modified the technique by splitting the peripheral cornea and placing the trephine more anteriorly (sclerocorneal trephining). However, this modification produced a thinner filtering bleb with a greater chance of late infection, and Sugar (205) advocated a return to the original, more posterior placement of the trephine, which he called limboscleral trephination (or trepanation). The subsequent experience of Sugar (206) and others supported the merit of this technique.

TECHNIQUE (FIG. 37.12). A 1.5- or 2.0-mm trephine blade is placed over the limbus just behind the corneolimbal junction. The trephine is tilted forward so that the anterior edge of the blade enters the anterior chamber first. Entry into the anterior chamber is usually indicated by a movement of the upper pupillary margin toward the trephine. The trephine button, which is hinged on the scleral side and may rotate forward due to prolapse of the iris, is excised by cutting across the hinge with scissors. As with other filtering procedures, care must be taken to avoid cutting into the ciliary body.

Thermal Sclerostomy (Scheie Procedure)

In 1924, Preziosi (207) described a filtering technique in which a limbal fistula was created by entering the anterior chamber angle with an electrocautery instrument. Scheie (208) later described a procedure which also utilized cautery but differed from the Preziosi operation in that a limbal scratch incision was first made, and the cautery was then used to retract the wound edges, thereby creating the fistula.

TECHNIQUE (FIG. 37.13). Light cautery is applied to the sclera in a 1×5 mm area behind the corneolimbal junction. A 5-mm limbal scratch incision is then made through the cauterized area, perpendicular to the scleral surface, and cautery is applied to the lips of the incision until the wound edges separate by at least 1 mm.

The escape of aqueous from the limbal incision may interfere with the application of cautery, and this can be partially avoided by stopping the initial scratch incision just

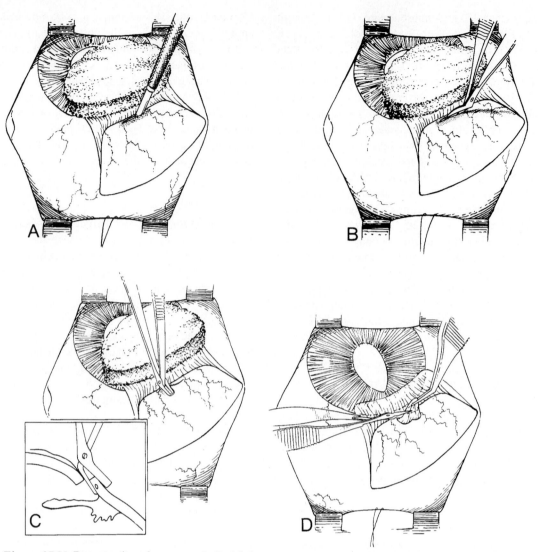

Figure 37.11. Posterior lip sclerectomy. **A.** Beveled incision into anterior chamber. **B.** Enlargement of limbal incision with scissors. **C.** Excision of full-thickness tissue from posterior lip of incision with sclerectomy punch. **D.** Peripheral iridectomy created as for all standard filtering procedures. (Portions reprinted by permission from Shields, MB: Trabeculectomy vs. full-thickness filtering operation for control of glaucoma. Ophthalmic Surg 11:498, 1980.)

before it enters the anterior chamber, applying cautery, and then completing the incision (209). In addition, bipolar cautery can be effectively used in the wet field. Another modification is to place a temporary suture across the fistula to avoid an early flat anterior chamber (210).

Iridencleisis

This procedure differs from the other forms of full-thickness filtering surgery in that a wedge of iris is incarcerated into the limbal incision in an effort to maintain a patent channel for aqueous outflow. This was once a popular procedure, but it lost favor partly due to the suspicion that the associated incidence of sympathetic ophthalmia was higher than with other filtering procedures. Although this fear was not substantiated, the operation never regained popularity.

NEWER LASER AND OTHER SCLEROSTOMY TECHNIQUES[c]

Laser Sclerostomy Ab Externo

Laser energy has also been used to create the fistula, most of which are full thickness. This can either be performed from either an ab externo or ab interno approach. The argon laser has been studied for the former approach (211), although the *holmium laser,* also referred to as THC:YAG (thulium, holmium, and chromium-doped yttrium-aluminum-garnet crystal) laser, has undergone the most extensive evaluation for laser sclerostomy ab externo. The laser operates in the

[c]Refer to M.B. Shields: Color Atlas of Glaucoma. Baltimore: Williams & Wilkins, 1998, Plate III17

near-infrared region with a wavelength of 2100 nm. A right-angle exit of the laser beam from the tip of the fiberoptic probe allows subconjunctival advancement of the probe from a small conjunctival incision to the limbus where the fistula is created. Rabbit studies supported the feasibility of the procedure (212, 213), and preliminary clinical trials provided encouraging short-term results (214, 215). Longer followup, however, revealed estimated probabilities of success of approximately 65% at 1 year (216, 217) and 57% at 30 months (218). One small study revealed an estimated success of 31% at 9 months (219).

Failure of holmium laser ab externo sclerostomy appears to be related to occlusion of the external portion of the scle-rostomy by scar tissue, which was observed histologically in a trabeculectomy specimen that was excised 3 months after the holmium sclerostomy (220). Rabbit studies suggest it might be possible to improve the success rate by using pre-operative subconjunctival mitomycin-C (221), or by using an erbium:YAG laser, which creates a smaller thermal dam-age zone around the fistula (222). Another complication is early hypotony due to the full-thickness nature of the fistula, and performing the sclerostomy within a one-third-thickness corneal pocket beneath the conjunctiva has been suggested as a way to reduce this problem (223).

Other lasers that have been evaluated for laser scleros-tomy ab externo include a giant-pulsed (up to 200 W of peak

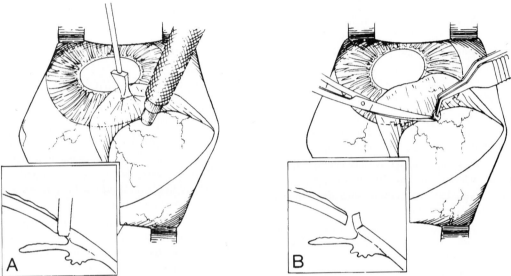

Figure 37.12. Limboscleral trephination. **A.** Trephine button partially excised by tilting the trephine an-teriorly. **B.** Completion of excision by cutting posterior attachment with scissors.

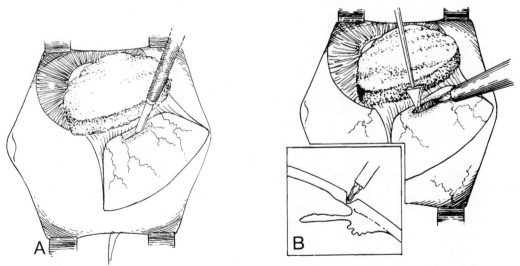

Figure 37.13. Thermal sclerostomy. **A.** Limbal incision created (may initially be partial- or full-thickness). **B.** Application of cautery to the lips of the incision to separate the wound edges. A par-tial-thickness incision is then extended into the anterior chamber and cautery is applied to the depths of the wound.

power at pulses of 20 or 40 msec) Nd:YAG laser (224), a picosecond Nd:YLF (yttrium-lithium-fluoride) 1053 nm laser (225, 226), a semiconductor diode laser (227), and a 193-nm excimer laser (228). Excimer lasers have also been used in a modified trabeculectomy to precisely remove scleral tissue overlying Schlemm's canal, leaving the trabecular meshwork intact (229, 230).

Laser Sclerostomy Ab Interno

In addition to creating full-thickness fistulas with laser energy from the external approach, lasers and other instruments are being evaluated to create sclerostomies ab interno, i.e., from the anterior chamber to the subconjunctival space. The main theoretic advantage of this technique is that it requires no dissection of the conjunctiva, which is elevated prior to creating the sclerostomy with a fluid injection over the surgical site, thereby reducing the risk of scarring and bleb failure. The first attempt at laser sclerostomy ab interno was made with a Q-switched neodymuim:YAG laser, focused into the anterior chamber angle through a special gonioprism (231–233). This was shown to be effective in creating a sclerostomy, but required very high levels of energy. Subsequent modifications involved staining the sclera with methylene blue dye by iontophoresis and using a pulsed dye laser with a wavelength of 660 nm, which is maximally absorbed by methylene blue (234–236). This concept is attractive since it would allow filtering surgery to be performed in the office with rapid postoperative recovery. However, further refinement is needed before it is likely to achieve widespread clinical acceptance.

Most attempts with laser sclerostomy ab interno have utilized contact laser probes, the tip of which is introduced into the anterior chamber via a limbal incision 180° from the sclerostomy site. The tip is passed across the anterior chamber to the trabecular meshwork where the sclerostomy is created (Fig. 37.14). This technique has been evaluated with continuous-wave neodymium:YAG lasers (237–240), high-energy argon blue-green laser (241, 242), and excimer (243), erbium (244), diode (245), and Nd:YLF (246) lasers. Rabbit studies of Nd:YAG, holmium, and erbium lasers indicate that increasing wavelengths are associated with decreasing thermal damage around the sclerostomy, which would theoretically decrease subconjunctival scarring and filtration failure (247, 248).

A modification of laser sclerostomy ab interno is the creation of a small lamellar corneal incision near the sclerostomy through which the laser probe is introduced. Using a straight probe holmium laser and adjunctive subconjunctival mitomycin-C, this technique appeared to be promising in a preliminary rabbit study (249).

Other Internal Sclerostomy Techniques

Internal sclerostomies have also been successfully performed with an automated trephine (250, 251), and bipolar cautery (252) and diathermy (253) probes. It is likely that other instruments and techniques will be evaluated in the future, as this promising approach to glaucoma filtering surgery continues to evolve.

PREVENTION AND MANAGEMENT OF COMPLICATIONS[d]

The following complications may occur with any filtering procedure, although some operations and techniques appear to provide certain advantages over others. We first consider the complications in general and then compare the merits of the various filtering procedures. It is helpful to think of these complications in three phases: intraoperative, early postoperative, and late postoperative.

Intraoperative Complications

Tearing or Buttonholing the Conjunctival Flap

The conjunctiva may be inadvertently torn or cut during preparation or closure of the flap. This complication can be minimized by gentle handling of the tissues as outlined earlier in this chapter. When it does occur, it may be possible to close the defect using fine suture on a round, tapered needle. Nylon suture has been used for this purpose (254), although 10–0 polyglycolic acid or polyglactin has the advantage of being absorbable. With small holes the tissue can be puckered together with a figure eight or mattress suture, while a large tear may require a running suture. Tissue adhesive (255) and light bipolar cautery may also be used to close small holes, but these methods are less reliable than suturing.

Hemorrhage

Episcleral bleeding is particularly common in glaucoma patients who have been on long-term antiglaucoma medication. It can be managed with irrigation or light cautery, and should be under control before the anterior chamber is entered. Once inside the eye, inadvertent cutting of the ciliary body may cause brisk bleeding. Cauterization is difficult in these cases, although the intraocular, bipolar units at a low setting are usually effective. Alternative management involves gentle, sustained pressure over the fistula with a sponge or a large air bubble in the anterior chamber. A choroidal, or expulsive, hemorrhage is a particularly devastating complication that usually results from sudden reduction in the IOP with rupture of a large choroidal vessel. The most important step in the management of these cases is immediate closure of the fistula. Some surgeons will make a scleral incision in the inferior temporal quadrant to allow the blood to drain from this site until it stops spontaneously, although the value of this approach has not been substantiated.

[d]Refer to M.B. Shields: Color Atlas of Glaucoma. Baltimore: Williams & Wilkins, 1998, Plates III25–26.

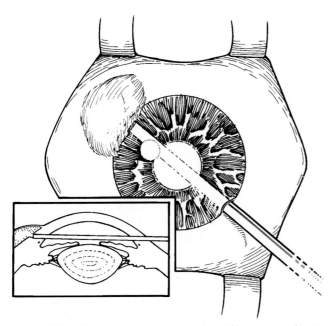

Figure 37.14. Internal sclerostomy. A laser fiberoptic probe tip or automated trephine is inserted into the anterior chamber through a limbal stab incision and is used to create a full-thickness fistula beneath elevated conjunctiva 180° from the entry site.

Hemorrhage into the lens has also been reported as a rare complication of glaucoma surgery (256).

Choroidal Effusion

This complication may occur during glaucoma filtering surgery, especially in eyes with prominent episcleral vessels, as in cases of Sturge-Weber syndrome (257). The suprachoroidal fluid in these cases contains very little protein (18% of plasma concentration), suggesting that a pressure differential drives fluid and small molecules from choroidal capillaries into extravascular spaces (258). This complication is usually recognized by a sudden shallowing of the anterior chamber during the operation or by the rotation of ciliary processes through the iridectomy and into the surgical fistula. If severe, it can be managed by making a scleral incision to release the suprachoroidal fluid (257).

Other Intraoperative Complications

Vitreous loss may occur during creation of the fistula or iridectomy, due to rupture of the lens zonules and hyaloid membrane, which usually results from excessive manipulation. The vitreous should be removed from the surgical site with sponges and scissors or a vitrectomy instrument. *Lens injury* may remain limited to the surgical site if it is small, while larger injuries may cause gradual widespread extension or acute cataract formation, occasionally with severe uveitis (259). *Stripping of Descemet's membrane* during glaucoma surgery with subsequent corneal edema has also been reported (260). The *scleral flap* may be inadvertently

torn from its limbal hinge, in which case it can be reattached with 10–0 nylon mattress sutures (261) or, if the flap is too thin, it can be replaced with donor sclera (262).

Early Postoperative Complications

During the first few days or weeks after a filtering procedure, the complications most often faced by the surgeon are either an IOP that is too low (hypotony) or too high. In either case, the anterior chamber may be shallow to flat or deep. It is important to be familiar with the mechanisms that can lead to the resulting four categories of complications and how they can be managed.

Hypotony and Flat Anterior Chamber

A low, often unrecordable, IOP is common during the early postoperative period, and is typically associated with a shallow anterior chamber. The anterior chamber is usually shallowest on postoperative day 2 or 3 and gradually deepens over the next 2 weeks (263). It is important to distinguish between a *shallow anterior chamber* with iridocorneal touch and a *flat anterior chamber* with cornea-lens touch since the management and prognosis differ significantly (264). In the former situation, the cornea is typically clear and the iris stroma has not been flattened by the gentle touch with the cornea (Fig. 37.15). In most of these eyes the anterior

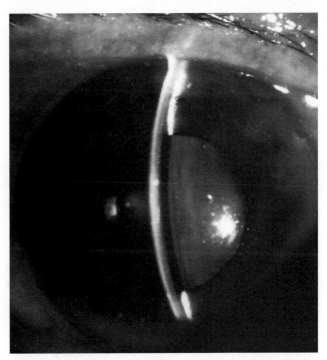

Figure 37.15. Slitlamp appearance of shallow anterior chamber in early postoperative period following a trabeculectomy showing iridocorneal touch with separation between cornea and lens. (Reprinted by permission from Stewart, WC, Shields, MB: Management of anterior chamber depth after trabeculectomy. Am J Ophthalmol 106:41, 1988.)

chamber will deepen spontaneously with time and requires no special management beyond the usual postoperative care. The prolonged shallow anterior chamber may be associated with a reduced corneal endothelial cell count (265) and some synechiae formation (266). However these sequelae do not usually influence the long-term outcome and must be weighed against the risk of interfering with the bleb function by premature intervention. If the shallow chamber persists beyond the first week or two, measures to reform the anterior chamber are usually indicated. With a truly flat anterior chamber, however, in which the cornea is swollen and the iris stroma is flattened, immediate postoperative management is required to avoid a poor surgical result.

As in all cases, the best way to deal with a potential complication is to take steps to avoid it. Careful wound closure, as discussed earlier in this chapter, is one such step toward avoiding a flat anterior chamber. Another measure that was discussed earlier is the injection of a viscoelastic into the anterior chamber. Most studies have shown that this does not reduce the incidence of flat anterior chambers when injected at the end of the filtering procedure (18, 19),

although deepening the anterior chamber with sodium hyaluronate at the beginning of the operation and maintaining the chamber depth throughout the procedure may result in deeper chambers postoperatively (20, 21).

When hypotony and a flat anterior chamber do occur, the first step is to determine the cause and then take the appropriate steps to correct it. We now consider these causes and how they can be managed.

CONJUNCTIVAL DEFECT. If there is an obvious hole in the conjunctival flap or a leak at the wound edge, it may be possible to achieve spontaneous closure with a pressure patch (Fig. 37.16). A fusiform-shaped cotton ball can be placed over the lid in the area of the fistula and held in place with the gauze pads to act as a tamponade. If this type of pressure dressing is used, the patient should be kept awake, with the fellow eye open and looking straight ahead, since the Bell's phenomenon of sleep may place the tamponade over the center of the cornea. Examination several hours later (the pressure patch is usually left on from morning until evening) often reveals closure of the defect

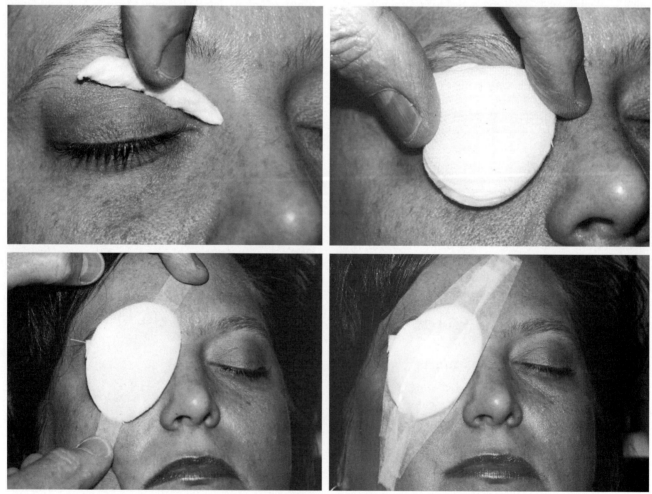

Figure 37.16. Pressure patch technique for eye with flat anterior chamber due to excessive filtration in early postoperative period. **A.** Fusiform-shaped cotton ball placed over upper lid in location corresponding to surgical fistula. **B.** Folded eye pad placed just below brow. **C.** Second, open eye pad positioned. **D.** Multiple strips of tape applied with moderate tension.

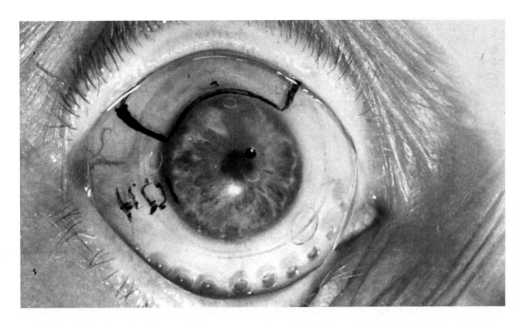

Figure 37.17. Simmons shell with tamponade positioned over surgical site prior to application of pressure patch for management of filtering bleb with leak or excessive filtration. (Courtesy of Richard J. Simmons, M.D.)

and reformation of the anterior chamber. If the leaking defect persists, however, a scleral shell tamponade (Simmons shell) (267), symblepharon-ring (268), or large diameter (20.5-mm) therapeutic soft contact lens (269) may be effective. With the Simmons shell, the tamponade portion is placed over the defective area (Fig. 37.17) and secured with a tight pressure dressing. The dressing should be changed daily with examination of the eye through the shell, but the shell can be left in place for 3 days, which gives the defect more time to heal. In some cases, placing a bandage contact lens beneath the shell provides improved patient comfort. If patching with a shell or lens is also not successful, some surgeons have found that the leak can be closed with cyanoacrylate tissue adhesive (270, 271), possibly covered by a collagen shield (272), autologous fibrin glue (273, 274), or blue-green argon laser applications after pretreatment of the bleb with rose bengal (275). Other cases may require suturing of the defect (254, 276) or, when the defect is large, it may be necessary to develop a new conjunctival flap from tissue posterior to the defect (277) or free conjunctival autografts (278, 279).

EXCESSIVE FILTRATION. In other cases, there may be no apparent conjunctival defect or wound leak, but filtration may simply be excessive due to a large fistula or an exceptionally large filtering bleb. It is in this regard that trabeculectomies are felt to offer one advantage over full-thickness filtering procedures, since the protective scleral flap minimizes excessive filtration. With the advent of antimetabolite adjunctive therapy, however, there is a tendency for increased flow of aqueous around the scleral flap and through the conjunctival bleb, and overfiltration has again become a common early postoperative complication. To minimize this risk, as discussed earlier in this chapter, some surgeons choose to increase the protective aspect of a trabeculectomy by using multiple nylon sutures for tight closure of the scleral flap.

Sutures can be selectively cut postoperatively with a laser if filtration is inadequate (42, 280). Other surgeons prefer to secure the scleral flap with releasable sutures, which can be removed postoperatively as needed (43–47, 281).

If the early postoperative period is complicated by excessive filtration with a flat anterior chamber and corneal decompensation, the first step is usually firm patching of the eye, as described above, often with the addition of the Simmons shell or other tamponading device. If the chamber depth cannot be maintained after several days, and especially if corneal decompensation is present, surgical intervention is usually indicated. It may be sufficient to deepen the anterior chamber with balanced salt solution, sodium hyaluronate (282), a large air bubble (283), or a gas such as perfluoropropane (284) or sulfur hexafluoride. The air and gases are more toxic than balanced salt solution or viscoelastics and can cause cataract formation (284–286). A rabbit study, however, suggests that 15% perfluoropropane or 50% sulfur hexafluoride are no more toxic than air and may be beneficial and relatively safe in reforming persistently flat anterior chambers (286).

SEROUS CHOROIDAL DETACHMENTS. Anterior chamber deepening alone may not be sufficient if large choroidal detachments are also present. Fluid commonly collects in the suprachoroidal space in hypotonus eyes. Hypotony is generally felt to contribute to the mechanism of choroidal detachments, although additional factors, such as inflammation and venous congestion, also appear to be important (287). The fluid in the detachments is high in protein (67% of plasma concentration), suggesting that a pressure differential causes fluid with small- and medium-size protein molecules to pass from choroidal capillaries to extravascular spaces (258, 288). The choroidal detachment apparently prolongs the hypotony by reducing aqueous production and possibly by increasing uveoscleral outflow.

Most serous choroidal detachments resolve spontaneously along with the normal rise in IOP during the first few postoperative days or weeks. If limited in size and duration, they do not interfere with the long-term outcome of trabeculectomy surgery (289), and it is usually only necessary to drain them when they are associated with a persistent flat anterior chamber or if a choroidal hemorrhage is suspected (290). The technique involves draining the suprachoroidal fluid through sclerotomies in the two inferior quadrants and deepening the anterior chamber with a balanced salt solution or viscoelastic.

Much less commonly, a *serous retinal detachment* may occur after glaucoma filtering surgery, presumably by a mechanism similar to that for choroidal detachments (291). These typically resolve spontaneously, although the patient may not regain the full preoperative visual acuity.

Hypotony and Deep Anterior Chamber

A lower than normal IOP during the first week or two after trabeculectomy usually does not constitute a complication, provided there are no related problems, such as wound leak, excessive inflammation, flat anterior chamber or posterior pole abnormality. If the hypotony persists, however, it can lead to one of the most serious complications, which has been referred to as *hypotony maculopathy*. The typical fundus findings include fine macular striae radiating from the fovea, often with more extensive choroidal folds and tortuous retinal vessels and occasional disc swelling, but no evidence of vascular leakage. The visual acuity is markedly reduced. Not all patients with subnormal IOP will develop the maculopathy, and risk factors for the complication includes young age, myopia, and the preoperative use of carbonic anhydrase inhibitors (292, 293). The hypotony can occur with any filtering surgery technique, although the incidence has increased with the adjunctive use of antimetabolites, as discussed earlier in this chapter. It has been reported with 5-FU (292, 293), but has been especially prevalent with adjunctive *mitomycin-C,* which appears to be influenced by the concentration and exposure time of the drug (294).

As previously discussed, the best approach to the problem is prevention by minimizing the use of antimetabolites and employing tight wound closure. When the complication does occur it is difficult to treat. Standard measures, such as pressure patching or the application of trichloroacetic acid or cryotherapy to the bleb, are rarely effective. Some success has been reported with the injection of autologous blood into the bleb (295–298). The application of high-energy, thermal-pulsed Nd:YAG laser to the base of the bleb has also been reported to be effective in some patients (437). When these measures are not successful, surgical revision of the filtering procedure is usually indicated. Reported surgical approaches have included resuturing the scleral flap (299) and donor scleral patch grafting (300, 301). Another effective technique is to excise the filtering bleb, undermine adjacent conjunctiva, and pull it down to the limbus to create a new filtering bleb (156). It is not clear how long an eye can tolerate hypotony maculopathy before the visual loss is irreversible, but return of good vision has been reported when the overfiltration was reversed within 6 months of the onset of the complication (299).

Elevated Intraocular Pressure and Flat Anterior Chamber

An elevated IOP with a flat anterior chamber in the early postoperative course suggests one of three mechanisms: (a) malignant (ciliary block) glaucoma, (b) an incomplete iridectomy with pupillary block, or (c) a delayed suprachoroidal hemorrhage. The diagnosis and management of these conditions was considered in Chapter 23, and the following are a few additional details regarding the delayed hemorrhage.

DELAYED SUPRACHOROIDAL HEMORRHAGES. Delayed suprachoroidal hemorrhages following filtering surgery typically present during the first few postoperative days with severe pain, occasional nausea, and a marked reduction in vision. The IOP is usually, but not always, elevated, the anterior chamber is shallow or flat, and large choroidal detachments, often with central touch, are present. Based on retrospective studies, the complication is uncommon, occurring in less than 2% of most large series (302–305). However, in a prospective ultrasonographic evaluation of 158 patients after filtering surgery, delayed suprachoroidal hemorrhage was detected in 11 (7%), suggesting that most cases go clinically unrecognized (306). In addition, the incidence goes up considerably with certain risk factors, especially aphakia and vitrectomy (302–306). In one series of 305 filtering procedures, the overall incidence of delayed suprachoroidal hemorrhage was 1.6%, but this rose to 13% in aphakic eyes, and to 33% of aphakic, vitrectomized eyes (304). Not all cases require surgical correction, and in those that do it is best to wait until the clotted blood has lysed. In one series, monitored by echography, the mean time for clot lysis was 14 days and the mean duration of central retinal apposition was 15 days (307). The visual prognosis is worse with associated retinal detachment and 360° suprachoroidal hemorrhage, both of which constitute indications for surgical intervention (308), along with kissing choroidal detachments, vitreous incarceration (309), and vitreoretinal adhesions (310). Surgical intervention is usually limited to drainage of the hemorrhage through anterior sclerostomies, with vitrectomy reserved for vitreous incarceration (309) or vitreoretinal adhesions (310).

Elevated Intraocular Pressure and Deep Anterior Chamber

An elevated IOP with a deep anterior chamber indicates inadequate filtration due to (a) obstruction of the fistula by iris, ciliary processes, lens, or vitreous, or (b) an absent or poorly functioning filtering bleb. Chances of the former complication may be minimized during surgery by making an adequate fistula and iridectomy and by avoiding excessive surgical manipulation. When faced with a high pressure and deep anterior chamber, the possibility of obstruction of the fistula should first be evaluated by gonioscopy. If iris or ciliary processes are obstructing the fistula, it may be possible to retract the tissue with the application of low-energy argon laser therapy. If the internal obstruction cannot be eliminated, it is usually necessary to resume antiglaucoma medication and possibly to revise the procedure or repeat it at a later date. If fistula obstruction is not found, attention must then be given to bleb failure which, as discussed earlier in this chapter, is the most common cause of failure in glaucoma filtering surgery (78).

MANAGEMENT OF THE FAILING BLEB. The filtering bleb in these cases is typically low to flat and heavily vascularized with no microcysts (Fig. 37.18). The operation is doomed to failure unless immediate, aggressive steps are taken. Corticosteroid therapy should be increased, such as drops every 1–2 hours, occasionally with the addition of subconjunctival steroids. As previously noted, subconjunctival 5-FU may also be effective even if started several days after the surgery (122).

Intermittent application of *digital pressure* should also be used in an attempt to expand the subconjunctival space by forcing aqueous into it. This is usually performed by applying steady pressure with the index fingers to the inferior sclera through the lower lid for approximately 15 seconds (Fig. 37.19). If the digital pressure lowers the tension and ex-

pands the bleb, the patient may be instructed to perform the procedure at home several times each day. A modification of digital pressure, especially following trabeculectomy, involves pressing an anesthetic-moistened applicator beside the edge of the scleral flap (311). If the IOP cannot be lowered by digital pressure, the next step is usually laser suture lysis (312–315) or removal of a releasable suture. The argon laser is most commonly used for suture lysis, with typical settings of 50 μm, 0.02–0.1-second duration, and 300–1000 mW of power (315), although a lower energy of 250 mW and 0.02 second has also been reported to be effective (313). Other lasers may also be effective, including krypton (315) and diode (314), and a laser lens holder has been developed for performing diode laser suture lysis in children under anesthesia (314). If suture lysis or release is not effective, or if a blood/fibrin clot appears to be obstructing the fistula, intracameral *tissue plasminogen activator* may be beneficial (316–319). The recommended intracameral dosage is 6–12.5 μg (319). A subconjunctival dose of 25 μg was also reported to be successful in releasing a trabeculectomy flap that appeared to be adherent to its scleral bed (326).

When these measures fail, glaucoma medications should be resumed. Revision of a flat, vascularized bleb has a low chance of success, but can be tried. In most cases, a repeat filtering procedure with adjunctive mitomycin-C or 5-FU will eventually be required.

ENCAPSULATED FILTERING BLEB. These blebs, which have also been called Tenon's capsule cysts (321) and high bleb phase (322), are characterized by a highly elevated, smooth-domed bleb with large vessels, but intervening avascular

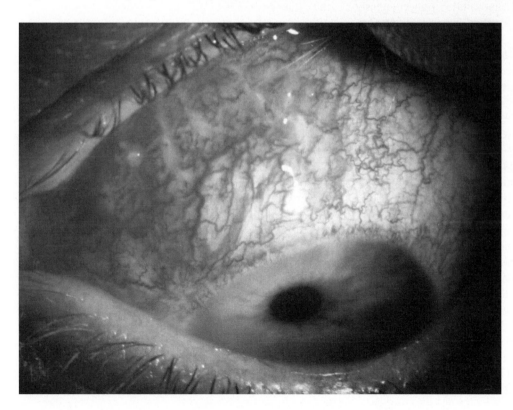

Figure 37.18. Typical appearance of a failing filtering bleb characterized by a low-to-flat, heavily vascularized conjunctiva.

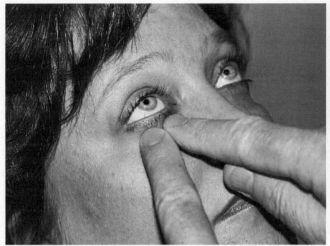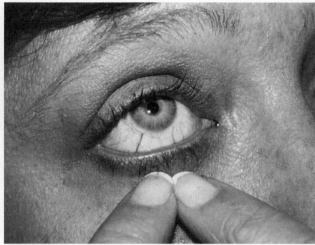

Figure 37.19. Digital pressure for eye with failing filtering bleb. **A.** Application of pressure by physician. **B.** Application of pressure by patient.

spaces and no microcysts (Fig. 37.20). Movement of the conjunctiva will reveal a second, stationary set of vessels beneath the conjunctiva, which is in the layer of fibrous tissue that lines the bleb. It is important to distinguish this type of bleb from the typical failing bleb, as previously discussed. Both are associated with an elevated IOP and deep anterior chamber in the early postoperative period, but the prognosis and management differ significantly.

Encapsulated blebs are common, occurring in 10–14% of reported series (321–323). These observations were made in the 1980s, raising the question as to whether treatment modalities that became popular during that time, such as β-adrenergic inhibitors and argon laser trabeculoplasty, might be responsible for the apparent increase in this complication. As previously discussed, long-term topical glaucoma therapy may be a risk factor for failure of trabeculectomy (90, 91), and it has been associated with increased inflammation of the conjunctiva and Tenon's capsule following filtering surgery (324). However, no clear cause-and-effect relationship has been established between any glaucoma drug and encapsulated blebs. Reports are conflicting regarding the influence of argon laser trabeculoplasty (325, 326). Adjunctive 5-FU may reduce the incidence of encapsulated blebs (327), although mitomycin-C may actually increase it, with a reported incidence of 29% in one series (328).

The encapsulated bleb usually appears during the first postoperative month. In managing them, it is important to be aware that most will begin functioning well within another few months. It is generally agreed that the mainstay of treatment is to resume glaucoma medication until the improvement occurs (329). Opinions differ, however, as to whether steroids and digital pressure should be used. One study suggested that prolonged steroid therapy may actually increase the incidence of encapsulated blebs (330), and it has been postulated that digital pressure may further reduce aqueous flow through the encapsulated bleb by compressing the subconjunctival layer of tissue (322). Those blebs that fail to re-

spond to conservative medical management may be restored surgically. One such technique is called *needling,* in which a needle, e.g., 25–30-gauge, is passed beneath the conjunctiva about 5–10 mm from the bleb, is used to balloon up the conjunctiva, and is then used to puncture and incise the fibrous episcleral tissue (331). An effective modification is to inject 5 mg of 5-FU (0.5 cc of 10 mg/ml) subconjunctivally at the time of the needling (332–334), although higher dosages should be avoided since they can cause corneal endothelial toxicity (335). A more involved, but possibly more definitive, technique is to dissect the conjunctiva from the mound of fibrous tissue, completely excise the latter, and resuture the conjunctiva (336).

Other Early Postoperative Complications

UVEITIS AND HYPHEMA. Anterior uveitis is seen to some degree during the early postoperative period in all patients. It is routinely managed with topical corticosteroids and a mydriatic-cycloplegic. When the inflammation is excessive (3+ flare and cell or fibrinoid iritis), increasing the frequency of the steroids to every hour or two is usually sufficient, and only rarely is stronger anti-inflammatory therapy required. Hyphema is less common and is usually managed conservatively with elevation of the head and limited activity. One study showed that the incidence of hyphema was 18% if the fistula was kept anterior to scleral spur, but rose to 56% if the excision of the fistula was extended posterior to scleral spur (337).

DELLEN. Dellen adjacent to large filtering blebs may occur during the early or late postoperative period. Most heal uneventfully with tear film replacements, although some may progress to corneal ulcers (338).

LOSS OF CENTRAL VISION. Loss of central vision (snuff out syndrome) may occur after glaucoma filtering surgery. Most studies have shown this to be uncommon (339–343). In one study of 508 eyes of 440 patients, snuff out occurred in four eyes (0.8%) (342). Risk factors included older age, preoperative macular splitting in the visual field, and severe hypotony. Although a small central island or split fixation is generally not considered to be a contraindication to glaucoma filtering surgery (339–343), it has been emphasized that it is a significant risk in predisposed patients (344), and the patient should be made aware of the risk and efforts should be made to minimize postoperative hypotony.

OCULAR DECOMPRESSION RETINOPATHY. Ocular decompression retinopathy is a term that was used to describe seven eyes of four patients who developed intraretinal hemorrhages immediately after trabeculectomies (345). An especially high preoperative IOP, with sudden decompression and alteration in the configuration of the lamina cribrosa may lead to retinal vein obstruction and cause this complication.

Late Postoperative Complications

Late Failure of Filtration

The most common late complication of any filtering procedure is eventual failure to maintain a low IOP. This may develop within months to years after an initially successful operation. It is hard to predict, based on the appearance of the bleb, which cases will ultimately fail, although persistent inflammation, as well as pre- and postoperative factors that predispose to an inflammatory response, appear to play an important role (346).

The mechanism of failure may be closure of the fistula (347), although it is more commonly related to scarring and cyst-like formation within the bleb (336, 346, 348). A histopathologic study of failed blebs revealed a marked inflammatory response, abundant fibroblasts, and deposition of new collagen within the first few months after surgery (346). In those eyes that failed in the later postoperative period, a hypocellular capsule of fibrous tissue lined by a thick layer of fibrin was seen beneath relatively normal conjunctiva and Tenon's capsule (346).

These cases rarely respond to digital pressure or pharmacologic agents to suppress inflammation or fibrosis. When the pressure cannot be controlled medically, and the bleb appears to be encapsulated, it may be possible to revise the bleb with the surgical techniques previously described (331–334, 336). Transconjunctival argon laser photocoagulation has also been used to remove visible subconjunctival pigmented tissue in full-thickness filtering procedures (349), and a Q-switched neodymium:YAG laser has been reported to be successful in cutting episcleral fibrous tissue through the conjunctiva in failed trabeculectomies or full-thickness filters (350, 351).

When gonioscopic evaluation suggests that the procedure has failed due to closure of the fistula by membranous tissue, it may be possible to reestablish patency by incising the tissue with a knife or needle (347) or with a spatula and monopolar diathermy probe (352) from an ab interno approach. It may also be possible to remove the obstructing element with laser surgery. Argon laser treatment has been reported to be effective for this purpose when the membrane is pigmented (353, 354), while pulsed neodymium:YAG lasers have been used successfully to eliminate nonpigmented tissue from the fistula (351, 355–357), or to loosen or penetrate the scleral flap through the fistula (358). These techniques, however, are usually only successful in those eyes with previously well-established filtering blebs (357).

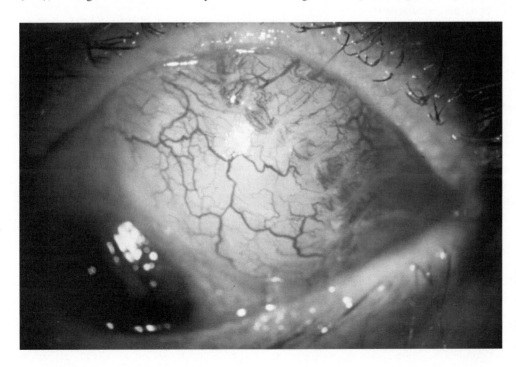

Figure 37.20. Typical appearance of an encapsulated bleb characterized by an elevated, smooth-domed conjunctiva with large vessels but intervening avascular areas and no microcysts.

When the above measures are not effective in reestablishing a failed filtering procedure, it is usually necessary to revise the bleb with incisional surgery or to repeat the operation in another quadrant with adjunctive mitomycin-C or 5-FU. Revision is usually more successful when dealing with encapsulated blebs as opposed to those that are flat and scarred down to underlying episclera (359).

A Leaking Filtering Bleb

A bleb wall that has become too thin may rupture, leading to loss of the anterior chamber and possible endophthalmitis. The defects are usually small, and the Siedel test is often helpful in confirming the leak. In some cases, the defect can be closed with tissue adhesive, although pressure patching with a Simmons shell (360, 361) or a collagen shield (362) may be more effective. When these measures fail, surgical revision by creation of a new conjunctival flap from tissue posterior to the defect may be required. Histologic examination of 10 leaking filtering blebs revealed an epithelial tract running from the surface of the bleb to the episclera in eight cases, and it was suggested that the bleb should be excised before bringing down the new flap to prevent epithelial downgrowth (363).

Endophthalmitis

Endophthalmitis is usually associated with a thin-walled filtering bleb (364, 365). It was once felt to be more common with full-thickness procedures, although it has also been reported following trabeculectomies (365–367). The incidence of endophthalmitis in one study was the same between thermal sclerostomy and trabeculectomy (368). With the increased use of adjunctive antimetabolites, the frequency of endophthalmitis with trabeculectomy appears to be on the rise (369). The risk of endophthalmitis in eyes with filtering blebs makes it imperative that any evidence of external infection, such as conjunctivitis, be treated aggressively. Eyes with very thin blebs require especially close observation for the possibility of rupture and subsequent endophthalmitis. Some surgeons elect to use prophylactic topical antibiotics in these cases, although a survey of members of the American Glaucoma Society revealed that 66% never use prophylactic antibiotics, and 28% only do so in selected cases (370). In the same paper, cultures of 41 patients on long-term topical antibiotic therapy in one eye revealed no significant difference in type of organisms between fellow eyes.

BLEBITIS. Infection following glaucoma filtering surgery rarely occurs in the early postoperative, but tends to have a late onset months or years after the surgery. It typically begins as a bleb infection (blebitis), in which the bleb is milky white and surrounded by intense conjunctival injection. There are usually variable degrees of anterior chamber reaction, but the vitreous is clear (371). Suggested treatment includes hospitalization, intravenous antibiotic therapy, and hourly topical fortified cefazolin and gentamicin (371). With prompt, aggressive therapy at this stage, the prognosis for visual recovery is much better than for fulminant endophthalmitis.

FULMINANT ENDOPHTHALMITIS. The majority of these cases are caused by virulent organisms such as Gram-negative rods and streptococci, which require prompt, aggressive management (372). When vitreous involvement is present or suspected, a recommended approach is to establish the diagnosis with aqueous and vitreous aspirates, and then to begin treatment with high-dose, broad-spectrum parenteral and periocular antibiotics such as gentamicin and cefazolin, and intravitreal antibiotics such as vancomycin and gentamicin, adjusting the treatment if necessary, according to culture and sensitivity results (372–375). In the Endophthalmitis Vitrectomy Study, which involved endophthalmitis after cataract surgery or secondary intraocular lens implant, a vitrectomy (as opposed to a vitreous tap or biopsy) was only beneficial in eyes with initial light perception vision, and systemic antibiotics were of no benefit (376). Corticosteroid therapy should also be used after antibiotic therapy has been established.

Cataracts

Cataracts are reported to occur in approximately one-third of eyes after filtering surgery (339, 377, 378). The mechanism of this complication is uncertain, but possible factors include (a) patient age, (b) duration of miotic therapy, (c) surgical manipulation, (d) postoperative iritis, (e) prolonged flat anterior chamber, and (f) nutritional changes (377–379).

Other Late Postoperative Complications

OVERHANGING FILTERING BLEBS. In some cases, a large bleb may gradually extend down over the cornea, possibly due to the effect of lid movements (Fig. 37.21). In some cases, these can be reduced by applying argon laser energy to the bleb (380), while others require incisional surgical correction by lifting the bleb from the cornea with an iris spatula, excising it near the limbus, and suturing the free edges (381).

SPONTANEOUS HYPHEMA. Spontaneous hyphema may occur weeks to years after filtering surgery (382). The bleeding may come from one of the cut ends of Schlemm's canal (383) or from abnormal vessels near the internal portion of the fistula (384). Bimanual bipolar diathermy has been suggested to treat bleeding from the anterior chamber angle (385), although argon laser photocoagulation may be more effective in these cases.

HYPOTONY AND CILIOCHOROIDAL DETACHMENT. Hypotony and ciliochoroidal detachment may occur at any time after a filtering procedure (386–388). Some may be chronic and recurrent (387) and inflammation is frequently present (387, 388). Other apparent risk factors include drugs that can incite ocular inflammation and aqueous suppressants (386, 387). Management in these cases involves discontinuation of the responsible drugs and aggressive anti-inflammatory therapy. Cataracts are common with this condition and cataract extraction may be associated with resolution of the choroidal detachments (387). Tearing of the retinal pigment epithelium has been reported as a sequela of hypotony and choroidal or serous retinal detachment after glaucoma surgery (389).

CORNEAL CHANGES. Corneal endothelial cell count has been shown to be reduced after glaucoma filtering surgery (390–391), which is influenced by early postoperative iridocorneal touch (390), but not by the use of adjunctive mitomycin-C (391). The trabeculectomy procedure can also alter corneal topography (392, 393), although it may be undetectable without topographic analysis (392) and usually does not persist (393).

EYELID CHANGES. Upper eyelid retraction after glaucoma filtering surgery was described in two patients, and was thought to result from the adrenergic effect of aqueous humor on Mueller's muscle (394). Ptosis has also been reported following glaucoma surgery, and may be related to surgical trauma to the levator muscle and adjacent tissue (395, 396).

SYMPATHETIC OPHTHALMIA. Sympathetic ophthalmia following glaucoma surgery is a rare complication. Studies suggest that this is not related to the type of operation, but rather to the preoperative condition of the eye, in that it occurs more commonly when operating on a blind, painful eye (397).

OUTCOMES OF FILTERING PROCEDURES

Trabeculectomy Versus Full-thickness Procedures

As previously noted, most surgeons today prefer some form of trabeculectomy, rather than a full-thickness procedure. Studies which have specifically compared trabeculectomies and full-thickness operations have shown comparable glaucoma control (398, 399). Some surveys suggested slightly better IOP control with full-thickness procedures (38, 400–404), although these studies were prior to the advent of adjunctive antimetabolite therapy.

Long-term Outcomes with Trabeculectomy

A number of series were reported in the late 1970s and 1980s regarding the outcomes of various forms of trabeculectomy. In general, the IOP results were comparable to those that had been previously described for various full-thickness procedures, with variable reductions in the incidence of complications (405–410). More recent studies, with followups of up to

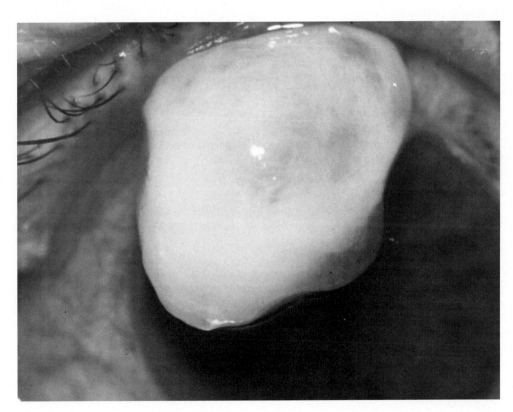

Figure 37.21. Excessive filtering bleb extending over cornea as a late complication of glaucoma filtering surgery.

12 years, show a gradual decline in the probability of successful IOP control over time, although the actual numbers vary considerably (411–413). One study of 75 patients, followed 6–12 years, revealed IOP control of 21 mm Hg or less in 90% at both 5 years and the final visit (411), while in another study of 43 eyes of patients with chronic open-angle glaucoma, 67% maintained an IOP below 21 mm Hg during a 7–10 year followup (412). Yet a third study, in which success was defined as an IOP of 20 mm Hg or less and a minimum reduction of 20%, revealed a probability of success after a single operation of 48% and 40% at 3 and 5 years, respectively (413). Of greater significance is visual field outcomes. One study of 54 patients revealed further loss of visual field in 28% during the first 5 years (414), while another study of 239 patients followed up to 10 years, revealed progressive glaucomatous damage in 25%, 30%, 43%, and 58% at 1, 2, 5, and 10 years, respectively (415). Consistent with previous reports, the reported incidence of cataract formation ranged from 22% to 38% (411, 412, 415).

Outcomes in High-Risk Populations

It is generally felt that glaucoma control among *black patients* is poorer than in white populations for most filtering procedures, although this has not been substantiated in all studies. With regard to trabeculectomies in black individuals, the reported success rates have mostly been in the same range as those for white patients (416–420), although some series have revealed less than 75% success with standard trabeculectomies (52, 421, 422). One study suggested that the explanation for the difference in outcome, if it truly exists, may be an increase in macrophages and fibroblasts and a decrease in mast cells and goblet cells in the conjunctiva of black patients as compared to that of white patients obtained at the time of filtering surgery (422). Some surgeons have noted improved pressure control in black patients when the trabeculectomy technique is modified to enhance filtration around the scleral flap (52, 423). Comparative studies of trabeculectomies and full-thickness filtering procedures within black populations have given conflicting results (404, 424–426).

It is reasonably well-established that *children* do worse with filtering procedures in general (427), including trabeculectomies (428–430). One study found no evidence that trabeculectomy is better than other procedures for advanced pediatric glaucomas (431), although these results may change with the addition of adjunctive antimetabolite therapy. Young patients, in the range of 15–40 years, have outcomes comparable to older adults (432), unless additional risk factors are present (433).

Aphakia is another factor which has an adverse influence on all filtering procedures, including trabeculectomies (434, 435). Patients with advanced chronic open-angle glaucoma also have a worse outcome than the general glaucoma population, with approximately one-third requiring a second operation within 3 years (436). In all of these high-risk cases,

however, the use of adjunctive antimetabolite therapy appears to improve the surgical outcome.

SUMMARY

Glaucoma filtering procedures lower the IOP by providing a limbal fistula through which aqueous humor drains into a subconjunctival space and subsequently filters through the conjunctiva to the tear film or is absorbed by surrounding tissues. The standard filtering techniques utilize common principles with regard to preparation of the conjunctival flap and the iridectomy. They differ primarily according to the method of creating the fistula, with the earlier procedures utilizing a full-thickness fistula, while the technique most commonly used today incorporates a guarded fistula beneath a partial-thickness scleral flap (trabeculectomy). Considerable attention has been given to the pharmacologic modulation of wound healing to minimize bleb failure. An alternative approach, which is also under evaluation, involves creation of a full-thickness fistula ab interno, usually with the use of laser energy, without dissection of a conjunctival flap. Complications may be encountered during filtering operations (e.g., tearing the conjunctival flap, hemorrhage, and choroidal effusion), as well as in the early postoperative period (e.g., hypotony, pressure elevation, uveitis, and hemorrhage), or late postoperative course (e.g., bleb failure, bleb leak, endophthalmitis, and cataracts).

REFERENCES

1. Migdal, C, Hitchings, R: The developing bleb: effect of topical anti-prostaglandins on the outcome of glaucoma fistulising surgery. Br J Ophthalmol 67:655, 1983.
2. Addicks, EM, Quigley, HA, Green, WR, Robin, AL: Histologic characteristics of filtering blebs in glaucomatous eyes. Arch Ophthalmol 101:795, 1983.
3. Benedikt, O: The effect of filtering operations. Klin Monatsbl Augenheilkd 170:10, 1977.
4. Kronfeld, PC: The chemical demonstration of transconjunctival passage of aqueous after antiglaucomatous operations. Am J Ophthalmol 35:38, 1952.
5. Galin, MA, Baras, I, McLean, JM: How does a filtering bleb work? Trans Am Acad Ophthalmol Otol 69:1082, 1965.
6. Teng, CC, Chi, HH, Katzin, HM: Histology and mechanism of filtering operations. Am J Ophthalmol 47:16, 1959.
7. Vesti, E, Raitta, C: Trabeculectomy at the inferior limbus. Acta Ophthalmol 70:220, 1992.
8. Luntz, MH: Trabeculectomy using a fornix-based conjunctival flap and tightly sutured scleral flap. Ophthalmology 87:985, 1980.
9. Faggioni, R: Trabeculectomy with conjunctival flap in the fornix: 12 months' follow-up. Klin Monatsbl Augenheilkd 182:385, 1983.
10. Brincker, P, Kessing, SV: Limbus-based versus fornix-based conjunctival flap in glaucoma filtering surgery. Acta Ophthalmol 70:641, 1992.
11. Shuster, JN, Krupin, T, Kolker, AE, Becker, B: Limbus- vs. fornix-based conjunctival flap in trabeculectomy. A long-term randomized study. Arch Ophthalmol 102:361, 1984.
12. Traverso, CE, Tomey, KF, Antonios, S: Limbal- vs. fornix-based conjunctival trabeculectomy flaps. Am J Ophthalmol 104:28, 1987.

13. Reichert, R, Stewart, W, Shields, MB: Limbus-based versus fornix-based conjunctival flaps in trabeculectomy. Ophthalmic Surg 18: 672, 1987.

14. Agbeja, AM, Dutton, GN: Conjunctival incisions for trabeculectomy and their relationship to the type of bleb formation. A preliminary study. Eye 1:738, 1987.

15. Grehn, F, Mauthe, S, Pfeiffer, N: Limbus-based versus fornix-based conjunctival flap in filtering surgery. A randomized prospective study. Int Ophthalmol 13:139, 1989.

16. Kapetansky, FM: Trabeculectomy, or trabeculectomy plus tenectomy: a comparative study. Glaucoma 2:451, 1980.

17. Miller, KN, Blasini, M, Shields, MB, Ho, C-H: A comparison of total and partial tenonectomy with trabeculectomy. Am J Ophthalmol 111:323, 1991.

18. Hung, SO: Role of sodium hyaluronate (Healonid) in triangular flap trabeculectomy. Br J Ophthalmol 69:46, 1985.

19. Teekhasaenee, C, Ritch, R: The use of PhEA 34c in trabeculectomy. Ophthalmology 93:487, 1986.

20. Wand, M: Viscoelastic agent and the prevention of post-filtration flat anterior chamber. Ophthalmic Surg 19:523, 1988.

21. Wand, M: Intraoperative intracameral viscoelastic agent in the prevention of postfiltration flat anterior chamber. J Glau 3:101, 1994.

22. Raitta, C, Vesti, E: The effect of sodium hyaluronate on the outcome of trabeculectomy. Ophthalmic Surg 22:145, 1991.

23. Barak, A, Alhalel, A, Kotas, R, Melamed, S: The protective effect of early intraoperative injection of viscoelastic material in trabeculectomy. Ophthalmic Surg 23:206, 1992.

24. Freedman, J: Iridectomy technique in trabeculectomy. Ophthalmic Surg 9:45, 1978.

25. Liss, RP, Scholes, GN, Crandall, AS: Glaucoma filtration surgery: new horizontal mattress closure of conjunctival incision. Ophthalmol Surg 22:298, 1991.

26. Wise, JB: Mitomycin-compatible suture technique for fornix-based conjunctival flaps in glaucoma filtration surgery. Arch Ophthalmol 111:992, 1993.

27. Sugar, HS: Experimental trabeculectomy in glaucoma. Am J Ophthalmol 51:623, 1961.

28. Cairns, JE: Trabeculectomy. Preliminary report of a new method. Am J Ophthalmol 5:673, 1968.

29. Rich, AM, McPherson, SD: Trabeculectomy in the owl monkey. Ann Ophthalmol 5:1082, 1973.

30. Spencer, WH: Histologic evaluation of microsurgical glaucoma techniques. Trans Am Acad Ophthalmol Otol 76:389, 1972.

31. Schmitt, H: Histological examination on disks obtained by goniotrephining with scleral flap. Klin Monatsbl Augenheilkd 167: 372, 1975.

32. Taylor, HR: A histologic survey of trabeculectomy. Am J Ophthalmol 82:733, 1976.

33. Lalive d'Epinay, S, Reme, C, Witmer, R: Influence of different topographical locations of trabeculectomy specimens on regulation of intraocular pressure and the quality of the filtering bleb. Klin Monatsbl Augenheilkd 182:387, 1983.

34. Cairns, JE: Trabeculectomy. Trans Am Acad Ophthalmol Otol 75:1395, 1971.

35. Linner, E: Aqueous outflow routes following trabeculectomy. New Trends Ophthalmol 7:173, 1992.

36. Shields, MB, Shelburne, JD, Bell, SW: The ultrastructure of human limbal collagen. Invest Ophthalmol Vis Sci 16:864, 1977.

37. Shields, MB, Bradbury, MJ, Shelburne, JD, Bell, SW: The permeability of the outer layers of limbus and anterior sclera. Invest Ophthalmol Vis Sci 16:866, 1977.

38. Shields, MB: Trabeculectomy vs. full-thickness filtering operation for control of glaucoma. Ophthalmic Surg 11:498, 1980.

39. Benedikt, O: The mode of action of trabeculectomy. Klin Monatsbl Augenheilkd 167:679, 1975.

40. Benedikt, O: Demonstration of aqueous outflow patterns of normal and glaucomatous human eyes through the injection of fluorescein

41. Blok, MDW, Greve, EL, Dunnebier, EA, et al: Scleral flap sutures and the development of shallow or flat anterior chamber after trabeculectomy. Ophthalmic Surg 24:309, 1993.

42. Hoskins, HD Jr, Migliazzo, C: Management of failing filtering blebs with the argon laser. Ophthalmic Surg 15:731, 1984.

43. Ritch, R, Potash, SD, Liebmann, JM: A new lens for argon laser suture lysis. Ophthalmic Surg 25:126, 1994.

44. Johnstone, MA, Wellington, DP, Ziel, CJ: A releasable scleral-flap tamponade suture for guarded filtration surgery. Arch Ophthalmol 111:398, 1993.

45. Hsu, C-T, Yarng, S-S: A modified removable suture in trabeculectomy. Ophthalmic Surg 24:579, 1993.

46. Kolker, AE, Kass, MA, Rait, JL: Trabeculectomy with releasable sutures. Arch Ophthalmol 112:62, 1994.

47. Maberley, D, Apel, A, Rootman, DS: Releasable "U" suture for trabeculectomy surgery. Ophthalmic Surg 25:251, 1994.

48. Krasnov, MM: A modified trabeculectomy. Ann Ophthalmol 6: 178, 1974.

49. Clemente, P: Goniotrepanation with triangular scleral flap. Klin Monatsbl Augenehilkd 177:455, 1980.

50. Dellaporta, A: Experiences with trepano-trabeculectomy. Trans Am Acad Ophthalmol Otol 79:362, 1975.

51. David, R, Sachs, U: Quantitative trabeculectomy. Br J Ophthalmol 65:457, 1981.

52. Welsh, NH: Trabeculectomy with fistula formation in the African. Br J Ophthalmol 56:32, 1972.

53. Schumer, RA, Odrich, SA: A scleral tunnel incision for trabeculectomy. Am J Ophthalmol 120:528, 1995.

54. Van Buskirk, EM: Trabeculectomy without conjunctival incision. Am J Ophthalmol 113:145, 1992.

55. Cioffi, GA, Van Buskirk, EM: Corneal trabeculectomy without conjunctival incision. Extended follow-up and histologic findings. Ophthalmology 100:1077, 1993.

56. Watson, PG: Surgery of the glaucomas. Br J Ophthalmol 56: 299, 1972.

57. Watson, PG, Barnett, F: Effectiveness of trabeculectomy in glaucoma. Am J Ophthalmol 79:831, 1975.

58. Hollwich, F, Fronimopoulos, J, Junemann, G, et al: Indication, technique and results of goniotrephining with scleral flap in primary chronic glaucoma. Klin Monatsbl Augenheilkd 163: 513, 1973.

59. Papst, W, Brunke, R: Goniotrepanation as a second fistulizing procedure. Klin Monatsbl Augenheilkd 176:915, 1980.

60. Smith, BF, Schuster, H, Seidenberg, B: Subscleral sclerectomy: a double-flap operation for glaucoma. Am J Ophthalmol 71:884, 1971.

61. Vasco-Posada, J: Glaucoma: esclerectomia subescleral. Arch Soc Am Oftal Optom 6:235, 1967.

62. Tomey, KF, Shammas, IV: Single snip trabeculectomy using a specially designed punch. Ophthalmic Surg 17:816, 1986.

63. Soll, DB: Intrascleral filtering procedure for glaucoma. Am J Ophthalmol 75:390, 1973.

64. Schimek, RA, Williamson, WR: Trabeculectomy with cautery. Ophthalmic Surg 8:35, 1977.

65. McGuigan, LJB, Luntz, MH, Freedman, J, Harrison, R: The role of subscleral Scheie procedure in glaucoma surgery. Ophthalmic Surg 17:802, 1986.

66. Beckman, H, Fuller, TA: Carbon dioxide laser scleral dissection and filtering procedure for glaucoma. Am J Ophthalmol 88:73, 1979.

67. Krasnov, MM: Sinusotomy. Foundation, results, prospects. Trans Am Acad Ophthalmol Otol 76:368, 1972.

68. Nesterov, AP: Role of the blockade of Schlemm's canal in pathogenesis of primary open-angle glaucoma. Am J Ophthalmol 70: 691, 1970.

69. Ellingson, BA, Grant, WM: Trabeculotomy and sinusotomy in enucleated human eyes. Invest Ophthalmol 11:21, 1972.

solution in the anterior chamber. Graefes Arch Clin Exp Ophthalmol 199:45, 1976.

70. Zimmerman, TJ, Kooner, KS, Ford, VJ, et al: Effectiveness of non-penetrating trabeculectomy in aphakic patients with glaucoma. Ophthalmic Surg 15:44, 1984.

71. Zimmerman, TJ, Kooner, KS, Ford, VJ, et al: Trabeculectomy vs. non-penetrating trabeculectomy: a retrospective study of two procedures in phakic patients with glaucoma. Ophthalmic Surg 15:734, 1984.

72. Weber, PA, Keates, RH, Opremcek, EM, et al: Two-stage neodymium-YAG laser trabeculotomy. Ophthalmic Surg 14:591, 1983.

73. Hara, T, Hara, T: Deep sclerectomy with Nd:YAG laser trabeculotomy ab interno: two-stage procedure. Ophthalmic Surg 19:101, 1988.

74. Lee, P-F, Shihab, ZM, Fu, Y-A: Modified trabeculectomy: a new procedure for neovascular glaucoma. Ophthalmic Surg 11:181, 1980.

75. Herschler, J, Agness, D: A modified filtering operation for neovascular glaucoma. Arch Ophthalmol 97:2339, 1979.

76. L'Esperance, FA Jr, Mittl, RN, James, WA Jr: Carbon dioxide laser trabeculostomy for the treatment of neovascular glaucoma. Ophthalmology 90:821, 1983.

77. Sinclair, SH, Aaberg, TM, Meredith, TA: A pars plana filtering procedure combined with lensectomy and vitrectomy for neovascular glaucoma. Am J Ophthalmol 93:185, 1982.

78. Maumenee, AE: External filtering operations for glaucoma: the mechansim of function and failure. Trans Am Ophthalmol Soc 58:319, 1960.

79. Kornblueth, W, Tenebaum, E: The inhibitory effect of aqueous humor on the growth of cells in tissue cultures. Am J Ophthalmol 42:70, 1956.

80. Herschler, J, Claflin, AJ, Fiorentino, G: The effect of aqueous humor on the growth of subconjunctival fibroblasts in tissue culture and its implications for glaucoma surgery. Am J Ophthalmol 89:245, 1980.

81. Radius, RL, Herschler, J, Claflin, A, Fiorentino, G: Aqueous humor changes after experimental filtering surgery. Am J Ophthalmol 89:250, 1980.

82. Jampel, HD: Ascorbic acid is cytotoxic to dividing human Tenon's capsule fibroblasts. A possible contributing factor in glaucoma filtration surgery success. Arch Ophthalmol 108:1323, 1990.

83. Tripathi, RC, Borisuth, NSC, Tripathi, BJ: Growth factors in the aqueous humor and their therapeutic implications in glaucoma and anterior segment disorders of the human eye. Drug Dev Res 22:1, 1991.

84. Jampel, HD, Roche, N, Stark, WJ, Roberts, AB: Transforming growth factor-β in human aqueous humor. Curr Eye Res 9:963, 1990.

85. Albrink, WS, Wallace, AC: Aqueous humor as a tissue culture nutrient. Proc Soc Exp Biol Med 77:754, 1951.

86. Ledbetter, SR, Hatchell, DL (Van Horn), O'Brien, WJ: Secondary aqueous humor stimulates the proliferation of cultured bovine corneal endothelial cells. Invest Ophthalmol Vis Sci 24:557, 1983.

87. Joseph, JP, Grierson, I, Hitchings, RA: Chemotactic activity of aqueous humor. A cause of failure of trabeculectomies? Arch Ophthalmol 107:69, 1989.

88. Gwynn, DR, Stewart, WC, Hennis, HL, et al: The influence of age upon inflammatory cell counts and structure of conjunctiva in chronic open-angle glaucoma. Acta Ophthalmol 71:691, 1993.

89. McMillan, TA, Stewart, WC, Hennis, HL, et al: Histologic differences in the conjunctiva of black and white glaucoma patients. Ophthalmic Surg 23:762, 1992.

90. Lavin, MJ, Wormald, RPL, Migdal, CS, Hitchings, RA: The influence of prior therapy on the success of trabeculectomy. Arch Ophthalmol 108:1543, 1990.

91. Broadway, DC, Grierson, I, O'Brien, C, Hitchings, RA: Adverse effects of topical antiglaucoma medication. II. The outcome of filtration surgery. Arch Ophthalmol 112:1446, 1994.

92. Johnson, DH, Yoshikawa, K, Brubaker, RF, Hodge, DO: The effect of long-term medical therapy on the outcome of filtration surgery. Am J Ophthalmol 117:139, 1994.

93. Broadway, DC, Grierson, I, O'Brien, C, Hitchings, RA: Adverse effects of topical antiglaucoma medication. I. The conjunctival cell profile. Arch Ophthalmol 112:1437, 1994.

94. Baudouin, C, Garcher, C, Haouat, N, et al: Expression of inflammatory membrane markers by conjunctival cells in chronically treated patients with glaucoma. Ophthalmology 101:454, 1994.

95. Gwynn, DR, Stewart, WC, Pitts, RA, et al: Conjunctival structure and cell counts and the results of filtering surgery. Am J Ophthalmol 116:464, 1993.

96. Brandt, JD, Wittpenn, JR, Katz, LJ, et al: Conjunctival impression cytology in patients with glaucoma using long-term topical medication. Am J Ophthalmol 112:297, 1991.

97. Cunliffe, IA, McIntyre, CA, Rees, RC, Rennie, IG: Pilot study on the effect of topical adrenergic medications on human Tenon's capsule fibroblasts in tissue culture. Br J Ophthalmol 79:70, 1995.

98. Broadway, DC, Grierson, I, Stürmer, J, Hitchings, RA: Reversal of topical antiglaucoma medication effects on the conjunctiva. Arch Ophthalmol 114:262, 1996.

99. Nguyen, KD, Lee, DA: Effect of steroids and nonsteroidal antiinflammatory agents on human ocular fibroblast. Invest Ophthalmol Vis Sci 33:2693, 1992.

100. McGuigan, LJB, Cook, DJ, Yablonski, ME: Dexamethasone, D-penicillamine, and glaucoma filter surgery in rabbits. Invest Ophthalmol Vis Sci 27:1755, 1986.

101. Starita, RJ, Fellman, RL, Spaeth, GL, et al: Short- and long-term effects of postoperative corticosteroids on trabeculectomy. Ophthalmology 92:938, 1985.

102. Roth, SM, Spaeth, GL, Starita, RJ, et al: The effects of postoperative corticosteroids on trabeculectomy and the clinical course of glaucoma: five-year follow-up study. Ophthalmic Surg 22:724, 1991.

103. Araujo, SV, Spaeth, GL, Roth, SM, Starita, RJ: A ten-year follow-up on a prospective, randomized trial of postoperative corticosteroids after trabeculectomy. Ophthalmology 102:1753, 1995.

104. Giangiacomo, J, Dueker, DK, Adelstein, E: The effect of preoperative subconjunctival triamcinolone administration on glaucoma filteration. I. Trabeculectomy following subconjunctival triamcinolone. Arch Ophthalmol 104:838, 1986.

105. Cantor, LB, Phillips, CA, Kramer, D, et al: Effect of topical flurbiprofen on trabeculectomy. J Glau 4:98, 1995.

106. Blumenkranz, MS, Claflin, A, Hajek, AS: Selection of therapeutic agents for intraocular proliferative disease. Cell culture evaluation. Arch Ophthalmol 102:598, 1984.

107. Khaw, PT, Ward, S, Porter, A, et al: The long-term effects of 5-fluorouracil and sodium butyrate on human Tenon's fibroblasts. Invest Ophthalmol Vis Sci 33:2043, 1992.

108. Gressel, MG, Parrish, RK II, Folberg, R: 5-Fluorouracil and glaucoma filtering surgery: I. An animal model. Ophthalmology 91:378, 1984.

109. Heuer, DK, Parrish, RK II, Gressel, MG, et al: 5-Fluorouracil and glaucoma filtering surgery. II. A Pilot study. Ophthalmology 91:384, 1984.

110. Heuer, DK, Parrish, RK, II, Gressel, MG, et al: 5-Fluorouracil and glaucoma filtering surgery. III. Intermediate follow-up of a pilot study. Ophthalmology 93:1537, 1986.

111. The Fluorouracil Filtering Surgery Study Group: Fluorouracil filtering surgery study one-year follow-up. Am J Ophthalmol 108:625, 1989.

112. 5-FU Study Group: Three-year follow-up of the fluorouracil filtering surgery study. Am J Ophthalmol 115:82, 1993.

113. Weinreb, RN: Adjusting the dose of 5-fluorouracil after filtration surgery to minimize side effects. Ophthalmology 94:564, 1987.

114. Ruderman, JM, Welch, DB, Smith, MF, Shoch, DE: A randomized study of 5- fluorouracil and filtration surgery. Am J Ophthalmol 104:218, 1987.

115. Araie, M, Shoji, N, Shirato, S, Nakano, Y: Postoperative subconjunctival 5-fluorouracil injections and success probability of trabeculectomy in Japanese. Results of 5-year follow-up. Jpn J Ophthalmol 36:158, 1992.

116. Goldenfeld, M, Krupin, T, Ruderman, JM, et al: 5-fluorouracil in initial trabeculectomy. A prospective, randomized, multicenter study. Ophthalmology 101:1024, 1994.

117. Whiteside-Michel, J, Liebmann, JM, Ritch, R: Initial 5-fluorouracil trabeculectomy in young patients. Ophthalmology 99:7, 1992.

118. Bansal, RK, Gupta, A: 5-fluorouracil in trabeculectomy for patients under the age of 40 years. Ophthalmic Surg 23:278, 1992.

119. Zalish, M, Leiba, H, Oliver, M: Subconjunctival injection of 5-fluorouracil following trabeculectomy for congenital and infantile glaucoma. Ophthalmic Surg 23:203, 1992.

120. Wilson, RP, Steinmann, WC: Use of trabeculectomy with postoperative 5-fluorouracil in patients requiring extremely low intraocular pressure levels to limit further glaucoma progression. Ophthalmology 98:1047, 1991.

121. Tsai, JC, Feuer, WJ, Parrish, RK, II, Grajewski, AL: 5-fluorouracil filtering surgery and neovascular glaucoma. Long-term follow-up of the original pilot study. Ophthalmology 102:887, 1995.

122. Krug, JH, Jr, Melamed, S: Adjunctive use of delayed and adjustable low-dose 5-fluorouracil in refractory glaucoma. Am J Ophthalmol 109:412, 1990.

123. Hefetz, L, Keren, T, Naveh, N: Early and late postoperative application of 5-fluorouracil following trabeculectomy in refractory glaucoma. Ophthalmic Surg 25:715, 1994.

124. Heuer, DK, Gressel, MG, Parrish, RK, II, et al: Topical fluorouracil. II. Postoperative administration in an animal model of glaucoma filtering surgery. Arch Ophthalmol 104:132, 1986.

125. Kando, M, Araie, M: Iontophoresis of 5-fluorouracil into the conjunctiva and sclera. Invest Ophthalmol Vis Sci 30:583, 1989.

126. Hasty, B, Heuer, DK, Minckler, DS: Primate trabeculectomies with 5-fluorouracil collagen implants. Am J Ophthalmol 109:721, 1990.

127. Finkelstein, I, Trope, GE, Heathcote, JG, et al: Further evaluation of collagen shields as a delivery system for 5-fluorouracil: histopathological observations. Can J Ophthalmol 26:129, 1991.

128. Lee, DA, Flores, RA, Anderson, PJ, et al: Glaucoma filtration surgery in rabbits using bioerodible polymers and 5-fluorouracil. Ophthalmology 94:1523, 1987.

129. Gould, L, Trope, G, Cheng, Y-L, et al: Fifty:fifty poly (DL glycolic acid-lactic acid) copolymer as a drug delivery system for 5-fluorouracil: a histopathological evaluation. Can J Ophthalmol 29:168, 1994.

130. Blandford, DL, Smith, TJ, Brown, JD, et al: Subconjunctival sustained release 5-fluorouracil. Invest Ophthalmol Vis Sci 33:3430, 1992.

131. Skuta, GL, Assil, K, Parrish, RK, II, et al: Filtering surgery in owl monkeys treated with the antimetabolite 5-fluorouridine 5'-monophosphate entrapped in multivesicular liposomes. Am J Ophthalmol 103:714, 1987.

132. Alvarado, JA: The use of a lipsome-encapsulated 5-fluoroorotate for glaucoma surgery: I. Animal studies. Trans Am Ophthalmol Soc 87:489, 1989.

133. Smith, MF, Sherwood, MB, Doyle, JW, Khaw, PT: Results of intraoperative 5-fluorouracil supplementation on trabeculectomy for open-angle glaucoma. Am J Ophthalmol 114:737, 1992.

134. Egbert, PR, Williams, AS, Singh, K, et al: A prospective trial of intraoperative fluorouracil during trabeculectomy in a black population. Am J Ophthalmol 116:612, 1993.

135. Cunliffe, IA, Longstaff, S: Intra-operative use of 5-fluorouracil in glaucoma filtering surgery. Acta Ophthalmol 71:739, 1993.

136. Feldman, RM, Dietze, PJ, Gross, RL, Oram, O: Intraoperative 5-fluorouracil administration in trabeculectomy. J Glau 3:302, 1994.

137. Chen, C-W: Enhanced intraocular pressure controlling effectiveness of trabeculectomy by local application of mitomycin c. Trans Asia-Pac Acad Ophthalmol 9:172, 1983.

138. Jampel, HD: Effect of brief exposure to mitomycin c on viability and proliferation of cultured human tenon's capsule fibroblasts. Ophthalmology 99:1471, 1992.

139. Madhavan, HN, Rao, SB, Vijaya, L, Neelakantan, A: In vitro sensitivity of human tenon's capsule fibroblasts to mitomycin c and its correlation with outcome of glaucoma filtration surgery. Ophthalmic Surg 26:61, 1995.

140. Khaw, PT, Doyle, JW, Sherwood, MB, et al: Prolonged localized tissue effects from 5-minute exposures to fluorouracil and mitomycin c. Arch Ophthalmol 111:263, 1993.

141. Smith, S, D'Amore, PA, Dreyer, EB: Comparative toxicity of mitomycin c and 5-fluorouracil in vitro. Am J Ophthalmol 118:332, 1994.

142. Bergstrom, TJ, Wilkinson, WS, Skuta, GL, et al: The effects of subconjunctival mitomycin-c on glaucoma filtration surgery in rabbits. Arch Ophthalmol 109:1725, 1991.

143. Palmer, SS: Mitomycin as adjunct chemotherapy with trabeculectomy. Ophthalmology 98:317, 1991.

144. Skuta, GL, Beeson, CC, Higginbotham, EJ, et al: Intraoperative mitomycin versus postoperative 5-fluorouracil in high-risk glaucoma filtering surgery. Ophthalmology 99:438, 1992.

145. Katz, GJ, Higginbotham, EJ, Lichter, PR, et al: Mitomycin c versus 5-fluorouracil in high-risk glaucoma filtering surgery. Extended follow-up. Ophthalmology 102:1263, 1995.

146. Kitazawa, Y, Kawase, K, Matsushita, H, Minobe, M: Trabeculectomy with mitomycin. A comparative study with fluorouracil. Arch Ophthalmol 109:1693, 1991.

147. Lamping, KA, Belkin, JK: 5-fluorouracil and mitomycin c in pseudophakic patients. Ophthalmology 102:70, 1995.

148. Mermoud, A, Salmon, JF, Murray, AND: Trabeculectomy with mitomycin c for refractory glaucoma in blacks. Am J Ophthalmol 116:72, 1993.

149. Prata, JA Jr, Neves, RA, Minckler, D, et al: Trabeculectomy with mitomycin c in glaucoma associated with uveitis. Ophthalmic Surg 25:616, 1994.

150. Susanna, R Jr, Oltrogge, EW, Carani, JCE, Nicolela, MT: Mitomycin as adjunct chemotherapy with trabeculectomy in congenital and developmental glaucomas. J Glau 4:151, 1995.

151. Yamamoto, T, Ichien, M, Suemori-Matsushita, H, Kitazawa, Y: Trabeculectomy with mitomycin c for normal-tension glaucoma. J Glau 4:158, 1995.

152. Costa, VP, Moster, MR, Wilson, RP, et al: Effects of topical mitomycin c on primary trabeculectomies and combined procedures. Br J Ophthalmol 77:693, 1993.

153. Mirza, GE, Karakucuk, S, Dogan, H, Erkilic, K: Filtering surgery with mitomycin-C in uncomplicated (primary open angle) glaucoma. Acta Ophthalmol 72:155, 1994.

154. Kupin, TH, Juzych, MS, Shin, DH, et al: Adjunctive mitomycin c in primary trabeculectomy in phakic eyes. Am J Ophthalmol 119:30, 1995.

155. Costa, VP, Wilson, RP, Moster, MR, et al: Hypotony maculopathy following the use of topical mitomycin c in glaucoma filtration surgery. Ophthalmic Surg 24:389, 1993.

156. Shields, MB, Scroggs, MW, Sloop, CM, Simmons, RB: Clinical and histopathologic observations concerning hypotony after trabeculectomy with adjunctive mitomycin c. Am J Ophthalmol 116:673, 1993.

157. Hietz, H, Brunner, R, Addicks, K, Krieglstein, GK: Histopathology of an avascular filtering bleb after trabeculectomy with mitomycin-c. J Glau 2:266, 1993.

158. Nuyts, RMMA, Felten, PC, Pels, E, et al: Histopathologic effects of mitomycin c after trabeculectomy in human glaucomatous eyes with persistent hypotony. Am J Ophthalmol 118:225, 1994.

159. Mietz, H, Addicks, K, Diestelhorst, M, Krieglstein, GK: Extraocular application of mitomycin c in a rabbit model: cytotoxic effects on the ciliary body and epithelium. Ophthalmic Surg 25:240, 1994.

160. Kee, C, Pelzek, CD, Kaufman, PL: Mitomycin c suppresses aqueous humor flow in cynomolgus monkeys. Arch Ophthalmol 113:239, 1995.

161. Derick, RJ, Pasquale, L, Quigley, HA, Jampel, H: Potential toxicity of mitomycin c. Arch Ophthalmol 109:1635, 1991.

162. Morrow, GL, II, Stein, RM, Heathcote, JG, et al: Ocular toxicity of mitomycin c and 5-fluorouracil in the rabbit. Can J Ophthalmol 29:268, 1994.

163. Mégevand, GS, Salmon, JF, Scholtz, RP, Murray, AND: The effect of reducing the exposure time of mitomycin c in glaucoma filtering surgery. Ophthalmology 102:84, 1995.

164. Bank, A, Allingham, RR: Application of mitomycin c during filtering surgery. Am J Ophthalmol 116:377, 1993.

165. Shin, DH, Reed, SY, Swords, RC, et al: Cellulose sponge punch for controlled mitomycin application. Arch Ophthalmol 112:1624, 1994.

166. Flynn, WJ, Carlson, DW, Bifano, SL: Mitomycin trabeculectomy: the microsurgical sponge difference. J Glau 4:86, 1995.

167. Prata, JA Jr, Minckler, DS, Baerveldt, G, et al: Site of mitomycin-c application during trabeculectomy. J Glau 3:296, 1994.

168. Prata, JA Jr, Minckler, DS, Koda, RT: Effects of external irrigation on mitomycin-c concentration in rabbit aqueous and vitreous humor. J Glau 4:32, 1995.

169. Litin, BS, Jones, MA, Kwong, EM, Herschler, J: Effect of antineoplastic drugs on cell proliferation—individually and in combination. Ophthalmic Surg 16:34, 1985.

170. Lee, DA, Goodwin, LT Jr, Panek, WC, et al: Effects of cytosine arabinoside-imprgnated bioerodible polymers on glaucoma filtration surgery in rabbits. J Glau 2:96, 1993.

171. Chu, JL, Shields, SR, Netland, PA: Enhancement of filtration surgery with cytosine arabinoside and reversal of toxicity with 2'-deoxycytidine. Curr Eye Res 13:839, 1994.

172. Salas-Prato, M, Assalian, A, Mehdi, AZ, et al: Inhibition by rapamycin of PDGF- and bFGF-induced human tenon fibroblast proliferation in vitro. J Glau 5:54, 1996.

173. Xu, Y, Yang, GH, Gin, WM, et al: Effect of subconjunctival daunorubicin on glaucoma surgery in rabbits. Ophthalmic Surg 24:382, 1993.

174. del Vecchio, PJ, Bizios, R, Holleran, LA, et al: Inhibition of human scleral fibroblast proliferation with heparin. Invest Ophthalmol Vis Sci 29:1272, 1988.

175. Joseph, JP, Grierson, I, Hitchings, RA: Taxol, cytochalasin B and colchicine effects on fibroblast migration and contraction: a role in glaucoma filtration surgery? Curr Eye Res 8:203, 1989.

176. Wilkerson, M, Fulcher, S, Shields, MB, Foulks, GN, Hatchell, DL, Houston, LL: Inhibition of human subconjunctival fibroblast proliferation by immunotoxin. Invest Ophthalmol Vis Sci 33:2293, 1992.

177. Gillies, M, Su, T, Sarossy, M, Hollows, F: Interferon-alpha 2b inhibits proliferation of human Tenon's capsule fibroblasts. Graefes Arch Clin Exp Ophthalmol 231:118, 1993.

178. Gillies, MC, Goldberg, I, Young, SH, Su, T: Glaucoma filtering surgery with interferon-α-2b. J Glau 2:229, 1993.

179. Nevárez, JA, Parrish, RK, II, Heuer, DK, et al: The effect of beta irradiation on monkey Tenon's capsule fibroblasts in tissue culture. Curr Eye Res 6:719, 1987.

180. Khaw, PT, Ward, S, Grierson, I, Rice, NSC: Effect of β radiation on proliferating human Tenon's capsule fibroblasts. Br J Ophthalmol 75:580, 1991.

181. Miller, MH, Grierson, I, Unger, WG, Hitchings, RA: The effect of topical dexamethasone and preoperative beta irradiation on a model of glaucoma fistulizing surgery in the rabbit. Ophthalmic Surg 21:44, 1990.

182. Miller, MH, Joseph, NH, Wishart, PK, Hitchings, RA: Lack of beneficial effect of intensive topical steroids and beta irradiation of eyes undergoing repeat trabeculectomy. Ophthalmic Surg 18:508, 1987.

183. Miller, MH, Rice, NSC: Trabeculectomy combined with β irradiation for congenital glaucoma. Br J Ophthalmol 75:584, 1991.

184. Fourman, S, Vaid, K: Effects of tissue plasminogen activator on glaucoma filter blebs in rabbits. Ophthalmic Surg 20:663, 1989.

185. Fourman, S, Wiley, L: Tissue plasminogen activator modifies healing of glaucoma filtering surgery in rabbits. Ophthalmic Surg 22:718, 1991.

186. Ozment, RR, Laiw, Z-C, Latina, MA: The use of tissue plasminogen activator in experimental filtration surgery. Ophthalmic Surg 23:22, 1992.

187. Latina, MA, Belmone, SJ, Park, C, Crean, E: Gamma-interferon effects on human fibroblasts from Tenon's capsule. Invest Ophthalmol Vis Sci 32:2806, 1991.

188. Lee, Y-C, Park, M-H, Baek, N-H: Effect of gamma-interferon on fibroblast proliferation and collagen synthesis after glaucoma filtering surgery in white rabbits. Kor J Ophthalmol 5:59, 1991.

189. Nguyen, KD, Hoang, AR, Lee, DA: Transcriptional control of human Tenon's capsule fibroblast collagen synthesis in vitro by gamma-interferon. Invest Ophthalmol Vis Sci 35:3064, 1994.

190. Assil, KK, Saperstein, D, Weinreb, RN, Chojkier, M: Inhibition of collagen synthesis in human episcleral fibroblasts by calcium ionophore A23187. J Glau 4:41, 1995.

191. McGuigan, LJB, Mason, RP, Sanchez, R, Quigley, HA: D-Penicillamine and beta-aminopropionitrile effects on experimental filtering surgery. Invest Ophthalmol Vis Sci 28:1625, 1987.

192. Fourman, S: Effects of aminoproprionitrile on glaucoma filter blebs in rabbits. Ophthalmic Surg 19:649, 1988.

193. LaGrange, F: Iridectomie et sclerectomie combinees dans le traitement du glaucome chronique. Procede nouveau pour l'etablissement de la cicatrice filtrante (1). Arch d'Opht 26:481, 1906.

194. Holth, S: Sclerectomie avec la pince emporte-piece dans le glaucome, de preference apres incision a la pique. Ann d'Ocul 142:1, 1909.

195. Berens, C: Iridocorneosclerectomy for glaucoma. Am J Ophthalmol 19:470, 1936.

196. McPherson, SD Jr, McCurdy, D: Anterior posterior lip sclerectomy. Proc Ann Staff Conf McPherson Hosp 13:19, 1974.

197. Gershen, HJ: Lateral lip sclerectomy. Arch Ophthalmol 86:534, 1971.

198. Iliff, CE, Haas, JS: Posterior lip sclerectomy. Am J Ophthalmol 54:688, 1962.

199. Regan, EF: Scleral cautery with iridectomy—an experimental study. Trans Am Ophthalmol Soc 61:219, 1963.

200. Gass, JDM: Anterior lip sclerectomy. A microsurgical technique for filtering operation for control of glaucoma. Ann Ophthalmol 2:355, 1970.

201. Henry, JC, Krupin, T, Wax, MB, Feitl, ME: A modified scleral punch for filtration surgery. Am J Ophthalmol 108:740, 1989.

202. Elliot, RH: A preliminary note on a new operative procedure for the establishment of a filtering cicatrix in the treatment of glaucoma. Ophthalmoscope 7:804, 1909.

203. Fergus, F: Treatment of glaucoma by trephining. Br Med J 2:983, 1909.

204. Elliot, RH: Sclero-corneal trephining in the operative treatment of glaucoma. London, George Pulman and Sons, 1913.

205. Sugar, HS: Limboscleral trephination. Am J Ophthalmol 52:29, 1961.

206. Sugar, HS: Limboscleral trepanation. Eleven years' experience. Arch Ophthalmol 85:703, 1971.

207. Preziosi, CL: The electro-cautery in the treatment of glaucoma. Br J Ophthalmol 8:414, 1924.

208. Scheie, HG: Retraction of scleral wound edges as a fistulizing procedure for glaucoma. Am J Ophthalmol 45:220, 1958.

209. Viswanathan, B, Brown, IAR: Peripheral iridectomy with scleral cautery for glaucoma. Arch Ophthalmol 93:34, 1975.

210. Shaffer, RN, Hetherington, J Jr, Hoskins, HD Jr: Guarded thermal sclerostomy. Am J Ophthalmol 72:769, 1971.

211. Litwin, RL: Successful argon laser sclerostomy for glaucoma. Ophthalmic Surg 10:22, 1979.

212. Hoskins, HD Jr, Iwach, AG, Drake, MV, et al: Subconjunctival THC:YAG laser limbal sclerostomy ab externo in the rabbit. Ophthalmic Surg 21:589, 1990.

213. Onda, E, Jikihara, S, Kitazawa, Y, et al: Determination of an appropriate laser setting for THC-YAG laser sclerostomy ab externo in rabbits. Ophthalmic Surg 23:198, 1992.

214. Hoskins, HD Jr, Iwach, AG, Vassiliadis, A, et al: Subconjunctival THC:YAG laser thermal sclerostomy. Ophthalmology 98:1394, 1991.

215. Saheb, NE: Short-term results of holmium laser sclerostomy in patients with uncontrolled glaucoma. Can J Ophthalmol 28:317, 1993.

216. Iwach, AG, Hoskins, HD, Jr, Drake, MV, Dickens, CJ: Subconjunctival THC:YAG ("holmium") laser thermal sclerostomy ab externo. A one-year report. Ophthalmology 100:356, 1993.

217. Bonomi, L, Perfetti, S, Marraffa, M, et al: Subconjunctival THC:YAG laser sclerostomy for the treatment of glaucoma: preliminary data. Ophthalmic Surg 24:300, 1993.

218. Iwach, AG, Hoskins, HD Jr, Drake, MV, Dickens, CJ: Update of the subconjunctival THC:YAG (holmium) laser sclerostomy ab externo clinical trial: 30-month report. Ophthalmic Surg 25:13, 1994.

219. Onda, E, Ando, H, Honbe, K, et al: Holmium-YAG laser sclerostomy ab externo for glaucoma filtering surgery. Jpn J Clin Ophthalmol 46:1555, 1992.

220. Feldman, RM, Oram, S, Gross, RL, et al: Histopathologic characteristics of failed holmium laser sclerostomy. Am J Ophthalmol 116:766, 1993.

221. Wang, T-H, Hung, PT, Ho, T-C: THC:YAG laser sclerostomy with preoperative mitomycin-c subconjuntival injection in rabbits. J Glau 2:260, 1993.

222. Wetzel, W, Scheu, M: Laser sclerostomy ab externo using mid infrared lasers. Ophthalmic Surg 24:6, 1993.

223. Fliegler, RJ, Mastrobattista, J, Luntz, MH: Subconjunctival THC:YAG laser sclerostomy under a partial-thickness corneal flap. Ophthalmic Surg 25:28, 1994.

224. Barak, A, Rosner, M, Solomon, A, et al: Use of the giant-pulse Nd:YAG laser for ab-externo sclerostomy in rabbits and humans. Ophthalmic Surg 26:68, 1995.

225. Cooper, HM, Schuman, JS, Puliafito, CA, et al: Picosecond neodymium:yttrium lithium fluoride laser sclerectomy. Am J Ophthalmol 115:221, 1993.

226. Park, SB, Kim, JC, Aquavella JV: Nd:YLF laser sclerostomy. Ophthalmic Surg 24:118, 1993.

227. Karp, CL, Higginbotham, EJ, Griffin, EO: Adjunctive use of transconjunctival mitomycin-c in ab externo diode laser sclerostomy surgery in rabbits. Ophthalmic Surg 25:22, 1994.

228. Allan, BDS, van Saarloos, PP, Cooper, RL, Constable, IJ: 193-nm excimer laser sclerostomy in pseudophakic patients with advanced open angle glaucoma. Br J Ophthalmol 78:199, 1994.

229. Seiler, T, Kriegerowski, M, Bende, T, Wollensak, J: Partial external trabeculectomy. Klin Monatsbl Augenheilkd 195:216, 1989.

230. Brooks, AMV, Samuel, M, Carroll, N, et al: Excimer laser filtration surgery. Am J Ophthalmol 119:40, 1995.

231. March, WF, Gherezghiher, T, Koss, MC, Nordquist, RE: Experimental YAG laser sclerostomy. Arch Ophthalmol 102:1834, 1984.

232. March, WF, Gherezghiher, R, Koss, MC, et al: Histologic study of a neodymium-YAG laser sclerostomy. Arch Ophthalmol 103:860, 1985.

233. Gherezghiher, T, March, WF, Koss, MC, Nordquist, RE: Neodymium-YAG laser sclerostomy in primates. Arch Ophthalmol 103:1543, 1985.

234. Latina, MA, Dobrogowski, M, March, WF, Birngruber, R: Laser sclerostomy by pulsed-dye laser and goniolens. Arch Ophthalmol 108:1745, 1990.

235. Latina, MA, Melamed, S, March, WF, et al: Gonioscopic ab interno laser sclerostomy. A pilot study in glaucoma patients. Ophthalmology 99:1736, 1992.

236. Melamed, S, Solomon, A, Neumann, D, et al: Internal sclerostomy using laser ablation of dyed sclera in glaucoma patients: a pilot study. Br J Ophthalmol 77:139, 1993.

237. Federman, JL, Wilson, RP, Ando, F, Peyman, GA: Contact laser: thermal sclerostomy ab interna. Ophthalmic Surg 18:726, 1987.

238. Higginbotham, EJ, Kao, G, Peyman, G: Internal sclerostomy with the Nd:YAG contact laser versus thermal sclerostomy in rabbits. Ophthalmology 95:385, 1988.

239. Javitt, JC, O'Connor, SS, Wilson, RP, Federman, JL: Laser sclerostomy ab interno using a continuous-wave Nd:YAG laser. Ophthalmic Surg 20:552, 1989.

240. Wilson, RP, Javitt, JC: Ab interno laser sclerostomy in aphakic patients with glaucoma and chronic inflammation. Am J Ophthalmol 110:178, 1990.

241. Jaffe, GJ, Mieler, WF, Radius, RL, et al: Ab interno sclerostomy with a high-powered argon endolaser. Clinicopathologic correlation. Arch Ophthalmol 107:1183, 1989.

242. Adachi, M, Ohya, T, Hirata, Y, et al: Internal sclerostomy with a high-powered argon laser. Acta Soc Ophthalmol Jpn 95:657, 1991.

243. Berlin, MS, Rajacich, G, Duffy, M, et al: Excimer laser photoablation in glaucoma filtering surgery. Am J Ophthalmol 103:713, 1987.

244. Shields, SR, Netland, PA, Chu, JL, et al: Transcorneal erbium laser sclerostomy: towards a guarded laser sclerostomy technique. J Glau 4:391, 1995.

245. Karp, CL, Higginbotham, EJ, Edward, DP, Musch, DC: Diode laser surgery. Ab interno and ab externo versus conventional surgery in rabbits. Ophthalmology 100:1567, 1993.

246. Oram, O, Gross, RL, Severin, TD, et al: Gonioscopic ab interno Nd:YLF laser sclerostomy in human cadaver eyes. Ophthalmic Surg 26:136, 1995.

247. Özler, SA, Hill, RA, Andrews, JJ, et al: Infrared laser sclerostomies. Invest Ophthalmol Vis Sci 32:2498, 1991.

248. Hill, RA, Özler, SA, Baerveldt, G, et al: Ab-interno neodymium:YAG versus erbium:YAG laser sclerostomies in a rabbit model. Ophthalmic Surg 23:192, 1992.

249. Chi, TSK, Berríos, RR, Netland, PA: Holmium laser sclerostomy via corneal approach with transconjunctival mitomycin-c in rabbits. Ophthalmic Surg 26:353, 1995.

250. Brown, RH, Denham, DB, Bruner, WE, et al: Internal sclerectomy for glaucoma filtering surgery with an automated trephine. Arch Ophthalmol 105:133, 1987.

251. Brown, RH, Lynch, MG, Denham, DB, et al: Internal sclerectomy with an automated trephine for advanced glaucoma. Ophthalmology 95:728, 1988.

252. Au, Y-K, Reynolds, MD, Chadalavada, R, Misra, RP: Bipolar cautery and internal thermal sclerostomy in a rabbit model. Ophthalmic Surg 23:188, 1992.

253. Brown, SVL, Higginbotham, EJ, Griffin, EO, et al. Ab interno sclerostomy using a goniodiathermy instrument. Ophthalmic Surg 25:112, 1994.

254. Petursson, GJ, Fraunfelder, FT: Repair of an inadvertent buttonhole or leaking filtering bleb. Arch Ophthalmol 97:926, 1979.

255. Awan, KJ, Spaeth, PG: Use of isobutyl-2-cyanoacrylate tissue adhesive in the repair of conjunctival fistula in filtering procedures for glaucoma. Ann Ophthalmol 6:851, 1974.

256. Ferry, AP: Hemorrhage into the lens as a complication of glaucoma surgery. Am J Ophthalmol 81:351, 1976.

257. Bellows, AR, Chylack, LT Jr, Epstein, DL, Hutchinson, BT: Choroidal effusion during glaucoma surgery in patients with prominent episcleral vessels. Arch Ophthalmol 97:493, 1979.

258. Bellows, AR, Chylack, LT Jr, Hutchinson, BT: Choroidal detachment. Clinical manifestation, therapy and mechanism of formation. Ophthalmology 88:1107, 1981.

259. Swan, KC, Lindgren, TW: Unintentional lens injury in glaucoma surgery. Trans Am Ophthalmol Soc 78:55, 1980.

260. Kozart, DM, Eagle, RC Jr: Stripping of Descemet's membrane after glaucoma surgery. Ophthalmic Surg 12:420, 1981.

261. Riley, SF, Smith, TJ, Simmons, RJ: Repair of a disinserted scleral flap in trabeculectomy. Ophthalmic Surg 24:349, 1993.

262. Riley, SF, Lima, FL, Smith, TJ, Simmons, RJ: Using donor sclera to create a flap in glaucoma filtering procedures. Ophthalmic Surg 25:117, 1994.

263. Kao, SF, Lichter, PR, Musch, DC: Anterior chamber depth following filtration surgery. Ophthalmic Surg 20:332, 1989.

264. Stewart, WC, Shields, MB: Management of anterior chamber depth after trabeculectomy. Am J Ophthalmol 106:41, 1988.

265. Fiore, PM, Richter, CU, Arzeno, G, et al: The effect of anterior chamber depth on endothelial cell count after filtration surgery. Arch Ophthalmol 107:1609, 1989.

266. Phillips, CI, Clark, CV, Levy, AM: Posterior synechiae after glaucoma operations: Aggravation by shallow anterior chamber and pilocarpine. Br J Ophthalmol 71:428, 1987.

267. Simmons, RJ, Kimbrough, RL: Shell tamponade in filtering surgery for glaucoma. Ophthalmic Surg 10:17, 1979.

268. Hill, RA, Aminlari, A, Sassani, JW, Michalski, M: Use of a symblepharon ring for treatment of over-filtration and leaking blebs after glaucoma filtration surgery. Ophthalmic Surg 21:707, 1990.

269. Blok, MDW, Kok, JHC, van Mil, C, et al: Use of the megasoft bandage lens for treatment of complications after trabeculectomy. Am J Ophthalmol 110:264, 1990.

270. Zalta, AH, Wieder, RH: Closure of leaking filtering blebs with cyanoacrylate tissue adhesive. Br J Ophthalmol 75:170, 1991.

271. Graham, SL, Goldberg, I: Cyanoacrylate adhesive closure of wound leaks following fornix-based trabeculectomy with adjunct 5-fluorouracil. J Glau 2:297, 1993.

272. Weber, PA, Baker, ND: The use of cyanoacrylate adhesive with a collagen shield in leaking filtering blebs. Ophthalmic Surg 20:284, 1989.

273. Graham, SL, Murray, B, Goldberg, I: Closure of fornix-based post-trabeculectomy conjunctival wound leaks with autologous fibrin glue. Am J Ophthalmol 114:221, 1992.

274. Asrani, SG, Wilensky, JT: Management of bleb leaks after glaucoma filtering surgery. Use of autologous fibrin tissue glue as an alternative. Ophthalmology 103:294, 1996.

275. Hennis, HL, Stewart, WC: Use of the argon laser to close filtering bleb leaks. Graefes Arch Clin Exp Ophthalmol 230:537, 1992.

276. Palmer, RM, Burgoyne, CF: Applications for a corneal mattress suture in anterior limbal wound repairs. Ophthalmic Surg 25:726, 1994.

277. Sugar, HS: Treatment of hypotony following filtering surgery for glaucoma. Am J Ophthalmol 71:1023, 1971.

278. Buxton, JN, Lavery, KT, Liebmann, JM, et al: Reconstruction of filtering blebs with free conjunctival autografts. Ophthalmology 101:635, 1994.

279. Wilson, MR, Kotas-Neumann, R: Free conjunctival patch for repair of persistent late bleb leak. Am J Ophthalmol 117:569, 1994.

280. Savage, JA, Condon, GP, Lytle, RA, Simmons, RJ: Laser suture lysis after trabeculectomy. Ophthalmology 95:1631, 1988.

281. Cohen, JS, Osher, RH: Releasable suture in filtering and combined procedures. In: Shields, MB, Pollack, IP, Kolker, AE, eds. Perspectives in glaucoma. Thorofare, NJ, Slack, Inc., 1988, p. 157.

282. Fisher, YL, Turtz, AI, Gold, M, et al: Use of sodium hyaluronate in reformation and reconstruction of the persistent flat anterior chamber in the presence of severe hypotony. Ophthalmic Surg 13:819, 1982.

283. Stewart, RH, Kimbrough, RL: A method of managing flat anterior chamber following trabeculectomy. Ophthalmic Surg 11:382, 1980.

284. Franks, WA, Hitchings, RA: Intraocular gas injection in the treatment of cornea-lens touch and choroidal effusion following fistulizing surgery. Ophthalmic Surg 21:831, 1990.

285. Asamoto, A, Yablonski, ME: Posttrabeculectomy anterior subcapsular cataract formation induced by anterior chamber air. Ophthalmic Surg 24:314, 1993.

286. Lee, DA, Wilson, MR, Yoshizumi, MO, Hall, M: The ocular effects of gases when injected into the anterior chamber of rabbit eyes. Arch Ophthalmol 109:571, 1991.

287. Brubaker, RF, Pederson, JE: Ciliochoroidal detachment. Surv Ophthalmol 27:281, 1983.

288. Chylack, LT Jr, Bellows, AR: Molecular sieving in suprachoroidal fluid formation in man. Invest Ophthalmol Vis Sci 17:420, 1978.

289. Stewart, WC, Crinkley, CMC: Influence of serous suprachoroidal detachments on the results of trabeculectomy surgery. Acta Ophthalmol 72:309, 1994.

290. Fourman, S: Management of cornea-lens touch after filtering surgery for glaucoma. Ophthalmology 97:424, 1990.

291. Lavin, M, Franks, W, Hitchings, RA: Serous retinal detachment following glaucoma filtering surgery. Arch Ophthalmol 108:1553, 1990.

292. Stamper, RL, McMenemy, MG, Lieberman, MF: Hypotonous maculopathy after trabeculectomy with subconjunctival 5-fluorouracil. Am J Ophthalmol 114:544, 1992.

293. Seah, SKL, Prata, JA Jr, Minckler, DS, et al: Hypotony following trabeculectomy. J Glau 4:73, 1995.

294. Zacharia, PT, Deppermann, SR, Schuman, JS: Ocular hypotony after trabeculectomy with mitomycin c. Am J Ophthalmol 116:314, 1993.

295. Wise, JB: Treatment of chronic postfiltration hypotony by intrableb injection of autologous blood. Arch Ophthalmol 111:827, 1993.

296. Nuyts, RMMA, Greve, EL, Geijssen, HC, Langerhorst, CT: Treatment of hypotonous maculopathy after trabeculectomy with mitomycin c. Am J Ophthalmol 118:322, 1994.

297. Leen, MM, Moster, MR, Katz, LJ, et al: Management of overfiltering and leaking blebs with autologous blood injection. Arch Ophthalmol 113:1050, 1995.

298. Smith, MF, Magauran, RG, III, Betchkal, J, Doyle, JW: Treatment of postfiltration bleb leaks with autologous blood. Ophthalmology 102:868, 1995.

299. Cohen, SM, Flynn, HW Jr, Palmberg, PF, et al: Treatment of hypotony maculopathy after trabeculectomy. Ophthalmic Surg Lasers 26:435, 1995.

300. Haynes, WL, Alward, WLM: Rapid visual recovery and long-term intraocular pressure control after donor scleral patch grafting for trabeculectomy-induced hypotony maculopathy. J Glau 4:200, 1995.

301. Clune, MJ, Shin, DH, Olivier, MMG, Kupin, TH: Partial-thickness scleral-patch graft in revision of trabeculectomy. Am J Ophthalmol 115:818, 1993.

302. Gressel, MG, Parrish, RK, Heuer, DK: Delayed nonexpulsive suprachoroidal hemorrhage. Arch Ophthalmol 102:1757, 1984.

303. Ruderman, JM, Harbin, TS Jr, Campbell, DG: Postoperative suprachoroidal hemorrhage following filtration procedures. Arch Ophthalmol 104:201, 1986.

304. Givens, K, Shields, MB: Suprachoroidal hemorrhage after glaucoma filtering surgery. Am J Ophthalmol 103:689, 1987.

305. Canning, CR, Lavin, M, McCartney, ACE, et al: Delayed suprachoroidal haemorrhage after glaucoma operations. Eye 3:327, 1989.

306. Rockwood, EJ, Kalenak, JW, Plotnik, JL, et al: Prospective ultrasonographic evaluation of intraoperative and delayed postoperative suprachoroidal hemorrhage from glaucoma filtering surgery. J Glau 4:16, 1995.

307. Chu, TG, Cano, MR, Green, RL, et al: Massive suprachoroidal hemorrhage with central retinal apposition. A clinical and echographic study. Arch Ophthalmol 109:1575, 1991.

308. Reynolds, MG, Haimovici, R, Flynn, HW Jr, et al: Suprachoroidal hemorrhage. Clinical features and results of secondary surgical management. Ophthalmology 100:460, 1993.

309. Le Mer, Y, Renard, Y, Allagui, M: Secondary management of suprachoroidal hemorrhages. Graefes Arch Clin Exp Ophthalmol 231:351, 1993.

310. Freeman, WR, Schneiderman, TE, Weinreb, RN, Baerveldt, G: Hemorrhagic choroidal detachment with anterior vitreoretinal adhesions. Ophthalmic Surg 22:670, 1991.

311. Traverso, CE, Greenidge, KC, Spaeth, GL, Wilson, RP: Focal Pressure: a new method to encourage filtration after trabeculectomy. Ophthalmic Surg 15:62, 1984.

312. Pappa, KS, Derick, RJ, Weber, PA, et al: Late argon laser suture lysis after mitomycin c trabeculectomy. Ophthalmology 100:1268, 1993.

313. Haynes, WL, Alward, WLM, McKinney, JK: Low-energy argon laser suture lysis after trabeculectomy. Am J Ophthalmol 117:800, 1994.

314. Beck, AD, Lynch, MG, Noe, R, Brown, RH: The use of a new laser lens holder for performing suture lysis in children. Arch Ophthalmol 113:140, 1995.

315. Morinelli, EN, Sidoti, PA, Heuer, DK, et al: Laser suture lysis after mitomycin c trabeculectomy. Ophthalmology 103:306, 1996.

316. Ortiz, JR, Walker, SD, McManus, PE, et al: Filtering bleb thrombolysis with tissue plasminogen activator. Am J Ophthalmol 106:624, 1988.

317. Tripathi, RC, Tripathi, BJ, Bornstein, S, et al: Use of tissue plasminogen activator for rapid dissolution of fibrin and blood clots in the eye after surgery for glaucoma and cataract in humans. Drug Dev Res 27:147, 1992.

318. Koerner, F, Boehnke, M: Clinical use of recombinant plasminogen activator for intraocular fibrinolysis. Ger J Ophthalmol 1:354, 1992.

319. Lundy, DC, Sidoti, P, Winarko, T, Minckler, D, Heuer, DK: Intracameral tissue plasminogen activator after glaucoma surgery. Indications, effectiveness, and complications. Ophthalmology 103:274, 1996.

320. Piltz, JR, Starita, RJ: The use of subconjunctivally administered tissue plasminogen activator after trabeculectomy. Ophthalmic Surg 25:51, 1994.

321. Sherwood, MB, Spaeth, GL, Simmons, ST, et al: Cysts of Tenon's capsule following filtration surgery. Medical management. Arch Ophthalmol 105:1517, 1987.

322. Scott, DR, Quigley, HA: Medical management of a high bleb phase after trabeculectomies. Ophthalmology 95:1169, 1988.

323. Richter, CU, Shingleton, BJ, Bellows, AR, et al: The development of encapsulated filtering blebs. Ophthalmology 95:1163, 1988.

324. Sherwood, MB, Grierson, I, Millar, L, Hitchings, RA: Long-term morphologic effects of antiglaucoma drugs on the conjunctiva and Tenon's capsule in glaucomatous patients. Ophthalmology 96:327, 1989.

325. Schoenleber, DB, Bellows, AR, Hutchinson, BT: Failed laser trabeculoplasty requiring surgery in open-angle glaucoma. Ophthalmic Surg 18:796, 1987.

326. Feldman, RM, Gross, RL, Spaeth, GL, et al: Risk factors for the development of Tenon's capsule cysts after trabeculectomy. Ophthalmology 96:336, 1989.

327. Oh, Y, Katz, LJ, Spaeth, GL, Wilson, RP: Risk factors for the development of encapsulated filtering blebs. The role of surgical glove powder for 5-fluorouracil. Ophthalmology 101:629, 1994.

328. Campagna, JA, Munden, PM, Alward, WLM: Tenon's cyst formation after trabeculectomy with mitomycin c. Ophthalmic Surg 26:57, 1995.

329. Shingleton, BJ, Richter, CU, Bellows, AR, Hutchinson, BT: Management of encapsulated filtration blebs. Ophthalmology 97:63, 1990.

330. Loftfield, K, Ball, SF: Filtering bleb encapsulation increased by steroid injection. Ophthalmic Surg 21:282, 1990.

331. Pederson, JE, Smith, SG: Surgical management of encapsulated filtering blebs. Ophthalmology 92:955, 1985.

332. Ewing, RH, Stamper, RL: Needle revision with and without 5-fluorouracil for the treatment of failed filtering blebs. Am J Ophthalmol 110:254, 1990.

333. Hodge, W, Saheb, N, Balazsi, G, Kasner, O: Treatment of encapsulated blebs with 30-gauge needling and injection of low-dose 5-fluorouracil. Can J Ophthalmol 27:233, 1992.

334. Shin, DH, Juzych, MS, Khatana, AK, et al: Needling revision of failed filtering blebs with adjunctive 5-fluorouracil. Ophthalmic Surg 24:242, 1993.

335. Mazey, BJ, Siegel, MJ, Siegel, LI, Dunn, SP: Corneal endothelial toxic effect secondary to fluorouracil needle bleb revision. Arch Ophthalmol 112:1411, 1994.

336. Van Buskirk, EM: Cysts of Tenon's capsule following filtration surgery. Am J Ophthalmol 94:522, 1982.

337. Konstas, AGP, Jay, JL: Modification of trabeculectomy to avoid postoperative hyphaema. The "guarded anterior fistula" operation. Br J Ophthalmol 76:353, 1992.

338. Soong, HK, Quigley, HA: Dellen associated with filtering blebs. Arch Ophthalmol 101:385, 1983.

339. O'Connell, EJ, Karseras, AG: Intraocular surgery in advanced glaucoma. Br J Ophthalmol 60:124, 1976.

340. Lawrence, GA: Surgical treatment of patients with advanced glaucomatous field defects. Arch Ophthalmol 81:804, 1969.

341. Lichter, PR, Ravin, JG: Risks of sudden visual loss after glaucoma surgery. Am J Ophthalmol 78:1009, 1974.

342. Costa, VP, Smith, M, Spaeth, GL, et al: Loss of visual acuity after trabeculectomy. Ophthalmology 100:599, 1993.

343. Martinez, JA, Brown, RH, Lynch, MG, Caplan, MB: Risk of postoperative visual loss in advanced glaucoma. Am J Ophthalmol 115:332, 1993.

344. Aggarwal, SP, Hendeles, S: Risk of sudden visual loss following trabeculectomy in advanced primary open-angle glaucoma. Br J Ophthalmol 70:97, 1986.

345. Fechtner, RD, Minckler, D, Weinreb, RN, et al: Complications of glaucoma surgery. Ocular decompression retinopathy. Arch Ophthalmol 110:965, 1992.

346. Hitchings, RA, Grierson, I: Clinicopathological correlation in eyes with failed fistulizing surgery. Trans Ophthalmol Soc UK 103:84, 1983.

347. Swan, KC: Reopening of nonfunctioning filters—simplified surgical techniques. Trans Am Acad Ophthalmol Otol 79:342, 1975.

348. Cohen, JS, Shaffer, RN, Hetherington, J Jr, Hoskins, D: Revision of filtration surgery. Arch Ophthalmol 95:1612, 1977.

349. Kurata, F, Krupin, T, Kolker, AE: Reopening filtration fistulas with transconjunctival argon laser photocoagulation. Am J Ophthalmol 98:340, 1984.

350. Rankin, GA, Latina, MA: Transconjunctival Nd:YAG laser revision of failing trabeculectomy. Ophthalmic Surg 21:365, 1990.

351. Latina, MA, Rankin, GA: Internal and transconjunctival neodymium:YAG laser revision of late failing filters. Ophthalmology 98:215, 1991.

352. Simmons, RB, Simmons, RJ: A better way to manage a failing filter. Rev Ophthalmol 82(Nov):82, 1995.

353. Ticho, U, Ivry, M: Reopening of occluded filtering blebs by argon laser photocoagulation. Am J Ophthalmol 84:413, 1977.

354. Van Buskirk, EM: Reopening filtration fistulas with the argon laser. Am J Ophthalmol 94:1, 1982.

355. Praeger, DL: The reopening of closed filtering blebs using the neodymium:YAG laser. Ophthalmology 91:373, 1984.

356. Dailey, RA, Samples, JR, Van Buskirk, EM: Reopening filtration fistulas with the neodymium:YAG laser. Am J Ophthalmol 102:491, 1986.

357. Oh, Younghyun, Katz, LJ: Indications and technique for reopening closed filtering blebs using the Nd:YAG laser—a review and case series. Ophthalmic Surg 24:617, 1993.

358. Cohn, HC, Whalen, WR, Aron-Rosa, D: YAG laser treatment in a series of failed trabeculectomies. Am J Ophthalmol 108:395, 1989.

359. Durcan, FJ, Cioff, GA, Van Buskirk, EM: Same-site revision of failed filtering blebs. J Glau 1:2, 1992.

360. Ruderman, JM, Allen, RC: Simmons' tamponade shell for leaking filtration blebs. Arch Ophthalmol 103:1708, 1985.

361. Melamed, S, Hersh, P, Kersten, D, et al: The use of glaucoma shell tamponade in leaking filtration blebs. Ophthalmology 93:839, 1986.

362. Fourman, S, Wiley, L: Use of a collagen shield to treat a glaucoma filter bleb leak. Am J Ophthalmol 107:673, 1989.

363. Sinnreich, Z, Barishak, R, Stein, R: Leaking filtering blebs. Am J Ophthalmol 86:345, 1978.

364. Hattenhauer, JM, Lipsich, MP: Late endophthalmitis after filtering surgery. Am J Ophthalmol 72:1097, 1971.

365. Ashkenazi, I, Melamed, S, Avni, I, et al: Risk factors associated with late infection of filtering blebs and endophthalmitis. Ophthalmic Surg 22:570, 1991.

366. Lobue, TD, Deutsch, TA, Stein, RM: Moraxella nonliquefaciens endophthalmitis after trabeculectomy. Am J Ophthalmol 99:343, 1985.

367. Phillips, WB, II, Wong, TP, Bergren, RL, et al: Late onset endophthalmitis associated with filtering blebs. Ophthalmic Surg 25:88, 1994.

368. Freedman, J, Gupta, M, Bunke, A: Endophthalmitis after trabeculectomy. Arch Ophthalmol 96:1017, 1978.

369. Ticho, U, Ophir, A: Late complications after glaucoma filtering surgery with adjunctive 5-fluorouracil. Am J Ophthalmol 115:506, 1993.

370. Wand, M, Quintiliani, R, Robinson, A: Antibiotic prophylaxis in eyes with filtration blebs: survey of glaucoma specialists, microbiological study, and recommendations. J Glau 4:103, 1995.

371. Brown, RH, Yang, LH, Walker, SD, et al: Treatment of bleb infection after glaucoma surgery. Arch Ophthalmol 112:57, 1994.

372. Mandelbaum, S, Forster, RK, Gelender, H, Culbertson, W: Late onset endophthalmitis associated with filtering blebs. Ophthalmology 92:964, 1985.

373. Kanski, JJ: Treatment of late endophthalmitis associated with filtering blebs. Arch Ophthalmol 91:339, 1974.

374. Stern, GA, Engel, HM, Driebe, WT, Jr: The treatment of postoperative endophthalmitis. Results of differing approaches to treatment. Ophthalmology 96:62, 1989.

375. Olk, RJ, Bohigian, GM: The management of endophthalmitis: diagnostic and therapeutic guidelines including the use of vitrectomy. Ophthalmic Surg 18:262, 1987.

376. Endophthalmitis Vitrectomy Study Group: Results of the endophthalmitis vitrectomy study. A randomized trial of immediate vitrectomy and of intravenous antibiotics for the treatment of postoperative bacterial endophthalmitis. Arch Ophthalmol 113: 1479, 1995.

377. Sugar, HS: Cataract and filtering surgery. Am J Ophthalmol 69: 740, 1970.

378. Chauvaud, D, Clay-Fressinet, C, Pouliquen, Y, Offret, G: Opacification of the lens after trabeculectomy. Arch Ophthalmol (Paris) 36:379, 1976.

379. Vesti, E: Development of cataract after trabeculectomy. Acta Ophthalmol 71:777, 1993.

380. Fink, AJ, Boys-Smith, JW, Brear, R: Management of large filtering blebs with the argon laser. Am J Ophthalmol 101:695, 1986.

381. Scheie, HG, Guehl, JJ III: Surgical management of overhanging blebs after filtering procedures. Arch Ophthalmol 97:325, 1979.

382. Harris, LS, Galin, MA: Delayed spontaneous hyphema following successful sclerotomy with cautery in three patients. Am J Ophthalmol 72:458, 1971.

383. Namba, H: Blood reflux into anterior chamber after trabeculectomy. Jpn J Ophthalmol 27:616, 1983.

384. Wilensky, JT: Late hyphema after filtering surgery for glaucoma. Ophthalmic Surg 14:227, 1983.

385. Michels, RG, Rice, TA: Bimanual bipolar diathermy for treatment of bleeding from the anterior chamber angle. Am J Ophthalmol 84: 873, 1977.

386. Vela, MA, Campbell, DG: Hypotony and ciliochoroidal detachment following pharmacologic aqueous suppressant therapy in previously filtered patients. Ophthalmology 92:50, 1985.

387. Berke, SJ, Bellows, R, Shingleton, BJ, et al: Chronic and recurrent choroidal detachment after glaucoma filtering surgery. Ophthalmology 94:154, 1987.

388. Burney, EN, Quigley, HA, Robin, AL: Hypotony and choroidal detachment as late complications of trabeculectomy. Am J Ophthalmol 103:685, 1987.

389. Laatikainen, L, Syrdalen, P: Tearing of retinal pigment epithelium after glaucoma surgery. Graefes Arch Clin Exp Ophthalmol 225: 308, 1987.

390. Smith, DL, Skuta, GL, Lindenmuth, KA, et al: The effect of glaucoma filtering surgery on corneal endothelial cell density. Ophthalmic Surg 22:251, 1991.

391. Pastor, SA, Williams, R, Hetherington, J, et al: Corneal endothelial cell loss following trabeculectomy with mitomycin c. J Glau 2: 112, 1993.

392. Rosen, WJ, Mannis, MJ, Brandt, JD: The effect of trabeculectomy on corneal topography. Ophthalmic Surg 23:395, 1992.

393. Hugkulstone, CE: Changes in keratometry following trabeculectomy. Br J Ophthalmol 75:217, 1991.

394. Putterman, AM, Urist, MJ: Upper eyelid retraction after glaucoma filtering procedures. Ann Ophthalmol 7:263, 1975.

395. Alpar, JJ: Acquired ptosis following cataract and glaucoma surgery. Glaucoma 4:66, 1982.

396. Deady, JP, Price, NJ, Sutton, GA: Ptosis following cataract and trabeculectomy surgery. Br J Ophthalmol 73:283, 1989.

397. Shammas, HF, Zubyk, NA, Stanfield, TF: Sympathetic uveitis following glaucoma surgery. Arch Ophthalmol 95:638, 1977.

398. Drance, SM, Vargas, E: Trabeculectomy and thermosclerectomy: a comparison of two procedures. Can J Ophthalmol 8:413, 1973.

399. Lewis, RA, Phelps, CD: Trabeculectomy v thermosclerostomy. A five-year follow-up. Arch Ophthalmol 102:533, 1984.

400. Spaeth, GL, Joseph, NH, Fernandes, E: Trabeculectomy: a re-evaluation after three years and a comparison with Scheie's procedure. Trans Am Acad Ophthalmol Otol 79:349, 1975.

401. Spaeth, GL, Poryzees, E: A comparison between peripheral iridectomy with thermal sclerostomy and trabeculectomy: a controlled study. Br J Ophthalmol 65:783, 1981.

402. Watkins, PH Jr, Brubaker, RF: Comparison of partial-thickness and full-thickness filtration procedures in open-angle glaucoma. Am J Ophthalmol 86:756, 1978.

403. Blondeau, P, Phelps, CD: Trabeculectomy vs. thermosclerostomy. A randomized prospective clinical trial. Arch Ophthalmol 99: 810, 1981.

404. Wilson, MR: Posterior lip sclerectomy vs. trabeculectomy in West Indian blacks. Arch Ophthalmol 107:1604, 1989.

405. Wilson, P: Trabeculectomy: Long-term follow-up. Br J Ophthalmol 61:535, 1977.

406. D'Ermo, F, Bonomi, L, Doro, D: A critical analysis of the long-term results of trabeculectomy. Am J Ophthalmol 88:829, 1979.

407. Zaidi, AA: Trabeculectomy: a review and 4-year follow-up. Br J Ophthalmol 64:436, 1980.

408. Jerndal, T, Lundstrom, M: 330 trabeculectomies. A long time study (3–5½ years). Acta Ophthalmol 58:947, 1980.

409. Mills, KB: Trabeculectomy: a retrospective long-term follow-up of 444 cases. Br J Ophthalmol 65:790, 1981.

410. Inaba, Z: Longterm results of trabeculectomy in the Japanese: An analysis of life table method. Jpn J Ophthalmol 26:361, 1982.

411. Popovic, V, Sjostrand, J: Long-term outcome following trabeculectomy: I. Retrospective analysis of intraocular pressure regulation and cataract formation. Acta Ophthalmol 69:299, 1991.

412. Akafo, SK, Goulstine, DB, Rosenthal, AR: Long-term post-trabeculectomy intraocular pressures. Acta Ophthalmol 70:312, 1992.

413. Nouri-Mahdavi, K, Brigatti, L, Weitzman, M, Caprioli, J: Outcomes of trabeculectomy for primary open-angle glaucoma. Ophthalmology 102:1760, 1995.

414. Popovic, V, Sjostrand, J: Long-term outcome following trabeculectomy: II. Visual field survival. Acta Ophthalmol 69:305, 1991.

415. Törnqvist, G, Drolsum, LK: Trabeculectomies. A long-term study. Acta Ophthalmol 69:450, 1991.

416. Freedman, J, Shen, E, Ahrens, M: Trabeculectomy in a Black American glaucoma population. Br J Ophthalmol 60:573, 1976.

417. Ferguson, JG Jr, MacDonald, R Jr: Trabeculectomy in blacks: a two-year follow-up. Ophthalmic Surg 8:41, 1977.

418. David, R, Freedman, J, Luntz, MH: Comparative study of Watson's and Cairn's trabeculectomies in a black population with open angle glaucoma. Br J Ophthalmol 61:117, 1977.

419. BenEzra, D, Chirambo, MC: Trabeculectomy. Ann Ophthalmol 10:1101, 1978.

420. Stewart, WC, Reid, KK, Pitts, RA: The results of trabeculectomy surgery in African-American versus white glaucoma patients. J Glau 2:236, 1993.

421. Miller, RD, Barber, JC: Trabeculectomy in black patients. Ophthalmic Surg 12:46, 1981.

422. Broadway, D, Grierson, I, Hitchings, R: Racial differences in the results of glaucoma filtration surgery: are racial differences in the conjunctival cell profile important? Br J Ophthalmol 78:466, 1994.

423. Thommy, CP, Bhar, IS: Trabeculectomy in Nigerian patients with open-angle glaucoma. Br J Ophthalmol 63:636, 1979.

424. Sandford-Smith, JH: The surgical treatment of open-angle glaucoma in Nigerians. Br J Ophthalmol 62:283, 1978.

425. Bakker, NJA, Manku, SI: Trabeculectomy versus Scheie's operation: a comparative retrospective study in open-angle glaucoma in Kenyans. Br J Ophthalmol 63:643, 1979.

426. Kietzman, B: Glaucoma surgery in Nigerian eyes: a five-year study. Ophthalmic Surg 7:52, 1976.

427. Cadera, W, Pachtman, MA, Cantor, LB, et al: Filtering surgery in childhood glaucoma. Ophthalmic Surg 15:319, 1984.

428. Stewart, RH, Kimbrough, RL, Bachh, H, Allbright, M: Trabeculectomy and modifications of trabeculectomy. Ophthalmic Surg 10:76, 1979.

429. Kolozsvari, L: Trabeculectomy in cases of buphthalmos. Klin Monatsbl Augenheilkd 183:503, 1983.

430. Gressel, MG, Heuer, DK, Parrish, RK II: Trabeculectomy in young patients. Ophthalmology 91:1242, 1984.

431. Beauchamp, GR, Parks, MM: Filtering surgery in children: barriers to success. Ophthalmology 86:170, 1979.

432. Costa, VP, Katz, LJ, Spaeth, GL, et al: Primary trabeculectomy in young adults. Ophthalmology 100:1071, 1993.

433. Sturmer, J, Broadway, DC, Hitchings, RA: Young patient trabeculectomy. Assessment of risk factors for failure. Ophthalmology 100:928, 1993.

434. Levene, RZ: Glaucoma filtering surgery factors that determine pressure control. Trans Am Ophthalmol Soc 82:282, 1984.

435. Heuer, DK, Gressel, MG, Parrish, RK II, et al: Trabeculectomy in aphakic eyes. Ophthalmology 91:1045, 1984.

436. Salmon, JF: The role of trabeculectomy in the treatment of advanced chronic angle-closure glaucoma. J Glau 2:285, 1993.

437. Mary Lynch, M.D., personal communication.

DRAINAGE IMPLANT SURGERY[a]

In an attempt to maintain patency of a drainage fistula in glaucoma filtering operations, a wide variety of foreign materials have been implanted in the eye, extending from the anterior chamber to a subconjunctival space. These were once referred to as setons, because the implants consisted of solid structures, such as threads, wires, or hairs, that were placed in a wound to form a track or fistula. These procedures were uniformly unsuccessful in maintaining a patent fistula. Newer devices, however, which utilize tubes that drain into external reservoirs, have been shown to have clinical benefit. In this chapter, we review the more commonly used drainage implant devices, the surgical techniques of implantation, the complications and their management, and the comparative merits and indications for this group of glaucoma surgical procedures.

IMPLANT DESIGNS

All modern drainage implant devices have the same basic design, which consists of a plastic tube that extends from the anterior chamber (or, in some cases, the vitreous cavity) to a plate, disc, or encircling element beneath conjunctiva and Tenon's capsule. The devices differ according to the size and shape of the external component and the materials from

which that component and the tube are constructed. One of the most fundamental design differences, however, is whether the device has an open, unobstructed drainage tube or one that contains a pressure-regulating valve.

Open Tube Implants

Molteno Implant

This is the prototype drainage implant device and has had the longest and most extensive clinical experience, since it was introduced by Molteno in 1969 (1). The original design consists of a *single-plate* of thin acrylic with a diameter of 13 mm and an area of 135 mm (2) (Fig. 38.1). A silicone tube, with an external diameter of 0.63 mm and an internal diameter of 0.30 mm, connects to the upper surface of the plate. The plate has a thickened rim, which is perforated to allow suturing to the sclera.

Subsequent modifications addressed various problems encountered with the original design. Success rates with single-plate Molteno implantation for glaucomas with poor surgical prognoses (aphakic/pseudophakic eyes, prior failed filters, neovascular glaucoma, and patients younger than 3 years of age) ranged from 25% to 46% in one study, but rose to 40% to 71% with implantation of a second plate (2). A *double-plate* Molteno implant combines two plates, one of which is attached to the silicone tube in the anterior

[a]Refer to M.B. Shields: Color Atlas of Glaucoma. Baltimore: Williams & Wilkins, 1998, Plates III37–41.

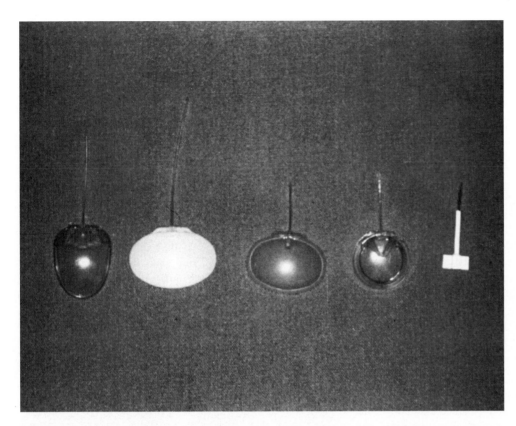

Figure 38.1. Glaucoma drainage implant devices. From *left* to *right*: Ahmed glaucoma valve, 200-mm² Baerveldt implant, Krupin eye valve with disc, dual-chamber Molteno implant, OptiMed implant. (Reprinted with permission from Prata, JA Jr, Mérmoud, A, LaBree, L, Minckler, DS: In vitro and in vivo flow characteristics of glaucoma drainage implants. Ophthalmology 102:894, 1995).

chamber, while a second tube connects the two plates, giving an increased surface area of 270 mm² (3). In a randomized trial of single-plate versus double-plate implants, the latter provided better intraocular pressure (IOP) control, but was associated with a greater risk of complications, most of which were related to hypotony (4). Another modification, which addresses the problem of hypotony, is the *dual-chamber,* single-plate implant, in which a V-shaped "pressure ridge" on the upper surface of the plate encases an area of 10.5 mm² around the opening of the silicone tube (5). In concept, the pressure ridge and overlying Tenon's capsule regulate the flow of aqueous into the main bleb cavity during the early postoperative period, thereby minimizing excessive filtration and hypotony. The validity of this concept was supported in one study of 40 consecutive patients (6).

The mechanism by which Molteno implants, and presumably the other drainage implant devices, control the IOP relates to a fibrous capsule that forms around the plate (Figs. 38.2 and 38.3). Studies of monkey eyes with single-plate Molteno implants indicate that the capsule functions by a passive mechanism, shunting the flow of aqueous humor (7). Latex microspheres passed freely through the capsule, but concentrated in the extracapsular space, suggesting that the capsule limits the filtration rate. The microspheres were also observed in the episcleral wall of the capsule, indicating that all surfaces contribute to filtration. This is consistent with echographic studies in human eyes, which reveal bleb formation on both sides of the plate in successful cases (8) (Fig. 38.4). Histopathologic studies of human eyes that were enucleated 2–6 years after Molteno implant

surgery revealed patent tubes with no appreciable anterior chamber reaction and minimal inflammatory reaction in the outer layers of the bleb wall (9).

Schocket Tube Shunt

Schocket and associates (10, 11) developed a technique in which a silicone, or Silastic, tube is extended from the anterior chamber to a 360° encircling #20 or #31 silicone band, as used in retinal detachment repair, which functioned in developing the reservoir for aqueous drainage. Modifications have included insertion of the tube into a band extending for only 90° beneath two rectus muscles (12), or into the preexisting encircling band in eyes with glaucoma after scleral buckling surgery (13). A long Krupin-Denver valve implant (discussed later under "Krupin Implants") has also been used in combination with a 180° scleral band (14).

Two randomized trials compared Schocket tube shunts to double-plate Molteno implants. Despite the fact that the Schocket shunt typically provides a larger surface area of the reservoir than the Molteno implants, the latter provided lower final IOPs in both studies (15, 16).

Baerveldt Implant

The unique feature of this series of nonvalved drainage implants is the large surface area of the plates, which are designed in such a way that they can be implanted through a one-quadrant conjunctival incision (Fig. 38.1). A silicone tube is attached to a barium-impregnated silicone plate

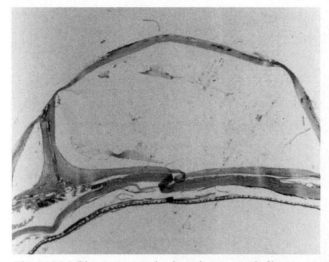

Figure 38.2. Photomicrograph of monkey eye with fibrous capsule surrounding a single-plate Molteno implant (lost in processing). A tongue of fibrous tissue has extended through a suture hole, connecting the two walls of the capsule. (Courtesy of Donand S. Minckler, M.D.)

with a surface area of 200 mm^2 (20 × 13 mm), 350 mm^2 (32 × 14 mm), or 500 mm^2 (36 × 17.5 mm) (17). In a rabbit study, the 200 mm^2 device and modified plates with surface areas of 100 mm^2 and 50 mm^2 were implanted and studied at 3 and 12 weeks for calculated resistance to flow (18). The results demonstrated a direct relationship between the surface area of the implants and the filtering capacity of their surrounding capsule.

The 350-mm^2 Baerveldt implant was compared with the double-plate Molteno implant in 34 patients with uncontrolled, complicated glaucoma, which revealed comparable IOP control with the two devices (19). However, the larger plates may be associated with more frequent postoperative complications, which will be discussed later in this chapter.

Valved Drainage Implants

Krupin Implants

The concept of a one-way valve, that opens at a predetermined IOP level to avoid the early postoperative complications of excessive drainage and hypotony, was introduced by Krupin and associates in 1976 (20). The original *Krupin-Denver valve* was composed of an internal Supramid tube cemented to an external Silastic tube (20). The valve-effect was created by making slits in the closed external end of the Silastic tube. The tube was short, extending only a few millimeters subconjunctivally, and had no external plate. Although preliminary experience was encouraging (21, 22), fibrosis eventually closed the subconjunctival portion of the valved tube (23), which led to failure in most cases.

In a subsequent technique, a long Krupin-Denver drainage tube, with the same one-way valve design, was attached to a 180° Schocket-type scleral explant, as previously described (14). This led to development of the *Krupin Eye*

Valve with Disc, which is the design in current use (Fig. 38.1). A Silastic tube is attached to an oval Silastic disc, conformed to the curvature of the globe, 13 × 18 mm, with 1.75-mm high side walls (24). The valve at the distal end of the tube is the same design as in the earlier Krupin implants and is manometrically calibrated to open at pressures between 10 and 12 mm Hg and close between 8 and 10 mm Hg.

Ahmed Glaucoma Valve

In this valved drainage implant design, a silicone tube is connected to a silicone sheet valve which is held in a polypropylene body (Fig. 38.1) (25). The body has a surface area of 180 mm^2 (16 × 13 mm) and is 1.9 mm thick. The valve mechanism consists of two thin silicone elastomer membranes, 8 mm long and 7 mm wide, which create a venturi-shaped chamber. Because the inlet cross-section of the chamber is wider than the outlet, a pressure differential is created which enables the valve to remain open even with a small pressure differential between the anterior chamber and sub-

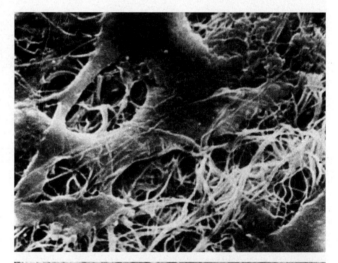

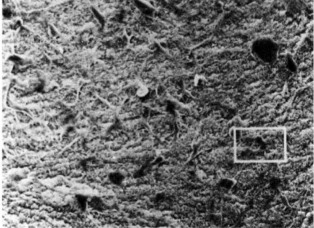

Figure 38.3. Scanning electron micrograph at low *(below)* and higher magnification *(inset)* of inner surface of fibrous capsule surrounding Molteno implant in human eye, removed during surgical revision. In the higher magnification, the surface is an open collagen mesh with a sparse population of probable fibroblasts. (Courtesy of Donald S. Minckler, M.D.)

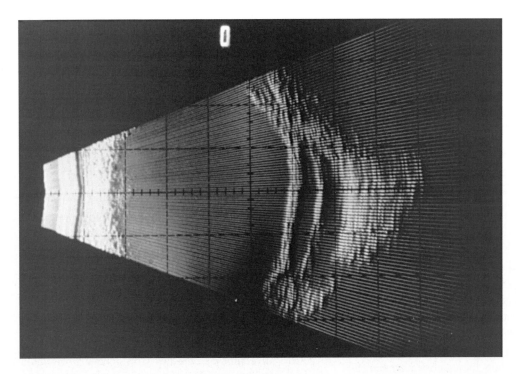

Figure 38.4. B-scan ultrasound of a functioning bleb around a Baerveldt implant in a human eye. The plate is represented by the middle echo, surrounded by echolucent fluid on both sides. The flattening of the adjacent eye wall is characteristic. (Courtesy of Donald S. Minckler, M.D.)

conjunctival space. The valve is designed to open with an IOP of 8 mm Hg.

Other Valved Implants

Other valved implants include the *Joseph tube* (silicone tube with slit valve in its side, calibrated to open between 4 and 20 mm Hg, attached to a 9-mm-wide silicone rubber strap) (26), the *OptiMed implant* (180–200 microtubules in a $3 \times 2 \times 2$ mm polymethylmethacrylate box, which allows aqueous to escape into periocular space) (27) (Fig. 38.1), and the *White pump shunt* (which has a surface area of 80 mm^2 and a mechanism that allows pumping of the reservoir to maintain patency of the tube) (28, 29).

The Krupin, Baerveldt, Ahmed, and OptiMed implants were compared in vitro and in vivo in rabbits (27). In air, the Krupin and Ahmed implants had opening pressures of 7.2 and 9.2 mm Hg and closing pressures of 3.9 and 5.2 mm, respectively. The OptiMed implant had the highest resistance values, with in vivo IOPs of 19.6 ± 5.6 mm Hg, compared to 7.5 ± 0.8 mm Hg with the Ahmed implant. In another study, comparing the clinical results of Joseph implants with Schocket-type implants and Molteno implants, the Joseph implants provided slightly lower IOPs and had significantly fewer failures than the Schocket devices, although the Molteno implants provided the lowest pressures at 12 months among eyes with successful IOP control (30).

SURGICAL TECHNIQUES

Basic Principles

The following techniques have been described for implantation of a single-plate Molteno device (31) (Fig. 38.5). Although certain variations are required for the different implant designs, these basic surgical principles apply in general to all drainage implant devices.

A fornix-based conjunctival flap is created in the superotemporal or superonasal quadrant. Whenever possible, the superonasal quadrant should be avoided, especially with the larger plate designs, to reduce the risk of inducing strabismus, which is discussed later (32). It has also been shown that the Ahmed implant, when placed in the superonasal quadrant, may come within 1 mm of the optic nerve (33). Since it is necessary to have surgical exposure to or beyond the equator of the globe, radial relaxing incisions should be placed on one or both sides of the conjunctival flap. Adequate surgical exposure is also dependent on proper placement of the bridle suture(s). One technique is to isolate the two rectus muscles on either side of the surgical site, after blunt dissection of Tenon's capsule from the episclera, and pass 4–0 silk sutures beneath each muscle. Alternatively, a partial-thickness, clear cornea suture of 6–0 silk can be placed near the surgical site and attached to the drape beneath the eye.

Spatulated needles with 8–0 silk suture are threaded through the two anterior positional holes of the external plate, and the plate is then tucked into sub-Tenon's space posteriorly and sutured to sclera with the anterior border 9–10 mm posterior to the limbus. Variations of this technique are obviously required for different plate designs. Implants with plates of larger circumferential dimensions, such as the Baerveldt, must be tucked under adjacent rectus muscles, while Schocket-type designs require dissection of one or more additional quadrants, depending on the extent of the encircling band. In the case of the Ahmed implant, which has larger anterior-posterior dimensions, it may be advisable not to extend the anterior border of the plate more than 8 mm behind the limbus.

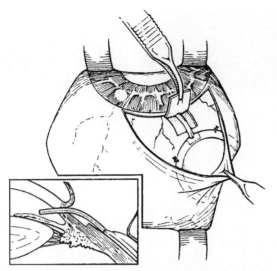

Figure 38.5. Basic technique of inserting Molteno implant. Silicone tube is inserted into anterior chamber via needle track and is connected to a subconjunctival acrylic plate that is attached to the sclera near the equator.

Before inserting the tube into the anterior chamber, a 6 × 8-mm partial-thickness, limbus-based scleral flap, as described in Chapter 37 for the trabeculectomy procedure, is dissected. A paracentesis is next made at the limbus in the inferotemporal quadrant with a sharp tapered blade. The anterior chamber is then entered beneath the scleral flap with a 21–23-gauge needle parallel to the iris plane. The angle at which the needle enters the anterior chamber is critical, since it is important that the tube, which will pass through this needle track, vault between cornea and iris, without touching either structure. The tube is cut, bevel up, to permit its extension 2–3 mm into the anterior chamber. With valved implants, it is advisable to irrigate balanced salt solution through the tube to ensure that the valve opens properly. The tube is then inserted into the anterior chamber via the needle track, using nontoothed forceps, and is secured to the sclera with a loose 9–0 or 10–0 nylon suture. The scleral flap is approximated at the two posterior corners with 10–0 nylon suture, and the conjunctiva-Tenon's capsule flap is secured at the limbus with wing sutures of 10–0 nylon or synthetic absorbable suture. The anterior chamber is then deepened with balanced salt solution via the paracentesis, and the tube is checked for proper position in the anterior chamber.

Subconjunctival steroids and antibiotics are injected at the completion of the procedure in a quadrant away from the surgical site. The basic postoperative management is the same as that described in Chapter 37 for filtering surgery, with topical steroid-antibiotic and mydriatic-cycloplegic preparations for the first several weeks.

Modifications of Basic Technique

Despite the use of a protective scleral flap, the tube will occasionally erode through both the scleral and conjunctival flaps at the limbus. To avoid this potential complication, most surgeons will suture a rectangle of preserved donor sclera of approximately 5 × 7 mm over the tube at the limbus. Processed pericardium is also available commercially for this purpose.

A common complication that has been encountered with the nonvalved implants is excessive filtration and hypotony in the early postoperative period. A variety of tube ligatures and stents have been used to minimize this problem and are discussed later under "Complications: Prevention and Management." Another surgical modification that has been used to address this issue is a two-stage approach, in which the tube is placed in the conjunctival space in the first stage. After the fibrous capsule has had time to develop, the tube is inserted into the anterior chamber in the second stage.

Another potential complication, as with all filtration procedures, is failure due to excessive fibrosis. A rabbit study was performed with bilateral implantation of 200 mm² Baerveldt implants, in which one eye was exposed intraoperatively to mitomycin-C 0.5 mg/ml for 5 minutes (34). The mitomycin-C-treated eyes had lower IOPs and higher perfusion rates at 2, 4, and 6 weeks, and histologic examination revealed thinner fibrous capsules with delayed maturation and less inflammatory infiltrate. Alternatively, subconjunctival 5-fluorouracil might be used postoperatively, although the value of either antimetabolite with drainage implant surgery has yet to be proven in clinical trials.

In aphakic (or possibly pseudophakic) eyes, in which a vitrectomy has been performed, it is also possible to insert the tube through a pars plana incision into the vitreous cavity. This has the advantage of keeping the tube away from the cornea and iris and reducing the risk of epithelial downgrowth.

COMPLICATIONS: PREVENTION AND MANAGEMENT

Hypotony

Until the fibrous capsule has developed around the external plate to regulate aqueous flow, the open, valveless tube implants, as noted earlier, provide very low resistance to flow, and hypotony in the early postoperative course is a frequent and serious complication. By far the best way to deal with this potential complication is prevention by temporarily obstructing the tube lumen. A wide variety of techniques have been described to achieve this goal. One basic technique is suture ligation of the tube. An 8–0 monofilament nylon suture can be tied around the intraocular portion of the tube and cut 7–10 days later with an argon laser (35), or a releasable nylon suture can be placed around the portion of the tube beneath the scleral flap with one end of the suture externalized on the cornea for later removal (36). A variation of the releasable suture is placement of a 6–0 absorbable (e.g., polyglactin) suture around a 5–0 Prolene suture and the tube near the plate, with one end of the Prolene suture near the limbus for subsequent removal (37). Others have described combining an absorbable suture ligature with the injection of perfluropropane in aphakic, vitrectomized eyes (38).

Another basic technique to minimize early hypotony is temporary occlusion of the tube lumen with a stent. A 5–0 nylon suture can be threaded into the tube at the plate end and secured with one or two absorbable sutures around the tube (39, 40). The exposed end of the nylon suture is positioned subconjunctivally near the limbus for subsequent removal. Biodegradable stents such as collagen lacrimal plugs (41), or 4–0 chromic suture (42), have also been evaluated, but have been less satisfactory because they do not always dissolve. Some surgeons combine stent occlusion with longitudinal slits in the tube to provide early IOP control (43), and a laboratory study indicated that a slit-valve of 2.0 mm appears to provide an opening pressure of around 10 mm Hg (44).

Yet another alternative to minimize the risk of early postoperative hypotony is the use of a valved implant.

Elevated Intraocular Pressure

Drainage implant procedures can also be complicated by elevated IOP in either the early or late postoperative period. In the early period, the tube may become obstructed by fibrin, blood, iris tissue, or vitreous. Reported techniques to open the occluded tube have included irrigation of the tube with balanced salt solution using a 30-gauge cannula through a paracentesis incision (45), the use of Nd:YAG (46) or Nd:YLF (47) lasers to open occluded tubes, and the intracameral injection of tissue plasminogen activator (0.1 cc of 5–13 µg) to dissolve a fibrin clot (48, 49). Late IOP elevation, especially when the intraocular portion of the tube appears to be patent, is usually due to an excessively thick fibrous capsule. It may be beneficial in these cases to thin or remove a portion of the capsule beneath the conjunctival flap. It has also been reported that topical corticosteroid therapy can cause IOP elevation despite the presence of a functioning drainage implant (50).

Ocular Motility Disturbance

As previously noted, implants with larger plates, especially when implanted in the inferonasal quadrant, can interrupt extraocular muscle function and cause strabismus and diplopia (32). Characteristic patterns are exotropia, hypertropia, heterotropia, or limitation of ocular rotations (51–55), although a Brown's superior oblique tendon-like syndrome has also been described (32, 56). While the complication is usually associated with the larger plates, such as the 350-mm² Baerveldt implant (51, 52, 56) and the Krupin valve with disc (53, 54), it may also occur with smaller plates, such as the single-plate or double-plate Molteno implants, especially in children (55). Corrective measures may require removal of the implant, replacement with a smaller plate design, or transfer to the superotemporal quadrant,

which will usually, although not always (53), relieve the diplopia.

Loss of Visual Acuity

In one series of 41 patients after Molteno implant surgery, the incidence of reduced visual acuity was 22%, with hypotony and shallow anterior chambers being the most commonly associated events (57). Other reported mechanisms of visual loss include retinal detachment (57–60), vitreous hemorrhage (57, 58), cystoid macular edema (58), and operating microscope-induced retinal phototoxicity (61).

Other Complications

Serial corneal endothelial cell counts in 19 patients after uneventful Molteno implants revealed slight, clinically insignificant progressive cell loss (62). Epithelial downgrowth is uncommon, but is a potential risk, especially with tubes inserted at the limbus. Epithelial invasion into the fibrous capsule with persistent aqueous leak was described in four patients during the early postoperative course following Baerveldt implant surgery (63). Sterile hypopyon was reported in seven patients after removal of 4–0 chromic suture stents (64), and sterile endophthalmitis was described in two patients approximately one month after discontinuation of postoperative corticosteroid therapy (65).

OUTCOMES AND INDICATIONS

Long-term Outcomes

Outcome studies have been reported for the more commonly used drainage implant devices. The following data were derived from "long-term" followups (usually a mean of 12 months or more) of overall study populations in which "success" was typically defined as a low-end cutoff of 5–6 mm Hg and a high-end of 21–22 mm Hg with or without medication. In three trials with Molteno implants, the success rates were 73–74% with a mean (66) or minimum (67) followup of 18 months and 57% with a mean followup of 44 months (68). A study of 82 black patients treated with Molteno implants and followed for a mean of 30 months gave a similar success rate of 72% (69). With Schocket-type implants, reported success rates were 91% with a mean followup of 10 months (12) and 81% with a 17.5-month mean followup (70), but fell to 30% at 36 months in one study, using lifetable methods (71). Reported success with Baerveldt implants was 93% and 88% for 350-mm² and 500-mm² implants, respectively, using 18-month lifetable analysis (72), although two other studies reported 72% success with a minimum of 6 months (73) or a mean of 13.6 months (74) followup. Studies with the Krupin valve and disc revealed 6- and 12-month lifetable success rates of 84% and 66%, respectively (75), while another group found an 80% success rate with a mean followup of 25 months (24). One study with the Ahmed valve revealed a cumulative probability of success at 12 months of 78% (25). The visual acuity improved or remained within one Snellen line of the preoperative value in 62–87% of the various studies, which is undoubtedly influenced by the relative proportion of glaucoma types in each study.

Indications

Drainage implant surgery is typically reserved for those eyes in which trabeculectomy with adjunctive antimetabolite therapy has either failed or is felt to have a very low chance of success. The latter includes young patients, and individuals with neovascular glaucoma, glaucoma associated with uveitis, glaucoma in aphakic or pseudophakic, and eyes with other prior surgery, such as vitreoretinal surgery and penetrating keratoplasty. Success rates vary with the different underlying disorders.

Young Patients

In pediatric patients (1 month to 13 years), with a wide range of developmental glaucomas, the reported success was 80% in one study using Molteno or Baerveldt implants (76), and 56% in another with Molteno implants (77). In patients under 21 years of age, reported success was 62% with Molteno implants at a mean of 22.7 months (78), and 93% and 86% at 6 and 12 months (lifetable analysis), respectively, with Baerveldt implants (79). In all of these cases, the need for repeat surgery is common.

Neovascular Glaucoma

Molteno implants have been successful in some eyes with neovascular glaucoma (80), although the success declines with time. In one study, the success rates were 62.1%, 52.9%, 43.1%, 30.8%, and 10.3% at 1, 2, 3, 4, and 5 years, respectively (81). Experience with the Baerveldt implant revealed 12- and 18-month lifetable success rates of 79% and 56%, respectively (82).

Previous Ocular Surgery

As previously noted, a failed trabeculectomy, especially when the conjunctiva is tightly scarred down in both superior quadrants, could be an indication for a drainage implant procedure. In addition, other types of ocular surgery may cause such conjunctival scarring that an implant will have a better chance than a trabeculectomy. Both Molteno (83) and Baerveldt (84) implants have been effective for *glaucomas associated with aphakia* or *pseudophakia*. The Molteno implant has also been used with some success in eyes with epithelial downgrowth (85). The Molteno and Schocket implants have both been used in association with pars plana vitrectomy in eyes with *vitreoretinal disorders* (86). The same two devices have also been used with some success in eyes following *penetrating keratoplasty* (87, 88), although failure may be high, occurring in 42% of one study (88). The Molteno implant has also been used with success in eyes with prior *cyclocryotherapy* (89).

COMPARISONS WITH ALTERNATIVE PROCEDURES

In patients with glaucomas that are at high risk of surgical failure, as described earlier, the surgeon usually must choose between a filtering operation with adjunctive antimetabolites, a drainage implant procedure, or a cyclodestructive operation. Most studies that have compared these surgical options have used the Molteno implant as the drainage implant device.

In one study, trabeculectomy without an adjunctive antimetabolite was compared to single-plate Molteno implants in patients with glaucoma associated with uveitis, which revealed 1- and 2-year lifetable success rates of 81% and 73%, respectively, with trabeculectomies, and 79% and 79%, respectively, with Molteno implants (90). A comparison of trabeculectomy with postoperative 5-fluorouracil and single-plate Molteno implants also revealed no significant differences in IOP outcome at 6 months postoperatively (91). However, when trabeculectomy with intraoperative mitomycin-C (0.3 mg/ml for 5 minutes) was compared to single-plate Molteno implants in high-risk glaucoma patients, the former procedure provided significantly greater IOP reduction at 12 months (success rates of 81.4% and 60.5%, respectively) (92). In each of these studies, the types of complications differed between the two procedures, as previously discussed, but they tended to be more frequent with the drainage implant operations.

Noncontact Nd:YAG cyclophotocoagulation was performed in 45 patients with advanced, uncontrolled glaucoma and the results were compared to that of 45 matched patients who underwent drainage implant surgery (Schocket, Joseph, or double-plate Molteno implants) (93). Success rates (IOP <21 mm Hg) at 1 year were 87% and 69% for the implant and laser procedures, respectively, although a large number of implant patients required further glaucoma surgery (35% vs. 22%, respectively). There was also a higher incidence of serious complications among the implant patients (17% vs. 9%, respectively) and a reduction in visual acuity at 1 year was greater in the implant group (33% vs. 11%, respectively).

SUMMARY

Drainage implant devices have been successful in maintaining patency of the fistula in glaucoma filtering operations since the development of tubes that drain into external reservoirs. Implant designs differ according to the size and shape of the external plate and whether the tube is open (Molteno, Schocket, and Baerveldt) or valved (Krupin, Ahmed, Joseph, OptiMed, White). The basic surgical technique involves implantation of one end of the tube in the anterior chamber, with the other attached to a plate near the equator. A fibrous capsule develops around the plate, which regulates the aqueous flow. Complications include hypotony, elevated IOP, ocular motility disturbance, and loss of visual acuity. Indications for drainage implant surgery include previous failed filters, young patients, neovascular glaucoma, glaucoma associated with uveitis, and glaucomas following cataract and other ocular surgery. Within this high-risk group, implant surgery was not as effective in controlling the IOP as trabeculectomy with mitomycin-C, but was somewhat more effective than cyclophotocoagulation.

REFERENCES

1. Molteno, ACB: New implant for drainage in glaucoma: clinical trial. Br J Ophthalmol 53:606, 1969.
2. Lloyd, MA, Sedlak, T, Heuer, DK, et al: Clinical experience with the single-plate Molteno implant in complicated glaucomas. Update of a pilot study. Ophthalmology 99:679, 1992.
3. Molteno, ACB: The optimal design of drainage implants for glaucoma. Trans Ophthalmol Soc NJ 33:39, 1981.
4. Heuer, DK, Lloyd, MA, Abrams, DA, et al: Which is better? One or two? A Randomized clinical trial of single-plate versus double-plate Molteno implantation for glaucomas in aphakia and pseudophakia. Ophthalmology 99:1512, 1992.
5. Molteno, ACB: The dual chamber single plate implant—its use in neovascular glaucoma. Aust NZ J Ophthalmol 18:431, 1990.
6. Freedman, J: Clinical experience with the Molteno dual-chamber single-plate implant. Ophthalmic Surg 23:238, 1992.
7. Wilcox, MJ, Minckler, DS, Ogden, TE: Pathophysiology of artificial aqueous drainage in primate eyes with Molteno implants. J Glau 3:140, 1994.
8. Lloyd, MA, Minckler, DS, Heuer, DK, et al: Echographic evaluation of glaucoma shunts. Ophthalmology 100:919, 1993.
9. Rubin, B, Chan, C-C, Burnier, M, et al: Histopathologic study of the Molteno glaucoma implant in three patients. Am J Ophthalmol 110:371, 1990.
10. Schocket, SS, Lakhanpal, V, Richards, RD: Anterior chamber tube shunt to an encircling band in the treatment of neovascular glaucoma. Ophthalmology 89:1188, 1982.
11. Schocket, SS, Nirankari, VS, Lakhanpal, V, et al: Anterior chamber tube shunt to an encircling band in the treatment of neovascular glaucoma and other refractory glaucomas: a long-term study. Ophthalmology 92:553, 1985.
12. Omi, CA, De Almeida, GV, Cohen, R, et al: Modified Schocket implant for refractory glaucoma. Experience of 55 cases. Ophthalmology 98:211, 1991.
13. Sidoti, PA, Minckler, DS, Baerveldt, G, et al: Aqueous tube shunt to a pre-existing episcleral encircling element in the treatment of complicated glaucomas. Ophthalmology 101:1036, 1994.
14. Krupin, T, Ritch, R, Camras, CB, et al: A long Krupin-Denver valve implant attached to a 180° scleral explant for glaucoma surgery. Ophthalmology 95:1174, 1988.
15. Wilson, RP, Cantor, L, Katz, LJ, et al: Aqueous shunts. Molteno versus Schocket. Ophthalmology 99:672, 1992.
16. Smith, MF, Sherwood, MB, McGorray, SP: Comparison of the double-plate Molteno drainage implant with the Schocket procedure. Arch Ophthalmol 110:1246, 1992.
17. Lloyd, MAE, Baerveldt, G, Heuer, DK, et al: Initial clinical experience with the Baerveldt implant in complicated glaucomas. Ophthalmology 101:640, 1994.
18. Prata, JA Jr, Santos, RCR, LaBree, L, Minckler, DS: Surface area of glaucoma implants and perfusion flow rates in rabbit eyes. J Glau 4:274, 1995.
19. Smith, MF, Doyle, JW, Sherwood, MB: Comparison of the Baerveldt glaucoma implant with the double-plate Molteno drainage implant. Arch Ophthalmol 113:444, 1995.
20. Krupin, T, Pados, SM, Becker, B, Newkirk, JB: Valve implants in filtering surgery. Am J Ophthalmol 81:232, 1976.
21. Krupin, T, Kaufman, P, Mandell, A, et al: Filtering valve implant surgery for eyes with neovascular glaucoma. Am J Ophthalmol 89:338, 1980.
22. Krupin, T, Kaufman, P, Mandell AI, et al: Long-term results of valve implants in filtering surgery for eyes with neovascular glaucoma. Am J Ophthalmol 95:775, 1983.
23. Folberg, R, Hargett, NA, Weaver, JE, McLean, IW: Filtering valve implant for neovascular glaucoma in proliferative diabetic retinopathy. Ophthalmology 89:286, 1982.
24. The Krupin Eye Valve Filtering Surgery Study Group: Krupin eye valve with disk for filtration surgery. Ophthalmology 101:651, 1994.
25. Coleman, AL, Hill, R, Wilson, MR, et al: Initial clinical experience with the Ahmed glaucoma valve implant. Am J Ophthalmol 120:23, 1995.
26. Joseph, NH, Sherwood, MB, Trantas, G, Hitchings, RA, Lattimer, J: A one-piece drainage system for glaucoma surgery. Trans Ophthalmol Soc UK 105:657, 1986.
27. Prata, JA Jr, Mérmoud, A, LaBree, L, Minckler, DS: In vitro and in vivo flow characteristics of glaucoma drainage implants. Ophthalmology 102:894, 1995.
28. White, TC: A new implantable ocular pressure relief device: a preliminary report. Glaucoma 7:289, 1985.
29. Chihara, E, Kubota, H, Takanashi, T, Nao-i, N: Outcome of white pump shunt surgery for neovascular glaucoma in Asians. Ophthalmic Surg 23:666, 1992.
30. Lavin, MJ, Franks, WA, Wormald, RPL, Hitchings, RA: Clinical risk factors for failure in glaucoma tube surgery. Arch Ophthalmol 110:480, 1992.
31. Melamed, S, Fiore, PM: Molteno implant surgery in refractory glaucoma. Surv Ophthalmol 34:441, 1990.
32. Prata, JA Jr, Minckler, DS, Green, RL: Pseudo-Brown's syndrome as a complication of glaucoma drainage implant surgery. Ophthalmic Surg 24:608, 1993.
33. Leen, MM, Witkop, GS, George, DP: Anatomic considerations in the implantation of the Ahmed glaucoma valve. Arch Ophthalmol 114:223, 1996.
34. Prata, JA Jr, Minckler, DS, Mermoud, A, Baerveldt, G: Effects of intraoperative mitomycin-C on the function of Baerveldt glaucoma drainage implants in rabbits. J Glau 5:29, 1996.
35. Liebmann, J, Ritch, R: Intraocular suture ligature to reduce hypotony following Molteno seton implantation. Ophthalmic Surg 23:51, 1992.
36. Sayyad, FE, El-Maghraby, A, Helal, M, Amayem, A: The use of releasable sutures in Molteno glaucoma implant procedures to reduce postoperative hypotony. Ophthalmic Surg 22:82, 1991.
37. Kooner, KS, Goode, SM: Removable ligature during Molteno implant procedure. Am J Ophthalmol 114:102, 1992.
38. Franks, WA, Hitchings, RA: Injection of perfluoropropane gas to prevent hypotony in eyes undergoing tube implant surgery. Ophthalmology 97:899, 1990.
39. Latina, MA: Single stage Molteno implant with combination internal occlusion and external ligature. Ophthalmic Surg 21:444, 1990.
40. Susanna, R Jr: Modifications of the Molteno implant and implant procedure. Ophthalmic Surg 22:611, 1991.
41. Stewart, W, Feldman, RM, Gross, RL: Collagen plug occlusion of Molteno tube shunts. Ophthalmic Surg 24:47, 1993.
42. Ball, SF, Herrington, RG: Long-term retention of chromic occlusion suture in glaucoma seton tubes. Arch Ophthalmol 111:1993.

43. Sherwood, MB, Smith, MF: Prevention of early hypotony associated with Molteno implants by a new occluding stent technique. Ophthalmology 100:85, 1993.

44. Brooks, SE, Dacey, MP, Lee, MB, Baerveldt, G: Modifications of the glaucoma drainage implant to prevent early postoperative hypertension and hypotony: a laboratory study. Ophthalmic Surg 25:311, 1994.

45. Krawitz, PL: Treatment of distal occlusion of Krupin eye valve with disk using cannular flush. Ophthalmic Surg 25:102, 1994.

46. Fiore, PM, Melamed, S: Use of neodymium:YAG laser to open an occluded Molteno tube. Ophthalmic Surg 20:53, 1989.

47. Oram, O, Gross, RL, Severin, TD, et al: Opening an occluded Molteno tube with the picosecond neodymium-yttrium lithium fluoride laser. Arch Ophthalmol 112:1023, 1994.

48. Pastor, SA, Schumann, SP, Starita, RJ, Fellman, RL: Intracameral tissue plasminogen activator: management of a fibrin clot occluding a Molteno tube. Ophthalmic Surg 24:853, 1993.

49. Sidoti, PA, Morinelli, EN, Heuer, DK, et al: Tissue plasminogen activator and glaucoma drainage implants. J Glau 4:258, 1995.

50. Mermoud, A, Salmon, JF: Corticosteroid-induced ocular hypertension in draining Molteno single-plate implants. J Glau 2:32, 1993.

51. Muñoz, M, Parrish, RK, II: Strabismus following implantation of Baerveldt drainage devices. Arch Ophthalmol 111:1096, 1993.

52. Smith, SL, Starita, RJ, Fellman, RL, Lynn, JR: Early clinical experience with the Baerveldt 350-mm² glaucoma implant and associated extraocular muscle imbalance. Ophthalmology 100:914, 1993.

53. Çardakli, UF, Perkins, TW: Recalcitrant diplopia after implantation of a Krupin valve with disc. Ophthalmic Surg 25:256, 1994.

54. Frank, JW, Perkins, TW, Kushner, BJ: Ocular motility defects in patients with the Krupin valve implant. Ophthalmic Surg 26:228, 1995.

55. Christmann, LM, Wilson, ME: Motility disturbances after Molteno implants. J Pediatr Ophthalmol Strabismus 29:44, 1992.

56. Ball, SF, Ellis, GS Jr, Herrington, RG, Liang, K: Brown's superior oblique tendon syndrome after Baerveldt glaucoma implant. Arch Ophthalmol 110:1368, 1992.

57. Melamed, S, Cahane, M, Gutman, I, Blumenthal, M: Postoperative complications after Molteno implant surgery. Am J Ophthalmol 111:319, 1991.

58. Lotufo, DG: Postoperative complications and visual loss following Molteno implantation. Ophthalmic Surg 22:650, 1991.

59. Huna, R, Melamed, S, Hirsh, A, Treister, G: Retinal detachment adherent to posterior chamber IOL after Molteno implant surgery. Ophthalmic Surg 21:854, 1990.

60. Waterhouse, WJ, Lloyd, MAE, Dugel, PU, et al: Rhegmatogenous retinal detachment after Molteno glaucoma implant surgery. Ophthalmology 101:665, 1994.

61. Kramer, T, Brown, R, Lynch, M, et al: Molteno implants and operating microscope-induced retinal phototoxicity. A clinicopathologic report. Arch Ophthalmol 109:379, 1991.

62. McDermott, ML, Swendris, RP, Shin, DH, et al: Corneal endothelial cell counts after Molteno implantation. Am J Ophthalmol 115:93, 1993.

63. Sidoti, PA, Minckler, DS, Baerveldt, G, et al: Epithelial ingrowth and glaucoma drainage implants. Ophthalmology 101:872, 1994.

64. Ball, SF, Loftfield, K, Scharfenberg, J: Molteno rip-cord suture hypopyon. Ophthalmic Surg 21:407, 1990.

65. Heher, KL, Lim, JI, Haller, JA, Jampel, HD: Late-onset sterile endophthalmitis after Molteno tube implantation. Am J Ophthalmol 114:771, 1992.

66. Airaksinen, PJ, Aisala, P, Tuulonen, A: Molteno implant surgery in uncontrolled glaucoma. Acta Ophthalmol 68:690, 1990.

67. Price, FW Jr, Wellemeyer, M: Long-term results of Molteno implants. Ophthalmic Surg 26:130, 1995.

68. Mills, RP, Reynolds, A, Emond, MJ, et al: Long-term survival of Molteno glaucoma drainage devices. Ophthalmology 103:299, 1996.

69. Freedman, J, Rubin, B: Molteno implants as a treatment for refractory glaucoma in black patients. Arch Ophthalmol 109:1417, 1991.

70. Spiegel, D, Shrader, RR, Wilson, RP: Anterior chamber tube shunt to an encircling band (Schocket procedure) in the treatment of refractory glaucoma. Ophthalmic Surg 23:804, 1992.

71. Watanabe, J, Sawaguchi, S, Iwata, K: Long-term results of anterior chamber tube shunt to an encircling band in the treatment of refractory glaucomas. Acta Ophthalmol 70:766, 1992.

72. Lloyd, MA, Baerveldt, G, Fellenbaum, PS, et al: Intermediate-term results of a randomized clinical trial of the 350- versus the 500-mm² Baerveldt implant. Ophthalmology 101:1456, 1994.

73. Hodkin, MJ, Goldblatt, WS, Burgoyne, CF, et al: Early clinical experience with the Baerveldt implant in complicated glaucomas. Am J Ophthalmol 120:32, 1995.

74. Siegner, SW, Netland, PA, Urban, RC Jr, et al: Clinical experience with the Baerveldt glaucoma drainage implant. Ophthalmology 102:1298, 1995.

75. Fellenbaum, PS, Almeida, AR, Minckler, DS, et al: Krupin disk implantation for complicated glaucomas. Ophthalmology 101:1178, 1994.

76. Netland, PA, Walton, DS: Glaucoma drainage implants in pediatric patients. Ophthalmic Surg 24:723, 1993.

77. Nesher, R, Sherwood, MB, Kass, MA, et al: Molteno implants in children. J Glau 1:228, 1992.

78. Hill, RA, Heuer, DK, Baerveldt, G, et al: Molteno implantation for glaucoma in young patients. Ophthalmology 98:1042, 1991.

79. Fellenbaum, PS, Sidoti, PA, Heuer, DK, et al: Experience with the Baerveldt implant in young patients with complicated glaucomas. J Glau 4:91, 1995.

80. Ancker, E, Molteno, ACB: Molteno drainage implant for neovascular glaucoma. Trans Ophthalmol Soc UK 102:122, 1982.

81. Mermoud, A, Salmon, JF, Alexander, P, et al: Molteno tube implantation for neovascular glaucoma. Long-term results and factors influencing the outcome. Ophthalmology 100:897, 1993.

82. Sidoti, PA, Dunphy, TR, Baerveldt, G, et al: Experience with the Baerveldt glaucoma implant in treating neovascular glaucoma. Ophthalmology 102:1107, 1995.

83. Ancker, E, Molteno, ACB: Surgical treatment of chronic aphakic glaucoma with the Molteno plastic implant. Klin Monatsbl Augenheilkd 177:365, 1980.

84. Varma, R, Heuer, DK, Lundy, DC, et al: Pars plana Baerveldt tube insertion with vitrectomy in glaucomas associated with pseudophakia and aphakia. Am J Ophthalmol 119:401, 1995.

85. Fish, LA, Heuer, DK, Baerveldt, G, et al: Molteno implantation for secondary glaucomas associated with advanced epithelial ingrowth. Ophthalmology 97:557, 1990.

86. Gandham, SB, Costa, VP, Katz, LJ, et al: Aqueous tube-shunt implantation and pars plana vitrectomy in eyes with refractory glaucoma. Am J Ophthalmol 116:189, 1993.

87. McDonnell, PJ, Robin, JB, Schanzlin, DJ, et al: Molteno implant for control of glaucoma in eyes after penetrating keratoplasty. Ophthalmology 95:364, 1988.

88. Sherwood, MB, Smith, MF, Driebe, WT Jr: Drainage tube implants in the treatment of glaucoma following penetrating keratoplasty. Ophthalmic Surg 24:185, 1993.

89. Wellemeyer, ML, Price, FW Jr: Molteno implants in patients with previous cyclocryotherapy. Ophthalmic Surg 24:395, 1993.

90. Hill, RA, Nguyen, QH, Baerveldt, G, et al: Trabeculectomy and Molteno implantation for glaucomas associated with uveitis. Ophthalmology 100:903, 1993.

91. Bluestein, EC, Stewart, WC: Trabeculectomy with 5-fluorouracil vs. single-plate Molteno implantation. Ophthalmic Surg 24:669, 1993.

92. Sayyad, FE, Helal, M, Elsherif, Z, El-Maghraby, A: Molteno implant versus trabeculectomy with adjunctive intraoperative mitomycin-C in high-risk glaucoma patients. J Glau 4:80, 1995.

93. Noureddin, BN, Wilson-Holt, N, Lavin, M, et al: Advanced uncontrolled glaucoma. Nd:YAG cyclophotocoagulation or tube surgery. Ophthalmology 99:430, 1992.

CYCLODESTRUCTIVE SURGERY[a]

All of the operations discussed in the preceding chapters lower the intraocular pressure (IOP) by improving the rate of aqueous outflow. An alternative approach is to reduce the rate of aqueous production by partially eliminating the function of the ciliary processes. These techniques are rarely the first operation of choice, because the results are hard to predict and the complication rate is high due to damage to adjacent ocular structures and the influence of a pronounced inflammatory response. However, the cyclodestructive procedures constitute a valuable adjunct in our surgical armamentarium for cases in which other operations have repeatedly failed or are felt to be contraindicated.

OVERVIEW OF CYCLODESTRUCTIVE PROCEDURES

Cyclodestructive operations differ according to (a) the destructive energy source and (b) the route by which the en-

ergy reaches the ciliary processes. In the 1930s and 1940s, several energy sources were evaluated, including diathermy, beta irradiation, and electrolysis, although only cyclo-diathermy achieved clinical acceptance. Cryotherapy was introduced in the 1950s and became the most commonly used cyclodestructive procedure. However, subsequent experience with laser cyclophotocoagulation showed clear advantages over other techniques, and it has become the preferred cyclodestructive operation. Other, more recently evaluated cyclodestructive techniques include therapeutic ultrasound and microwave cyclodestruction.

Each of the energy sources noted above may be delivered by the transscleral route, in which the destructive element passes through conjunctiva, sclera, and ciliary muscle before reaching the ciliary processes. Transscleral cyclodestructive operations have the advantages of being nonincisional and

[a]Refer to M.B. Shields: Color Atlas of Glaucoma. Baltimore: Williams & Wilkins, 1998, Plates III42–49.

relatively quick and easy. However, significant disadvantages include the inability to visualize the processes being treated and damage to adjacent tissue, leading to unpredictable results and frequent complications. With the advent of laser energy as the cyclodestructive element, alternative delivery routes are possible, including transpupillary and intraocular.

EARLY CYCLODESTRUCTIVE PROCEDURES

Penetrating Cyclodiathermy

Weve (1) introduced the concept of cyclodestructive surgery in 1933, using nonpenetrating diathermy to produce selective destruction of ciliary processes. Vogt (2, 3) modified the technique by using a diathermy probe which penetrated the sclera, and this became the standard cyclodestructive procedure. The technique involved penetration of the sclera 2.5–5 mm from the corneolimbal junction with a 1.0–1.5-mm electrode, and the application of a diathermy current of 40–45 mA for 10–20 seconds (3). This could be done with or without preparation of a conjunctival flap. One or two rows of diathermy lesions were generally placed several millimeters apart for approximately 180°. The mechanism of permanent IOP reduction was probably cell death within the ciliary body (4). In addition, it may be that the more posteriorly placed lesions created a draining fistula in the region of the pars plana.

Early reports of experience with cyclodiathermy were encouraging (5, 6). However, subsequent study revealed a low success rate and a significant incidence of hypotony. In a review of 100 cases, 5% had lasting, useful reduction in IOP, while about the same number developed phthisis (7). Results undoubtedly vary with the technique, and experience with a newer one-pole diathermy unit was said to be encouraging (8).

Other Early Cyclodestructive Procedures

Beta Irradiation Therapy

In 1948, Haik and coworkers (9) reported the experimental application of radium over the ciliary body in rabbit eyes and in one clinical case. Although this was shown to produce a reduction in the vascular supply of the ciliary body, it also caused damage to the lens, and the technique was never adopted for clinical use.

Cycloelectrolysis

Berens and coworkers (10), in 1949, described a technique which employed the use of low frequency galvanic current to create a chemical reaction within the ciliary body. This led to the formation of sodium hydroxide, which is caustic to the tissue of the ciliary body. Although this was shown in rabbit studies to produce destruction of ciliary processes

(11), the procedure did not seem to have significant advantages over penetrating cyclodiathermy and never achieved widespread clinical popularity.

Cyclocryotherapy

The use of a freezing source as the cyclodestructive element was suggested by Bietti (12) in 1950. Cyclocryotherapy was generally felt to be somewhat more predictable and less destructive than penetrating cyclodiathermy and gradually replaced the latter technique as the most commonly used cyclodestructive operation. It is still used by many surgeons, especially where laser technology is not available.

Mechanism of Action

PHYSICAL PRINCIPLES OF CRYOSURGERY (13). The ability of a freezing source, or cryogen, to freeze tissue depends on the degree to which it removes heat, which is a function of the boiling point of the source. For example, liquid nitrogen boils at $-195.6°$ C and is an excellent cryogen. When the freezing source is applied to a tissue, a hemispherical iceball will develop, composed of different thermogradients, or temperature zones. The temperature at any point within the iceball depends upon (a) the distance from the cryogen, with gradually increasing temperatures at progressively greater distances due to a resupplying of heat by blood vessels, and (b) the rate of freezing, with a rapid freeze producing colder temperatures near the edge of the growing iceball.

BIOLOGIC PRINCIPLES OF CRYOSURGERY (13). There are two phases of cryoinjury-induced in vivo cell death. Initially, freezing of extracellular fluid concentrates the remaining solutes, which leads to cellular dehydration and is the probable mechanism of cell death associated with a slow freeze. When the rate of cooling is rapid, intracellular ice crystals develop. Although these crystals are not always lethal to the cell, a slow thaw leads to the formation of larger crystals, which are highly destructive to the cell by an uncertain mechanism. Maximum cell death is achieved with a rapid freeze and a slow thaw. A second and later mechanism of cryo-induced cell death is a superimposed hemorrhagic infarction, which results from obliteration of the microcirculation within the frozen tissue. Ischemic necrosis is the histologic hallmark of cryoinjured tissue.

CYCLOCRYOTHERAPY. Cyclocryotherapy presumably destroys the ability of ciliary processes to produce aqueous humor by the biphasic mechanism of intracellular ice crystal formation and ischemic necrosis as outlined above. Animal studies have revealed significant differences between the temperature of the cryoprobe and the temperature within the treated tissues (14, 15). In living eyes, a temperature of $-60°$ C to $-80°$ C over the sclerolimbal area was shown to produce a temperature of approximately $-10°$C at the tips of the ciliary processes after a lag of 20–30 seconds (15). The latter temperature is near the minimum thermogradient at which cryoinjury normally occurs (15). Ciliary body blood flow in rabbits is reduced 50–60% when treated with −80°C cryoapplications for 60 seconds (16). Histologic studies of eyes treated with cyclocryotherapy show destruction of vascular, stromal, and epithelial elements of the ciliary processes with replacement by fibrous tissue (4, 15, 17, 18). Ciliary epithelium has been observed to regenerate in monkeys, but not in human eyes (18).

In addition to lowering the IOP, cyclocryotherapy may provide relief of pain by the destruction of corneal nerves. Wallerian degeneration of corneal nerve fibers was observed in rabbits following cyclocryotherapy, although regeneration began within 9–16 days (19).

Techniques

CRYOINSTRUMENTS. Either nitrous oxide or carbon dioxide gas cryosurgical units may be used. The diameters of the more commonly used cryoprobe tips range from 1.5 to 4 mm, and it has been suggested that 2.5 mm may be optimum for cyclocryotherapy (20). A modified cryoprobe with a curved 3 × 6-mm tip has been developed to reduce the number of applications required (21). An automatic timer to monitor the duration of each application has also been described (22).

CRYOPROBE PLACEMENT. With the 2.5-mm tip, placement of the anterior edge of the probe 1 mm from the corneolimbal junction temporally, inferiorly, and nasally, and 1.5 mm superiorly is believed to concentrate the maximum freezing effect over the ciliary processes (Figs. 39.1–39.3) (20). It has also been suggested that transillumination may be helpful by delineating the pars plicata (23, 24), although this is

not usually necessary unless the anatomic landmarks are distorted, as with buphthalmos. The cryoprobe should be applied with firm pressure on the sclera, since this may reduce ciliary blood flow, thereby contributing to faster penetration of the iceball to the ciliary processes (20). A device has been described which indicates the applicator contact pressure continuously during therapy, both optically and acoustically (25).

NUMBER OF CRYOAPPLICATIONS. Most surgeons treat two to three quadrants, with three to four cryoapplications per quadrant. A study in cats showed that graded cyclocryotherapy of 90°, 180°, or 270° produced graded destruction of the

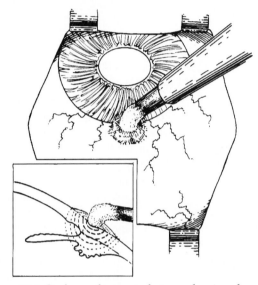

Figure 39.1. Cyclocryotherapy technique, showing placement of probe and shape of iceball *(inset).*

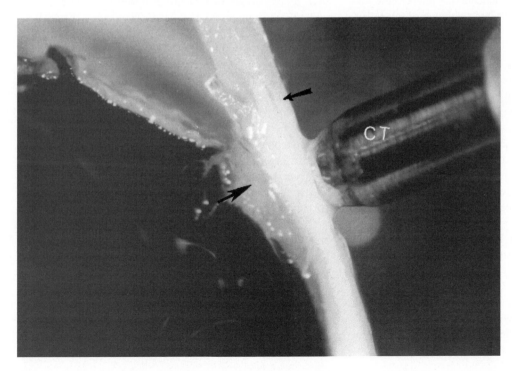

Figure 39.2. Section of human autopsy eye showing placement of cryoprobe tip (CT) in relation to ciliary body *(large arrow)* and anterior limbus *(small arrow).*

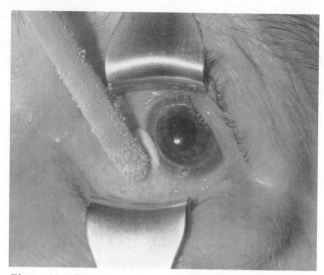

Figure 39.3. Typical appearance of iceball during cyclocryotherapy.

ciliary epithelium and proportionally related changes in IOP and aqueous humor dynamics (26). The number of cryolesions may be based to a degree on preoperative parameters, such as the type of glaucoma, the IOP level, and the number of previous cyclocryotherapy procedures. It has also been shown that younger patients generally require a larger number of cryoapplications than older individuals to achieve satisfactory pressure reduction (27). However, there are no precise guidelines by which an individual patient's response to therapy can be predicted, and it is best to err on the side of undertreatment rather than to run the risk of phthisis. One recommended approach is to limit each treatment session to six applications or less over 180° of the globe (23).

FREEZING TECHNIQUE. Studies indicate that temperature levels warmer than −60° C to −80° C or a duration of freeze less than 60 seconds does not provide adequate destruction of the ciliary process, while values much greater than these increase the risk of phthisis (20). Most surgeons, therefore, prefer −60° C to −80° C applications for 60 seconds (23, 24, 28). As previously noted, a rapid freeze and slow, unassisted thaw produce the maximum cell death (13). Opinions differ as to the value of repeating the freeze in the same site. In the cryosurgical management of tumors, multiple freeze/thaw cycles have been shown to produce increasingly greater tissue destruction (13). However, this does not necessarily imply optimum treatment, and no clear-cut advantage of the freeze-thaw-freeze technique has been shown for cyclocryotherapy. If the initial procedure does not adequately lower the IOP after approximately 1 month, cyclocryotherapy may be repeated one or more times as required. In one series of 61 eyes, 14 required two or more procedures (28).

POSTOPERATIVE MANAGEMENT. For approximately the first 24 hours, the patient may experience intense pain, and strong analgesics are often required. It has been noted that subconjunctival steroids at the end of the procedure also minimize the postoperative pain (23). In addition, frequent topical corticosteroids and a cycloplegic-mydriatic should be used routinely starting on the day of surgery. Since the IOP may remain elevated for a day or more after the treatment, it is advisable to keep the patient on the preoperative antiglaucoma medications, with the exception of miotics, until a pressure reduction is observed.

Complications

TRANSIENT INTRAOCULAR PRESSURE RISE. A marked rise in IOP may occur during cyclocryotherapy and in the early postoperative period. In one study, pressures of 60–80 mm Hg were recorded during the freezing phase, with return to baseline during the thawing phase (29). The authors felt this component of IOP elevation was due to volumetric changes, possibly related to scleral contraction, and they described a technique for controlling the complication with manometric regulation of the pressure during surgery. They also noted a second IOP rise that averaged 50 mm Hg and peaked 6 hours after the procedure. The mechanism for this component of the IOP elevation is unclear, but is probably associated with the marked inflammatory response. Gonioscopic evaluation after cyclocryotherapy revealed frozen aqueous humor in the anterior chamber angle (30), with the obvious consequences that this may have on the remaining conventional outflow system.

UVEITIS. Uveitis occurs in all cases and is usually intense, with the frequent formation of a fibrin clot. One study suggests that the inflammation is prostaglandin-induced and might be minimized by pretreatment with aspirin (31). However, a comparison of topical flurbiprofen, dexamethasone, and placebo suggested that cyclocryotherapy-induced inflammation is hard to control with any topical medication (32). A study in rabbits showed that an injection of heparin into the anterior chamber significantly reduced fibrin clots following cyclocryotherapy (33). A chronic aqueous flare usually persists due to permanent disruption of the blood-aqueous barrier (34), but this does not require treatment.

PAIN. Pain, as previously noted, may be intense after cyclocryotherapy and may last for days. It is most likely a consequence of the IOP elevation and inflammation, both of which should be treated vigorously along with the use of strong analgesics.

HYPHEMA. Hyphema is a common complication, especially in eyes with neovascular glaucoma, and usually clears with conservative management.

HYPOTONY. A major disadvantage of all cyclodestructive procedures is that nothing can be done to reverse the hypotony or phthisis, if this should occur. Although this complication is less common with cyclocryotherapy than with cyclo-diathermy (28), it does occur and is best avoided by treating a limited area each time. It is far better to repeat the treatment several times than to produce phthisis by overtreatment.

OTHER COMPLICATIONS. Other complications associated with cyclocryotherapy include choroidal detachment, which may lead to a flat anterior chamber (35). Intravitreal neovascularization from the ciliary body, with vitreous hemorrhage may follow cyclocryotherapy (36, 37), and may regress after panretinal photocoagulation (37). Anterior segment ischemia has been reported in eyes with neovascular glaucoma following 360° of cyclocryotherapy (38). Proliferation of retinal glial cells and pigment epithelial cells has been observed in rabbit eyes after cyclocryotherapy (39). A subretinal fibrosis has been reported in one clinical case (40). Other complications that have been reported include lens subluxation (41) and sympathetic ophthalmia (42, 43). Ocular rigidity in rabbit studies was found to be low initially, but then rose significantly after approximately 2 weeks, which is important to consider if indentation tonometry is being used (44).

Indications

Cyclocryotherapy is usually reserved for situations in which other glaucoma operations have repeatedly failed or in which the surgeon wishes to avoid incisional surgery. Conditions in which this procedure has been reported to have particular value include glaucoma after a penetrating keratoplasty (45, 46), chronic open-angle glaucoma in aphakia (27, 47), and congenital glaucoma (48, 49). Cyclocryotherapy is felt by some surgeons to be useful in the management of neovascular glaucoma (50, 51), although others feel that the main benefit of the surgery in this and other disorders is relief of pain (52–55).

TRANSSCLERAL CYCLOPHOTOCOAGULATION

In 1961, Weekers and associates (56) employed light as the cyclodestructive element, using the transscleral application of xenon-arc photocoagulation over the ciliary body. As with other operations that utilize light energy, however, it was the introduction of the laser that eventually led to the clinical application of cyclophotocoagulation. In 1969, Vucicevic and associates (57) reported the use of a *ruby laser* to perform transscleral cyclophotocoagulation in rabbits, with an adjunctive cytochemical agent to enhance laser absorption by the ciliary body. Other reports of transscleral laser cyclophotocoagulation followed (58–60), and in 1984, Beckman and Waeltermann (61) reported a 10-year experience with 241 eyes treated by transscleral ruby laser cyclophotocoagulation. Their overall rate of IOP control was 62%, with 86% in eyes with glaucoma in aphakia and 53%

in eyes with neovascular glaucoma. Chronic hypotony occurred in 41 eyes, with phthisis in 17 cases, although most eyes retained their preoperative level of vision. However, it was not until the availability of specially designed *neodymium:YAG* and, subsequently, *semiconductor diode* lasers that widespread interest developed in transscleral cyclophotocoagulation.

Instruments

Neodymium:YAG Lasers

Neodymium:YAG (Nd:YAG) lasers, with a wavelength of 1064 nm, are useful for transscleral cyclophotocoagulation because they traverse the sclera with relatively low absorption and scatter. They may be operated in either a pulsed, free-running, thermal mode, or a continuous-wave mode, and may be delivered by either a noncontact, slitlamp system, or a contact probe, fiberoptic system.

PULSED, THERMAL MODE. The Microruptor 2 (MR2; H.S. Meridian, formerly Lasag) provides slitlamp delivery in the free-running, thermal mode with 20-msec pulses. It has two additional features that are needed to perform transscleral cyclophotocoagulation: (a) an adjustable offset between the focal points of the helium-neon aiming beam and the therapeutic beam, so the latter can be set at a predetermined distance inside the eye when aiming on the conjunctiva (Fig. 39.4), and (b) high energy levels of up to 8–9 J. This instrument is no longer commercially available, but is the unit on which much of the early clinical experience is based. The Model gLase 106 (Sunrise Technologies), a contact delivery, short-pulse (1.0 msec), high-peak, high-energy (800 mJ/pulse) Nd:YAG laser, has also been evaluated in rabbit studies (62).

CONTINUOUS-WAVE MODE. The SLT CL60 (Surgical Laser Technologies) provides contact probe delivery in a continuous-wave mode of 0.1–10 seconds. A 2.2-mm sapphire-tipped, hand-held probe, which is focused at 1.5–2 mm in air, is coupled to a fiberoptic delivery system. The unit can provide powers in excess of 10 W. (Note that energy in joules equals power in watts times duration in seconds.) The SLT is the unit on which most of the early experience with contact, continuous-wave Nd:YAG transscleral cyclophotocoagulation is based. A subsequent instrument, the Microruptor 3 (MR3) also provides continuous-wave Nd:YAG laser energy, which can be delivered by either a 600-μm, flat-tip, quartz fiber probe or a slitlamp.

Semiconductor Diode Lasers

Although semiconductor diode lasers, with a range of wavelengths between 750 and 850 nm, do not traverse the sclera as efficiently as Nd:YAG lasers, they have the advantage of

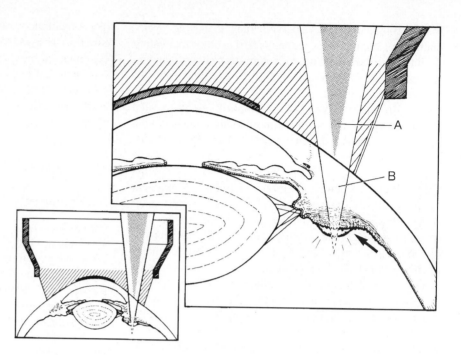

Figure 39.4. Noncontact transscleral Nd:YAG cyclophotocoagulation through a contact lens, showing HeNe aiming beam *(A)* focused on conjunctiva with therapeutic Nd:YAG beam *(B)* offset deep into ocular tissues and producing disruption of the ciliary epithelium *(arrow).*

greater absorption by uveal melanin. In addition, they have the advantage of solid-state construction with compact size, low maintenance requirements, and no special requirement for electric outlet or water-cooling.

The Oculight SLx (Iris Medical Instruments) is a continuous-wave, contact delivery diode laser with a wavelength of 810 nm, a maximum power output of 2.5–3.0 W, and a maximum duration of 9.9 seconds (63–65). The probe (G-Probe) consists of a 600 μm quartz fiberoptic, protruding 0.7 mm from a handpiece, which is fabricated to center the fiberoptic 1.2 mm behind the surgical limbus and parallel to the visual axis (Fig. 39.5) (65). The back of the G-Probe pushes the lid away from the surgical site, and the sides can be used to aide in spacing the laser applications (Fig. 39.6).

The Microlase (Keeler Instruments), with a wavelength of 780–830 nm, is a noncontact diode laser that attaches to a slitlamp (66). It provides a maximum power of 1200 mW and a maximum duration of 990 msec, with spot sizes of 100–500 μm. The Multilase is a similar laser, but provides contact delivery through a fiberoptic probe with a 1.7-mm tip, housed in a 3.0-mm casing, with a variable focus that produces a minimum spot size of 0.25 μm (67).

Krypton Lasers

Transscleral cyclophotocoagulation has also been performed with a retinal krypton laser, delivered by a contact probe. The shorter wavelength results in poorer scleral transmission but better uveal pigment absorption than with the Nd:YAG laser, and histologic lesions in rabbits were similar with the two lasers (68). Successful clinical results were reported, using 4–5 J of energy, 10-second exposures, and firm compression with the probe (69, 70).

Theories of Mechanism

The mechanism by which transscleral cyclophotocoagulation lowers IOP is not fully understood. The prevailing theory is that it reduces aqueous production by damaging the pars plicata, although it is not clear whether this is due to direct destruction of the ciliary epithelium or reduced vascular perfusion. Still other investigators suggest that the primary mechanism may be increased outflow through an effect on the pars plana. The following are studies that support these various theories.

Evidence for Reduced Aqueous Production

Initial rabbit studies showed that the transscleral application of Nd:YAG laser energy in the noncontact, free-running mode could damage the ciliary body and lower the IOP (71, 72). Histologic examination showed selective destruction of the ciliary epithelium (72, 73). In one study, the disrupted epithelium was elevated in a blister-like effect with sparing of ciliary muscle, sclera and conjunctiva (72). Another study showed damage to associated ciliary vessels in the immediate postoperative phase, followed by marked atrophy of the ciliary processes over the subsequent 4–8 weeks (73). An incomplete regeneration of the epithelial layers and capillary network correlated with the level of sustained IOP reduction (74). This histologic response was seen in pigmented rabbits, but not albinos (75), and it is presumed that the laser energy is absorbed by melanin granules and converted to heat, which creates the observed response.

Similar histologic changes have been described in rabbits treated with the contact, continuous-wave Nd:YAG laser, although there appears to be more of a coagulative necrosis of the epithelial layers (76) than is seen with the free-running mode.

Studies of human autopsy eyes revealed structural changes of the ciliary body similar to those seen in rabbits. The gross appearance of lesions created by the noncontact, free-running Nd:YAG laser was a white elevation of the ciliary epithelium (77). The histologic correlate was a blister-like elevation of the epithelial layers from the adjacent stroma with marked disruption primarily of the pigmented epithelium, but minimal change in the ciliary muscle and sclera in the path of the laser beam (Fig. 39.7) (78, 79). In contrast, the histologic appearance of lesions created by the contact, continuous-wave Nd:YAG laser was a smaller, more coagulative effect on the epithelium with less of the blister-like elevation (79, 80). One study showed a more full-thickness thermal effect, including sclera (79), while

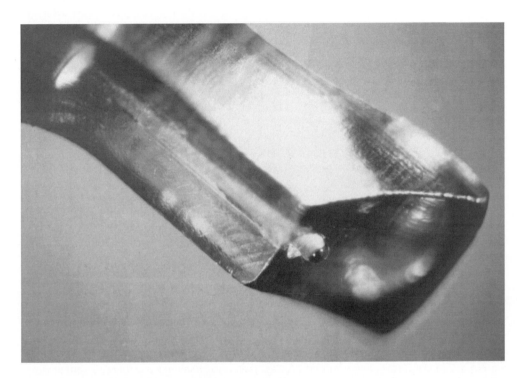

Figure 39.5. G-Probe for contact transscleral semiconductor diode laser cyclophotocoagulation. Note protrusion of rounded quartz fiberoptic tip from footplate of handpiece. (Courtesy of Mr. Theodore A. Boutacoff.)

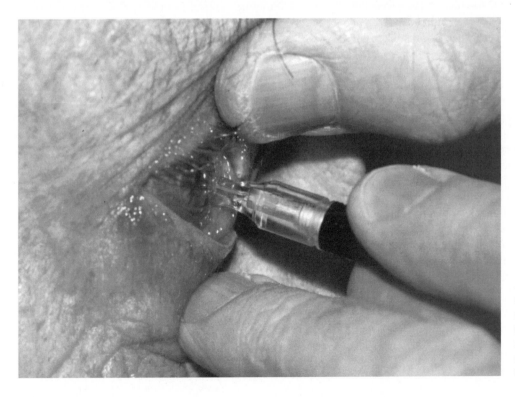

Figure 39.6. Transscleral diode cyclophotocoagulation, showing use of G-Probe to position fiberoptic 1.2 mm from surgical limbus and to space adjacent laser applications.

Figure 39.7. Light microscopic view of human autopsy eye treated with noncontact, free-running transscleral Nd:YAG cyclophotocoagulation showing blister-like elevation of disrupted ciliary epithelium (*black arrows*) with minimal ciliary muscle and scleral damage (*white arrows*). Defect on scleral surface was created by needle with India ink to mark center of laser track after laser application. (Reprinted with permission from Hampton, C, Shields, MB: Transscleral neodymium-YAG cyclophotocoagulation. A histologic study of human autopsy eyes. Arch Ophthalmol 106:1121, 1988.)

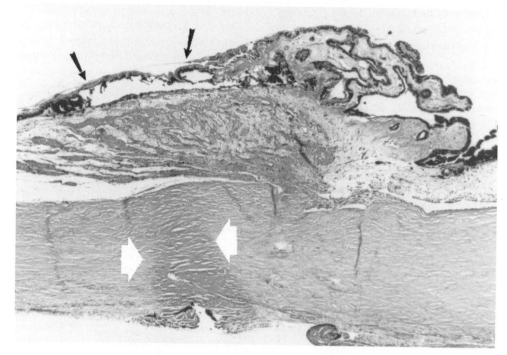

another showed no scleral alteration (80). A videographic study of human autopsy eyes also showed that shorter duration Nd:YAG laser exposures caused greater tissue disruption, while the more prolonged, continuous-wave exposures produced a more coagulative, shrinkage-like lesion (81).

Histologic studies have also been performed on human eyes that were enucleated at some point after transscleral Nd:YAG cyclophotocoagulation. In one series of eyes treated with the noncontact, free-running Nd:YAG laser a few days before scheduled enucleation, the structural changes were the same as those seen in human autopsy eyes with the addition of fibrin and scant inflammatory cells between the disrupted epithelial layers and stroma (82). No changes in ciliary body vasculature were observed. A clinicopathologic study of three eyes enucleated 2 weeks, 8 weeks, and 17 months after noncontact Nd:YAG cyclophotocoagulation, revealed destruction of the nonpigmented and pigmented ciliary epithelium, occlusion of capillaries and stromal necrosis, with subsequent hyperplasia of the epithelial layers, fibrosis and near total atrophy of the ciliary processes (83). Histologic evaluation of another eye, that had received the same laser treatment 70 days before enucleation for hypotony and pain, revealed pigment disruption and granulomatous inflammation of the ciliary body (84). Two eyes treated with contact, continuous-wave Nd:YAG transscleral cyclophotocoagulation one day before enucleation for melanomas revealed epithelial necrosis and partial capillary thrombosis of the ciliary body with slight scleral damage (85).

Evidence for Increased Aqueous Outflow

While the above studies confirm that transscleral cyclophotocoagulation can destroy tissues of the pars plicata, most likely by a direct effect on the ciliary epithelium, this does not prove that direct destruction of the pars plicata is an essential element in the mechanism of IOP reduction. Other studies have shown that more posteriorly placed lesions over the pars plana or even peripheral retina also lower the IOP (86–89). The explanation for this observation could be reduced aqueous production due to the inflammatory response (86), although it is not likely that this would be a sustained effect. An alternative explanation is enhanced aqueous outflow, either by transscleral filtration (87–91) or uveoscleral outflow (90, 91). In a monkey study of contact, continuous-wave Nd:YAG cyclophotocoagulation, in which right eyes were treated over the pars plicata, 1 mm behind the limbus, and left eyes were treated over the pars plana, 3 mm behind the limbus, IOP reduction occurred in both eyes, but returned to baseline by 8 weeks in the former group, while the latter maintained IOP reduction for the 6-month observation period (90). Histology of the latter eyes suggested enhanced uveoscleral outflow by showing tracer elements in enlarged extracellular spaces of the ciliary stroma from the anterior chamber to the suprachoroidal space. In a similar clinical trial in which laser applications were placed either 1.5 mm or 3.0–4.0 mm behind the limbus, the latter group had a higher percentage of eyes with sustained IOP reduction, although they also received more than twice as many laser applications (91). In another clinical trial, using noncontact Nd:YAG cyclophotocoagulation, in which all treatment parameters were kept constant except for laser placement either 1.5 or 3.0 mm posterior to the limbus, the former group had significantly lower IOP and required fewer retreatments during a 6-month followup (92).

In summary, the most likely mechanism of IOP lowering by transscleral Nd:YAG cyclophotocoagulation is reduced aqueous production through destruction of ciliary epithelium. However, alternative possibilities, including reduced inflow due to ciliary vascular disruption or chronic inflammation, or increased outflow due to pars plana/transscleral outflow or enhanced uveoscleral outflow, have not been ruled out.

Techniques

Pre- and Postoperative Management

Unlike most other glaucoma laser procedures, the intraoperative pain associated with transscleral cyclophotocoagulation is such that retrobulbar anesthesia is usually required, although this has been omitted by some surgeons with the contact, continuous-wave technique (85). Also, unlike most other laser procedures, as well as other transscleral cyclodestructive procedures, postoperative IOP rise is not a frequent problem, and special pre- and postoperative measures such as the use of topical apraclonidine are usually not necessary.

Postoperative inflammation can be a significant problem, requiring special prophylactic measures. One approach is to give a subconjunctival injection of a short-acting steroid at the end of the procedure and to prescribe topical atropine and steroid for approximately 10 days (93). Preoperative glaucoma medications are continued, except for miotics, until IOP reduction allows discontinuation. Postoperative pain is typically mild, and a weak analgesic is usually sufficient. Intraocular pressure is usually checked a few hours after the procedure, the following day, and thereafter as required.

Laser Settings and Protocols

The histologic studies with human eyes, as previously described, have been used to establish protocols for clinical trials. However, preferred settings differ among surgeons, and the optimum protocols have yet to be established.

ND:YAG NONCONTACT, THERMAL MODE. This technique utilizes the MR2 with a set pulse of 20 msec and a maximum offset between the aiming and therapeutic beams, which is 3.6 mm in air. As previously noted, opinions differ regarding placement of laser lesions, but most agree that focusing on conjunctiva 0.5–1.5 mm behind the limbus is optimum for damaging the pars plicata (77, 78, 82). Preferred energy levels also vary, with those reported ranging from 2 to 8 J (93–98). In a prospective trial of 89 patients, randomized to receive either 4 or 8 J of laser energy, there was a trend toward better IOP control with the higher energy level (98). The only significant difference was greater anterior chamber reaction during the early postoperative period in the 8-J group, although there was no significant difference in final visual acuities between the two groups.

With the patient seated at the laser slitlamp, and the eye fixed in the primary position, the laser beam will be slightly tangential to the scleral surface. The laser beam can be applied directly to the conjunctiva, although contact lenses have been designed for this operation. One is designed to maintain lid separation, compress and blanch the conjunctiva, and provide measurements from the limbus (99), while another is a glass cylinder with a truncated cone that is pressed against the conjunctiva (100). When compared to identical protocols without a contact lens, the use of the former lens did not alter the histologic findings in human autopsy eyes (101), nor did it appear to influence the results in a clinical trial, except for a higher incidence of phthisis (102). Nevertheless, it is likely that these lenses allow more laser energy to reach the ciliary body in the living eye by thinning and blanching the conjunctiva, as well as by reducing backscatter at the air-tissue interface, and lower laser settings may be advisable when using either lens. The total number of laser applications also varies among surgeons, with most reported protocols ranging from 30 to 40 evenly-spaced lesions for 360° (93–98). One study compared 180° to 360° treatments and showed that the latter provided IOP control with fewer repeat procedures and less major complications (103).

ND:YAG CONTACT, CONTINUOUS-WAVE. This technique has been performed primarily with the SLT, using exposure times of 0.5–0.7 second. The laser focus is fixed by the design of the probe tip, which is held perpendicular to the surface of the conjunctiva with the anterior edge of the probe 0.5–1.5 mm behind the limbus. Power settings vary considerably among surgeons with a range of approximately 4–9 W (4 W at 0.5 second provides an energy of 2 J, while 9 W at 0.7 second delivers 6.3 J) (104, 105). A study with human autopsy eyes suggested that black patients require less energy than white patients to produce comparable lesions, presumably due to differences in ciliary epithelial pigmentation (106). The reported number of applications also varies considerably from 16 for 360° (104) to 32–40 for 360° with sparing of the 3 and 9 o'clock positions (105). Similar protocols can be used with the MR3. In a rabbit study, comparing the SLT and MR3, settings of 3.0 W for 0.5 second and 3.2 W for 0.5 second, respectively, produced comparable ciliary body destruction in acute experiments, while 30 applications for 360° with these settings were equally effective in lowering the IOP in longitudinal experiments (107).

SEMICONDUCTOR DIODE, CONTINUOUS-WAVE. With the Oculight SLx, the G-Probe footplate is placed on conjunctiva with the short side adjacent to the limbus, which positions the fiberoptic tip 1.2-mm behind the limbus. Initial settings are 1750 mW and 2 seconds (65). If a popping sound is heard with the initial application, the power is reduced by increments of 250 mW until no pop is heard. If no pop is heard with the initial application, the power is increased by the same increments until the sound is heard and then reduced by one increment. Videographic studies of human autopsy eyes have shown that this audible indicator represents excessive tissue destruction, while a power setting one increment below this level is believed to provide optimum tissue damage (108). The laser applications are spaced circumferentially by placing the side of the G-Probe footplate adjacent to the indentation mark of the previous fiberoptic placement (Fig. 39.6). The original protocol involved 17–19 applications for 270° (65), although 24 applications for 360° may provide more effective IOP reduction. This procedure can be performed with the patient supine or reclining in an examination chair or positioned at a standard slit-lamp.

With the Microlase slitlamp attachment, the laser beam is focused on the conjunctiva 1 mm behind the surgical limbus and then defocused internally 1 mm, as measured by a millimeter ruler at the base of the biomicroscope (109). With settings of 1200 mW and 990 msec, 40–45 applications are placed for 360°. With the Multilase contact diode laser, the anterior margin of the probe casing is positioned at the surgical limbus, which places the center of the fiberoptic 1.5 mm posterior to the limbus (67). The settings and protocol are otherwise the same as described for the Microlase.

Clinical Experience

General Results

Transscleral cyclophotocoagulation, as with other cyclodestructive procedures, is typically reserved for patients with refractory forms of glaucoma, such as glaucomas in aphakia or pseudophakia, neovascular glaucoma, glaucomas associated with inflammation, and eyes with multiple failed filtering procedures or following penetrating keratoplasty. With Nd:YAG lasers in either the noncontact, pulsed,

thermal mode (93–98, 102, 110–116) or the contact, continuous-wave mode (104, 105, 117, 118), transscleral cyclophotocoagulation in general provides satisfactory IOP reduction in approximately two-thirds or more of the cases following the initial treatment session, with most of the remainder coming under control with one or more retreatments. Similar results have also been reported from preliminary experiences with both noncontact (109, 119) and contact (65, 120) transscleral diode cyclophotocoagulation. Maximum pressure reduction is typically achieved in 1 month, and it is usually desirable to wait at least this long before retreating. Results differ somewhat according to the type of glaucoma. In general, patients with glaucoma in aphakia or pseudophakia have more favorable results, while those with neovascular glaucoma tend to do less well. Patients with glaucoma following penetrating keratoplasty have good IOP response to Nd:YAG cyclophotocoagulation, although graft failure is a problem in some cases (121, 122). Contact transscleral Nd:YAG cyclophotocoagulation has also been shown to be beneficial in pediatric patients with refractory glaucoma (123).

Complications

In the immediate postoperative period, laser application sites may be seen as white conjunctival burns, especially with the noncontact technique, which can be minimized by blanching the conjunctiva with a contact lens (Fig. 39.8) (102). These burns and the associated mild conjunctival hyperemia typically resolve in a few days. Anterior chamber flare and cell are seen in all cases. This is usually mild-to-moderate, although some patients may develop fibrin clots or hypopyon. Hyphema may also be seen, especially in patients with neovascular glaucoma. The inflammatory re-

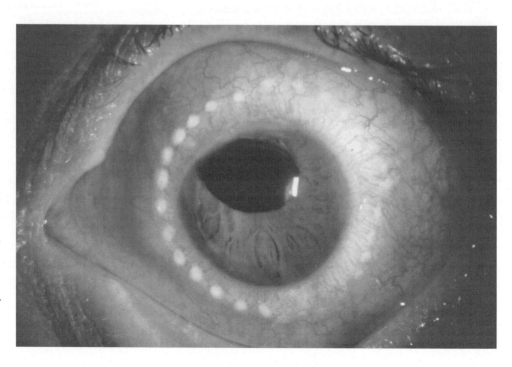

Figure 39.8. Slitlamp view of conjunctival burns immediately after noncontact, free-running transscleral Nd:YAG cyclophotocoagulation. Note the larger lesions on the *left* half, in which the procedure was performed without a contact lens, compared to the *right* side in which the lens was used.

sponse is transient and is routinely managed with postoperative subconjunctival and subsequent topical steroids. Many patients are left with a chronic flare due to a breakdown in the blood-aqueous barrier, but this does not require chronic treatment. A transient IOP rise occurs in a small percentage of patients, and is usually not of significance (124). Nevertheless, it is advisable to check the pressure a few hours after the procedure and on the following day. Postoperative pain also tends to be mild, with many patients requiring no analgesic, and rarely more than a mild pain reliever during the first 24 hours. In summary, inflammation, transient IOP elevation, and pain are all significantly less than is typically encountered with cyclocryotherapy.

Other reported complications have included hypotony with choroidal detachments and a flat anterior chamber (125), vitreous hemorrhages, and cataracts. Several cases of sympathetic ophthalmia have been reported in association with transscleral cyclophotocoagulation (126–130). In most cases, the treated eye had undergone prior incisional surgery, and the sympathizing eyes responded promptly to steroid therapy. In one series of 500 patients, treated with noncontact transscleral Nd:YAG cyclophotocoagulation, no case of sympathetic ophthalmia was observed (116). Nevertheless, the surgeon should be alert for this possibility. Cases of malignant glaucoma have also been described following Nd:YAG cyclophotocoagulation (131, 132).

The most significant complication associated with transscleral cyclophotocoagulation is loss of visual acuity. Some degree of visual loss may occur in as high as 50% of cases. In many cases this appears to be associated with the underlying disorder, such as a retinopathy or keratopathy. However, it is felt that at least half of the cases of visual reduction are a direct result of the laser treatment (116). The precise mechanisms of the latter are not fully understood, but likely causes include macular edema associated with the inflammatory response and possibly a direct phototoxic effect. In any case, until the explanations for this complication and its treatment are better understood, it is advisable to use transscleral cyclophotocoagulation with caution in eyes with good visual potential.

Influence of Treatment Variables

EXPOSURE DURATIONS. As previously noted, histologic and in vitro videographic studies of transscleral Nd:YAG cyclophotocoagulation have revealed an influence of exposure duration on tissue responses of the ciliary body. The thermal mode (20 msec) produces an explosive, blister-like lesion, while the continuous-wave mode (usually 0.5–2.0 seconds) produces a more gradual contraction and coagulation of the tissue (77–81). The variable tissue response to different exposure times also appears to influence the degree of anterior chamber reaction. Using a rabbit model to evaluate the inflammatory response to continuous-wave Nd:YAG cyclophotocoagulation (133), a shorter exposure duration of 0.2 second, as compared to 2 seconds (with the power ad-

justed in both cases to provide a constant energy of 2 J) was associated with greater tissue disruption and inflammation (134). In clinical practice, however, these differences appear to be less significant, since similar results have been reported with 20 msec thermal modes (93–98, 102, 110–116) and 0.7 second (700 msec) continuous-wave (104, 105, 117, 118) Nd:YAG cyclophotocoagulation.

ND:YAG VERSUS DIODE WAVELENGTHS. As previously noted, semiconductor diode lasers have the physical advantages of being compact and portable with no special electric outlet or water-cooling requirements and with solid-state construction that is relatively durable and requires minimal maintenance. The different wavelengths of the Nd:YAG (1064 nm) and diode (750–850 nm) lasers also impart variable biologic effects, with the latter having less effective scleral transmission and increased light scattering, but greater absorption by melanin. In a videographic study of human autopsy eyes, comparing contact transscleral continuous-wave Nd:YAG and diode cyclophotocoagulation, the former produced more prominent whitening and contraction of the ciliary epithelium, while the latter seemed to produce a deeper tissue contraction. The histologic correlate was predominant coagulation and disruption of the ciliary epithelium with the Nd:YAG laser, while the diode treatment was associated with less epithelial effect and more coagulative response in the ciliary muscle. These findings are consistent with other studies, which revealed coagulative changes in the ciliary epithelium, stroma, and vasculature of human autopsy eyes in response to diode cyclophotocoagulation (135), as well as deeper, more extensive tissue damage, when compared to similar energy levels of Nd:YAG treatment in both rabbit (136) and preenucleation human (137) eyes. However, the latter study revealed similar lesions at lower energy levels (137), and another videographic study of human autopsy eyes revealed similar ciliary body responses to noncontact Nd:YAG and diode laser applications (138). Preliminary clinical trials with transscleral diode cyclophotocoagulation suggest less visual loss than with the Nd:YAG procedures (65, 109, 119, 120), although larger comparative trials are needed to establish the relative merits of these two techniques.

CONTACT VERSUS NONCONTACT DELIVERY. Contact delivery systems with both Nd:YAG and diode lasers have the advantages of allowing treatment with the patient either sitting or supine. The latter is especially advantageous when performing the surgery on children under anesthesia. However, there are certain potential disadvantages with the use of contact probes. As noted in Chapter 37, full-thickness sclerostomies can be created with laser probes, and this is obviously to be avoided with transscleral cyclophotocoagulation. Inadvertent sclerostomies have been reported with both diode (65) and Nd:YAG (139) contact cyclophotocoagulation. This complication appears to occur primarily with flat-tipped fiberoptics, probably due to accumulation of

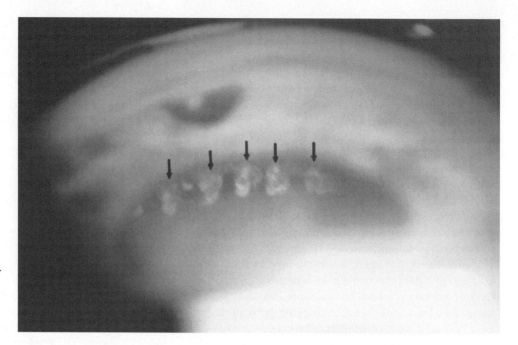

Figure 39.9. Gonioscopic view of ciliary processes *(arrows)* during transpupillary cyclophotocoagulation. Exposure of processes in this eye is due to retraction of iris by fibrovascular membrane of neovascular glaucoma.

carbonized tissue, which increases the temperature of the fiber tip (140). It is minimized by the use of rounded, well-polished tips, which are incorporated into most contact probe designs, although even these should be inspected before and periodically during treatment to make sure they are free of mucous or other debris. Another important consideration in avoiding excessive surface temperature is to keep the eyeball moist, to maintain appropriate tissue-fiberoptic contact.

Another disadvantage of contact delivery is the variability of tissue response. Factors influencing this variable include probe pressure, probe diameter, and time of probe contact, all of which alter scleral transparency and, thereby, effect the percentage of laser energy reaching the ciliary body (141, 142). Probe designs to standardize pressure include footplates to control the depth of fiberoptic indentation (65), and spring-loaded devices to control fiberoptic pressure (141, 142). In a study of 315 enucleated porcine eyes, these two design concepts and a manually-controlled probe were evaluated with Nd:YAG cyclophotocoagulation (143). Considerable variability in size and severity of ciliary epithelial lesions was observed with all three probe designs, although the probe controlling depth of fiberoptic indentation produced the least variability.

Comparisons with Alternative Procedures

Comparisons of transscleral Nd:YAG cyclophotocoagulation to cyclocryotherapy in both rabbits (144) and humans (145) have revealed insignificant differences in IOP responses, but less tissue destruction (144) and fewer complications (145) with the laser treatments. Based on these and other reports of the various cyclodestructive operations, it is now believed that transscleral cyclophotocoagulation is the cyclodestructive procedure of choice.

As discussed in Chapter 38, a comparison of noncontact transscleral Nd:YAG cyclophotocoagulation to several drainage implant devices revealed better IOP control with the latter techniques (146). Although the laser group had less visual loss in that study, the loss of visual acuity with all transscleral cyclophotocoagulation procedures remains an important concern. In general, filtering surgery with adjunctive antimetabolite therapy or drainage implant surgery is preferred in patients with good visual potential, although transscleral cyclophotocoagulation offers a reasonable alternative in the high risk glaucoma population, especially when the visual potential is poor.

OTHER ROUTES OF CYCLOPHOTOCOAGULATION

Transpupillary Cyclophotocoagulation

In 1971, Lee and Pomerantzeff (147) introduced the concept of argon laser cyclophotocoagulation via a transpupillary approach. Histopathologic studies in rabbit (147) and human (148) eyes confirmed the ability of direct laser application to selectively destroy ciliary processes.

Transpupillary cyclophotocoagulation is limited to those eyes in which a sufficient number of ciliary processes can be visualized gonioscopically. This is not possible in most eyes, especially those in which long-term miotic therapy prevents wide dilatation. However, situations such as a large iridectomy or retraction of the iris, as in advanced neovascular glaucoma, may provide adequate visualization of ciliary processes (Fig. 39.9). Special contact lenses with scleral depressors have been developed to rotate the processes into better view. Typical argon laser settings are 0.1–0.2 second, 100–200 μm, and an energy level that is sufficient to produce white discoloration, as well as a brown concave burn, often with pigment dispersion and/or gas bubbles (usually 700–1000 mW). All visible portions of the ciliary process should be treated, which typically requires 3–5 applications per process. All visible processes should be treated up to a total of 180°. Additional processes can be treated at subsequent sessions if required.

The reported results with transpupillary cyclophotocoagulation have been variable (149–154). Those cases in which the procedure fails may be due, in part, to the number of ciliary processes that can be visualized and treated (151) and to the intensity of the laser burns to each process (149). However, the number of treated processes and the intensity of treatment do not always correlate with the extent of the IOP reduction (154). Another factor which may contribute to failure of transpupillary cyclophotocoagulation is the angle at which the processes are visualized gonioscopically. Even with scleral indentation, only the anterior tips of the ciliary ridges are usually exposed, preventing destruction of the entire ciliary process (Fig. 39.10) (154).

Intraocular Cyclophotocoagulation

An alternative to transscleral and transpupillary cyclophotocoagulation in eyes with glaucoma in aphakia, or possibly pseudophakia, is intraocular cyclophotocoagulation, using an endophotocoagulator through a pars plana incision. Visualization with this technique can usually be accomplished by the transpupillary route or with endoscopic visualization.

Intraocular Cyclophotocoagulation with Transpupillary Visualization

Vitreoretinal surgeons have reported the use of argon laser endophotocoagulators via a pars plana incision for the treatment of retinal disorders under transpupillary visualization (155–157). During the course of a vitrectomy in an aphakic eye, it is possible to lower the IOP and use scleral indentation to bring the ciliary processes into transpupillary view for the purpose of cyclophotocoagulation with the intraocular laser probe (158–160).

After performing the vitrectomy, the vitreous instrument is removed and the endophotocoagulator is inserted through the same cannula. Scleral indentation in the opposite quadrants is then used to bring several ciliary processes into view, and the tip of the laser probe is positioned 2–3 mm from the processes (Fig. 39.11). With an exposure time of 0.1–0.2 second, laser therapy is applied to individual ciliary processes, using an energy level that is sufficient to produce a white reaction and a shallow tissue disruption (usually 1000 mW). Three to five laser exposures are then applied to each process in the two quadrants opposite the entry site.

In one large series, three-fourths of the eyes had an IOP of 21 mm Hg or less with or without medications after one or two treatments, with an average followup of 13 months (160). The primary value of this procedure is as an adjunct to pars plana vitrectomy in eyes with refractory glaucoma.

Intraocular Cyclophotocoagulation with Endoscopic Visualization

An ocular endoscope was modified for intraocular cyclophotocoagulation by attaching a laser fiberoptic, con-

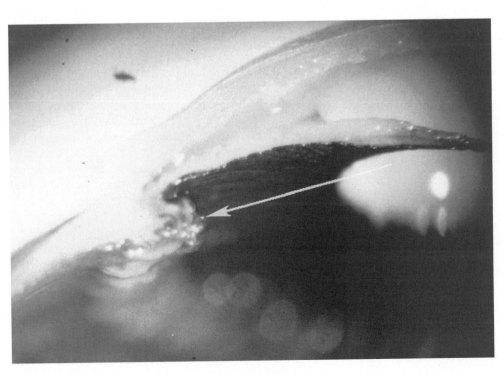

Figure 39.10. Section of human autopsy eye showing angle of ciliary process visualization during transpupillary cyclophotocoagulation (*arrow*), which provides view of only the anterior tip of the process. (Reprinted with permission from Shields, MB: Cyclodestructive surgery for glaucoma: past, present and future. Trans Am Ophthalmol Soc 83:285, 1985.)

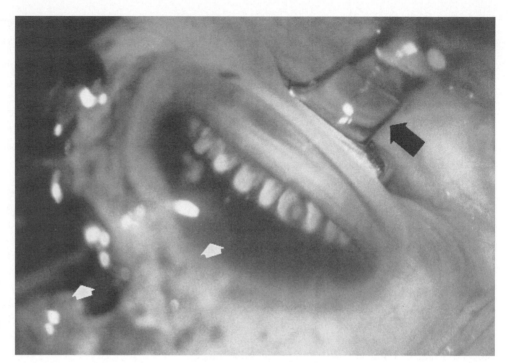

Figure 39.11. Intraocular cyclophotocoagulation with transpupillary visualization. Ciliary processes are brought into view with scleral depressor *(black arrow)* and treated with laser endophotocoagulator *(white arrows)* via a pars plana incision. (Reprinted with permission from Shields, MB: Cyclodestructive surgery for glaucoma: Past, present and future. Trans Am Ophthalmol Soc 83:285, 1985.)

nected to a continuous-wave argon laser, to the tip of the instrument (158, 161, 162). This allowed direct visualization of ciliary processes via the pars plana incision with simultaneous application of the laser energy. In a study with monkeys, treated with a lensectomy, anterior vitrectomy, and endoscopic cyclophotocoagulation, histopathologic evaluation of the treated ciliary processes revealed variable degrees of epithelial layer destruction and late fibrosis of the ciliary processes (161). A preliminary clinical trial demonstrated the ability of this technique to reduce IOP by selective photodestruction of ciliary processes (162).

An ophthalmic laser microendoscope has also been developed which houses fiberoptics for a video monitor, diode laser endophotocoagulation, and illumination in a 20-gauge probe (163). Preliminary experience in 10 patients with neovascular glaucoma, in whom a vitrectomy and lensectomy had been previously performed or was combined with the endoscopic cyclophotocoagulation, revealed favorable results with this instrument (164).

OTHER CYCLODESTRUCTIVE PROCEDURES

Therapeutic Ultrasound

In 1964, Purnell and associates (165) introduced the concept of using focused transscleral ultrasonic radiation to produce localized destruction of the ciliary body in rabbit eyes. Coleman and coworkers, in 1985, reported the results of rabbit studies (166) and preliminary clinical trials (167) with high-intensity focused ultrasound.

The basic technique involves an immersion applicator with which an average of six to seven exposures of ultrasound are delivered at an intensity level of 10 kW/cm^2 for 5 seconds each to scleral sites near the limbus (167, 168). In addition to reducing aqueous inflow by destruction of ciliary epithelium, the authors postulated that this procedure may improve aqueous outflow by selective thinning of scleral collagen and by separation of the ciliary body from the sclera. The histologic evaluation of a human eye enucleated 8 months after therapeutic ultrasound revealed localized destruction of the ciliary epithelial layers, profound atrophy of the ciliary muscle, and loss of scleral collagen (169). A contact ultrasound applicator was subsequently developed, which uses a distensible rubber membrane that can be inflated to control the stand-off distance relative to the surface of the eye. When compared to the immersion technique in rabbit and porcine eyes, the lesions in the sclera and ciliary body were similar when the same focal position was used, while deeper focusing resulted in less superficial damage (170).

Several clinical trials of therapeutic ultrasound in patients with refractory glaucomas, similar to those described in studies of other cyclodestructive procedures, have revealed IOP reduction to the low 20s or less in one-half to two-thirds of the cases 6–12 months after a single treatment (168, 171, 172). In a multicenter study involving 880 eyes, success (IOP between 6 and 22 mm Hg) after a single treatment was 48.7% at 6 months (173). With retreatments as required, the success rate rose to 79.3% at 1 year. The most common complication was an immediate postoperative IOP rise and mild iritis. Scleral thinning was observed in 2.5%, and phthisis in 1.1%. Decreased visual acuity occurred in approximately 20% of the cases.

Transscleral Microwave Cyclodestruction

The direct application of high-frequency electromagnetic radiation over the conjunctiva in rabbits produced heat-induced damage to the ciliary body with relative sparing of the conjunctiva and sclera (174). In rabbits with experimentally induced glaucoma, the procedure was successful in reducing IOP in all treated eyes for 4 weeks (175).

Excision of the Ciliary Body

In addition to the use of many cyclodestructive elements, as described earlier, other surgeons have sought to reduce aqueous production by removal of a portion of the ciliary body. Several studies have revealed reasonable success and complication rates with this basic approach in eyes with unusually refractory glaucomas (176–178).

SUMMARY

Cyclodestructive operations lower the IOP by partially eliminating the function of the ciliary processes, thereby reducing aqueous production. Destructive sources for the more commonly used procedures have included diathermy, cryogens, laser, and ultrasound. Each of these energy sources are delivered by the transscleral route, which provides a simple, quick, nonincisional technique, but is associated with unpredictable results and a high rate of complications. With transscleral laser energy as the cyclodestructive source, tissue destruction can be more precise, with a significant reduction in complications, although visual loss remains an important consideration. The use of laser energy also allows the alternative delivery routes of transpupillary and intraocular cyclophotocoagulation.

REFERENCES

1. Weve, H: Die Zyklodiatermie das Corpus ciliare bei Glaukom. Zentralbl Ophthalmol 29:562, 1933.
2. Vogt, A: Versuche zur intraokularen Druckherabsetzung mittels Diatermieschadigung des Corpus ciliare (Zyklodiatermiestichelung). Klin Monatsbl Augenheilkd 97:672, 1936.
3. Vogt, A: Cyclodiathermypuncture in cases of glaucoma. Br J Ophthalmol 24:288, 1940.
4. Edmonds, C, de Roetth, A Jr, Howard, GM: Histopathologic changes following cryosurgery and diathermy of the rabbit ciliary body. Am J Ophthalmol 69:65, 1970.
5. Albaugh, CH, Dunphy, EB: Cyclodiathermy. Arch Ophthalmol 27:543, 1942.
6. Stocker, FW: Response of chronic simple glaucoma to treatment with cyclodiathermy puncture. Arch Ophthalmol 34:181, 1945.
7. Walton, DS, Grant, WM: Penetrating cyclodiathermy for filtration. Arch Ophthalmol 83:47, 1970.
8. Nesterov, AP, Egorov, EA: Transconjunctival penetrating cyclodiathermy in glaucoma. J Ocul Ther Surg July-Aug:216, 1983.
9. Haik, GM, Breffeilh, LA, Barber, A: Beta irradiation as a possible therapeutic agent in glaucoma. Am J Ophthalmol 31:945, 1948.
10. Berens, C, Sheppard, LB, Duel, AB Jr: Cycloelectrolysis for glaucoma. Trans Am Ophthalmol Soc 47:364, 1949.
11. Sheppard, LB: Retrociliary cyclodiathermy versus retrociliary cycloelectrolysis. Effects on the normal rabbit eye. Am J Ophthalmol 46:27, 1958.
12. Bietti, G: Surgical intervention on the ciliary body. New trends for the relief of glaucoma. JAMA 142:889, 1950.
13. Wilkes, TDI, Fraunfelder, FT: Principles of cryosurgery. Ophthalmic Surg 10:21, 1979.
14. de Roetth, A Jr: Ciliary body temperatures in cryosurgery. Arch Ophthalmol 85:204, 1971.
15. Quigley, HA: Histological and physiological studies of cyclocryotherapy in primate and human eyes. Am J Ophthalmol 82:722, 1976.
16. Green, K, Hull, DS, Bowman, K: Cyclocryotherapy and ocular blood flow. Glaucoma 1:141, 1979.
17. Ferry, AP: Histopathologic observations on human eyes following cyclocryotherapy for glaucoma. Trans Am Acad Ophthalmol Otol 83:90, 1977.
18. Smith, RS, Boyle, E, Rudt, LA: Cyclocryotherapy. A light and electron microscopic study. Arch Ophthalmol 95:284, 1977.
19. Wener, RG, Pinkerton, RMH, Robertson, DM: Cryosurgical induced changes in corneal nerves. Can J Ophthalmol 8:548, 1973.
20. Prost, M: Cyclocryotherapy for glaucoma. Evaluation of techniques. Surv Ophthalmol 28:93, 1983.
21. Machemer, R: Modified cryoprobe for retinal detachment surgery and cyclocryotherapy. Am J Ophthalmol 83:123, 1977.
22. Machemer, R, Lashley, R: Automatic timer for cryotherapy. Am J Ophthalmol 83:125, 1977.
23. Bellows, AR: Cyclocryotherapy: Its role in the treatment of glaucoma. Perspect Ophthalmol 4:139, 1980.
24. Wesley, RE, Kielar, RA: Cyclocryotherapy in treatment of glaucoma. Glaucoma 3:533, 1980.
25. Matthes, R, Koza, K-D, Heber, G, Matthaus, W: A new device for glaucoma cryotherapy. Klin Monatsbl Augenheilkd 195:100, 1989.
26. Higginbotham, EJ, Lee, DA, Bartels, SP, et al: Effects of cyclocryotherapy on aqueous humor dynamics in cats. Arch Ophthalmol 106:396, 1988.
27. Brindley, G, Shields, MB: Value and limitations of cyclocryotherapy. Graefes Arch Clin Exp Ophthalmol 224:545, 1986.
28. Bellows, AR, Grant, WM: Cyclocryotherapy in advanced inadequately controlled glaucoma. Am J Ophthalmol 75:679, 1973.
29. Caprioli, J, Sears, M: Regulation of intraocular pressure during cyclocryotherapy for advanced glaucoma. Am J Ophthalmol 101:542, 1986.
30. Strasser, G, Haddad, R: Gonioscopic changes after cyclocryocoagulation. Klin Monatsbl Augenheilkd 187:343, 1985.
31. Chavis, RM, Vygantas, CM, Vygantas, A: Experimental inhibition of prostaglandin-like inflammatory response after cryotherapy. Am J Ophthalmol 82:310, 1976.
32. Hurvitz, LM, Spaeth, GL, Zakhour, I, et al: A comparison of the effect of flurbiprofen, dexamethasone, and placebo on cyclocryotherapy-induced inflammation. Ophthalmic Surg 15:394, 1984.
33. Johnson, RN, Balyeat, E, Stern, WH: Heparin prophylaxis for intraocular fibrin. Ophthalmology 94:597, 1987.
34. Haddad, R: Cyclocryotherapy: experimental studies of the breadkown of the blood-aqueous barrier and analysis of a long term follow-up study. Wien Klin Wochenschr 93(Suppl 126):3, 1981.
35. Kaiden, JS, Serniuk, RA, Bader, BF: Choroidal detachment with flat anterior chamber after cyclocryotherapy. Ann Ophthalmol 11:1111, 1979.
36. Goldberg, MF, Ericson, ES: Intravitreal ciliary body neovascularization. Ophthalmic Surg 8:62, 1977.
37. Gieser, RG, Gieser, DK: Treatment of intravitreal ciliary body neovascularization. Ophthalmic Surg 15:508, 1984.

38. Krupin, T, Johnson, MF, Becker, B: Anterior segment ischemia after cyclocryotherapy. Am J Ophthalmol 84:426, 1977.

39. Yamishita, H, Sears, ML: Complications of cyclocryosurgery. Glaucoma 2:273, 1980.

40. Kao, SF, Morgan, CM, Bergstrom, TJ: Subretinal fibrosis following cyclocryotherapy. Arch Ophthalmol 105:1175, 1987.

41. Pearson, PA, Baldwin, LB, Smith, TJ: Lens subluxation as a complication of cyclocryotherapy. Ophthalmic Surg 20:445, 1989.

42. Sabates, R: Choroiditis compatible with the histopathologic diagnosis of sympathetic ophthalmia following cyclocryotherapy of neovascular glaucoma. Ophthalmic Surg 19:176, 1988.

43. Harrison, TJ: Sympathetic ophthalmia after cyclocryotherapy of neovascular glaucoma without ocular penetration. Ophthalmic Surg 24:44, 1993.

44. Paterson, CA, Paterson, EF, Briggs, SA: Experimental cryosurgery. Effect upon ocular rigidity and intraocular pressure. Arch Ophthalmol 86:425, 1971.

45. West, CE, Wood, TO, Kaufman, HE: Cyclocryotherapy for glaucoma pre- or postpenetrating keratoplasty. Am J Ophthalmol 76:485, 1973.

46. Binder, PS, Abel, R Jr, Kaufman, HE: Cyclocryotherapy for glaucoma after penetrating keratoplasty. Am J Ophthalmol 79:489, 1975.

47. Bellows, AR, Grant, WM: Cyclocryotherapy of chronic open-angle glaucoma in aphakic eyes. Am J Ophthalmol 85:615, 1978.

48. Frucht-Pery, J, Feldman, ST, Brown, SI: Transplantation of congenitally opaque corneas from eyes with exaggerated buphthalmos. Am J Ophthalmol 107:655, 1989.

49. Al Faran, MF, Tomey, KF, Al Mutlaq, FA: Cyclocryotherapy in selected cases of congenital glaucoma. Ophthalmic Surg 21:794, 1990.

50. Feibel, RM, Bigger, JF: Rubeosis iridis and neovascular glaucoma. Evaluation of cyclocryotherapy. Am J Ophthalmol 74:862, 1972.

51. Klein, J, Kuechle, HJ: Cryotherapy of the ciliary body in cases of secondary glaucoma with poor prognosis. Klin Monatsbl Augenheilkd 179:470, 1981.

52. Faulborn, J, Birnbaum, F: Cyclocryotherapy of haemorrhagic glaucoma: clinical long time and histopathologic results. Klin Monatsbl Augenheilkd 170:651, 1977.

53. Krupin, T, Mitchell, KB, Becker, B: Cyclocryotherapy in neovascular glaucoma. Am J Ophthalmol 86:24, 1978.

54. Caprioli, J, Strang, SL, Spaeth, GL, Poryzees, EH: Cyclocryotherapy in the treatment of advanced glaucoma. Ophthalmology 92:947, 1985.

55. Benson, MT, Nelson, ME: Cyclocryotherapy: a review of cases over a 10-year period. Br J Ophthalmol 74:103, 1990.

56. Weekers, R, Lavergne, G, Watillon, M, et al: Effects of photocoagulation of ciliary body upon ocular tension. Am J Ophthalmol 52:156, 1961.

57. Vucicevic, ZM, Tsou, KC, Nazarian, IH, et al: A cytochemical approach to the laser coagulation of the ciliary body. Mod Probl Ophthalmol 8:467, 1969.

58. Smith, RS, Stein, MN: Ocular hazards of transscleral laser radiation: II. Intraocular injury produced by ruby and neodymium lasers. Am J Ophthalmol 67:100, 1969.

59. Beckman, H, Kinoshita, A, Rota, AN, Sugar, HS: Transscleral ruby laser irradiation of the ciliary body in the treatment of intractable glaucoma. Trans Am Acad Ophthalmol Otol 76:423, 1972.

60. Beckman, H, Sugar, HS: Neodymium laser cyclocoagulation. Arch Ophthalmol 90:27, 1973.

61. Beckman, H, Waeltermann, J: Transscleral ruby laser cyclocoagulation. Am J Ophthalmol 98:788, 1984.

62. Iwach, AG, Drake, MV, Hoskins, HD Jr, et al: A new contact neodymium:YAG laser for cyclophotocoagulation. Ophthalmic Surg 22:345, 1991.

63. Peyman, GA, Naguib, KS, Gaasterland, D: Transscleral application of a semiconductor diode laser. Laser Surg Med 10:569, 1990.

64. Schuman, JS, Jacobson, JJ, Puliafito, CA, et al: Experimental use of semiconductor diode laser in contact transscleral cyclophotocoagulation in rabbits. Arch Ophthalmol 108:1152, 1990.

65. Gaasterland, DE, Pollack, IP: Initial experience with a new method of laser transscleral cyclophotocoagulation for ciliary ablation in severe glaucoma. Trans Am Ophthalmol Soc 90:225, 1992.

66. Hennis, HL, Assia, E, Stewart, WC, et al: Transscleral cyclophotocoagulation using a semiconductor diode laser in cadaver eyes. Ophthalmic Surg 22:274, 1991.

67. Stroman, GA, Stewart, WC, Hamzavi, S, et al: Contact versus noncontact diode laser transscleral cyclophotocoagulation in cadaver eyes. Ophthalmic Surg Lasers 27:60, 1996.

68. Immonen, I, Suomalainen, V-P, Kivelä, T, Viherkoski, E: Energy levels needed for cyclophotocoagulation: a comparison of transscleral contact cw-YAG and krypton lasers in the rabbit eye. Ophthalmic Surg 24:530, 1993.

69. Immonen, IJR, Puska, P, Raitta, C: Transscleral contact krypton laser cyclophotocoagulation for treatment of glaucoma. Ophthalmology 101:876, 1994.

70. Kivelä, T, Puska, P, Raitta, C, et al: Clinically successful contact transscleral krypton laser cyclophotocoagulation. Long-term histopathologic and immunohistochemical autopsy findings. Ar Ophthal 113:1447, 1995.

71. Wilensky, JT, Welch, D, Mirolovich, M: Transscleral cyclocoagulation using a neodymium:YAG laser. Ophthalmic Surg 16:95, 1985.

72. Devenyi, RG, Trope, GE, Hunter, WH: Neodymium-YAG transscleral cyclocoagulation in rabbit eyes. Br J Ophthalmol 71:441, 1987.

73. England, C, van der Zypen, E, Fankhauser, F, Kwasniewska, S: Ultrastructure of the rabbit ciliary body following transscleral cyclophotocoagulation with the free-running Nd:YAG laser: Preliminary findings. Lasers Ophthalmol 1:61, 1986.

74. van der Zypen, E, England, C, Fankhauser, F, Kwasniewska, S: The effect of transscleral laser cyclophotocoagulation on rabbit ciliary body vascularization. Graefes Arch Clin Exp Ophthalmol 227:172, 1989.

75. Cantor, LB, Nichols, DA, Katz, LJ, et al: Neodymium-YAG transscleral cyclophotocoagulation. The role of pigmentation. Invest Ophthalmol Vis Sci 30:1834, 1989.

76. Brancato, R, Leoni, G, Trabucchi, G, Trabucchi, E: Transscleral contact cyclophotocoagulation with Nd:YAG laser CW: experimental study on rabbit eyes. Int J Tiss Reac 9:493, 1987.

77. Fankhauser, F, van der Zypen, E, Kwasniewska, S, et al: Transscleral cyclophotocoagulation using a neodymium YAG laser. Ophthalmic Surg 17:94, 1986.

78. Hampton, C, Shields, MB: Transscleral neodymium-YAG cyclophotocoagulation. A histologic study of human autopsy eyes. Arch Ophthalmol 106:1121, 1988.

79. Schubert, HD: Noncontact and contact pars plana transscleral neodymium:YAG laser cyclophotocoagulation in postmortem eyes. Ophthalmology 96:1471, 1989.

80. Allingham, RR, de Kater, AW, Bellows, AR, Hsu, J: Probe placement and power levels in contact transscleral neodymium:YAG cyclophotocoagulation. Arch Ophthalmol 108:738, 1990.

81. Prum, BE Jr, Shields, SR, Simmons, RB, et al: The influence of exposure duration in transscleral Nd:YAG laser cyclophotocoagulation. Am J Ophthalmol 114:560, 1992.

82. Blasini, M, Simmons, R, Shields, MB: Early tissue response to transscleral neodymium:YAG cyclophotocoagulation. Invest Ophthalmol Vis Sci 31:1114, 1990.

83. Marsh, P, Wilson, DJ, Samples, JR, Morrison, JC: A clinicopathologic correlative study of noncontact transscleral Nd:YAG cyclophotocoagulation. Am J Ophthalmol 115:597, 1993.

84. Shields, SM, Stevens, JL, Kass, MA, Smith, ME: Histopathologic findings after Nd:YAG transscleral cyclophotocoagulation. Am J Ophthalmol 106:100, 1988.

85. Brancato, R, Leoni, G, Trabucchi, G, Cappellini, A: Probe placement and energy levels in continuous wave neodymium-YAG contact transscleral cyclophotocoagulation. Arch Ophthalmol 108:679, 1990.

86. Schubert, HD, Federman, JL: The role of inflammation on CW Nd:YAG contact transscleral photocoagulation and cryopexy. Invest Ophthalmol Vis Sci 30:543, 1989.

87. Schubert, HD, Federman, JL: A comparison of CW Nd:YAG contact transscleral cyclophotocoagulation with cyclocryopexy. Invest Ophthalmol Vis Sci 30:536, 1989.

88. Schubert, HD, Agarwala, A, Arbizo, V: Changes in aqueous outflow after in vitro neodymium: Yttrium aluminum garnet laser cyclophotocoagulation. Invest Ophthalmol Vis Sci 31:1834, 1990.

89. Schubert, HD, Agarwala, A: Quantitative CW Nd:YAG pars plana transscleral photocoagulation in postmortem eyes. Ophthalmic Surg 21:835, 1990.

90. Liu, G-J, Mizukawa, A, Okisaka, S: Mechanism of intraocular pressure decrease after contact transscleral continuous-wave Nd:YAG laser cyclophotocoagulation. Ophthalmic Res 26:65, 1994.

91. Ando, F, Kawai, T: Transscleral contact cyclophotocoagulation for refractory glaucoma: comparison of the results of pars plicata and pars plana irradiation. Lasers Light Ophthalmol 5:143, 1993.

92. Crymes, BM, Gross, RL: Laser placement in noncontact Nd:YAG cyclophotocoagulation. Am J Ophthalmol 110:670, 1990.

93. Hampton, C, Shields, MB, Miller, KN, Blasini, M: Evaluation of a protocol for transscleral neodymium:YAG cyclophotocoagulation in one hundred patients. Ophthalmology 97:910, 1990.

94. Devenyi, RG, Trope, GE, Hunter, WH, Badeeb, O: Neodymium:YAG transscleral cyclocoagulation in human eyes. Ophthalmology 94:1519, 1987.

95. Badeeb, O, Trope, GE, Mortimer, C: Short-term effects of neodymium-YAG transscleral cyclocoagulation in patients with uncontrolled glaucoma. Br J Ophthalmol 72:615, 1988.

96. Klapper, RM, Wandel, T, Donnenfeld, E, Perry, HD: Transscleral neodymium:YAG thermal cyclophotocoagulation in refractory glaucoma. A preliminary report. Ophthalmology 95:719, 1988.

97. Trope, GE, Ma, S: Mid-term effects of neodymium:YAG transscleral cyclocoagulation in glaucoma. Ophthalmology 97:73, 1990.

98. Shields, MB, Wilkerson, MH, Echelman, DA: A comparison of two energy levels for noncontact transscleral neodymium:YAG cyclophotocoagulation. Arch Ophthalmol 111:484, 1993.

99. Shields, MB, Blasini, M, Simmons, R, Erickson, PJ: A contact lens for transscleral Nd:YAG cyclophotocoagulation. Am J Ophthalmol 108:457, 1989.

100. Dürr, U, Henchoz, P-D, Fankhauser, F, et al: Results and methods of transscleral laser cyclodestruction: a new contact lens for use with non-contact systems. Lasers Light Ophthalmol 3:123, 1990.

101. Simmons, RB, Blasini, M, Shields, MB, Erickson, PJ: Comparison of transscleral neodymium:YAG cyclophotocoagulation with and without a contact lens in human autopsy eyes. Am J Ophthalmol 109:174, 1990.

102. Simmons, RB, Shields, MB, Blasini, M, et al: Transscleral Nd:YAG laser cyclophotocoagulation with a contact lens. Am J Ophthalmol 112:671, 1991.

103. Hardten, DR, Brown, JD: Transscleral neodymium:YAG cyclophotocoagulation: comparison of 180-degree and 360-degree initial treatments. Ophthalmic Surg 24:181, 1993.

104. Brancato, R, Giovanni, L, Trabucchi, G, Pietroni, C: Contact transscleral cyclophotocoagulation with Nd:YAG laser in uncontrolled glaucoma. Ophthalmic Surg 20:547, 1989.

105. Schuman, JS, Puliafito, CA, Allingham, RR, et al: Contact transscleral continuous wave neodymium:YAG laser cyclophotocoagulation. Ophthalmology 97:571, 1990.

106. Coleman, AL, Jampel, HD, Javitt, JC, et al: Transscleral cyclophotocoagulation of human autopsy and monkey eyes. Ophthalmic Surg 22:638, 1991.

107. Guo, KL, Karp, CL, Higginbotham, EJ, et al: Comparative efficacy of the SLT versus LASAG Nd:YAG delivery systems in rabbits. J Glau 4:268, 1995.

108. Simmons, RB, Prum, BE Jr, Shields, SR, et al: Videographic and histologic comparison of Nd:YAG and diode laser contact transscleral cyclophotocoagulation. Am J Ophthalmol 117:337, 1994.

109. Hennis, HL, Stewart, WC: Semiconductor diode laser transscleral cyclophotocoagulation in patients with glaucoma. Am J Ophthalmol 113:81, 1992.

110. Kalenak, JW, Parkinson, JM, Kass, MA, Kolker, AE: Transscleral neodymium:YAG laser cyclocoagulation for uncontrolled glaucoma. Ophthalmic Surg 21:346, 1990.

111. Balazsi, G: Noncontact thermal mode Nd:YAG laser transscleral cyclocoagulation in the treatment of glaucoma. Intermediate follow-up. Ophthalmology 98:1858, 1991.

112. Wright, MM, Grajewski, AL, Feuer, WJ: Nd:YAG cyclophotocoagulation: outcome of treatment for uncontrolled glaucoma. Ophthalmic Surg 22:279, 1991.

113. Heidenkummer, H-P, Mangouritsas, G, Kampik, A: Clinical application and results of Nd-YAG-cyclophotocoagulation in refractory glaucoma. Klin Monatsbl Augenheilkd 198:174, 1991.

114. Al-Ghamdi, S, Ol-Obeidan, S, Tomey, KF, Al-Jadaan, I: Transscleral neodymium:YAG laser cyclophotocoagulation for end-stage glaucoma, refractory glaucoma, and painful blind eyes. Ophthalmic Surg 24:526, 1993.

115. Baez, KA, Ulbig, MW, McHugh, D, et al: Long-term results of ab externo neodymium:YAG cyclophotocoagulation. Ger J Ophthalmol 3:395, 1994.

116. Shields, MB, Shields, SE: Noncontact transscleral Nd:YAG cyclophotocoagulation: a long-term follow-up of 500 patients. Trans Am Ophthalmol Soc 92:271, 1994.

117. Schuman, JS, Bellows, AR, Shingleton, BJ, et al: Contact transscleral Nd:YAG laser cyclophotocoagulation. Midterm results. Ophthalmology 99:1089, 1992.

118. Kermani, O, Mons, B, Kirchhof, B, Krieglstein, GK: Contact cw-Nd:YAG laser cyclophotocoagulation for treatment of refractory glaucoma. Ger J Ophthalmol 1:74, 1992.

119. Hawkins, TA, Stewart, WC: One-year results of semiconductor transscleral cyclophotocoagulation in patients with glaucoma. Arch Ophthalmol 111:488, 1993.

120. Ulbig, MW, McHugh, D, McNaught, A, Hamilton, P: Contact diode laser cyclo-photocoagulation for refractory glaucoma. A pilot study. Ger J Ophthalmol 3:212, 1994.

121. Hardten, DR, Brown, JD, Holland, EJ: Results of neodymium:YAG laser transscleral cyclophotocoagulation for postkeratoplasty glaucoma. J Glau 2:241, 1993.

122. Threlkeld, AB, Shields, MB: Noncontact transscleral Nd:YAG cyclophotocoagulation for glaucoma after penetrating keratoplasty. Am J Ophthalmol 120:569, 1995.

123. Phelan, MJ, Higginbotham, EJ: Contact transscleral Nd:YAG laser cyclophotocoagulation for the treatment of refractory pediatric glaucoma. Ophthalmic Surg Lasers 26:401, 1995.

124. Trope, GE, Murphy, PH: Immediate pressure effects of Nd:YAG cyclocoagulation. Am J Ophthalmol 112:603, 1991.

125. Maus, M, Katz, LJ: Choroidal detachment, flat anterior chamber, and hypotony as complications of neodymium:YAG laser cyclophotocoagulation. Ophthalmology 97:69, 1990.

126. Edward, DP, Brown, SVL, Higginbotham, E, et al: Sympathetic ophthalmia following neodymium:YAG cyclotherapy. Ophthalmic Surg 20:544, 1989.

127. Brown, SVL, Higginbotham, E, Tessler, H: Sympathetic ophthalmia following Nd:YAG cyclotherapy. Ophthalmic Surg 21:736, 1990.

128. Lam, S, Tessler, HH, Lam, BL, Wilensky, JT: High incidence of sympathetic ophthalmia after contact and noncontact neodymium:YAG cyclotherapy. Ophthalmology 99:1818, 1992.

129. Pastor, SA, Iwach, A, Nozik, RA, et al: Presumed sympathetic ophthalmia following Nd:YAG transscleral cyclophotocoagulation. J Glau 2:30, 1993.

130. Bechrakis, NE, Müller-Stolzenburg, NW, Helbig, H, Foerster, MH: Arch Ophthalmol 112:80, 1994.

131. Hardten, DR, Brown, JD: Malignant glaucoma after Nd:YAG cyclophotocoagulation. Am J Ophthalmol 111:245, 1991.

132. Wand, M, Schuman, JS, Puliafito, CA: Malignant glaucoma after contact transscleral Nd:YAG laser cyclophotocoagulation. J Glau 2:110, 1993.

133. Nasisse, MP, McGahan, MC, Shields, MB, et al: Inflammatory effects of continuous-wave neodymium:yttrium aluminum garnet laser cyclophotocoagulation. Invest Ophthalmol Vis Sci 33:2216, 1992.

134. Echelman, DA, Nasisse, MP, Shields, MB, et al: Influence of exposure time on inflammatory response to neodymium:YAG cyclophotocoagulation in rabbits. Arch Ophthalmol 112:977, 1994.

135. Schuman, JS, Noecker, RJ, Puliafito, CA, et al: Energy levels and probe placement in contact transscleral semiconductor diode laser cyclophotocoagulation in human cadaver eyes. Arch Ophthalmol 109:1534, 1991.

136. Brancato, R, Leoni, G, Trabucchi, G, Cappellini, A: Histopathology of continuous wave neodymium:yttrium aluminum garnet and diode laser contact transscleral lesions in rabbit ciliary body. Invest Ophthalmol Vis Sci 32:1586, 1991.

137. Brancato, R, Trabucchi, G, Verdi, M, et al: Diode and Nd:YAG laser contact transscleral cyclophotocoagulation in a human eye: a comparative histopathologic study of the lesions produced using a new fiber optic probe. Ophthalmic Surg 25:607, 1994.

138. Assia, EI, Hennis, HL, Stewart, WC, et al: A comparison of neodymium:yttrium aluminum garnet and diode laser transscleral cyclophotocoagulation and cyclocryotherapy. Invest Ophthalmol Vis Sci 32:2774, 1991.

139. Beadles, KA, Smith, MF: Inadvertent sclerostomy during transscleral Nd:YAG cyclophotocoagulation. Am J Ophthalmol 118:669, 1994.

140. Stolzenburg, S, Kresse, S, Müller-Stolzenburg, NW: Thermal side reactions during in vitro contact cyclophotocoagulation with the continuous wave Nd:YAG laser. Ophthalmic Surg 21:356, 1990.

141. Rol, P, Barth, W, Schwager, M, et al: Devices for the control of laser transmission across the sclera during transscleral photocoagulation. Ophthalmic Surg 23:459, 1992.

142. Fankhauser, F, Kwasniewska, S, Dürr, U, et al: A new instrument for controlling pressure exerted on the sclera during contact Nd:YAG laser cyclodestruction. Ophthalmic Surg 23:465, 1992.

143. Echelman, DA, Stern, RA, Shields, SR, et al: Variability of contact transscleral neodymium:YAG cyclophotocoagulation. Invest Ophthalmol Vis Sci 36:497, 1995.

144. Higginbotham, EJ, Harrison, M, Zou, X: Cyclophotocoagulation with the transscleral contact neodymium:YAG laser versus cyclocryotherapy in rabbits. Ophthalmic Surg 22:27, 1991.

145. Suzuki, Y, Araie, M, Yumita, A, Yamamoto, T: Transscleral Nd:YAG laser cyclophotocoagulation versus cyclocryotherapy. Graefes Arch Clin Exp Ophthalmol 229:33, 1991.

146. Noureddin, BN, Wilson-Holt, N, Lavin, M, et al: Advanced uncontrolled glaucoma. Nd:YAG cyclophotocoagulation or tube surgery. Ophthalmology 99:430, 1992.

147. Lee, P-F, Pomerantzeff, O: Transpupillary cyclophotocoagulation of rabbit eyes. An experimental approach to glaucoma surgery. Am J Ophthalmol 71:911, 1971.

148. Bartl, G, Haller, BM, Wocheslander, E, Hofmann, H: Light and electron microscopic observations after argon laser photocoagulation of ciliary processes. Klin Monatsbl Augenheilkd 181:414, 1982.

149. Lee, P-F: Argon laser photocoagulation of the ciliary processes in cases of aphakic glaucoma. Arch Ophthalmol 97:2135, 1979.

150. Bernard, JA, Haut, J, Demailly, Ph, et al: Coagulation of the ciliary processes with the argon laser. Its use in certain types of hypertonia. Arch Ophthalmol (Paris) 34:577, 1974.

151. Merritt, JC: Transpupillary photocoagulation of the ciliary processes. Ann Ophthalmol 8:325, 1976.

152. Lee, P-F, Shihab, Z, Eberle, M: Partial ciliary process laser photocoagulation in the managment of glaucoma. Lasers Surg Med 1:85, 1980.

153. Klapper, RM, Dodick, JM: Transpupillary argon laser cyclophotocoagulation. Doc Ophthalmol Proc 36:197, 1984.

154. Shields, S, Stewart, WC, Shields, MB: Transpupillary argon laser cyclophotocoagulation in the treatment of glaucoma. Ophthalmic Surg 19:171, 1988.

155. Fleishman, JA, Schwartz, M, Dixon, JA: Argon laser endophotocoagulation. An intraoperative trans-pars plana technique. Arch Ophthalmol 99:1610, 1981.

156. Peyman, GA, Salzano, TC, Green, JL: Argon endolaser. Arch Ophthalmol 99:2037, 1981.

157. Landers, MB, Trese, MT, Stef'ansson, E, Bessler, M: Argon laser intraocular photocoagulation. Ophthalmology 89:785, 1982.

158. Shields, MB: Cyclodestructive surgery for glaucoma: past, present and future. Trans Am Ophthalmol Soc 83:285, 1985.

159. Patel, A, Thompson, JT, Michels, RG, Quigley, HA: Endolaser treatment of the ciliary body for uncontrolled glaucoma. Ophthalmology 93:825, 1986.

160. Zarbin, MA, Michels, RG, de Bustros, S, et al: Endolaser treatment of the ciliary body for severe glaucoma. Ophthalmology 95:1639, 1988.

161. Shields, MB, Chandler, DB, Hickingbotham, D, Klintworth, GK: Intraocular cyclophotocoagulation. Histopathologic evaluation in primates. Arch Ophthalmol 103:1731, 1985.

162. Shields, MB: Intraocular cyclophotocoagulation. Trans Ophthalmol Soc UK 105:237, 1986.

163. Uram, M: Ophthalmic laser microendoscope endophotocoagulation. Ophthalmology 99:1829, 1992.

164. Uram, M: Ophthalmic laser microendoscope ciliary process ablation in the management of neovascular glaucoma. Ophthalmology 99:1823, 1992.

165. Purnell, EW, Sokollu, A, Torchia, R, Taner, N: Focal chorioretinitis produced by ultrasound. Invest Ophthalmol 3:657, 1964.

166. Coleman, DJ, Lizzi, FL, Driller, J, et al: Therapeutic ultrasound in the treatment of glaucoma. I. Experimental model. Ophthalmology 92:339, 1985.

167. Coleman, DJ, Lizzi, FL, Driller, J, et al: Therapeutic ultrasound in the treatment of glaucoma. II. Clinical applications. Ophthalmology 92:347, 1985.

168. Burgess, SEP, Silverman, RH, Coleman, DJ, et al: Treatment of glaucoma with high-intensity focused ultrasound. Ophthalmology 93:831, 1986.

169. Margo, CE: Therapeutic ultrasound. Light and electron microscopic findings in an eye treated for glaucoma. Arch Ophthalmol 104:735, 1986.

170. Polack, PJ, Iwamoto, T, Silverman, RH, et al: Histologic effects of contact ultrasound for the treatment of glaucoma. Invest Ophthalmol Vis Sci 32:2136, 1991.

171. Maskin, SL, Mandell, AI, Smith, JA, et al: Therapeutic ultrasound for refractory glaucoma: a three-center study. Ophthalmic Surg 20:186, 1989.

172. Valtot, F, Kopel, J, Haut, J: Treatment of glaucoma with high intensity focused ultrasound. Int Ophthalmol 13:167, 1989.

173. Silverman, RH, Vogelsang, B, Rondeau, MJ, Coleman, DJ: Therapeutic ultrasound for the treatment of glaucoma. Am J Ophthalmol 111:327, 1991.

174. Finger, PT, Smith, PD, Paglione, RW, Perry, HD: Transscleral microwave cyclodestruction. Invest Ophthalmol Vis Sci 31:2151, 1990.

175. Finger, PT, Moshfeghi, DM, Smith, PD, Perry, HD: Microwave cyclodestruction for glaucoma in a rabbit model. Arch Ophthalmol 109:1001, 1991.

176. Freyler, H, Scheimbauer, I: Excision of the ciliary body (Sautter procedure) as a last resort in secondary glaucoma. Klin Monatsbl Augenheilkd 179:473, 1981.

177. Demeler, U: Ciliary surgery for glaucoma. Trans Ophthalmol Soc UK 105:242, 1986.

178. Welge-Lussen, L, Stadler, G: Results with a modified ciliary body excision to reduce intraocular pressure. Klin Monatsbl Augenheilkd 189:199, 1986.

Chapter 40

SURGICAL APPROACHES FOR COEXISTING GLAUCOMA AND CATARACT[a]

I. Indications
    A. Predicting visual potential
    B. Cataract extraction alone
    C. Filtering surgery alone (two-stage approach)
    D. Combined cataract extraction and glaucoma surgery

II. Techniques
    A. Cataract surgery in eyes with glaucoma
    B. Cataract extraction after filtering surgery
    C. Combined cataract and glaucoma surgery
        1. Guarded fistula and cataract extraction
        2. Adjunctive use of antimetabolites
        3. Other combined techniques

In the management of a patient with a cataract, for which extraction is indicated, and coexisting glaucoma, there are three basic surgical approaches: (a) cataract extraction alone; (b) glaucoma filtering surgery alone, followed by cataract removal at a later date (two-stage approach); and (c) combined cataract and glaucoma surgery as a single procedure. Combined procedures have certain advantages and disadvantages in comparison with the other two options. As compared to cataract surgery alone, combined procedures have a greater risk of complications such as increased inflammation, hyphema, hypotony, shallow anterior chambers, and choroidal detachments, but have the advantage of less early intraocular pressure (IOP) rise. As compared to a filtering operation alone, with or without subsequent cataract extraction, the combined procedures usually have a lower chance of long-term glaucoma control, but have the obvious advantage of one operation instead of two. For these reasons, the surgeon should consider each of the basic surgical options and select the approach that seems to be most appropriate for each individual patient. However, with advances in both cataract and glaucoma surgery, success rates with combined procedures have improved and relative indications have shifted. We first review the general indications for the three basic surgical approaches and then consider how advances in surgical techniques are influencing the relative indications for these procedures.

INDICATIONS

Predicting Visual Potential

In each case, it is assumed that a cataract is present for which extraction is indicated, independent of the glaucoma. However, the visual significance of the cataract is often difficult to determine in an eye with both a cataract and glaucoma, in which it is hard to know how much the glaucoma is contributing to the reduced vision. Several instruments have been developed to help predict the anticipated postoperative visual acuity. One focuses a miniaturized Snellen visual acuity chart on the retina (Potential Acuity Meter or PAM) while others project stripe patterns from either a laser or white light (Visometer) source. In one study, the Visometer gave more accurate predictions than the PAM in cataract patients with open-angle glaucoma, even with glaucomatous field loss (1). In other studies, the PAM was accurate if the glaucomatous damage was mild-to-moderate and the postoperative visual acuity was 20/40 to 20/50 or better, whereas the results with

[a]Refer to M.B. Shields: Color Atlas of Glaucoma. Baltimore: Williams & Wilkins, 1998, Plates III50–54.

advanced visual field loss or a worse postoperative vision were not reliable (2, 3). Automated perimetry was found to be useful in predicting whether the vision would be better or worse than 20/40. Combining this with the use of the PAM further increased the predictive value (3).

When it is decided that cataract surgery is needed, the selection of the specific surgical approach is based primarily on the status of the glaucoma.

Cataract Extraction Alone

When the IOP is under good control on a low dose of well-tolerated medication, most surgeons prefer a cataract extraction alone. However, cataract extraction with a posterior chamber intraocular lens implantation can be associated with a significant IOP rise during the early postoperative course in patients with preexisting glaucoma, especially with extracapsular techniques (4–9). In one study of extracapsular cataract extraction and posterior chamber lens implantation, more than half of the patients had pressures greater than 25 mm Hg 2–3 hours postoperatively (6). In another study, comparing extracapsular extraction to phacoemulsification, a significant increase in IOP during the first 5–7 hours after surgery was seen in approximately 20% of the former group, compared to 11% with phacoemulsification using a sclerocorneal suture and 4.7% with phacoemulsification and a sutureless scleral tunnel (9). Although the pressure can usually be brought under control within the first few postoperative days, patients with advanced glaucomatous damage before surgery may suffer additional, irreversible loss of vision during this time. Therefore, moderate-to-advanced glaucomatous optic atrophy and visual field loss may argue against cataract surgery alone, despite the preoperative level of IOP, although the risk may be less with phacoemulsification techniques.

Several studies have also looked at the IOP course in the intermediate and late postoperative periods following cataract surgery in patients with preexisting glaucoma. In general, the extracapsular techniques with posterior chamber implants were shown to be tolerated better than intracapsular procedures (5, 10), although postoperative glaucoma control could be a significant problem with either technique. During the first 2–4 months after extracapsular surgery, many glaucoma patients will have pressures above the preoperative baseline, while the IOP in others may be unchanged or even improved (10–13). Patients with preexisting open-angle glaucoma were found to have a small reduction in mean IOP and to require fewer medications 1–2 years after extracapsular cataract surgery (14–16). A similar trend has been seen in glaucoma patients following phacoemulsification and lens implantation. In one series of 51 patients, the mean IOP was reduced 4.1 mm Hg at 6 months and 3.8 mm Hg at 2 years (17). However, this trend may reverse with time (18), and cataract surgery alone should not be relied upon as a means of treating uncontrolled glaucoma. On the other hand, when the IOP is well-controlled on a low dose of well-tolerated medication with mild glaucomatous damage, cataract surgery alone, es-

pecially phacoemulsification with posterior chamber intraocular lens implantation, appears to be a reasonable choice.

Filtering Surgery Alone

When the glaucoma is uncontrolled despite maximum tolerable medical therapy and laser trabeculoplasty, the surgical procedure of choice is the one which has the greatest chance of providing long-term IOP control. In most cases, this is a filtering operation performed alone. In some patients, eliminating the need for miotic therapy postoperatively will improve the vision enough to delay the need for cataract surgery. In other cases, the cataract can be removed 4–6 months later, once the filtering bleb is well-established, as the second part of a two-stage approach. In one study, patients who underwent the two-stage procedure had a greater percentage of long-term IOP reduction than those who had cataract surgery alone or a combined cataract-glaucoma operation (8). In another study of 21 patients undergoing extracapsular cataract extraction with posterior chamber lens implantation in eyes with established filtering blebs and followed for a minimum of 48 months, the IOP rose an average of 3.5 mm Hg, with six eyes requiring resumption of medical therapy and two requiring repeat filtering surgery (19). With newer techniques of phacoemulsification via a clear cornea incision, it may be that these results will be further improved.

Combined Cataract Extraction and Glaucoma Surgery

Between the two extremes noted above, i.e., those patients with good glaucoma control and those with uncontrolled glaucoma which poses an immediate threat to vision, there is a third group of patients with borderline glaucoma status for whom a combined procedure may be indicated. There is often a fine line of judgment involved in selecting these cases, although the following situations are some in which such an approach might be preferred: (a) glaucoma under borderline control, despite maximum tolerable medical therapy and laser trabeculoplasty; (b) adequate IOP control, but significant drug-induced side effects; (c) adequate IOP control on well-tolerated medical therapy, but advanced glaucomatous optic atrophy; or (d) uncontrolled glaucoma, but an urgent need to restore vision or when two operations are not feasible.

The rationale for a combined procedure, as opposed to cataract surgery alone, in eyes with good IOP control but advanced damage, is the risk of a transient pressure rise in the early postoperative period, as previously discussed. Even if laser trabeculoplasty has achieved good IOP control, it may still be necessary to combine glaucoma surgery with the cataract extraction, since a good response to laser therapy before cataract surgery does not guarantee postoperative pressure control (20). Studies have shown that the early postoperative pressure rise is significantly less after a combined procedure than after cataract extraction alone (7, 8), and this was probably the primary benefit of the combined surgery during the era of extracapsular cataract surgery, when long-term glaucoma control following combined procedures was less predictable. However, with the advent of small incision cataract surgery and the adjunctive use of antimetabolites with the filtering surgery (discussed later in this chapter), the long-term results of combined procedures have improved, and the relative indications for this surgical option have expanded. Nevertheless, there is still a role for each of the three basic surgical options, the selection of which depends not only on the status of the individual patient, but also on the results that each surgeon experiences with the various operations.

TECHNIQUES

Cataract Surgery in Eyes with Glaucoma

In some cases, the cataract operation can be performed in the surgeon's usual manner, with no special measures for the co-existing glaucoma. A common problem with cataract surgery in the glaucomatous eye, however, is the irreversible *miosis* from chronic miotic therapy. This became more important with the advent of extracapsular cataract extraction and especially phacoemulsification, in which adequate pupillary dilatation is needed to perform the surgery safely and effectively. A wide variety of techniques have been described to surgically enlarge the pupil. One approach is to make a sector iridotomy above, often with two inferior sphincter-otomies (21), or multiple sphincterotomies and a peripheral iridectomy (22). If a sector iridotomy is made, some surgeons will elect to close it with sutures after implanting the lens (23, 24), although it can be left open if the lens haptics are rotated horizontally away from the iridotomy. One study compared patients with sutured and unsutured sector iridotomies and found no difference in glare sensitivity (25).

Several microiris retractors have been developed to mechanically enlarge a miotic pupil (26–28). A flexible nylon hook with a Silastic sleeve (27) has proven to be especially useful for cataract surgery (Fig. 40.1). Other techniques include mechanical stretching of the pupil (29), a variety of iris suture techniques (30–32), and a maneuver of tucking the iris pillars of a sector iridectomy (33). It has also been suggested that phacoemulsification can be performed through a pupil of 4 mm or more if the capsulorhexis is intact and the nucleus is fractured into small segments in the capsule (34), although this obviously depends on the skill of the surgeon.

Viscoelastic substances, such as hyaluronic acid, should be used with caution in eyes with glaucoma. They are especially useful during the anterior capsulotomy, not only for maintaining a deep anterior chamber, but also for providing some additional pupillary dilatation. However, they increase the risk of an early postoperative IOP rise and should be thoroughly aspirated and irrigated from the eye by the end of the procedure. If pupillary constriction is needed after lens implantation, intracameral *carbachol* may be preferable to acetylcholine, since the former is reported to be associ-

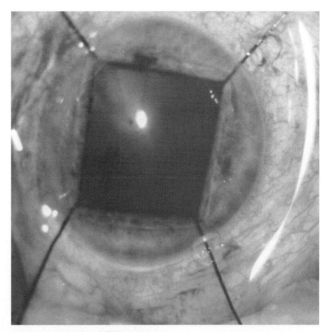

Figure 40.1. Four flexible iris retractors, inserted through clear cornea stab incisions, are used to dilate a chronically-miotic pupil during combined cataract and glaucoma surgery.

ated with better early postoperative pressure control (35). In another study, a combination of intraoperative acetylcholine and postoperative acetazolamide was more effective in preventing an acute IOP rise than either medication alone (36).

Selection of the proper *intraocular lens* is also important in eyes with glaucoma. Posterior chamber lenses appear to be very well tolerated, whereas anterior chamber lenses should, in most cases, be avoided in glaucomatous eyes. However, when loss of capsular support precludes the standard implantation of a posterior chamber lens, the surgeon usually must decide between a sutured posterior chamber lens or an anterior chamber lens. Several techniques have been described for the former option (37–40), most of which utilize the basic principle of passing two 10–0 prolene sutures, attached to the lens haptics, through the ciliary sulcus and sclera, and securing them beneath conjunctival and partial-thickness scleral flaps. These can all be difficult techniques, however, especially if they are not performed frequently, and it has been reported that the much easier procedure of implanting a semiflexible, one-piece, open-loop anterior chamber intraocular lens is associated with reasonable long-term IOP control in most glaucomatous eyes (41).

Cataract Extraction After Filtering Surgery

When extraction of the cataract becomes necessary in an eye with a functioning filtering bleb, the cataract incision should be positioned to maximize bleb survival. Some surgeons have preferred to make the incision inferiorly (42–44), while others have preferred a clear corneal incision superiorly (Fig. 40.2) (44–47) or a temporal limbal incision (48), the latter of which is especially useful if the filtering surgery

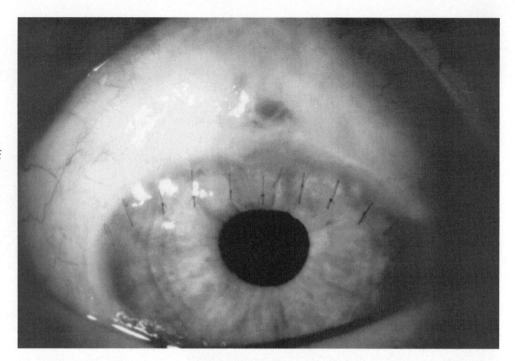

Figure 40.2. Slitlamp view of eye with functioning glaucoma filtering bleb in which extracapsular cataract extraction and posterior chamber lens implantation were performed through a clear corneal incision to preserve the preexisting bleb. (Reprinted with permission from Ritch R, Shields MB, Krupin T, eds. The glaucomas. 2nd ed. St. Louis, CV Mosby, 1996, p. 1751.)

was performed in the superior nasal quadrant. These basic methods are generally comparable with regard to preserving function of the filtering bleb, although most eyes will have a slightly higher IOP postoperatively, and many will require more glaucoma medication.

With the advent of small incision cataract surgery, using phacoemulsification and foldable posterior chamber intraocular lenses, the clear corneal incision technique, with or without a corneal suture, has become an ideal approach to cataract surgery in the eye with an established filtering bleb. Some surgeons prefer to use a temporal corneal incision, although a superior-temporal or superior-nasal incision (depending on the location of the filtering bleb) has the advantages of allowing the surgeon to operate in a more customary position (Fig. 40.3).

Combined Cataract and Glaucoma Surgery

Early combined operations that utilized full-thickness filtering procedures were associated with an increased risk of a transient shallow or flat anterior chamber, which often led to significant complications in the inflamed, aphakic eye. For this reason, most combined operations have employed a glaucoma procedure that is less likely to cause loss of the anterior chamber.

A cyclodialysis was used in combined procedures for many years, with reports of good results (49–52). However, in one large series, an analysis of the postoperative course suggested that the IOP reduction in many cases was due to the effect of the cataract surgery, rather than the cyclodialysis (51). Since this effect may be lost with the newer techniques of wound closure, and considering the unpredictable nature of cyclodialysis, most surgeons now prefer some form of guarded fistula for combined procedures.

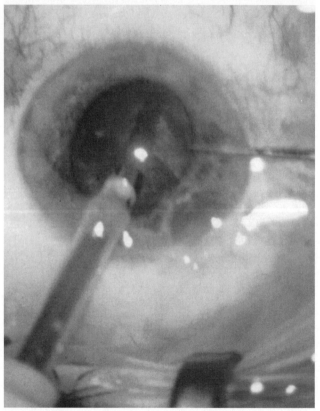

Figure 40.3. Intraoperative view during phacoemulsification and foldable posterior chamber intraocular lens implantation via superior-temporal clear corneal incision in eye with established filtering bleb in superior-nasal quadrant.

Guarded Fistula and Cataract Extraction

The protective scleral flap over a limbal fistula, which reduces the chances of an early postoperative flat anterior chamber, makes the guarded filtering operation particularly desirable for combined procedures. Several techniques were described for combining a *trabeculectomy* with intracapsular cataract surgery during the 1970s (53–57), but it was not until the popularity of *extracapsular cataract extraction* and posterior chamber intraocular lens implantation (the "triple procedure") in the 1980s that combined trabeculectomy and cataract extraction began to provide reasonably consistent long-term glaucoma control (58–65).

The basic approach involves preparation of the partial-thickness scleral flap and limbal fistula in the usual manner, followed by extension of the corneoscleral incision from either side of the fistula. Alternatively, the cataract incision can be made in clear cornea, anterior to the trabeculectomy site (65). After a standard extracapsular lens extraction and implantation of the posterior chamber lens, both scleral flap and corneoscleral or corneal incision are closed with multiple sutures. The conjunctival flap is closed in the manner described for glaucoma filtering procedures (Chapter 37). A limbal-based versus fornix-based conjunctival flap has not been found to influence the outcome of combined trabeculectomy and extracapsular cataract surgery (61, 63). The use of topical apraclonidine 1% before, immediately after, and 12 hours after surgery has been shown to decrease larger IOP elevations in eyes undergoing combined extracapsular cataract extraction and trabeculectomy (66).

A simplified technique for creating a guarded fistula in conjunction with cataract surgery is to prepare a very beveled corneoscleral incision and create the fistula in the posterior lip of the incision with a scleral punch or scissors (Fig. 40.4). When the corneoscleral incision is approximated, the anterior lip of the incision covers the fistula, in the same manner as a trabeculectomy (Fig. 40.5). The procedure was originally described in conjunction with intra-

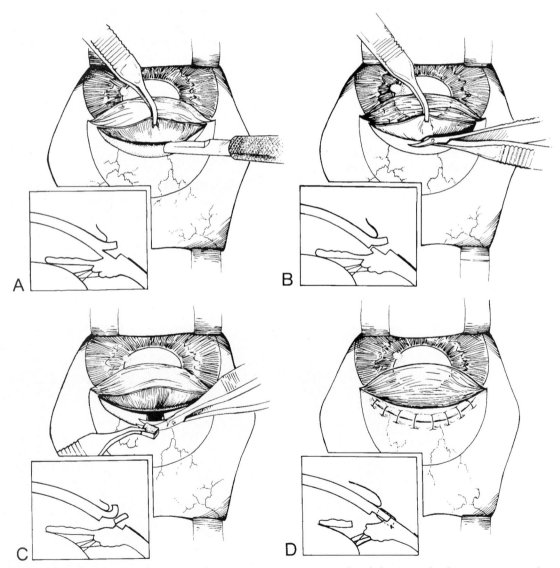

Figure 40.4. Guarded sclerectomy and extracapsular cataract extraction. **A.** A beveled corneoscleral incision is created. **B.** The incision is extended full thickness with corneoscleral scissors. **C.** After cataract extraction and posterior chamber intraocular lens implantation, the glaucoma drainage fistula is created in the posterior lip of the corneoscleral incision. **D.** Approximation of the incision brings the anterior lip as a guard over the fistula.

capsular cataract surgery (67, 68), and was later modified for extracapsular techniques (8, 21, 69). A comparison of limbal-based versus fornix-based conjunctival flaps revealed similar long-term IOP control and visual acuity, but better early postoperative pressure control with the limbal-based flaps (69). The procedure has been referred to as a *guarded sclerectomy* (21), although it only represents a modification of the basic trabeculectomy concept. The long-term results of the procedure are comparable to those with combined trabeculectomy and cataract extraction, although the guarded sclerectomy may require less surgical manipulation.

Phacoemulsification has increasingly become the preferred cataract technique for combined procedures during the 1990s and appears to be associated with further improvement in the long-term success rates. The procedure can be combined with a standard *trabeculectomy*, utilizing the fistula for the cataract incision (70). The incision may be 6 mm with a rigid intraocular lens or 3 mm with a foldable lens. The latter has been shown to have a significantly lower incidence of postoperative complications and better visual acuity in the early postoperative period (71). Alternatively, the trabeculectomy can be performed in the standard manner, with the phacoemulsification and foldable lens implantation through a separate temporal corneal incision (72). The scleral tunnel incision, that is commonly used with routine phacoemulsification, allows application of the *guarded sclerectomy* concept, in that the fistula can be excised from the posterior lip of the incision, leaving the anterior lip of the tunnel to cover the fistula (73) (Fig. 40.6).

Several studies have compared phacoemulsification to extracapsular cataract extraction in combination with a guarded filtering procedure, with the general results that the former is associated with fewer complications, improved long-term IOP control, and a better visual outcome (74–76).

Another study compared combined phacoemulsification and trabeculectomy in patients with controlled IOP preoperatively to trabeculectomy alone in patients with uncontrolled IOP and showed no significant difference in glaucoma control after one year (77).

Adjunctive Use of Antimetabolites

Another factor that may be associated with the improved long-term IOP control with combined procedures is the adjunctive us of antimetabolites to minimize excessive fibrosis. The first of these to be evaluated was *5-fluorouracil* (5-FU), which is typically administered as several postoperative subconjunctival injections. Although preliminary experience with combined extracapsular cataract extraction and trabeculectomy suggested some benefit (78), subsequent studies showed no significant difference with or without adjunctive 5-FU (79, 80). Studies with combined phacoemulsification and trabeculectomy also showed little (81) or no (82) benefit to 5-FU. When intraoperative *mitomycin-C* was used in conjunction with combined phacoemulsification and trabeculectomy, the IOP was controlled at 6–12 months postoperatively (83, 84), although a prospective trial, comparing eyes with and without mitomycin-C, revealed no significant differences in the IOP or visual outcomes (85).

Other Combined Techniques

Techniques have been described in which a *trabeculotomy* is performed through a radial incision at 12 o'clock adjacent to a partial-thickness corneoscleral incision before extending the incision full-thickness for the cataract surgery (17, 86). Phacoemulsification has also been combined with holmium *laser sclerostomy* using either an ab interno (87) or ab externo (88) approach.

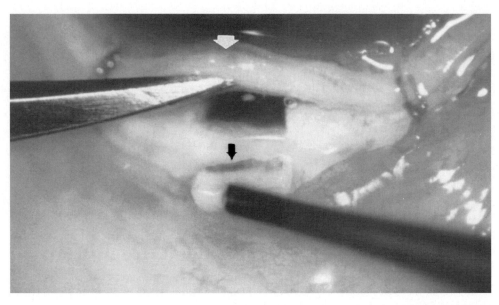

Figure 40.5. Intraoperative view during guarded sclerectomy and extracapsular cataract extraction showing excision of fistula *(arrow)* from posterior lip of corneoscleral incision. (Reprinted with permission from Ritch R, Shields MB, Krupin T, eds. The glaucomas. St. Louis, CV Mosby, 1989, p. 705.)

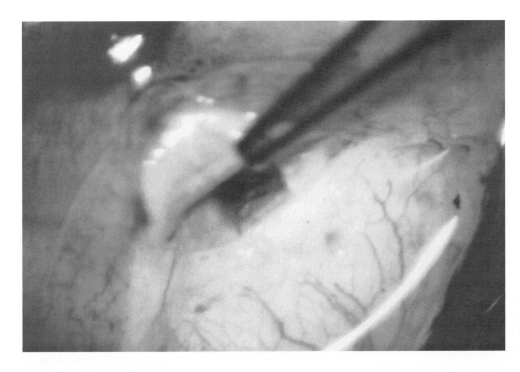

Figure 40.6. Intraoperative view during guarded sclerectomy and phacoemulsification showing excision of fistula from posterior lip of scleral tunnel incision.

SUMMARY

In an eye with a cataract, for which extraction is felt to be indicated, and coexisting glaucoma, the surgical approach is based primarily on the status of the glaucoma. In some cases, cataract extraction alone may be sufficient, whereas other eyes may require filtering surgery alone with cataract surgery at a later date. In other patients, a combined glaucoma and cataract operation may be the procedure of choice. The preferred technique for the glaucoma portion of a combined procedure is usually some form of guarded filtering surgery, and the combination of phacoemulsification with a guarded filtering procedure, possibly in conjunction with antimetabolite therapy, appears to have improved the long-term success rate of the combined procedure.

REFERENCES

1. Spurny, RC, Zaldivar, R, Belcher, CD, III, Simmons, RJ: Instruments for predicting visual acuity. A clinical comparison. Arch Ophthalmol 104:196, 1986.
2. Asbell, PA, Chiang, B, Amin, A, Podos, SM: Retinal acuity evaluation with the potential acuity meter in glaucoma patients. Ophthalmology 92:764, 1985.
3. Stewart, WC, Connor, AB, Hunt, HH: Prediction of postoperative visual acuity in patients with total glaucomatous cupping using the potential acuity meter and automated perimetry. Ophthalmic Surg 24:730, 1993.
4. McGuigan, LJB, Gottsch, J, Stark, WJ, et al: Extracapsular cataract extraction and posterior chamber lens implantation in eyes with preexisting glaucoma. Arch Ophthalmol 104:1301, 1986.
5. Vu, MT, Shields, MB: The early postoperative pressure course in glaucoma patients following cataract surgery. Ophthalmic Surg 19:467, 1988.
6. Gross, JG, Meyer, DR, Robin, AL, et al: Increased intraocular pressure in the immediate postoperative period after extracapsular cataract extraction. Am J Ophthalmol 105:466, 1988.
7. Krupin, T, Feitl, ME, Bishop, KI: Postoperative intraocular pressure rise in open-angle glaucoma patients after cataract or combined cataractfiltration surgery. Ophthalmology 96:579, 1989.
8. Murchison, JF Jr, Shields, MB: An evaluation of three surgical approaches for coexisting cataract and glaucoma. Ophthalmic Surg 20:393, 1989.
9. Lagrèze, W-DA, Bömer, TG, Funk, J: Effect of surgical technique on the increase in intraocular pressure after cataract extraction. Ophthalmic Surg Lasers 27:169, 1996.
10. Hansen, TE, Naeser, K, Rask, KL: A prospective study of intraocular pressure four months after extracapsular extraction with implantation of posterior chamber lenses. J Cataract Refract Surg 13:35, 1987.
11. Brown, SVL, Thomas, JV, Budenz, DL, et al: Effect of cataract surgery on intraocular pressure reduction obtained with laser trabeculoplasty. Am J Ophthalmol 100:373, 1985.
12. Savage, JA, Thomas, JV, Belcher, CD III, Simmons, RJ: Extracapsular cataract extraction and posterior chamber intraocular lens implantation in glaucomatous eyes. Ophthalmology 92:1506, 1985.
13. McMahan, LB, Monica, ML, Zimmerman, TJ: Posterior chamber pseudophakes in glaucoma patients. Ophthalmic Surg 17:146, 1986.
14. Radius, RL, Schultz, K, Sobocinski, K, et al: Pseudophakia and intraocular pressure. Am J Ophthalmol 97:738, 1984.
15. Handa, J, Henry, JC, Krupin, T, Keates, E: Extracapsular cataract extraction with posterior chamber lens implantation in patients with glaucoma. Arch Ophthalmol 105:765, 1987.
16. Cinotti, DJ, Fiore, PM, Maltzman, BA, et al: Control of intraocular pressure in glaucomatous eyes after extracapsular cataract extraction with intraocular lens implantation. J Cataract Refract Surg 14:650, 1988.
17. Gimbel, HV, Meyer, D, DeBroff, BM, et al: Intraocular pressure response to combined phacoemulsification and trabeculotomy ab externo versus phacoemulsification alone in primary open-angle glaucoma. J Cataract Refract Surg 21:653, 1995.
18. Sponagel, LD, Gloor, B: Does implantation of posterior chamber lenses lower intraocular pressure? Klin Monatsbl Augenheilk 188:495, 1986.

19. Dickens, MA, Cashwell, LF: Long-term effect of cataract extraction on the function of an established filtering bleb. Ophthalmic Surg Lasers 27:9, 1996.

20. Galin, MA, Obstbaum, SA, Asano, Y, et al: Laser trabeculoplasty and cataract surgery. Trans Ophthalmol Soc UK 104:72, 1984.

21. Shields, MB: Combined cataract extraction and guarded sclerectomy. Reevaluation in the extracapsular era. Ophthalmology 93:366, 1986.

22. Kolker, AE, Stewart, RH, LeBlanc, RP: Cataract extraction in glaucomatous patients. Arch Ophthalmol 84:63, 1970.

23. Saito, Y, Kiboshi, H: A new intra-anterior chamber iris suturing method. Am J Ophthalmol 105:701, 1988.

24. Whitsett, JC, Stewart, RH: A new technique for combined cataract/glaucoma procedures in patients on chronic miotics. Ophthalmic Surg 24:481, 1993.

25. Cahane, M, Glovinsky, Y, Blumenthal, M: Effect of a resutured iridotomy on glare disability in glaucoma patients having cataract surgery. J Cataract Refract Surg 17:58, 1991.

26. McCuen, BW, II, Hickingbotham, D, Tsai, M, de Juan, E Jr: Temporary iris fixation with a micro-iris retractor. Arch Ophthalmol 107:925, 1989.

27. de Juan, E Jr, Hickingbotham, D: Flexible iris retractor. Am J Ophthalmol 111:776, 1991.

28. Fuller, DG, Wilson, DL: Translimbal iris hook for pupillary dilation during vitreous surgery. Am J Ophthalmol 110:577, 1990.

29. Miller, KM, Keener, GT Jr: Stretch pupilloplasty for small pupil phacoemulsification. Am J Ophthalmol 115:107, 1994.

30. Murray, TG, Abrams, GW: A new self-sealing needle for iris suture fixation. Arch Ophthalmol 108:746, 1990.

31. Freeman, WR, Feldman, ST, Munguia, D, et al: The prethreaded pupillary dilating (Torpedo) suture for phakic and aphakic eyes. Arch Ophthalmol 110:564, 1992.

32. Gaudric, A: Transpupillary continuous suture for intraoperative mydriasis. Am J Ophthalmol 115:670, 1993.

33. Johnstone, MA: The iris tucking maneuver in cataract surgery for glaucoma patients with miotic pupils. Am J Ophthalmol 113:586, 1992.

34. Gimbel, HV: Nucleofractis phacoemulsification through a small pupil. Can J Ophthalmol 27:115, 1992.

35. Ruiz, RS, Rhem, MN, Prager, TC: Effects of carbachol and acetylcholine on intraocular pressure after cataract extraction. Am J Ophthalmol 107:7, 1989.

36. West, J, Burke, J, Cunliffe, I, Longstaff, S: Prevention of acute postoperative pressure rises in glaucoma patients undergoing cataract extraction with posterior chamber lens implant. Br J Ophthalmol 76:534, 1992.

37. Hu, BV, Shin, DH, Gibbs, KA, Hong, YJ: Implantation of posterior chamber lens in the absence of capsular and zonular support. Arch Ophthalmol 106:416, 1988.

38. Stark, WJ, Gottsch, JD, Goodman, DF, et al: Posterior chamber intraocular lens implantation in the absence of capsular support. Arch Ophthalmol 107:1078, 1989.

39. Lindquist, TD, Agapitos, PJ, Lindstrom, RL, et al: Transscleral fixation of posterior chamber intraocular lenses in the absence of capsular support. Ophthalmic Surg 20:769, 1989.

40. Sayyad, FE, Helal, M, El Sherif, Z, et al: Trabeculectomy combined with transscleral sutured posterior chamber lens in the management of glaucoma in aphakia. Middle East J Ophthalmol 1:9, 1993.

41. Bergman, M, Laatikainen, L: Intraocular pressure level in glaucomatous and nonglaucomatous eyes after complicated cataract surgery and implantation of an AC-IOL. Ophthalmic Surg 23:378, 1992.

42. Baloglou, P, Matta, C, Asdourian, K: Cataract extraction after filtering operations. Arch Ophthalmol 88:12, 1972.

43. Simmons, RJ, Thomas, JV, Singh, OS, Taheri, N: Surgical indications and options in the management of coexisting glaucoma and cataract. Glaucoma 4:92, 1982.

44. Kass, MA: Cataract extraction in an eye with a filtering bleb. Ophthalmology 89:871, 1982.

45. Oyakawa, RT, Maumenee, AE: Clear-cornea cataract extraction in eyes with functioning filtering blebs. Am J Ophthalmol 93:294, 1982.

46. Wocheslander, E, Bartl, G: Follow-up examinations after trabeculectomy and cataract surgery. Klin Monatsbl Augenheilkd 183:323, 1983.

47. Binkhorst, CD, Huber, C: Cataract extraction and intraocular lens implantation after fistulizing glaucoma surgery. Am Intra-ocular Implant Soc J 7:133, 1981.

48. Antonios, SR, Traverso, CE, Tomey, KF: Extracapsular cataract extraction using a temporal limbal approach after filtering operations. Arch Ophthalmol 106:608, 1988.

49. Galin, MA, Baras, I, Sambursky, J: Glaucoma and cataract. A study of cyclodialysis-lens extraction. Am J Ophthalmol 67:522, 1969.

50. Shemleva, VV, Mukhina, EA: Combined cataract extraction and cyclodialysis. Vestn Oftalmol 85:30, 1972.

51. Shields, MB, Simmons, RJ: Combined cyclodialysis and cataract extraction. Trans Am Acad Ophthalmol Otol 81:286, 1976.

52. McAllister, JA, Spaeth, GL: Intracapsular cataract extraction with cyclodialysis. A useful procedure. Klin Monatsbl Augenheilkd 184:283, 1984.

53. Dellaporta, A: Combined trepano-trabeculectomy and cataract extraction. Trans Am Ophthalmol Soc 69:113, 1971.

54. Rich, W: Cataract extraction with trabeculectomy. Trans Ophthalmol Soc UK 94:458, 1974.

55. Jerndal, T, Lundstrom, M: Trabeculectomy combined with cataract extraction. Am J Ophthalmol 81:227, 1976.

56. Stewart, RH, Loftis, MD: Combined cataract extraction and thermal sclerostomy versus combined cataract extraction and trabeculectomy. Ophthalmic Surg 7:93, 1976.

57. Johns, GE, Layden, WE: Combined trabeculectomy and cataract extraction. Am J Ophthalmol 88:973, 1979.

58. Percival, SPB: Glaucoma triple procedure of extracapsular cataract extraction, posterior chamber lens implantation, and trabeculectomy. Br J Ophthalmol 69:99, 1985.

59. Ohanesian, RV, Kim, EW: A prospective study of combined extracapsular cataract extraction, posterior chamber lens implantation, and trabeculectomy. Am Intra-ocular Implant Soc J 11:142, 1985.

60. Jay, JL: Extracapsular lens extraction and posterior chamber intraocular lens insertion combined with trabeculectomy. Br J Ophthalmol 69:487, 1985.

61. Simmons, ST, Litoff, D, Nichols, DA, et al: Extracapsular cataract extraction and posterior chamber intraocular lens implantation combined with trabeculectomy in patients with glaucoma. Am J Ophthalmol 104:465, 1987.

62. Raitta, C, Tarkkanen, A: Combined procedure for the management of glaucoma and cataract. Acta Ophthalmol 66:667, 1988.

63. McCartney, KL, Memmen, JE, Stark, W, et al: The efficacy and safety of combined trabeculectomy, cataract extraction, and intraocular lens implantation. Ophthalmology 95:754, 1988.

64. Neumann, R, Zalish, M, Oliver, M: Effect of intraocular lens implantation on combined extracapsular cataract extraction with trabeculectomy: A comparative study. Br J Ophthalmol 72:741, 1988.

65. Longstaff, S, Wormald, RPL, Mazover, A, Hitchings, RA: Glaucoma triple procedures: efficacy on intraocular pressure control and visual outcome. Ophthalmic Surg 21:786, 1990.

66. Robin, AL: Effect of topical apraclonidine on the frequency of intraocular pressure elevations after combined extracapsular cataract extraction and trabeculectomy. Ophthalmology 100:628, 1993.

67. Spaeth, GL, Sivalingam, E: The partial-punch: A new combined cataract-glaucoma operation. Ophthalmic Surg 7:53, 1976.

68. Shields, MB: Combined cataract extraction and glaucoma surgery. Ophthalmology 89:231, 1982.

69. Murchison, JF Jr, Shields, MB: Limbal-based vs. fornix-based conjunctival flaps in combined extracapsular cataract surgery and glaucoma filtering procedure. Am J Ophthalmol 109:709, 1990.

70. Hansen, LL, Hoffmann, F: Combination of phacoemulsification and trabeculectomy—results of a retrospective study. Klin Monatsbl Augenheilk 190:478, 1987.

71. Lyle, WA, Jin, JC: Comparison of a 3- and 6-mm incision in combined phacoemulsification and trabeculectomy. Am J Ophthalmol 111:189, 1991.

72. Weitzman, M, Caprioli, J: Temporal corneal phacoemulsification combined with separate-incision superior trabeculectomy. Ophthalmic Surg 26:271, 1995.

73. Shingleton, BJ, Kalina, PH: Combined phacoemulsification, intraocular lens implantation, and trabeculectomy with a modified scleral tunnel and single-stitch closure. J Cataract Refract Surg 21:528, 1995.

74. Wishart, PK, Austin, MW: Combined cataract extraction and trabeculectomy: phacoemulsification compared with extracapsular technique. Ophthalmic Surg 24:814, 1993.

75. Stewart, WC, Crinkley, CMC, Carlson, AN: Results of trabeculectomy combined with phacoemulsification versus trabeculectomy combined with extracapsular cataract extraction in patients with advanced glaucoma. Ophthalmic Surg 25:621, 1994.

76. Shingleton, BJ, Jacobson, LM, Kuperwaser, MC: Comparison of combined cataract and glaucoma surgery using planned extracapsular and phacoemulsification techniques. Ophthalmic Surg Lasers 26:414, 1995.

77. Stewart, WC, Crinkley, CMC, Carlson, AN: Results of combined phacoemulsification and trabeculectomy in patients with elevated preoperative intraocular pressures. J Glau 4:164, 1995.

78. Cohen, JS: Combined cataract implant and filtering surgery with 5-fluorouracil. Ophthalmic Surg 21:181, 1990.

79. Hennis, HL, Stewart, WC: The use of 5-fluorouracil in patients following combined trabeculectomy and cataract extraction. Ophthalmic Surg 22:451, 1991.

80. Wong, PC, Ruderman, JM, Krupin, T, et al: 5-Fluorouracil after primary combined filtration surgery. Am J Ophthalmol 117:149, 1994.

81. Hurvitz, LM: 5-FU-supplemented phacoemulsification, posterior chamber intraocular lens implantation, and trabeculectomy. Ophthalmic Surg 24:674, 1993.

82. O'Grady, JM, Juzych, MS, Shin, DH, et al: Trabeculectomy, phacoemulsification, and posterior chamber lens implantation with and without 5-fluorouracil. Am J Ophthalmol 116:594, 1993.

83. Munden, PM, Alward, WLM: Combined phacoemulsification, posterior chamber intraocular lens implantation, and trabeculectomy with mitomycin C. Am J Ophthalmol 119:20, 1995.

84. Joos, KM, Bueche, MJ, Palmberg, PF, et al: One-year follow-up results of combined mitomycin C trabeculectomy and extracapsular cataract extraction. Ophthalmology 102:76, 1995.

85. Shin, DH, Simone, PA, Song, MS, et al: Adjunctive subconjunctival mitomycin C in glaucoma triple procedure. Ophthalmology 102:1550, 1995.

86. McPherson, SD Jr: Combined trabeculotomy and cataract extraction as a single operation. Trans Am Ophthalmol Soc 74:251, 1976.

87. Kendrick, RM, Kollarits, CR: Combined cataract-glaucoma surgery using the THC:YAG (holmium) laser ab interno without gonioscopy. Ophthalmic Surg 23:697, 1992.

88. Terry, S: Combined no-stitch phacoemulsification cataract extraction with foldable silicone intraocular implant and Holmium laser sclerostomy followed by 5-FU injections. Ophthalmic Surg 23:218, 1992.

INDEX

Page numbers in *italics* denote figures; those followed by *t* denote tables.

Truly Visionary

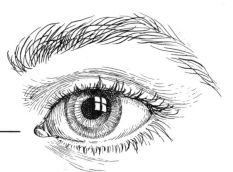

Textbook of Glaucoma, *Fourth Edition*

M. Bruce Shields, MD

This thorough revision of an outstanding text is a must for the ophthalmologist. Written by one of the leading names in glaucoma, the text presents the full scope of the disorder with updates that reflect the most current thinking.
1998/608 pages/0-683-07693-0

Color Atlas of Glaucoma

M. Bruce Shields, MD

The perfect companion to the *Textbook*, this atlas is devoted to both medical and surgical management of glaucoma with coverage of basic aspects, clinical forms, and medical/surgical issues. The bountiful color illustrations enhance and reinforce the comprehensive companion text.
1998/0-683-07696-5

Chandler and Grant's Glaucoma,
Fourth Edition

David L. Epstein, MD, R. Rand Allingham, MD, and Joel S. Shuman, MD

In addition to exploring the mechanisms behind clinical observation, this text provides specifics on how to treat the individual patient in the office. There is a wealth of practical information applicable to day-to-day work, emphasizing the best new strategies for therapy—as well as potential future directions—the fourth edition is the perfect answer to streamlining the ophthalmologist's clinical decision-making every day.
1997/670 pages/484 illustrations/0-683-02808-1

Ocular Differential Diagnosis,
Sixth Edition

Frederick Hampton Roy, MD, FACS

This latest edition is a concise, user-friendly resource organized by region of the eye. It provides rapid access to diagnosis based on signs and symptoms. The book also includes comprehensive lists of diagnoses and drugs associated with various ophthalmic disorders. Section editors in each subspecialty ensures accuracy and quality of content and terminology.
1996/753 pages/135 illustrations/0-683-07415-6

Printed in US   3/97   SHIETBIA   ➡   S7B245

Try them for 30 days.   If not completely satisfied, return them within 30 days at no further obligation (US and Canada only). There's no risk to you.

From the US call: 1-800-638-0672
From Canada call: 1-800-665-1148
From outside the US and Canada call: 410-528-4223
From the UK and Europe call: 44 (171) 385-2357
From Southeast Asia call: (852) 2610-2339
All other countries call: 410-528-4223
Also available from your local health sciences bookstore.

E-mail: custserv@wwilkins.com
Home page: http://www.wwilkins.com

Williams & Wilkins
A WAVERLY COMPANY
351 West Camden Street
Baltimore, Maryland 21201-2436 U.S.A.

Yes, I want to add these selections to my ophthalmology library.

Please send me:

_____ Epstein: Chandler & Grant's Glaucoma, 4th ed.
(0-683-02808-1).....................................$125.00
_____ Roy: Ocular Differential Diagnosis, 6th ed.
(0-683-07415-6).......................................$65.00
_____ Shields: Textbook of Glaucoma, 4th ed.
(0-683-07693-0)....................................$110.00
_____ Shields: Color Atlas of Glaucoma
(0-683-07696-5)....................................$149.00

30 day guarantee - See details above
Payment options
❑ Check enclosed (plus $5.00 handling)
❑ Bill me (plus postage and handling)
❑ Charge my credit card (plus postage and handling)
    Card No. _____
    Exp. Date _____
❑ VISA ❑ MasterCard ❑ American Express ❑ Discover
Signature or p.o.#_____

CA, IL, MA, MD, NY, & PA residents add state sales tax. Prices are subject to change without notice. Prices valid in the U.S. only.

Name _____
Address _____
City/State/Zip _____
Phone (_____)_____fax (_____)_____
Specialty/Profession _____
E-mail address _____

From the US call: 1-800-638-0672
From Canada call: 1-800-665-1148
From outside the US and Canada call: 410-528-4223
From the UK and Europe call: 44 (171) 385-2357
From Southeast Asia call: (852) 2610-2339
All other countries call: 410-528-4223

Williams & Wilkins • A WAVERLY COMPANY
351 West Camden Street, Baltimore, MD 21201-2436 U.S.A.

Printed in US   3/97   SHIETBIA   ➡   S7B245   A